Manual of Dietetic Practice
Second Edition

Manual of Dietetic Practice

Editorial Group
on behalf of the British Dietetic Association

Chairman Greta Walton
Chairman British Dietetic Association 1983–5
Alison Black
Celia Firmin
Christine Russell
Briony Thomas
Jacki Tredger

Editor Briony Thomas

The British Dietetic Association was founded in 1936 to advance the science and practice of dietetics and to promote the training and continuing education of dietitians.

Today it is established as the only society to represent the interest of qualified practitioners in the United Kingdom and is recognized as such throughout the world.

Manual of Dietetic Practice

Second Edition

Edited for
The British Dietetic Association by

Briony Thomas BSc, PhD, SRD

Formerly Research Nutritionist
Unit for Metabolic Medicine
Department of Medicine
Guy's Hospital
London

Foreword by

Dame Barbara Clayton DBE

Honorary President
British Dietetic Association

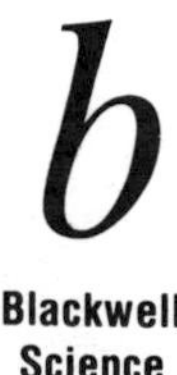

Blackwell
Science

Editorial Offices:
Osney Mead, Oxford OX2 0EL
25 John Street, London WC1N 2BL
23 Ainslie Place, Edinburgh EH3 6AJ
238 Main Street, Cambridge, Massachusetts 02142, USA
54 University Street, Carlton, Victoria 3053, Australia

Other Editorial Offices:
Arnette Blackwell SA
1, rue de Lille
75007 Paris
France

Blackwell Wissenschafts-Verlag GmbH
Kurfürstendamm 57
10707 Berlin
Germany

Blackwell MZV
Feldgasse 13
A-1238 Wien
Austria

First published 1988
Reprinted 1989
Second edition 1994
Reprinted 1994 (twice)

Set by Setrite Typesetters Ltd.
Printed and bound in Great Britain by The University Press, Cambridge.

DISTRIBUTORS

Marston Book Services Ltd
PO Box 87
Oxford OX2 0DT
(*Orders*: Tel: 01865 791155
Fax: 01865 791927
Telex: 837515)

USA
Blackwell Science, Inc.
238 Main Street
Cambridge, MA 02142
(*Orders*: Tel: 800 759-6102
617 876-7000)

Canada
Times Mirror Professional Publishing Ltd
130 Flaska Drive
Markham, Ontario L6G 1B8
(*Orders*: Tel: 800 268-4178
Fax: 416 470-6739)

Australia
Blackwell Science Pty Ltd
54 University Street,
Carlton, Victoria 3053
(*Orders*: Tel: 03 347-5552)

A catalogue record for this book is available from the British Library

ISBN 0-632-03003-8

Library of Congress
Cataloging in Publication Data

Manual of dietetic practice/edited
for the British Dietetic Association by Briony Thomas; foreword by Dame Barbara Clayton. — 2nd ed.
p. cm.
Includes bibliographical references and index.
ISBN 0-632-03003-8
1. Diet in disease. 2. Diet therapy. I. Thomas, Briony.
II. British Dietetic Association.
[DNLM: 1. Dietetics. 2. Diet Therapy.
3. Nutrition. WB 400
M294 1994]
RM216.M295 1994
615.8′54 — dc20
DNLM/DLC
for Library of Congress 93-20867
CIP

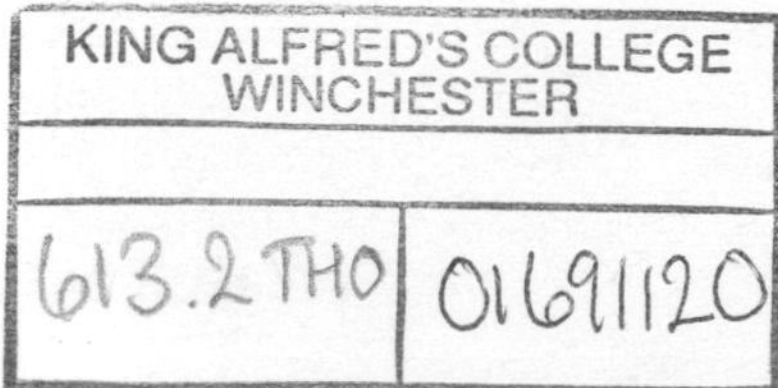

Contents

List of contributors

RACHEL ABRAHAM BSc SRD *Senior Dietitian, Northwick Park Hospital, Harrow.*

CHERIE BB AMBASNA BSc SRD *Formerly Chief Dietitian, The Middlesex Hospital, London.*

ANNIE S ANDERSON BSc PhD SRD *Research Fellow, University of Glasgow Department of Human Nutrition.*

ALISON ANDERTON BSc SRD *Senior Renal Dietitian, St Peter's Hospital/The Middlesex Hospital, London.*

CHRISTINE BALDWIN BSc SRD *Senior Dietitian, King's College Hospital, London.*

JANE BEBELL BSc SRD *Chief Dietitian, BHB Community Health Care NHS Trust.*

NAOMI BECKLES WILLSON BSc Dip Diet SRD *Paediatric Dietitian, Westminster Children's Hospital, London.*

SUE BENNETT SRD *Senior Renal Dietitian, Leicester General Hospital.*

SHEILA BINGHAM BSc SRD PhD *Senior Scientist, Dunn Clinical Nutrition Centre, Cambridge.*

ALISON E BLACK BSc SRD FBDA FIFST *Senior Scientific Officer, Dunn Clinical Nutrition Centre, Cambridge.*

GERALDINE M BLEAKNEY SRD Dip H.Ed *Head of Health Promotion Programmes, Dept Public Health Medicine, Eastern Health and Social Services Board, Belfast.*

DIANE BRIGG SRD *Clinical Manager – Nutrition and Dietetic Services, Ormskirk District General Hospital, Lancashire.*

CATHERINE BRYAN BSc SRD *Senior 1 (HIV) Dietitian, Westminster Hospital, London.*

ANDREW D CARVER BSc SRD *Senior Dietitian, Royal Edinburgh Hospital.*

ISSY COLE-HAMILTON BSc SRD *Dietitian, London.*

CATHERINE COLLINS BSc SRD *Senior Dietitian (ITU), St George's Hospital, Tooting, London.*

MOIRA DIXON BSc SRD *Director of Dietetic Services, Bradford Hospitals (NHS) Trust.*

ROSEMARY A DODDS BSc SRD *Research Dietitian, Unit for Metabolic Medicine, United Medical and Dental Schools, Guy's Campus, London SE1.*

PHYLLIS M EATON BA BSc SRD *Senior Dietitian, Dept of Geriatric Medicine, Dudley Road Hospital, Birmingham.*

JANE ELY BSc SRD *Paediatric Dietitian, King's College Hospital, London.*

DR SJ EVANS BSc DCC PhD C Chem FRSC *Consultant Clinical Biochemist, General Hospital, Northampton.*

JULIE FENTON SRD MHCIMA *Senior Dietitian, Normansfield, Teddington, Middlesex.*

CELIA FIRMIN BSc SRD *Manager – Nutrition and Dietetic Service, Leeds Community and Mental Health Services NHS Trust.*

MARGARET SN GELLATLY SRD *Honorary Dietary Adviser, Prader-Willi Syndrome Association (UK), Formerly District Dietitian, Mid-Essex Health Authority.*

CYNTHIA GOMES BSc SRD *Formerly District Dietitian, The Middlesex Hospital, London.*

AZMINA GOVINDJI BSc SRD *Chief Dietitian and Head of Diet Information Service, British Diabetic Association, London.*

MIRANDA GREG BSc SRD *Senior Dietitian, Chelsea and Westminster Hospital, London.*

JANE GRIFFIN BSc SRD *Consultant Sports Dietitian, Ealing, London.*

CAROLINE HADFIELD BSc SRD *Chief Renal Dietitian, St Mary's Hospital, Portsmouth.*

RICHARD HAWORTH M Phil, ACP, M Coll P, SRD *Head of Division of Nutrition and Dietetics, Glasgow Caledonian University.*

FRANCES HAY SRD *Senior Dietitian, Services for People with Learning Disabilities, Portsmouth.*

MARY HERITAGE BSc LCSLT *Senior Speech and Language Therapist, Nottingham City Hospital.*

PAT HOWARD SRD *Head of Nutrition and Dietetic Services, Bristol Royal Infirmary.*

PATRICIA M HULME BSc SRD *Head of Nutrition and Dietetic Services, Northwick Park Hospital, Harrow.*

MAUREEN HUNTER BSc MBA SRD *Rehabilitation Services Manager, The Royal Marsden Hospital, London and Surrey.*

RUTH JAMES BSc SRD *Chief Dietitian, John Radcliffe Hospital, Oxford.*

SARAH JEAN-MARIE BSc SRD *Community Dietitian, Royal London Hospital.*

SUSAN A JEBB BSc PhD SRD *Scientist, MRC Dunn Clinical Nutrition Centre, Cambridge.*

KAREN JEFFEREYS SRD *Chief Dietitian, Services for People with Learning Disabilities, Portsmouth.*

SHEILA D KENNEY BSc SRD *Senior Dietitian, Westminster Hospital, London.*

PETER KING BSc PhD SRD *Senior Dietitian, St Lawrence Hospital, Chepstow, Gwent.*

MARGARET S LAWSON MSc Cert Ed PhD SRD *Senior Lecturer in Paediatric Nutrition, Institute of Child Health and Head of Dietetic Services, The Hospitals for Sick Children, London.*

ANITA MACDONALD BSc SRD *Head of Dietetic Services, Birmingham Children's Hospital.*

RUTH MARKS BSc SRD *Dietitian, London.*

JACKIE MOORES BSc SRD *Community Dietitian, Chapel Allerton Clinic, Leeds.*

TINA MORLEY BSc MBA SRD *Clinical Audit Adviser (Formerly District Dietitian), North Warwickshire NHS Trust.*

MARGARET MURPHY BSc PhD *Lecturer in Nutrition, University of Surrey.*

ALISON M NICHOLLS BSc MPhil SRD *Senior Lecturer, Cardiff Institute of Higher Education, Cardiff.*

MARY O'KANE BSc SRD *Senior Dietitian, The General Infirmary, Leeds.*

GILL PAGE BSc SRD *Senior Dietitian, Nottingham City Hospital.*

CAROLYN PATCHELL BSc SRD *Chief Paediatric Dietitian, The Children's Hospital, Birmingham.*

SUSAN PATTEN SRD *Chief IV Dietitian, Queen Elizabeth Hospital, King's Lynn (Formerly Senior Dietitian, Westminster Children's Hospital).*

CLAIRE PLESTER BSc SRD *Research Dietitian, The Royal Infirmary, Edinburgh.*

MAGGIE PRICE BSc SRD *Senior Dietitian, Ely Hospital, Cardiff.*

LYNNE RADBONE BSc SRD *Senior Dietitian, Addenbrooke's Hospital, Cambridge.*

ROSEMARY RICHARDSON MSc SRD *Lecturer, Queen Margaret College, Edinburgh.*

ALEXANDRA RIORDAN BSc SRD *Formerly Research Dietitian, Dept of Gastroenterology, Addenbrooke's Hospital, Cambridge.*

SYLVIA ROBERT SARGEANT SRD *Consultant Dietitian, Brentford, Middlesex.*

LIANE S ROE AB MPH RD *Research Nutritionist, Dept of Public Health and Primary Care, University of Oxford.*

KATHLEEN ROSS BSc SRD *Senior Dietitian, Royal Aberdeen Children's Hospital.*

CHRISTINE RUSSELL SRD *Head of Nutrition, Cow & Gate Nutricia Ltd.*

ROSEMARY SEDDON SRD *Freelance Dietitian, Ruislip, Middlesex.*

ELIZABETH SIMPSON SRD *Freelance Dietitian, Chorleywood, Herts.*

JOHN STANTON BSc SRD *Chief Dietitian, Booth Hall Children's Hospital, Manchester.*

JENNIE STARR BSc Dip Diet SRD *Dietetic Services Manager, Eastbourne and County Healthcare NHS Trust.*

FIONA STEVEN BSc SRD MHSM *Chief Dietitian, Western Infirmary/Gartnavel General Hospitals Unit, Glasgow.*

CAROLYN SUMMERBELL SRD PhD *Lecturer in Nutrition, St Bartholomew's Hospital Medical College, London.*

BRIONY THOMAS BSc SRD PhD *Freelance Nutritionist, Surrey. Formerly Research Nutritionist, Unit for Metabolic Medicine, Guy's Hospital, London.*

DENISE THOMAS M Phil SRD *Chief Dietitian, St James Hospital, Portsmouth.*

JACKI TREDGER BSc SRD PhD *Lecturer in Dietetics, University of Surrey.*

KATHRYN F TWINE BSc SRD *Chief Dietitian, The Radcliffe Infirmary, Oxford.*

ERNEST WALTON MD FRCPath *Consultant Pathologist, Formerly of North Tees General Hospital, Stockton on Tees.*

RAE WARD BSc SRD *Consultant Dietitian, The Coeliac Society of the United Kingdom.*

AILSA WELCH BSc SRD *Information Scientist, The Royal Society of Chemistry, Cambridge.*

GILLIAN WHEELER BSc SRD *Manager, Nutrition and Dietetic Service, Northampton Health Authority.*

CHRISTINE M WILLIAMS BSc PhD *Lecturer in Human Nutrition, University of Surrey.*

RICHARD C WILSON BSc SRD *Director of Nutrition and Dietetics, King's College Hospital, London.*

HAZEL A WITTE SRD *Unit Dietitian, Aberdeen Royal Infirmary.*

SUSAN WOODS BSc SRD *Senior Dietitian, Services for People with Learning Disabilities, Portsmouth.*

Acknowledgements

Miss R Abraham, *Northwick Park Hospital, Harrow, Middlesex.*

Martha Annan, *Chief Dietitian, Maidstone Hospital, Kent.*

Mrs Barbara Baigent B Pharm MR Pharm.

Dr CJ Bates, *MRC Dunn Nutrition Centre, Cambridge.*

Dr John Berkeley, *Roxburghe House, Aberdeen.*

Miss PJ Brereton, *Dietetic Advisor, Northwick Park Hospital, Harrow, Middx.*

Valerie Campbell, *Senior Dietitian, St George's Hospital, London.*

Dr Roger Chapman, *Consultant Gastroenterologist, John Radcliffe Hospital, Oxford.*

Mei Ngoh Chang, *Dietitian, London.*

Dr TJ Cole, *MRC Dunn Nutrition Centre, Cambridge.*

Mrs Mary Cooper, *Community Dietitian, St Mary's Hospital, Leeds.*

Professor TJ David, *Department of Child Health, University of Manchester and Hon Consultant Physician, Booth Hall Children's Hospital.*

Dr PSW Davies, *MRC Dunn Nutrition Centre, Cambridge.*

Dietitians of the Liver Interest Group of the British Dietetic Association.

Dr MG Dunnigan, *Stobhill General Hospital, Glasgow.*

MR P Edmond, *Director Scottish Spinal Injury Service, Glasgow.*

Dr M Elia, *MRC Dunn Nutrition Centre, Cambridge.*

Professor DR Fraser, *Professor of Animal Science, University of Sydney, Australia.*

Angela M. Greenwood, *Community Dietitian, Dewsbury District Hospital.*

Mrs Janet B Henderson, *Stobhill General Hospital, Glasgow.*

Anne Heughan, *Nutritionist, Coronary Prevention Group, London.*

Bridie Holland BSc SRD, *Senior Information Scientist, The Royal Society of Chemistry, Cambridge.*

Paula Hunt, *Nutritionist/Dietitian, HEA Primary Care Unit, Oxford.*

Dr JO Hunter, *Consultant Physician, Addenbrooke's Hospital, Cambridge.*

Dr BM Laurance, *Formerly Consultant Physician, Queen Elizabeth Hospital for Sick Children, London.*

Mrs Nancy Mately, *Secretary, Cardiff Royal Infirmary.*

Dr Martin B Mattock, *Principal Biochemist, Unit for Metabolic Medicine, Guy's Hospital, London.*

Rekha Naidu BSc SRD, *Consultant Dietitian, Gaborone, Botswana.*

Lynne Peace, *Spinal Injuries Dietitian, Stoke Mandeville Hospital.*

Caroline Penman, *Senior Dietitian, City Hospital, Edinburgh.*

Dr B Pentland, *Consultant Physician, Brain Injuries Rehabilitation Unit, Edinburgh.*

Miss Rosemary Richardson MSc SRD, *Queen Margaret College, Edinburgh.*

Dr J Reeve, *Northwick Park Hospital, Harrow.*

The Research Committee of the British Dietetic Association.

Dr AS Ritch, Hon Secretary, *British Geriatrics Society.*

S Springfield, *University Hospital, London.*

Rhoda Sutherland SRD, *Dietitian, Southampton.*

Dr DI Thurnham, *MRC Dunn Nutrition Centre, Cambridge.*

Georgina West, *Diet Department, British Diabetic Association, London.*

Gabrielle Williams, *District Dietitian, Halton General Hospital, Cheshire.*

Foreword

It is a great pleasure to write the Foreword to the second edition of a *Manual of Dietetic Practice* which has proved so successful and popular with working dietitians and students not only in Britain but in other English-speaking countries. The Editor, Dr Briony Thomas, and most of the contributors to this second edition are dietitians. The format remains much the same but everything has been updated or re-written and new chapters concerned with such subjects as AIDS and Terminal Care have been added. This Manual is extraordinarily thorough. Most chapters commence with a brief account of the scientific basis for the practical recommendations. The latter are very detailed and a holistic approach to the care of the individual is evident.

Although the Manual is primarily for dietitians, it has much to contribute to the knowledge and skills of other health professionals, including doctors and nurses. The Manual represents a great achievement on the part of the British Dietetic Association which is increasingly providing leadership and information in the public domain. With the publication of *Health of the Nation* which places such emphasis on good nutrition in the maintenance of health and the prevention of disease, the role of dietitians assumes ever greater importance. The British Dietetic Association can be proud of this Manual and all that it is doing in the field of nutrition.

Dame Barbara Clayton, DBE
Honorary Research Professor
in Metabolism
University of Southampton

Introduction

The first edition of the *Manual of Dietetic Practice* received an enthusiastic response from dietitians. The aim of the book had been to provide comprehensive and essentially practical guidance on all aspects of dietetics – from the promotion of health to the management of disease. Much to the relief to those who had produced it, the *Manual* appeared to fulfil this objective. All levels of the dietetic profession, from students to the most senior, seemed to find it of value. Above all, it was a pleasure to hear that the book was actually being *used*, and not just gathering dust on a bookshelf.

However, as with any scientific textbook, the passage of time meant that parts of the text became out-of-date and it was clear that a new edition would be welcomed. All sections of the *Manual* have therefore been updated and many of them completely re-written and expanded. In response to requests from dietitians, coverage of subjects such as AIDS/HIV disease, brain and spinal injuries and pressure sores has been included. To save space, a few topics which appeared to be little used or which will be covered in the forthcoming *Textbook of Paediatric Dietetic Practice* have been omitted.

The format of the *Manual* has remained much as before although the book has been divided into 7 main sections, rather than 6, as a number of topics have been brought together under the new heading of 'Acute trauma'. For those who are unfamiliar with the layout:

Section 1 General Dietetic Principles and Practice
Discusses the basic 'tools of the trade' required by every dietitian. This section covers the principles of healthy eating, the assessment of nutritional requirements, intake and status, and the practical aspects of advising and feeding patients.

Section 2 Foods and Nutrients
This is a compendium of information about foods, food components and nutrients. It can be used a reference source by itself but it also complements other sections (particularly those on 'Therapeutic Dietetics') by providing practical details of specific dietary manipulations (e.g. sodium restriction or an increased fibre intake). This avoids the need for constant repetition of dietary details throughout the book.

Section 3 Nutritional Needs of Population Subgroups
Discusses the nutritional needs and problems of particular sections of the population i.e. the factors which may be relevant to a person's age, ethnic origin, degree of physical or learning ability or income. The information may be helpful when giving guidance to individuals or groups of people. It may also be useful for preparing educational material for the general public or health care professionals.

Section 4 Therapeutic Dietetics for Disease States
Looks at the dietetic management of clinical disorders. The order in which topics are presented has been rearranged slightly and coverage of subjects such as food intolerance and cancer have been moved into this section. As before, readers are cross-referred to other sections for specific details of dietary manipulations or practical aspects of enteral or parenteral feeding.

Section 5 Dietetic Management of Acute Trauma
Covers the metabolic consequences of acute injury and discusses the nutritional implications of brain or spinal injury, burns and surgery. Management of pressure sores is also included in this section.

Section 6 Investigative Procedures
Discusses metabolic balance diets, diagnostic tests and dietetic research.

Section 7 Appendices
Contains ready reference information on conversion factors, clinical reference ranges, addresses and abbreviations. Anthropometric and BMR tables, food portion sizes and compositional data on proprietary nutritional products have also been moved to the Appendices to make them easier to find.

While every effort has been made to ensure that the information given in this book is correct, those involved in the book's production cannot accept liability for any errors which may have inadvertently occurred, nor the consequences of them. We would particularly like to stress that compositional details of manufactured products (e.g. specialist feeds) are given for guidance only; obviously the formulation of such products is likely to change and dietitians must ensure that they are using up-to-date information before recommending their use for patients.

We have also endeavoured to obtain the necessary permission to use all copyright material reproduced in this book. If any omissions have occurred in this respect, or incorrect acknowledgements given, we offer our sincere apologies and will rectify this at the earliest opportunity.

Producing a book of this nature is an enormous undertaking and involves many people. An enormous debt of gratitude is owed to the contributors who have worked so hard to transcribe their practical expertise into written material. Mention must also be made of some of our former authors who, for various reasons, were unable to contribute to this edition but some of whose work remains within the revised text. These are: Avril Aslett-Bentley, Carol Bowyer, Mary Cooper, Pat Crooks, Wendy Doyle, Liz Eeley, Diane Holdsworth, Susan Howie, Jennifer King, Carol Logan, Sue Lupson, Jill Metcalfe, Lesley Michael, Marion Noble, Jenny Salmon, Doug Scott, Diane Spalding, Pat Torrens and Steve Wootton. Other people who have given us valuable help and advice are listed in the Acknowledgements. Grateful thanks are also due to John Grigg and the British Dietetic Association for supporting the project, and to Richard Miles and the production staff at Blackwell Science for their encouragement and patience. I hope that those who use this book will find that the efforts of those who have created it have been worthwhile.

Briony Thomas
Editor

Section 1 General dietetic principles and practice

1.1 Basic principles of a healthy diet

1.1.1 Perspective

Man has been preoccupied since the earliest times with the relationship between food and health. Complex classifications of foods according to their 'elemental qualities' survived in orthodox teaching for almost 2000 years. Only over the past 200 years, with the development of the science of nutrition, has it become possible to make quantitative recommendations about the amount and type of food (the diet) which should be eaten to maintain health.

1.1.2 Essential nutrients

One of the first principles of healthy eating is that the requirement for the essential nutrients – amino acids, vitamins, inorganic nutrients, essential fatty acids and energy – must be met. Most foods contain a variety of nutrients but, as nearly all are deficient in one or more, requirements for essential nutrients are most likely to be met if a wide variety of foods is eaten in moderation. It is sometimes stated that energy requirement – and therefore energy intake – is the cornerstone of every diet. However, although intakes of energy yielding nutrients are highly correlated with total energy intake, there are only small or negative correlations between energy intake and other nutrients (Table 1.1). Good sources of vitamin C for example are generally low in energy.

In general the essential nutrients are to be found in greater amounts and in more bioavailable forms in animal products such as meat, fish, cheese, eggs and milk. Hence these food groups, together with vegetables and fruit, have traditionally been emphasized in guidelines for healthy eating particularly for those at most risk of classic deficiency disease – the young, the elderly and pregnant or breast feeding women. However, in Westernized countries the occurrence of malnutrition, as judged by poor growth rates or frank clinical symptoms, is now rare and confined to well-defined circumstances – for example certain ethnic minority groups. In present-day urban societies, it is the major life-threatening conditions of middle and later life in which diet is now recognized to be of crucial importance.

1.1.3 Current problems

In most Western countries, coronary heart disease accounts for more deaths and more premature deaths than any other single cause. Mortality from CHD in the UK is amongst the highest in the world. Though genetic variation in apolipoproteins is important in determining susceptibility to coronary heart disease, about half the risk is attributable to smoking, high blood pressure and raised serum cholesterol concentrations, with the last two being profoundly affected by diet. Hypertension, which is a risk factor for stroke, is related to alcohol consumption, obesity, high dietary sodium intake, and reduced intakes of potassium and possibly calcium and magnesium (DHHS 1988). Relative risk of stroke is increased fourfold in people with usual diastolic blood pressures of 105 mm Hg and above (WHO 1990).

In cancer, attributable risk from diet for all sites is estimated to be 35%, although at the major sites of breast, bowel and stomach the contribution from diet is substan-

Table 1.1 Correlation coefficients between dietary variables in 16-day weighed records from 160 free-living women aged 50–65 (Source: Bingham *et al* 1994)

a) *Absolute intakes*	Fat	Protein	Starch	Sucrose	NSP	Retinol	Carotene	Vitamin C	Alcohol
Total energy	0.86	0.68	0.57	0.67	0.28	0.21	−0.02	0.17	0.19
Fat		0.48	0.38	0.41	0.01	0.26	−0.12	0.02	0.09
Protein			0.35	0.42	0.44	0.19	0.24	0.32	0.14
Starch				0.28	0.31	0.07	−0.09	−0.01	−0.11
Sucrose					0.28	0.09	0.14	0.31	−0.25
NSP						0.03	0.48	0.60	0.00
Retinol							−0.09	0.09	0.00
Carotene								0.45	−0.04
Vitamin C									0.07

b) *Intakes as a percentage of total calories*	Fat (% calories)	Protein (% calories)	Carbohydrate (% calories)
Total calories	0.18	−0.45	0.00

tially greater (Doll and Peto 1981). In addition low non-starch polysaccharide (NSP) intake and hence low stool weight is associated with greater risk of constipation, diverticular disease, gallstones and cancer. For constipation alone, about 0.5 million patients consult their general practitioners in England and Wales (DoH 1991b). Sucrose is one of the main risk factors for dental caries and some estimates suggest that new cases of non-insulin dependent diabetes (NIDDM) could be halved by preventing obesity in middle aged adults (DHHS 1988).

1.1.4 Practical recommendations

This substantial potential contribution of diet to health and to prevention of disease has been recognized in recent publications (WHO 1990; DoH 1991a; DoH 1991b). Dietary Reference Values (DRV) for fat, non-starch polysaccharides (NSP), starch, non-milk extrinsic sugars (NMES) and sodium are substantially different from present-day levels. These are discussed further in Section 1.2, but Table 1.2 shows present-day intakes in relation to WHO (1990) values and the DRVs. Substantial differences are evident. To meet these goals, on average saturated fat needs to be reduced by 40%, total fat by 13% and sodium by 50%. Present consumption of non-milk extrinsic sugars is uncertain, but consumption level estimates, after allowance for non-food use, are 15% total energy (BNF 1987), so that intakes should decrease by one third. Other sugar and starch intakes need to increase by one third, and NSP intakes by 50% on average. Vegetable and fruit consumption needs to double.

Table 1.3 sets out possible ways in which average diets could be altered to meet the DRVs; 50% of this increase in NSP could be brought about by a doubling of vegetable

Table 1.2 Dietary changes that will improve health in the UK

Dietary component	Present intake[1]	DRV[2]	WHO Population goals[3]
Percentage total energy from total fat	38	33	15–30
Percentage total energy from saturated fat	16	10	0–10
Non-milk extrinsic sugars, % total energy	15[4]	10	0–10
Starch and other sugars, % total energy	28	37	50–70
NSP, g per day	12	18	16–24
Vegetables and fruit, g per day	208	380[5]	400
Sodium intake, mmol per day	150	70	100

[1] Gregory *et al* (1990)
[2] DoH (1991b)
[3] WHO (1990)
[4] BNF (1987)
[5] Bingham (1991)

Table 1.3 Possible change in average consumption of foods to achieve proposed targets for 2005

Food	Present[1] intake g	Possible change to g	*Contributions to required alterations in:* Saturated fatty acids g	NME sugars g	NSP g	Starch & other sugars g	*Increase* or *decrease*
Wholemeal and other bread	43	110	—	—	2.2	50	2.5
White bread	65	85	—	—	0.3	10	1.3
Vegetables	135	270	—	—	3.0	11	2.0
Fruit	73	110	—	—	0.3	4	1.5
Potatoes	132	200	—	—	0.8	13	1.5
Biscuits, cakes, puddings	80	40	2.4	8	—	—	0.5
Whole milk to semi-skimmed	164	164	2.0	—	—	—	1.0
Saturated spreads to low fat	10	10	4.0	—	—	—	1.0
Leaner meat	150	150	3.0	—	—	—	1.0
Chips, crisps and lower fat	62	31	1.2	—	—	—	0.5
Chocolate	9	5	0.7	2	—	—	0.5
Sugar, preserves	23	12	—	12	—	—	0.5
Beverages, soft drinks	100	50	—	3	—	—	0.5
Total			−13g	−25g	+6.5g	+88g*	

* Includes allowance for the reduction in sources of non-milk extrinsic sugars
[1] Gregory *et al* (1990)

intake from present consumption levels of 135 to 270 g per day. There is emerging evidence that high vegetable intakes are particularly effective in the provision of anti-oxidants important in the prevention of stroke and CHD, and of cancer of the stomach, bowel, oesophagus and lung (Section 2.6.2). A doubling of vegetable intake will make up the 20 mmol shortfall between recommended levels of 90 mmol per day potassium and present intakes of 70 mmol per day (Gregory *et al* 1990; DoH 1991a). In addition, vegetables are major sources of folate and hence of particular value in the prevention of neural tube defects. Starch consumption would need to increase substantially to compensate for reduced energy from non-milk extrinsic sugars and fat, and would most usefully be derived from bread. If this were mainly wholemeal bread, the goal for NSP would easily be met. Salt levels in bread need to be reduced, however, to avoid an increase in non-discretionary consumption. At present bread and cereal products supply 40% of total non-discretionary intake. Overall reduction in the sodium content of manufactured and processed food will be necessary, since intakes from non-discretionary sources are in the region of 120 mmol per day, 50 mmol greater than the DRV. The rest of the increase in starch and intrinsic sugars would be derived from potato and fruit consumption.

Towards reducing the intake of saturated fatty acids by about 13 g, a simple change from full fat to semi-skimmed milk and from full fat to low fat spreads will reduce fat consumption by 6 g. A change from average fat to lean meat and substitution with fish might achieve a further 3 g reduction, and halving consumption of biscuits, cakes, puddings, chips, crisps and chocolate (which currently supply 24% of the total intake of saturated fatty acids) would achieve the remaining 4 g. Consumption of soft drinks and table sugar would need to be halved to make the necessary 25 g reduction in non-milk extrinsic sugars. By definition, half the population will need to make more and half make less than these changes, with older age groups requiring greater changes because serum cholesterol concentrations, body weight, and saturated fat consumption are all greater in these groups than in 25–34 year old (Gregory *et al* 1990).

1.1.5 Feasibility of achieving targets

It is clear from Section 1.1.3 that a substantial improvement in health would result if DRV and WHO population goals were achieved. The population target levels are all compatible with a diet comprised of normal food and are already being consumed by other populations or have been met in the UK in the past. However, dietitians have a major role to play in instigating these changes which have been endorsed by the British Dietetic Association (BDA 1991). This role encompasses education throughout schools, colleges, institutions, the media, patients, the general community, health professionals and even workers in the food industry. A consistent message, combined with government action in education, health, agriculture and industry, is essential for achieving change and consequent benefits to health for all of the community.

References

Bingham S (1991) Dietary aspects of a health strategy for England. *Br Med J* **303**, 353–5

Bingham SA, Gill C, Welch A, Day K, Cassidy A, Khan KT, Snagd MJ, Key TJA, Roe L and Day NE (1994) Comparison of dietary assessment methods in nutritional epidemiology: weighed records versus 24 hour recalls, food frequency questionnaires and estimated diet records. *Br J Nutr* (submitted).

British Dietetic Association (1991) *Response to 'The Health of the Nation'.* BDA, Birmingham.

British Nutrition Foundation (1987) *Task force on sugars and syrups.* BNF, London.

Department of Health (1991a) *Committee on Medical Aspects of Food Policy. Dietary Reference Values for food energy and nutrients for the United Kingdom,* Rep Hlth Soc Subj **41**, HMSO, London.

Department of Health (1991b) *The Health of the Nation.* HMSO, London.

Department of Health and Human Services (1988) *Surgeon General's report on nutrition and health.* Washington DC, DHHS (Publication 88–50 210).

Doll R and Peto R (1981) Quantitative estimates of avoidable risks of cancer in the US today. *J Natl Cancer Inst* **66**, 1192–308.

Gregory J, Foster K, Tyler H and Wiseman M (1990) *The dietary and nutritional survey of adults.* HMSO, London.

World Health Organization (1990) *Diet, nutrition and the prevention of chronic diseases. WHO Tech Rep Ser No 797.* WHO Geneva.

1.2 Dietary reference values and recommended dietary allowances

1.2.1 Definition

Guidance on the adequacy of diets of populations is required for many purposes, and standards against which measured intakes can be compared are published by most governments and by the World Health Organization (WHO 1985), the British Nutrition Foundation (BNF 1989) and the National Research Council (NRC 1989). These standards have been called Recommended Daily Amounts (RDA), defined as 'the average amount of the nutrient which should be provided per head in a group of people if the needs of practically all members of the group are to be met' (DHSS 1979). In an earlier report, they were called Recommended Daily Intakes (RDI), defined as 'the amount sufficient, or more than sufficient, for the nutritional needs of practically all healthy persons in a population' (DHSS 1969). Both these definitions attempted to make it clear that these values refer only to population estimates and, because of the physiological differences between individuals, should not be used alone for judging the adequacy of individual diets (see below).

In the latest report of the Committee on Medical Aspects (COMA) of Food Policy (DoH 1991), the single RDA figures have been replaced by three standards, called Dietary Reference Values (DRV). These are defined in Table 1.4. The Reference Nutrient Intake (RNI) is equivalent to RDA or RDI values. Note that the DRVs for energy are Estimated Average Requirements (EARs), since it is clearly inappropriate to add on extra provision to allow for individual variation in energy requirement without adverse effect on energy balance in the population concerned. Similarly the DRVs for the main energy yielding nutrients, fats, sugars and starches, and for NSP (dietary fibre) are also given as population averages.

Table 1.4 Definition of Dietary Reference Values (DRVs)

EAR	*Estimated Average Requirement* The average requirement for a nutrient for a class of individuals
RNI	*Reference Nutrient Intake* Nutrient values two standard deviations greater than the EAR. Assuming a normal population distribution, this covers the needs of at least 97.5% of the population. Intakes above this amount will almost certainly be adequate for both populations and individuals within that population
LNRI	*Lower Reference Nutrient Intake* Nutrient values two standard deviations less than the EAR. Intakes below this amount will almost certainly be inadequate for both populations and individuals within that population

1.2.2 Derivation of DRVs

In deriving DRVs, the EAR is first established from physiological criteria, which include data on intakes needed to maintain circulating enzyme levels in the body, intakes associated with freedom from signs or symptoms of deficiency disease, and energy expenditure. Allowances are also made for the bioavailability of nutrients in food, and it is assumed that the DRVs for other nutrients are met. The DRVs only apply to groups of healthy people and may not be appropriate for some clinical conditions, such as infections and major gastrointestinal or metabolic disorders.

1.2.3 Individual advice

Because the RNI is set at two standard deviations above the EAR, the requirement of the majority of individuals would be lower than this. Nevertheless, it is prudent to give advice about diet to an individual whose intakes are shown to be habitually less than the RNI (see Section 1.1). Intakes less than the LNRI are almost certainly deficient. Because it is an average, half the class is expected to require more than the EAR for energy, and half less. In practice, a body weight which is in accordance with the ideal remains the best indication for the individual that requirements for energy expenditure are adequately balanced by energy intake (but see below).

1.2.4 Summary of DRVs

Detailed tables of the UK DRVs with background information on their derivation are published in a 200 page booklet, entitled *Dietary Reference Values for Food Energy and Nutrients for the UK*, Department of Health and Social Subjects No. 41, available from HMSO, 1991 price £11.50 (DoH 1991). This is required reading for all dietitians, and only a summary is given here.

Estimated average requirements for energy are given in Table 1.5. Two assumptions are made in these EARs. First, standard body weights (for example, 74 kg men, 60–63 kg women) have been used to calculate Basal Metabolic Rates (BMRs) using standard equations derived by Schofield *et al* (1985). The equations are given as an annex in the DRV Report (DoH 1991), and an average BMR for groups of people with body weights different

Table 1.5 Estimated Average Requirements (EARs) for Energy

Age	EARs MJ/d (kcal/d)	
	males	females
0–3 months	2.28 (545)	2.16 (515)
4–6 months	2.89 (690)	2.69 (645)
7–9 months	3.44 (825)	3.20 (765)
10–12 months	3.85 (920)	3.61 (865)
1–3 years	5.15 (1230)	4.86 (1165)
4–6 years	7.16 (1715)	6.46 (1545)
7–10 years	8.24 (1970)	7.28 (1740)
11–14 years	9.27 (2220)	7.92 (1845)
15–18 years	11.51 (2755)	8.83 (2110)
19–50 years	10.60 (2550)	8.10 (1940)
51–59 years	10.60 (2550)	8.00 (1900)
60–64 years	9.93 (2380)	7.99 (1900)
65–74 years	9.71 (2330)	7.96 (1900)
75+ years	8.77 (2100)	7.61 (1810)
Pregnancy		+0.80* (200)
Lactation:		
1 month		+1.90 (450)
2 months		+2.20 (530)
3 months		+2.40 (570)
4–6 months (Group 1)**		+2.00 (480)
4–6 months (Group 2)		+2.40 (570)
>6 months (Group 1)		+1.00 (240)
>6 months (Group 2)		+2.30 (550)

* Last trimester only

** Group 1: Women who practise exclusive or almost exclusive breast feeding until the baby is 3–4 months old.

Group 2: Women whose intention is that breast milk should provide the primary source of nourishment for the baby for 6 months or more.

DoH (1991). Information reproduced with the permission of the Controller of Her Majesty's Stationery Office

Table 1.6 Reference Nutrient Intakes for Protein

Age	Reference Nutrient Intake[a] g/d
0–3 months	12.5[b]
4–6 months	12.7
7–9 months	13.7
10–12 months	14.9
1–3 years	14.5
4–6 years	19.7
7–10 years	28.3
Males:	
11–14 years	42.1
15–18 years	55.2
19–50 years	55.5
50+ years	53.3
Females:	
11–14 years	41.2
15–18 years	45.0
19–50 years	45.0
50+ years	46.5
Pregnancy[c]	+6
Lactation[c]	
0–4 months	+11
4+ months	+8

[a] These figures, based on egg and milk protein, assume complete digestibility

[b] No values for infants 0–3 months are given by WHO. The RNI is calculated from the recommendations of COMA

[c] To be added to adult requirement through all stages of pregnancy and lactation

DoH (1991). Information reproduced with the permission of the Controller of Her Majesty's Stationery Office

from the average can be calculated if wished. A ready reference BMR table based on these equations is given in Appendix 4, Tables 7.40 and 7.41. Individual estimates are subject to variability of approximately ±10%. Having established BMR energy requirements, an allowance is then added on for activity. Most sedentary populations expend only about 40% more energy in excess of the BMR, so that the values in Table 1.5 are equal to the calculated BMR times 1.4. Within the average of 10.6 MJ for men, however, the range would vary from 9.3 MJ in men weighing only 60 kg to as much as 17 MJ in groups of 85 kg men with activity levels of 2.2 times the BMR. Detailed tables for all classes of the population are given in the Report (DoH 1991).

The RNIs for protein are given in Table 1.6. These are based on the EAR sufficient to maintain nitrogen balance, and are less than the previously published values (DHSS 1979) which were based on usual dietary intakes.

Tables 1.7 and 1.8 show RNIs for most vitamins and minerals. Vitamin C RNIs are somewhat greater than previous RDAs, and vitamin A levels rather less. Calcium levels are substantially greater than previously, as are RNIs for iron in women of childbearing age. There are new estimates of RNIs for phosphorus, magnesium, zinc, copper, selenium and iodine. The RNIs of 70 mmol sodium and 90 mmol potassium were based on the need to reduce blood pressure levels in the UK population. Since the RNI is much less than the current intake of 150 mmol Na per day, and the RNI of 90 mmol is greater than the current intake of 70 mmol, these DRVs have important implications for the present UK diet, and for the work of dietitians in achieving them.

Insufficient information was available for establishing RNIs for pantothenic acid, biotin, vitamin E, vitamin K, manganese, molybdenum, chromium and fluoride. Guidance on safe intakes is shown in Table 1.9.

Major differences between current intakes and the DRVs for fat, fatty acids, starch, NSP (fibre) and sugars have also emerged (see Table 1.10). The percentage of energy from saturated fatty acids is presently about 16%, and a reduction to 10% is required to reduce present levels of serum cholesterol from 5.8 mmol/l towards the desirable level of 5.2 mmol/l. Monounsaturated fats and polyunsaturates (including the essential fatty acids) should remain at pres-

Table 1.7 Reference Nutrient Intakes for Vitamins

Age	Thiamin	Riboflavin	Niacin (nicotinic acid equivalent)	Vitamin B6	Vitamin B12	Folate	Vitamin C	Vitamin A	vitamin D
	mg/d	mg/d	mg/d	mg/d[†]	µg/d	µg/d	mg/d	µg/d	µg/d
0–3 months	0.2	0.4	3	0.2	0.3	50	25	350	8.5
4–6 months	0.2	0.4	3	0.2	0.3	50	25	350	8.5
7–9 months	0.2	0.4	4	0.3	0.4	50	25	350	7
10–12 months	0.3	0.4	5	0.4	0.4	50	25	350	7
1–3 years	0.5	0.6	8	0.7	0.5	70	30	400	7
4–6 years	0.7	0.8	11	0.9	0.8	100	30	500	—
7–10 years	0.7	1.0	12	1.0	1.0	150	30	500	—
Males									
11–14 years	0.9	1.2	15	1.2	1.2	200	35	600	—
15–18 years	1.1	1.3	18	1.5	1.5	200	40	700	—
19–50 years	1.0	1.3	17	1.4	1.5	200	40	700	—
50+ years	0.9	1.3	16	1.4	1.5	200	40	700	**
Females									
11–14 years	0.7	1.1	12	1.0	1.2	200	35	600	—
15–18 years	0.8	1.1	14	1.2	1.5	200	40	600	—
19–50 years	0.8	1.1	13	1.2	1.5	200	40	600	—
50+ years	0.8	1.1	12	1.2	1.5	200	40	600	**
Pregnancy	+0.1***	+0.3	*	*	*	+100	+10	+100	10
Lactation:									
0–4 months	+0.2	+0.5	+2	*	+0.5	+60	+30	+350	10
4+ months	+0.2	+0.5	+2	*	+0.5	+60	+30	+350	10

* No increment ** After age 65 the RNI is 10 µg/d for men and women *** For last trimester only [†] Based on protein providing 14.7 per cent of EAR for energy

DoH (1991). Reproduced with the permission of the Controller of Her Majesty's Stationery Office

Table 1.8a Reference Nutrient Intakes for Minerals (SI Units)

Age	Calcium	Phosphorus[1]	Magnesium	Sodium[2]	Potassium[3]	Chloride[4]	Iron	Zinc	Copper	Selenium	Iodine
	mmol/d	mmol/d	mmol/d	mmol/d	mmol/d	mmol/d	µmol/d	µmol/d	µmol/d	µmol/d	µmol/d
0–3 months	13.1	13.1	2.2	9	20	9	30	60	5	0.1	0.4
4–6 months	13.1	13.1	2.5	12	22	12	80	60	5	0.2	0.5
7–9 months	13.1	13.1	3.2	14	18	14	140	75	5	0.1	0.5
10–12 months	13.1	13.1	3.3	15	18	15	140	75	5	0.1	0.5
1–3 years	8.8	8.8	3.5	22	20	22	120	75	6	0.2	0.6
4–6 years	11.3	11.3	4.8	30	28	30	110	100	9	0.3	0.8
7–10 years	13.8	13.8	8.0	50	50	50	160	110	11	0.4	0.9
Males											
11–14 years	25.0	25.0	11.5	70	80	70	200	140	13	0.6	1.0
15–18 years	25.0	25.0	12.3	70	90	70	200	145	16	0.9	1.0
19–50 years	17.5	17.5	12.3	70	90	70	160	145	19	0.9	1.0
50+ years	17.5	17.5	12.3	70	90	70	160	145	19	0.9	1.0
Females											
11–14 years	20.0	20.0	11.5	70	80	70	260[5]	140	13	0.6	1.0
15–18 years	20.0	20.0	12.3	70	90	70	260[5]	110	16	0.8	1.1
19–50 years	17.5	17.5	10.9	70	90	70	260[5]	110	19	0.8	1.1
50+ years	17.5	17.5	10.9	70	90	70	160	110	19	0.8	1.1
Pregnancy	*	*	*	*	*	*	*	*	*	*	*
Lactation:											
0–4 months	+14.3	+14.3	+2.1	*	*	*	*	+90	+5	+0.2	*
4+ months	+14.3	+14.3	+2.1	*	*	*	*	+40	+5	+0.2	*

* No increment [1] Phosphorus RNI is set equal to calcium in molar terms [2] 1 mmol sodium = 23 mg [3] 1 mmol potassium = 39 mg [4] Corresponds to sodium 1 mmol = 35.5 mg [5] Insufficient for women with high menstrual losses where the most practical way of meeting iron requirements is to take iron supplements

DoH (1991). Reproduced with the permission of the Controller of Her Majesty's Stationery Office

Table 1.8b Reference Nutrient Intakes for Minerals (SI Units) (continued)

Age	Calcium mg/d	Phosphorus[1] mg/d	Magnesium mg/d	Sodium mg/d[2]	Potassium mg/d[3]	Chloride[4] mg/d	Iron mg/d	Zinc mg/d	Copper mg/d	Selenium μg/d	Iodine μg/d
0–3 months	525	400	55	210	800	320	1.7	4.0	0.2	10	50
4–6 months	525	400	60	280	850	400	4.3	4.0	0.3	13	60
7–9 months	525	400	75	320	700	500	7.8	5.0	0.3	10	60
10–12 months	525	400	80	350	700	500	7.8	5.0	0.3	10	60
1–3 years	350	270	85	500	800	800	6.9	5.0	0.4	15	70
4–6 years	450	350	120	700	1100	1100	6.1	6.5	0.6	20	100
7–10 years	550	450	200	1200	2000	1800	8.7	7.0	0.7	30	110
Males											
11–14 years	1000	775	280	1600	3100	2500	11.3	9.0	0.8	45	130
15–18 years	1000	775	300	1600	3500	2500	11.3	9.5	1.0	70	140
19–50 years	700	550	300	1600	3500	2500	8.7	9.5	1.2	75	140
50+ years	700	550	300	1600	3500	2500	8.7	9.5	1.2	75	140
Females											
11–14 years	800	625	280	1600	3100	2500	14.8[5]	9.0	0.8	45	130
15–18 years	800	625	300	1600	3500	2500	14.8[5]	7.0	1.0	60	140
19–50 years	700	550	270	1600	3500	2500	14.8[5]	7.0	1.2	60	140
50+ years	700	550	270	1600	3500	2500	8.7	7.0	1.2	60	140
Pregnancy	*	*	*	*	*	*	*	*	*	*	*
Lactation:											
0–4 months	+550	+440	+50	*	*	*	*	+6.0	+0.3	+15	*
4+ months	+550	+440	+50	*	*	*	*	+2.5	+0.3	+15	*

* No increment
[1] Phosphorus RNI is set equal to calcium in molar terms
[2] 1 mmol sodium = 23 mg
[3] 1 mmol potassium = 39 mg
[4] Corresponds to sodium 1 mmol = 35.5 mg
[5] Insufficient for women with high menstrual losses where the most practical way of meeting iron requirements is to take iron supplements

DoH (1991). Reproduced with the permission of the Controller of Her Majesty's Stationery Office

Table 1.9 Safe intakes

Nutrient	Safe intake*
Vitamins:	
Pantothenic acid	
adults	3–7 mg/d
infants	1.7 mg/d
Biotin	10–200 μg/d
Vitamin E	
men	above 4 mg/d
women	above 3 mg/d
infants	0.4 mg/g polyunsaturated fatty acids
Vitamin K	
adults	1 μg/kg/d
infants	10 μg/d
Minerals:	
Manganese	
adults	about 1.4 mg (26 μmol)/d
infants and children	above 16 μg (0.3 μmol)/kg/day
Molybdenum	
adults	50–400 μg/d
infants, children and adolescents	0.5–1.5 μg/kg/d
Chromium	
adults	above 25 μg (0.5 μmol)/d
children and adolescents	0.1–1.0 μg (2–20 μmol)/kg/d
Fluoride (for infants only)	0.05 mg (3 μmol)/kg/d

* A level or range of intake at which there is no risk of deficiency, and below a level where there is a risk of undesirable effects.

DoH (1991). Reproduced with the permission of the Controller of Her Majesty's Stationery Office

ent levels of 12% and 6% respectively, so that overall there has to be a reduction in total fat consumption from present day levels of 38% to 33% total energy.

Non-milk extrinsic sugars (NMES) consumption is also recommended to decrease on average for present day levels to 10% total energy because of their established contribution to dental caries. The remainder of the energy supply (37%) should be made up with other sugars and starch.

Non-starch polysaccharides (NSP) need also to increase from present day levels of 12 g to 18 g per day in order that stool weight should increase from 100 to 125 g per day. Low stool weight is associated with increased risk of constipation, diverticular disease, gallstones and bowel cancer.

The DRVs will therefore entail major changes to the UK diet, in the order of a 50% increase in NSP intake, and a 40% reduction in saturated fat consumption. These are of the same order as those recently recommended by WHO (1990). The dietitian has a crucial role in instigating these changes by advising on choice of foods that will fulfil the DRVs. Some suggestions are given in Section 1.1.4.

Table 1.10 Dietary Reference Values for fat and carbohydrate for adults as a percentage of daily total energy intake (percentage of food energy)

	Individual minimum	Population average	Individual maximum
Saturated fatty acids		10 (11)	
Cis-polyunsaturated fatty acids		6 (6.5)	10
	n−3 0.2		
	n−6 1.0		
Cis-monounsaturated fatty acids		12 (13)	
Trans fatty acids		2 (2)	
Total fatty acids		30 (32.5)	
TOTAL FAT		33 (35)	
Non-milk extrinsic sugars	0	10 (11)	
Intrinsic and milk sugars and starch		37 (39)	
TOTAL CARBOHYDRATE		47 (50)	
NON-STARCH POLYSACCHARIDE (g/d)	12	18	24

The average percentage contribution to total energy does not total 100% because figures for protein and alcohol are excluded. Protein intakes average 15 per cent of total energy which is above the RNI. It is recognised that many individuals will derive some energy from alcohol, and this has been assumed to average 5 per cent approximating to current intakes. However the Panel allowed that some groups might not drink alcohol and that for some purposes nutrient intakes as a proportion of food energy (without alcohol) might be useful. Therefore average figures are given as percentages both of total energy and, in parenthesis, of food energy.

DoH (1991). Reproduced with the permission of the Controller of Her Majesty's Stationery Office

References

British Nutrition Foundation (1989) *Recommended Dietary Allowances. What are they and how should they be used?* Briefing Paper 19. BNF, London.

Department of Health (1991) *Dietary Reference Values for food energy and nutrients for the United Kingdom.* Rep Hlth Soc Subj 41. HMSO, London.

Department of Health and Social Security (1969) *Recommended intakes of nutrients for the UK.* Rep Hlth Soc Subj 120, HMSO, London.

Department of Health and Social Security (1979) *Recommended Daily Amounts of food energy and nutrients for groups of people in the UK.* Rep 15, Hlth Soc Subj HMSO, London.

National Research Council (1989) *Recommended dietary allowances*, 10e. National Academic Press, Washington, DC.

Schofield WN, Schofield C and James WPT (1985) BMR – review and prediction. *Hum Nutr: Clin Nutr* **39** (Supplement), 1–96.

World Health Organization (1985) *Energy and protein requirements.* Tech Rep Ser 724. WHO, Geneva.

World Health Organization (1990) *Diet, nutrition and the prevention of chronic diseases.* Tech Rep Ser 797. WHO, Geneva.

1.3 Normal nutrient intakes

1.3.1 Normal intakes

Knowledge of the expected normal range of nutrient intakes of different age and sex groups is useful:

1 to give guidance on whether the intake of a given individual is abnormally high or low.

2 to establish the level which may be regarded as *high* or *low* for research purposes or in planning therapeutic diets.

Tables 1.11 and 1.12 show the mean ± s.d., 10th, 50th and 90th centiles of nutrient intakes in several age/sex groups, as reported in studies conducted by the DHSS during 1968 to 1971 (Darke *et al* 1980) and by Gregory *et al* during 1986–87 (1990). (The 10th centile is the value such that 10% of the population studied had lower intakes and 90% had higher intakes.)

Table 1.12 includes a majority of the nutrients listed in McCance and Widdowson's *The Composition of Foods* (Paul and Southgate 1978). Figures for the intake of lesser B vitamins however must be regarded as provisional (Cooke 1983; Black *et al* 1985).

Nutrient intake is related to total energy intake. Therefore, to help in assessing the probable ranges of usual intakes for nutrients not shown in the tables, Fig. 1.1 is included. This shows how the energy intakes of all the age/sex groups in Tables 1.11 and 1.12 relate to each other. Thus, for example, since the range of energy intakes of girls aged 10–11 is only a little less than that of women aged 18–55, then the intakes of other nutrients are likely to have a range similar to that of 18–55 year old women.

Extremes of nutrient intakes recorded in seven day surveys are not *usual* intakes of those individuals. In any short survey some people will be studied during periods of intake either lower or higher than their own average (*usual*) intake. In addition there is a bias to under-estimation of food intake in many dietary surveys. When evaluating the *usual* diet of a single individual, reported nutrient intakes that are more than one standard deviation from the population mean should be treated with caution. Energy intakes should be carefully evaluated against the likely energy requirements of that individual. (see Section 2.1.3 Energy requirements, and 2.1.4 Prescribing energy intakes). Nutrient intakes are related to the total amount of food eaten. Therefore, if energy intake has been under-reported, nutrient intakes may also have been under-reported.

1.3.2 Dietary composition and nutrient intake

The nutrient density of a diet is the vitamin and mineral content per unit of energy, usually expressed per 1000 kcal

Table 1.11a–h The mean daily intake, standard deviation, 10th, 50th and 90th centiles for total energy and selected nutrients obtained by seven day weighed dietary studies in 1967 to 1971

a) Age 12–23 months

	Boys (n = 149)					Girls (n = 154)				
	Mean	SD	10th centile	50th centile	90th centile	Mean	SD	10th centile	50th centile	90th centile
Energy: MJ	5.05	1.22	3.54	4.90	6.49	4.74	1.16	3.42	4.58	6.09
kcal	1207	291	847	1172	1551	1133	277	817	1094	1454
Total protein (g)	37.8	10.4	25.6	36.5	52.2	35.3	9.4	25.0	33.8	44.9
Animal protein (g)	27.4	8.6	16.2	26.7	39.4	26.0	8.7	16.3	25.1	35.1
Fat (g)	51.2	15.2	33.8	49.2	70.6	48.7	13.6	32.5	46.8	65.2
Carbohydrate (g)	157	42	104	154	214	146	42	101	141	197
Calcium (mg)	744	233	459	725	1041	704	272	445	656	958
Iron (mg)	7.0	3.4	3.6	6.3	10.8	6.5	3.1	3.6	5.7	9.9
Retinol equiv. (μg)	821	570	334	616	1641	798	623	287	566	1698
Thiamin (mg)	0.63	0.32	0.40	0.55	0.89	0.57	0.20	0.36	0.52	0.78
Riboflavin (mg)	1.21	0.66	0.71	1.11	1.77	1.10	0.46	0.67	1.01	1.54
Nicotinic acid (mg)	6.56	5.54	3.45	5.53	10.09	5.78	3.01	3.20	4.99	8.17
Pyridoxine (mg)	0.65	0.34	0.41	0.60	0.87	0.60	0.21	0.39	0.57	0.80
Ascorbic acid (mg)	42.6	34.9	13.3	28.4	90.6	41.0	31.3	14.3	32.2	87.8
Cholecalciferol (μg)	3.14	3.85	0.46	1.44	8.14	3.84	4.96	0.42	1.64	10.47

b) Age 24–35 months

	Boys (n = 206)					Girls (n = 201)				
	Mean	SD	10th centile	50th centile	90th centile	Mean	SD	10th centile	50th centile	90th centile
Energy: MJ	5.73	1.49	4.08	5.49	7.50	5.37	1.30	4.11	5.09	6.85
kcal	1370	357	975	1312	1793	1284	310	983	1217	1636
Total protein (g)	39.7	10.9	26.8	38.6	52.0	38.5	10.5	27.6	37.1	50.4
Animal protein (g)	27.4	9.0	17.8	26.3	37.2	27.1	8.7	18.2	25.8	37.7
Fat (g)	57.9	17.8	37.3	56.0	78.8	55.5	16.0	40.0	53.5	73.7
Carbohydrate (g)	182	51	127	174	240	167	42	121	160	211
Calcium (mg)	678	216	425	669	890	660	210	439	620	877
Iron (mg)	6.8	2.4	4.5	6.2	9.2	6.4	2.5	4.0	5.8	9.3
Retinol equiv. (μg)	656	430	300	496	1155	704	635	274	496	1285
Thiamin (mg)	0.65	0.25	0.42	0.60	0.90	0.68	0.51	0.39	0.61	0.91
Riboflavin (mg)	1.06	0.33	0.68	0.99	1.45	1.04	0.39	0.65	0.94	1.66
Nicotinic acid (mg)	7.08	3.15	4.17	6.38	10.94	6.80	3.16	3.97	6.17	10.27
Pyridoxine (mg)	0.70	0.20	0.44	0.67	0.97	0.66	0.20	0.43	0.63	0.88
Ascorbic acid (mg)	36.3	31.0	14.3	25.3	63.7	38.8	37.9	13.1	26.2	80.4
Cholecalciferol (μg)	2.29	3.02	0.45	1.24	5.55	2.63	4.57	0.44	1.21	6.38

c) Age 36–47 months

	Boys (n = 276)					Girls (n = 262)				
	Mean	SD	10th centile	50th centile	90th centile	Mean	SD	10th centile	50th centile	90th centile
Energy: MJ	6.40	1.58	4.68	6.20	8.44	5.80	1.49	4.40	5.51	7.44
kcal	1529	378	1119	1481	2016	1387	355	1051	1317	1777
Total protein (g)	43.9	12.1	29.9	42.3	59.1	39.2	10.5	28.3	37.6	51.8
Animal protein (g)	29.4	9.6	18.9	28.6	41.0	26.6	11.3	17.2	25.3	36.2
Fat (g)	64.0	20.2	43.6	61.3	86.7	58.6	18.6	40.6	54.1	82.2
Carbohydrate (g)	204	49	149	198	259	186	48	138	180	239
Calcium (mg)	704	225	448	665	964	618	202	397	594	856
Iron (mg)	7.4	2.6	4.8	7.1	10.1	6.7	2.1	4.3	6.3	9.1
Retinol equiv. (μg)	764	630	318	576	1425	636	458	297	491	1185
Thiamin (mg)	0.75	0.27	0.47	0.69	1.08	0.64	0.24	0.43	0.60	0.87
Riboflavin (mg)	1.16	0.39	0.71	1.11	1.62	1.00	0.36	0.61	0.95	1.37
Nicotinic acid (mg)	8.26	3.35	4.88	7.46	12.23	7.29	3.04	4.47	6.90	10.30
Pyridoxine (mg)	0.77	0.23	0.51	0.73	1.03	0.69	0.20	0.48	0.66	0.92
Ascorbic acid (mg)	40.0	34.4	16.0	27.2	84.0	35.8	30.9	14.0	25.3	77.1
Cholecalciferol (μg)	1.94	2.62	0.46	1.16	3.80	1.94	2.59	0.49	1.04	4.34

d) Age 10–11 years

	Boys (n = 163)					Girls (n = 158)				
	Mean	SD	10th centile	50th centile	90th centile	Mean	SD	10th centile	50th centile	90th centile
Energy: MJ	9.08	1.63	6.99	9.13	11.03	8.02	1.56	6.02	7.86	10.20
kcal	2169	390	1670	2181	2634	1916	372	1437	1879	2438
Total protein (g)	62.4	12.5	45.5	62.0	78.8	55.4	11.3	42.3	54.5	70.5
Animal protein (g)	39.1	9.9	25.8	39.0	51.4	35.6	9.2	24.2	35.0	49.2
Fat (g)	90.7	19.6	67.7	90.4	115.3	82.8	19.9	61.1	80.0	106.8
Carbohydrate (g)	292	58	224	292	366	252	52	183	253	318
Calcium (mg)	899	231	588	904	1172	787	224	495	778	1080
Iron (mg)	10.8	2.6	7.9	10.7	14.3	9.7	2.3	7.0	9.5	12.3
Retinol equiv. (μg)	893	548	409	724	1497	812	453	379	707	1363
Thiamin (mg)	1.03	0.28	0.72	1.00	1.40	0.88	0.21	0.60	0.84	1.14
Riboflavin (mg)	1.43	0.40	0.91	1.42	1.95	1.24	0.36	0.83	1.17	1.76
Nicotinic acid (mg)	11.19	3.13	7.85	10.45	15.94	9.57	2.46	6.62	9.28	12.40
Pyridoxine (mg)	1.16	0.24	0.85	1.16	1.47	1.05	0.23	0.78	1.02	1.35
Ascorbic acid (mg)	48.5	24.4	26.5	42.7	72.0	46.2	23.4	25.6	41.1	68.7
Cholecalciferol (μg)	1.66	1.02	0.82	1.44	2.52	1.44	0.74	0.72	1.30	2.22

e) Age 14–15 years

	Boys (n = 390)					Girls (n = 401)				
	Mean	SD	10th centile	50th centile	90th centile	Mean	SD	10th centile	50th centile	90th centile
Energy: MJ	10.25	2.47	7.28	10.16	13.44	8.00	1.90	5.61	7.98	10.19
kcal	2451	589	1739	2427	3210	1911	454	1340	1907	2435
Total protein (g)	71.2	17.4	48.8	71.0	94.2	57.2	13.9	40.9	56.1	73.6
Animal protein (g)	42.0	13.3	25.2	41.5	58.9	35.1	11.6	22.0	33.1	49.1
Fat (g)	101.8	28.2	66.6	98.7	137.7	84.7	23.0	57.4	83.4	111.3
Carbohydrate (g)	330	87	224	329	445	243	64	160	242	320
Calcium (mg)	870	299	503	841	1261	667	238	393	623	1007
Iron (mg)	12.4	3.5	8.3	12.0	17.1	10.1	2.7	7.0	9.8	13.0
Retinol equiv. (μg)	860	610	382	711	1358	780	574	329	628	1423
Thiamin (mg)	1.17	0.35	0.77	1.14	1.59	0.92	0.50	0.63	0.87	1.19
Riboflavin (mg)	1.48	0.57	0.83	1.40	2.20	1.13	0.71	0.66	1.07	1.63
Nicotinic acid (mg)	13.31	4.22	8.66	12.87	18.04	10.53	5.06	7.17	10.05	13.55
Pyridoxine (mg)	1.40	0.35	0.97	1.38	1.82	1.17	0.53	0.80	1.12	1.49
Ascorbic acid (mg)	53.3	29.2	27.5	49.4	76.6	48.8	27.9	26.0	42.4	77.6
Cholecalciferol (μg)	2.11	1.67	0.70	1.68	3.78	1.81	1.38	0.61	1.43	3.33

f) Age 65–74 years

	Men (n = 213)					Women (n = 225)				
	Mean	SD	10th centile	50th centile	90th centile	Mean	SD	10th centile	50th centile	90th centile
Energy: MJ	9.82	2.44	6.70	9.81	12.58	7.48	1.91	5.11	7.47	9.79
kcal	2347	582	1600	2344	3006	1788	456	1220	1784	2339
Total protein (g)	74.8	17.8	53.8	72.3	96.3	59.2	14.4	42.3	58.4	77.6
Animal protein (g)	50.9	13.9	34.7	48.9	68.1	41.1	11.6	26.3	40.5	53.3
Fat (g)	110.0	32.8	68.5	109.2	150.3	87.4	26.3	55.0	84.6	121.4
Carbohydrate (g)	267	75	175	266	355	200	61	128	195	277
Calcium (mg)	911	282	574	885	1249	796	244	487	790	1063
Iron (mg)	12.2	3.3	8.2	12.1	16.4	9.4	2.6	6.4	9.1	12.9
Retinol equiv. (μg)	1142	686	513	958	2007	1027	676	490	815	1747
Thiamin (mg)	1.05	0.35	0.68	1.01	1.40	0.82	0.23	0.56	0.78	1.11
Riboflavin (mg)	1.55	0.48	0.96	1.46	2.16	1.27	0.42	0.78	1.19	1.78
Nicotinic acid (mg)	16.91	7.42	9.89	14.58	26.97	11.49	4.56	7.12	10.30	17.50
Pyridoxine (mg)	1.37	0.41	0.90	1.31	1.90	1.01	0.28	0.70	0.96	1.38
Ascorbic acid (mg)	42.8	26.0	17.3	38.0	72.2	40.5	27.8	15.9	32.4	74.1
Cholecalciferol (μg)	3.34	3.26	0.93	2.09	6.64	2.32	2.18	0.66	1.60	4.38

g) Age 75+ years

	Men (n = 179)					Women (n = 204)				
	Mean	SD	10th centile	50th centile	90th centile	Mean	SD	10th centile	50th centile	90th centile
Energy: MJ	8.80	2.31	5.94	8.78	11.60	6.81	1.72	4.59	6.78	9.00
kcal	2103	551	419	2098	2771	1627	410	1097	1619	2149
Total protein (g)	67.6	18.4	43.5	67.5	87.5	53.6	13.0	34.9	54.0	69.8
Animal protein (g)	45.9	14.1	28.2	44.7	64.1	37.4	10.4	22.9	37.6	50.1
Fat (g)	97.9	29.2	65.0	95.8	137.4	77.6	22.0	53.8	75.0	105.0
Carbohydrate (g)	244	73	154	240	327	187	59	112	183	255
Calcium (mg)	883	302	503	852	1253	726	253	418	698	1008
Iron (mg)	10.9	3.2	6.5	10.6	14.9	8.5	2.5	5.4	8.4	11.7
Retinol equiv. (μg)	1094	741	512	880	1892	888	588	404	729	1387
Thiamin (mg)	0.93	0.29	0.56	0.90	1.27	0.74	0.23	0.48	0.72	1.02
Riboflavin (mg)	1.40	0.51	0.80	1.34	2.06	1.13	0.39	0.66	1.09	1.71
Nicotinic acid (mg)	13.55	5.04	7.76	12.48	19.51	10.18	3.80	6.18	9.35	14.33
Pyridoxine (mg)	1.18	0.36	0.72	1.17	1.58	0.93	0.27	0.62	0.91	1.27
Ascorbic acid (mg)	37.7	23.1	13.8	33.7	60.8	33.7	20.0	12.3	29.2	58.7
Cholecalciferol (μg)	2.68	2.13	0.75	1.96	5.42	2.09	1.79	0.63	1.48	4.39

h) Pregnant women in the 6th–7th month of pregnancy (n = 435)

	Mean	SD	10th centile	50th centile	90th centile
Energy: MJ	9.01	2.10	6.35	9.04	11.60
kcal	2152	503	1517	2159	2771
Total protein (g)	70.5	16.7	49.6	70.3	92.3
Animal protein (g)	47.8	14.3	31.0	46.8	65.6
Fat (g)	97.9	26.4	65.1	96.6	130.6
Carbohydrate (g)	260	69	172	264	344
Calcium (mg)	959	320	547	946	1363
Iron (mg)	11.7	3.1	8.2	11.5	15.4
Retinol equiv. (μg)	1269	975	516	961	2485
Thiamin (mg)	1.04	0.28	0.70	1.03	1.38
Riboflavin (mg)	1.60	0.67	0.92	1.51	2.30
Nicotinic acid (mg)	14.30	5.30	8.88	13.41	20.34
Pyridoxine (mg)	1.27	0.32	0.88	1.24	1.66
Ascorbic acid (mg)	54.9	24.7	28.0	49.7	89.0
Cholecalciferol (μg)	2.28	2.01	0.76	1.66	4.40

From: Darke *et al* (1980). Reproduced with permission from *Br J Nutr.*

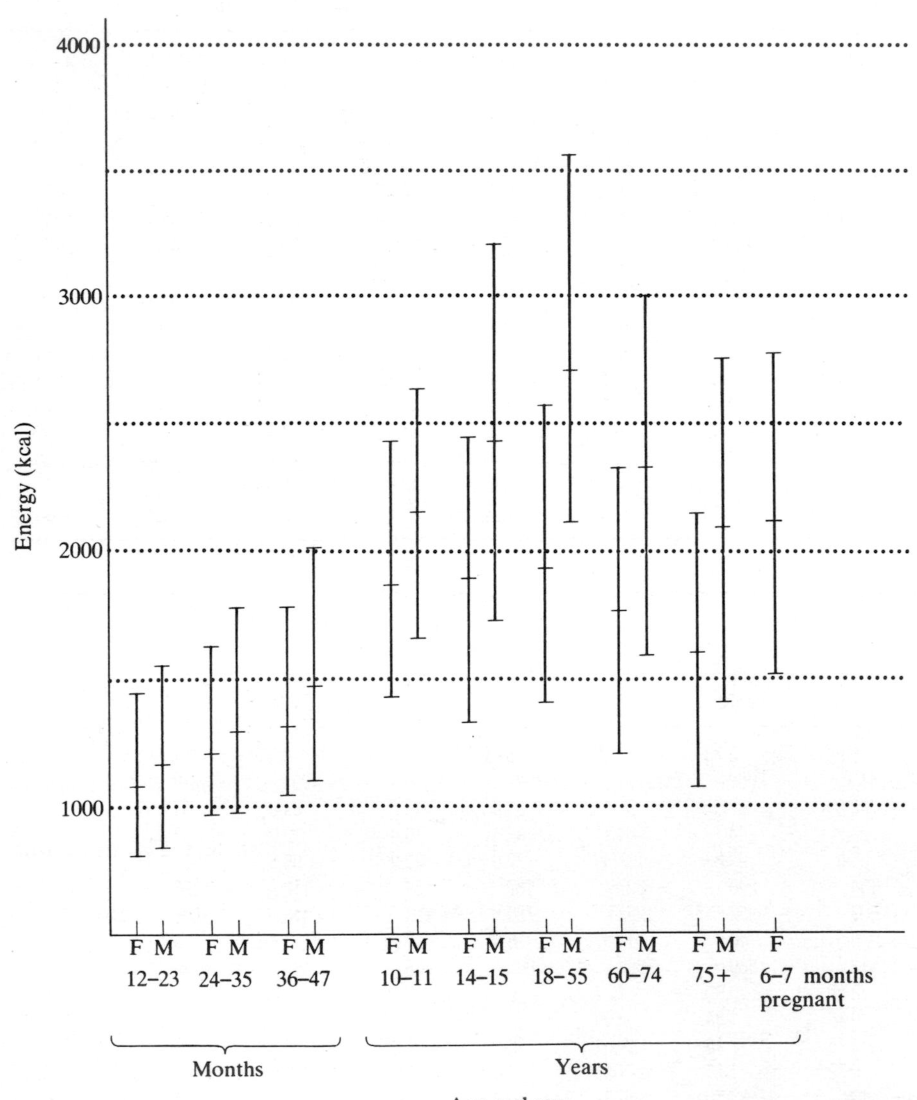

Fig. 1.1 Range (10th, 50th and 90th centiles) of energy intakes in different age and sex groups (Darke *et al* 1980; Nelson and Paul, personal communication

Table 1.12 The mean daily intake, standard deviation, lower 2.5, 50, and upper 2.5 centiles for total energy and selected nutrients obtained by seven day weighed dietary survey, 1986–87 (Compiled from Gregory *et al* 1990)

Nutrient	Men (n = 1007)					Women (n = 1110)				
	Mean	SD	2.5 centile	50 centile	97.5 centile	Mean	SD	2.5 centile	50 centile	97.5 centile
Energy MJ	10.29	2.49	5.59	10.25	15.20	7.06	1.82	3.36	7.10	10.84
Energy kcal	2450.0	593	1330	2440	3620	1680	433	800	1690	2580
Protein g	84.7	20.8	47.1	84.0	129.1	62.0	15.3	31.8	61.8	92.3
Total fat g	102.3	28.0	49.8	101.8	155.8	73.5	22.7	31.3	73.3	124.5
Saturated fatty acids g	42.0	13.2	19.1	40.7	69.4	31.1	10.7	11.8	30.5	54.6
n-3 PUFA g	1.95	0.66	0.79	1.83	3.74	1.35	0.67	0.53	1.26	2.68
n-6 PUFA g	13.8	6.26	5.1	12.6	29.0	9.6	4.66	3.1	8.8	21.3
Monounsaturated fatty acids g	31.4	8.90	15.6	30.9	49.5	22.1	7.00	10.0	21.8	37.1
P/S ratio	0.40	0.23	0.16	0.35	0.87	0.38	0.20	0.15	0.34	0.85
Cholesterol mg	390	148	151	375	741	280	107	98	269	511
Total carbohydrate g	272	79	131	268	435	193	60	83	192	314
Total sugars g	115	49	37	109	224	86	37	25	84	171
Starch g	156	46	69	152	258	106	33	42	106	172
Fibre g	24.9	8.9	10.3	23.8	44.8	18.6	6.7	7.5	17.9	33.5
Alcohol g	25.0	31.3		14.4		6.9	10.3		2.3	
Iron mg	13.7	4.9	6.5	13.2	25.7	10.5	4.3	4.6	9.8	21.1
Calcium mg	937	307	409	917	1597	726	260	266	716	1299
Sodium mg	3376	982	1551	3320	5600	2351	683	1131	2313	3724
Chloride mg	5179	1470	2464	5115	8510	3573	1023	1723	3536	5598
Potassium mg	3187	824	1724	3143	4816	2434	700	1200	2410	4017
Magnesium mg	323	102	156	312	548	237	83	105	226	441
Phosphorus mg	1452	382	782	1429	2310	1072	303	511	1054	1719
Copper mg	1.59	0.66	0.74	1.48	3.44	1.23	0.67	0.56	1.12	2.79
Zinc mg	11.4	3.6	5.7	10.9	19.0	8.4	2.7	3.6	8.2	13.6
Iodine μg	237	102	96	225	418	171	73	63	161	355
Retinol μg	1226	1747	190	602	6564	1058	1583	134	463	5698
Carotene μg	2414	1975	247	1895	7563	2129	1832	197	1696	6523
Retinol equivalents μg	1628	1836	290	1012	6964	1413	1633	249	810	6159
Thiamin mg	1.70	0.66	0.79	1.65	2.87	1.24	0.33	0.55	1.22	2.06
Riboflavin mg	2.08	0.66	0.92	2.00	3.65	1.57	0.67	0.59	1.50	2.94
Niacin equivalents mg	39.9	10.9	21.6	39.2	62.2	28.5	8.0	13.7	28.1	46.4
Vitamin B_6 mg	2.48	0.99	1.20	2.38	4.47	1.57	0.67	0.71	1.54	2.62
Vitamin B_{12} μg	7.2	5.6	2.4	5.7	22.9	5.2	4.3	1.3	3.9	17.8
Folate μg	311	102	145	300	555	213	70	91	208	368
Biotin μg	38.9	14.8	15.1	37.8	69.7	28.3	14.0	9.8	26.4	56.3
Pantothenic acid mg	6.3	2.0	2.9	6.1	10.5	4.5	1.3	2.1	4.4	7.7
Vitamin C mg	66.5	39.6	19.1	57.6	170.9	62.0	39.3	13.6	52.6	161.4
Vitamin D μg	3.43	2.64	0.51	2.87	9.92	2.51	1.67	0.43	2.17	6.89
Vitamin E mg	9.9	4.6	3.5	9.3	19.5	7.2	3.3	2.5	6.7	15.2

(or per 5 MJ); it provides a useful measure of dietary quality. In certain circumstances when energy intake is low, it is important to maximize the nutrient density.

Total micronutrient intake is governed by total food intake which, in turn, is governed in the long term by energy requirements. There is probably a relationship between energy and nutrient requirements such that a small healthy person has lower than average requirements for both energy and micronutrients. However, when appetite is small and nutrient requirements are above average, as in the elderly or sick, or when food intake has been deliberately restricted, as on reducing diets, the micronutrient density should be maximized.

Table 1.13 shows the RNI for adult women expressed as the nutrient density in diets of average energy requirement (1940 kcal) and in diets of 1500, 1200 and 1000 kcal. This is compared with the actual nutrient densities in diets as reported by women in poor economic circumstances (Gregory *et al* 1990) and of dietitians (Cole-Hamilton *et al* 1986). The latter have the highest nutrient densities found in diet studies and the figures for Week 2, when the dietitians were making strenuous efforts to eat according to dietary guidelines, are likely to be the maximum achievable in real diets without supplementation. (It should be noted however that the energy intake in Week 2 is low and that the subjects had failed to compensate for the energy lost in reducing fat intake. Had they done so the densities would probably have been lower.)

Table 1.13 Nutrient density per 1000 kcal in reported diets of adult women

Nutrient	RNI[1] expressed as nutrient density	RNI expressed as required density in low energy diets			Household receiving benefits (Gregory *et al* 1990)	Unemployed head of household (Gregory *et al* 1990)	Dietitians Week 1 (Cole-Hamilton *et al* 1986)	Dietitians Week 2 (Cole-Hamilton *et al* 1986)
Energy intake, kcal	1940	1500	1200	1000	1560	1640	1902	1679
Nutrient density								
Vitamin A μg	309	400	584	600	833	539	811	1459
Thiamin mg	0.41	0.53	0.67	0.80	0.75	0.71	0.68	0.83
Riboflavin mg	0.57	0.73	0.92	1.1	0.89	0.8	1.05	1.19
Niacin equivalents mg	6.7	8.7	10.8	13.0	16.4	16.0	18.4	22.0
Vitamin B_6 mg	0.62	0.80	1.00	1.20	0.93	0.89	0.84	1.07
Vitamin B_{12} μg	0.77	1.00	1.25	1.50	3.36	2.33	3.15	3.57
Folate μg	103	133	167	200	120	117	121	148
Vitamin C mg	21	27	33	40	30	36	56	66
Iron mg	7.63	9.87	12.3	14.8	5.44	6.27	7.89	10.1
Calcium mg	361	467	583	700	361	397	533	542
Sodium mg	824	1067	1333	1600	1392	1421	1352	1422
Potassium mg	1840	2333	2917	3500	1287	1395	1746	2174
Magnesium mg	139	180	225	270	128	135	202	271
Phosphorus mg	284	367	458	550	579	601	760	909
Copper mg	0.62	0.80	1.00	1.20	0.63	0.66	0.95	1.19
Zinc mg	3.61	4.67	5.83	7.00	4.67	4.62	5.68	6.85

[1] As given by Department of Health (1991)

Table 1.14 The contribution of foods to vitamin C intake

	Parsley	Milk	Oranges
Portion weight (g)	1	30	80
× frequency	1/month	8/day	2/week
× content /100 g	130	1.5	50
= intake per day (mg)	0.04	3.6	11.4

The households receiving benefit had low densities for folate, iron, potassium and magnesium. Again, the reported energy intake is low and there was probably an element of under-eating or under-reporting due to the effort of keeping diet records. This was most likely to occur for snack foods. True nutrient densities could have been lower. The dietitians achieved the RNI for all nutrients except potassium. This demonstrates that it is possible to achieve the RNI even with relatively low energy intakes.

Dietary nutrient density is increased (a) by decreasing the proportion of the diet that comes from fat and from sugar, and (b) by increasing the amounts of fruit and vegetables consumed. This may not always be acceptable, and there may be a case for routine vitamin/mineral supplementation to hospital patients whose requirements – particularly in infectious or post-traumatic states – are known to be increased and whose appetites are small (Hackett *et al* 1979; Todd *et al* 1984), and also to the elderly in institutional care.

The contribution which an individual food makes to nutrient intake depends on three factors:

1 The nutrient content per 100 g.
2 The size of the portion eaten.
3 The frequency of consumption.

Therefore, it is not sufficient, when identifying foods to increase or reduce intake, to simply run the eye down the tables of content per 100 g. The other two factors also have to be considered. This is illustrated in Table 1.14. Parsley contains almost three times as much vitamin C as oranges, but makes a negligible contribution to total intake, while milk, containing 1/33rd as much makes a significant contribution.

Table 2.29 (in Section 2.6 on Vitamins) lists some 130 foods with their vitamin content per portion. This highlights those foods that make most contribution to vitamin intake for each individual portion consumed.

References

Black AE, Paul AA and Hall C (1985) Footnotes to food tables 2. The underestimation of intakes of lesser B vitamins by pregnant and lactating women as calculated using the fourth edition of McCance and Widdowson's *The Composition of Foods*. *Hum Nutr: Appl Nutr* **39A**, 19–22.

Cole-Hamilton I, Gunner K, Leverkus C and Starr J (1986) A study among dietitians and adult members of their households of the practicalities and implications of following proposed dietary guidelines for the UK. *Hum Nutr: Appl Nutr* **40A**, 365–89.

Cooke JR (1983) Food composition tables – analytical problems in the collection of data. *Hum Nutr: Appl Nutr* **37A**, 441–7.

Darke SJ, Disselduff MM and Try GP (1980) Frequency distributions of mean daily intakes of food energy and selected nutrients obtained during nutrition surveys of different groups of people in Great Britain between 1968 and 1971. *Br J Nutr* **44**, 243–52.

Department of Health (1991) *Dietary Reference Values for food energy and nutrients for the United Kingdom*. Rep. Hlth Soc. Subj 41. HMSO, London.

Gregory J, Foster K, Tyler H and Wiseman M (1990) *Dietary survey of British adults*. HMSO, London.

Hackett AF, Yeoung CK and Hill GL (1979) Eating patterns in patients recovering from major surgery – a study of voluntary food intake and energy balance. *Br J Surg* **66**, 415–8.

Paul AA and Southgate DAT (1978) McCance and Widdowson's *The Composition of Foods*. HMSO, London.

Todd EA, Hunt P, Crowe PJ and Royle GT (1984) What do patients eat in hospital? *Hum Nutr: Appl Nutr* **38A**, 294–7.

1.4 Food tables

1.4.1 Available food tables

UK food tables

The UK food tables are those of McCance and Widdowson's *The Composition of Foods* and of the associated supplement series (see Table 1.15). These publications are produced by the Royal Society of Chemistry (RSC) and the Ministry of Agriculture Fisheries and Food (MAFF) who work in collaboration to update the UK food tables. The supplements, each based on one or more food group, are produced as a series and, to date, the RSC and MAFF have published supplements for *Cereals and Cereal Products* (1988), *Milk Products and Eggs* (1989), *Vegetables, Herbs and Spices* (1991), *Fruit and Nuts* (1992) and *Vegetable Dishes* (1992). The supplements provide the most detailed information in terms of numbers of foods and nutrients in these food groups. In time, the supplement series will be extended to cover all food groups. The fifth edition of McCance and Widdowson's *The Composition of Foods* (Holland *et al* 1991) is the core publication for the food tables and has been produced so that the data can be used alone or in conjunction with the supplements. The fifth edition gives the main nutrients for a whole range of foods and includes some 'new' foods, which are not reported in the supplement publications. The introduction and appendices in the fifth edition give an explanation of the ways in which the tables are derived and guidelines for their use.

A computerized National Nutrient Databank has been developed by the RSC so that the data are available as computer files in addition to the printed publications. The

Table 1.15 The UK food tables

Publication	Publisher
McCance and Widdowson's *The Composition of Foods*, fifth edition. Holland B, Welch AA, Unwin ID, Buss DH, Paul AA, Southgate DAT (1991)	Royal Society of Chemistry, Cambridge
Supplements to '*The Composition of Foods*'	
First supplement to McCance and Widdowson's The Composition of Foods, fourth edition: Amino acid composition (mg per 100 g food) and fatty acid composition (g per 100 g food). Paul AA, Southgate DAT, Russell J (1980)	HMSO, London and Royal Society of Chemistry, Cambridge
Second supplement to McCance and Widdowson's The Composition of Foods, fourth edition: Immigrant foods. Tan SP, Wenlock RW, Buss DH (1985)	HMSO, London and Royal Society of Chemistry, Cambridge
Third supplement to McCance and Widdowson's The Composition of Foods, fourth edition: Cereals and Cereal Products. Holland B, Unwin ID, Buss DH (1988)	Royal Society of Chemistry, Cambridge
Fourth supplement to McCance and Widdowson's The Composition of Foods, fourth edition: Milk Products and Eggs. Holland B, Unwin ID, Buss DH (1989)	Royal Society of Chemistry, Cambridge
Fifth supplement to McCance and Widdowson's The Composition of Foods, fourth edition: Vegetables, Herbs and Spices. Holland B, Unwin ID, Buss DH (1991)	Royal Society of Chemistry, Cambridge
First supplement to McCance and Widdowson's The Composition of Foods, 5th edition: Fruit and Nuts. Holland B, Unwin ID, Buss DH (1992)	Royal Society of Chemistry, Cambridge
Second supplement to McCance and Widdowson's The Composition of Foods, fifth edition: Vegetable Dishes. Holland B, Welch A, Buss DH (1992)	Royal Society of Chemistry, Cambridge
Additional food table publications	
Food Labelling Data for Manufacturers (1992)	Royal Society of Chemistry, Cambridge
Nutrient Content of Food Portions Davies J and Dickerson J (1991)	Royal Society of Chemistry, Cambridge
The Food Number Index. Companion to the Composition of Foods and its supplements (1992)	Royal Society of Chemistry, Cambridge

Nutrient Databank data is used in several nutrient analysis programs for use on personal computers, see Section 1.5, Computers in Dietetics.

Within the UK, specialist food tables are available for use by manufacturers of food, for food labelling. The values in these specialist tables are based on *The Composition of Foods* and have been calculated using the general conversion factors given in the EC Directive on Nutrition Labelling of Foodstuffs (1990). However, the main UK food tables should still be used for research and general work by nutritionists and dietitians, as more specific and accurate factors are used to produce the nutrient values.

Abbreviated sets of food tables such as the *Nutrient Content of Food Portions* (Davies and Dickerson 1991) and those in the *Manual of Nutrition* (MAFF 1985) are also available but contain limited numbers of foods and nutrients. In the *Nutrient Content of Food Portions*, nutrients are given for average portion sizes of food and not per 100 g as in the main tables. However, these abbreviated food tables are not adequate for detailed dietary work and may sometimes be misleading. Without sufficient foods being included in reference tables, the lack of a full range of data can lead to misinterpretation, particularly by inexperienced users of food tables.

Other food tables

Table 1.16 shows a selection of food tables from other countries.

Table 1.16 A selected list of other food tables

Title	Available from
Composition of Foods Watt BK, Merrill AL (1975) Agricultural Handbook No 8 Revisions of Agricultural Handbook No 8 8–1 Dairy and egg products (1976) 8–2 Spices and herbs (1977) 8–3 Baby foods (1978) 8–4 Fats and oils (1979) 8–5 Poultry products (1979) 8–6 Soups, sauces and gravies (1980) 8–7 Sausages and luncheon meats (1981) 8–8 Breakfast cereals (1982) 8–9 Fruits and fruit juices (1982) 8–10 Pork products (1983) 8–11 Vegetable and vegetable products (1984) 8–12 Nut and seed products (1984) 8–13 Beef products (1986) (revised, 1990) 8–14 Beverages (1986) 8–15 Fin fish and shellfish products (1987) 8–16 Legumes and legume products (1986) 8–17 Lamb, veal, and game products (1989) 8–18 Baked products (in preparation) 8–19 Snacks and sweets (1991) 8–20 Cereal grains and pasta (1989) 8–21 Fast foods (1988) 1989 Supplement (first) 1990 (96 new and revised items) 1990 Supplement (second) 1991 (114 new and revised items) 1991 Supplement (third) (in preparation)	Superintendent of Documents, US Government Printing Office, Washington DC 20402, USA
Composition of Foods, Australia, Volume 1. Cashel K, English R, Lewis J (1989) Department of Community Services and Health, Canberra *Additional volumes* Vol. 2 Cereals and cereal products (English *et al* 1990) Vol. 3 Dairy products, eggs and fish (Lewis and English 1990) Vol. 4 Fats and oils, processed meat, fruit and vegetables (English and Lewis, 1990) Vol. 5 Nuts and legumes, beverages, miscellaneous foods (Lewis and English, 1990)	Dept of Community Services and Health GPO Box 9848 Canberra ACT 2601 Australia
Food composition and nutrition tables 1989/90, 4th revised and completed edition. Souci-Fachman-Kraut (1989). Wissenschaftliche Verlagsgesellschaft mbH, Stuttgart.	Wissenschaftliche Verlagsgesellschaft mbH, Postfach 40, D-7000 Stuttgart Germany

1.4.2 Using the food tables

Before using any set of food tables it is essential to read the introduction. It is important to know how the values in the tables have been selected and the criteria which were used to evaluate them. Care should be taken when comparing values from different sets of food tables because the definition and expression of the nutrients may not always be the same. Different conversion factors may have been used to prepare the values, e.g. to calculate protein from nitrogen or to convert the major nutrients to total energy. The same nutrient may be quoted in different ways, e.g. carbohydrate can be expressed as monosaccharide equivalents, actual weights or 'by difference' (see Holland *et al* 1991). Monosaccharide equivalents, the usual form of expression in UK food tables, give higher values for disaccharide and polysaccharide sugars than when expressed as actual weight (see Holland *et al* 1991). Figures for carbohydrate 'by difference' are obtained by subtracting measured weights of the main proximates from the total weight of the food and may include the contribution from any dietary fibre present as well as errors from the other analyses. Different analytical techniques may have been used for the same nutrient to provide the values in different sets of tables.

The values in food tables are generally averages of representative samples of food or selected values from literature surveys. Like any other biological material, the composition of a particular food can vary considerably. Certainly the nutrient values quoted in food tables cannot be regarded as having the accuracy of atomic weight determinations or be used as such. Several factors may cause the actual value of samples of food and the nutrient values in the food tables to differ. These factors include biological variability, variations in recipes and cooking practices and food storage conditions. A more detailed explanation is given in *The Composition of Foods* (Holland *et al* 1991). In practice, the UK food table values will usually be representative of most foods because they are updated regularly and great care is taken in the preparation of the tables. For instance, 'market share' information is used to assess which foods are included, and foods for analysis are obtained using a well-defined protocol. Nutritional composition data needs to be regularly updated because foods themselves change. The range and types of foods available steadily increase; new products are constantly being developed and old ones reformulated. The composition of apparently traditional foods can change and alterations in food composition may also result from the introduction of new plant varieties, importation from different countries, and changes in processing techniques and fortification practices. For these reasons it is advisable to use the most recent nutrient data available, so that the values will be the best reflection of the current food supply.

A measure of the variation in nutrient composition in foods is given in some tables as the standard deviation. Calculations can be made to find the coefficient of variation of foods (see Cameron and van Staveren 1988). In general the relative importance of nutrient variation in foods gets smaller as the number of foods consumed during the day increases. So that where there might be some uncertainty attached to the nutrient values of only a few foods calculated using foods tables, the effect of this uncertainty becomes less important as the number of foods eaten during a day increases. Thus, for instance, in a typical African diet where only a few foods may be eaten during the day (maybe 3–5), and where individual foods vary widely in their water content, the calculated food table values will be unlikely to be a good reflection of true nutrient intake (Cameron and van Staveren 1988). Conversely in Western diets where a number of very different food items are eaten, agreement is likely to be good. For a metabolic diet based on very few foods, duplicates of the actual foods concerned must be prepared for direct laboratory analysis.

Where studies have been made to compare the average intake of individuals eating their normal diet, with values from food tables and from analysed duplicate diets kept over the same period of time, random errors introduced ranged from 2–20% for individual estimates of protein, fat, carbohydrate, iron and calcium, depending on the nutrient studied and the number of observations (Bingham 1987). In general, the nutrient intake calculated from food tables and from direct analysis will tend to agree more closely if a greater variety of foods is recorded in the daily diet, or if the length of time individuals are asked to keep records is extended, or if the numbers of individuals chosen to represent a population average is increased. For nutrients which are present in moderate amounts in most foods, the length of recording time required to provide a good estimate of nutrient intake will be less than for a nutrient which is concentrated in only a few foods. For instance, to provide the accuracy necessary to compare an individual with a physiological characteristic (e.g. energy expenditure), seven days of weighed records may be necessary to assess energy and protein intakes, assuming that ±10% standard error is acceptable. It may be possible to observe people with very stable eating habits for a shorter time but those with greater variation may require longer. For most other nutrients the recording period would need to be longer than for energy and protein, particularly for those concentrated in only a few foods. For example, vitamin C may require 36 days of recording to be within ±10% of the true intake. This topic has been discussed in greater detail by Bingham (1987) and Cameron and van Staveren (1988).

Some nutrients may be less well-reflected in food tables than others due to external factors which affect food such as cooking and fortification practices. Some samples of these are potassium, calcium, iron, chloride, iodine, β-carotene and vitamin C (see Holland *et al* 1991). If accurate information concerning the intake of these nutrients is required, great attention must be paid to the details of foods consumed. Salt consumption is usually underestimated using food tables because it is difficult to know how much salt is added when food is eaten. Therefore, salt intake is most accurately assessed by analysis of complete 24-hour urine samples (see Section 2.7.1) although for planning low-sodium diets the UK food table values are adequate.

Bioavailability affects many nutrients to some degree and is defined as the proportion of a nutrient capable of being absorbed and available for use or storage (Bender 1989). In the UK food tables, allowance has been made for the reduced activities of the different forms of three of the vitamins (i.e. for retinol, carotenoid and tocopherol fractions), but for most other nutrients the values quoted are the actual amounts present. Although it is known that other nutrients are absorbed and utilized with varying degrees of efficiency, there is currently insufficient information with which to modify the UK tables. When using other food tables it is worth checking whether any of the nutrient values have been modified to account for their bioavailability.

There are errors which can be made when using food table data in nutrient analysis programs, for example:

1 missing nutrient values in food composition tables may be treated as zero values during calculation, resulting in an underestimation of nutrient intake (missing values in the UK food tables are shown by an N flag indicating that there may be significant quantities of a nutrient present but no reliable information on the amount is available);

2 errors may be made in the measurement, recording and estimation of food weights;

3 the food chosen for coding may be incorrect or inappropriate – this can happen for many reasons, one of them being a lack of familiarity with local food names;

4 there may be incorrect entry of food code numbers into the computing system.

Nutrient intakes should never be reported with a greater apparent precision than that of the published values.

References

Bender AE (1989) Nutritional significance of bioavailability. In *Nutrient availability: chemical and biological aspects* Southgate DAT, Johnson IT and Fenwick GR (Eds) Special publication No 72. Royal Society of Chemistry, Cambridge. pp. 3–9.

Bingham SA (1987) The dietary assessment of individuals; methods, accuracy; new techniques and recommendations. *Nutr Abs Rev (Series A)* **57**, 705–42.

Cameron ME and van Staveren WA (1988) *Manual on methodology for food consumption studies*. Oxford University Press, Oxford.

Cashel K, English R and Lewis J (1989) *Composition of foods, Australia*. Vol 1. Department of Community Services and Health, Canberra.

Davies J and Dickerson J (1991) *Nutrient Content of Food Portions*. Royal Society of Chemistry, Cambridge.

EC Council Directive of 24 September 1990 on Nutrition labelling for foodstuffs (90/496/EEC). *Official Journal of the European Communities* **No L 276/41**.

English R, Lewis J and Cashel K (1990) *Cereals and cereal products*. Vol 2. Department of Community Services and Health, Canberra.

English R and Lewis J (1990) *Fats and oils, processed meat, fruit and vegetables*. Vol 4. Department of Community Services and Health, Canberra.

Food Labelling Data for Manufacturers (1992) Royal Society of Chemistry, Cambridge.

Holland B, Unwin ID and Buss DH (1988) *Third supplement to McCance and Widdowson's* The Composition of Foods, 4e: *Cereals and cereal products*. Royal Society of Chemistry, Cambridge.

Holland B, Unwin ID and Buss DH (1989) *Fourth supplement to McCance and Widdowson's* The Composition of Foods, 4e: *Milk products and eggs*. Royal Society of Chemistry, Cambridge.

Holland B, Welch AA, Unwin ID, Buss DH, Paul AA and Southgate DAT (1991b) *McCance and Widdowson's* The Composition of Foods 5e. Royal Society of Chemistry, Cambridge.

Holland B, Unwin ID and Buss DH (1991a) *Fifth supplement to McCance and Widdowson's* The Composition of Foods, 4e: *Vegetables, herbs and spices*. Royal Society of Chemistry, Cambridge.

Holland B, Unwin ID and Buss DH (1992) *First supplement to McCance and Widdowson's* The Composition of Foods, 5e: *Fruit and nuts*. Royal Society of Chemistry, Cambridge.

Lewis J and English R (1990) *Nuts and legumes, beverages, miscellaneous foods*. Vol 5. Department of Community Services and Health, Canberra.

Lewis J and English R (1990) *Dairy products, eggs and fish*. Vol 3. Department of Community Services and Health, Canberra.

Ministry of Agriculture Fisheries and Food (1985) *Manual of Nutrition*. HMSO, London.

Paul AA, Southgate DAT and Russell J (1980) *First supplement to McCance and Widdowson's* The Composition of Foods, 4e: *Amino acid composition (mg per 100 g food) and fatty acid composition (g per 100 g food)*. HMSO, London.

Souci SW, Fachmann W and Kraut H (1989) *Food composition and nutrition tables 1989/90*. 4e revised and completed. Wissenschaftliche Verlagsgesellschaft mbH, Stuttgart.

Tan SP, Wenlock RW and Buss DH (1985) *Second supplement to McCance and Widdowson's* The Composition of Foods, 4e: *Immigrant foods*. HMSO, London.

Watt BK and Merrill AL (1975) *Composition of foods: raw, processed, prepared*. Agriculture Handbook No 8, US Dept of Agriculture, Washington DC.

1.5 Computers in dietetics

Computers can be used in all aspects of dietetics and are valuable tools in the clinical, educational and management areas of dietetic work (Howard and Hall 1981; Morley 1984; Bassham *et al* 1990; Evans 1992). They can store, retrieve and manipulate information which 'the user' provides. They do this using a specially designed set of instructions – the 'program'. Computers vary in size from the older large mainframes and the newer lap-top and personal microcomputers which can now store vast amounts of information. It is beyond the scope of this section to explain the difference between these types of computers and the different software as these are continually developing and changing. It is suggested that the novice in this area reads any recent paperback on this topic available at high street bookshops. These books also explain computer jargon. Some books are specifically targeted at medical practice (see further reading at the end of this section). For those dietitians working in the NHS a useful handbook on *Information Technology in Healthcare* is produced by the Institute of Health Services Management (1991a) and is updated regularly. There are computer courses run for dietitians by training departments in the NHS and other educational bodies such as Salford University (Bassham and Fletcher 1986), and local education institutions.

The advantages of computers are that:

1 They can manipulate data much faster than the human brain.

2 They are more accurate and reliable (provided they are operated and programmed correctly).

3 They can perform complex tasks (e.g. handle many variables and collate different sets of data rapidly).

4 They can cope with increasing volumes of data.

5 They can store information in a small space.

It must be remembered, however, that they cannot think for themselves and are only as good as the data which is put into them and the programs (or software) which are used to run them. Their disadvantages include:

1 High initial cost.

2 Dependence on technology.

3 The necessity of support for the users.

4 Lack of flexibility.

5 Lack of suitable programs.

Computers have been used by dietitians internationally (Youngwirth 1983) and continue to be used (Williams and Burnet 1984) in all aspects of dietetic work, from data storage to nutrition education (Dennison *et al* 1991). A summary of the main areas of application is included in Table 1.17. Although there are now many different types of computers on the market, there is still little software available specifically for dietitians in the UK, although the range in the USA is much wider. Many general business programs can, however, be adapted for dietetic purposes. These programs include spreadsheets (complex calculation

Table 1.17 Use of computers by dietitians

USE	PROGRAM DETAILS
Dietary computation	
Dietary analysis	Most based on McCance and Widdowson food tables. Commercial software available, both specific and linked with catering. Some dietetic departments have developed their own. Smaller programs with limited foods available
Dietary assessment	Few available, e.g. for assessment of requirements in nutritional support
Dietary construction	Collation/construction of diets, e.g. choosing foods rich in a nutrient, or involving detailed diets, such as PKU/ketogenic diets
Dietetic management	Especially workload analysis • overall dietetic workload, e.g. FIP (Morley 1992) • caseload/priorities (Scott 1988) • Körner packages, e.g. COMCARE
Education/training Staff/patients	Computer assisted learning packages (CAL) both commercial and tutoring or authoring systems used. Range from 'fun' games to student tutorials
Interview/counselling	Very few programs available, but other programs could be adapted
Information storage	Application of *database* packages for • patient records/lists • manufactured product information • special feeds/regimens • standard recipes/menus
Administration	Using business packages, e.g. word processing, spreadsheets, planners, etc. for • diet sheets/product lists • reports • appointments/records • budgets/stock control
Research	Specific programs written for projects. Statistical packages available, questionnaire analysis.
Links with other systems	Patient administration systems – links with hospital mainframe. Commercial links, e.g. Prestel, Micronet, Food databanks.

packages), databases (large filing and retrieval systems) and authoring systems (computer assisted learning) (Morley 1986). A list of programs which are of use in dietetics is available from the British Dietetic Association and has been compiled by the Research Committee (BDA 1991). The NHS has a 'Register of Computer Applications' (contact East Anglian Regional Health Authority, Union Lane, Chesterton, Cambridge CB4 1RF; on-line access is available via Telecom Gold). Unfortunately, to date few dietetic packages are on this register. The American Journal of Dietetic Software contains a list of dietetic software and is published annually. The Journal of the American Dietetic Association also publishes monthly updates on computers and software showing a range of applications.

Programs unique to dietetics fall into three main categories:

1 Dietary Computation Systems (including nutrient analysis and dietary assessment).
2 Dietetic Management Systems (including workload/statistical systems).
3 Education/Training packages.

All other types of programs are adaptations of general business/management packages. Dietetic specific packages are described below.

1.5.1 Dietary computation systems

Nutritional analysis programs

The process of assessing the nutrient content of any diet involves:

- establishing the foods eaten and the quantities, either from a pre-determined menu or by dietary assessment (see Section 1.7);
- looking up each individual food in food tables and calculating the amounts of each nutrient provided by the given weight of the food;
- totalling the amounts of each nutrient obtained from all the foods;
- converting the total intake to amounts per day (or other set period of time).

These calculations are simple but laborious and time-consuming when done by hand and lend themselves to computerisation (Bassham *et al* 1984). Nutrient analysis systems have been developed over the past 20 years and vary from programs with limited analysis of up to 100 foods to those which will handle the full 'McCance and Widdowson' food tables (Holland *et al* 1991). The latter are able to analyse at least 950 foods for over 40 nutritional factors, including fatty acids and amino acids. Programs can be used for the analysis of the intake of a single person on a special diet over a specified period, or the total nutrient content of the hospital menu over a monthly cycle, or large numbers of diet records obtained from surveys.

The principle advantages of using computers for detailed diet analysis are as follows.

a) It saves time and gives more reliable results. Research has shown that direct entry into a microcomputer saves more time and is more accurate than indirect entry by manual coding and using computer operators (Sheppard *et al* 1990).
b) The intake of many nutrients can be calculated as easily as the intake of one or two. Taking advantage of this facility may therefore enable a better total clinical assessment to be made.
c) Updating the food database is often easier, and manufactured products can be included.
d) The system can be used in menu planning and could be linked with catering departments for monitoring stores, food uptake and costings.
e) Usage in collation of diet sheets and food lists.
f) The system can be updated easily with new issues of food tables, as these are available on disk from the Royal Society of Chemistry.
g) Analysis can be compared with 'reference' values. These can be recommended daily allowances, and most dietary analysis packages now have been updated to include the newer dietary reference values (DoH 1991). Some programs allow users to define their own reference values for specific projects.

Most computerized nutrient analysis programs follow a format similar to that outlined in Fig. 1.2. Any analysis program must have an accurate food and nutrient database. Care must also be taken over the use of the database in any of these programs especially as many people are inclined to believe that everything produced by a computer must be correct. Whether calculated by computer or by hand, the values obtained for nutrient content of the diet are only as accurate as the method of dietary assessment used to establish the food eaten (see Section 1.6) If McCance and Widdowson food tables are being used, thought must be given as to how to cope with trace values, estimated values and 'no data' values. Consideration must also be given to the handling of composite dishes in programs using food groups. Setting up a computerized food database can be difficult, time-consuming and requires expertise (Bassham and Stanton 1984), and only a few programmers or dietitians have attempted it. The early programs relied on a paper tape from HMSO containing food data (Russell 1978) and this was used to put together programs for hospital and university mainframe computers (Brereton *et al* 1973; McConnell and Wilson 1976; Walsh 1976; Day 1980; Lowell and Mechie 1983). These programs are now largely out of date and are not available commercially. They often used batch processing and were not available on-line. They have been replaced by programs for microcomputers most of which are available commercially and are summarized in Table 1.18.

Some of the programs listed in Table 1.18 also have

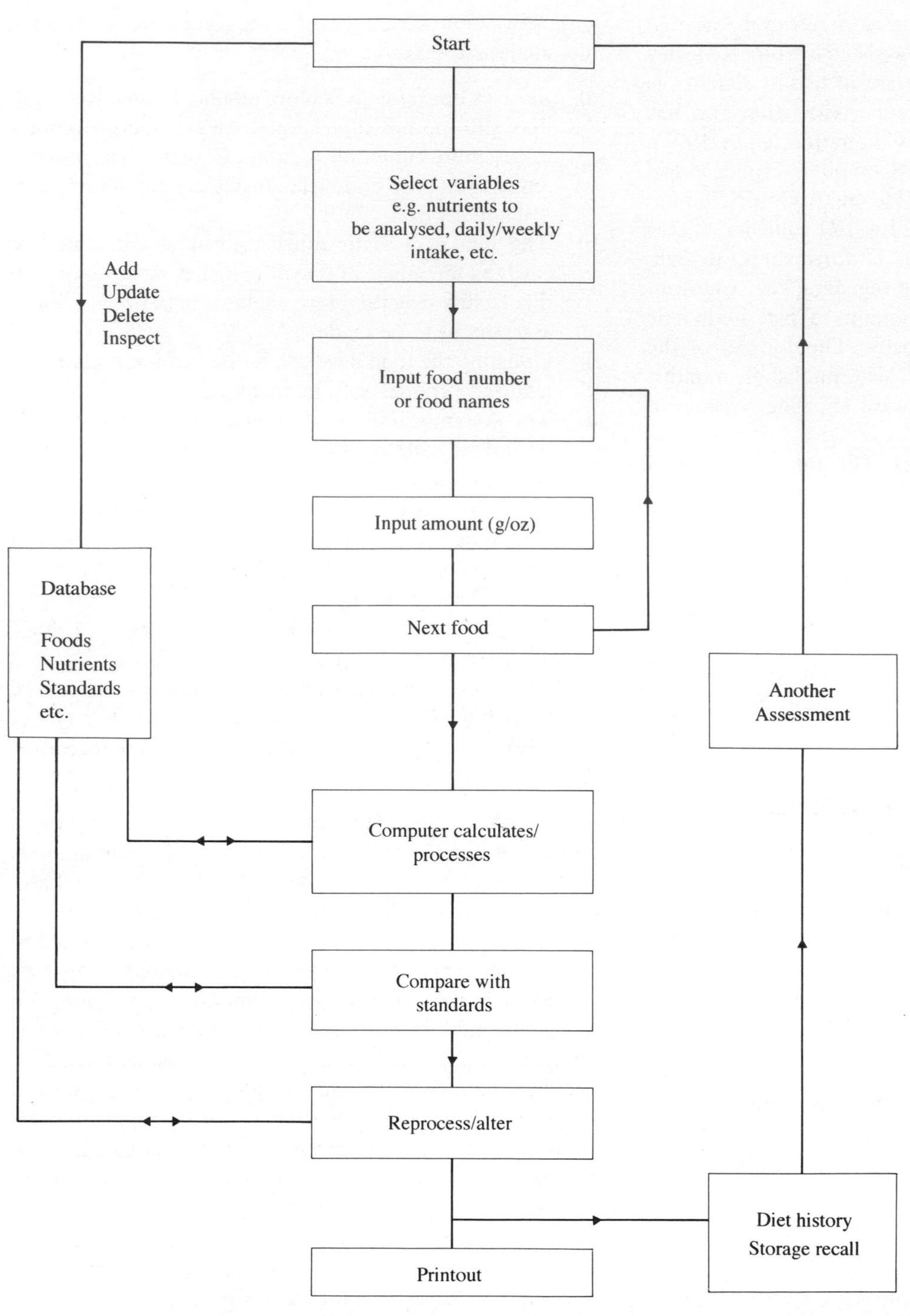

Fig. 1.2 Flowchart of 'typical' diet analysis program

additional facilities to straight nutrient analysis, such as comparing results with standards, e.g. dietary reference values. Others have additional information in the database, for example the nutrient composition of cooked dishes published in the supplements to McCance and Widdowson (Wiles *et al* 1980) or immigrant food information (Tan *et al* 1985). Some of these programs have been developed further especially to make use of the data produced. Graphical outputs and report-writer facilities and better/integrated file handling have been added (in the 'Microdiet' package for example), or interview questionnaire developments such as 'Diet Q'.

With any program it is essential to check that it meets the user's specific requirements, and to try it out before purchasing it. Table 1.19 is a guide to what to look for in a nutritional analysis program.

As well as programs based on the complete McCance and Widdowson food tables, there are some which allow

Table 1.18 Nutritional analysis programs available for purchase

Program (Supplier)	Reference
Comp-Eat (Lifeline Nutritional Services London)	Brambleby and Carlson (1988)
Dietplan-5 (Forestfield Software Ltd Horsham)	
Diet 2000 (Computing Department Brunel University)	Clarke (1989)
Diet Manager (Fretwell Downing Ltd Sheffield)	
Foodbase (Institute of Brain Chemistry Hackney Hospital)	
Microdiet (University of Salford)	Bassham *et al* (1984)
Superdiet II (Computing Unit University of Surrey)	
Diet Q (Tinuviel Software Bristol)	

- All programs have McCance and Widdowson food tables (Holland *et al* 1991) as their database, except Diet Q (which should include these in the future). All programs that use McCance and Widdowson Food Tables 5th Edition have to be licensed with the Royal Society of Chemistry, who produce the food tables and supplements in computer readable form.
- Some older programs have recently come off the market and are no longer available for purchase, e.g. 'Nutrical' (Hall *et al* 1984), or are being updated/changed, e.g. UNIDAP.
- Full program details, including contact names, addresses, telephone numbers and costs are available in the British Dietetic Association's 'Computer software' listing (BDA 1991).

analysis of about 100 foods for five to eight different nutrients. Other programs have been written to run on microcomputers for use in schools. Some enterprising software firms now produce very simple analysis programs for use on home computers; again there are some details in the BDA software list. In the future it may be possible to work out the total nutrient content of a meal whilst it is being cooked in the kitchen, especially as some electronic scales now contain details of food composition.

Table 1.19 Checklist for assessing a nutrient analysis program (Adapted from Hoover and Perloff 1981)

General	Can the system be updated/who will do this? What back up/support will there be if the system goes wrong? Will it work with other systems? Check compatibility e.g. with catering systems Cost of updates/developments Training offered?
Input	How is this done? Are food names or food numbers used? Can a food number be found if needed? Are standard portions indicated? Can different units, e.g. ounces or grams, be used?
Analysis	Will it analyse all nutrients including micronutrients? How does it cope with values for which there is no information in the database? Does it compare with standards, e.g. dietary reference values? Can these be altered? Will it do costings? Will it work out nutrients in terms of — Total amount/percentage total? — Percentage energy intake? — Percentage of a pre-defined standard? — Per portion/100 kcal/100 g/kg body weight/unit cost? — Ratios, e.g. polyunsaturated: saturated fatty acids? Will it give exchanges, food groups, or type? Does it have conversion factors/averaging factors? How accurate is the analysis? What is the error?
Output	What format is used — is this clear? Will it give complete analysis per meal/day/week? Can you select individual nutrients to be displayed? How does it show zero values/estimates/trace amounts on the printout? Can you use different output formats, e.g. bar graphs, pie charts etc?
Database	Where does the data come from — which food tables have been used? Can you add/delete nutrients or foods or add/delete manufactured products? Can you list the database? Can you set your own standards/recommended daily intakes/dietary goals? Does it cope with mixed dish recipes? Can you store/recall information, e.g. diet histories? How is it updated as new information is published?

Dietary assessment and construction

There have been several developments on the use of computers to replace some of the more detailed and laborious calculations needed to assess an individual's nutritional requirements after nutritional assessment. The majority of these programs have been developed for either nutritional support or paediatric special diets, often in-house using a variety of programs. Some diet and nutritional support product companies have supported this objective and helped with development. Few of these packages are available commercially and only occasionally are they used on a wide scale. Some were developed for hand-held computers (Colley *et al* 1985) and, in the USA, are more usually found on the local hospital computer network (Evans 1992).

More recently there have been developments to 'construct diets' using computers. This has been possible given the individual requirements and access to a food database and other information such as food preferences, frequency of meals etc. These programs are still in their infancy but are being looked at, for example, by the University of

Salford for diabetes and renal disease, especially in the research arena (Poyser 1990; Fletcher and Soden 1991).

1.5.2 Education and training

The potential for the use of computers as an educational tool for nutrition and special diets has not yet been realized. There are a few programs available, especially for schools, on general nutrition and attempts have been made to use computers interactively to obtain diet histories (Wise 1986) followed by diet analysis with written feedback. These programs are not widely available but have been used in some health promotion campaigns both here (Bray and Kemm 1986) and overseas (Dennison *et al* 1991).

Computer assisted learning packages have also been used to inform patients about special diets. Some have been developed for diabetes, and some insulin companies now use these in marketing; it is hoped to develop diabetic packages further. The NHS has a computer assisted learning programme, developed in conjunction with the NHS Training Authority, called TEACH (IHSM 1991a). This would lend itself to education of patients, clients, dietitians and students.

1.5.3 Dietetic management systems

The publishing of the work of the NHS Körner steering groups by the Department of Health and Social Security in 1984, highlighted the need for accurate information on NHS workload. These reports proposed 'minimum data sets' for different professional groups. The requirements for data collection for dietetics were published in the fourth Körner Report (DHSS 1984) and defined the data to be collected about dietetic contacts with patients, and dietetic workload. Although there was discussion about the appropriateness of some of the data items suggested, it meant that for the first time there was the potential to provide standard data nationally on aspects of dietetic services. Due to the amount of data that needed to be collected, many health districts looked into computerization of this information. Some opted for their own systems; others developed regional systems – e.g. FIP (Financial Information Project) in the West Midlands, which was then adapted and is now used in other regions (Morley 1992). Others bought in commercial packages such as COMCARE. This has been the biggest growth area in dietetic computer applications over the past five years. Some of these systems were developed by dietetic departments to include additional data, for example dietetic treatment and outcomes (Morley 1992) or care level analysis (Scott 1988). These programs could be developed into total information systems for dietetic services (see Section 1.5.4, below).

With the recent changes due to the NHS and Community Care Act, information requirements have and will continue to change. New minimum data sets are being produced (Evans 1991) under the proposals of Working Paper 11 'Framework for Information Systems: The Next Steps' (DoH Information Management Group 1990). New data manuals are being produced; the first one (Manual 1) on hospital services has been published (NHS Management Executive 1991) and Manual 3 will contain information on 'Paramedical and Cross-sectional Services'.

These systems are now linking with others primarily set up for resource management initiatives (National Dietetic Managers Committee 1991; IHSM 1991b), including collaborative care planning and case-mix analysis. These systems attempt to document the workload attributable to patients (individual or groups of diagnostically related patients) during a hospital stay. (Rowson 1989). They can then be linked to hospital systems and those used for medical and clinical audit (DoH 1990).

1.5.4 Total dietetic systems

In the USA and Canada, systems for dietetic services have developed out of catering systems as the two departments are usually managed and financed together. These systems have in some cases covered the breadth of the 'computer needs' of clinical dietetic services. They do not include many community applications although could be adapted to do so. These programs cover clinical workload, scheduling, diet ordering, appointments, word processing, statistics and nutrient analysis. Developments linked to catering systems to include dietetic aspects such as meal/diet ordering have been slow to be developed in the UK.

A total dietetic system was proposed by dietitians in Scotland (Sub-Committee on Dietetics 1988), but unfortunately this is not yet available. However, new proposals for NHS systems, such as HISS (Hospital Information Support Systems) could incorporate dietetic services systems.

1.5.5 Data Protection Act

The Data Protection Act (1984) came into force in 1985 and by the middle of 1986 all computers which held personal data about individuals for practice, private or research purposes had to be registered with the Registrar (NHS Training Authority 1985). It is important therefore, that dietitians using computers register under this Act. For those working in the NHS registration is usually collective at district or unit level and further information is available from district or area health boards who usually have a designated officer for the Act. There is also a wealth of material explaining the implications of the Act (National Health Service Computer Policy Committee 1984; The Data Protection Act 1985; Morley 1986).

1.5.6 The future

There has been enormous expansion in the application of

computers in all areas of health care, both from the clinical and management perspective. This ranges from expert systems in medical areas to total hospital management systems. Recent changes in the NHS have meant that accurate information is now essential and the use of computers to help collect, collate and interpret this data is vital. Health services are starting to integrate and network these systems into a comprehensive information system across areas of health care (Cross 1992), and this should include dietetics.

The future will see the continued growth of computer developments, especially with the use of lap-tops (potentially saving some secretarial time) and the use of computerized information for contracting/service agreements and workload management. There are also many developments that will impact on dietetic services such as developments in catering systems and ward ordering. There will be development of communication systems and patient information systems to include caseload analysis, resource usage and clinical audit. Dietitians need to be aware of this and develop systems that integrate with these where appropriate. As systems in the USA and other countries are further ahead, it is useful to stay in contact with what is happening internationally (Evans 1992).

Further reading

British Dietetic Association (1986) *Computer guide for dietitians*, British Dietetic Association, Birmingham.

Norris D, Skilbeck C, Hayward A and Torpy D (1985) *Microcomputers in clinical practice*. John Wiley, Chichester.

Steward T and Willis A (1989) *Computers – a guide to choosing and using*. Oxford University Press, Oxford.

British Journal of Health Care Computing. Published ten times per year.

References

Bassham S and Fletcher LR (1986) Computer appreciation training for dietitians. *Hum Nutr: Appl Nutr* **39A**, 400–406.

Bassham S, Fletcher LR and Soden P (1990) Scientific uses of computers in dietetic departments. *Medical Informatics* **40**, 7–10.

Bassham S, Fletcher LR and Stanton RJH (1984) Dietary analysis with the aid of a microcomputer. *J Microcomp Applic* **7**, 279–89.

Bassham S and Stanton RHJ (1984) Something to add. *British Dietetic Association ADviser* **12**, 19–20.

Brambleby P and Carlson E (1988) PC for diet analysis. *Br J of Healthcare Computing*. **October**, 39.

Bray AJ and Kemm JR (1986) Use of computer administered healthy eating quiz for data collection and health promotion. *Proc Nutr Soc* **45**, 86.

Brereton P, Healy MJR and Pittaway M (1973) A simple computerized system for dietary calculations. *Nutrition(London)* **3**, 200–205.

British Dietetic Association Research Committee (1991) *Computer Software*, Fehily A (Ed) BDA Birmingham.

Clarke M (1989) Computerized dietary analysis: a truly interactive approach. *J Hum Nutr Dietet* **2**, 287–93.

Colley CM, Fleck A and Howard JP (1985) Pocket computers: a new aid to nutritional support. *Br Med J* **290**, 1403–6.

Cross M (1992) Against all the odds. *Health Service Journal* **April 30**, 34–6.

Data Protection Act (1984) HMSO, London.

Data Protection Registrar (1985) *Guidelines No. 1 on the Data Protection Act*. Springfield House, Water Lane, Wilmslow.

Day KC (1980) Recipe – a computer program for calculating the nutrient content of foods. *J Hum Nutr* **34**, 181–7.

Dennison KF, Dennison D and Ward JY (1991) Computerized nutrition program. Effect on nutrient intake of senior citizens. *J Am Dietet Assoc* **91**, 1431–3.

Department of Health (1990) *Guide to computing systems for medical audit* – EL(90) MB/81. DoH, London.

Department of Health (1991) *Dietary Reference Values for food, energy and nutrients for the United Kingdom*. Report 41 on Health and Social Subjects. HMSO, London.

Department of Health Information Management Group (1990) *Framework for information system: the next steps*. HMSO, London.

Department of Health and Social Security (1984) Steering Group on Health Service Information: *Fourth Report to the Secretary of State (Körner Report IV)*. HMSO, London.

Evans E (1991) Standard issue. *Br J Health Care Computing* **8(5)**, 20–22.

Evans S (1992) Evolution of computer applications in dietetics in the USA. *BDA ADviser*, **Spring**, 6–14.

Fletcher LR and Soden PM (1991) Diet construction using linear programming. *Diabetes Nutr Metab* **4(1)** Supplement 1, 169–74.

Hall L, Carter D, Pettit B, Pettit S and Springford J (1984) Chips in the dietetic department. *British Dietetic Association ADviser* **13**, 21–2.

Holland B, Welch AA, Unwin ID, Buss DH, Paul AA and Southgate DAT (1991) *The Composition of Foods* 5th edition. Royal Society of Chemistry, Cambridge.

Hoover LW and Perloff BP (1981) *Model for review of nutrient database system capabilities*. University of Missouri Press, Missouri.

Howard JP and Hall L (1981) *A review of the use of computers in dietetic departments*. Unpublished.

Institute of Health Services Management (1991a) *Information technology in health care* 12e. Longman, Essex.

Institute of Health Services Management (1991b). 'Resource Management' Section B93 in *Information technology in health care* 12e. pp. B9.3–01–B9.3–11. Longman, Essex.

Lowell JP and Mechie JR (1983) Computerized dietary calculations: an interactive approach updated. *Hum Nutr: Appl Nutr* **37A**, 36–40.

McConnell FG and Wilson A (1976) Computerized nutritional analysis in the dietetic department of a teaching hospital. *J Hum Nutr* **30**, 405–13.

Morley T (1984) Why compute? *British Dietetic Association ADviser* **13**, 19–20.

Morley T (1986) *Computer Guide for Dietitians*. British Dietetic Association Research Committee, Birmingham.

Morley T (1992) The uses of a patient based dietetic data collection system. *J Hum Nutr Dietet* **5**, 399–407.

NHS Management Executive (1991) *The Data Manual*, Model 1 – Hospital Services. HMSO, London.

National Dietetic Managers Committee of the BDA (1991) *Resource Management*, Briefing Paper 1. British Dietetic Association, Birmingham.

National Health Service Computer Policy Committee (1984) *Data protection guidelines for NHS authorities*. Centre for Information Technology, Birmingham.

National Health Service Training Authority (1985) *Data Protection Act – resource pack*. National Computing Centre Ltd, NHSTA, Bristol.

Poyser J (1990) Simulated Teaching. *Br J of Health Care Computing*. **May**, 12–16.

Rowson J (1989) Resource management: the London way. *Br J of Health Care Computing*. **October**, 16–17.

Russell J (1978) *The paper tape version of McCance and Widdowson'* The Composition of Foods. HMSO, London.

Scott DW (1988) Evaluation of Dietetic Activity Analysis (DAA) *J Hum Nutr Diet* **1**, 59–70.

Sheppard AM, Coles KJ, Fehily AM and Holliday RM (1990) A direct data entry system for processing dietary records: comparison with manual coding. *J Hum Nutr Dietet* **3**, 209–214.

Sub-committee on Dietetics of the National Paramedical Consultative Committee (1988) *Computing in Dietetic Departments*. Scottish Home and Health Deparment, Edinburgh.

Tan SP, Wenlock RW and Buss DH (1985) *Immigrant foods*. Second supplement to McCance and Widdowson's *The Composition of Foods*. HMSO, London.

Walsh KA (1976) Computerized dietary calculation; an interactive approach. *J Hum Nutr* **30**, 395–403.

Wiles SJ, Nettleton PA, Black AE and Paul AA (1980) The nutrient composition of some cooked dishes eaten in Britain: a supplementary food composition table. *J Hum Nutr* **34**, 189–223.

Williams CS and Burnet LW (1984) Future applications of the micro-computer in dietetics. *Hum Nutr: Appl Nutr* **38A**, 99–109.

Wise A (1986) Interactive computer programs for applied nutrition education. *Hum Nutr: Appl Nutr* **39A**, 407–14.

Youngwirth J (1983) The evolution of computers in dietetics: a review. *J Am Diet Assoc* **82**, 62–7.

1.6 Dietary assessment methodology

1.6.1 Methods

There are five basic methods in use for assessing dietary intake in free-living individuals, which were first described 50–60 years ago. Two are records of actual consumption, made at the time of eating food, one with weights of food established by the subjects themselves (Widdowson 1936), and the other with estimated weights of food (Youmans *et al* 1942). The other three methods attempt to assess diet in the recent past by asking subjects about their food intake the previous day, the 24-hour recall (Wiehl 1942), or over the past few weeks or months, the diet history (Turner 1940). The diet history may be used in an attempt to estimate intake in the distant past. Questionnaires may be used to assess usual diet, either recent or distant past, but are usually devised for completion by the subjects concerned without supervision (Wiehl and Reed 1960) and are rarely used in clinical work.

1.6.2 Accuracy

Accurate results from these methods require a high degree of skill and care on the part of the dietitian. The reason for this is that a number of errors are introduced at each stage of dietary assessment and the net result may be a systematic bias or large random deviations from the true mean. Large random error will entail numerous observations before individuals are classified correctly for their average nutrient intake, and systematic errors invalidate individual comparisons with standards such as, for example, the Dietary Reference Value.

1.6.3 Aims

At the outset of a dietary investigation it is essential to establish which nutrients are of interest and how accurate the results are required to be, due to the effect of normal day to day variation in nutrient intake (see below). All results are dependent on (1) the degree of co-operation from the subjects and their ability to give accurate reports or records of their dietary habits, and (2) on adequate food tables (Section 1.4). Food tables cannot be used to measure salt consumption; urine analysis is a preferable method (see subsection 'validity'). Methods for present or recent past dietary assessment, and retrospective dietary investigations are discussed below.

1.6.4 Choice of method

In theory the most accurate method available is the *weighed dietary record* where the weights of all food and beverages consumed are recorded. This requires a robust and convenient set of scales weighing up to 2 kg and accurate to ±1 g which can be given to the subject for use at home. Scales with a taring facility should be avoided because this often causes confusion. People should be given a demonstration of how to weigh a meal on to their normal plates, recording the cumulative weights, and then be asked to repeat the demonstration themselves. Once they have grasped the essence of the technique, a notebook and a set of simple instructions should be provided and the need for adequate details of recipes, brand names and foods consumed away from home explained. Electronic scales with an automatic recording facility can help with illiterate groups. The PETRA scales (available from Cherlyn Electronics, Kings Court, King's Hedges Road, Cambridge, England) record a spoken description of the item and the weight (undisclosed to the volunteer) on to a cassette; this is later played back through a special console. The FRED system (available from BC Systems Ltd, 35 Harford Street, Trowbridge, Wilts., England) uses condensed food tables of 95 items, each represented by a separate key on a small desktop computer/scales. The keys can be labelled with pictograms, and weight is recorded automatically, undisclosed to the operator. It must be emphasized to subjects that they must continue with their normal dietary habits, and not change their usual menu or amounts of foods whilst keeping the record. Subjects should be visited at home or asked to return to the clinic to check that they have understood all the instructions and are keeping the record correctly.

If only energy and energy yielding nutrients are to be assessed, a seven day record is sufficient if an accuracy of ±10% standard error is acceptable (Table 1.20). This is equivalent to a range of 20 g protein (40 g at $p < 0.05$) assuming an average of 100 g/day. As can be seen from the table, vitamins, minerals and fibre require longer periods of observation, at least 14 days. These do not have to be obtained over a single period of time and four records each of four days duration would be an acceptable compromise. People with stable food habits, and therefore with lower than average within-person coefficients of variation, can be observed for shorter periods, while longer investigations are necessary in those with erratic eating patterns in order to obtain a satisfactory level of precision.

Table 1.20 The effect of day to day variation on the precision of estimates of the average nutrient intake

Item	Average* within person variation %	% standard error† of a 7-day record average	Number of days†† of records necessary to be ±10% of the average
Energy	23	9	5
Carbohydrate	25	9	6
Protein	27	10	7
Fat	31	12	10
Dietary fibre	31	12	10
Calcium	32	12	10
Iron	35	13	12
Thiamin	39	15	15
Riboflavin	44	17	19
Cholesterol	52	20	27
Vitamin C	60	23	36

* Data from up to 19 population samples in Britain, USA, Canada, Israel and others (Bingham 1987).

† †† Calculated from % standard error (se) $= \frac{cv\%}{\sqrt{n}}$ and $n = \frac{cv^2}{\%se^2}$ (Balogh *et al* 1971).

The main disadvantage with the weighed food record is that it is a tedious procedure for the subject if conventional written records are used and hence it requires a considerable amount of co-operation. In studies of groups of patients (e.g. monitoring dietary compliance or effectiveness) there is always a risk that a high level of non-participation may introduce an element of bias; those who are unable or unwilling to take part may well have different dietary habits from those who do participate. Government surveys using this method do however achieve high response rates of 80% from randomly selected population samples (Gregory *et al* 1990). Thus, the seven or more days weighed food record can be used to obtain accurate data from population samples.

Another method of assessing dietary intake from a subject's point of view is *the unweighed food record* where the quantity of food is estimated by description using models, standard portions, food replicas and household measures. However, this technique is more demanding for the dietitian who either needs to become skilled in interpreting these descriptions or to use a computer data base incorporating them. There is a risk that individuals may consistently under- or overestimate their portion sizes, hence introducing systematic errors. Dietary assessments using this method are likely to be less accurate than those derived from weighed records, but may be more readily obtainable from the patients. At least 14 days of records need to be obtained if minerals and vitamins are to be assessed, as detailed above.

The most important, and most commonly used, method in clinical work is the *diet history* which aims to assess the usual nutrient intake by means of dietary questioning. A full dietary history may take as much as $1\frac{1}{2}$ hours to complete properly, although a shortened version is often adequate for the purpose of advising on dietary modification. Practical details have been described in the original publication (Turner 1940). However, because the accuracy of the dietary history is so dependent on the interviewing techniques and method of questioning used to obtain the information, these aspects are discussed in Section 1.7.

Recent studies have shown that intakes assessed by diet history appear to be greater than those obtained from records (Bingham 1987) probably because subjects tend to overestimate how often they consume foods. Nutritionists experienced in taking diet histories can correct for this overestimation with a factor based on the probable numbers of meals eaten during the period of time covered (Callmer, personal communication). Nevertheless, patients are rarely able to recall their food intake with accuracy. Turner (1940) noted that the results from a diet history did not show absolute agreement with those from weighed records, and the dietitian using the diet history should be aware of the approximate amount of error involved. Turner's studies suggested that, for example, protein intakes assessed by the two methods were likely to differ by 32 g on average (standard deviation of difference 16%).

An assessment of the usual diet of a patient based on a single 24-hour recall is not recommended if an accurate estimate of nutrient intake is required; this method tends to be associated with systematic underestimation of food intake and fails to take account of daily variations in dietary habits. At best, it can only give a rough idea of the type of food consumed and approximate meal pattern. Unfortunately, owing to constraints on time, this method of dietary investigation is one on which many dietitians have to rely in clinical practice. If this is unavoidable then dietitians should at least be aware of the limited nature of any information obtained in this way.

1.6.5 Validity

No matter how carefully done, dietary assessments using any of the above methods rely on information given to the dietitian by the patient. Where there is any doubt of the veracity of a report, for example when investigating an obese or anorectic patient, an independent check is needed.

Energy expenditure can now be measured by a non-invasive technique and has been used to validate estimates of energy intake (Livingstone *et al* 1990; Black *et al* 1993). Whilst this technique of direct measurement by the doubly-labelled water technique is too expensive for routine use, an indirect method can give some indication of the accuracy of energy intake measurements. This (and the 24 hour urine method described below) relies on the assumption that body weight is constant during the period of investigation. Negative energy (and protein) balances will obviously occur if patients are unable to eat, or are slimming.

As an indirect estimate of energy expenditure, Basal Metabolic Rate (BMR) can be calculated from body weight using the modified Schofield equations (see Section 2.1.2).

Ready reference tables for these are given in Appendix 4. Total energy expenditure can then be calculated using the relevant physical activity ratio (see Section 2.1.3). For most sedentary population groups this is 1.4. Since energy intake should match expenditure, the dietary intake value can also be expressed as a rate of BMR. Estimates markedly less than 1.4 are likely to be wrong for a group of individuals.

This method is of uncertain accuracy for individuals, although if sufficient days of observation are available, dietary intake to BMR ratios of less than 1.2 are unphysiological in the absence of weight loss. Above this, there is a range of possible values depending partly on energy expenditure, because physical activity ratios can be as high as 2.2 over the 24 hour period. In addition, there is a range of individual values in BMR in relation to weight of about 10% coefficient of variation.

Another check is the 24-hour urinary nitrogen output, which can be compared with the reported nitrogen (protein) intake (Isaksson 1980). Urine nitrogen should not exceed dietary intake and should be within the range of 81 ±5% standard deviation (Bingham and Cummings 1985). In a Swedish study (Warnold *et al* 1978), the reported dietary intake of obese patients obtained from a diet history was only 46 g protein (7 g nitrogen), whereas their actual intake estimated from 24-hour urinary nitrogen output was 87 g protein, a two-fold difference, or 190% of the supposed dietary intake. Diabetic subjects have been shown to have a tendency to report their prescribed diet rather than their actual food intake as monitored by their 24-hour urine nitrogen output (Steen *et al* 1977). When 24-hour urine collections are used in this way, or for the assessment of salt consumption, their completeness must be assured by using the para-amino-benzoic acid (PABA) check method. Patients are given an oral dose of PABA and the amount recovered in the urine is an index of the completeness of the urine collection (Bingham and Cummings 1983).

1.6.6 Retrospective dietary assessments

The dietitian may be asked to obtain an assessment of a patient's eating habits in the distant past for diagnostic or research purposes in conditions with a prolonged latent period. In this case, a diet history interview referring patients back to around the time in question may be undertaken. However, a number of recent studies have shown that individuals' reports of past dietary habits are strongly biased towards those of the present (Byers *et al* 1983; Jensen *et al* 1984; Rohan and Potter 1984); people cannot remember their dietary habits of several years ago. Estimates of past dietary habits may therefore be misleading.

1.6.7 Dietary survey methodology in research and epidemiology

This is a highly specialized field and dietitians are advised to consult the following publications (Marr 1971; Black 1982; Black *et al* 1983; 1991; 1993; Bingham 1985; 1987; 1991; Goldberg *et al* 1991) or recommend them to clinicians, before undertaking survey work of either groups or individuals.

References

Balogh M, Kahn HA and Medalie JH (1971) Random repeat 24-hour dietary recalls. *Am J Clin Nutr* **24**, 304–10.

Bingham S (1985) Aspects of dietary survey methodology. *BNF Bull* **10**(44), 90–103.

Bingham S (1987) The dietary assessment of individuals; methods, accuracy, new techniques and recommendations. *Nutr Abstr Rev* **57**, 705–742.

Bingham S (1991) Validation of dietary assessment through biomarkers. In *Biomarkers of Dietary Exposure* Kok FJ and Van't Veer (Eds) Smith-Gordon, London. pp. 41–52.

Bingham S and Cummings JH (1983) The use of PABA as a marker to validate the completeness of 24-hour urine collections in man. *Clin Sci* **64**, 629–35.

Bingham S and Cummings JH (1985) Urine nitrogen as an independent validatory measure of the dietary intake. *Am J Clin Nutr* **42**, 1276–89.

Black AE (1982) The logistics of dietary surveys. *Hum Nutr: Appl Nutr* **36A**, 85–94.

Black AE, Cole TJ, Wiles SJ and White F (1983) Daily variation in food intake of infants from 2–18 months. *Hum Nutr: Appl Nutr* **37A**, 448–58.

Black AE, Goldberg GR, Jebb SA, Livingstone MBE and Prentice AM (1991) Critical evaluation of energy intake data using fundamental principles of energy physiology. 2. Evaluating the results of dietary surveys. *Eur J Clin Nutr* **45**, 583–99.

Black AE, Prentice AM, Goldberg GR, Jebb SA, Bingham SA, Livingstone MBE and Coward WA (1993) Measurements of total energy expenditure provide insights into validity of dietary measurements of energy intake. *J Am Dietet Assoc* **93**(5), 572–9.

Byers TE, Randall I, Marshall JR, Rzepka TF, Cummings KM and Graham S (1983) Dietary history from the distant past. *Nutr Cancer* **5**, 69–77.

Goldberg GR, Black AE, Jebb SA, Cole TJ, Murgatroyd PR, Coward WA and Prentice AM (1991) Critical evaluation of energy intake data using fundamental principles of energy physiology. 1 Derivation of cut-off values to identify under-recording. *Eur J Am Nutr* **45**, 569–81.

Gregory J, Foster K, Tyler H and Wiseman M (1990) *The dietary and nutritional survey of adults*. HMSO, London.

Isaksson B (1980) Urinary nitrogen output as a validity test in dietary surveys. *Am J Clin Nutr* **33**, 4–12.

Jensen OM Wahrendorf J, Rosenquist A and Geser A (1984) The reliability of questionnaire-derived historic dietary information and temporal stability of food habits in individuals. *Am J Epidemiol* **120**, 281–90.

Livingstone MBE, Prentice AM, Strain JJ, Coward WA, Black AE, Barker ME, McKenna PG and Whitehead RG (1990) Accuracy of weighed dietary records in studies of diet and health. *Br Med J* **300**, 708–712.

Marr JW (1971) Individual dietary surveys: purposes and methods. *World Rev Nutr Diet* **13**, 105–64.

Rohan TE and Potter JO (1984) Retrospective assessment of dietary intake. *Am J Epidemiol* **120**, 876–7.

Steen B, Isaksson B and Svanborg A (1977) Intake of energy and nutrients in 70 year old males and females in Gothenburg, Sweden. *Acta Med Scand* [Supp 1] **611**, 39–86.

Turner D (1940) The estimation of the patient's home dietary intake. *J Am Diet Assoc* **16**, 875–81.

Warnold I, Carlgren G and Krotkiewski M (1978) Energy expenditure and body composition during weight reduction in hyperplastic obese women. *Am J Clin Nutr* **31**, 750–63.
Widdowson EM (1936) A study of English diets by the individual method. Part I. Men. *J Hyg* **36**, 269–92.
Wiehl DG (1942) Diets of a group of aircraft workers in Southern California. *Millbank Memorial Fund Quarterly* **20**, 329–66.
Wiehl DG and Reed R (1960) Development of new or improved methods for epidemiologic investigation. *Am J Public Health* **50**, 824–8.
Youmans JB, Patton EW and Kern R (1942) Surveys of the nutrition of populations. *Am J Public Health* **32**, 1371–9.

1.7 Dietary assessment in clinical practice

The following are practical guidelines for assessing the dietary intake of individuals prior to giving therapeutic dietary advice or guidance on healthy eating.

1.7.1 Preparation for the assessment of dietary intake

Reason for the assessment

The reason for the assessment must be clear as this will determine the methodology. For example, 'Is it part of a research study?' If it is, there will be a detailed protocol to ensure all assessments are carried out in a standardized way. Alternatively, the assessment may be part of the evidence used in clarifying a diagnosis. For example, 'Is the observed anaemia related to poor diet?'. The assessment will look at overall energy intake as this relates to iron intake but will concentrate on major sources of iron, vitamin C, folate, fibre, rather than sugar or fat intakes. The assessment may be one of a series in the same patient looking at dietary compliance. For example, assessment of the diet of a person with diabetes may look specifically at energy balance meal by meal, day by day, as well as sugar and fat intake, both type and quantity.

Reasons for the dietary assessment should be given either verbally or in writing to the person concerned. Instructions for completing a food diary or checklist prior to interview may also need to be given.

Background information relevant to the assessment

This may be obtained from case notes, the referral letter or may have to be obtained directly from the person. This information is needed to identify any special factors to be taken into consideration when obtaining the diet information and assessing the information.

Obtaining information

This can be more difficult and hence time-consuming if the person has difficulties in communicating, for example deafness, English as a second language, learning difficulties. The presence of a relative or carer may be necessary if the diet assessment is to be valid. There may need to be a change in the method of data collection from verbal to written.

Assessing information

This requires knowledge of any clinical problem, known or suspected, current or recent medication prescribed or self-administered, and accuracy of the information obtained (i.e. the reliability of responses).

The environment for the assessment

A setting which is free of interruption and acknowledges the exchange of confidential information is ideal but frequently not available to dietitians – be they hospital or community based. Hospital wards are full of disruptions (as indeed can be outpatient clinics not least of all due to telephones and 'bleeps'). The patient's home is a good setting but is only used in a small proportion of assessments.

Duration of the assessment

Following through good interview techniques and the questioning required to obtain information can take at least half an hour, often longer for a full diet history. In a long interview, a break in the questioning at a suitable time to allow a mental rest is helpful to both the dietitian and the person providing the information.

Recording information

Accurate and complete recording of information collected is essential. Dietitians use forms developed to meet their needs and these may differ from department to department and on the assessment required. Forms should record all essential patient/client personal and medical information. Most forms are designed with a checklist and cross-check facility. For example:

- Meal pattern through the day;
- Food frequency checklist.

The result of the assessment should be recorded to complete the form and make it available for further evaluation or audit (see Table 1.21).

1.7.2 The diet history – steps in obtaining dietary information

It is the outcome which is important – to ensure that the diet information is collected in the most effective and accurate way, ideally with both parties enjoying and learning

Table 1.21 Suggested sections to include in forms for taking diet histories

Patient/client information	Personal details Consultant/GP/other referring agent Medical and social information
Diet history	Meal pattern *e.g.* Breakfast } Time/place Mid-morning } Midday } Differences – week days Mid-afternoon } weekends Evening } During evening } Effect of employment – During night } shifts
	Food frequency and portion size *e.g.* covering major foods and liquids from all food groups able to identify sources – fat, sugar, fibre, alcohol – vitamin C, iron, calcium
Other relevant details	Date, Cooking methods (including salt) Finances
Results	

from the experience. As the dietitians become more experienced they are able to develop their own style and are able to vary their approach to suit the individual.

A detailed diet history requires probing for the variety of foods eaten, the quantities eaten and the cooking methods. For a broader diet history, food habits and patterns, with some detail related to specific foods, will be required.

The following steps need to be included but not necessarily in the order shown.

- Establish the daily meal pattern and expand into the weekly pattern. Take the respondent through a day to find out the pattern of meals, snacks and drinks throughout a typical week. Question how this is affected by being at work, at home, or away from home, by sharing food or drinks with visitors.
- Twenty-four hour recall can be used to start obtaining details of the types of food eaten and is often easier for the respondent to remember. This can be expanded to find out other examples of meals eaten over a seven day period.
- Establish the quantities of food eaten; the degree of accuracy required will depend on why the assessment is being undertaken. Twenty-four hour recall can assist this process. Use of food models, photographs of foods, food packages can all assist respondents to remember the details of their diet. This can be difficult if the respondent has little to do with shopping or cooking and, in such cases, the assessment can only be very general and descriptive.
- Establish recipes of composite dishes or brand names of specific foods or prepared meals used.
- Cross-check the information obtained during the interview using a variety of methods. For example, getting the respondent to confirm details when the dietitian summarizes the details or asking the respondent to describe food frequency which can then be checked against the details of the history. Food models can also help in the cross-checking. This procedure is more important when a detailed and quantitative diet assessment is required.
- Check there is sufficient detail, if required, to code food for detailed analysis.

1.7.3 Problems encountered when taking diet histories and assessing results

Assumptions about responses

It is easy to transfer the dietitian's own eating patterns to other people. It is important to check what the respondent means by, for example, 'lean fried fish'. Is it bought from a fish and chip shop? Is it a pre-packed frozen product? Or is it fresh fish cooked at home? Is it battered, breadcrumbed, shallow-, deep-fat or stir-fried?

Inadequate record keeping

It is important to have forms that enable all details to be recorded easily and clearly at the time. Copying out rough notes is time-consuming and can result in inaccuracies. A second dietitian should be able to use the information and produce a very similar assessment.

Poor interview technique

This can result in the respondent getting bored and giving inaccurate responses to speed up the process. A variety of styles of questioning, short breaks in questioning and watching for signs of fatigue, especially in sick patients, will improve the quality of the assessment.

Reliability

The more irregular the eating pattern, the harder it is to obtain a reliable diet history. Respondents may not be entirely truthful and the dietitian should have strategies for dealing with this situation if it is exposed.

Bias is introduced into the respondent's memory during a diet history with respect to:

- overestimation of 'proper' meals;
- under-remembering snacks and drink and alcohol;
- memory being weighted to the previous seven days.

1.7.4 Analysis of the information

Assessment of food intake

Depending on the reason for taking the diet history, the food intake may be assessed or analysed in a variety of ways:

1 By relating the food intake to a daily food guide.
2 By using knowledge of food composition to make a judgement about some aspects of the diet (e.g. the adequacy of fibre intake or the likely contribution of the diet to dental caries).
3 By using a table of approximate food values to make a crude calculation of the intake of one or more dietary constituents.
4 By using detailed tables of food composition to calculate the intake of specific nutrients.

The first three points are relevant to the brief diet history and the latter point to the full diet history.

Assessment of nutrient intake

Nutrient intake = nutrient content of food × portion weight × frequency of consumption.

A good illustration of this is to compare the relative contributions of parsley and milk to vitamin C intake:

Parsley provides	150 mg vitamin C/100 g
	× 1 g portion
	× once/week
	= 0.2 mg/day
Milk provides	1.5 mg vitamin C/100 g
	× 30 g portion
	× eight/day
	= 3.6 mg/day

The food code used to derive nutritional data from food tables should be that which best represents the food described by the respondent. Quantities should have been checked thoroughly by the end of the interview.

1.7.5 Interpretation of the information

The results should be interpreted by considering the limitations by the method, the judgement on the quality of information obtained, and the variability of individual nutritional requirements. It is meaningless to report results to the nearest mg of calcium or g of protein. It is also more realistic to give results as a range of ±20% on the calculated value.

An individual's intake cannot meaningfully be compared directly with DRVs which are standards for group intake.

The written interpretation of the results must be expressed concisely and clearly. Where appropriate, suggestions should be made for correcting dietary problems. These may be passed immediately to the respondent in the form of dietary advice.

1.7.6 Evaluation

It is important to review the whole process by which dietary assessment is obtained in order to improve and increase confidence in the following:

1 The interview process.
2 The validity of the information collected.
3 The reliability of the information collected. Can two dietitians get the same result from the respondent and can a single dietitian get the same result on two occasions with the same patient?
4 The development of a standardized but flexible process for diet history and assessment.

1.8 Dietary modification

The dietitian is educated and trained to 'interpret and communicate the science of nutrition to enhance the quality of life of individuals and groups in health and disease, by using principles from the health and social sciences . . . 'Dietitians enable people to take a personal responsibility for their health by making more appropriate choices about food and life style' (*Towards the Twenty First Century*, British Dietetic Association 1991).

Whether giving dietary advice to a patient or carrying out a project which includes teaching others about food choices and healthy eating, dietitians draw on all their skills to communicate the scientific detail in ways appropriate to their 'audience'. There are two stages to this process, the principles of dietary modification and the presentation of dietary modification information. These will be considered separately but, obviously, they inter-relate in day-to-day practice.

1.8.1 Principles of dietary modification

Table 1.22 details the knowledge, skills and attitudes required to carry out the processes of dietary modification. Not all of these elements will necessarily apply in every dietary modification; however it is essential that all three elements are available within a dietetic service to ensure the quality of the work. The resulting information must be converted into a form of use which is appropriate for a dietitian's patients, clients or public audiences.

Table 1.22 Principles of dietary modification for therapeutic purposes and for the promotion of healthy eating

Knowledge	The dietitian should know the: – standards for dietary modification based on up-to-date knowledge of medical and dietetic research e.g. quantitative and/or qualitative – issues for consideration to maintain overall dietary adequacy whilst adhering to the dietary modification required, e.g. short-term/long-term consequences; effects in child or adult – basic facts of the dietary modification as used in education. e.g. exchange systems, 'free from' foods, food groups – support systems for dietary modification from within dietetic service and other agencies, e.g. social workers, lay groups, research charities
Skills	The dietitian should be able to: – manipulate scientific knowledge of diet therapy into dietary information accessible to patients or the general public, e.g. production of dietary information, whether visual, tape, video, computer – counter the effects of limitations imposed both by diet modification and the individual or client group involved, e.g. food preferences, financial considerations, effects of culture, effect of age – calculate, to the required degree of accuracy, the nutrient content of the dietary modification
Attitudes	The dietitian should demonstrate commitment to: – continuing education to maintain standards of dietetic practice – evaluating the outcome of dietary modification by auditing their work against standards and by communicating findings

1.8.2 Presentation of dietary modification information

Qualitative methods

All detailed dietary manipulations need to be presented with choices, clear guidelines, menu guidance and supporting information such as advice on suitable manufactured foods. It is the dietitian who can make this information practical and usable by categorizing the details so that the patient (or client) is not presented with endless 'lists'. Information should be offered in a way which avoids the 'good foods – bad foods' categories. Patients/clients should be encouraged to understand the key relationship between a food and a diet; the value of a food depends on the amount of nutrient (or food component) in the food and the frequency with which the food is consumed.

Dietitians are frequently faced with patients or clients who are 'feeling guilty' about eating certain foods supposed not to be 'good'. Interpreting dietary modification in a sensible way is essential to help with compliance, both short and long term. Dietary changes are more likely to be followed if clear explanations and simple instructions are provided as to why the diet has to be changed. Patients forget a large proportion of orally presented information, and the results of communication can be improved with written information which gives clear explanations and simple instructions. However, it is also known that there are problems with written material in that it may not be read or understood. Table 1.23 gives examples of presenting qualitative dietary modification information.

Dietitians use a variety of methods – oral, visual and written – to maximize the effectiveness of communication. Dietary education entails a lot more than 'giving a diet sheet' or 'chatting about healthy eating'.

Table 1.23 Presentation of information for dietary modification

QUALITATIVE METHODS	EXAMPLES
Commonly asked questions and answers	What is ? Answer -----
Rules or guidelines	Six steps to Healthy Eating
Checklists	√ box as you make the change in your diet
'Dos and Don'ts'	Weight control advice *Do* – try to reduce your sweet tooth; use artificial sweeteners to help if you need them *Don't* – add sugar to your drinks or breakfast cereals or cooking
Desirable food choices	Lipid lowering diet Highly desirable – eat daily; Suitable – eat occasionally; Best avoided Food groups, e.g. cereals e.g. dairy
Elimination diet with replacement foods	Milk free diet Exclude all sources of dairy produce, i.e. milk, yogurt, butter, cheese, cream, ice cream, etc. Replace milk with milk substitute, e.g. (named examples given) Replace spreading fat with, e.g. . . .
QUANTITATIVE METHODS	**EXAMPLES**
Menu plan	Calculated content for nutrients as required, e.g. high protein, high energy
High and low foods (with definitions)	Low potassium diet: High potassium foods } Based on agreed content per normal serving Low potassium foods }
Exchanges	Protein (2 g–6 g) Carbohydrate (10 g multiples) Phenylalanine (20 mg and 50 mg) Energy (calories e.g. 40, 70, 200); Fat (7 g)
Quizzes	Based on rating system, e.g. Healthy Eating categories Fat, sugar, salt, fibre
SUPPLEMENTARY INFORMATION	Manufactured foods Shopping advice – read the label Cooking methods Recipes
PRESENTATION CONSIDERATIONS	Professionally produced – printer or 'in house' computer Use of hand written information Format of leaflets, size, number of folds, pages, etc. Use of pictures or drawings or diagrams Readability of text Posters Displays Tapes – sound and video

Quantitative methods

There are often essential for constructing therapeutic diets, for example dietary treatment of phenylketonuria, chronic renal failure, or in the provision of nutrition support (oral, enteral or parenteral). It is the remit of the dietitian to ensure that the effect of a change of quantity in one or more nutrients or dietary components does not result in dietary imbalance.

Levels of nutrients in a diet

The absolute level of a nutrient in a therapeutic diet is ideally established by reference to the desired biochemical/

physiological/clinical effect. Thus, a low protein diet for a patient in renal failure contains a level of protein only as low as is necessary to keep blood urea at acceptable levels while maintaining nitrogen balance. Alternatively, a statistical definition can be made. Thus, an intake which is more than two standard deviations away from the average is likely to occur in less than 5% of a given population and can be classified as low if below and high if above the average intake. For example, Bingham (1979) defines low fibre diets as follows: 'The standard deviation of fibre intakes in a random British population aged 20–80 years was ± 5.2 g/day with a mean of 20 g/day. A low dietary fibre diet would therefore contain 10 g of dietary fibre or less on this basis'.

Where there is no biochemical or other yardstick then a 'low X' diet usually implies a level which is as low as is practicable and acceptable in terms of usual eating patterns. The generally accepted nutrient levels in low or high therapeutic diets will be found in the relevant clinical sections.

Constructing therapeutic diets

There are two basic methods of constructing quantified therapeutic diets:

1 Using an exchange system which delivers a fixed amount of nutrient per food portion.

2 Quantifying the portion size of foods and the frequency of their consumption.

Exchange systems The desired level of intake is specified and the diet is constructed from an exchange list, i.e. the size of the portion of each food containing a given amount of the nutrient is defined and the patient is allowed a specified number of these portions. For example, a 40 g protein diet may be constructed from 5×6 g protein exchanges and 5×2 g protein exchanges plus unlimited quantities of foods virtually free from protein. This method is used typically for controlled diets where there are biochemical parameters which are influenced by diets which have an immediate impact on symptoms, e.g. renal disease.

Regulation via portion control and food consumption frequency
The diet is constructed from normal sized portions of foods but those foods which have the highest content of a particular nutrients per portion are excluded from the diet. However, frequency of consumption must also be taken into account and it may be necessary to limit the number of portions of foods of moderate content of the given nutrient if they are eaten very frequently, e.g. bread, milk and butter. The amount of the given nutrient in the diet is thus allowed to achieve an unspecified, but lower than habitual, intake. This method is used typically when diet is a key component of a multi-factorial condition, e.g. coronary heart disease.

Table 1.23 gives examples of ways in which quantitative dietary modification information may be presented.

Reference

Bingham SA (1979) Low residue diets: a reappraisal of their meaning and content. *J Hum Nutr* **33**, 516.

1.9 Giving dietary advice

The following section attempts to identify the principal knowledge, skills and attitudes required to give dietary advice. It can only provide an overview and further reading and study should be undertaken to expand on all the areas noted. *Psychology* offers many insights into practices which are likely to result in successful communication and increased compliance. *Sociology* can provide insight into values which govern social action, and attitudes and beliefs relating to health and illness.

1.9.1 What is the dietitian trying to do?

As the 'giving of dietary advice' is one of our fundamental roles, it is essential that dietitians seek to establish measurable outcomes for this work. These outcomes need to show what dietitians can achieve and, if necessary, they can be examined and compared with the outcomes of others 'giving dietary advice' – for example, doctors and practice nurses. A common work situation for dietitians is to be with a patient or a group of people about whom they have only a small amount of background information. A dietitian's skill lies in making a quick and continuous assessment of the situation and in tailoring actions to meet the needs of that individual or group. This may involve:

- Establishing rapport and building a confidential, trusting, helping relationship;
- Addressing any immediate anxieties held by the patient and helping to give a clear understanding of what is happening;
- Assessing dietary, social and behavioural circumstances;
- Providing dietary education and setting realistic and achievable goals;
- Establishing a system for reinforcement, follow-up and support;
- Involving the person and their family/carers in support.

This work is carried out in the knowledge of the following.

- The dietitian and the patient or the group might have very different views of what needs to be done. This often results from poor levels of knowledge about food/nutrition, and about illness/health, and lack of agreement over the problem being addressed.
- Recall is often limited to the first issues raised and concentration span can be very short. A few clear messages, backed up with relevant written and visual material, may improve recall and enable behaviour change.
- Knowing what to do is a long way from actually doing it. A dietitian must discover what motivates a person to change behaviour and maintain the change; this will depend on that person's beliefs and values. Non-compliance has to be accepted by the dietitian as the outcome for some people. There are some factors which even the most experienced dietitian cannot influence.

Table 1.24 details the knowledge, skill and attitude components which are relevant to the principles of giving dietary advice.

1.9.2 How are dietitians trying to give dietary advice?

Dietitians need to consider four key areas when giving dietary advice:

1 Factors affecting an individual's food choice.
2 Communication of dietary advice.
3 Consideration of behaviour modification.
4 Motivation.

Factors affecting an individual's food choice

Factors affecting the food choice of an individual include:

- Cultural background;
- Religious or ethical beliefs;
- Taste preferences;
- Income;
- Lifestyle;
- Social conventions;
- Family/peer group pressures;
- Advertising;
- Knowledge/beliefs about food and diet.

Failure to take account of these and other factors will result in impractical dietary advice being offered.

Availability and cost of food

There have been many changes in food retailing over the last decade including the growth of supermarkets away from main shopping centres, the increasingly limited range of more expensive foods in small local shops, (even though the shop may be able to offer small packs for single households), and further limitations on door to door deliveries, such as milk. This can be contrasted with advances in food manufacturing, for example the rapid growth of

Table 1.24 Principles of giving dietary advice for therapeutic purposes or the promotion of healthy eating

This takes into account the different situations in which dietary advice might be given	
i.e. one-to-one / small or large group / written information	to patients/clients/carers / public / media setting
Knowledge	The dietitian should know the – Nutritional composition of common foods – Major and significant food sources of nutrients or other food components, e.g. lactose – Nutritional requirements (DRVs) of all client groups – Standards and procedures relating to dietary modifications.
Skills	The dietitian should be able to – Assess current diet and eating patterns to the required degree of accuracy, using accepted standards, i.e. quantitative or qualitative skills – Assess personal (social, financial) and medical factors which relate to ability to understand and adhere to dietary modification – Apply knowledge of principles of behaviour change and motivate 'clients' – Apply knowledge of education/learning in a variety of ways in a variety of settings – Communicate effectively with individuals, groups, both verbally and in writing – Monitor all activity and evaluate outcome for the dietitian and the 'client', i.e. dietary effectiveness and compliance
Attitudes	The dietitian should demonstrate – Confidence and competence to practise – Equity of approach, i.e. non-judgemental and understanding of cultural and social attitudes – Professional relationships with 'clients' – Commitment to enabling 'clients' to make informed choices

cook-chill ready meals and convenience food generally. There is a need for nutritionally sound, cheap, convenience foods which, currently, is not met.

Cultural influences

(See also Section 3.9, Black and Ethnic Minority Communities)

Among the strongest determinants of food choice are cultural factors. These include peer group pressures, social conventions, religious practices, the status value afforded to different foods, the influence of other members of the household and individual lifestyles.

Every dietitian is familiar with instances of, for example, the child who is ridiculed or feels ostracized for taking wholemeal bread to school or for not buying an ice cream on the way home; the business executive who 'has' to eat rich meals when entertaining clients; the Muslim child who cannot get suitable school meals; the demeaning associations of eating large amounts of bread and potatoes as an indication of poverty; the woman who always cooks chips for the whole household because that is all 'he' will eat and the teenagers who 'do not have time' to eat a sit down meal because they are 'far too busy'. These, and many other cultural factors, are compounded by economic considerations (see Section 3.8, Low Income Groups).

Psychological influences

For many people the strongest influence over their eating behaviour is psychological. Food, especially sweet food, is often used as an important form of reward or punishment for children. Some may be given sweets by parents as a means of dealing with their own feelings of guilt, caused, perhaps, by the conflict between the necessity for many mothers to go out to work and the condemnation from society in general for doing so. For many adults, compulsive eating is a way of finding comfort during depression, loneliness and boredom. Anorexia nervosa can be a way of coping with hate or anger towards a parent or fear of maturity. Whatever the cause, the problem is unlikely to be resolved by dietary advice — although in some cases it can be part of the solution.

Individual choices and preferences

Every individual has personal food preferences and tastes. These may change from time to time but will affect what is eaten at a given time. Taste preferences are based primarily on the flavour, colour, texture and smell of food but may also be based on association of a certain food with an unpleasant incident. On the whole, tastes are acquired early in life but are subject to many other influences. Dietitians need to take personal preferences into account whenever advice is being given. Moral and political convictions may also influence the foods people buy and eat. The most common examples of this are vegetarianism, veganism, or not eating products from countries with particular political regimes.

Knowledge and information

In order for people to have more control over what they eat, they must be informed. Information on its own, however, is not sufficient. People also need to know how to evaluate that information and to act upon it.

Information about food and nutrition comes from a wide variety of sources including friends, relatives, teachers, health professionals, advertisements, magazine and newspaper articles, promotions and food manufacturers. It is wide-ranging and can be inconsistent, confusing, often inaccurate and open to misinterpretation. Dietitians should be aware of the diversity of information that the general public receives and the impact that some of it, particularly television advertisements, can have.

Communication of dietary advice

The way information is given and received in one-to-one or group situations is the subject of many books and much research. Dietitians often refer to interviews, group work and counselling as the main activities, but these terms hide a spectrum of other activities such as listening skills, planning a learning experience, changing behaviour, evaluating outcome.

Dietitians act as counsellors in that they assist individuals to make decisions by offering new ways of dealing with or adjusting to food-related problems. Because of the social and psychological issues involved, dietitians often find themselves moving into non-nutritional areas, for example, stress-related problems, and lifestyle behaviours of smoking, drinking and exercise. It is important that dietitians are clear about their own attitudes and values. Most want 'to help' or 'do something useful' for people. It is important that the dietitian does not 'take over' in the sense of controlling the situation, nor give too much advice and place the patient or client in a dependent relationship. Dietitians can be affected by apparent failures if they have shown too much personal responsibility for a patient or client's situation.

Dietary counselling has to incorporate skills of questioning, active listening, and non-verbal communication.

Questioning

A friendly tone indicates a wish to understand and assist. Ideally, questions should enable the respondent to report their situation. These are called *open questions* and are often used at the opening of interviews as they are less threatening. For example, 'Can you tell me about your eating habits?'

Frequently, open questions will be more specific. For example, 'Can you tell me about any snacks you eat?' The respondent can control the interview by the answer.

Closed questions can also be helpful providing they do not limit the respondent's answer. For example, 'Who cooks the meals at home?' Some closed questions can have 'Yes' or 'No' answers. For example, 'Do you eat wholemeal bread?' The interviewer can remain more in control with these shorter answer closed questions but may appear as unfriendly and disinterested to the respondent.

Many questions result in follow-on questions. These can show the respondent that their answers are being carefully considered. If the respondent is reluctant then more *probing questions* may be needed. For example, 'Please tell me more about that'. Non verbal cues, for example, 'Oh!' or 'Uh huh' can encourage more information to be given.

The form of questioning which must be avoided is asking *leading questions*. For example, 'What do you eat for tea – meat and two vegetables?'. This can reveal judgements already made and create hostility and poor response. The interviewer must be able to sense when too many questions have been asked by watching for responses, both verbal and non-verbal. Sensitive areas should also be noted.

Active listening

These are skills which dietitians need to develop if they are to improve communication in any situation.

Paraphrase and summarize what has been said to show understanding or seek agreement of the situation. For example, 'So, you have breakfast cereal five days a week, but something cooked on Saturday and Sunday'. *Reflection* of what has been said by repeating in a supportive manner what the respondent has said. For example, 'Is this what you are saying . . .?' This can include identifying inconsistencies.

Non-verbal communication

Non-verbal communication can be more influential than verbal communication, to reinforce or contradict the verbal message. Key areas are facial expression, body language and gestures, eye contact, and tone of voice. These can be used by the interviewer, and dietitians must be aware of their own non-verbal communication. Non-verbal communication must also be observed in the respondent.

Facial expression can show inner feelings. For example, a smiling but not grinning face can welcome whereas a look of surprise at a response might inhibit. Glancing at a watch displays an obvious impatience for the interview to be ended.

Body language and gestures including distance between people, have a greater effect than is often appreciated. For example, a recoil at an offered hand shake or folded arms, sitting back in a chair.

Eye contact is essential to build rapport, especially in group settings. Until good eye contact is established, little useful communication can take place.

Tone of voice can often 'give away' a wide range of feelings, from emotion and stress to disinterest. Over-reaction in the interviewer can aggravate the situation.

Evaluation of communication

Dietitians should review the outcome of communication, whether interviews are one-to-one or group sessions. Trying to remember details is difficult so tape recorders or a peer can be used to facilitate this process. Group discussions on how each member communicates different messages can lead to improved communication.

Behaviour modification

Dietitians have been able to work with and learn from psychologists to provide strategies for helping their clients to modify or change their eating habits. Many of these can appear very simple and need to be reinforced and supported if new behaviours are to be learned. Dietitians have used strategies without fully acknowledging their psychological basis.

'Be positive'	Focusing on foods allowed rather than those disallowed.
'Goal setting'	Acknowledging that change takes time with short, medium and long term goals.
'Self-monitoring'	Keeping food diaries to identify the behaviour and factors which affect behaviour, i.e. what food was eaten, how much, when, where, with whom and with what feelings.
'Shopping lists'	Advising never to shop on an empty stomach. Always using a list and keeping to it.
'Reduce nibbling'	Throwing away leftovers immediately Re-arranging the kitchen food storage Writing notices in cupboards or on tins
'Reward systems'	Agreeing reward for achieved behaviour, not necessarily food (e.g. new clothes, bouquet of flowers) Praise from family, friends Financial reward/penalty.

It is important that communication allows identification of problem eating behaviours and that dietitians offer practical help to modify behaviours.

Motivation

Motivation is a complex subject and needs consideration for each individual. Some people can motivate themselves but most require to be challenged, some even 'threatened', to achieve results. Food behaviours are difficult to change because of the many factors affecting and controlling food choice. Dietitians know people do change their behaviour and maintain the change.

Knowledge

Knowledge is a key factor but is not sufficient on its own to motivate a person to change.

Interest/belief

Interest and belief in the role of diet in their health are essential to create change, including the extent to which individuals believe that:

- they are susceptible to disease/illness (e.g. coronary heart disease);
- the disease would affect their life and lifestyle (e.g. symptoms of overweight);
- the benefits from changes in behaviour outweigh the barriers to change (e.g. sugar consumption and teeth).

Perceptions

Perceptions about diets and dietitians must be considered and addressed. For example, that healthy diets are 'expensive', 'you need to be a good cook', 'you cannot eat the foods you like'.

Support

Support to continue changing behaviour from those involved with the patient/client is important to success. A good example is a sponsored slim with clear goals and regular support. Within families, support may require others to change their behaviours or expectations. The involvement of friends and carers in the dietary education process can be vital to some, but less important and possibly inhibiting to others.

It is important to address the complexity of changing habits, the denial of a problem by some patients/clients and the long term goal which improving diet may offer in contrast with the immediate enjoyment of current eating behaviours. Dietitians may need personal support from psychologists to address some of their feelings when trying to support patients, especially those with more complex problems.

1.9.3 Which teaching aids help a dietitian give dietary advice?

Table 1.23 (see Section 1.8, above) lists the different ways in which dietary information can be organized and presented, usually as printed information. There are many other aids which can support advice given on a one-to-one basis, in formal lectures or in groups.

Writing boards, flip charts, flannel boards, magnetic boards and overhead projectors can be used to illustrate and clarify points while the dietitian is speaking, in response to questions or for recording the main points of discussions. The writing and pictures must be clear and legible for the person furthest away and must complement the teaching.

Food models, actual foods and food packets make the best teaching aids. People can recognize them immediately and relate to them in a personal way. Posters, slides and photographs are also useful but have limitations. When using slides in particular it is easy to lose some contact with the audience because of the need for dimmed lights.

Tape slides, videos and films can be useful but care is needed to ensure that they do not replace the teaching but complement it. Videos are particularly useful because they can be stopped and repeated, picking up on specific points of interest to the group.

1.9.4 How do dietitians choose the most appropriate teaching methods?

Teaching should not be confused with learning. An individual or a group can be 'taught' for example, which foods to increase when increasing fibre in the diet, but unless the learner(s) take(s) an active part in learning then the information 'taught' will not be related to changing behaviour.

Decision on the teaching method will depend upon:

1 Subject, e.g. conceptual, factual, controversial;
2 Audience, e.g. individual or group or mass audience;
3 Style, e.g. formal or informal, passive or interactive;
4 Current knowledge and experiences of the individuals or group;
5 Resources available, including facilities, educational resources, finance and time.

Working with individuals

Much dietetic work, whether related to therapeutic diets or nutrition education, will take place on a one-to-one basis and the format of dietary information has already been discussed, as have methods of assessing dietary intake advice. Put these together with giving dietary advice, and the expertise of a dietitian can be seen.

As with motivation, dietitians have many strategies to enhance learning which they build into their teaching.

Clear objectives established and shared with the learner, using terms such as 'to recall', 'to use', 'to explain', which describe the outcome or results of the learning experience.

Awareness of readiness to learn by recognizing when the learner is unreceptive because of tiredness, anxiety, lack of knowledge or motivation; and acknowledging that most people have a concentration span of 5–10 minutes.

Providing a good learning environment. This can be as simple as allowing sufficient time, without interruptions, in a pleasant and, if necessary, confidential atmosphere. Equally important is using language understood by the learner and controlling the amount of information to be included.

Establishing a sequence to the learning experience. This includes establishing the learner's starting level of understanding (i.e. 'knowing the audience') and building on what exists, working through a 'checklist' of knowledge, skills to be learned over a period of time, moving on when learning has been demonstrated.

Encouraging success. This includes setting realistic goals, rewarding even verbally correct responses or behaviour, ignoring incorrect responses or behaviour.

Providing activities to ensure learning. Learning by doing can include bringing food items to the teaching session, participating in the learning by planning a menu, or describing how they would react in example situations.

Providing support and offering reinforcement over time through follow-up for patients, fixed time reviews, update sessions, etc.

Evaluation of progress so learner and teacher can adapt the teaching methods to maintain progress and address new, additional learning needs.

Group work

Individuals act in different ways depending on whether they are alone, with one or a few others, or in a larger group. 'Group dynamics' must be recognized and considered by dietitians intending to use groups for teaching. There are skills to learn in making groups effective, for example acting as facilitator. This may take place after a dietitian has given a presentation of information or set a problem to solve. Facilitating new or established groups involves:

1 Providing a suitable environment, for example by arrangement of chairs.
2 Encouraging 'ice breaking' activities, e.g. introductions, etc.
3 Helping the group establish its 'ground rules', e.g. responsibility to contribute, commitment to the agreed outcome.
4 Remaining as a guide to the group process and not participating.
5 Encouraging all members to contribute and controlling over-talkative participants.
6 Providing open questions to move the group forward.
7 Providing summaries of progress to keep the group to task.

No two groups are exactly alike for reasons over which the dietitian has no control, so it is essential to evaluate work done by groups and explore whether this is the most effective way of teaching in that situation.

The media

The largest groups and the widest audiences are reached by dietitians via the mass media. The same basic principles of communication apply. For most dietitians, the mass media will include access to local newspapers, local radio and television. Dietitians are also working at national levels, through the BDA Public Relations activity, or freelance work or consultancy. All forms of mass media are becoming increasingly interested in health issues.

Writing press releases

Press releases are one of the most useful ways for dietitians to communicate with the media. Press rooms receive dozens of press releases everyday and many of the articles in any newspaper are taken from them. There are a few basic principles which should be applied when writing press releases. All press releases must be typed, preferably with wide margins, and double spaced. They must give information about what is happening and why, who is doing it, and where and when it is happening. The first two sentences are the most important and should contain all the main points. The rest of the press release should concentrate on giving facts and information. Quotations from people involved in the event are also useful. All press releases must give the name and telephone number of a contact person who is available and able to give more details to interested journalists. They should also have a simple title, designed to help the news editor spot the interest of the story.

Writing articles for newspapers and magazines

Articles will need to reflect the style of the paper or magazine, in choice of language, use of cartoons, pictures, etc. It is important that dietitians are clear about their brief and establish their degree of control over what is finally published.

Responding to the press

If a dietitian is contacted unexpectedly by the press, great care should be taken over what is said via the telephone. Authors and people who comment on issues have very little control over what is finally published. On the whole, however, the media are sympathetic towards issues raised by or involving dietitians and do not deliberately try to denigrate the profession or misrepresent the issues.

Television and radio interviews

Media interviews may be live or recorded; either way it is essential to be well prepared. If invited to an interview, the dietitian will have some idea of the issues to be discussed. It is important to have a few main points to put across – the number will depend on the amount of time – and to keep to these as far as possible. The whole experience can be nerve-racking but this can be minimised by thorough preparation. It is worth remembering that when listening to the interview later, it always sounds better than it seemed at the time!

1.9.5 How do dietitians know when they have been successful?

It is essential that dietitians evaluate both the process of giving dietary advice, including the quality of all aspects of communication, and the outcome of dietary advice, i.e. the changes in the behaviour of our patients, clients or public.

The system within which dietary advice is being given may have ascribed service standards, for example inpatient service in a hospital, outpatient clinic routine, group sessions for dietary education. These would determine the educational time and support resources available. This should enable the dietitian to deliver a good service to most patients or groups.

The dietary advice being offered is also likely to have standards ascribed covering philosophy of treatment, priority of messages, education material available, education process over time, and measurable outcome.

Table 1.25 clearly states the steps which are critical for the success of permanent dietary change. These criteria can be used to evaluate what the patient has been able to achieve and to assess compliance.

It is important that the outcomes of dietary education are included within the auditing of care of conditions with an important dietary component – such as diabetes, treatment of raised lipids and nutrition support. This will enable multidisciplinary audit to show the role and benefit of nutrition and dietetic intervention.

Dietitians need to carry out more research into the effectiveness of different methods of giving dietary advice to support their practice.

Table 1.25 Steps in patient behaviour that are critical for the success of permanent dietary management

1. The person acknowledges that he has a problem, e.g. diabetes
2. The person accepts that diet is a sole or adjunctive method of helping to solve this problem, e.g. control the diabetes
3. The person participates in assessing his current dietary pattern, social environment, thoughts, beliefs and feelings
4. The person acknowledges that successful dietary change will require an extended period of time
5. The person participates in developing an overall strategy and in setting long term goals regarding e.g. diabetes and diet
6. The person participates in planning each step of dietary change
7. The person makes each dietary change
8. The person participates in assessing whether he has succeeded in making each change
9. The person participates in assessing his attainment of e.g. diabetic control
10. The person participates in devising a plan for maintaining dietary changes as goals are approached

(after Tillotson *et al* 1984)

Further reading

Davidson C, Kowalska AZ, Nutman PNS and Pearson GC (1987) Dietitian-patient communication: a critical appraisal and approach to training. *Hum Nutr: Appl Nutr* **41A**, 381–9.

Fehily AM, Vaughan-Williams E, Shiels K, Williams AHK, Horner M *et al* (1991) Factors influencing compliance with dietary advice: the Diet and Reinfarction Trial (DART) *J Hum Nutr Dietet* **4**, 33–42.

Fieldhouse P (1979) An interview model for use in dietetic training. *J Hum Nutr* **33**, 206–210.

Gowers E (1984) *The complete plain words*. Penguin Books, London.

Halli B and Calabrese RJ (1986) *Communication and education skills, the dietitian's guide*. Lea and Febiger, Philadelphia.

Ley P (1988) *Communicating with patients*. Chapman and Hall, London.

References

Inner London Education Authority (1985) *Nutrition guidelines*. Heinemann Education, London.

Tillotson JL, Winston MC and Hall Y (1984) Critical behaviours in the management of hypertension. *J Am Dietet Assoc* **84**, 290.

1.10 Measurements of body composition

Measurements of body composition can provide useful information in addition to that obtained from weight and height alone. They may be used cross-sectionally, with reference to appropriate standards, to assess body composition in relation to a statistical normality, or longitudinally to measure changes in response to a change in diet, exercise patterns, or disease.

The only direct method of measuring body composition is chemical analysis of cadavers. A variety of *in-vivo* techniques exist for measuring one or more compartments of the body – fat, water, lean tissue or bone – but all are indirect. The accuracy of each method depends on the validity of the underlying assumptions. Whilst these assumptions are broadly true for healthy adults, they may not be true in clinical situations where gross aberrations of body composition, particularly water, may exist.

The choice of method for a given situation is determined by many factors including cost, access to facilities, subject co-operation and the numbers of subjects to be studied. In general the most practical method will rarely be the most accurate. It is therefore extremely important to consider the sensitivity of the method employed before drawing conclusions.

Commonly it is assumed that the body is composed of two compartments. These may be *either* fat and fat-free mass (FFM) *or* adipose tissue and lean body mass (LBM). The two systems should not be used interchangeably. Fat refers to chemically defined fat and FFM is the remainder of the body. Adipose tissue is that tissue which can be separated from the body by dissection. It contains small amounts of water, protein, potassium etc. in addition to fat. LBM is the remainder of the body after the removal of adipose tissue.

Reviews of techniques for measuring body composition may be found in Lukaski (1987) and Coward *et al* (1988).

1.10.1 Bedside methods

These are methods suited for use outside the laboratory, either in the community or at the bedside. All are relatively cheap, simple to perform and non-invasive. However as they all depend on regression equations derived from studies in which this technique has been compared with an accepted 'reference' method (usually densitometry), accuracy is compromised for convenience.

Weight and height

Weight may be simply, and with due care, accurately measured. Fewest errors are generally incurred using well calibrated digital scales. Height is best measured using a precisely positioned wall mounted stadiometer.

Various indices of obesity have been devised based on weight and height measurements. The most commonly used is the Quetelet Index or Body Mass Index (BMI), which is calculated as:

$$\frac{\text{Weight (kg)}}{\text{Height}^2\text{(m)}}$$

This assumes that all excess weight is excess fat. This is broadly true for the average population but invalid at extremes of body composition. For example, in highly trained athletes the apparent excess weight is likely to be lean tissue. Errors will also be incurred as a result of alterations in hydration or reductions in stature due to kyphosis.

A BMI of 18–25 is considered to be the desirable range for both men and women (Table 1.26). A BMI between 25 and 30 represents Grade I obesity, 30–40 Grade II, and upwards of 40, Grade III (Garrow 1981). BMI can also be expressed as percent body fat using a variety of simple prediction equations. For example:

Males: % fat = (1.281 BMI) – 10.13
Females: % fat = (1.480 BMI) – 7.0

Table 1.26 gives the range of weight/height^2 expressed in the Metropolitan Life Insurance Tables (1983).

Table 1.26 The range of the weight-height index (W/H^2) calculated from the 'desirable' weights for heights given by the Metropolitan Life Insurance Tables, 1983

		Small frame	Medium frame	Large frame
Men	1.58 m	23.2–24.3	22.7–25.6	25.0–27.4
	1.93 m	19.6–21.4	20.7–22.7	22.0–25.2
Women	1.48 m	21.3–23.2	22.8–25.4	24.7–27.6
	1.83 m	18.8–20.6	20.2–22.1	21.6–24.5

Weights are expressed as kg with an adjustment of 2.3 kg for men and 1.4 kg for women to obtain weight without clothes. Heights are expressed in metres; 2.5 cm were subtracted to obtain height without heels

Skinfold thicknesses

Principle

The method is derived from measurements of body density (see Section 1.9.2, Densitometry). Equations have been derived in which skinfold thicknesses measured at predetermined sites can be used to predict total body fat as determined by densitometry. This assumes, firstly, that subcutaneous fat is a constant proportion of total body fat and, secondly, that the chosen measurement sites also have a constant relationship to total body fat. One of the best known set of equations are those of Durnin and Womersley (1974). A useful review of the value of assessing body fat from skinfolds is provided by Schemmel (1980).

Differences in fat distribution either between individuals or in one individual studied at two points in time will lead to errors. Most equations are age and sex specific. The relationship of skinfolds with age is due to the increase in the proportion of body fat which is deposited internally rather than subcutaneously. Changes in the fat-free mass, particularly concerning the skeleton will exert both an age and sex specific effect, for example, the marked decrease in bone mineral in women after the menopause.

Practicalities

Skinfold thickness is measured by pinching a fold of skin plus subcutaneous fat between a pair of Harpenden skinfold calipers (Table 1.27). The ends of the calipers are of standard area and are applied at a standard pressure. Since subcutaneous fat is compressible when the full pressure of the caliper is applied, the observed reading will initially fall rapidly followed by a slow drift downwards. This is a particular problem in the obese where a further problem is that the jaws of the calipers may not be wide enough to encompass the fat fold.

The correct anatomical site is difficult to establish and in some cases the site may be inaccessible due to burns, bandages etc. Measurements made by different observers may vary substantially, but experienced observers can produce results reproducible to within 0.2 kg fat. Wherever possible all measurements should be made by a single observer. However, where this is impractical and more than one observer is involved, it is essential that they frequently make measurements on the same subject to standardize their technique and check the agreement of the results. Between and within observer variation has been studied by Womersley and Durnin (1973) and Branson *et al* (1982).

Table 1.27 Standard sites and techniques for skinfold thickness measurements

Triceps skinfold	With arm bent at right-angles, the length from the tip of the acromion process on the scapula to the olecranon process of the ulna is measured and the mid-point marked. With the arm hanging loosely by the side, the skinfold at the mid-point level on the back of the arm over the triceps muscle is picked up between the thumb and forefinger of the left hand. The calipers are placed on the skinfold just below the fingers, the fingers removed, and a reading taken
Biceps	As for the triceps, but over the biceps muscle on the front of the arm
Subscapular	About 1 inch in and below the angle of the scapula towards the midline and at an angle of approximately 45 to the spine along the natural line of skin cleavage
Supra-iliac	Midway between the anterior superior iliac spine crest and the lowest point of the ribs, horizontal to the floor, or just above the iliac crest in the mid-axillary line
	A fuller account of the technique can be found in Tanner and Whitehouse (1962), Weiner and Lourie (1969) and Owen (1982)

Skinfold standards

Standard tables exist for the interpretation of skinfold data for both children and adults and the technique could be applied for example in the assessment of the prevalence of obesity in a population. However its value in assessing changes in an individual is limited by the insensitivity of the technique. Realistically body fat will have to change by several kilograms in order to accurately identify this change on the basis of skinfold thickness measurements. Tables of skinfold standards are given in Appendix 3, Tables 7.35–7.38.

Impedance/resistance

Principle

Whole-body impedance or resistance is a relatively new technique for the measurement of body composition. Four self-adhesive surface electrodes are placed on the non-dominant side of the body midway between the radial and ulnar processes, between the medial and lateral maleoli, the metacarpophalangeal joint of the index finger and the metatarsophalangeal joint of the big toe. A small current is then passed across the electrodes (typically 800 μAmps, 50 kHz) and the voltage drop across the body measured. Resistance can then be calculated from Ohm's Law:

$$\text{Resistance} = \frac{\text{Voltage}}{\text{Current}}$$

Impedance is the sum of resistance plus reactance. In the body the reactive component is sufficiently small to be ignored and resistance can be used as an approximation for impedance.

Fat is a poor conductor of the applied current whereas lean tissue with its water and electrolyte content is highly conductive. The method therefore measures total body water (TBW). Fat-free mass (FFM) is estimated from TBW by assuming that it is 73% water. Body fat is determined by subtracting the estimate of FFM from total body weight. The error on this measurement therefore includes errors on the measurement of body weight, the assumed hydration of fat-free mass and the measurement of impedance.

For subjects with abnormalities of water balance, care should be taken when extrapolating from measurements of total body water to fat-free mass or fat as the hydration fraction is likely to be much more variable than in the healthy population.

The contribution of different segments of the body to whole-body impedance varies due to differences in body geometry and particularly cross-sectional area. For example, an arm represents only 4% of body weight yet contributes 46% to the total body impedance, whereas the trunk which is 46% of body weight contributes 10% to total body impedance. This is important as the contribution of a given change in impedance to the whole-body measurement will depend on the body segment in which this change occurs (Fuller and Elia 1989). Similarly changes in the relationship of intracellular to extracellular water, or in the concentration of electrolytes, will also cause deviations in the relationship between the measured impedance and total body water (see Jebb and Elia 1991).

Practicalities

The necessary equipment is basically cheap, but the cost of commercial systems has been elevated by the inclusion of a large collection of computer software to calculate body composition. It is important not to be distracted by the technology when considering the value of this method, since the calculations are straightforward and can easily be performed with a calculator, if not a pen and paper! The technique is associated with considerably less inter-observer error than are skinfold thicknesses. Table 1.28 shows the observer variation for several different body composition techniques when conducted under rigorous research conditions with attention to the standardisation of the methods. The variation is likely to be greater in everyday clinical practice. The positioning of the electrodes is important, but the sites are well defined anatomical landmarks which are easily located. In large scale surveys with multiple observers impedance may be a sensible choice. Impedance measurements are probably more acceptable to subjects than skinfold thicknesses and most subjects are impressed by the technology!

Table 1.28 Residual coefficient of variation (cv) for body fat mass (kg) measured by six observers (Fuller *et al* 1991)

Method	cv (%)
Height and weight	1.1
Skinfolds (mm)	4.6
Impedance (ohms)	2.6
NIRI	4.2

Infra-red interactance (NIRI)

Principle

The body is irradiated with a beam of near infra-red radiation. The pattern of the reflected radiation is influenced by the absorption characteristics of the underlying tissue. Currently only one commercial instrument is available (Futrex 5000) which employs two wavelengths of light at 940 and 950 nm. Prediction equations interpret the optical density measurements to produce an estimate of body fat.

Practicalities

Measurements are made at a single site at the midpoint of the upper arm over the biceps muscle. This assumes that the tissue composition at this site reflects that of the whole body. The prediction equations also employ weight, height, sex and a subjective assessment of activity in order to calculate body composition. In comparison with densitometry it appears to be less accurate than other bedside measurements and there is more associated observer error than with the impedance technique (Table 1.28).

1.10.2 Research methods

The following methods are all more accurate than the bedside methods and make fewer assumptions, but all have practical limitations in terms of the capital cost and the availability of equipment and technical expertise.

Densitometry

Principle

This method was first described by Behnke *et al* in 1942 and today it remains one of the most widely used techniques for the measurement of body composition. It is generally regarded as the reference method against which other methods are evaluated.

The method assumes that the body is composed of two compartments – Body fat and fat-free mass which have a densities of 0.9 kg/l and 1.1 kg/l respectively. Thus, if the density of the body is known, the proportion which is fat can be calculated from Siri's equation (1956):

$$\%\text{Fat} = \left\{\frac{(4.95) - 4.50}{\text{d}}\right\} \times 100$$

where d = body density.

Body fat has a relatively constant density, but fat-free mass is a very heterogeneous compartment comprising protein, water, bone and glycogen which, if it is to have a constant density, must exist in a fixed proportion. This is not always the case. For example water balance is known to fluctuate at different times of day and to change rapidly in situations such as exercise or following excessive alcohol intake; bone density varies between sexes, races and with age. Such deviations lead to errors in the estimate of body composition.

Practicalities

The density of a body is equivalent to the mass in air divided by its volume. The mass of the subject in air can be conventionally measured by weighing, whilst volume is measured as the difference between the weight of the subject in air and the weight under water. Lung volume is measured at the time of the measurement using standard techniques (e.g. helium dilution, oxygen dilution or nitrogen washout) and subtracted from the body volume measurement. Gut volume is not measured directly but radiological studies suggest that for a fasted subject it is approximately 100 ml, which must also be deducted.

Densitometry facilities are only available in a limited number of centres. Many subjects are unable to co-operate with the rigorous procedure and it is unsuitable for the very young, old or infirm. However the method is well accepted by more subjects than might be expected, and after careful instruction the procedure takes less than ten minutes.

Total body water

Principle

The measurement of total body water is based on a dilution principle. The subject drinks a dose of labelled water and, after a delay for it to equilibrate with body water, a sample of body fluid (blood, urine or saliva) is taken to measure the dilution of the administered dose. The dilution principle may be simplified to:

Amount of dose given = Concentration per ml in body fluid × Total body weight

Today, the tracers of choice are ^2H_2O or $H_2^{18}O$ which are stable and non-radioactive. The former is more commonly used on account of cost.

This method again divides the body into two compartments, fat and fat-free mass. It is assumed that the fat compartment is anhydrous and that fat-free mass is hydrated to a known and constant extent, usually 73% for a healthy subject. Thus if total body water can be measured, lean tissue mass can be calculated and fat mass obtained by difference from body weight.

Unfortunately the reference figure of 73% is merely an estimate based on the results of limited cadaver analyses and animal desiccations. The degree of hydration of lean tissue is extremely variable, both within and between individuals. Adipose tissue is known to contain a small amount of water and as the degree of adiposity increases the water content also rises. In the clinical environment where many patients may have abnormalities of water balance, manifest as oedema or dehydration, the hydration fraction is even more difficult to assess and is likely to cover a broader range than that seen in the healthy population.

Practicalities

Subjects are required only to drink a dose of labelled water and collect a urine or saliva sample so in theory this method can be performed on all subjects in all locations. The analysis of the samples however requires access to sophisticated facilities (e.g. mass spectrometer) and considerable expertise.

Total body potassium

Principle

The natural gamma emitting isotope of potassium ^{40}K can be measured *in-vivo* using a whole-body counter. Assuming that ^{40}K represents a fixed proportion of total body potassium, it can be used to give an estimate of total body potassium. The method then assumes that potassium exists only in fat-free tissues at a known and constant concentration, hence it is possible to use the measured ^{40}K to estimate fat-free mass (Forbes *et al* 1961).

However potassium is not evenly distributed, more is found in muscle than other lean tissues. Its concentration varies with age, both during growth and development and after maturity and also with adiposity.

Practicalities

Few centres have access to whole-body counters to measure ^{40}K. The measurement takes time to perform (approximately 90 minutes at Addenbrooke's Hospital, Cambridge) during which the subject is enclosed in a well shielded counter connected only by an intercom to the observer. It is therefore unsuitable for patients in need of acute medical care.

Dual energy X-ray absorptiometry (DEXA)

Principle

This method uses a rectilinear scanner with an X-ray source which emits low dose X-rays at two different energies. A detector system measures the X-rays transmitted through the body. Using two different wavelengths two simultaneous equations can be derived to calculate two compartments – bone and soft tissue. The same principles can then be extended to resolve the soft tissue into fat and fat-free mass (Mazess *et al* 1984).

The technique is reproducible with repeated estimates of fat and fat free mass (as a % of body weight) within 1% of each other. Additionally this technique is able to divide the body into segments (e.g. trunk, right and left legs etc.), which gives an indication of regional body composition.

Data from this technique is at present limited but encouraging and shows good agreement with densitometry and deuterium dilution techniques, although the results may be less accurate at the extremes of body composition (e.g. anorexia nervosa or gross obesity) than for normal weight individuals. Currently results from different machines may vary due to differences in both hardware and software.

Practicalities

The procedure is straightforward and non-invasive. Subjects lie still on a bed as the scanning arm passes over them which takes approximately 20 minutes. Modern machines give a minute radiation dose (approx 0.02–0.05 mRem, versus 40 mRem for a chest X-ray) so it is suitable for use in most groups of subject, including children. Subjects are not separated from the investigator, and it is possible to perform repeated scans to measure changes in body composition. The equipment is expensive but may be available in some hospitals.

Multi-compartment models

A sophisticated analysis of body composition can be obtained by combining measurements of bone mineral (from DEXA), total body water (from dilution techniques) and body volume (from density) in a model which comprises four compartments – bone mineral, water, fat and the remaining fat-free mass. Details of this approach have been described by Fuller *et al* (1992).

Imaging techniques

Imaging techniques may also be considered to be multicompartmental models. *X-rays* can be used to look at regional fat distribution and so forth, but the radiation dose and poor image quality have restricted its use for whole-body analysis. *Computed tomography (CT)* offers improved resolution, although also with a significant radiation hazard. Radiation risks become particularly significant for longitudinal studies and are clearly inappropriate for vulnerable subsets of the population. However CT scans can provide useful compositional data on subjects undergoing repeated scans for other clinical purposes. If specific sites are chosen, regional changes can be studied or even extrapolated to whole-body measurements. So far CT scanning has mostly been used for the measurement of intra-abdominal and subcutaneous fat. *Magnetic resonance imaging (MRI)* is based on the principle that certain nuclei with intrinsic magnetic properties align themselves along the direction of a magnetic field when a radio frequency wave is passed through the body. As the radio wave is turned off the nuclei revert back to their original position, emitting the energy that they had absorbed earlier. This emission can be detected and, from its frequency and intensity, images of tissues can be constructed. There is no associated radiation therefore allowing repeated measurements on any group of subjects.

Imaging techniques are able to assess the size of individual organs or tissues as well as providing information about adipose tissue or muscle and its distribution. Whole-body scans can be used to assess the mass of adipose tissue or muscle. Such techniques offer a uniquely direct approach to the estimation of particular body compartments. The disadvantages are that they are expensive, time-consuming and, in the case of CT scanning, involve a not inconsiderable radiation dose to the subject. These techniques are unlikely to be used routinely but they may act as useful reference methods in some circumstances.

References

Behnke AR, Feen BG and Welham WC (1942) The specific gravity of healthy men: body weight/volume as an index of obesity. *JAMA* **118**, 495–8.

Branson RS, Vaucher YE, Harrison GG, Vargas M and Thies C (1982) Inter and intra-observer reliability of skinfold thickness measurements in newborn infants. *Hum Biol* **54**, 137–43.

Coward WA, Parkinson SA and Murgatroyd PR (1988) Body composition measurements for nutrition research. *Nutr Res Rev* **1**, 115–24.

Durnin JVGA and Womersley J (1974) Body fat assessed from total body density and its estimation from skinfold thickness: measurements on 481 men and women aged from 16 to 72 years. *Br J Nutr* **32**, 77–97.

Forbes GB, Gallup J and Hursh JB (1961) Estimation of total body fat from potassium-40 counting. *Science* **133**, 101–102.

Fuller NJ and Elia M (1989) Potential use of bioelectrical impedance of the 'whole-body' and of body segments for the assessment of body composition: comparison with densitometry and anthropometry. *Eur J Clin Nutr* **43**, 779–91.

Fuller NJ, Jebb SA, Goldberg GR, Pullicino E, Adams C and Cole TJ (1991) Inter-observer variability in the measurement of body composition. *Eur J Clin Nutr* **45**, 43–9.

Fuller NJ, Jebb SA, Laskey A, Coward WA and Elia M (1992) Four-component model for the assessment of body composition in humans; comparison with alternative methods, and evaluation of the density and hydration of fat-free mass. *Clin Sci* **82**, 687–93.

Garrow JS (1981) *Treat obesity seriously: a clinical manual.* pp. 27–9. Churchill Livingstone, Edinburgh.

Jebb SA and Elia M (1991) Assessment of changes in total body water in patients undergoing renal dialysis using bioelectrical impedance analysis. *Clin Nut* **10**, 81–4.

Lukaski HC (1987) Methods for the assessment of human body composition: traditional and new. *Am J Clin Nutr* **46**, 537–56.

Mazess RB, Peppler WW and Gibbons M (1984) Total body composition by dual photon (^{153}Gd) absorptiometry. *Am J Clin Nutr* **40**, 834–9.

Metropolitan Life (1983) *Metropolitan Life Insurance Company Statistical Bulletin* **64**, 1–9.

Owen GM (1982) Measurement, recording and assessment of skinfold thickness in childhood and adolescence: report of a small meeting. *Am J Clin Nutr* **35**, 629–38.

Schemmel R (1980) The assessment of obesity. In *Nutrition, physiology and obesity*. Schemmel R (Ed) pp. 1–23. CRC Press, Boca Raton, Florida.

Tanner JM and Whitehouse RH (1962) Standards for subcutaneous fat in British children. Percentiles for thickness of skinfolds over triceps and below scapula. *Br Med J* **1**, 446–50.

Weiner JS and Lourie JA (1969) *Human biology: A guide to field methods*. IBP Handbook No 9. Blackwell Scientific Publications, Oxford.

Womersley J and Durnin JVGA (1973) An experimental study on variability of measurements of skinfold thickness in young adults. *Hum Biol* **45**, 281–92.

1.11 The assessment of nutritional status in clinical situations

1.11.1 General considerations

Assessment of nutritional status is usually undertaken for three reasons:

1 To confirm a diagnosis of undernutrition.

2 To identify the reasons for the presence of undernutrition.

3 To provide a way of monitoring the effectiveness of nutritional support.

Many changes take place in the body in the presence of undernutrition and a multitude of tests have been described which attempt to quantify them. Since nutritional assessment may be undertaken in a variety of settings, it is important to select indicators which are relatively simple to use and which do not need sophisticated resources. This may sometimes mean sacrificing precision for practicality although any test should always be reliable, reproducible and relevant – both to the clinician and to the patient. The following points are important.

- No single nutritional index should be considered in isolation – there are many reasons for abnormal results apart from undernutrition.
- When an element of subjectivity is involved (e.g. anthropometric measurements), and repeated measurements are to be done on a longitudinal basis, tests should always be performed by the same observer.
- Biochemical 'nutritional markers' may often reflect dietary intake rather than long term nutritional status. Fasting samples can sometimes give more reliable results (e.g. glucose, proteins, potassium, vitamins).
- By contrast, certain homeostatic mechanisms can mean that body stores may be nutrient-depleted before circulating levels show any measurable decrease (e.g. zinc, calcium).
- Great care is needed when assessing children – particularly neonates – and specific parameters must be applied. The risk of nutritional deficiencies occurring is increased during times of accelerated growth.

1.11.2 Assessing the nature and extent of nutritional depletion

Nutritional depletion can be caused by an inadequate nutritional intake or a failure to digest, absorb and/or utilize nutrients. Any of these can result from disease.

Clinical examination

The usefulness of good clinical observation and assessment must not be underestimated. An experienced practitioner should be able to identify patients as normal, moderately or severely malnourished (Baker *et al* 1982). Some clinical signs associated with undernutrition are summarized in Table 1.29.

Body weight and weight loss

A simple yet frequently under used index of body mass is body weight. Patients should be weighed in hospital or light clothing on *accurate* weighing scales. Actual body weight may then be compared with either the patient's usual body weight or ideal body weight (Metropolitan Life 1983).

Percentage weight loss is a useful indicator of nutritional status (Table 1.30) and may be calculated using the formula:

$$\% \text{ Weight loss} = \frac{\text{(Usual weight} - \text{Actual (or ideal) weight)}}{\text{Usual weight}} \times 100$$

It is also helpful to relate this to time and a weight loss of 10% or more during the preceding three months should be considered a cause for concern.

When measuring body weight one should consider the possible presence of the following.

- **Obesity** – this may mask significant reductions in lean body mass. One way to detect obesity is to estimate Body Mass Index (BMI) (Garrow 1981). However, this measurement may be misleading in the 'very lean' or oedematous individual (Table 1.31).
- **Oedema** – this will also distort weight and may be caused by disease, drug therapy or by nutritional support (particularly if parenteral regimens are prescribed). It is important to remember that short term weight changes more usually reflect alterations in fluid balance.

The patient's weight should be recorded on admission and most patients should then be weighed regularly thereafter (usually once or twice a week unless otherwise prescribed). The results can be compared with ideal weight for height tables (Metropolitan Life 1983). However, these tables have been criticised as they are, in themselves, self-

Table 1.29 Physical signs associated with nutritional depletion. Christakis (1979). Reproduced with permission

Organ system	Physical signs	Nutrient deficiency
Hair	Becomes fine, dull, dry, brittle, stiff, straight; becomes red in Blacks, then lighter in colour; may be 'bleached' in Whites ('flag sign'); is easily and painlessly pluckable; outer one third of eyebrow may be sparse in hypothyroidism (cretinism, iodine deficiency or other causes)	Protein-energy
Nails	Ridging, brittle, easily broken, flattened, spoon shaped, thin, lustreless	Iron
Face	Brown, patchy, pigmentation of cheeks Parotid enlargement 'Moon face'	Protein-energy
Eyes	Photophobia; poor twilight vision; loss of shiny, bright, moist appearance of eyes; xerosis of bulbar conjunctivae; loss of light reflex; decreased lacrimation; keratomalacia (corneal softening), corneal ulceration which may lead to extrusion of lens; Bitot's spot (frothy white or yellow spots under bulbar conjunctivae)	Vitamin A
	Palpebral conjunctivae are pale	Iron or Folate
	Circumcorneal capillary injection with penetration of corneal limbus	Riboflavin
	Tissue at external angles of both eyes which is red and moist. Angular blepharitis (or palpebritis)	Riboflavin Pyridoxine
	Optic neuritis	B12
Nose	Nasolabial dyssebacea (exfoliation, inflammation, excessive oil production and fissuring of sebaceous glands, which are moist and red). May be found at angles of eyes, ears or other sites	Riboflavin
	Nasolabial seborrhoea	Pyridoxine
Lips	Cheilosis, inflammation of the mucous membranes of the lips and the loss of the clear differentiation between the mucocutaneous border of the lips	Riboflavin
Gums	Interdental gingival hypertrophy	Vitamin C
	Gingivitis	Vitamin A, Niacin Riboflavin
Mouth	Angular stomatitis; cheilosis; angular scars	Riboflavin
	Apthous stomatitis	Folic acid
Tongue	Atrophic lingual papillae, sore, erythematous	Iron
	Glossitis, painful, sore	Folic acid
	Magenta in colour, atrophic lingual papillae; filiform and fungiform papillae hypertrophy	Riboflavin
	Scarlet; raw; atrophic lingual papillae; fissures	Niacin
	Glossitis	Pyridoxine
Teeth	Caries	Fluoride
	Mottled enamel, fluorosis	Fluoride (excessive)
	Caries	Phosphorus
	Malposition; hypoplastic line across upper primary incisors becomes filled with yellow-brown pigment; caries then occurs and tooth may break off	Protein-energy
Neck	Neck mass (goitre)	Iodine
Skin	Xerosis (dryness of skin)	Vitamin A
	Follicular hyperkeratosis ('goose-flesh,' 'sharkskin,' 'sand-paper skin') keratotic plugs arising from hypertrophied hair follicles. Acneiform lesions	
	Perifollicular petechiae which produce a 'pink halo' effect around coiled hair follicles intradermal petechiae, purpura, ecchymoses due to capillary fragility. Haemarthroses; cortical haemorrhages of bone visualizable on X-ray	Vitamin C
	Intracutaneous haemorrhages; gastrointestinal haemorrhage	Vitamin K
	Pallor	Iron, folic acid
	Pallor; icterus	B12

Table 1.29 *contd.*

Organ system	Physical signs	Nutrient deficiency
	Erythema early, vascularization, crusting, desquamation. Increased pigmentation (even in Blacks), thickened, inelastic, fissured, especially in skin exposed to sun; becoming scaly, dry, atrophic in intertrigenous areas, maceration and abrasion may occur. 'Necklace of Casals' in neckline exposed to sun; Malar and supraorbital pigmentation	Niacin
	Oedema (pitting), 'Flaky paint': dermatosis, Hyperkeratosis or 'Crazy pavement' dermatosis	Protein-energy
	Hyperpigmentation	
	Scrotum dermatitis erythema, hyperpigmentation	Niacin
Vulva	Vulvovaginitis and chronic mucocutaneous candidiasis	Iron
Skeletal	Osteoporosis (in association with low protein intake and fluoride deficiency)	Calcium
	Epiphyseal enlargement, painless.	Vitamin D
	Beading of ribs ('Rachitic Rosary').	
	Delayed fusion of fontanelies, craniotabes. Bowed legs, frontal or parietal bossing of skull. Deformities of thorax (Harrison's Sulcus, pigeon breast).	
	Osteomalacia (adults)	
	Subperiosteal haematoma. Epiphyseal enlargement, painful	Vitamin C
Muscular	Hypotonia	Vitamin D
	Muscle wasting; weakness, fatigue, inactivity; loss of subcutaneous fat	Protein-energy
	Intramuscular haematoma	Vitamin C
	Calf muscle tenderness; weakness	Thiamin
Central Nervous System	Apathy (kwashiorkor); irritability (marasumus); Psychomotor changes.	Protein
	Hyporeflexia; foot and wrist drop. Hypesthesia, parasthesia	Thiamin
	Psychotic behaviour (dementia)	Niacin
	Peripheral neuropathy, symmetrical sensory and motor deficits, especially in lower extremities. Drug resistant convulsions (infants). Dementia, forgetfulness	Pyridoxine
	Areflexia. Extensor plantar responses. Loss of position and vibratory sense. Ataxia, paresthesias	B_{12}
	Tremor, convulsions, behavioural disturbances	Magnesium
Liver	Hepatomegaly (fatty infiltration)	Protein-energy
Gastrointestinal	Anorexia, flatulence, diarrhoea	B_{12}
	Diarrhoea	Niacin, Protein-energy
Cardiovascular	Tachycardia, congestive heart failure (high output type), cardiac enlargement, electrocardiographic changes	Thiamin

Reproduced with permission from Christakis (1979)

selective. It is often more practical to use the patient's admission weight as a baseline measurement.

Finally, it is important to remember that total body weight does not differentiate between tissues and it may be necessary to perform other measurements to assess body composition in more detail.

Dietary history

The dietary or nutritional history is one of the most important tools in the assessment of nutritional status. Many factors must be considered when recording a dietary intake (Section 1.7) and it is often the dietitian who is able to confirm a diagnosis of undernutrition. In some cases, a dietary history may reveal previously unsuspected nutritional depletion. A history should, therefore, provide information about energy and nitrogen intake as well as giving details of nutrients such as electrolytes (e.g. potassium), minerals (e.g. iron, calcium) trace metals and vitamins. It is also important to remember the interrelationships of these nutrients. Suspicion of any nutritional deficiency should be highlighted together with appropriate advice on the restoration of an adequate nutritional intake (with recommendations for pharmaceutical supplementation, if this is considered necessary). Moreover, the dietary history is also a useful tool in identifying individual patients who may be nutritionally 'at risk'. These could include patients undergoing gastrointestinal surgery, radio-

Table 1.30 Indicators of nutritional depletion (Jelliffe 1966; Bishop *et al* 1981)

Parameter	Normal range	Depletion		
		Mild	Moderate	Severe
Body weight	100% (i.e. usual weight for height)	95–100%	90–95%	<90%
Mid arm muscle circumference[†]	100% Male = +25.3 cm *or* ++28.7 cm[†] Female = +23.2 cm *or* ++22.0 cm	80–90%	60–80%	<60%
Triceps skinfold thickness[†]	100% Male = +12.5 mm *or* ++12.0 mm[†] Female = +16.5 mm *or* ++23.0 mm	80–90%	60–80%	<60%
Grip strength	100% Male = 40 kg* Female = 27.5 kg*	85%	75–85%	<75%
Creatinine: height index	100%	80–95%	60–80%	<60%
Serum albumin[§]	35–45 g/l	30–35 g/l	25–30 g/l	<25 g/l
Serum transferrin[§]	200–300 mg/100 ml	150–200 mg/100 ml	100–150 mg/100 ml	<100 mg/100 ml
Total lymphocyte[§] count	1500–3500/mm^3	1200–1500/mm^3	800–1200/mm^3	<800/mm^3

* This measurement is affected by age
[†] See Appendix 3 for discussion of the different values given
\+ from Jellife (1966)
[§] Remember that these parameters are all more likely to reflect the disease state rather than nutritional status
++ from Bishop *et al* (1981)

Table 1.31 Body mass index

$$\text{Body Mass Index (Quetelet Index)} = \frac{\text{Weight (kg)}}{\text{Height (m)}^2}$$

Interpretation of data obtained
<20 = Long term hazard to health
20–24.9 = Desirable
25–29.9 = Overweight
30–39.9 = Obese
<40 = Severe obesity, morbid obesity

therapy and/or chemotherapy as well as some patients with neurological disease or those being repeatedly fasted for various clinical investigations (Table 1.32).

Clinical measurements of body composition (See also Section 1.9)

Many tests have been devised which provide a quantitative estimate of the body's fat and protein stores.

Fat stores (see also Section 1.9.2, second paragraph)

Using the tables of Durnin and Womersley (1974) an estimation of the fat stores at skinfold sites (triceps, biceps, subscapular and iliac crest) enables an assessment of fat mass to be made. However, in the bed-bound, hospitalized patient a single measurement of triceps skinfold thickness is a useful method of estimating endogenous fat stores. This measurement can then be compared with standard tables (Appendix 3, Tables 7.36 and 7.37).

When measuring arm anthropometry it is important to use robust and reliable calipers on the subject's non-dominant arm. In order to minimize inter-observer variation, only one observer should make the anthropometric measurements (Heymsfield and Casper 1987), and initial values should be recorded on admission as a baseline.

Skeletal muscle mass

Mid-arm muscle circumference (MAMC) This is derived from the mid-upper arm circumference (MUAC) and triceps skinfold thickness (TSF) using the formula:

Table 1.32 Clinical factors to consider when taking a dietary history

Whether there is an underlying disease state
Whether there is impairment in organic function
Whether undernutrition is present and, if so, its extent and duration
Whether there are likely to be any drug-nutrient interactions
Whether there is an increased requirement for any nutrient and, if so, which and why?
Whether the present situation is likely to change and, if so, will this affect the nutritional status?

$$MAMC(cm) = MUAC(cm) - (TSF (mm) \times 0.314)$$

This measurement gives an estimate of the skeletal muscle mass.

Dynamometry It has been suggested that grip strength is a useful index of muscle function (Griffith and Clark 1984). Using a hand grip dynamometer, values from the subject are expressed as a percentage of the standard (Table 1.30). This technique is limited by the fact that grip strength may be affected by training, local debility and age.

Bioelectrical Impedance Analysis (BIA) (see also Section 1.10.1, paragraph on Impedance/Resistance) Impedance is the resistance and reactance to a small alternating circuit current. This technique gives an estimation of lean body mass and, by subtraction from body weight, fat mass. The main body compartment which allows conduction of an electric current is the lean tissue containing water and electrolytes. The fat will act as an insulator. The resistance component is mainly dependent on the amount of electrolyte-containing water within the body. In contrast, the reactive component is mainly a function of the cell membranes. Therefore, sequential BIA (using reliable equipment) permits assessment of the changes taking place in an individual's lean body mass and body cell mass (Fearon *et al* 1992). These measurements, however, are of limited use in patients with grossly abnormal fluid balance (e.g. dehydration, ascites).

Visceral proteins

The visceral protein compartment is responsible for tissue function, protein synthesis and immune competence. The first two functions can be assessed by monitoring the serum concentration of transport proteins synthesized by the liver. However, subnormal levels of serum proteins are affected more by the presence of disease, stress or trauma than by the individual's nutritional status (Fleck 1988).

Serum albumin This long half-life (18 days) serum protein is a commonly used marker of nutritional status and is more affected by the presence of disease, stress and hepatic function than by undernutrition (O'Keefe and Dicker 1988; Klein 1990). It is worth noting that the same mediators that cause the albumin level to fall in inflammatory disease also cause a rise in acute phase protein levels, for example C-reactive protein (CRP). This fact allows identification of hypoalbuminaemia as a result of an inflammatory response. For example, a patient with a normal CRP (<10 mg/l) and a low serum albumin (<30 g/l) suggests undernutrition. Conversely, an elevated CRP (>10 mg/l) with a low serum albumin is indicative of an acute phase response.

Serum transferrin (TF) This has a shorter half-life than albumin and is considered to be a more sensitive marker of nutritional status. However, it is also affected by all the previously listed factors. Measurements may be made directly or by calculation from the total iron binding capacity (TIBC) using the formula:

$$\text{Serum TF} = (\text{TIBC} \times 0.8) - 43$$

Note: Several authors recommend that local figures should be used in this calculation since a variety of procedures exist for measuring both TIBC and transferrin.

Rapid turnover proteins These include thyroxin binding prealbumin and retinol binding protein which have a very high turnover rate and are extremely sensitive. They are not usually appropriate indicators of nutritional depletion in the clinical situation and are rarely available as routine biochemical indices.

Immune competence

It has been suggested that immune competence may be used as an index of nutritional depletion (Shizgal 1981; Chandra 1983; 1990). Delayed cutaneous hypersensitivity to recall antigens such as mumps and also total lymphocyte count have been used as nutritional markers. However, as with visceral protein, they are affected by factors other than nutrition. For example, patients with neoplastic disease, jaundice or diabetes may be anergic and yet they may have normal nutritional status.

Note: Total lymphocyte count (TLC) may be calculated using the formula:

$$\text{TLC} = \frac{\%\ \text{lymphocytes} \times \text{WBC}}{100}$$

Nitrogen balance

An immediate assessment of protein balance can be made by estimating the nitrogen content of a *complete* 24 hour urine collection and relating this to nitrogen intake (Table 1.33). These measurements may need to be modified if the patient has large nitrogen losses from any other sources such as burns or fistulae. However, nitrogen balance only measures the present state and is more often used when *monitoring* nutritional support. It does not necessarily reflect nutritional status.

Table 1.33 Calculation of nitrogen balance

Nitrogen input = g protein consumed in 24 hours ÷ 6.25
Nitrogen output = g urinary urea nitrogen excreted in 24 hours + 2–4 g*
Nitrogen balance = Nitrogen input − nitrogen output
This should be 0 to +1

* 2–4 g to allow for obligatory nitrogen losses in faeces, sweat, etc.

Summary

The tests which have been described can be considered as general indicators of nutritional status. If a deficiency of a particular nutrient (e.g. an individual vitamin or mineral) is suspected, then an appropriate and specific test can be used provided any constraints which may apply are borne in mind.

The assessment of nutritional status forms a useful basis from which to plan subsequent treatment. No individual indicator is exclusively or uniquely related to nutritional status. A combination of tests should therefore be applied to measure body composition and function and the results interpreted with caution. It is also important to remember the inherent difficulties associated with relating general standards to individual patients.

Nutritional assessment is an important component of clinical care and audit. The key to the successful management of the nutritionally 'at risk' patient is to be aware of the fact that depletion may exist (Roubenoff *et al* 1982). This will help to ensure that relevant tests are carried out to confirm the diagnosis and that subsequent therapy is appropriately planned and managed. The importance of longitudinal measurements in the management of patients cannot be overemphasized.

Further reading

Blackburn GL, Bistrian BR, Maini BS, Schiamm HT and Smith MF (1977) Nutritional and metabolic assessment of the hospitalised patient. *J Parent Ent Nutr* **1**, 11–12.

Elia M and Lunn PG (1989) The place of some newer techniques in studies of nutrition in the hospitalised patient. *J Hum Nut Diet* **2**, 85–94.

Goode AW (1981) The scientific basis of nutritional assessment. *Br J Anaesth* **53**(2), 161–7.

Grant JP, Custer PB and Thurlow J (1981) Current techniques of nutritional assessment. *Surg Clin North Am* **61**(3), 437–63.

Haw MP, Bell SJ, Blackburn GL (1991) Potential of parenteral and enteral nutrition in inflammation and immune dysfunction: a new challenge for dietitians. *J Am Diet Assoc* **91**, 701–706, 709.

Jeejeebhoy KN (1990) Assessment of nutritional assessment. *J Parent Ent Nutr* **14**(5), 193S–6S.

Jensen T, Englert DM and Dudrick S (1983) *Nutritional assessment – a manual for practitioners*. Prentice Hall, London.

McMahon M and Bistrian BR (1990) The physiology of nutritional assessment in protein calorie malnutrition. *Disease a month* **7**, 375–417.

Starker PM (1990) Nutritional assessment of the hospitalised patient. *Advances in Nutritional Research* **8**, Draper HH (Ed) pp. 109–118. Plenum Press, New York.

Whicher JT and Dieppe PA (1985) Acute phase proteins. *Clinical Immunology and Allergy* **5**(3), 425–46.

Wright R and Heymsfield S (1984) *Nutritional Assessment*. Blackwell Scientific Publications, Oxford.

References

Baker JP, Detsky AS, Wesson DE *et al* (1982) A comparison of clinical judgement and objective measurements. *N Engl J Med* **306**, 969–88.

Bishop CW, Bowen PE and Ritchey SJ (1981) Norms for nutritional assessment of American adults by upper arm anthropometry. *Am J Clin Nutr* **34**, 2530–9.

Chandra RK (1983) Nutrition, immunity and infection: Present knowledge and future directions. *Lancet* **1**, 688–91.

Chandra RK (1990) The relationship between immunology, nutrition and disease in elderly people. *Age and Ageing* **19**, S25–31.

Christakis G (1979) How to make a nutritional diagnosis without really trying. *J Flor Med Assoc* **66**(4), 349–56.

Durnin JVGA and Wolmersley J (1974) Body fat assessed from total body density and its estimation from skinfold thickness: measurements on 481 men and women aged from 16 to 72 years. *Br J Nutr* **32**, 77–97.

Fearon KCH, Richardson RA, Hannan J *et al* (1992) Bioelectrical Impedance Analysis in the measurements of the body composition of surgical patients. *Br J Surg* (In press)

Fleck A (1988) Plasma proteins as nutritional indicators in the perioperative period. *Brit J Clin Prac* Suppl 63, Vol **42**(12), 20–24.

Garrow JS (1981) *Treat obesity seriously: a clinical manual*. pp 27–9. Churchill Livingstone, Edinburgh.

Griffith CDM and Clark RG (1984) A comparison of the 'Sheffield' prognostic index with forearm muscle dynamometry in patients from Sheffield undergoing major abdominal and urological surgery. *Clin Nut* **3**, 147–51.

Heymsfield SB and Casper K (1987) Anthropometric assessment of the adult hospitalised patient. *J Parent Ent Nutr* **11**(5), 36S–41S.

Jelliffe DB (1966) *The assessment of the nutritional status of the community*. pp. 442. WHO, Geneva.

Klein S (1990) The myth of serum albumin as a measure of nutritional status. *Gastroenterology* **99**(6), 1845–6.

Metropolitan Life (1983) *Metropolitan Life Insurance Company Statistical Bulletin* **64**, 1–9.

O'Keefe SJD and Dicker J (1988) Is plasma albumin concentration useful in the assessment of the nutritional status of hospital patients? *Eur J Clin Nut* **42**, 41–5.

Roubenoff R, Roubenoff RA, Preto J, Balke W (1987) Malnutrition among hospitalised patients: a problem of physician awareness. *Arch Int Med* **147**, 1462–5.

Shizgal HM (1981) Nutrition and immune function. *Surg Ann* **13**, 15–29.

1.12 Estimation of nutritional requirements for the provision of nutritional support

1.12.1 General considerations

The aim of nutritional support, whether in a healthy or sick individual, is to provide enough of the essential nutrients to promote and maintain health. Various sets of tables have been compiled to facilitate these calculations when considering healthy populations. However, several factors can influence nutritional requirements – even in the healthy person. These include age, sex and activity as well as the use of various drugs which can alter the requirement for specific nutrients – especially if they are taken on a long term basis (see Section 2.10).

The presence of disease can modify nutritional requirements further, particularly with respect to energy and nitrogen but also for other nutrients. Initial research to identify the precise nutritional needs of sick patients has been subsequently consolidated (Bistrian *et al* 1976; Hill *et al* 1977; Hill *et al* 1991; Lennard-Jones 1992).

It is essential that each patient is considered on an individual basis. In every instance the same procedure should be followed (Fig. 1.3). The aim of nutritional support is to minimize losses by restoring and maintaining the normal homeostatic processes within the body.

Basic objectives

Achieving nitrogen equilibrium or positive nitrogen balance

Where possible, positive nitrogen balance should be achieved in order to protect lean body mass and visceral protein status (e.g. serum levels of transport proteins), thus enabling immune competence to be maintained and the functions of the vital organs, particularly the liver, to be preserved.

Prevention or minimization of weight loss

The rate and degree of weight loss have long been recognized as major determining factors in the incidence of post-trauma mortality (Studley 1936). In general, patients should **not** be prescribed weight reducing regimens while they are acutely ill, even if they are overweight. An exception may be made in the case of severely obese patients.

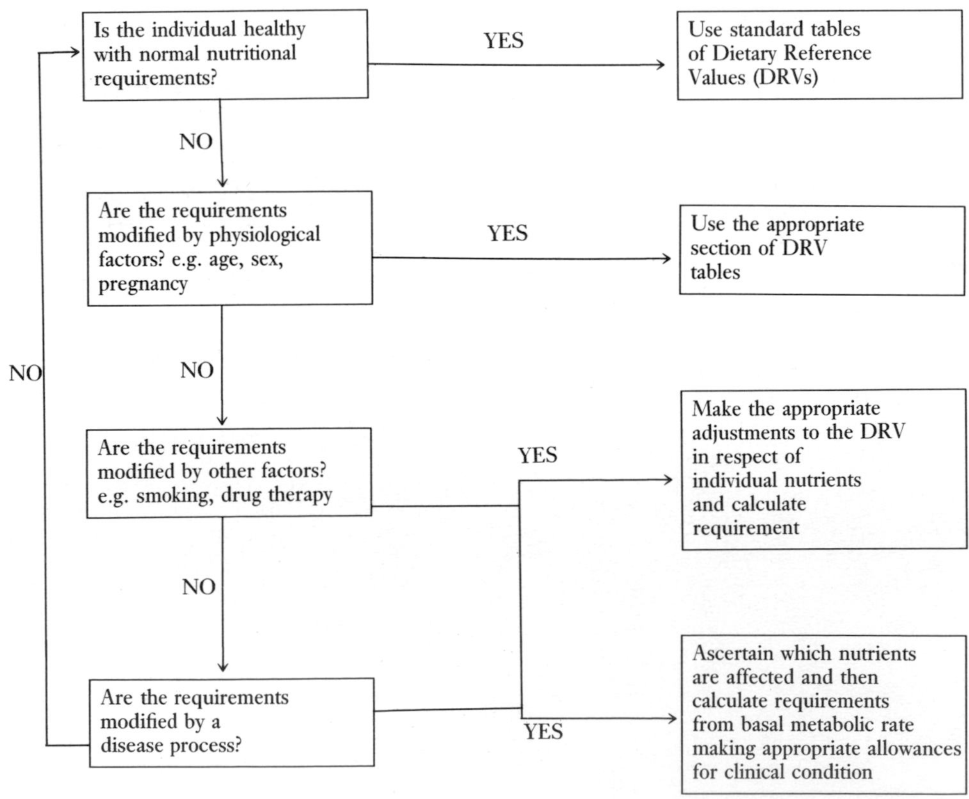

Fig. 1.3 Initial estimation of nutritional requirements.

Provision of sufficient minerals and vitamins

Adequate provision of all minerals, trace elements and vitamins is required to enable optimal substrate metabolism to take place.

Maintenance of fluid balance

Maintenance of fluid balance is crucial to renal, cardiovascular and respiratory function.

Prevention of overfeeding

Overfeeding can result in metabolic and other clinical problems including obesity (Solomon and Kirby 1990). Moreover, overfeeding will also reduce the cost-effectiveness of nutritional support.

Other considerations

There are, of course, many other nutritionally related functions which also have to be considered – including the maintenance of essential systems such as the nervous system. The needs of children merit special consideration; these are outlined in Sections 3.2–3.5.

Whatever the category of the patient being considered for nutritional support, it must not be forgotten that tissue maintenance and/or repletion cannot be achieved if there is a deficiency of any single nutrient. It is also important to remember that there are some patients in whom the nutritional requirement for a particular substrate may exceed their ability to handle it (for example, nitrogen requirements in the critically ill, particularly if there are concurrent extrarenal losses). It is not possible therefore to meet the requirement and, in the short term, it is unnecessary to do so.

Effects of injury

Hormonal changes

Hormonal changes affect nutritional requirements and must be taken into consideration. The hormonal response to injury has been well reviewed by Wilmore (1977) and Woolfson (1978). It is discussed further in Section 5.1. In brief, the initial metabolic response to injury is an increase in the secretion of catabolic hormones (glucagon, cortisol and the catecholamines) which stimulate glycogenolysis and gluconeogenesis and hence increase the available supply of glucose. Insulin secretion, although initially inhibited by high levels of catecholamines, is also increased during the 'catabolic' phase of injury but, paradoxically, there is often coexistent hyperglycaemia caused by insulin 'resistance'. These changes should not be confused with the changes which occur during starvation (Table 1.34).

Table 1.34 Comparison of the effects of starvation and injury (Woolfson 1978)

	Starvation	Injury
Metabolic rate	Decreased	Increased
Weight	Slow loss	Rapid loss
Energy	Almost all from fat	80% from fat. Remainder from protein
Nitrogen	Losses reduced	Losses increased
Hormones	Early small increases in catecholamines, glucagon, cortisol, hGH, then slow fall	Increases in catecholamines, glucagon, cortisol, hGH
	Insulin decreased	Insulin increased but relative insulin deficiency
Water and sodium	Initial loss. Later retention	Retention

The metabolic response to injury

Currently, this is the subject of much clinical research. The role of specific amino acids (notably glutamine and the branched chain amino acids) is being examined and the presence of glutamine is being confirmed as an essential substrate for the maintenance of the intestinal mucosa (Lacey and Wilmore 1990). In the absence of enteral feeding, the integrity of the mucosa is compromised and there follows a translocation of bacteria into the systemic circulation (Mainous *et al* 1991). This can initiate and/or modify the 'acute phase' response and is mediated through cytokine metabolism (Haw *et al* 1991). This, in turn, may affect both the immune response and the response to inflammation (via prostaglandin synthesis).

Assessment of nutritional status

It is necessary to assess the present nutritional status of the patient so that future nutritional requirements can be determined. Particular attention should be paid to clinical appearance, weight loss (particularly if this has occurred during the previous three months) and nitrogen balance (see Section 1.11).

1.12.2 Calculation of nutritional requirements

Energy requirements

One of the two principal nutritional changes which occur in illness relates to the requirement for energy (the other being the need for nitrogen). The energy requirement is dependent upon the Basal Metabolic Rate (BMR). This is the amount of energy which is needed to maintain physiological equilibrium while lying at rest in the fasted state and it can be measured by using indirect calorimetry (Jequier 1987). However, it may be difficult to make these measurements (e.g. in critically ill patients) and so prediction equations are widely used.

Calculation of the BMR (see Section 2.1.2, for more detailed discussion)

There are numerous prediction equations based on weight and height or surface area. The two most commonly used in the past were the Harris-Benedict equation (1919) and the Robertson and Reid (1952) standards (BMR per m^2). However, the equations that should now be used in *clinical situations* are those of Schofield *et al* (1985). There are twelve equations – by sex and six age groups – for calculating BMR from weight or from weight and height. The differences made by including height in the equation are unimportant for practical purposes. The equations for calculating BMR from weight alone are given in Table 1.35 and a look-up table of BMR by sex, and weight in Table 1.36. The latter however is not applicable to individuals over 60 years of age. For discussion of BMR equations see Elia (1992).

For healthy individuals, the Schofield equations were modified by the COMA committee on DRVs by excluding some results derived from studies in Third World countries. These are the more appropriate equations to use for healthy people and are given in Section 2.1. An extensive look-up table using the modified Schofield equations is given in Appendix 4, Tables 7.40 and 7.41. The Robertson and Reid (1952) standards and the Harris-Benedict (1919) equations are also given (for reference) in Appendix 4.

Prediction equations are derived from indirect calorimetry of healthy individuals, so their use in hospitalized patients may be inappropriate. They are used as a first step in calculating the energy requirements in a number of disease states.

Table 1.35 Equations for estimating basal metabolic rate from weight (*m*, male *f*, female). (BMR is expressed in MJ/24h; weight in kg; sample size is given as *n*, multiple correlation as R; standard error of the estimate as s.e.) (Schofield 1985). Reproduced with permission

Children:	*n*	R	s.e.
under 3 years			
m BMR = 0.249 wt − 0.127	162	0.95	0.2925
f BMR = 0.244 wt − 0.130	137	0.96	0.2456
3–10 years			
m BMR = 0.095 wt + 2.110	338	0.83	0.2803
f BMR = 0.085 wt + 2.033	413	0.81	0.2924
10–18 years			
m BMR = 0.074 wt + 2.754	734	0.93	0.4404
f BMR = 0.056 wt + 2.898	575	0.80	0.4661
Adults: 18–30 years			
m BMR = 0.063 wt + 2.896	2879	0.65	0.6407
f BMR = 0.062 wt + 2.036	829	0.73	0.4967
30–60 years			
m BMR = 0.048 wt + 3.653	646	0.60	0.6997
f BMR = 0.034 wt + 3.538	372	0.68	0.4653
Over 60 years			
m BMR = 0.049 wt + 2.459	50	0.71	0.6865
f BMR = 0.038 wt + 2.755	38	0.68	0.4511

Table 1.36 Standard basal metabolic rates for individuals of both sexes (Schofield 1985). Reproduced with permission

Body weight (kg)	MJ/24 h *m*	MJ/24 h *f*	Body weight (kg)	MJ/24 h *m*	MJ/24 h *f*	Body weight (kg)	MJ/24 h *m*	MJ/24 h *f*
3	0.5	0.6	31	5.0	4.6	59	6.7	5.6
4	0.8	0.8	32	5.0	4.6	60	6.8	5.6
5	1.0	1.0	33	5.1	4.7	61	6.8	5.7
6	1.2	1.3	34	5.2	4.7	62	6.9	5.7
7	1.5	1.6	35	5.2	4.8	63	7.0	5.8
8	1.8	1.8	36	5.3	4.8	64	7.0	5.8
9	2.0	2.1	37	5.4	4.8	65	7.0	5.9
10	2.3	2.3	38	5.5	4.9	66	7.1	5.9
11	2.6	2.6	39	5.5	4.9	67	7.1	6.0
12	2.8	2.8	40	5.6	4.9	68	7.2	6.0
13	3.0	3.0	41	5.6	5.0	69	7.2	6.0
14	3.2	3.2	42	5.7	5.0	70	7.3	6.1
15	3.4	3.4	43	5.8	5.0	71	7.3	6.1
16	3.6	3.5	44	5.8	5.1	72	7.3	6.1
17	3.7	3.6	45	5.9	5.1	73	7.4	6.2
18	3.8	3.7	46	6.0	5.1	74	7.4	6.2
19	3.9	3.8	47	6.0	5.2	75	7.5	6.2
20	4.0	3.9	48	6.1	5.2	76	7.5	6.3
21	4.1	3.9	49	6.1	5.2	77	7.6	6.3
22	4.2	4.0	50	6.2	5.3	78	7.6	6.3
23	4.3	4.0	51	6.3	5.3	79	7.7	6.4
24	4.4	4.1	52	6.3	5.3	80	7.7	6.4
25	4.5	4.2	53	6.4	5.4	81	7.7	6.5
26	4.6	4.2	54	6.4	5.4	82	7.8	6.5
27	4.7	4.3	55	6.5	5.4	83	7.8	6.6
28	4.7	4.4	56	6.6	5.5	84	7.8	6.6
29	4.8	4.5	57	6.6	5.5	85	7.9	6.6
30	4.9	4.5	58	6.7	5.5			

Not applicable to the elderly

For men over 60 years use BMR = 0.049 (wt) + 2.46, or BMR = 0.038 (wt) + 4.07 (ht) − 3.49

For women over 60 years use BMR = 0.038 (wt) + 2.76, or BMR = 0.033 (wt) + 1.92 (ht) + 0.07

Table 1.37 Activity and injury factors for estimation of energy requirements (Long 1984)

Basal energy Expenditure* × activity factor × injury factor	
Activity factors	
Patients confined to bed	× 1.2
Patients out of bed	× 1.3
Injury factors	
Minor surgery	× 1.20
Skeletal trauma	× 1.35
Major sepsis	× 1.60
Severe thermal burn**	× 2.10

* See Section 2.1.2 for calculation of basal energy expenditure (or basal metabolic rate).

** See also Section 5.4.

Estimation of energy requirement from BMR

Several authors have proposed standards to meet the increased energy requirements generated by a variety of disease states. The most commonly used are the percentage

Fig. 1.4 A general method for estimating the approximate energy and protein (N) requirements in adult patients receiving artificial nutritional support (Elia 1990). Reproduced from *Medicine International* 1990; 82: 3392–96 by courtesy of the Medicine Group (Journals) Ltd.

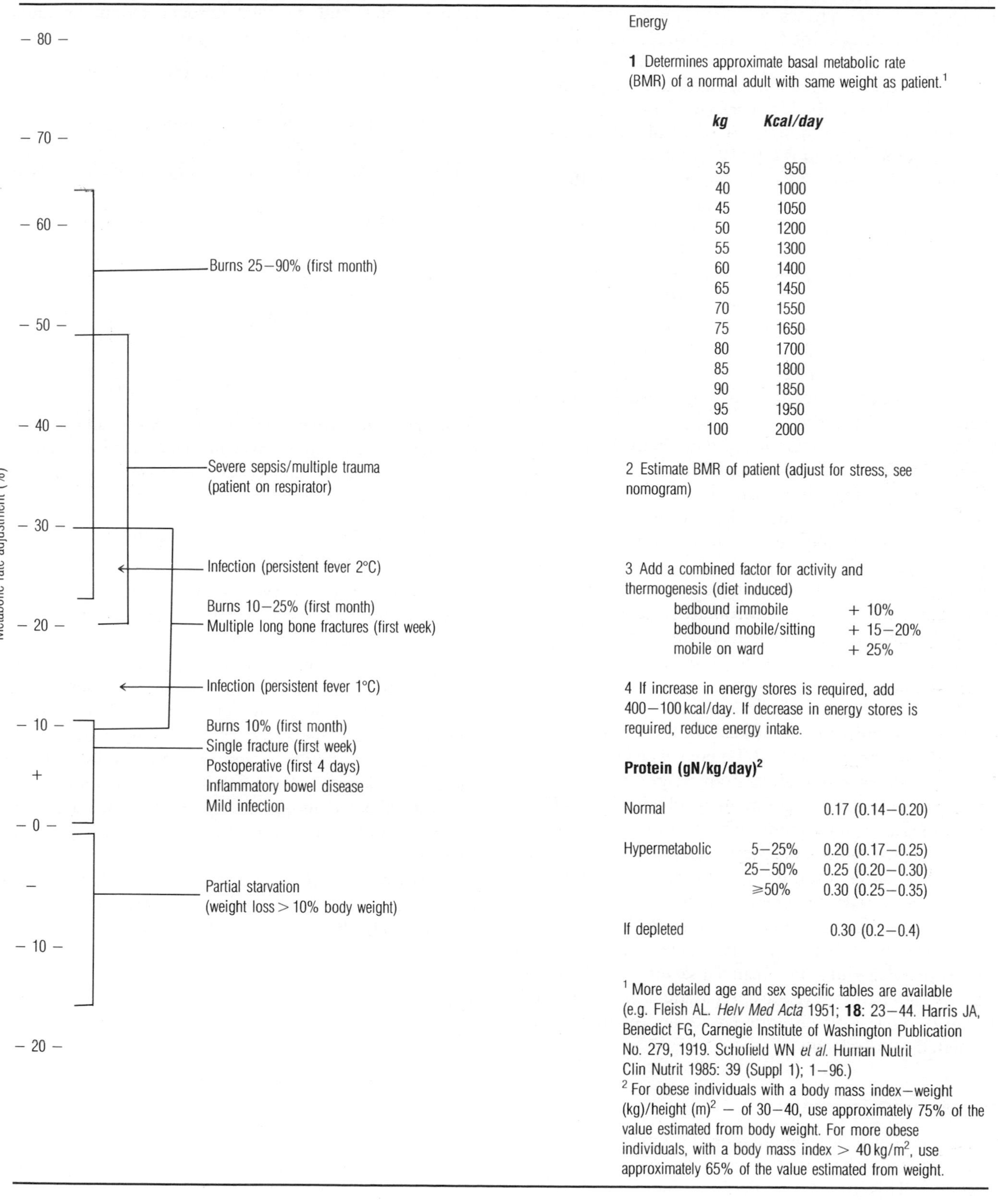

Energy

1 Determines approximate basal metabolic rate (BMR) of a normal adult with same weight as patient.[1]

kg	***Kcal/day***
35	950
40	1000
45	1050
50	1200
55	1300
60	1400
65	1450
70	1550
75	1650
80	1700
85	1800
90	1850
95	1950
100	2000

2 Estimate BMR of patient (adjust for stress, see nomogram)

3 Add a combined factor for activity and thermogenesis (diet induced)

bedbound immobile	+ 10%
bedbound mobile/sitting	+ 15–20%
mobile on ward	+ 25%

4 If increase in energy stores is required, add 400–100 kcal/day. If decrease in energy stores is required, reduce energy intake.

Protein (gN/kg/day)[2]

Normal		0.17 (0.14–0.20)
Hypermetabolic	5–25%	0.20 (0.17–0.25)
	25–50%	0.25 (0.20–0.30)
	⩾50%	0.30 (0.25–0.35)
If depleted		0.30 (0.2–0.4)

[1] More detailed age and sex specific tables are available (e.g. Fleish AL. *Helv Med Acta* 1951; **18**: 23–44. Harris JA, Benedict FG, Carnegie Institute of Washington Publication No. 279, 1919. Schofield WN *et al.* Human Nutrit Clin Nutrit 1985: 39 (Suppl 1); 1–96.)

[2] For obese individuals with a body mass index—weight (kg)/height $(m)^2$ — of 30–40, use approximately 75% of the value estimated from body weight. For more obese individuals, with a body mass index > 40 kg/m^2, use approximately 65% of the value estimated from weight.

additions to BMR proposed by Wilmore (1977) or the injury and activity factors devised by Long (1984) (Table 1.37). Elia (1990) has described how these factors can be considered collectively when calculating energy requirements (Fig. 1.4). Specific formulae have also been devised in respect of thermal injury (see Section 5.4) and the collective effects of infection on nutritional requirements have been well described (Scrimshaw, 1991).

The daily energy requirement is calculated by making further modifications to the BMR as follows:

1 Specific dynamic effect of feeding = BMR + 10%
2 Activity (if Long's factors are not used)
  (a) On ventilator = BMR − 15%
  (b) Unconscious = BMR
  (c) Bed-bound and awake = BMR + 10%
  (d) Sitting in a chair = BMR + 20%
  (e) Walking around ward = BMR + 30%
3 Allowance for weight gain = +300 kcal/day. This will lead to a gain of up to 1 kg/week, a realistic target for most patients. Sudden fluctuations in weight usually represent changes in fluid balance.
4 Pyrexia − each 1°C increase in body temperature produces a 10−12% rise in the BMR.

The ambient temperature affects energy requirements. This is only relevant if the patient is nursed in anything other than a thermoneutral environment (23−26°C). Patients nursed in a cooler area have to expend more energy to maintain their body temperature. Conversely, patients nursed in warmer environments, such as intensive care units, need less energy to maintain their temperature.

Another, less precise, method of calculating energy requirements is to allocate an arbitrary allowance of energy based on weight and clinical condition:

1 Normal requirement = 30 kcal/kg body weight/day.
2 Moderate stress = 35 kcal/kg body weight/day.
3 Severe stress = 40 kcal/kg body weight/day.

The figures for energy requirements obtained from these calculations are often significantly lower than those quoted in the standard tables of Dietary Reference Values (DoH 1991). The latter, of course, are devised for groups of healthy individuals and may not be appropriate when considering acutely ill patients in hospital. The calculated figures are also often lower than those used in current clinical practice and some financial savings may be made, particularly when intravenous preparations are being used, if the feeding regimens are based on the individual's calculated requirements.

Nitrogen requirements

Patients do not have a requirement for nitrogen *per se*, but for amino acids which are the substrates needed for protein synthesis. This may be particularly important if oral or tube feeding regimens are being considered when it may be more difficult to achieve an appropriately balanced intake of amino acids (Bell *et al* 1991). The aim of nutritional support is to achieve a state of nitrogen balance where the input and output are equal. This should be monitored carefully and can be assessed by measuring the nitrogen input and the total nitrogen output (including urinary, faecal and any other losses).

Nitrogen excretion in g is approximately equal to:

$$\text{g urinary urea excreted in 24 hours} \times \frac{28^*}{60} \times \frac{6^{**}}{5}$$

* The molecular weight of urea is 60 of which 28 parts are nitrogen.
** Approximately 80% of the total urinary nitrogen is urea.

For practical purposes this formula can be condensed to:

$$\text{Nitrogen excretion in g} = \frac{\text{mmol urinary urea excreted in 24 hours}}{30}$$

Some laboratories may not be able to measure total nitrogen excretion and some hospitals consider this to be expensive, time-consuming and unnecessary. Urinary urea output can be measured instead and the following formula applied:

$$\text{mmol urinary urea excreted in 24 hours} \div 5 = \text{g protein lost per 24 hours}$$

Many factors affect nitrogen requirements including the previous nutritional status of the patient (a nutritionally depleted or stressed patient may only retain 50% of the nitrogen which is given) and the presence of concurrent infection (Scrimshaw 1991). It is not always either possible or practical to give all the nitrogen which is required especially during the early days following a trauma. All nitrogen losses should be considered carefully including those from faeces and any fistulae or burned areas. The greatest amount of nitrogen is lost 3−5 days after accidental injury or during the peak response to sepsis or burns (Table 1.38).

Nutritional support can be based either on these figures as described above or on arbitrary energy-nitrogen ratios (Table 1.39). It is also possible to estimate nitrogen

Table 1.38 Protein requirements during peak catabolic response in patients following injury or during infection (Wilmore 1977)

Patient group	Condition	g/kg/day	
		Protein	Nitrogen
Normal	Average level of exercise	0.5−1.0	0.08−0.16
Mildly stressed	Elective operation	0.7−1.1	0.11−0.18
Moderately stressed	Major operations, infections, fractures	1.5−2.0	0.24−0.32
Severely stressed	Multiple injuries, fractures, major burns	2.0−4.0	0.32−0.64

Table 1.39 Commonly used energy: nitrogen ratios

	Total	Non-nitrogen
	Energy : Nitrogen	Energy : Nitrogen
Normal individuals	250–350 : 1	225–325 : 1
Convalescence	200 : 1	175 : 1
Mild catabolism	150 : 1	125 : 1
Moderate catabolism	125 : 1	100 : 1
Severe catabolism	100 : 1	75 : 1

requirements based on 24 hours urinary urea excretions by using a graph. Whichever method is used, it is important to monitor nitrogen balance carefully to ensure optimal nutritional support. Nitrogen input should never be less than 0.16 g/kg body weight and 0.20 g/kg body weight has been proposed as the optimum intake for severely injured patients immediately post-trauma (Larsson *et al* 1990).

It is not always possible to measure nitrogen output in patients who have renal failure. The rate of urea nitrogen production can be estimated by referring to serum urea concentrations. Calculation of nitrogen output in anuric patients with renal failure is as follows:

$$\text{g urea nitrogen produced per day} = [(\text{Urea 2} - \text{Urea 1}) \times W \times 0.6 + (W \text{ gain} \times \text{Urea 2})] \times 0.028$$

Urea 1 = serum urea at start of period (mmol/l)
Urea 2 = serum urea at end of period (mmol/l)
0.6 = factor to estimate total body water
W = weight in kg

Mineral requirements

This covers the provision of the major electrolytes (sodium and potassium), minerals and trace elements. This is an area of continuing research and reference to the current literature will be helpful.

Sodium

In the presence of normal renal function and fluid balance the basic requirement is 1.0 mmol Na^+ per kg body weight. Some specific surgical procedures can increase this e.g. extensive small bowel resection, and the requirement may be as much as 100 mmol Na^+ per litre when patients are being tube fed (Spiller *et al* 1987).

Potassium

This is needed to maintain the patency of the 'sodium pump' as well as to ensure that the intake of nitrogen is used effectively. The basic requirement is 5.0–6.0 mmol K^+ per g nitrogen. In the presence of depletion and/or catabolism a further 2 mmol K^+ per g nitrogen should be given (up to a maximum of 9 mmol K^+ per g nitrogen). This requirement needs to be carefully monitored and may need modification in the presence of cardiac impairment or renal failure.

Other minerals and trace elements

These are normally prescribed according to the Dietary Reference Values and customary clinical practice. It is important to remember that both minerals and trace elements are essential substrates for the metabolic processes and that any deficiency may limit the recovery process.

Vitamin requirements

Vitamins are usually administered according to the Dietary Reference Values and customary clinical practice. This may mean that some vitamins need only be given on a weekly or monthly basis (including vitamins A, D, B and folic acid). The actual dosage may vary but it is useful to remember that enough should be given to cover not only the DRV but also any expected losses during administration. This is particularly important in parenteral regimens (see Section 1.15).

Certain procedures may modify the requirement for particular vitamins. These include chemotherapy (B vitamins), surgery (vitamins C and vitamin K) and anticoagulant therapy (vitamin K). On the whole it is appropriate to give more rather than less of the water soluble vitamins since they are cheap, particularly in tablet form, and any moderate excess is excreted in the urine. If a complete supplement is prescribed, the contents of individual vitamins should not exceed the Dietary Reference Values.

Fluid requirements

Although not a nutrient as such, the maintenance of fluid balance is often one of the most important aspects of the management of the acutely ill patient (see Section 2.9). This is particularly critical in the presence of tissue breakdown (e.g. malnutrition or gross sepsis) which may result in an increase in the total body water. It is important to check body weight and serum osmolality regularly (daily if necessary) to monitor any changes in gross fluid balance. Since the fluid requirement is an integral part of the estimation and provision of nutritional support, it must be considered in this context and it will be necessary to know the exact water content of a feeding regimen.

Summary

The provision of appropriate nutritional support is an essential component of patient management. The estimate of nutritional requirements must necessarily include this. Requirements are influenced by many factors, each of which must be considered carefully on an individual basis. Once nutritional therapy has been commenced it is important to monitor the patient regularly and carefully. As the clinical condition changes, so will the requirement for nutritional support and all regimens should be constructed with this in mind.

Further reading

Caldwell MD and Kennedy-Caldwell C (1981) Normal nutritional requirements. *Surg Clin North Am* **61**(3), 489–507.

Cunningham JJ (1990) Factors contributing to increased energy expenditure in thermal injury: a review of studies employing indirect calorimetry. *J Parent Ent Nutr* **14**(6), 649–56.

Curren PW, Richmond D, Marvin J and Baxter CR (1974) Dietary requirements of patients with major burns. *J Am Diet Assoc* **65**(4), 415–7.

Dudrick SJ (Ed) (1991) *Current strategies in surgical nutrition*. WB Saunders, Philadelphia.

Elwyn DH (1980) Nutritional requirements of adult surgical patients. *Crit Care Med* **8**(1), 9–20.

Hill GL and Church J (1984) Energy and protein requirements of general surgical patients requiring intravenous nutrition. *Br J Surg* **71**, 1–9.

Karran SJ and Alberti KGMM (Eds) (1980) *Practical nutritional support*. Pitman Medical, Tunbridge Wells.

Kielanowski J (1976) Energy cost of protein deposition. In *Protein metabolism and nutrition*, Cole DJA, Boorman KN, Buttery PJ, Lewis D, Neal RJ and Swan H (Eds) pp. 207–15. Butterworths, London.

Kinney JM (1975) Energy requirements of the surgical patient. In *Manual of surgical nutrition* Ballinger WF *et al* (Eds) pp. 223–35. WB Saunders, Philadelphia.

Kinney JM and Borum PR (Eds) (1989) *Perspectives in Clinical Nutrition*. Urban and Schwarzenberg, Baltimore.

Merritt RJ, Sinatra FR and Smith GA (1983) Nutritional support of the hospitalised child. In *Advances in nutritional research* Vol 5. Draper HH (Ed) pp. 77–103. Plenum Press, New York.

Paauw JD, McCarnish MA, Dean RE and Duellette TR (1984) Assessment of caloric needs in stressed patients. *J Am Coll Nutr* **3**, 51–9.

Shenkin A (1988) Clinical aspects of vitamin and trace element metabolism. *Clinical Gastroenterology* **2**(4), 765–98. Baillière Tindall, London.

Stonor HB (1982) Assessment of energy expenditure. *Proc Nutr Soc* **41**, 349–53.

Sutherland AB (1976) Nitrogen balance and nutritional requirement in the burn patient: a reappraisal. *Burns* **2**, 238–44.

Tweedle DEF (1982) *Metabolic care*. Churchill Livingstone, Edinburgh.

Wilmore DW (1974) Nutrition and metabolism following thermal injury. *Clin Plast Surg* **1**(4), 603–19.

Whicher JT and Dieppe P (1985) Acute Phase Proteins. *Clinical Immunology and Allergy* **3**, 425–46.

References

Bell SJ, Bistrian BR, Ainsley BM, Manji N, Lewis EJ, Joyce C and Blackburn GL (1991) A chemical score to evaluate the protein quality of commercial parenteral and enteral formulas: Emphasis on patients with liver failure. *J Am Diet Assoc* **91**(5), 586–589.

Bistrian BR, Blackburn GL, Vitale J, Cochran D and Naylor J (1976) Prevalence of malnutrition in general medical patients. *J Am Diet Assoc* **235**(15), 1567–70.

Department of Health (1991) Committee on Medical Aspects of Food Policy. *Dietary Reference Values for food energy and nutrients for the United Kingdom*. HMSO, London.

Elia M (1990) Artificial nutritional support. *Medicine International* **82**, 3392–6.

Elia M (1992) Energy expenditure in the whole body. In *Energy metabolism. Tissue determinants and cellular corollaries*. Kinney JM and Tucker HN (Eds). Raven Press, New York.

Fleish A (1951) Le metabolisme basal standard et sa determination au moyen du 'metabocalculator'. *Helv Med Acta* **18**, 23.

Harris JA and Benedict FG (1919) *Biometric studies of basal metabolism in man*. Carnegie Institute, Washington.

Haw MP, Bell SJ and Blackburn GL (1991) Potential of parenteral and enteral nutrition in inflammation and immune dysfunction: a new challenge for dietitians. *J Am Diet Assoc* **91**, 701–706, 709.

Hill GL, Blackett RL, Pickford L, Burkinshaw L, Young GA, Warren JV, Schorah CJ and Morgan DB (1977) Malnutrition in surgical patients – an unrecognised problem. *Lancet* **1**, 689–92.

Hill GL, Witney GB, Christie PM and Church JM (1991) Protein status and metabolic expenditure determine the response to intravenous nutrition – a new classification of surgical malnutrition. *Br J Surg* **78**, 109–113.

Jequier E (1987) Measurements of energy expenditure in clinical nutritional assessment. *J Parent Ent Nutr* **11**(5), 86S–89S.

Lacey JM and Wilmore DW (1990) Is glutamine a conditionally essential amino acid? *Nutrition Reviews* **48**(8), 297–309.

Larsson J, Lennmarken C, Martensson J, Sandstedt S and Vinnars E (1990) Nitrogen requirements in severely injured patients. *Br J Surg* **77**, 413–16.

Lennard-Jones J (1992) *A positive approach to nutrition as treatment*. Kings Fund Centre, London.

Long CL (1984) The energy and protein requirements of the critically ill patient. In *Nutritional assessment*, Wright RA and Heymsfield S (Eds) pp. 157–81. Blackwell Scientific Publications, Boston.

Mainous M, Dazhong X, Qi Lu, Berg RD and Deitch EA (1991) Oral-TPN-induced bacterial translocation and impaired immune defenses are reversed by refeeding. *Surgery* **110**(2), 277–84.

Robertson JD and Reid DD (1952) Standards for the basal metabolism of normal people in Britain. *Lancet* **1**, 940–3.

Schofield WN, Schofield C and James WPT (1985) Basal metabolic rate – review and prediction, together with annotated bibliography of source material. *Hum Nutr: Clin Nutr* **39C**(Suppl 1), 5–96.

Scrimshaw NS (1991) Effect of infection on nutrient requirements. *J Parent Ent Nutr* **15**(6), 589–600.

Solomon SM and Kirby DF (1990) The refeeding syndrome: a review. *J Parent Ent Nutr* **14**(1), 90–96.

Spiller RC, Jones BJM and Silk DBA (1987) Jejunal water and electrolyte absorption from two proprietary feeds in man: importance of sodium content. *Gut* **28**, 681–7.

Studley HO (1936) Percentage weight loss in patients with chronic peptic ulcer. *J Am Diet Assoc* **106**, 458–60.

Wilmore DW (1977) *The metabolic management of the critically ill*. Plenum Medical Book Company, New York.

Woolfson AMJ (1978) Metabolic considerations in nutritional support. In *Developments in clinical nutrition*. Johnston IDA and Lee HA (Eds) pp. 35–47. MSC Consultants, Tunbridge Wells.

1.13 Enteral feeding

Enteral feeding can be defined as nutrition provided via the gastrointestinal tract. It includes nutrition taken orally or administered by enteric tube, though the term is generally reserved to refer to the latter.

Hull (1985) remarked that the 'GUT' may be considered as an acronym for 'God uses this' and adds 'present evidence comparing enteral with parenteral suggests he was right!' Hull has demonstrated that in terms of nutritional repletion the enteral route is as efficient as the parenteral. Moreover, enteral feeding has been shown to maintain intestinal structure and function (Shanbhogue *et al* 1986) and has the additional benefits of reduced cost and low risk of serious complications.

Numerous factors, both physiological and psychological, may cause or exacerbate anorexia in the hospitalized patient. Presentation of the food is also an important, yet often neglected, cause of food rejection. Many patients dislike institutional meals served in standard portions and presented at rigid times. Furthermore, there are periods when a patient may be 'nil by mouth' for example, preoperatively or in preparation for investigations. Hence, many hospitalized patients are at risk of becoming progressively malnourished, particularly those with chronic or debilitating disease (many of whom may also be malnourished on admission). Several authors have reported that 30–35% of hospitalized patients exhibit some degree of malnutrition (Bistrian *et al* 1974; 1976; Hill *et al* 1977) and surgical patients appear to be particularly at risk.

During the past two decades many workers have tried to demonstrate the benefits of providing nutritional support (Mullen *et al* 1980; Starker *et al* 1986; Buzby *et al* 1988). However, due to poor experimental design, studies suggesting that nutritional support may have a place in reducing morbidity and mortality have, so far, proved inconclusive. One of the few well controlled studies to show clear benefit from 'feeding' was that of Bastow *et al* 1983. This group considered a different 'end point' with nutrition, namely rehabilitation time. Malnourished individuals who received an additional 1000 kcal/day had a significantly shorter rehabilitation time than their non-tube fed counterparts. Current thinking suggests that, by improving organ function and immunocompetence, nutritional support may aid the recovery process and reduce the period required for convalescence (Allison 1988). Hence appropriate nutritional support may be cost effective by reducing the length and cost of hospitalization (PENG 1988).

The provision of adequate nutrition is therefore an important component of patient care. In the 'nutritionally at risk' patient with a functioning gut, nutritional support may be provided in a number of ways:

1 Normal food and drink.
2 Fortification of diet.
3 Sip feeds and nutritional supplements.
4 Tube feeds.

More than one feeding route may be used in an attempt to maximize intake.

1.13.1 Normal food and drink

For many patients adequate nutritional support may be provided by simple adaptation of the hospital menu. For example, a patient with multiple fractures, who has increased nutritional requirements and a good appetite, could be given larger portions and frequent snacks. Conversely, the patient who suffers from nausea, is unlikely to manage the traditional 'meat and two veg' hospital meal but may tolerate a sandwich and yoghurt. One should take into account any chewing or swallowing difficulties and ensure the meal is of a suitable consistency (e.g. soft or puréed as necessary). Good liaison between the dietetic department, nurses and catering staff is essential to ensure appropriate meals are provided.

1.13.2 Fortification of the diet

If a patient is able to eat a normal diet, but in quantities insufficient to meet his or her requirements, then fortification of the diet should be considered. The aim of fortification is to maximize the energy and/or nitrogen content of the diet without making the food unpalatable. Foods of low nutritional value (e.g. tea, squash, clear soup, jellies) should be discouraged unless suitably fortified. The diet can be fortified using high energy and nitrogen foods such as skimmed milk powder, cream, butter and milk. In addition a variety of proprietary products have been developed (Table 1.40); these have the advantage of a low electrolyte content and are therefore suitable for patients with renal and liver disease. Patients and carers need to be given full instructions regarding their use in order to optimize this form of nutritional supplementation (Morris *et al* 1990).

Patients requiring puréed or liquidized meals (e.g. those with oesophageal cancer or fractured jaw) often benefit from fortification of their diet as it is difficult for this group to achieve an adequate nutritional intake.

Table 1.40 Feed modules*

Carbohydrate sources	Protein sources	Fat sources
Caloreen (*P*) (Roussel)	Casilan (*P*) (Farley Health Products)	Calogen (*L*) (Scientific Hospital Supplies)
Maxijul (*P*/*L*) (Scientific Hospital Supplies)	Maxipro HBV (*P*) (Scientific Hospital Supplies)	Liquigen (*L*) (Scientific Hospital Supplies)
Polycal (*P*) (Cow and Gate Nutricia)	Promod (*P*) (Ross)	MCT oil (*L*) (Cow and Gate Nutricia, Bristol Myers, Scientific Hospital Supplies)
Polycose (*L*/*P*) (Ross)	Protifar (*P*) (Cow and Gate Nutricia)	Duocal (*L*/*P*) (Scientific Hospital Supplies)
Hycal (*L*) (Beecham)		
Fortical (*L*) (Cow and Gate Nutricia)		
Duocal (*L*/*P*) (Scientific Hospital Supplies)		

* Compositional details of these products are given in Appendix 6, Tables 7.44–7.46 inclusive.

L = Liquid *P* = Powder

1.13.3 Sip feeds and nutritional supplements

These products can be used to augment a patient's dietary intake or as a sole source of nutrition. Nutritional supplements are available in the form of sweet drinks, soups and puddings (Table 1.41). These products may be used to improve the nutritional intake of patients with increased requirements (e.g. burns and post-operative patients and those with multiple fractures).

Sip feeds are nutritionally complete and are available in tetrapacks or cans. The patient should be encouraged to taste the product before the supplementation level is quantified, and acceptance and uptake should be closely monitored. Most of these products are milk-based and some patients find it difficult to take the quantities recommended; although not nutritionally complete, a new sip feed based on fruit juice has been developed which may provide a useful alternative. In the elderly population, sip feeding has proved particularly effective. Recent work has demonstrated that this form of nutritional support is associated with an improved clinical outcome in both benign and malignant disease (Bolton *et al* 1990; Ek *et al* 1990; Larsson *et al* 1990).

1.13.4 Tube feeding

Tube feeding should be considered in patients with a functioning gut, who are unwilling or unable to meet their requirements orally. Guidelines for the use of enteral nutrition in the adult patient have been issued by The American Society of Parenteral and Enteral Nutrition (ASPEN 1987). In practice, the decision to tube feed is made by the clinician in consultation with the dietitian; each patient should be considered individually taking the clinical condition, treatment plan and nutritional state into account.

Currently, a wide range of tube feeds are commercially available. These may be administered nasogastrically, nasoduodenally or nasojejunally. Recently, there has been an upsurge of interest in providing nutrition via feeding gastrostomies and jejunostomies (Fig. 1.5).

Routes of administration

Ryles and Levin's tubes

Ryles and Levin's tubes are rigid wide bore nasogastric tubes designed for stomach drainage but which were commonly used in the early days of enteral feeding. They

Table 1.41 Proprietary sip feeds and supplements*

Complete sip feeds	High protein supplements*
Ensure (Ross)	Build Up (Carnation)
Ensure Plus (Ross)	Build Up Soup (Carnation)
Fresubin (Fresenius)	Complan (Farley Health)
Fortisip (Cow and Gate Nutricia)	Complan Soup (Farley Health)
Liquisorb (Merck)	Formance (Ross)
Liquisorbon MCT (Merck)	Fortimel (Cow and Gate Nutricia)
	Maxisorb Pudding (Scientific Hospital Supplies)
	Maxisorb Soup (Scientific Hospital Supplies)
	Protein Forte (Fresenius)
	Forti Pudding (Cow and Gate Nutricia)
	Provide (Fresenius)

* Compositional details of these products are given in Appendix 6, Table 7.46

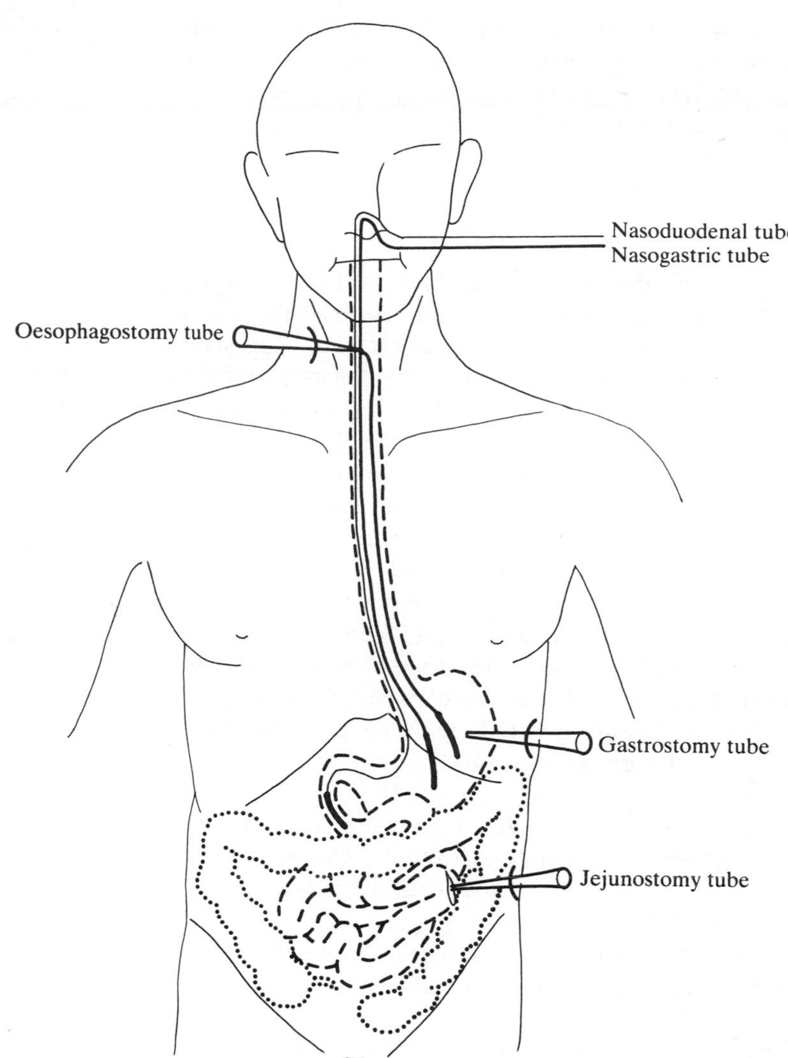

Fig. 1.5 Routes of enteral feeding

are uncomfortable for the patient, however, and can cause oesophageal ulceration. These feeding tubes have largely been replaced by fine bore nasogastric (ng) tubes. However, in patients at risk of aspiration (e.g. stroke patients) or where there is concern about gastric function (e.g. post-operatively), Ryle's and Levin's tubes may be preferred. Although a clinical decision, generally speaking these tubes should not be used for feeding patients for more than a few days. Patient comfort and acceptance are improved with passage of a fine bore ng tube. If concern about gastric function or aspiration remains then nasoduodenal or jejunal feeding may be considered.

Fine bore nasogastric tubes

These are the most commonly used feeding tubes. These tubes have small internal diameters (1–2 mm), are flexible and available in PVC for short term and in polyurethene for longer term feeding. Most of these tubes have a guidewire to assist intubation. Before commencing feeding it is very important that the tube position is checked. This may be done in a number of ways:

1 Injection of air into the tube and listening for bubbling noises with a stethoscope over the stomach.

2 Aspiration of gastric juices and testing with litmus.

3 Chest X-ray (all feeding tubes are radio-opaque).

The tube position should also be checked if the patient has a violent coughing fit, vomits, or is receiving chest physiotherapy. Policies and procedures to check tube position may vary in different health authorities.

Although the small diameter of these tubes increases patient comfort and tolerance, it also increases the risk of tube blockage, particularly with viscous feeds and/or slow infusion rates. Before feeding is commenced and between feeds, tubes should be flushed with 20–30 ml of sterile water in a 50 ml syringe (Taylor 1988).

Weighted tubes

These tend to be longer tubes (>100 cm) which may

facilitate duodenal intubation. This may be beneficial in patients with abnormal gastric function (e.g. post-operatively) or if there is any risk of aspiration. However, placement into the duodenum may need to be under direct vision or endoscopy.

Gastrostomy feeding

Traditionally this technique has been performed surgically and involves the creation of a tract between the stomach and the abdominal surface. Recent evidence suggests that endoscopic placement is preferable (Hollands *et al* 1989; Moran *et al* 1990) although patient selection must be appropriate (Ponsky and Gauderer 1989).

The siting of a percutaneous endoscopic gastrostomy (PEG) has a number of advantages over surgical placement. It does not involve a general anaesthetic or a laparotomy, it is cheaper and quicker to perform, has fewer complications and is easily removed. Gastrostomy feeding is considered more aesthetic than nasogastric, and there is a reduced risk of tube misplacement or blockage (Shike *et al* 1989). Gastrostomy placement is recommended for long term feeding. Tubes are generally replaced at 9–12 monthly intervals although one company has produced a tube which may be left *in situ* for five years (the Bower PEG system – Merck). The major indications are neurological disorders, head and neck cancer and cystic fibrosis. Contraindications include ileus, sepsis, ascites, Crohn's disease, clotting disorders and previous gastric surgery.

Gastrostomy feeding tubes may be used within 12–24 hours of placement, although some centres start feeding immediately following insertion.

Some gastrostomy kits include a 'button' version which is fitted once the tract has been formed. However the gastrostomy buttons are rather prone to leakage.

Jejunostomy feeding

Similar to a gastrostomy, this technique involves a tract between the jejunum and the abdominal surface. A feeding jejunostomy may be performed either surgically or endoscopically. Traditionally, Foley catheters have been used for jejunostomy feeding but more recently fine bore needle catheter jejunostomy kits have become available and are better suited. Endoscopic placement of a gastro-jejunostomy is possible and this involves the creation of a PEG through which the jejunostomy tube is introduced, and then endoscopically positioned in the jejunum (Westfall *et al* 1990) (Fig. 1.6). Contraindications are as for PEG insertion.

Jejunostomy feeding is appropriate when there is concern regarding aspiration or if there is abnormal gastric function. The most common indications for use are following major upper gastrointestinal surgery or hepato-biliary surgery. The jejunostomy can be sited surgically at the time of operation and used for feeding within 12 hours. Unlike the stomach and large bowel, the small intestine is functional within a few hours of surgery (Dunn *et al* 1980; Strickland and Greene 1986).

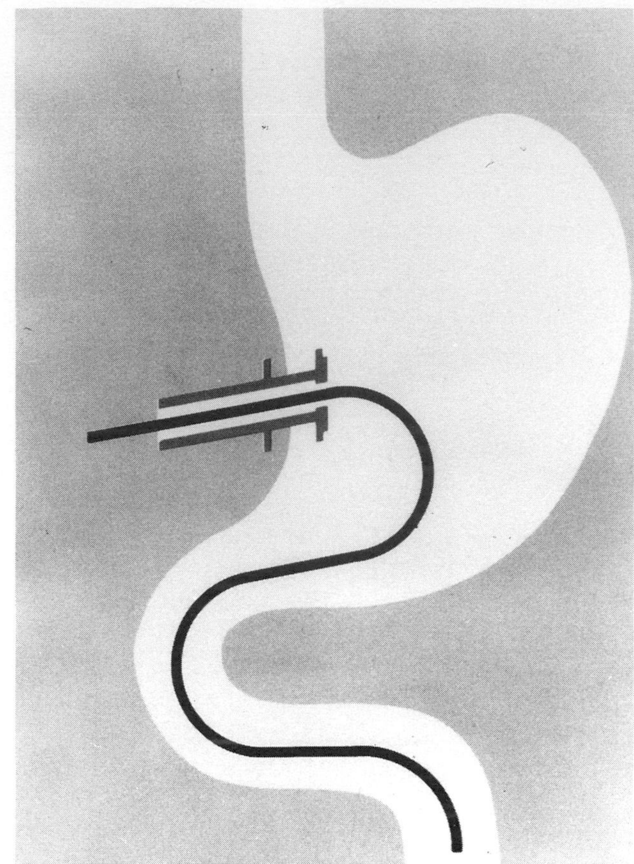

Fig. 1.6 Percutaneous endoscopic jejunostomy

For jejunostomies sited in the upper small bowel, a whole protein feed should be well tolerated (McIntyre *et al* 1986). However, if there is pancreatic or biliary insufficiency or if the jejunostomy has been sited in the lower small bowel, an elemental or peptide-based feed is indicated. Absorption and the integrity of the insertion should be checked by first administering water at 20–30 ml/hr over 12 hours; if tolerated, feeding may be commenced at a low volume (20–30 ml/hr). The volume of feed can then be increased gradually over the next 4–5 days until the required intake is achieved. Feeding should take place over a 24 hour period using an enteral feeding pump to control the flow rate. In order to help prevent blockage, flushing of the catheter every 4–6 hours with 10–20 ml of sterile water has been recommended (Russell 1984). Jejunostomy feeding is claimed to provide a safe, cost-effective alternative to TPN as a method of providing post-operative nutritional support (Fletcher and Little 1986). It is not however without its complications and patients must be carefully selected and monitored (Delany and Lundine 1988).

Tube feeds available

Hospital made tube foods

Early tube feeding regimens were prepared in hospital kitchens from mixtures of hospital food, dietary, vitamin and occasionally mineral supplements. Today these regimens are rarely used, because their preparation is time-consuming and no longer considered cost-effective. Additionally, there is an increased risk of microbial contamination and it is difficult to ensure the correct osmolarity and balance of trace elements. Occasionally it may be necessary to formulate modular feeds from individual sources of nitrogen, fat, etc. for patients with specific requirements (e.g. children with liver failure, see Section 4.12). These feeds should be prepared in very clean conditions by a well trained diet cook.

Commercially prepared tube feeds

A wide range of commercially prepared, nutritionally complete feeds are available. These are produced in liquid or powder form and packaged in bottles, cans or sachets.

Standard whole protein or polymeric feeds

These contain whole protein as their nitrogen source and carbohydrate and hydrolysed fat as the energy (Table 1.42). They are low lactose, low residue and have a relatively low osmolarity. They have been standardized to provide an energy content of 1 kcal/ml and their nitrogen content ranges from 5–7 g/l. They are suitable for most patients.

Starter feeds

These hypotonic feeds may be prepared by diluting standard formulae or are available commercially to reduce the risk of contamination. Their reduced osmolarity is thought to lower the incidence of osmotic diarrhoea; however, they also have a reduced nutritional content. The necessity for these feeds is debatable. Some authors believe that the use of starter regimens is unnecessary and serves only to prolong the time taken to achieve an adequate nutritional intake (Keohane *et al* 1984; Rees *et al* 1986).

High energy and nitrogen feeds

These products generally provide 1.5–2 kcal/ml and have an increased nitrogen content when compared with standard formulae. They tend to be hypertonic and consequently should be administered with caution initially. These feeds are useful in providing nutritional support for patients on a fluid restriction (e.g. those in cardiac failure or intensive care) and for overnight feeding when any additional fluids can be taken/administered during the day.

Table 1.42 Proprietary whole protein tube feeds*

Standard (1 kcal/ml)	High Energy/ Nitrogen	Fibre	Paediatric	Specialized Formulae
Clinifeed Favour (Clintec Nutrition)	Clinifeed 400 (Clintec Nutrition)	Enrich (Ross Laboratories)	Paediasure (Ross Laboratories)	Liquisorb MCT (Merck)
Clinifeed Iso (Clintec Nutrition)	Clinifeed Extra (Clintec Nutrition)	Fresubin Plus F (Fresenius)	Nutrison Paediatric (Cow and Gate Nutricia)	Nutrison low sodium (Cow and Gate Nutricia)
Ensure (Ross Laboratories)	Clinifeed Protein Rich (Clintec Nutrition)	Nutrison fibre (Cow and Gate Nutricia)		Nutrison low protein low minerals (Cow and Gate Nutricia)
Enteral 400 (Scientific Hospital Supplies)	Ensure Plus (Ross Laboratories)			Nutrison Soya (Cow and Gate Nutricia)
Fresubin (Fresenius)	High Energy Liquisorb (Merck)			Pre Nutrison (Cow and Gate Nutricia)
Isocal (Mead Johnson)	Nutrison Energy Plus (Cow and Gate Nutricia)			Pulmocare (Ross Laboratories)
Nutrison standard (Cow and Gate Nutricia)	Two Cal HN (Ross Laboratories)			Fresubin 750 (Fresenius)
Osmolite (Ross Laboratories)				Triosorbon (Merck)

* Compositional details of these products are given in Appendix 7, Table 7.56

Fibre feeds

Traditionally enteral formulae are low in residue and this characteristic is important for some patients such as those with fistulae. However, because dietary fibre has a number of clinical benefits (such as improving stool consistency) feeds supplemented with fibre (soy polysaccharide) have been produced. Since the fibre content of these feeds makes them more viscous it is recommended that they are administered via a tube of 1.5 mm internal diameter or greater, and with pump assistance. However, clinical trials which have examined the effect of fibre supplemented feeds on bowel function have proved inconclusive (Patil *et al* 1985; Hart and Dobb 1988). Moreover, the inclusion of dietary fibre into the feeding regimen may have a number of potential disadvantages. It may cause bloating and distension and can chelate with divalent cations such as calcium and magnesium (although most manufacturers supplement their fibre feeds accordingly). In summary the role of fibre in enteral formulae has not yet been clearly defined and more studies are required to clarify its potential uses (Silk 1989).

Specialized formulae

There are an increasing number of feeds available for specific clinical conditions. For example enteral feeds are now available for children, for long term feeding and for respiratory-compromised patients (Table 1.42). These feeds tend to be more expensive than standard products and their potential benefits require further evaluation before their use is advocated. Currently, the role of tissue-specific substances such as glutamine, branched chain amino acids, and polyunsaturated fatty acids is causing much interest and controversy in nutritional research; additional information on this topic may be found under further reading.

Elemental and peptide feeds

In the majority of patients, whole protein feeds are generally well tolerated even in the presence of a degree of gut malfunction (Payne-James *et al* 1988). However, with severe gut impairment (e.g. Crohn's exacerbation or post-pancreatectomy) a pre-digested formula may be indicated (Table 1.43). It has been shown that appropriate use of these feeds may reduce the requirement for TPN in certain conditions (Hamaoui *et al* 1990). Elemental diets have a low triglyceride content, but contain an increased proportion of medium chain triglycerides. The main energy source is provided from monosaccharides. The protein fraction is in the form of amino acids since it was originally thought that this was the most rapidly absorbed form of protein. It has since been demonstrated, however, that the absorption of short chain peptides is more efficient than that of amino acids (Silk *et al* 1979; 1980; Craft *et al* 1968).

Table 1.43 Proprietary peptide and elemental feeds*

Peptide	Elemental
Fresenius OPD (Fresenius)	E028 (Scientific Hospital Supplies)
MCT Pepdite 0–2† (Scientific Hospital Supplies)	Flexical (Bristol Myers)
MCT Pepdite 2+ (Scientific Hospital Supplies)	
Pepdite 0–2† (Scientific Hospital Supplies)	
Pepdite 2+ (Scientific Hospital Supplies)	
Peptamen (Clinitec)	
Pepti-2000 (Cow & Gate Nutricia)	
Peptisorb (Merck)	
Peptisorbon (Merck)	
Reabilan (Clintec Nutrition)	

† infant formulae

* Compositional details of these products are given in Appendix 7, Table 7.57

Moreover peptides produce a less hypertonic feeding solution and may reduce the incidence of osmotic diarrhoea (Adibi 1990). For these reasons, a range of peptide-based feeds is now available.

Choice of feeding regimen

Once an appropriate feed has been selected the patient's feeding regimen may be determined. This should be discussed with medical or nursing staff and then clearly outlined on suitable charts. There are a number of factors which should be considered, as detailed below.

Gut function

This may be adversely affected by periods of starvation, drugs, disease, surgery or treatment regimen (such as chemotherapy or radiotherapy). In these conditions, enteral feeding should be introduced slowly; gastric emptying should be established if NG or gastrostomy feeding is being used. A suitable starter regimen should be outlined which permits a gradual increase in the volume administered as tolerance improves.

Fluid requirements

Fluid balance is a priority and the feeding regimen must take into account any ongoing fluid overload, deficit or losses and any other sources of fluid. The volume of the feed delivered should be clearly displayed on the feeding/fluid chart.

Energy and nitrogen requirements

The estimation of energy and nitrogen requirements is discussed in Section 1.12. High energy and nitrogen feeds are available, alternatively the energy and nitrogen content of standard tube feeds can be altered using appropriate feed modules (Table 1.40).

Period of feeding

The period of feeding should be clearly stated on the feeding regimen, and fluid charts should be monitored to check appropriate feed administration. It is often useful to build a break into the feeding regimen to allow time for baths, physiotherapy, trips to X-ray etc. Overnight feeding may be used to supplement an inadequate oral intake and in an attempt to improve appetite. It also permits the patient to move freely during the day.

Elecrolyte status

Electrolyte imbalances are more often related to the patient's clinical condition and drug therapy than to the feed. Low sodium and electrolyte feeds are available but in practice it is more common to manipulate the volume of standard feeds or adjust drug therapy. The electrolyte content of the feeding regimen should be stated on the feeding chart.

Mineral status

Additional minerals may need to be given to patients with increased mineral losses, for example losses of magnesium and zinc in inflammatory bowel disease and other malabsorption states.

Nursing considerations

Close liaison with nursing colleagues is vital when initiating and in monitoring enteral nutrition. Commercially prepared feeds are preferable as they reduce demands on nursing time and minimize the risk of microbial contamination. Details of flushing procedures and the changing of giving sets etc. should be given on the feeding charts.

Cost

If possible, regimens should be tailored so that whole bottles/cans are used and feed does not have to be discarded. Good nursing care of enteral feeding tubes will also help control cost by reducing the need for frequent replacement.

Control of infusion rate

Bolus feeding

This technique involves the syringing of a volume of feed down a feeding tube at regular intervals. The relatively rapid administration of large volumes of feed is associated with an increased incidence of diarrhoea and abdominal discomfort when compared with continuous drip feeding. Today this traditional feeding technique is rarely employed; however it may still be useful as a method of administration in very restless or agitated patients who tend to disconnect feeding sets. No more than 250–300 ml should be given at any one time. The feed should be allowed to flow under gravity through an extension tube and given at room temperature.

Gravity feeding

Patients may be continuously drip fed by adjusting the roller clamp on the giving set. This involves calculating the drip rate, and adjusting it to administer the prescribed volume in a set time. This method of feed administration is more time-consuming and less accurate than pump assisted feeding.

Pump controlled feeding

A variety of enteral feeding pumps are currently available. These pumps are safe and simple to use provided appropriate training is given. They control the accuracy of flow delivery within ±10% of the expected volume (Torrance and Harrison 1988).

Administration reservoirs and sets

A range of feeding reservoirs and compatible giving sets are available. Some feeds may be administered directly from their container, thus the need to decant is avoided and the risk of microbial contamination is reduced. In order to avoid any risk of connecting an enteral feed to an intravenous line, the luer fitting on the giving set should be 'female'. The choice of administration set is primarily governed by cost, convenience and nurse preference.

Microbial aspects of tube feeding

The preparation of enteral feeds, whether hospital-made or commercially prepared, necessitates careful attention to aseptic technique. Pre-sterilized enteral feeds should be used (Bastow *et al* 1982) and should be administered via sterile giving sets using sterile water to dilute the feed if required. Any additives should be added aseptically. Hospital-made or powdered enteral feeds should be recon-

Table 1.44 Monitoring of tube feeding

Biochemistry	Fluid Balance	Nutritional Assessment	Nutritional Intake
Electrolytes	Fluid charts	Weight	Fluid charts
Urea	Weight	24 hr urine urea	Food charts
Liver function tests		Serum proteins	Diet history
Blood glucose		Anthropometry	Liaison with nursing staff
Urinalysis		Appearance	
Vitamin & mineral status		Mobility	

Table 1.45 Enteral feeding complications

Category	Feeding complications	Suggested remedies
Gastrointestinal side effects	Nausea and vomiting	**1** Anti-emetics **2** Nasoduodenal feeding **3** Reduce infusion rate **4** Reduce strength of feed
	Diarrhoea	**1** Anti-diarrhoeal agent e.g. codeine phosphate, loperamide **2** Discontinue broad spectrum antibiotics if possible **3** Reduce osmolarity of feed or if necessary strength **4** ? fibre containing feed **5** ? lactose-free feed **6** Reduce infusion rate (important if introducing feed into a starved gut) **7** Ensure good microbiological control (Anderton 1983)
	Constipation	**1** Appropriate enema, laxatives, bulking agents **2** Extra fluid **3** ? fibre containing feed **4** Keep patient mobile if possible
Aspiration (This feeding complication should be avoided rather than remedied by routine checking of tube position i.e. aspiration of gastric acid and testing with litmus paper)	Aspiration pneumonia	**1** Nasoduodenal or nasojejunal intubation **2** Wide bore tube and 4-hrly aspiration **3** Jejunostomy feeding if problem long term **4** Continuous pump controlled feeding **5** Prop patient's head up on pillows at night
	Large gastric aspirates	**1** Reduce volume of feed (to 20–30 ml/hr) with 4-hrly aspirates to check absorption **2** Parenteral nutrition may be required
Tube related	Tube blockage (regular flushing with sterile water should prevent this problem)	**1** Flushing with sterile water to which a pinch of sodium bicarbonate has been added **2** Avoid administering drugs via the feeding tube, if this is not possible ensure they are in a liquid form or very finely crushed. Flush tube before & after administration **3** Pancreatic enzyme solution has been shown to digest clots of feed (Marcuard and Perkins, 1988)
	NG tube withdrawal	**1** Tape tube securely to patient's face **2** Occasionally mits or splints have been used on children **3** Consider gastrostomy or jejunostomy placement if the problem is long term **4** Often the only answer is prompt replacement of the tube by medical staff
Metabolic	Hyperglycaemia	**1** Regular blood glucose monitoring and appropriate insulin therapy
	Abnormal liver function tests	**1** This is not usually due to the enteral feed (Richardson *et al* 1988) and will rarely require a reduction in feed volume or cessation of feeding

stituted with sterile equipment under very clean conditions (Anderton 1983). Giving sets and reservoirs should be discarded every 24 hours. For patients and their families involved in home enteral feeding, adequate training with appropriate verbal and written instruction should be provided (Anderton 1990).

Monitoring

Monitoring of nutritional support is important to detect potential feeding complications and in assessing the efficacy of the nutritional regimen. A number of studies have highlighted significant discrepancies between the volume of feed prescribed and that received (Abernathy *et al* 1989; Rees *et al* 1989; Robertson 1990). It is essential that this is closely monitored so nutrient intake can be accurately determined. Prior to feeding, and regularly throughout the feeding period, the patients should also undergo nutritional assessment (Table 1.44). The measurements made and their frequency of monitoring will depend on the individual patient, the patient's stability and the stage of feeding. Obviously, the critically ill patient will require much closer monitoring than the stable, home enterally fed patient.

Complications of tube feeding

Appropriate patient and equipment selection together with careful management should minimize feeding complications (Taylor 1989). Fortunately, serious complications (e.g. aspiration pneumonia) associated with enteral feeding are rare. Conversely, minor feeding complications are common; prompt recognition and, if necessary, treatment is an essential component of patient management.

The following points should be considered:

1 Patient selection (e.g. gastric emptying must be established in a patient before commencing ng feeding to help prevent vomiting).

2 Feeding route (e.g. gastrostomy feeding will prevent problems with tube withdrawal in long term feed patients).

3 Feeding equipment (e.g. tubes should be flushed regularly to help prevent blockage. Using fine bore tubes whenever possible will improve patient comfort and tolerance and reduce the risk of nasal necrosis and oesophageal erosions.

4 Feed composition (e.g. the selection of a peptide-based feed for a patient with malabsorption may minimize gastrointestinal losses and prevent abdominal distension). Hyperosmolar feeds should be introduced gradually to improve tolerance.

5 Regimen (e.g. reduced rate and gradual introduction in post-operative jejunostomy feeding will reduce the incidence of diarrhoea).

6 Monitoring (e.g. regular blood glucose monitoring and appropriate insulin therapy for glucose intolerant patients to reduce problems of hyperglycaemia).

Many dietetic departments have written enteral feeding policies which cover these points. It is important that dietitians liaise closely with nursing staff caring for the enterally fed patients, and that nurses are appropriately trained in using enteral feeding equipment.

If feeding complications do occur, prompt and appropriate action is essential (see Table 1.45). If possible, reduction of the flow rate or the strength of the feed should be avoided as this is likely to result in negative nitrogen/energy balance.

Home enteral nutrition

Home enteral feeding is an expanding field, with over 1300 new patients in the UK in 1990, and has been shown to improve quality of life in a variety of conditions. Primary indications include head and neck cancer (Campos *et al* 1990), cystic fibrosis (Moore *et al* 1986) and inflammatory bowel disease (Russell 1985; Blair *et al* 1986).

'Successful home enteral feeding is the result of careful co-ordination of a number of details, including comprehensive patient education, delivery of equipment and supplies and provision of follow-up nutrition care' (Skipper 1990). These aspects of care vary in different Health Authorities and the Parenteral and Enteral Nutrition Group of the British Dietetic Association has set up a home enteral feeding register to monitor this. During 1990, approximately 700 patients were reported as being discharged home on enteral feeding. It is important that dietitians throughout the U.K. register their patients in order to collate national data. A number of authors have also pointed out the importance of psychosocial aspects of home enteral feeding (Gulledge *et al* 1987; Heaphey 1987; Reeves-Garcia and Heyman 1988).

At present a variety of feeds are available on prescription, however the feeding equipment is not and must be financed by hospital or community budgets. A number of companies have recognized that home enteral feeding is an expanding market and provide a variety of services including training, delivery of feeds and equipment and servicing of pumps.

The aim of home enteral feeding should be to optimize the patient's quality of life whilst minimizing the inconvenience caused by the feeding regimen. If appropriate, the patient should be fed overnight to allow freedom of movement during the day (Bastow *et al* 1985) although portable feeding systems are available.

Discontinuing tube feeding

Wherever possible, nutritional support should be phased out gradually, once normal eating has resumed or improved. To ensure that an adequate energy and nitrogen intake is maintained, close dietetic involvement is essential. Patients in whom tube feeding is discontinued may benefit from sip feeding in addition to their normal diet until an adequate diet is taken.

Many patients leaving hospital are still on an inadequate

intake and regular follow-up at outpatient clinics or in the community is advisable wherever possible.

Further reading

Allison SP (1987) Nutrition support: efficacy versus cost. *Nutrition International* 3(1), 19–24.

Grimble G, Payne-James J, Rees and Silk D (1988) Physiology of digestion and absorption of enteral diets. *Intensive Therapy and Clinical Monitoring* **Dec**, 267–74.

Grimble G, Payne-James JJ, Rees R and Silk DBA (1989) Enteral nutrition: novel substrates. *Intensive Therapy and Clinical Monitoring* **Feb**, 51–7.

Hessov I (1988) Oral feeding after uncomplicated abdominal surgery. *Brit J Clin Pract* **42** (Suppl 63), 75–9.

Lacey JM and Wilmore DW (1990) Is glutamine a conditionally essential amino acid? *Nutrition Reviews* **48**(8), 297–308.

O'Sullivan KR and Mathias PM (1990) Analysis of selenium content in commercial dietetic products. *Eur J Clin Nutr* **44**, 235–40.

Payne-James J and Silk DBA (1990) Clinical nutrition support better control and assessment are needed. *Br Med J* **301**, 1–2.

Paediatric Group and PENG (1988) Paediatric enteral feeding solutions and systems. British Dietetic Association, Birmingham.

Pesola GE, Hogg JE, Yonnios T, MacConell RE and Carlon GC (1989). Isotonic nasogastric tube feedings: do they cause diarrhoea? *Crit Care Med* **17**(11), 1151–5.

Richardson RA and Shenkin A (1989) Enteral nutrition. *Current Opinion in Gastroenterology* **5**, 295–300.

Rombeau JL and Barot LR (1981) Enteral nutritional therapy. *Surg Clin North Am* **61**, 605–20.

Souba WW, Klimberg S, Plumley DA, Salloum RM, Flynn TC, Bland KI and Copeland EM (1990) The role of glutamine in maintaining a healthy gut and supporting the metabolic response to injury and infection. *J Surg Res* **48**, 383–99.

References

Abernathy GB, Heizer WD, Holcombe BJ, Raasch RH, Schlegel KE and Hak LJ (1989) Efficacy of tube feeding in supplying energy requirements of hospitalized patients. *J Parent Ent Nutr* **13**(4), 387–91.

Adibi SA (1990) Physiological significance and practical application of peptide transport in human intestine. *Nutrition* **6**(3), 267–8.

Allison SP (1988) Panel discussion. *Br J Clin Prac* **42**(12), Symposium Supplement 63, 69–72.

Anderton A (1983) Microbiological aspects of the preparation and administration of nasogastric and nasoenteric tube feeds in hospitals: a review. *Hum Nutr: Appl Nutr* **37A**, 426–40.

Anderton A (1990) Microbial aspects of home enteral nutrition. *J Hum Nutr Diet* **3**(6), 403–412.

ASPEN Board of Directors (1987) Guidelines for the use of enteral nutrition in the adult patient. *J Parent Ent Nutr* **11**(5), 435–9.

Bastow MD, Greaves P and Allison SP (1982) Microbial contamination of enteral feeds. *Hum Nutr: Appl Nutr* **36**(3), 213–17.

Bastow MD, Rawlings J and Allison SP (1983) Benefits of supplementary tube feeding after fractured neck of femur: a randomized controlled trial. *Br Med J* **287**, 1589–92.

Bastow D, Rawlings J and Allison SP (1985) Overnight nasogastric tube feeding. *Clin Nutr* **4**(1), 7–11.

Bistrian BR, Blackburn GL, Hallowell E and Heddle R (1974) Protein status of general surgical patients. *J Am Med Assoc* **230**, 858–60.

Bistrian BR, Blackburn GL, Vitale J, Cochran D and Naylor J (1976) Prevelence of malnutrition in general medical patients. *J Am Med Assoc* **235**, 1567–70.

Blair GK, Yaman M and Wossan DE (1986) Preoperative home elemental enteral nutrition in complicated Crohn's disease. *J Pediatr Surg* **21**(9), 769–71.

Bolton J, Shanon L, Smith V, Abbott R, Bell SJ, Stubbs L and Slevin ML (1990) Comparison of short-term and long-term palatability of six commercially available oral supplements. *J Hum Nutr Diet* **3**(5), 317–21.

Buzby GP, Knox LS, Crosby LO, Eisenberg JM, Hoakenson CM, McNeal GE, Page CP, Peterson OL, Reinhardt GF and Wilford WO (1988) Study protocol: a randomized clinical trial of total parenteral nutrition in malnourished surgical patients. *Am J Clin Nutr* **47**, 366–81.

Campos ACL, Butters M and Meguid HM (1990) Home enteral nutrition via gastrostomy in advanced head and neck cancer patients. *Head Neck Surg* **12**(2), 137–42.

Craft IL, Geddes D, Hyde CW, Wise IJ and Matthews DM (1968) Absorption and malabsorption of glycine and glycine peptides in man. *Gut* **9**, 425–37.

Delany HM and Lundine P (1988) Pros and cons of needle catheter jejunostomy. *Nutrition* **4**(2) 119–24.

Dunn EL, Moore EE and Bolus RW (1980) Immediate postoperative feeding following massive abdominal trauma – the catheter jejunostomy. *J Parent Ent Nutr* **4**(4), 393–5.

Ek AC, Larsson S, von Schenck H, Thorslund S, Unosson M and Bjurul P (1990) The correlation between energy, malnutrition and clinical outcome in an elderly hospital population. *Clin Nutr* **9**, 185–9.

Fletcher JP and Little JM (1986) A comparison of parenteral nutrition and early postoperative enteral feeding on the nitrogen balance after surgery. *Surgery* **100**(1), 21–4.

Gulledge AD, Sharp JW, Matarese LE, O'Neill and Steiger ME (1987) Psychosocial issues of home parenteral and enteral nutrition. *Nutr Clin Pract* **2**(5), 183–94.

Hamaoui E, Lefowitz R, Olender L, Kransnopolsky-Levine E, Favale M, Webb H and Hoover E (1990) Enteral nutrition in the early postoperative period: a new semi-elemental formula versus total parenteral nutrition. *J Parent Ent Nutr* **14**(5), 501–507.

Hart GK and Dobb GJ (1988) Effect of a fecal bulking agent on diarrhoea during enteral feeding in the critically ill. *J Parent Ent Nutr* **12**(5), 465–8.

Heaphey LL (1987) Psychosocial aspects of nutrition support: some observations. *Nutr Clin Pract* **2**(5), 181–2.

Hill GL, Blacket RL, Pickford L, Burkinshaw L, Young GA, Warren JV, Schorah CJ and Morgan DB (1977) Malnutrition in surgical patients. *Lancet* **i**, 689–92.

Hollands MJ, Fletcher JP and Young J (1989) Percutaneous feeding gastrostomy. *Med J Aust* **151**(6), 330–31.

Hull S (1985) Enteral versus parenteral nutrition support–rationale for increased use of enteral feeding. *Z Gastroenterologie* (Suppl) **23**, 55–63.

Keohane PP, Attrill H, Love M, Frost P and Silk DBA (1984) Relation between osmolality of diet and gastrointestinal side effects in enteral nutrition. *Br Med J* **288**, 678–80.

Larsson J, Unosson M, Ek AC, Nilsson L, Thorslund S and Bjurult (1990) Effect of dietary supplement on nutritional status and clinical outcome in 501 geriatric patients – a randomized study. *Clin Nutr* **9**, 179–84.

Marcuard SP and Perkins AM (1988) Clogging of feeding tubes. *J Parent Ent Nutr* **12**(4), 403–405.

McIntyre PB, Fitchew M and Lennard-Jones JE (1986) Patients with a high jejunostomy do not need a special diet. *Gastroenterology* **91**, 25–33.

Moore MC, Greene HL, Donald WD and Dunn GD (1986) Enteral tube feeding as adjunct therapy in malnourished patient with cystic fibrosis: a clinical study and literature review. *Am J Clin Nutr* **44**(1), 33–41.

Moran BJ, Taylor MB and Johnson CD (1990) Percutaneous endoscopic gastrostomy. *Br J Surg* **77**, 858–62.

Morris R, Hart K, Smith V, Shannon L, Bolton J, Abbott R, Alleyne M,

Plant H and Slevin ML (1990) A comparison of the energy supplements Polycal and Duocal in cancer patients. *J Hum Nutr Diet* **3**(3), 171–6.

Mullen JL, Buzby GP, Matthews DC, Smale BF and Rosato EF (1980) Reduction of operative morbidity and mortality by combined preoperative and postoperative nutrition support. *Ann Surg* **192**(5), 604–613.

Patil DH, Grimble GK, Keohane PP, Atrill PP, Love HM and Silk DB (1985) Do fibre containing enteral diets have advantages over existing low residue diets? *Clin Nutr* **4**(2), 67–71.

Payne-James JJ, Rees RGP, Grimble GK and Silk DBA (1988) Enteral nutrition: clinical application. *Intensive Therapy and Clinical Monitoring* **Nov**, 239–46.

Parenteral and Enteral Nutrition Group (1988) The management of nutritionally compromised patients in hospital – a discussion paper. British Dietetic Association, Birmingham.

Ponsky JL and Gauderer MW (1989) Percutaneous endoscopic gastrostomy: indications, limitations, techniques and results. *Wld J Surg* **13**(2), 165–70.

Rees RG, Keohane PP, Grimble GK, Frost PG, Attrill H and Silk DB (1986) Elemental diet administered nasogastrically without starter regimens to patients with inflammatory bowel disease. *J Parent Ent Nutr* **10**(3), 258–62.

Rees RGP, Cooper TM, Beetham R, Frost PG and Silk DBA (1989) Influence of energy and nitrogen contents of enteral diets on nitrogen balance: a double blind prospective controlled clinical trial. *Gut* **30**, 123–9.

Reeves-Garcia J and Heyman MB (1988) Survey of complications of paediatric home enteral tube feedings and discussion of developmental and psychosocial issues. *Nutrition* **4**(5), 375–9.

Richardson RA, Garden OJ and Shenkin A (1988) Enteral nutrition and liver function test abnormalities. *J Hum Nutr Diet* **1**(4), 227–32.

Robertson SM (1990) How much of the prescribed volume of enteral feed does the hospitalized patient actually receive? *J Hum Nutr Diet* **3**, 165–70.

Russell CA (1984) Fine needle jejunostomy feeding in patients with oesophageal or gastric carcinoma. *Appl Nutr* **11**, 1–7.

Russell RI (1985) Home enteral nutrition with formula diets. *Z Gastroenterol* **23**(Suppl), 94–7.

Shanbhogue LK, Bistrain BR and Blackburn GL (1986) Trends in enteral nutrition in the surgical patient. *J R Coll Surg Edinb* **31**(5), 267–73.

Shike M, Berner YN, Gerdes H, Gerold FP, Bloch A, Sessions R and Strong E (1989) Percutaneous endoscopic gastrostomy and jejunostomy for long-term feeding in patients with cancer of the head and neck. *Otolaryngology – Head and Neck Surgery* **101**(5), 549–54.

Silk DBA, Chung YC, Berger K, Conley K, Beigler M, Sleigenger MH, Spiller GA and Kim YS (1979) Comparison of oral feeding of peptide and amino acid meals in normal human subjects *Gut* **20**, 291–9.

Silk DBA, Fairclough PD, Clark ML, Hegarty JE, Marrs TC, Addison JM, Burston D, Clegg KM and Matthews DM (1980) Use of a peptide rather than free amino acid nitrogen source in chemically defined 'elemental' diets. *J Parent Ent Nutr* **4**(6), 548–53.

Silk DB (1989) Fibre and enteral nutrition. *Gut* **30**(2), 246–64.

Skipper A (1990) A survey of the role of the dietitian in preparing patients for home enteral feeding. *J Am Diet Assoc* **84**, 330–35.

Starker PM, Lasala PA, Askanazi J, Todd G, Hensle TW and Kinney JM (1986) The influence of preoperative TPN upon morbidity and mortality. *Surg Gynecol Obstet* **162**(6), 569–74.

Strickland GF and Greene FL (1986) Needle catheter jejunostomy for postoperative nutritional support. *South Med J* **79**(11), 1389–92.

Taylor SJ (1988) A guide to nasogastric feeding. *Professional Nurse* **August**, 439–42.

Taylor SJ (1989) Preventing complications in enteral feeding. *Professional Nurse*, **Feb**, 247–9.

Torrance AD and Harrison C (1988) A controlled study of the performance of five enteral feeding pumps. *J Hum Nutr Diet* **1**(1), 1–7.

Westfall SH, Andrus CH and Naunhheim KS (1990) Reproducible, safe jejunostomy replacement technique by a percutaneous endoscopic method. *Am Surg* **56**(3), 141–3.

1.14 Enteral feeding in paediatric patients

1.14.1 Basic considerations in paediatric patients

Nutritional support in children differs from that in adults in a number of ways. These are examined below.

Nutritional requirements

In paediatrics, estimations of energy and nutrient requirements have to allow for normal growth as well as all other metabolic needs (including any metabolic consequences of illness or injury) (Taylor *et al* 1987). This means that the nutritional requirements of a child can vary widely with age and circumstances and no single standard commercially available feed is able to meet the nutritional needs of all paediatric patients.

Nutritional problems are most likely to occur in infancy. Infants and children have fewer body reserves of all nutrients, particularly energy, than adults. For example, an adult has sufficient energy stores for approximately 90 days, a full-term infant for about 32 days but a pre-term infant may only have sufficient for 5 days (Heird 1977). If an infant or child is unable to feed orally, it is more critical for them that nutritional support is started quickly.

Interruption of normal feeding development

Normally during infancy and early childhood, new feeding skills are being learnt and developed. If an infant or young child is tube fed for a period of time during this critical period and no oral food or drink is consumed, it may adversely affect and delay normal feeding behaviour. In paediatrics it is therefore vital, wherever possible, that oral consumption at some level is encouraged.

Effects of malnutrition

In paediatrics, poor nutritional support may not only result in growth failure and inadequate growth, it may result in immunodeficiency, apathetic and withdrawn behaviour, widespread gastrointestinal dysfunction, reduced muscle power and myocardial dysfunction (Booth and MacDonald 1990).

1.14.2 Indications for enteral feeding in paediatric patients

There are five broad indications for enteral feeding in children. These are discussed below.

Inadequate energy and nutrient intake

Anorexia associated with chronic illness, or inability to eat adequate quantities of food, are common problems in paediatrics. Examples of patients requiring enteral feeding include infants with breathing difficulties associated with respiratory and cardiac disorders, infants and children with oro-facial malformations and oral-motor incoordination, where normal sucking and chewing mechanisms are impaired (Stapleford 1989). Children with degenerative disease who can no longer eat or drink, and children with chronic illnesses such as malignancy, cystic fibrosis and renal disease are also frequently enterally fed.

Increased nutritional requirements

Many infants and children with chronic or severe illnesses have a need for extra nutrients, particularly energy, but due to the anorexia associated with their disease are unable to meet their nutritional requirements by normal eating. Examples of such disease states include liver disease, cystic fibrosis and congenital heart disease. However, tube feeding is normally only initiated when a child struggles to gain weight and grow adequately on an oral diet. In many cases, the feed is given as an overnight continuous infusion so that the child can eat 'normally' during the day, and it will supply a varying percentage of the patient's nutritional needs depending on the child's clinical condition and overall appetite. It is often stated that overnight feeding will not decrease the appetite during the day (Stapleford 1989), but this still remains to be established in paediatrics.

Disease or injury to the oesophagus

Examples in paediatrics include oesophageal injury after ingestion of caustic soda chemicals or tracheo-oesophageal fistula.

Gastrointestinal disease

Infants and children with a very short bowel following resection may absorb nutrients more efficiently if their nutrition is given as continuous enteral feed rather than as intermittent bottle feeds. In addition, an elemental diet may be used in Crohn's disease to treat growth failure and induce remission of the disease. Elemental feeds are frequently given via a tube rather than orally due to the unpalatability of these feeds. Other indications for enteral feeding are children with severe oesophageal reflux, gastro-intestinal malformation and or malabsorption.

Metabolic disease

Infants and children with Type 1 glycogen storage disease need a continuous enteral feed overnight to avoid hypoglycaemia.

1.14.3 Choice of feed

The choice of feed is dependent upon the age, weight, activity and clinical condition of the child. There are four main categories of feeds: whole protein, protein hydrolysate, modular and elemental. Whole protein feeds are used primarily for children with a normal gut while protein hydrolysate, modular and elemental feeds are used for children with defective bowel function.

Whole protein feeds for patients with a normal gut

0–12 months

Infants less than four months of age can be given either expressed breast milk or an infant formula milk via the tube at a normal fluid requirement volume of 150–200 ml/kg. However, fat from breast milk may adhere to the inside of the tube and thereby reduce the energy content of the feed.

If infants are failing to thrive while taking maximum volumes of infant formula feed, *or* are over the age of four months, additional energy supplements need to be added. These are usually added in the form of glucose polymers or a fat emulsion, or a combination of both.

Initially, glucose polymers such as Maxijul (SHS), Polycal (Cow & Gate Nutricia) or Caloreen (Clintec) should be gradually introduced in 1 g/100 ml increments up to a maximum total carbohydrate feed concentration of 12 g/100 ml. (Normal infant milk carbohydrate concentration is 7 g/100 ml). An extra 5 g/100 ml of added carbohydrate will provide an additional 19 kcal/100 ml. Higher carbohydrate concentrations may cause osmotic diarrhoea. If further energy supplementation is required, a fat emulsion may also be added in 1.0 g/100 ml increments to a maximum total feed fat concentration of 5 g/100 ml. (Normal infant milk fat concentration is 3.5 g/100 ml.) An extra 1.5 g fat/100 ml will provide an additional 14 kcal/100 ml. A 50% long chain fat emulsion, such as Calogen (Scientific Hospital Supplies), is used in preference to a medium-chain triglyceride (MCT) emulsion (Booth and MacDonald 1990). MCT contains no essential fatty acids, will increase the osmolality of the feed and is associated with dicarboxylic aciduria (Henderson and Dear 1986). No more than 50% of the total energy should be provided by fat.

1–5 years (8–20 kg)

Until recently, there has been no whole protein standard enteral feed whose nutritional composition has been ideally suited to meet the nutritional needs of this age group; adult feeds are generally high in protein, sodium, potassium and have an inappropriate vitamin and mineral profile. Paediatric dietitians have either had to devise 'home-brew' feeds or modify the protein and electrolyte content of existing adult feeds by diluting them with water by up to 30% depending on the original feed composition, and making up the energy deficit by adding additional glucose polymer and a fat emulsion to produce a feed providing 100 kcal/100 ml. Neither the 'home-brew' or modified adult feed is ideal. Both carry a risk of microbiological contamination from the use of non-sterile ingredients and from the feed 'handlers' and utensils. Mistakes may occur both during the calculation and preparation of such feeds and both take additional time to prepare.

In 1988, the Paediatric Group and the Parenteral and Enteral Nutrition Group (PEN Group) of the BDA published a report giving recommendations for the composition of an enteral feed suitable for this age group. Partly as a result of this report there are now two paediatric enteral feeds which are available on prescription under ACBS listing for a number of indications. The composition of both these feeds compared with the Paediatric and PEN Group recommendations are given in Table 1.46.

Over 5 years (over 20 kg)

Any commercially available standard enteral feed is suitable given in appropriate volumes. However, care needs to be exercised when using high energy feeds for older children as these products are high in protein. They may be required for overnight enteral feeds for some older paediatric patients who need a high energy feed in a small volume. If these feeds are used, it is important to monitor overall protein intake to ensure this is not excessive.

Feeding paediatric patients with defective bowel function

Protein hydrolysate feeds

The majority of infants and young patients with protracted diarrhoea, short bowel syndrome, cow's milk protein enteropathy who need a tube feed can usually tolerate a commercially available standard protein-hydrolysate feed such as Nutramigen (Mead Johnson), Pregestimil (Mead Johnson), PeptiJunior (Cow & Gate Nutricia) or Pepdite 0–2 (SHS). If additional energy supplementation is needed, glucose polymers and an LCT fat emulsion, such as Calogen (SHS), is used as previously described but particular care is needed when adding extra carbohydrate to Nutramigen and Pregestimil as these are already high

Table 1.46 Composition of paediatric enteral feeds for the 1–5 year old group

		Paediatric Group and PEN Group Recommendations for the composition of a feed	Nutrison Paediatric	Paediasure
			Cow and Gate Nutricia per 100 ml	Ross Laboratories per 100 ml
Energy		100	101	100
Protein	g	2.6	2.7	3.0
Fat	g	4	4.5	5.0
Carbohydrate	g	14	12.2	11.0
Sodium	mmol	2.5	2.5	2.0
Potassium	mmol	2.5	2.1	3.3
Calcium	mg	55	80	98
Phosphorus	mmol	1.7	1.9	2.6
Magnesium	mg		15	20
Iron	mg	0.7	1.0	1.4
Zinc	mg	0.7	1.0	1.2
Manganese	mg	0.1	0.1	2.3
Selenium	μg	4	—	2.3
Molybdenum	μg	5	—	3.6
Copper	mg	0.1	0.1	0.1
Iodine	μg	6	6	9.6
Chromium	μg	4	—	3.0
Vitamin A	μg	35	40	79
Vitamin D	μg	0.7	1.0	1.28
Vitamin E	mg	0.4	0.6	2.3
Vitamin K	μg	2	2.0	3.8
Vitamin C	mg	3	4.5	10
Vitamin B1	mg	0.15	0.2	0.3
Vitamin B2	mg	0.2	0.2	0.2
Nicotinic Acid	mg	0.8	0.9	1.7
Vitamin B6	mg	0.09	0.1	0.3
Folic Acid	μg	12	15	37
Vitamin B12	μg	0.2	0.2	0.6
Pantothenic Acid	mg	0.3	0.3	1.0
Inositol	mg	15	—	8
Biotin	μg	6	7.0	32
Choline	mg	15	—	30

carbohydrate feeds (9.0 g/100 ml) and carbohydrate intolerance may be a problem.

Modular feeds

If protein hydrolysate feeds are not tolerated, it may be necessary to use a modular feed based on separate protein, fat, carbohydrate, vitamin and mineral components so the individual ingredients and their quantities used can be adapted to meet the specific needs and tolerances of an infant and child. The most common protein source used is the product Comminuted Chicken (Cow and Gate Nutricia) which is simply finely ground chicken meat in water. A variety of carbohydrates may be used, including glucose polymers, sucrose and glucose and either a long chain fat emulsion, such as Calogen (SHS), or a medium chain fat emulsion such as Liquigen (SHS), is added for the fat source. A comprehensive mineral and vitamin supplement is also given. The chief advantage of modular feeds is their flexibility; the ingredients can be changed or adjusted relatively easily. However, they are complex, require detailed calculations and accurate weighing and measuring facilities, and mistakes can be made in their calculation and preparation; it also takes several days to build the feed up to full strength. In addition, if Comminuted Chicken is given via a continuous enteral feed, the chicken fibres have a tendency to block the tube. To avoid this, Comminuted Chicken can be thickened with 0.5% Nestargel (Nestlé) but even with this adjustment it still will not pass through a size 6 Fg PVC Portex or a Silk polyurethane tube.

Elemental feeds

Elemental diets are used in children with Crohn's disease, multiple food intolerance, short gut syndrome and other malabsorption syndromes. With the exception of one infant preparation, Neocate (SHS), elemental preparations based on amino acids have been formulated for adults and are generally high in protein and different products vary widely in their content of electrolytes, vitamins and minerals. The elemental and semi-elemental feeds such as Elemental 028 (SHS) and Flexical (Bristol Myers) contain less protein than other similar feeds and have acceptable electrolyte, vitamin and mineral profiles, but these need matching to the specific nutritional requirements of the individual child being fed. Elemental 028 has a very high osmolality and would need careful introduction into a child's diet. These preparations are not palatable and usually need to be given via a nasogastric tube.

1.14.4 Feeding equipment

The administration enteral feeds which are given continuously should be controlled by an enteral feeding pump. Desirable features of a pump suitable for paediatrics include accuracy, a reliable alarm system and the delivery of feeds by 1 ml increments up to 50 ml/hour and thereafter in 5 ml or 10 ml increments. Ideally they should also be lightweight, portable and easy to use, but it is difficult to find all these features in any one pump. Until the ideal pump is developed, safety features and reliability must take top priority in paediatrics.

Either PVC or polyurethane nasogastric tubes are used for feeding. PVC tubes are used for short term feeding for children with swallowing difficulties and those who vomit repeatedly (e.g. patients on chemotherapy or with reflux). Polyurethane tubes are used for long term feeding.

1.14.5 Home enteral feeding

Many paediatric patients requiring enteral feeding are fed long term and parents need to be competent in all aspects of enteral feeding. Particular emphasis should be placed upon safety during parent training. The parents' teaching programme should include familiarization with the feeding equipment, safety aspects, any preparation of special feeds and a discussion on any problems they are likely to face at home. The child also needs to be psychologically prepared for enteral feeding and dolls and teddies with enteral tubes attached, photographs of other children receiving enteral feeds, colouring booklets, reward stickers and certificates are all helpful in making enteral feeding a more acceptable process (Holden 1990).

Where possible, the timing of enteral feeds is adjusted to meet the lifestyle of the patient, and feeds are frequently given overnight only. Older children are taught and encouraged to pass their own nasogastric tube and some prefer to remove this before going to school and repass it every night. There is increasing use of gastrostomy feeding in long term patients.

In a recent survey of 35 patients on home enteral feeding, no major complications such as aspiration, or entanglement in the tubing were found (Holden *et al* 1991). However, sleep disturbance particularly related to nocturia was common and vomiting, osmotic diarrhoea, gastro-oesophageal reflux and obesity can occur (Booth and MacDonald 1990). It is essential that good hospital and community support is provided for infants and children on home enteral feeding and that there is regular monitoring of growth, nutritional intake and food intolerance.

References

Booth IW and MacDonald A (1990) Nutrition. In *Paediatric Vade Mecum*, Insley JA (Ed) Edward Arnold, London.

Heird WC (1977) Feeding the premature infant human milk or artificial formula. *Am J Dis Childh* **131**, 468–9.

Henderson MJ and Dear PRF (1986) Dicarboxylic aciduria and medium chain triglyceride supplemented milk. *Arch Dis Childh* **61**, 610.

Holden C. (1990) Home enteral feeding. *Paediatric Nursing* **2**, 14–16.

Holden C, Puntis J, Charlton C and Booth IW (1991) Home enteral nutrition acceptability and safety. *Arch Dis Childh* **66**, 148–51.

Stapleford P (1989) Formula feeding. *Paediatric Nursing* **1**, 14–16.

Taylor C, Nunn T, Rangecroft L (1987) Parenteral nutrition for infants and children. In *Enteral and Parenteral Nutrition*, Grant A and Todd E (Eds) pp. 168–90. Blackwell Scientific Publications, Oxford.

1.15 Parenteral nutrition

Total parenteral nutrition (TPN) is a method of providing nutritional support to an individual whose gastrointestinal tract is either not functioning or is inaccessible. Nutrients are delivered directly into the circulatory system via a central venous catheter or via the peripheral veins. Other names for TPN are intravenous feeding (IV feeding) and, less commonly, intravenous hyperalimentation (IVH).

Total Parenteral Nutrition should be considered when:

- all methods and routes of enteral nutrition have been considered and are not deemed to be appropriate;
- complete rest of the gastrointestinal tract is required (e.g. for small bowel fistulae, acute exacerbation of inflammatory bowel disease, post small bowel surgery, anastomotic breakdown);
- the gastrointestinal tract is inaccessible, for example because of oesophageal stricture (when it is *not possible* to insert an enteral feeding tube);
- total nutrient requirements cannot be met using the enteral route due to limited absorption within the gastrointestinal tract (e.g. major burns, premature infants, following bone marrow transplantation, radiation enteritis, short bowel syndrome).

Parenteral nutrition support may be needed for the duration of an acute illness. In some chronic disease states such as short gut syndrome (caused by extensive small bowel resection), small bowel fistulae, some AIDS and cancer sufferers, TPN may be needed over a period of months or even for life. These patients will be taught how to care for and administer their own TPN at home (with considerable support and monitoring from the hospital).

Although TPN is an essential and potentially life-saving therapy, it is expensive and carries life-threatening complications (e.g. sepsis and metabolic disorders) so must be monitored and administered correctly. In evaluating the indications for TPN, it must be remembered that TPN rarely treats the underlying disease but may influence one of the secondary effects of that disease – malnutrition. Regardless of the underlying disease process, the decision to initiate TPN should be made on:

- the anticipated duration of inability to access the gut and/or absorb nutrients enterally;
- the degree of malnutrition;
- the degree of metabolic stress;
- the predicted outcome (prognosis) for the patient.

1.15.1 Central or peripheral feeding?

Once it has been established that the patient needs nutritional support (Fig. 1.7) and that the enteral route is not available then the decision between central and peripheral feeding should be made.

In the early days of TPN, glucose was used as the main non-protein energy source, leading to hypertonic feeding solutions (see Table 1.47). These solutions had to be administered via a central venous catheter in order to effect rapid dilution and reduce the risk of venotoxicity. IV fat emulsions are now available and used as a dense energy source. These emulsions are isotonic and therefore reduce the overall osmolality of the TPN solution (when administered with it). A less concentrated glucose source is therefore needed to provide additional energy which will reduce the osmolality of the TPN solutions. These changes have led to a number of centres investigating the peripheral route as an alternative to central vein catheterization for administering TPN.

When deciding on the optimal route for providing TPN the estimated duration of feeding should be assessed along with the individual's nutrient requirements. If TPN is likely to be needed for less than seven days (e.g. non complicated post-operative paralytic ileus) then peripheral feeding could be considered (at least in the early stages) until the patient's clinical progress and outcome can be assessed. If it is clear that the patient may need TPN for more than seven days (e.g. fistula), or their nutritional requirements are high (e.g. severe burns), most centres would insert a central feeding catheter; others have demonstrated the efficient management of peripheral nutrition as their standard route of parenteral feeding.

In hospitals where a multidisciplinary nutrition team is established with experienced clinicians available to insert the central feeding catheters, and designated nurses to

Table 1.47 Energy and osmolality of fats and glucose

		m.osmol/l	kcal/l
Fat emulsion	10%	250	1000 kcal/l
	20%	300	2000 kcal/l
Glucose	5%	277	200 kcal/l
	10%	555	400 kcal/l
	20%	1110	800 kcal/l
	50%	2775	2000 kcal/l

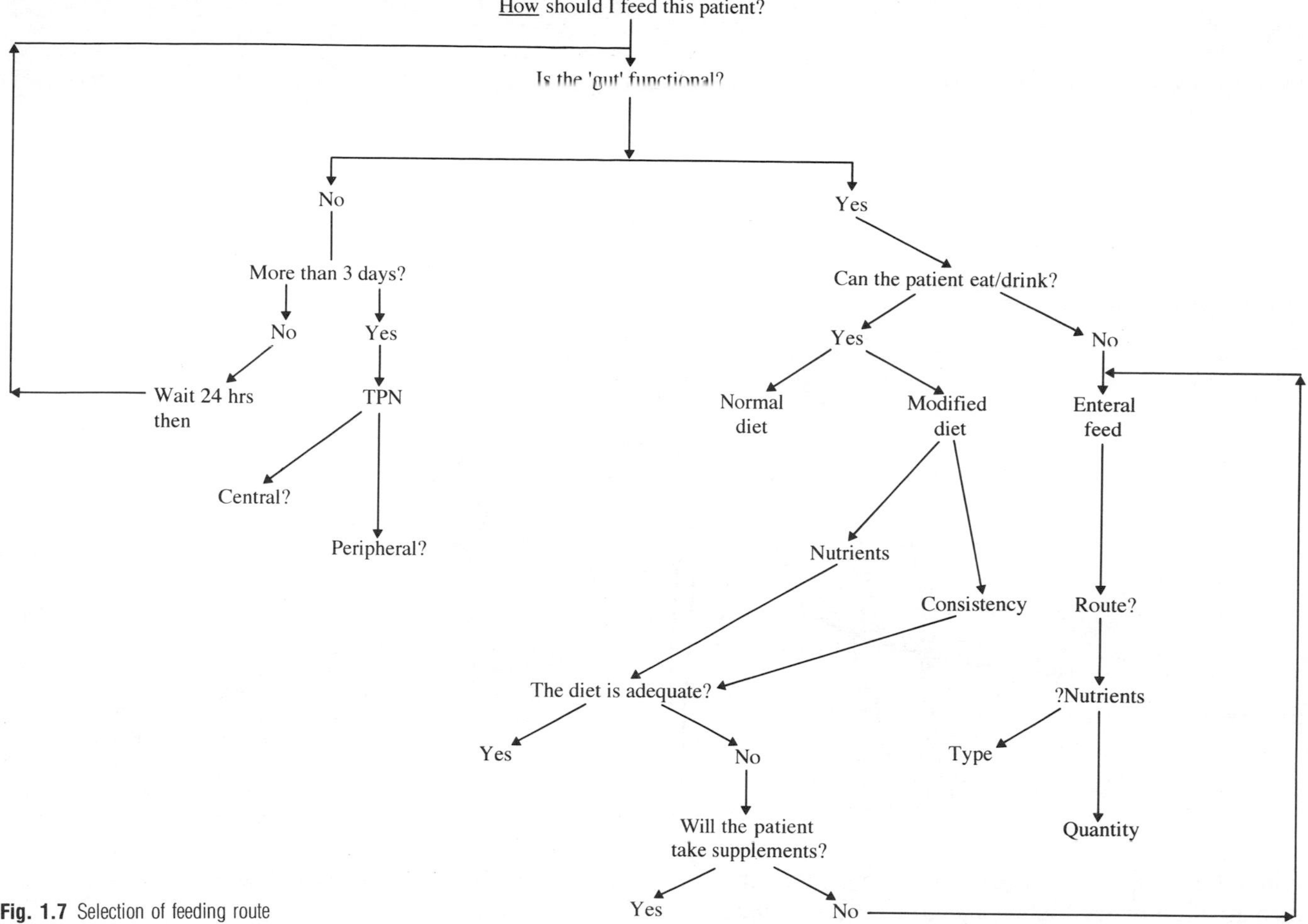

Fig. 1.7 Selection of feeding route

care for the catheters then the complications associated with central line feeding (Table 1.48) can be greatly reduced (Shanbhogue *et al* 1987).

1.15.2 Access

Establishing and maintaining suitable access to the circulation is essential for the successful management of TPN. This aspect, although of interest to dietitians (who should be aware of the procedures, practices and complications), is not their immediate concern and is not discussed in detail here (see Tweedle 1982; Silk 1983; Grant and Todd 1987).

Central vein cannulation is currently the most commonly used route for administering TPN. The central feeding catheter should be inserted aseptically via the subclavian

Table 1.48 Advantages and disadvantages of peripheral or central vein feeding

	Advantages	Disadvantages
Central vein feeding	No venotoxicity. Flexibility of nutrient content (fluid, electrolytes concentration) Once catheter is inserted no patient discomfort (catheter can remain *in situ* for months)	Needs a skilled clinician to insert catheter (complications include pneumothorax, haemothorax, arterial puncture, air embolus). High risk of catheter-related sepsis. High cost due to highly skilled manpower needed, solutions, catheters, X-ray.
Peripheral vein feeding	'Simple' insertion of peripheral catheter by junior doctor. Low risk of catheter-related sepsis. Less expensive. Low risk of complications of insertion.	Increased risk of occlusion phlebitis due to hypertonic solutions requiring regular resiting of catheter. Patient arm immobilized. Less flexibility of nutrients (requires volume >2500 ml). Extravasation can cause severe tissue necrosis and subsequent scarring. Requires continuous infusion.

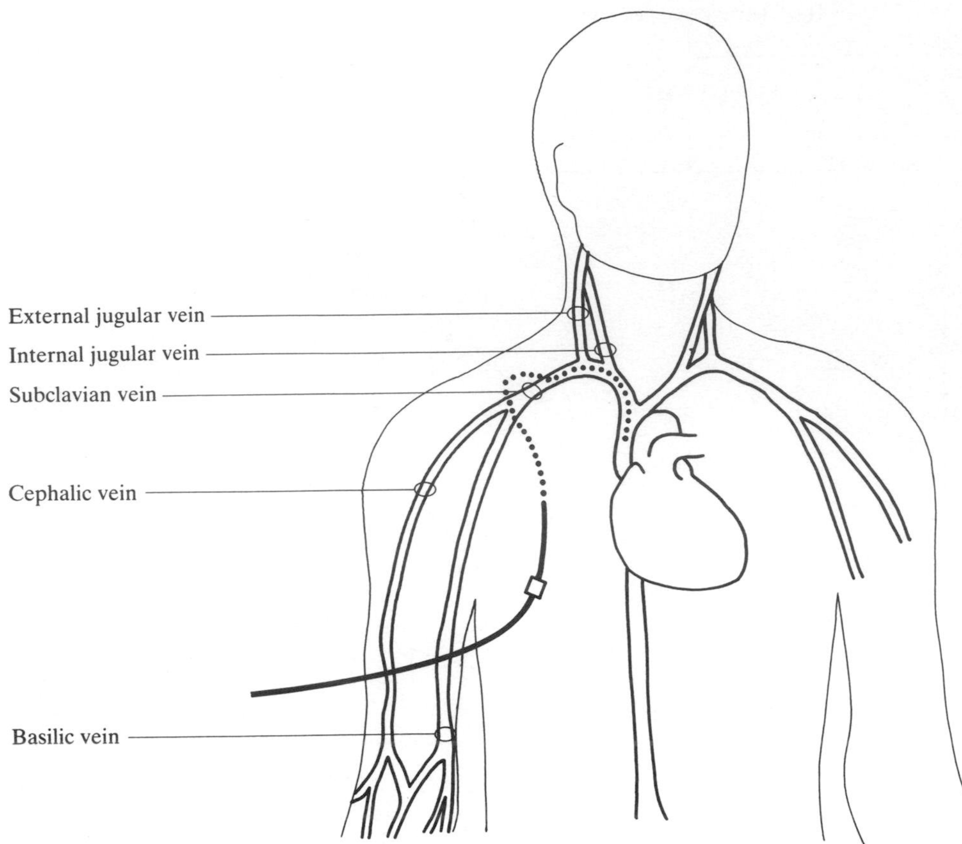

Fig. 1.8 Illustration of a feeding catheter inserted via the subclavian vein into the superior vena cava and tunnelled under the skin (dotted line). Other entry sites may be used as indicated.

vein into the superior vena cava (Fig. 1.8). The catheter is then usually tunnelled subcutaneously down onto the chest. This provides a flat surface so that a good occlusive sterile dressing can be applied to the catheter entry site and therefore reduce the risk of catheter infections. *The catheter should be used for the administration of TPN only.* Separate venous access is required for blood, plasma protein fraction, saline, drugs and CVP measurements. The administration of these via the TPN catheter will increase the risk of a catheter infection (Mughal 1989). In some cases, a double or triple lumen catheter may be inserted to enable the administration of drugs and monitoring of CVP simultaneously (e.g. for chemotherapy or ITU patients). Again one lumen should be identified, labelled and designated *for TPN use only* (Pemberton *et al* 1986).

Peripheral vein cannulation allows access to the central veins via a peripheral vein and has been shown to be an acceptable alternative to direct central vein cannulation (Hansell 1989). This is used particularly for short term feeding where the peripheral veins are viable and a fluid volume of more than 2500 ml over a 24 hour period can be tolerated.

1.15.3 Administration

Maintenance of a continuous flow rate is essential with parenteral nutrition in order to:

1 Control blood glucose (avoiding either hyperglycaemia or hypoglycaemia).
2 Avoid occlusion of the venous line especially with peripheral feeding.
3 Optimize the utilization of infused nutrients and to maintain fluid balance.

Various methods are used to maintain flow rate:

1 Mechanical controllers (e.g. clamps and other types of variable resistance devices).
2 Electro-mechanical devices (e.g. peristaltic pumps; flow controllers and volumetric pumps).

With the exception of the volumetric pumps, control of flow rate relies on counting the rate of drop flow. Because of the complex composition of parenteral nutrition solutions, the drop size differs from that of simple intravenous fluids on which the devices are calibrated (Allwood 1984a). A volumetric pump should be used to regulate TPN administration.

The feeding solutions may be administered using a three-litre bag containing the compounded daily regimen or using a multiple bottle system.

Disadvantages of using a multiple bottle system include:

1 Increased risk of infection due to several bottle changes/day.
2 Increased risk of hyper/hypoglycaemia due to changes in glucose concentration.
3 More nursing time required.
4 Increased risk of line blockage.

Disadvantages of using a Big Bag System may include:

1 Less rapid response to change in nutrient requirements.

2 More risk of compounding complications due to instability of nutrients in solutions. (Table 1.51, below).

1.15.4 Nutritional requirements

Requirements during parenteral nutrition for energy, nitrogen, fluid, sodium and potassium are quantitatively the same as those for enteral nutrition (see Section 1.13). There are however, notable differences with respect to the *qualitative* requirements for energy and nitrogen intake and these are discussed later.

Quantitative differences do exist in the requirements for certain mineral, trace elements and vitamins because there is, firstly, no loss due to absorptive capacity of the gastrointestinal tract and, secondly, a greater risk of overdosage exists. Table 1.49 gives suggested recommended daily intravenous intakes. They should only be used for guidance in selecting the most appropriate preparations from those available. A good review is given by Greene *et al* (1988). Actual requirements vary between individuals and there

Table 1.49 Suggested micronutrient requirements in parenteral nutrition

Nutrient	Infants 0–1 year (per kg body weight per day)		Children 1–15 years[1] (per kg body weight per day)	Adults[2] (per day)
	pre-term	full-term		
Ca (mmol)	1.5	1.0 –1.5	0.5 –1.0	7.7 –14.0
Mg (mmol)	0.3	0.15–0.3	0.1 –0.15	2.8 –28.0[3]
P (mmol)	0.5 –1.5	0.5 –1.5	0.12–0.4	10 –50
Fe (μmol)	2.0 –3.0	2.0 –3.0	1.0 –2.0	19.5 –70
Mn (μmol)	0.3 –1.0	0.3 –1.0	0.3	2.7 –14.4[4]
Zn (μmol)	2.0 –6.0	0.6 –2.3	0.3 –0.6 (1.5 for 1–5 years)	37.5 –100[3]
Cu (μmol)	0.4 –0.85	0.3 –0.4	0.1 –0.3	7.5 –22.5[4]
Cr (μmol)	0.01–0.02	0.01–0.02	0.01	0.19–2.9
Se (μmol)	0.04	0.04	0.4	0.4
Mo (μmol)	0.12	0.12		0.2
F (μmol)	1.3	1.3	0.7 –1.5	49 –105
I (μmol)	0.04	0.04	0.02–0.04	1.0
Thiamin (mg)	0.05–2.0	0.05–2.0	0.02–2.0	3.0
Riboflavin (mg)	1.0 –0.4	0.1 –0.4	0.03–0.4	3.6
Nicotinic acid (mg)	1.0 –4.0	1.0 –4.0	1.0 –4.0	40
Pyridoxine (mg)	0.1 –0.6	0.1 –0.6	0.03–0.6	4.0
Folic acid (μg)	20 –100	20 –50	3.0 –50.0	500[5]
Vitamin B12 (μg)	0.2 –5.0	0.2 –5.0	0.3 –5.0	5.0[5]
Vitamin B5 (mg)	1.0 –2.0	1.0 –2.0	0.2 –2.0	15.0
Biotin (μg)	30 –60	30 –60	5 –60	60 –200
Vitamin C (mg)	3 –20	3 –20	0.5 –25.0	100 –500
Vitamin A (μg)	100 –150	100 –150	10 –150	1000
Vitamin D (μg)	2.5 (max 10 μg/day)	2.5 (max 10 μg/day)	2.5 (max 10 μg/day)	5
Vitamin E (mg)	0.7 –1.0	0.7 –1.0	0.4 –1.0	7
Vitamin K (μg)	50 –150	50 –150	2.0 –150	20 –140[5]
Linoleic acid (μg)	0.5 –1.0	0.5 –1.0	0.3 –0.7	10 –50

[1] The wide variations in quoted requirements for children (1–15 years) are due to the variations caused by age differences and disease effects on requirements (see Grotte *et al* 1982).

[2] The higher requirements for adults indicate requirements for more catabolic patients.

[3] For increased gastrointestinal losses (adults): Additional zinc: 256 μmol/l, stool and ileostomy losses. 183 μmol/l, small bowel fistula losses. Additional chromium: 0.38 μmol/day. Total magnesium at least 10 mmol/day.

[4] Avoid high Cu and Mn intakes if there is biliary obstruction.

[5] Can be given as 15 mg folic acid, 1000 μg vitamin B12 and 10 mg vitamin K intramuscularly initially and weekly thereafter (Bradley *et al* 1978). This vitamin B12 and vitamin K dose may be adequate given monthly, but patients with prolonged prothrombin time (e.g. if also receiving antibiotics) may require more vitamin K; up to 10 mg/day (Hands *et al* 1985).

Requirements devised from the following sources: Jeejeebhoy *et al* (1973) Tovey *et al* (1977); Bradley *et al* (1978) Shenkin and Wretlind (1978); Wolfram *et al* (1978); Freund *et al* (1979); Strelling *et al* (1979); Wolman *et al* (1979); Ruberg and Mirtallo (1981); Shike *et al* (1981); Adamkin (1982); Grotte *et al* (1982); Innis and Allardyce (1983); Kien and Ganther (1983); Lockitch *et al* (1983); Friel *et al* (1984); Kingsnorth (1984); Quercia *et al* (1984); Hands *et al* (1985); Mock *et al* (1985); Russell (1985); Greene *et al* (1988).

are variable losses during mixing and administration of solutions (Table 1.51). Providing reasonable precautions are taken, the recommendations given in Table 1.49 will be adequate. However, meeting recommended intakes is no substitute for the regular assessment of patients for early signs of nutritional deficiencies or excesses (see below).

It is desirable to keep the number of additives in parenteral nutrition regimens to a minimum. The question inevitably arises of when to add micronutrients. Several factors need to be taken into account.

- The patients concerned are generally nutritionally depleted before starting nutritional support; this may have occurred over a period of several weeks or months.
- The disease process itself may increase turnover and losses of micronutrients or may impair their metabolism (e.g. folate).
- The availability of certain micronutrients may be impaired by the administration process (see below).

Whenever possible, deficiency states need to be corrected, and then complete nutritional support given from the start of parenteral feeding. It is not always necessary to give the nutrient daily in order to achieve the desired intake.

1.15.5 Sources of nutrients

The types of products used to provide a parenteral feeding regimen are summarized in Table 1.50.

Energy

The sources of energy in a parenteral nutrition regimen are carbohydrate and/or fat. (It is assumed, perhaps optimistically on occasions, that the amino acid content of parenteral regimen makes no contribution to its energy yield). There are important qualitative considerations to be taken into account when deciding which sources of energy to use.

Carbohydrate sources of energy

Glucose This is the preferred carbohydrate source. It is cheap, well metabolized by all tissues, has an established nitrogen sparing effect and serum levels can easily be monitored.

Fructose, sorbitol, xylitol and ethanol These all have established nitrogen sparing abilities, are less thrombophlebitic than glucose and do not readily result in hyperglycaemia. However, fructose and sorbitol produce lactate when metabolized which may precipitate lactic acidosis. Serum fructose levels cannot be monitored easily and they require metabolism by the liver to glucose before being utilized by other tissues for energy. More detailed discussion on the utilization of these energy substrates is given by Tweedle (1982), Silk (1983) and Grimble *et al* (1989).

Table 1.50 Types of products used in parenteral nutrition

Nutrient	Sources
Energy	Glucose solutions in concentrations from 5% to 70% Glucose/electrolyte solutions Some amino acid solutions also contain glucose, fructose, sorbitol and/or ethanol. Lipid emulsions of 10% or 20% (LCT or MCT/LCT)
Nitrogen	Crystalline amino acid solutions ranging in nitrogen concentrations from 5 g/l to 24 g/l Specialist amino acid solutions, e.g. branched chain amino acids, essential amino acids, paediatric formulations, isotonic solutions
Electrolytes and trace elements	Glucose/electrolyte/trace element solutions, e.g. Glucoplex, Nutracel Amino acid solutions may contain electrolytes and some trace elements Sodium chloride and acetate solutions Potassium, phosphate, calcium and magnesium additives The phospholipid emulsifier in lipid emulsions provides phosphate but usually in insufficient quantities for requirements Composite trace element additives, e.g. Addamel, Additrace, Ped-el, local preparations of single trace element additives
Vitamins	Composite additives, e.g. Solivito, Vitlipid adult/infant, Multibionta, Parentrovite, Multiple Vitamin Solution Individual vitamin preparations Intralipid provides some vitamin E and essential fatty acids
Albumin/plasma protein fraction	These may be given to compensate severe hypoproteinaemia and can comprise albumin, plasma protein fraction or blood. They should not be regarded as sources of nitrogen or trace elements when calculating intakes

Glucose polymers Glucose polymers may provide a way of reducing the osmolality of the TPN solution. This would enable more energy dense feeds to be given peripherally and reduce the incidence of phlebitis.

Research to date shows glucose polymers to be poorly utilized by the patient. High urinary losses of glucose suggest an upper limit of renal hydrolysis and the subsequent reabsorption of glucose. Further studies are continuing to find polymers that may be better utilized but, at present, glucose remains the carbohydrate energy source of choice.

Complications associated with the use of glucose

It should be noted that with very high glucose intakes (more than 40 kcal/kg/day) which saturate glucose oxidation, the excess is converted to fat (Grimble *et al* 1989). High carbohydrate intake may also increase carbon dioxide production, aggravating impaired respiration function causing difficulties in 'weaning' ventilated patients.

Excessive hepatic lipogenesis can produce 'fatty liver' or 'TPN liver'. This usually occurs when glucose is given as the sole energy source (Baker and Rosenberg 1986).

Septic and traumatized patients can develop peripheral insulin resistance due to the altered hormonal profile that is associated with stress (Stoner *et al* 1983; Lemoyne and Jeejeebhoy 1986). Decreased glucose utilization may occur if the TPN solution has a significant glucose load and is stopped suddenly instead of being gradually reduced.

Fat sources of energy

Whole body protein is restored more quickly when 15–40% of energy is supplied as lipid to depleted patients (Grimble *et al* 1989), than when glucose is the sole energy supply. Fat oxidation produces less carbon dioxide than carbohydrate oxidation. This will be of benefit to patients with respiratory distress syndrome as well as with the weaning of patients from a ventilator. Lipid emulsions are now widely used to provide 30–40% of total calories in TPN regimens. They are however, significantly more expensive than glucose solutions.

Long chain triglycerides Currently, lipid emulsions containing long chain triglycerides (LCT) are being used, however research is being undertaken to investigate the use of other novel lipid emulsions. Emulsions containing LCT have a limited ability to provide energy by direct oxidation and there are fears that excess fat may accumulate in the reticulo-endothelial system of some patients. This may lead to impaired clearance of systemic bacteria and it is therefore recommended that lipid is either given in the TPN bag or as an infusion over a period of not less than 20 hours rather than as a bolus infusion.

Medium chain triglycerides Medium Chain Triglyceride (MCT) is more rapidly oxidized than LCT leading to faster energy production and less risk of lipid deposition. MCT does not require carnitine for mitochondrial membrane transportation whereas LCT does. Stressed patients who are carnitine deficient will utilize MCT better than LCT. Infusion of excessive amounts of MCT may produce adverse side effects due to the toxicity of medium chain fatty acids (MCFA). For clinical use, lipid emulsions containing 50% MCT and 50% LCT are being devised to prevent accumulation of high levels of MCFA in plasma. This is still at the research stage and more clinical work is needed.

Research is also continuing into the use of LCT emulsions with optimal omega-3/omega-6 essential fatty acid ratios (see Section 2.3). Omega-6 essential fatty acids have potent vaso-active, broncho-active, chemotactic and muscle contractile properties. Omega-3 fatty acids have been shown to reduce platelet aggregation and may help prevent post-operative thrombosis. Fat emulsions with a high omega-3/omega-6 ratio may have benefits in moderating an excessive inflammatory response to trauma or sepsis.

At the present time it is recommended that a fat emulsion (LCT) is used to provide 30–40% of the total energy requirements in an all-in-one TPN mixture with glucose being the carbohydrate energy source. In some cases of respiratory distress or with peripheral feeding fat may provide up to 60% of the energy requirements.

In long term patients where LCT lipid emulsion is not used, then essential fatty acids must be given. (MCT does not contain these).

Intralipid (Kabi Pharmacia) contains linoleic acid and 500 ml infused twice a week should prevent essential fatty acid deficiency. If IV fat is contraindicated, then Press *et al* (1974) found that 230 ml sunflower oil rubbed daily into the flexor muscle of the forearm could provide sufficient linoleic acid to prevent deficiency symptoms.

Complications associated with the use of fat emulsions

There is less flexibility in the choice of nutrients when fat is included in the TPN bag. High concentrations of some nutrients and electrolytes may cause breakdown (cracking or creaming) of the lipid emulsion (Cripps 1984).

Lipid emulsions should be used with care in pre-term infants and neonates. Free fatty acids are released into the plasma following lipid infusion. These may compete with bilirubin for the binding sites on plasma albumin thus reducing bilirubin binding capacity (Whittington and Burckart 1982). The net result is an increase in free circulating bilirubin which may increase the risk of bilirubin encephalopathy (kernicterus). Bilirubin levels should be monitored and 10% lipid emulsion administered slowly over 24 hours and IV fat introduced at 0.5 g/kg increasing to a maximum of 3 g fat/kg (at 0.5 g/kg/day increments).

Pulmonary impairment has been reported as a temporary phenomenon following lipid infusion. This is thought to be due to a rapid infusion of lipid and can be overcome by including the fat emulsion in the TPN bag or giving it separately over more than 20 hours.

Nitrogen source

The choice of amino acid solution depends upon several issues, not all of which are nutritional. These include the following:

1 The concentration of nitrogen per litre of the amino acid solution.

2 The energy, electrolyte and mineral content of the amino acid solution.

3 An amino acid profile for optimum utilization.

4 Factors relevant to the safe and simple compounding of big bags by pharmacy especially if lipid is to be included. These include the nitrogen concentration, amino acid profile, pH, content of calcium and magnesium and total electrolyte concentration.

5 Cost.

All nitrogen sources currently sold in the UK for parenteral nutrition are crystalline amino acid solutions. The wide range of amino acid solutions available bears testimony to the unresolved debate on the optimum amino acid profile for parenteral nutrition. It is generally advised that the ratio of essential amino acid (g): to total nitrogen (g) (the E:T ratio) should be about 1:3, and the majority of solutions currently available meet this criterion. However in the sick patient and in the infant the concept of essential and non-essential amino acids must be questioned. Certain amino acids may not be essential in the strict sense but they may significantly improve the utilization of other amino acids.

Glycine Glycine has been much criticized as a cheap 'filler' amino acid. However, Kingsnorth *et al* (1980) found the half-life of glycine to be considerably shorter than that of alanine which is recognized as a most efficacious source of nitrogen (glutamate had an even shorter half-life). Nevertheless, large amounts of glycine or glutamic acid should not be given. The inclusion of arginine will prevent hyperammonaemia occurring when glycine is administered.

Cyst(e)ine Cyst(e)ine is reported to be essential for infants (Sturman *et al* 1970) and for patients with cirrhosis (Rudman *et al* 1981; Chawla *et al* 1984). There can be technical problems in measuring cyst(e)ine levels (Malloy *et al* 1983) and there are difficulties in maintaining a stable form of cyst(e)ine in amino acid solutions particularly in higher nitrogen concentrations. The cyst(e)ine argument remains unresolved, but any solution should contain either cyst(e)ine or an enhanced level of methionine as a precursor of cyst(e)ine. Additional methionine may increase folate requirements (Connor *et al* 1978).

Tyrosine The ability of infants and the very ill to synthesize tyrosine is questionable, but if it is not included in the mixture then additional phenylalanine should be given, although care is needed with levels of phenylalanine in solution as transient hyperphenylalaninaemia can occur.

Histidine Histidine is essential in infants as well as in the very ill and patients with renal failure.

Carnitine This is an important trimethylamine normally synthesized in the liver from lysine, methionine and glycine in the presence of ascorbic acid and pyridoxine. It has an important role in the oxidation of fatty acids by facilitating their transport across the mitochondrial membrane. Currently parenteral nutrition solutions do not contain carnitine. Carnitine synthesis may be impaired in sick patients (Tao and Yoshimura 1980) and in premature infants (Schmidt-Sommerfield *et al* 1983) and hence fat utilization may be reduced. Carnitine is being tested in current research programmes.

Safety however must come before optimum profile and all amino acids are individually toxic if administered in large enough dosages. There are two schools of thought:

1 To supply all amino acids since the conversion of 'essential' amino acids to 'non-essential' amino acids is in doubt in these patients.

2 To supply adequate amounts of important precursors (e.g. alanine) and avoid giving amino acids which may accumulate to toxic levels (e.g. glutamic acid and aspartic acid) or which may be unstable in solution (e.g. cyst(e)ine and tyrosine).

The amino acid profile is also of significance when the amino acid solution is to be mixed with lipid emulsions. Aspartic and glutamic acids may accelerate the coalescence of lipid particles, whereas arginine, lysine and histidine may help to maintain emulsion stability (Hardy *et al* 1982).

Amino acid solutions for special situations

Essential amino acids These have been advocated for patients in acute renal failure (Wilmore and Dudrick 1969). However, such patients have the same nutritional needs as others with similar medical or surgical problems. They do not require special amino acid formulations but they do require dialysis to allow full nutritional requirements to be met. Amino acid solutions without electrolytes may be useful in such situations.

Branched chain amino acids (BCAA) (i.e. valine, leucine and isoleucine) Patients with hepatic precoma or severe hepatic damage may benefit from a higher proportion of BCAA (Silk 1988). These amino acids, which are not metabolized by the liver directly but by the peripheral tissues, may also be of benefit to patients with severe burns or sepsis and possibly also severely traumatized patients. Currently, a 4% BCAA solution is available for use in conjunction with other amino acid solutions. Unfortunately, it is too dilute to be useful for the latter groups of patients.

Isotonic amino acid solutions These, when administered peripherally without additional energy, have been advocated as a means of achieving a positive nitrogen balance in the post-operative patient (Blackburn *et al* 1973). However, when healthy subjects are given intravenous amino acids alone, the level of ketones in the blood is less than that found in prolonged starvation, showing that gluconeogenesis of amino acids takes place in order to provide energy for cerebral tissues.

A second important observation which weakens Blackburn's hypothesis is that the administration of amino acids alone stimulates rather than suppresses the secretion of insulin and thus will inhibit lipogenesis. The clinical benefit of this method of nutritional support remains to be proven (Collins *et al* 1978).

Stability of solutions and availability of nutrients

Having overcome the hurdles of aseptic administration and the selection of appropriate nutritional substrate in correct quantities, it may be found that the compatibility of preparations will restrict what can be given to the patient. Much research has been done and much remains to be done in this field and the subject has been reviewed by Allwood (1984b). With present knowledge it should be possible to meet the needs of all patients. Problems may occur when big bags are prepared, especially if lipid emulsion is to be included. Care is also required when using additives in multiple bottle regimens. Pharmacy departments will have access to the necessary data but it is important that dietitians are aware of the problems involved as they affect nutrient availability. Three-litre bag formulations are complex chemical mixtures and many as yet unknown reactions and losses may occur. The main reasons for loss of nutrient availability or stability are as follows.

1 *Precipitation*, particularly of calcium phosphate, but folic acid may also cause precipitation.
2 *Photodegradation* can affect many nutrients to varying degrees (see Table 1.51). Artificial light is not of concern but daylight, even from a nearby window, can cause significant losses of vitamin A and riboflavin. The solution must also be protected from the intense ultra-violet light used in neonatal phototherapy.
3 *Oxidation*, principally of vitamin C (see Table 1.51).
4 *Degradation*.
5 *Adsorption* on to plastic bags and administration sets.
6 *Breakdown of fat emulsion*. This may result in irreversible lipid/water phase separation and can be caused by a high concentration of total electrolytes, in particular of divalent and trivalent cations. There are many other factors which may affect emulsion stability (Table 1.51).

1.15.6 Assessment

The patient's nutritional requirements should be calculated as described earlier in this chapter (Section 1.15.4) then adjustments made for either the IV administration of electrolytes or any additional electrolyte, mineral or fluid losses.

Hospitals may have their own range of TPN standard feeding regimens, with given amounts of nitrogen and energy. Individual flexibility is allowed for within the electrolyte content.

Hospitals with their own pharmacy compounding unit may manufacture their own TPN bags. Commercial companies also supply standard TPN regimens in three-litre bags to hospitals and patients at home on TPN according to the hospitals' prescription.

Anthropometric measurements are useful for monitoring the effects of nutrition support for long term patients (see Section 1.11).

1.15.7 Monitoring

Monitoring is necessary to detect and minimize complications of the TPN regimen. Some metabolic complications and suggested parameters for monitoring are given in Table 1.52. The frequency with which the patient should be monitored initially is suggested. In practice this depends upon the clinical condition of the patient, the nature of the feeding regimen and the results of previous measurements. A monitoring protocol should be prepared for each hospital in consultation with all concerned (including the laboratory staff) and adapted for each patient.

Fluid balance must be monitored daily. IV fluids that were given to maintain hydration should be stopped when TPN starts. Fluid charts must be accurately completed and show all fluid intake (IV drugs, oral, TPN) and all output (urine, stoma, fistula, blood loss). A daily weight chart is also essential to ensure the accuracy of fluid balance charts. One litre of fluid weighs approximately 1 kg and any rapid fluctuations in weight will be due to fluid change rather than alteration in body mass. Initially it is a good idea to ascertain the volume of IV fluid on which the patient has been maintained and then provide that volume of TPN. This should be roughly 35–45 ml/kg in the patient with a normal state of hydration with no clinical reason for altering the fluid requirements.

Long term or home TPN patients are generally more stable, and may be fed using cyclical feeding (e.g. feed is infused for 12 hours overnight at a suitably increased flow rate). This has been shown to reduce hepatic abnormalities and allows the patient to become more mobile. Care with rebound hypoglycaemia must be taken and, if necessary, the infusion rate reduced for two hours prior to stopping the TPN.

Table 1.51 Losses of nutrient availability in parenteral nutrition solutions

Nutrient	Nature of loss(es)	Possible causes of loss(es)	Preventative action(s)
Dextrose	None	None	None
Lipid	Flocculation (reversible) ↓ Coalescence (irreversible) ↓ Lipid/water phase separation Photodegradation of essential fatty acids	High total electrolyte concentration particularly divalent and trivalent cations Calcium affecting phospholipid emulsifier. Low pH from dextrose and amino acid content Over-dilution of emulsifier Exposure to intense phototherapy in neonatal units	Careful control over electrolyte content in bags Correct procedure in preparing bags Inclusion of certain amino acids in big bag regimens may aid stability Limit storage time of bags containing lipid Add only Vitlipid and Solivito to Intralipid bottles
Amino acids	Photodegradation of glycine, leucine, tryptophan, methionine and tyrosine	Long term exposure to daylight Exposure to intense phototherapy in neonatal units	Cover in storage
Trace elements	Precipitation of iron Other trace elements appear stable	Precipitation of iron phosphate when iron compounds are added to certain amino acid solutions (e.g. Synthamin)	Include 500 mg vitamin C in big bags Add trace element/iron additive to dextrose rather than to amino acid solution in multiple bottle regimen.
Electrolytes	Precipitation of calcium phosphate	Excessive calcium and phosphate concentrations Increasing pH. Sudden change of temperature (removing from refrigerator). Mixing of lipid emulsion in line with calcium/phosphate mixtures as may occur in infant feeding	Calcium (mmol/l) × Phosphate (mmol/l) not to exceed 185 Do not mix calcium with phosphate in multiple bottle regimens.
Vitamin A	Photodegradation	Short term exposure to daylight	Give sufficient Vitamin A for unavoidable loss Cover during storage and infusion Give in lipid containing bottle/bag Do not hang near a window
	Loss from solution	Acetate vitamin A ester absorbed on to plastic bag	Use palmitate vitamin A ester
Thiamin	Degraded	Metabisulphite in undiluted amino acid solutions Low pH	Give sufficient thiamin for unavoidable losses Use big bag *or* add to another component of regimen *or* add to amino acid solution not containing metabisulphite
Riboflavin	Photodegradation (up to 57%)	Exposure to daylight. Phototherapy	Add sufficient to cover unavoidable losses.
Pyridoxine	Photodegradation (small)	Exposure to direct sunlight	Protect from daylight
Vitamin K	Photodegradation	Exposure to daylight	Protect from daylight or give intramuscularly
Folic acid	Loss from solution Precipitation	Adsorption to plastic bags High calcium concentrations Increased risk if added to certain amino acid solutions pH less than 5.0	Add sufficient folic acid for unavoidable losses Watch calcium content in bag Give intramuscular folate weekly Avoid storing bags containing folate
Vitamin C	Oxidation	Dissolved oxygen introduced when filling big bags or absorbed through plastic bag Copper if added acts as a catalyst in vitamin C oxidation Low pH	Add sufficient vitamin C for unavoidable losses Give vitamin C and copper in separate bags e.g. alternate days *or* use a cystine/cysteine containing amino acid solution (inhibits catalytic action of copper) *or* add excess vitamin C (see also trace elements — preventing iron precipitation)

1.15.8 Complications

Complications associated with TPN can be divided into three categories: technical, infectious and metabolic. The possible technical complications of subclavian venous catheter insertion include pneumothorax, haemothorax, hydrothorax, venous or arterial laceration; brachial plexus or tracheal injury; and catheter or air embolus. The most frequent of these is pneumothorax which occurs in 2–3% of patients. Complications of line insertion are highly correlated with the skill and experience of the clinician involved (Mughal 1989).

Complications with long term indwelling catheters include line sepsis, thrombosis, vessel erosion and cardiac

Table 1.52 Monitoring of parenteral feeding

Biochemical monitoring	Serum haemoglobin	Daily and then weekly
	Serum sodium	Daily until stable. When the patient is losing more than 1 litre of fluid via a fistula/stoma it is better to compensate for this separately by using either Hartmans solution or 5% dextrose saline solution through a side arm or peripherally. This reduces the need for vast alterations to the basic TPN solution by providing the additional sodium and fluid requirements, needed to compensate for the losses. Low serum Na usually indicates fluid overload unless there are obvious sodium losses (e.g. small bowel fistula, high ileostomy, biliary leak)
	Serum potassium	Daily until stable. Remember to increase and monitor serum levels if insulin is being given
	Liver function tests	Alk Phos, AST initially. Then weekly unless abnormalities arise (see complications)
	Albumin	Short term TPN will *not* affect the serum albumin. A low level indicates trauma and/or fluid overload. Albumin, fresh frozen plasma (FFP) or Plasma Protein Fraction (PPF) can be given to increase the oncotic pressure in a patient with a low albumin (less than 30 mg/l). This may increase their albumin levels and help reverse peripheral oedema by encouraging fluid to move intracellularly
	Serum urea and creatinine	Initially, then weekly unless the patient develops renal failure
	Serum phosphate	Initially, then weekly. In the malnourished patient or the ITU patient where dextrose solution may be given for a few days the patient is likely to be phosphate depleted and refeeding will exacerbate this. Hypophosphataemia can cause muscular fatigue (particularly respiratory muscles) and poor oxygen uptake by the haemoglobin and therefore serum levels should be monitored and corrected
	Serum magnesium	Initially and then weekly. A lot of patients on TPN have gastrointestinal disease and or may have increased magnesium losses e.g. bone marrow transplantation, Crohn's disease, fistula, stoma
	Trace elements (Zn, S, Co, Mn)	Initially then three monthly in a stable long term patient. Catabolic patients may have 'falsely' high serum levels of some trace elements
Fluid balance		Daily fluid balance charts should be kept aiming for a positive balance of 500 ml in a non pyrexic patient. The pyrexic patient will require more fluid. Checks should be made for any alteration in fistula/stoma output or other fluid losses. A daily weight chart should be kept remembering that rapid changes will be due to fluid retention or loss. Checks should also be made for overt signs of fluid overload ('puffiness' of ankles, legs, 'tightness' of fingers). The dehydrated patient may complain of having a dry mouth or being very thirsty. Raised serum sodium, haemoglobin, urea with a normal creatinine may indicate the patient is dehydrated.
Urinary tests	Glucose	6-hourly urinalysis for glucose. If the urinalysis is positive then the serum glucose level should be monitored 6-hourly. If the serum level is consistently more than 11 mmol/l a sliding scale infusion of fast acting insulin should be considered
	24 hour urinary urea	Twice weekly when practical to assess nitrogen losses
	24-hour urinary sodium	Useful weekly to assess body's sodium status

arrhythmias. Sepsis is the most common long term complication and occurs in 2–7% of patients (Sitzman *et al* 1989). Sepsis is the only life threatening complication that occurs frequently and should be minimized by having strict protocols governing insertion and care of central venous catheters. Where possible, specially trained nursing staff should be employed to monitor these protocols, and thus achieve an acceptable sepsis rate.

Hepatic dysfunction

This may be seen after four weeks or longer on parenteral nutrition. There tends to be a characteristic pattern of an initial increase in the serum aspartate and alanine amino transferases followed by a mild progressive rise in alkaline phosphatase and eventually a rise in serum bilirubin. Clinically the patient may be seen to become jaundiced due to cholestasis. The phenomenon is generally reversible on cessation of feeding (Tweedle *et al* 1978). The cause is unclear but several possibilities have been suggested:

1 Cholestasis.
2 Excessive glucose intake leading to fatty liver.
3 Deficiency of essential fatty acids.
4 Continuous 24-hour feeding.
5 Suppression of trophic and/or secretion stimulant gut hormones.
6 Lithocholate toxicity.
7 Toxic breakdown products of tryptophan.
8 Choline deficiency.
9 Methionine deficiency.

In several reports, lipid has been withdrawn from the feeding regimen and an improvement in cholestasis has occurred (although it has not always been made clear whether the lipid was substituted with equicaloric quantities of glucose or whether the total energy intake was reduced). The type of energy substrate given is undoubtedly important in avoiding this complication (Buzby *et al* 1981). In a few infants developing cholestatic jaundice on long term TPN the problem has developed into a progressive disease leading to cirrhosis.

If hepatic changes are sufficient to give rise to clinical concern the following procedure is suggested:

1 Consider whether there is a non-nutritional cause (e.g. sepsis).
2 If glucose alone is being used for energy, then substitute 30–50% of energy with lipid.
3 If practical (i.e. in a stable patient), cyclical feeding (e.g. 12 hours out of 24 hours) can be tried.
4 Reduce the total energy intake by reducing lipid or glucose, maintain nitrogen intake and monitor.
5 If jaundice worsens, consider stopping feeding for 3–4 days and observe.
6 Consider giving a small amount of oral food, if allowed, as this may help reduce cholestasis.

Cholelithiasis

Cholelithiasis may be found in both adults and children receiving long term TPN. Prolonged TPN (over one year), ileal resection and lack of an oral intake are all major contributors to the formation of gallstones.

When possible a small oral intake should be maintained.

Polymyopathy

Polymyopathy with muscular pain and high serum creatinine and phosphate has been reported in long term TPN. This may be due to deficiency of essential fatty acids, or possibly selenium.

Metabolic bone disease

A metabolic bone disease characterized by skeletal pain and hypercalcuria has been reported in long term parenteral nutrition (Shike *et al* 1980; McCullough *et al* 1987). This syndrome is seen after at least three months of parenteral nutrition. A number of causes have been suggested in conflicting reports namely:

- Excess vitamin D intake (Shike *et al* 1980);
- Excess aluminium in solutions, especially casein hydrolysates (Klein *et al* 1980);
- High nitrogen intake particularly as part of a cyclic PN regimen (Vernejoul *et al* 1985).

A transient hypercalcuria occurring after one week of TPN and persisting for between one and four weeks was reported by Gordon *et al* (1984). This was not found to be related to calcium intake and was not considered to represent a major mineral metabolic problem.

Hypercholesterolaemia and hypertriglyceridaemia

Elevated serum levels of cholesterol and triglycerides have been reported in patients receiving TPN, but can be minimized by careful control of energy intake, lipid, carbohydrate balance and weight.

Deficiency of trace elements

Deficiencies of trace elements including zinc, copper, chromium and selenium have been reported. It is essential these are added and levels monitored especially in long term patients (Fleming 1989).

Deficiencies of vitamins

Deficiencies of vitamins A, E, B_{12}, and biotin have been reported (Husami and Abumrad 1986).

1.15.9 The nutrition team

It is essential that patients on TPN are closely monitored in order to minimise the risk of complications. Ideally, TPN patients should be overseen by a multidisciplinary nutrition team. This would normally consist of a consultant physician, surgeon or anaesthetist, experienced surgeons and anaesthetists who would insert all central feeding lines, a dietitian to assess nutritional requirements, a pharmacist to advise on compatibility of solutions, a biochemist, and a nursing sister to co-ordinate the team and ensure the lines are cared for properly. Liaison with an infection control nurse or consultant microbiologist is also beneficial.

The role of the dietitian in the nutrition team

The dietitian should be able to:

- Advise on the most appropriate method of feeding and ensure that TPN is not initiated when the enteral route could be used (see Fig. 1.7);
- Assess the patient's nutritional requirements (a clinical opinion is usually needed for determining fluid requirements);
- Monitor the patient's progress in conjunction with other team members;
- Ensure that enteral nutrition is introduced as early as possible and that the transition from TPN to enteral nutrition goes smoothly and effectively.

References

Adamkin DH (1982) Intravenous fat emulsions: a neonatologist's point of view. In *Current perspectives in the use of lipid emulsion*. Johnston IDA (Ed) pp. 1–10. MTP Press, Lancaster.

Allwood MC (1984a) Drop size of infusions containing fat emulsion. *Br J Parent Ther* 5, 113–6.

Allwood MC (1984b) Compatibility and stability of TPN mixtures in big bags. *J Clin Hosp Pharm* 9, 181–98.

Baker AL and Rosenberg IH (1986) Hepatic complications of total parenteral nutrition. *Am J Medicine* **82**, 489–97.

Blackburn GL, Flatt JP, Clowes GHA and O'Donnell TE (1973) Peripheral intravenous feeding with isotonic amino acid solutions. *Am J Surg* **125**, 447–54.

Bradley JA, King RFJG, Schorah CJ and Hill GL (1978) Vitamins in intravenous feeding: a study of water soluble vitamins in critically ill patients receiving intravenous nutrition. *Br J Surg* **65**, 492–4.

Buzby GP, Mullen JL, Stein P and Rosato EF (1981) Manipulation of TPN caloric substrate and fatty infiltration of the liver. *J Surg Res* **31**, 46–54.

Chawla RK, Lewis FW, Kutner MH, Bate DM, Roy RGB and Rudman D (1984) Plasma cysteine, cystine and glutathione in cirrhosis. *Gastroenterology* **87**, 770–6.

Collins JP, Oxby CB and Hill GL (1978) Intravenous amino acids and intravenous hyperalimentation as protein sparing therapy after major surgery: a controlled clinical trial. *Lancet* **i**, 788–91.

Connor H, Newton DJ, Preston FE and Woods HF (1978) Oral methionine as a cause of acute serum folate deficiency: its relevance to parenteral nutrition. *Postgrad Med J* **54**, 318–20.

Cripps AL (1984) Stability studies on Total Parenteral Nutrition mixtures containing fat emulsions. *Br J Pharmaceutical Practice* **June**, 187–95.

Fleming CR (1989) Trace element metabolism in adult patients requiring Total Parenteral Nutrition 1–3. *Am J Clin Nutr* **49**, 573–9.

Freund H, Atamain S and Fisher JE (1979) Chromium deficiency during total parenteral nutrition. *J Am Med Assoc* **241**, 496–8.

Friel JK, Gibson RS, Peliowski A and Watts J (1984) Serum zinc, copper and selenium concentrations in preterm infants receiving enteral nutrition or parenteral nutrition supplemented with zinc and copper. *J Paediatr* **104**, 763–8.

Gordon D, Allan A, Sim AJW and Shenkin A (1984) Transient hypercalciuria after commencing total intravenous nutrition. *Clin Nutr* 3, 215–9.

Grant A and Todd E (1988) *Enteral and parenteral nutrition* — a clinical handbook. Blackwell Scientific Publications, Oxford.

Greene HL, Hambridge KM, Schanler R and Tsang RC (1988) Guidelines for the use of vitamins, trace elements, calcium, magnesium, and phosphorus in infants and children receiving Total Parenteral Nutrition: Report of the Subcommittee on Paediatric Parenteral Nutrient Requirements from the Committee on Clinical Practice Issues of the American Society for Clinical Nutrition 1–3. *Am J Clin Nutr* **48**, 1324–42.

Grimble GK, Payne-James JJ, Rees RG and Silk DBA (1989) TPN: novel energy substrates. *Intensive Therapy and Clinical Monitoring* **10**(4), April, 108–113.

Grotte G, Meurling S and Wretlind A (1982) Parenteral nutrition. In *A textbook of paediatric nutrition* 2e McLaren DS and Burman D (Eds) pp. 228–54. Churchill Livingstone, London.

Hands LJ, Royle GT and Kettlewell MGW (1985) Vitamin K requirements in patients receiving total parenteral nutrition. *Br J Surg* **72**, 665–7.

Hansell DT (1989) Intravenous nutrition: the central or peripheral route? *Intensive Therapy and Clinical Monitoring* **June/July**, 184–90.

Hardy G, Cotter R and Dawe R (1982) The stability and comparative clearance of TPN mixtures with lipid. In *Current perspectives in the use of lipid emulsion*, Johnston IDA (Ed) pp. 63–82. MTP Press Ltd, Lancaster.

Husami T and Abumrad NJ (1986) Adverse metabolic consequences of nutritional support: micronutrients. *Surg Clin of N Am* **66**(5), 1049–69.

Innis SM and Allardyce DB (1983) Possible biotin deficiency in adults receiving long term total parenteral nutrition. *Am J Clin Nutr* **37**, 185–7.

Jeejeebhoy KN, Zohrab WJ, Langer B, Phillips MJ, Kuksis A and Anderson GH (1973) Total parenteral nutrition at home for 23 months without complications and with good rehabilitation. *Gastroenterology* **65**, 811–20.

Kien CL and Ganther HE (1983) Manifestations of chronic selenium deficiency in a child receiving total parenteral nutrition. *Am J Clin Nutr* **37**, 319–28.

Kingsnorth AN, Ross BD and Kettlewell M (1980) Cost effective parenteral feeding. *Lancet* **ii**, 1371.

Kingsnorth AN (1984) Trace elements in adult total parenteral nutrition. *Br J Parent Ther* **5**, 8–22.

Lemoyne M and Jeejeebhoy KN (1986) Total Parenteral Nutrition in the critically ill patient. *Chest* **89**(4), 568–75.

Lockitch G, Godolphin W, Pendray MR, Riddell D and Quigley G (1983) Serum zinc, copper, retinol binding protein, pre-albumin and ceruloplasmin concentrations in infants receiving intravenous zinc and copper supplementations. *J Paediatr* **102**, 304–308.

Malloy MH, Russin DK and Richardson CJ (1983) Cyst(e)ine measurements during total parenteral nutrition. *Am J Clin Nutr* **37**, 188–91.

McCullough ML and Hsu N (1987) Metabolic bone disease in home Total Parenteral Nutrition. *J Am Diet Assoc* **87**, 915–20.

Mock DM, Baswell DL, Baker H, Holman RT and Sweetman L (1985) Biotin deficiency complicating parenteral alimentation: diagnosis, metabolic repercussions and treatment. *J Paediatr* **106**, 762–9.

Mughal MM (1989) Complications of intravenous feeding catheters. *Br J Surg* **76**, 15–21.

Pemberton LB, Lyman B, Lander V and Covinsky J (1986) Sepsis from triple- vs single-lumen catheters during Total Parenteral Nutrition in surgical or critically ill patients. *Arch Surg* **121**, 591–4.

Press M, Hartop PJ and Prottey C (1974) Correction of essential fatty acid deficiency in man by the cutaneous application of sunflower seed oil. *Lancet* **i**, 597–9.

Quercia RA, Korn S, O'Neill D, Doughty JE, Ludwig M, Schweizer R and Sigman R (1984) Selenium deficiency and fatal cardiomyopathy in a patient receiving long term home parenteral nutrition. *Clin Pharm* **3**, 531–5.

Ruberg RL and Mirtallo J (1981) Vitamin and trace element requirements in parenteral nutrition: an update. *Ohio State Med J* **12**, 725–9.

Rudman D, Kutner M, Ansley J, Jansen R, Chippani J and Bain RP (1981) Hypotyrosinaemia, hypocystinaemia and failure to retain nitrogen during total parenteral nutrition of cirrhotic patients. *Gastroenterology* **81**, 1025–35.

Russell RI (1985) Magnesium requirements in patients with chronic inflammatory bowel disease receiving intravenous nutrition. *Br J Parent Ther* **6**, 86–94.

Schmidt-Sommerfield E, Penn D and Wolf H (1983) Carnitine deficiency in premature infants receiving total parenteral nutrition: effect of L-carnitine supplementation. *J Paediatr* **102**, 931–4.

Shanbhogue LKR, Chwals WJ, Weintraub M, Blackburn GL and Bistrian BR (1987) Parenteral nutrition in the surgical patient. *Br J Surg* **74**, 172–80.

Shenkin A and Wretlind A (1978) Parenteral nutrition. *World Rev Nutr Diet* **28**, 1–111.

Shike M, Harrison JE, Sturtridge WC, Tam CS, Bobecko PE, Jones G, Murray TM and Jeejeebhoy KN (1980) Metabolic bone disease in patients receiving long term total parenteral nutrition. *Ann Int Med* **92**, 343–50.

Shike M, Rouet M, Kurain R, Whitewell J, Stewart S and Jeejeebhoy KN (1981) Copper metabolism and requirements in total parenteral nutrition. *Gastroenterology* **81**, 290–7.

Silk DBA (1983) *Nutritional support in hospital practice*. Blackwell Scientific Publications, Oxford.

Silk DBA (1988) Parenteral nutrition in patients with liver disease. *J Hepatology* **7**, 269–77.

Sitzmann JV, Pitt HA and The Patient Care Committee of the American Gastroenterological Association (1989) Statement on Guidelines for Total Parenteral Nutrition. *Digest Dis & Sci* **34**(4), 489–96.

Stoner HB, Little RA, Frayn KN, Elebute AE, Tresaden J and Gross E (1983) The effect of sepsis on the oxidation of carbohydrate and fat. *Br J Surg* **70**, 32–5.

Strelling MK, Blackledge DG and Goodall HB (1979) Diagnosis and management of folate deficiency in low birth weight infants. *Arch Dis Childh* **54**, 271–7.

Sturman JA, Gaull G and Raiha NCR (1970) Absence of cystathionase in human fetal liver: is cystine essential? *Science* **169**, 74–6.

Tao RC and Yoshimura NN (1980) Carnitine metabolism and its application in parenteral nutrition. *J Parent Ent Nutr* **4**, 469–86.

Tovey SJ, Benton KGF and Lee HA (1977) Hypophosphataemia and phosphorus requirements during intravenous nutrition. *Postgrad Med J* **53**, 289–97.

Tweedle DEF, Skidmore FD, Gleave EN and Knass DA (1978) Nutritional support for patients undergoing surgery for cancer of the head and neck. In *Developments in clinical nutrition* Johnston IDA and Lee HA (Eds) pp. 59–69. MCS Consultants, Tunbridge Wells.

Tweedle DEF (1982) *Metabolic care*. Churchill Livingstone, Edinburgh.

Vernejoul MC de, Messing B, Modrowski D, Bielakoff J, Buisine A and Miravet L (1985) Multifactorial low remodelling bone disease during cyclic total parenteral nutrition. *J Clin Endocrinol Metab* **60**, 109–113.

Whittington PF and Burckart GT (1982) Changes in binding of bilirubin due to intravenous lipid emulsion. In *Current perspectives in the use of lipid emulsion*. Johnston IDA (Ed) pp. 15–28. MTP Press, Lancaster.

Wilmore DW and Dudrick SJ (1969) Treatment of acute renal failure with intravenous essential L-amino acids. *Arch Surg* **99**, 669–73.

Wolfram G, Eckart J, Walther B and Zollner N (1978) Factors influencing essential fatty acid requirement in total parenteral nutrition. *J Parent Ent Nutr* **2**, 634–9.

Wolman SL, Anderson GH, Marliss EB and Jeejeebhoy KN (1979) Zinc in total parenteral nutrition and metabolic effects. *Gastroenterology* **76**, 458–67.

1.16 Institutional feeding

This section of the manual describes, in outline, how the best institutions plan their food service. These notes may be used by the dietitian who is asked to comment upon or audit the food service of his or her own or another institution. If the procedures described have been carried out, the dietitian can be sure that the food service of an institution is likely to perform its function of providing adequate and enjoyable nutritional support.

At least 90% of clients in an institution rely entirely on the food offered for the majority of their nutrition. Dietitians working in hospitals and other institutions have an important responsibility to fulfill in ensuring that these nutritional needs are met.

The changes in the Health Service and in the provision of community care emphasize the need for a quality service to clients. At the same time the cost-effectiveness of all services is coming under close scrutiny. The cost-effectiveness of good quality food services has been overlooked in the past. The cost of institutional malnutrition is also being recognized (Mullen *et al* 1979; Jensen *et al* 1982; Bender 1984; Twomey and Patching 1985; Askanazi *et al* 1986; Haydock and Hill 1986; Robinson *et al* 1987; Reilly *et al* 1988). These changes mitigate to the advantage of dietitians and caterers seeking to improve the quality of food service.

For the purposes of this section, institutional feeding is a term which applies to food service in establishments where the organization is the sole or main provider of food for the residents i.e. hospitals, residential homes, nursing homes, hospices, prisons etc. Some of the principles discussed will also be relevant to other types of large scale catering such as industrial or educational catering. (School meals are discussed in Section 3.5.5).

Florence Nightingale was among those who, at the end of the last century, realized that the provision of wholesome food was essential for recovery from disease and the prevention of diet related disorders. Her maxim was that, 'Above all else a hospital should do the patient no harm'. This maxim must be the byword of those charged with the responsibility of providing food for the institutionalized and the aim should be to ensure that the food provided is nutritionally adequate.

Institutional feeding is a multidisciplinary function. It cannot be emphasized too strongly that every person involved in the 'food chain', from the ordering and delivery of provisions to the actual ingestion of food, has a vital role to play. One weak link in the chain will assure failure and, consequently, the risk of malnutrition with its associated morbidity and mortality (Bistrian *et al* 1976; Hill *et al* 1977).

1.16.1 The role of the dietitian and the catering manager

The dietitian's role

Growing awareness of the influence of food on the recovery and well-being of patients in hospitals at the beginning of this century ultimately led to the development of the profession of dietetics. The dietitian is a nutrition expert with the particular skill of translating nutritional knowledge into practical advice for the provision of food suitable for maintaining good health in all age groups, aiding recovery from disease and treating diet related conditions. This expertise can be used to assess the overall nutritional adequacy of menus and the suitability of food provided for specific groups.

The catering manager's role

The catering manager is expert in the production and distribution of food on a large scale. In particular the catering manager will be skilled in menu planning, food purchase, food production, food distribution, food service, personnel management, accounting, food hygiene, food handling, health and safety in kitchens and kitchen management. Caterers preparing meals for people who eat regularly in institutions must accept a high level of responsibility for the nutrition of those people.

The common purpose

The dietitian and the catering manager are both responsible for ensuring that nutritionally adequate and appetising food is provided in hospitals.

Many factors have affected this working relationship over the years. The shift in dietetics to an all graduate profession with a clinical/medical model of training and, more recently, pressures on hospital caterers brought about by competitive tendering and the development of contracts, the capital costs incurred as a result of the lifting of Crown Immunity in 1987 and the introduction of the Food Act in 1991, have tended to create tensions over priorities relating to the nutritional quality and quantity of hospital food.

The complementary nature of the roles and responsibilities of dietitian and catering manager must be clearly understood and used on a daily basis towards the common purpose of providing a quality catering service. This starts with menu planning.

1.16.2 Menu planning

General considerations

The menu is the blueprint for operations in any catering establishment (Taylor 1990). The nutritional value of the food and its suitability for the resident client group is determined by the menu. The dietitian wishing to influence the provision of food or audit food provision in an institution must check the menu.

The main elements to be considered in good menu planning are your clients and your situation.

Knowing your clients

What kind of catering service do your clients want, and what kind of catering service do they need? Never forget the old dietetic maxim, 'The nutritional value of food not eaten is nil'.

The following factors affect food choice and provision:

Age

Children have very different preferences to adults and elderly people. The age of the client group must be taken into account if nutritional needs and food preferences are to be met.

Sex

Nutritional needs and food preferences differ between men and women.

Ethnic and cultural mix

Food preferences are an important expression of ethnic and cultural identity. Catering for these needs is a vital part of institutional catering. Patients are already anxious about their surroundings particularly in hospital; the added stress of unfamiliar or unacceptable food is unnecessary because there is sufficient information available to caterers on ethnic and cultural food habits. The dietitian should provide specific details for the local client group (Hill 1990).

Food preferences

Food preferences are influenced by socioeconomic factors. The wide variety of restaurants from MacDonalds to Le Gavroche bear witness to this. It is important for the menu planner to know the socioeconomic mix of clients to be served.

Routine and formal audit of the needs and preferences of the client group is the best way of ensuring that a menu meets the needs of that group and continues to do so.

Effects of illness

Illness may itself affect appetite, sense of taste and food preference.

Therapeutic case mix

Every institution will, at some time, have to cater for clients who have conditions requiring some kind of therapeutic diet. The menu planner needs to know which diets are likely to be needed, in what quantity and how often. Common dietary needs for the management of obesity, diabetes and hyperlipidaemias should be incorporated in the main body of every institution's selective menu. There may also be demands specific to institutions with renal units or liver units etc., which can also be incorporated into the main menu. Catering for these needs separately is costly and unnecessary (DoH 1986) but this remains the case in many hospitals particularly those with bulk meal systems.

Nutritional needs

The Committee on Medical Aspects of Food Policy publishes its Dietary Reference Values (DoH 1991) particularly for those involved in planning menus and food supplies. The menu planner also needs to be aware of any extra requirements which are unique to the client group. For example, a menu planned for an orthopaedic unit or a burns unit must take account of the extra requirement for energy and other nutrients in these client groups.

Knowing your situation

The dietitian has little direct influence on the type of catering service offered. However it is vital that the dietitian understands the local situation and how it affects the food offered.

Scale of the operation

The requirements of a 1000 bed acute hospital are very different to those of nursing home with ten residents.

Budget

How much have you got to spend? This is an important question and one which the menu planner must ask. The caterer will have a daily or weekly provisions cost within which to work if the catering budget is to be managed.

Availability of supplies

Are provisions available at an affordable price? What proportion of fresh, tinned or frozen commodities are going to be used? Can suppliers deliver fresh food every day at a suitable price? Where are supplies going to be obtained? What guarantees of quality are there? What specifications for the quality of supplies (including nutritional quality) are going to be laid down? How are standards to be assured?

Storage facilities

The Food Act 1991 makes stringent requirements of institutional caterers with regard to the storage of food. The nutritional quality of food deteriorates rapidly if it is not stored properly. The menu planner must be familiar with the storage facilities available.

Kitchen equipment and facilities

The menu planner must ensure that there are enough ovens, steamers, stoves, *bain maries*, boilers, pots and pans to prepare the menu proposed. For example it may not be possible to have a roast main course and a baked pudding on at the same meal if there is insufficient oven space!

Staff skills

The profile and skill-mix of the staff available to store, prepare, cook, serve and distribute food must be well understood by the menu planner. To design a menu which cannot be produced is not a good idea. The staffing resources available must also be fully understood. One cannot supply a cooked breakfast for service at 7.30AM if the kitchen staff start work at 7.00AM.

Distribution system and equipment

If the food is to be cooked and served to the client immediately, as would be the case in a small residential home, then the problems of distribution are minimal and do not affect menu planning. In a large hospital, where the kitchen might be located in a different building to the client, the distribution methods have far more impact.

Keeping food hot for a long period of time while it is distributed will have a deleterious effect on its palatability and its nutrient content. The menu planner needs to be aware of this so that anticipated nutrient deficits can be compensated for, and so that unsuitable dishes are not used (e.g. scrambled eggs are unsuitable for hot distribution because suppuration will occur).

Logistics of distribution

In designing a menu which will be appropriate for the institution and its clients, the menu planner needs to understand the logistics of the distribution system. When do clients want their meals? How long will it take to deliver food from the kitchen to the point of service? How many distribution staff will be needed? Can temperature control be maintained? Are the enough lifts, trolley tugs, free routes to the points of service? Can the distribution equipment be returned to the kitchen in time to be prepared for the next meal? All these questions have an influence on the menu, its composition and its suitability for a particular institution.

Service method

If the food is to be served onto plates in the kitchen, the constraints imposed upon the menu planner are different to those that would apply if the food is to be distributed in bulk.

Service equipment

The menu planner must be aware of the service equipment available. It is no good planning a menu which needs a bowl for soup, a bowl for salad and a bowl for pudding if you don't have enough bowls. If food needs to be prepared in service equipment (e.g. mousse in ramekins), that equipment will not be available for use earlier in the day.

How to plan a menu

A great deal of information is required before one embarks upon planning a menu. It is a time-consuming task, but if it is approached in stages it becomes more manageable as it is a logical process.

Menu planning should not be done by committees. If too many people are involved, planning will be a long, drawn out and probably fruitless process. The catering manager should be the compiler of the menu (i.e. this should be the responsibility of one person). However there should be consultation with dietitians and nursing staff and the views of patients should also be incorporated.

The difference between a well designed menu and one which is badly planned is not always immediately apparent to the lay person. A badly planned menu will ensure not only that the food presented to the client is inappropriate and poor nutritionally, it will also be difficult to provide and will be uneconomic.

1 Information gathering

Get together all the information described above. The client groups and the catering system must be well understood before the menu planning process can be undertaken.

2 Healthy eating

Caterers providing food to clients in an institution have a responsibility for the health and well-being of those clients. It is important that an institution's menu provides a healthy food choice. This must not compromise those clients who need energy-dense food; extra sugar and fat may well be indicated for these clients who often have a poor appetite.

The emphasis must be on providing choice; in this way clients needing what might be regarded as 'unhealthy' foods can be catered for. Institutional food is eaten by a large proportion of the population at some time or another and it has an important part to play in the promotion of good health and the prevention of diet related disease.

3 *Recipes*

Gather together as many tried and tested recipes as possible, preferably sized appropriately for the client group. Recipes which have previously been nutritionally analysed and costed are a great help (DoH 1988; Robbins 1989). Recipes should include information about serving equipment, yield, preparation time and garnishes required.

4 *Menu structure*

This must meet the needs of the patients and be compatible with the catering system. How many meals are there to be each day? How many main courses at each meal? What starters are to be offered? How many staples (i.e. potatoes, rice, pasta etc.) are to be offered? What choice of vegetables is to be offered? Will a side salad be available at every meal? How many puddings are to be offered? Will this include ice cream and cheese and biscuits? What modified diets are going to come from the main menu? What ethnic and cultural needs are to be met from the main menu? How long is the menu cycle going to be? Table 1.53 illustrates a draft outline structure for a large hospital menu offering the minimum number of choices to allow a reasonable number of modified diets to be incorporated.

5 *Plan the menu*

Take time to fit the recipes carefully into the structure. It is important at this stage to be able to visualise the menu as a whole. Planning on a large wall chart is advisable as it is important at this stage to consider how dishes complement one another in colour, texture, taste and appearance. Day one of a 21 day menu cycle must not be the same as day 21!

6 *Costing*

If recipes have been pre-costed this process becomes simpler. A planning figure for cost must be used which takes account of waste, shrinkage and seasonal price fluctuations. The weather will also have an effect on cost; dishes such as ice cream and salads will be more popular in hot weather, baked puddings and roast dinners will be more popular in cold weather.

The popularity of dishes will also have a day to day impact on the overall cost of the menu. Popular cheap dishes can offset the cost of the occasional more expensive dish.

A carefully costed menu is essential for the management of an institution's catering budget.

7 *Nutritional assessment*

Once planned, the menu as a whole should be assessed for its nutritional content and its suitability for the client group. Table 1.54 provides guidance for provision in a general hospital environment. The dietitian assessing the menu may need to refer to the COMA report on Dietary Reference Values (DoH 1991) and devise criteria for the

Table 1.53 Outline structure of a menu for a large hospital

Breakfast	Lunch	Supper
Fruit juice	Fruit juice	Fruit juice
Fresh fruit	Soup	Soup
Wholemeal cereal	Main meat or fish dish	Main meat or fish dish
Low residue cereal	Soft dish (suitable for those with no teeth)	Snack dish
Porridge		Soft dish
	Vegan dish	Vegan dish
Wholemeal bread	Salad	Sandwich
White bread		
	Suitable staple	Suitable staple
Butter	Mashed potato	Mashed potato
Low fat spread		
	Vegetable 1	Vegetable 1
Boiled egg	Vegetable 2	Vegetable 2
Jam	Baked pudding	Baked pudding
Marmalade	Milk pudding	Milk pudding
	Custard	Ice cream
Milk	Fresh fruit	Cheese and biscuits

Table 1.54 Guide to nutrient content of a typical acute hospital menu

Nutrient	Minimum content	Could provide	Notes
Protein	50 g/day Main dishes should provide 12–18 g protein each	90 g/day	It must be remembered that protein provided with insufficient energy cannot be used for growth and repair
Fat			Every effort should be made to use unsaturated fats where possible and a choice of yellow fats including low fat spread should be offered
Carbohydrate			A variety of wholemeal staple foods should be provided to encourage the consumption of non-starch polysaccharide
Energy	1200 kcal/day	2500 kcal/day	Patients in hospital are *not* representative of the general population and may require food which has a high energy density — food which would not be considered advisable, in the long term, for the healthy adult population
Vitamin C	40 mg/day		Readily destroyed by most large scale food provision systems. Fresh fruit juice, fruit and salad vegetables should be provided. Vitamin C supplements should be considered for those patients deemed to be at risk of deficiency
Folate	200 μg/day		Readily destroyed by most large scale food provision systems. Supplementation for pregnant women should be considered because they are currently advised not to have liver, a rich source of folate (DoH 1990)
Vitamin D	10 μg/day		Supplementation should be considered for pregnant and lactating women because they are currently advised not to have liver, a rich source of vitamin D (DoH 1990)

particular client group against which the menu can be assessed. Once again, recipes which have already been nutritionally analysed are very useful at this stage.

It may be necessary to code dishes as to their suitability for particular modified diets, vegetarians etc. The coding definitions set out in the Department of Health's Recipe File (DoH 1988) are probably the most widely use (see Table 1.55).

8 Test the menu

Testing the menu is the next most important step. Inform

Table 1.55 Guide to the coding of dishes suitable for particular diets (DoH 1988)

Dishes suitable for:	Should contain:	Notes
Weight reducing diets	Main course ≤ 300 kcal Pudding 50–100 kcal	
Diabetic diets	<3 g sugar (non-milk extrinsic sugar)	The use of the 10 g carbohydrate exchange system in the management of the diabetic diet is currently the subject of much controversy. The reader should consult the British Diabetic Association Guidelines (1992) for further information. If carbohydrate exchanges are to be used then any dish containing more than 5 g carbohydrate should have its carbohydrate content declared in 10 g exchanges
Fat reduced diets	Main course ≤ 15 g fat Pudding < 5 g fat	If this declaration is to be used to guide patients who need to control their serum lipid levels then the fat used should be predominantly of a mono- or polyunsaturated nature. When used to reduce total fat content (e.g. for the management of fat malabsorption) the type of fat is not so critical

everyone affected that the menu is to be tested and organize a system by which clients can make their views known and understood.

9 Review the menu

Menus grow old and client groups change. An institution's menu should be audited monthly. Clients' comments and suggestions, statistics on waste and dish popularity and the comments of dietitians, nursing and other staff should be used to review and refine the menu. As this process continues it is important to look at the menu as a whole, at the very least annually; frequently reviewed menus can rapidly deteriorate both in their nutritional content and by gradually increasing in cost.

1.16.3 The food distribution chain

A brilliantly planned menu is worthless if the food is stone cold when it arrives at the patient's bedside. The dietitian and the caterer need to be in control of the entire chain of events which enables raw ingredients to be prepared, distributed and delivered into the client's stomach which is the only place from which one can be sure that food provided is likely to nourish.

The path from the supplier's delivery van to the patient/client's stomach is often referred to as the *food chain*. The dietitian must understand the full workings and limitations of the food chain if food service provision is to be effective. Fig. 1.9 illustrates the food chain in a typical hospital.

All institutions will have a food chain of some description and there are important points the dietitian must consider if the food supplied is to be of maximum benefit to the client. The next few points are particularly relevant to hospitals with 200 or more beds, although some issues are also pertinent to smaller institutions.

Storekeeping

The management of provisions stores is an important first step in ensuring that good quality, wholesome and nutritionally optimal food is available. Secure inventory control is a key part of overall budget management. Ingredients kitchens can also maintain tight quality control on production and the implementation of standard recipes.

Food production

Standard recipes are the key to quality control in the production of food in the kitchen. If food production staff are not using standard recipes then the nutritional value of the food and its cost will be unknown quantities.

Standard recipes should include:

- An ingredients list;
- A method of production including the containers to be used and the equipment required (oven temperatures etc.);
- An expected yield;
- Production time;
- Garnishes required;
- Serving equipment required;
- The nutritional content of the dish including its suitability for particular modified diets;
- The best standard recipes include a colour photograph of the finished product.

It is possible, using modern information technology, for sized, standard recipes to be produced daily for each dish on the menu. The ingredients and the recipe can be put together in the ingredients kitchen. Skilled cooks then spend the minimum of time carrying out the unskilled work of gathering together and preparing ingredients and can concentrate on the skilled job of food production.

Service staff

Staff serving food either in a central kitchen for subsequent distribution or nearer the point of consumption, need to be aware of portion sizes for each dish, garnishes required and serving equipment to be used. Food service is a very important part of the food chain; the first part of the digestion of food is the cephalic phase stimulated by the

Professions involved or influencing the food chain in a typical hospital

* General Managers
* Caterers
* Dietitians
* Nurses
* Medical staff

SUPPLIERS ⇨ STORES ⇨ KITCHEN ⇨ DISTRIBUTION ⇨ NURSING ⇨ PATIENT

The chain is as strong as its weakest link

Fig. 1.9 The food chain

sight and smell of a dish. The appearance of food is the first step towards it being consumed, all food service staff must be made aware of its importance.

Distribution of food

Food must be distributed as quickly as possible. Hot holding of food has disastrous consequences for its nutritional value, its appearance and its taste, and must be kept to a minimum. The timing and logistics of distribution must be carefully planned and monitored. The time taken to serve food to patients once it arrives on the ward must also be taken into account.

Food service

Serving food to patients in a hospital and monitoring their food consumption is a nursing responsibility. Those responsible for ward areas or residential areas must ensure that there are suitable surroundings for the consumption of food.

Staff must ensure that suitable eating aids and equipment are available for patients who need them. There must be sufficient staff available at meal times to help those patients who cannot eat unaided. Staff who are responsible for feeding patients should be properly trained and, ideally, should themselves have experienced being fed by another. Ward routine should be so organized as to allow staff sufficient time to carry out their feeding service without interruptions.

Food choice

Clients and patients in institutions must have a choice of food and that choice should be exercised as close to the time of service as possible. There must be a mechanism in place by which the views of the client group with regard to food service can be made known and acted upon promptly.

Audit

The entire food chain must have in place a mechanism for internal, continuous audit. An institution's food service should be integrated into the total quality management of the organization. Accurate records must be kept in provisions stores, kitchens, distribution points and food service points, which provide an audit trail for the investigation of problems and the monitoring of standards. A food standards monitoring group with recognized reporting mechanisms and client representation should oversee the process of audit.

1.16.4 Recent advances in technology

Food production and distribution

Cook freeze, cook chill and cook conserve are catering technologies which have allowed food production to be divorced from food service. Using these methods of food preservation, food production is not tied to meal times and may well be remote from the area of food service. This means that food production units can make more efficient use of staff and facilities and benefit from economies of scale when they produce food for several end users.

In each system, food is cooked and then preserved by freezing, chilling or pasteurization and chilling, respectively. The food can be distributed in this preserved state and 'finished' or 'regenerated' at the point of service.

Quality control of the entire process is critical to its success. The Department of Health has strict guidelines on the use of these methods of food service (DoH 1989). If control is poor it will be microbiologically unsafe and the nutritional value of the food will diminish.

Information technology

Catering management systems are now readily available 'off the shelf'. This application of computer systems greatly facilitates institutional feeding particularly in large institutions such as hospitals. Software now available enables:

- Interactive menu planning with automatic nutritional analysis and costing;
- Archiving of all information on the production of food, facilitating audit and forecasting for production and budget management purposes;
- Inventory and stock control;
- Implementation of standard recipes;
- Acquisition of patient/client food choice in 'real time' (i.e. very close to the time of service and not 24 hours or more in advance);
- Printing of personalized menus including the patient's name and location and offering only those dishes which are compatible with a patient's dietary management.

Many of the mundane operational tasks associated with institutional feeding can now be automated enabling caterers and dietitians more time to audit and assure the quality of the service.

Further reading

Pyke M (1974) *Catering science and technology*. John Murray, London.

References

Askanazi J, Hensle TW, Starker PM, Lockhart SH, Olsson C, Kinney JM (1986) Effect of immediate post-operative nutritional support on

length of hospitalization. *Ann Surg* **203**, 236–9.
Bender A (1984) Institutional malnutrition. *Br Med J* **288**, 92–3.
Bistrian BR, Blackburn GL, Vitale J, Cochran D, Naylor J (1976) Prevalence of malnutrition in general medical patients. *J Am Med Assoc* **235**, 1567–70.
British Diabetic Association (1992) Dietary recommendations for people with diabetes: an update for the 1990s. *Diabetic Medicine* **9**(2), 189–202.
Department of Health (1986) *Health service catering manual. Volume 1, Nutrition and modified diets* 3e. HMSO, London.
Department of Health (1988) *Catering for health: The recipe file.* HMSO, London.
Department of Health (1989) *Chilled and frozen guidelines on cook-chill and cook freeze catering systems.* HMSO, London.
Department of Health Press Release No:90/507 (1990) Women cautioned: Watch your vitamin A intake. Hazard Warning Circular 25 October 1990. HMSO, London.
Department of Health (1991) Dietary Reference Values for food energy and nutrients for the United Kingdom. Report on Health and Social Subjects 41. HMSO, London.
Haydock DA and Hill GL (1986) Impaired wound healing in surgical patients with varying degrees of malnutrition. *J Parent Ent Nutr* **10**, 550–54.
Hill GL, Pickford I, Young GA, Schorah CJ, Blackett RL, Burkinshaw L, Warren JV, Morgan DB (1977) Malnutrition in surgical patients: an unrecognized problem. *Lancet* **1**, 689–92.
Hill SE (1990) *More than rice and peas.* The Food Commission, London.
Jensen JE, Jensen TG, Smith TK, Johnson DA, Dudrick SJ (1982) Nutrition in orthopaedic surgery. *J Bone Joint Surg* **64A**(9), 1263–72.
Mullen JL, Gertner MH, Buzby GP, Goodhart CL, Rosato EF (1979) Implications of malnutrition in the surgical patient. *Arch Surg* **114**, 121–5.
Reilly JJ, Hull SF, Albert N, Waller A, Bringardener S (1988) Economic impact of malnutrition: a model system for hospitalized patients. *J Parent Ent Nutr* **12**, 371.
Robbins C (1989) *The healthy catering manual.* Dorling Kindersley, London.
Robinson G, Goldstein M, Levine GM (1987) The impact of nutritional status on DRG length of stay. *J Parent Ent Nutr* **11**, 49–51.
Taylor E and Taylor J (1990) *Mastering catering theory.* Macmillan Master Series. Macmillan Education, London.
Twomey PL and Patching SC (1985) Cost-effectiveness of nutritional support. *J Parent Ent Nutr* **9**, 3–10.

1.17 Food policy

During the 1980s, a number of scientific reports highlighted the relationship between diet and health (DHSS 1981; RCP 1981; RCP 1983; NACNE 1983; DHSS 1984; BMA 1986; DoH 1989). A food policy attempts to implement these recommendations within a particular population group or organization and thus promote better health via an appropriate diet.

A *policy* may be considered to be a statement of intent which has been endorsed by the highest authority within an organization and will therefore be incorporated into that organization's planning process. A *food policy* will often be in the form of a written statement outlining the dietary changes to be achieved, by whom and over what timescale. This may well be accompanied by an outline of the strategies to be employed for promoting dietary change and will form part of the management's health care strategy.

Food policies have been adopted by Health Authorities, private companies, local and education authorities throughout the country. Since a policy will have been endorsed by the organization's hierarchy, it will have advantages over localized 'one-off' initiatives by:

1 Promoting collaboration among relevant people in the planning and implementation processes.

2 Allowing coherent and sustained actions which can be referred to by changing personnel.

3 Being more likely to attract funding.

1.17.1 Development of food policies in the National Health Service

Health Authorities have a responsibility laid down by government to assess and provide for the health needs of the population (Acheson 1988). In 1986, a survey of Health Authorities and Health Boards in the UK investigated work being done on food policies (Gibson and Champion 1989). A follow-up survey in 1989 showed that 82% of these had a formally approved policy and a further 14% were developing or planning to develop one (Gibson *et al* 1990a).

The development of these policies has largely been the result of a grass-roots initiative since there has been no directive from central government to do so. The two reports which have been most influential in providing the impetus are those from the National Advisory Committee on Nutrition Education (NACNE 1983) and the Report on *Diet and Cardiovascular Disease* (DHSS 1984). The dietary goals or targets in food policies are usually based on these recommendations.

In the 1990s, there have been two documents which further justify the need for food policies. The COMA report on Dietary Reference Values (DoH 1991a) gives an essential update on required nutrient intakes for population groups within the UK. The Government's strategy on health has also been set out in the document *The Health of the Nation* (DoH 1991b).

1.17.2 Basis of a policy document

Food policy documents vary according to the local situation. The policy may simply be a statement of intent such 'a commitment to improve the nutritional status of the population in a particular area'. This can then be built upon and a strategy for implementation devised alongside it. There is no blueprint for a policy document.

It is worth considering, however, the points that a food policy document may cover. These include:

- A review of the scientific evidence supporting the need for dietary change;
- The aims and objectives of the policy;
- Target group(s) within the population;
- The dietary goals (targets) to be met;
- Timescale objectives;
- Translation of the dietary goals into practical catering/ healthy eating guidelines;
- Strategies for implementation;
- Methods for monitoring and evaluation;
- Financial resources, including manpower implications;
- Reference/supporting material.

The policy is likely to be drawn up by a working group with a predominance of dietitians and health promotion officers (Gibson and Champion 1989).

In 1989, 53% of Health Authorities/Health Boards had identified those responsible for co-ordinating policy implementation, usually dietetic or health promotion departments or the working group.

It is important to be aware of interests outside the immediate health service environment. The proceedings of the Food Network Conference (Hurren and Black 1991), organized jointly by the HEA and the BDA, clearly identify the range of interests that are involved. Food is big business.

1.17.3 Food policy aims

Most policies developed initially have been for healthy adults based on the NACNE and COMA goals and aim to:

- Provide information and/or education for consumers about the relationship between diet and health allowing informed choices to be made;
- Ensure that healthy food choices are available and enjoyable;
- Educate staff to support the policy principles and content.

Other groups within the population including children, pregnant and breast feeding women, low income families, elderly people, those of ethnic origin and hospital patients will need special consideration to take account of their specific needs.

1.17.4 Implementation

Within the NHS, a Health Authority will have a policy covering its catchment area. There are often two distinct areas of food policy work; that done in hospitals and that done in the community (Gibson and Champion 1989).

Much work has been carried out at Health Authority sites because the NHS is the largest employer in Britain and all staff (hospital and community) can be seen as potential educators. Additionally, the majority of State Registered dietitians work in the NHS and they are in the forefront of policy implementation.

With the increasing move to greater autonomy within the NHS, self-governing trusts will now be setting their own policies. This means that the issue of food policies must be considered on the basis of the purchaser-provider divide.

The *commissioning and purchasing* of health care is now the responsibility of Health Authorities.

The *providers* of health care generally fall into one of three categories:

1 Directly managed units.
2 NHS self-governing trusts.
3 Private health care facilities.

Thus now, and in the future, if Health Authorities wish patients to be given care in establishments giving a high priority to nutrition, it is likely that they will:

- Identify a nutrition policy they wish to see achieved;
- Require contracts to be awarded to providers who meet their nutritional specifications.

Policies for promoting health, including food issues, may well be the responsibility of persons charged with service quality issues on both the purchaser and provider side. At the present time, dietitians may be asked to advise both health care purchasers and providers.

Increasing pressure on dietetic departments and all service providers to generate an income can lead to problems. Money-making schemes which, for example, sell advertizing space on menu cards or allow burger bars and cake shops on hospital sites can undermine a food policy.

General aspects of implementation in hospital and community services

The policy

It is essential that all personnel involved in any specific action are in agreement with the translation of the dietary guidelines within the policy. Practical guidelines can still cause confusion if misinterpreted; for example, if unfamiliar cooking methods are incorrectly applied due to the lack of appropriate training. Within the community the policy adopted by some organizations may differ to that of the Health Authority. Any area of difference must be identified and discussed before any collaborative action is taken.

Outside initiatives affecting food policy work

Initiatives from organizations outside the Health Authority which aim to promote a healthy food choice should be considered when implementing an HA strategy since it may be beneficial to participate in other projects. Examples include the HEA's 'Look After Your Heart' Campaign (LAYH) of which the 'Heartbeat Award', 'Food for the Heart Month' and the 'Workplace Project' have been positive initiatives. The Regional Health Authority may also set targets at District HA level, such as working towards a reduction in deaths from heart disease and cancer.

Personnel

Before embarking on a project it is essential to know who will help. It is worth noting that lack of commitment and support by staff has been reported as a barrier to implementation (Montague 1986; Gibson *et al* 1990a), so it is important to involve those with a positive attitude.

Help is most likely to come from:

- Member(s) of the Food Policy team/working group;
- Community Health Council;
- Local key staff, both hospital and community based, (e.g. in management, catering, nursing, dietetics, medical — especially from the department of Public Health, health promotion, dentistry, primary health care team, local education, local authority, voluntary organizations, polytechnic/university).

The approach

The changes to be made may be low or high profile. For example a low profile change would include the substitution of semi-skimmed milk for whole milk and the change from frying to grilling in catering outlets without publicity. A high profile change might be the introduction of a new menu labelling scheme or a new food labelling scheme in a retail outlet with a high degree of publicity to promote and assist customer choice.

Involving consumers by using questionnaires, inviting clients to join planning groups or offering tasting days for a new menu items will allow consumer acceptability to be tested.

Resources

The resources needed for each action should be clearly identified. These may include staff time, teaching materials, cost of new products, reference material, accommodation. These must be known so that appropriate bids may be made for funding and the costs included in the evaluation of the policy. Lack of funding has repeatedly been reported as a barrier to implementation (Gibson *et al* 1990a).

Promotion

Numerous different activities have been carried out to promote food policies. Table 1.56 lists some suggestions which can be modified to meet local needs.

Specific aspects of implementation in hospitals

Meeting nutritional needs of hospital inpatients

Reports of malnutrition among hospital patients have shown the problems associated with meeting their nutritional needs (PENG 1990; Lennard-Jones 1992). It is essential that this is considered when implementing general healthy eating guidelines. A food policy has been shown to improve the diet of some patients (Wallis and Poulter 1988) but it is vital that any dietary intervention is monitored and evaluated to ensure that this is the case (Nelson 1989).

Table 1.56 Examples of activities for implementing a food policy
(It will be helpful to include a timetable of the planned events and to record the overall project cost)

Area of action	Target group	Key staff in implementation	Possible areas of training needed	Resources available/needed	Monitoring method
Staff training	Caterers Nurses Nursing auxillaries Medical staff Voluntary groups Primary health care team College of nursing Local authority staff	Dietitian Manager of appropriate service Health promotion	Importance of healthy eating to each group What the food policy means New ideas for catering Nutritional needs of patient/client groups	Staff time Accommodation	Numbers attending Questionnaires on knowledge/attitude
Recipe/menu development	Staff restaurants Patients meal service Workplace canteens	Catering Manager and staff Dietitian Patient/staff/client representatives	Recipe evaluation Menu adaptation Marketing Food choice/availability	Literature	Nutritional analysis Food choices Food costs Food wastage Food purchasing Satisfaction survey Laxative use
Positive marketing e.g. Healthy eating days Healthy eating weeks Quizzes Food fairs	Staff Patients Clients outside NHS General public	Health Promotion Officers Dietitians Caterers 'Local' key staff	Healthy eating message Practical meal ideas Tasting sessions	Teaching materials Money	Questionnaires Attendance numbers Media interest
Changes in food – Pricing – Availability – Sales	Vending machines Tuck shops Restaurants Luncheon clubs Snack bars Retail shops Workplaces Sporting outlets	Caterers Dietitians Finance departments Local retailers/businesses	Data collection and presentation	Support from other agencies	Recording of changes over period of survey
Production of educational material	Staff Public Other	Local staff/individuals involved in projects Health Promotion Officers Dietitian	According to project needs e.g. leaflets, video, poster, menucards	e.g. Retailers Companies Volunteers	Pre- and post-intervention changes

Catering and purchasing

A food policy can be a useful way of reminding a Health Authority of its responsibility when issuing contract specifications. The policy recommendations should be included in both Health Service contracts and catering contracts. Practical dietary information can thus be given on:

- Ingredients to be used;
- Cooking methods;
- Portion size;
- Frequency of items on the menus;
- Specific products necessary for therapeutic diets.

The mechanisms used to monitor the contract can check whether or not these specifications are met. The effects of any cost saving initiatives within the hospital services or catering budget may lead to undesirable changes as far as food policy implementation is concerned. Reductions in staff numbers, catering systems using food produced by outside food manufacturers, and a reduction in foods prepared on site may reduce the opportunity for developing recipes with favourable dietary modifications and reduce the food choices available.

The nutritional specification of food items on contract is worth investigating. These specifications are very rarely determined at District level but it is an issue which can be taken up at Regional level possibly via a Regional Dietitians' Group or Regional Supplies Offices Group.

1.17.5 Monitoring and evaluation

Evaluation is the process by which the effectiveness of the intervention is assessed (Gibson and Champion 1989). Evaluation reports may be used to promote the policy, raise awareness of the policy, provide information for deciding whether to continue, stop or modify a specific activity or for providing further funding. *Evaluation Methodologies for Food and Health Policies* (Gibson *et al* 1990b) is essential reading on this.

In respect of food policy work, it has been said that 'evaluation is heard but not seen' (Food Policy News 1985/86). Evaluation may seem a daunting task but by starting in a small way with one project it can be very worthwhile.

A necessary first step is to record baseline data against which changes resulting from the policy implementation can be measured. Although changes in morbidity and mortality may not be seen for 30 years or more, other factors can be measured. These include:

- Measurement of the activities of different departments involved in implementation;
- Changes in organizational practices;
- Changes in knowledge, attitudes and behaviour.

Such measurements may be made in different ways, for example:

- Recording changes in the purchasing pattern of organizations and individuals;
- Questionnaires and surveys;
- Nutritional analysis.

These measurements are then repeated at regular intervals (Yorkshire RHA 1986).

Useful addresses

Health Education Authority
Mabledon Place, London, WC1H 9TX
Community Nutrition Group,
British Dietetic Association, Birmingham
Food Policy News,
c/o Shire Lodge, The Old Stables,
East Langton, Leicestershire, LE16 7TW
Food Policy Research Department,
University of Bradford, Bradford, BD7 1DP
Public Health Alliance,
Room 204, Snow Hill House
10–15 Livery Street, Birmingham B3 2PE

Further reading

Booth D and Kemm JR (1992) *Promotion of healthier eating: how to collect and use information for planning, monitoring and evaluation*. HMSO, London.
DHSS (1988) *Catering for health. The recipe file*. HMSO, London.
Robbins C (1989) *The healthy catering manual*. Dorling Kindersley, London.

References

Acheson D (1988) *Public Health in England; the report of the committee of enquiry into the future development of the public health function*. HMSO, London.
British Medical Association (1986) *Diet, nutrition and health*. BMA, London.
DHSS (1981) *Prevention and health: Avoiding heart attacks*. HMSO, London.
DHSS (1984) Report on Health and Social Subjects No 28. *Diet and cardiovascular disease*. HMSO, London.
Department of Health (1989) Report on Health and Social Subjects 37. *Dietary sugars and human disease*. Committee on Medical Aspects of Food Policy. HMSO, London.
Department of Health (1991a) *Dietary Reference Values for food energy and nutrients for the United Kingdom*. Rep Health Soc Subj No 41. HMSO, London.
Department of Health (1991b) *The health of the nation*. HMSO, London.
Food Policy News (1985/86) London. Editorial. Evaluate or be lost.
Gibson L and Champion P (1989) *Results of the 1986 Food Health Policy Survey*. Health Education Authority, London.
Gibson L, Kallevik J and Hunt R (1990a) Food Health Policies. *The UK District Health Authority and Health Board National Study*. Progress Report. Health Education Authority, London.
Gibson L, Poulter J and Winkler J (1990b) Evaluation methodologies for food and health policies. *J Hum Nutr Dietet* 3, 55–9.
Hurren C and Black A (Eds.) (1991) *The food network. Achieving a healthy diet by the year 2000*. Smith-Gordon, London.
Lennard-Jones JE (1992) *A positive approach to nutrition as treatment*. King's Fund Centre, London.
Montague S (1986) Development of local food and health policies in Britain. *J Roy Soc Hlth* 4, 147–9.

National Advisory Committee on Nutrition Education (1983) *Proposals for nutritional guidelines for health education in Britain*. Health Education Council, London.

Nelson J (1989) Some food for thought. *The Health Service Journal* 99, 666–7.

Parental and Enteral Nutrition Group (PENG) (1990) The management of nutritionally compromised patients in hospital. A discussion paper. British Dietetic Association, Birmingham.

Royal College of Physicians of London (1981) *Report on the Medical Aspects of Dietary Fibre*. RCP, London.

Royal College of Physicians of London (1983) Obesity. *J Roy Coll Physcns* **17**, 3–58.

Wallis C and Poulter J (1988) Longitudinal study of food intake of psychiatric patients following food policy implementation. *J Hum Nutr Dietet* **1**, 23–8.

Yorkshire Regional Health Authority (1986) *Guidelines on formulating a food policy*. Yorkshire RHA, Harrogate.

Section 2 **Foods and nutrients**

2.1 Dietary energy

2.1.1 Fundamental principles

The fundamental principles of energy physiology, bomb calorimetry and the measurement of food energy, direct and indirect calorimetry for the measurement of energy expenditure and discussion of the regulation of body weight are to be found in Passmore and Eastwood (1986).

The fundamental principle of energy physiology and the regulation of body weight is

Energy intake = Energy Expenditure ± Changes in Body Stores.

Intake and expenditure are not balanced on a daily or even a weekly basis, but, if weight remains stable, then, over a period of time, energy intake must equal energy expenditure and energy requirements are determined by energy expenditure.

2.1.2 The components of energy expenditure

The components of energy expenditure are

1 Basal metabolic rate (BMR).

2 Energy expended above the resting rate due to physical activity.

3 Energy expended above the resting rate due to thermogenesis as a response to food intake, drugs or psychological influences.

Figure 2.1 shows the contribution made by these three components to the 24-hour energy expenditure of normal weight sedentary subjects and the factors that affect them (Jequier 1984).

Total energy expenditure (TEE)

Total energy expenditure may be measured in four ways.

Whole body calorimetry The subject is confined in a whole body calorimeter. This enables the energy expenditure under controlled conditions to be measured, but gives limited information on energy expenditure under free-living conditions. (See Passmore and Eastwood 1986, for the principles of calorimetry.)

Activity diary The subject keeps a minute by minute activity diary, and subsequently the times spent on individual activities are totalled and multiplied by the energy cost in kcal per minute. The latter may be taken from the literature or determined from measurements made on the subject under study. This technique has been much used by the leading energy physiologists and has provided valuable information on energy requirements. Keeping an activity diary is extremely tedious for the subject, however and the technique, except in the hands of dedicated researchers and highly committed subjects, is relatively crude.

The doubly-labelled water technique (DLW) A technique for measuring TEE in small mammals using the stable isotopes of ^2H and ^{18}O has been available since the 1950s. In the 1980s, improvements in the precision of isotope-ratio mass spectrometers reduced the costs making it financially viable for studies in humans. The subject takes a drink of water labelled with ^2H and ^{18}O and provides a single sample of urine for each of the next 10–20 days. The level of isotope in the body water is measured in the daily urine samples using mass spectrometry. The isotopes distribute themselves throughout the body water and enter the metabolic pool. Deuterium leaves the body in water, and oxygen 18 leaves in both water and carbon dioxide. The difference between the rates of disappearance of the two isotopes permits calculation of the carbon dioxide produced and hence, using classical respirometry equations, of the energy expended. For more detail see Prentice (1986).

Since TEE by DLW is measured over 10–20 days, it represents energy expenditure integrated over a relatively long time period unlike the usually very short measurements obtained by calorimetry. It is an ideal field technique and has provided new insights into the energy expenditure of free-living subjects. The technique is however expensive and requires sophisticated laboratory back-up.

The technique has been validated against calorimetry in 13 studies by four independent research groups. Accuracy (agreement between means) is 1–3% and precision (standard deviation of differences between DLW and calorimetry) is 2–8%. In one laboratory, the coefficient of variation (CV) of repeated measurements on the same subject was ±8.5% (Prentice and Black unpublished). This includes both the measurement error and the biological variation in week to week activities.

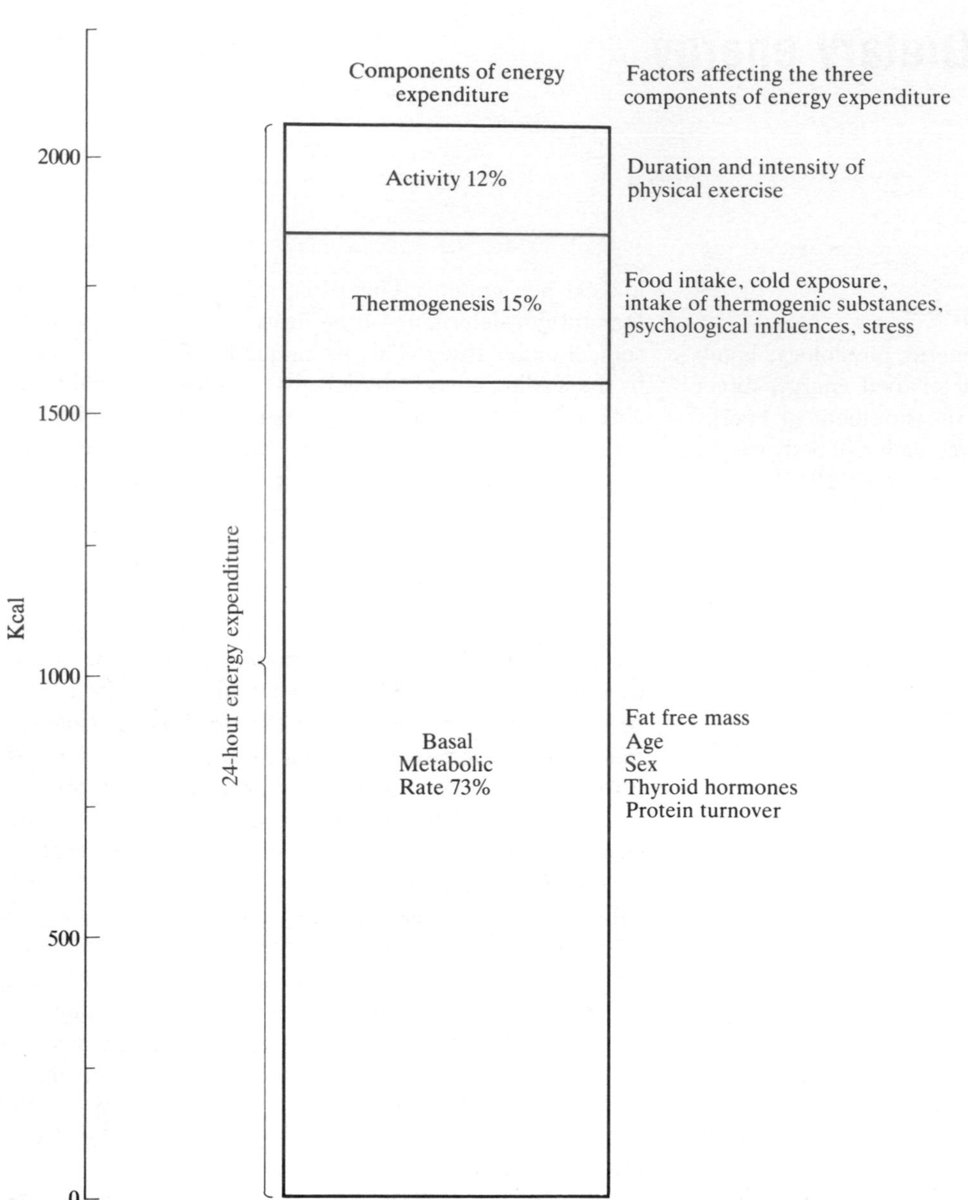

Fig. 2.1 Factors affecting the three components of energy expenditure.

Heart rate monitoring The subject has electrodes attached to his or her chest over a period of time; these pick up the electrical impulses generated by the heart. The heart beats are 'collected' by radio monitors similar to wrist watches. Since the heart rate is proportional to the level of activity an estimate of energy expenditure over a period of time can be obtained. Each subject has to be personally 'calibrated' by measurement of the heart rate while lying, sitting, standing, and cycling at graded and increasing workloads. The major limitation of this technique is that heart rate is not sensitive to changes in energy expenditure at the low levels of activity that constitute most of a sedentary lifestyle. The technique is more fully described by Spurr *et al* (1988).

Basal metabolic rate (BMR)

The BMR is a standardized measurement. It is the energy expenditure (expressed per 24 hours) measured immediately upon waking, in a state of complete physical rest, 13 hours after the last meal, with the subject lying awake and completely still and in a thermoneutral temperature. It requires therefore that the subject sleep in the place where the measurement is made. Under highly standardized and controlled conditions the CV for BMR measurements made on the same individual on repeated occasions is around ±2%.

The conditions for a true BMR measurement may not always be obtainable. The Resting Metabolic Rate (RMR) is any other measurement of resting metabolism under conditions that approximate to the above. A frequent compromise is to bring the subject to the place of measurement early in the morning in a fasting state and to ensure at least half an hour of relaxed rest before making the measurement.

A number of equations exist for predicting BMR, also several sets of 'standards' derived from them. Since BMR is the major component of energy expenditure and is the basis of the Dietary Reference Values (DRVs) for energy (see below), it is important to understand the limitations of the equations. These have been comprehensively reviewed by Elia (1992).

The equations are derived from samples of individuals on whom BMR has been measured. For an individual of a given age, sex, weight and height the various equations may give predicted values for the BMR that differ by anything from 2% to 20%. The differences may appear in particular age-sex groups or there may be also systematic differences between standards (illustrated in Fig. 2.2).

Reasons for differences between standards probably include both methodological and biological differences in the data used to derive them. These include:

1 Whether individuals were measured once only or on several occasions;

2 Differences in equipment used, for example whether a hood or mouthpiece was used to collect expired air;

3 Different environmental temperatures used;

4 Whether body weight did or did not include street clothes;

5 Equations used to calculate energy expenditure from gaseous exchange are rarely specified and may be different;

6 Variable proportions of subjects at the extremes of body composition (i.e. with high or low BMI);

7 Race;

8 Varying numbers of subjects.

Differences between standards are complicated by the use of surface area in some equations and weight and height in others. Surface area is itself usually predicted by equations based on weight and height and therefore compounds the errors in the calculation of BMR. Standards based on surface area include those of Aub and Dubois, Boothby and colleagues (Mayo Clinic), Robertson and Reid, Fleish, and Quenouille and colleagues none of which are widely used today.

The equations of Harris and Benedict (1919) were based on weight and height and have remained widely used particularly in clinical practice. They were derived from measurements on only 239 subjects although covering a range of body size and composition. Benedict himself acknowledged that the equations overestimate BMR, and in 24 studies reviewed by Elia (1992) the mean per cent deviation of measured BMR from the Harris and Benedict prediction was −5.8% for men and −7.2% for women; in only two out of 44 groups was the deviation positive.

The most recent standards based on weight and substantial numbers of subjects are those of Schofield *et al* (1985). These authors reviewed the literature on BMR for the FAO/WHO/UNU (1985) committee on energy and protein requirements. Technically acceptable results were extracted from the literature for 7549 individuals and used to derive equations for predicting BMR from body weight for six age ranges: 0−3, 3−10, 10−18, 18−30, 30−60,

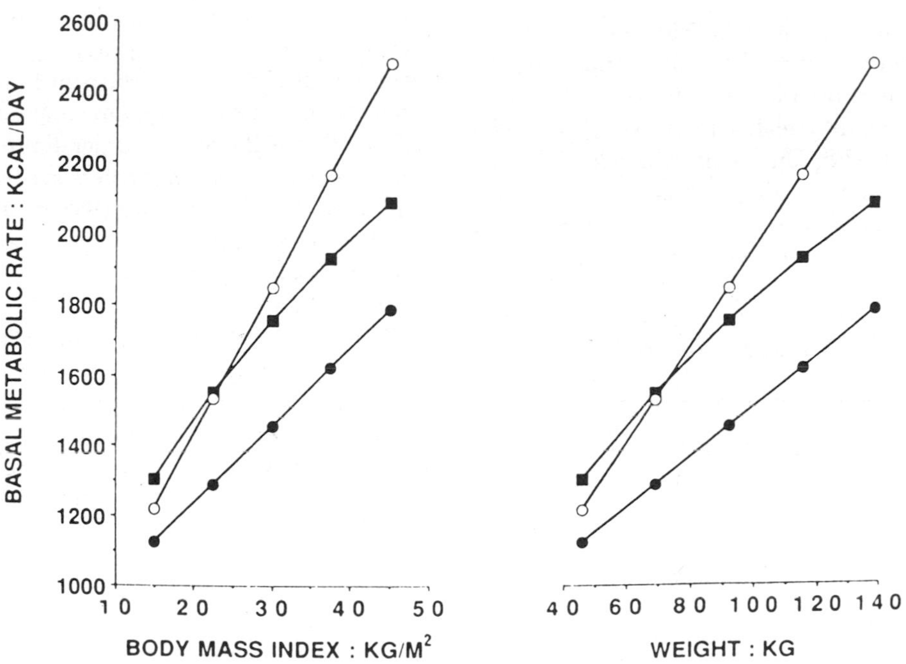

Fig. 2.2 Prediction of basal metabolic rate in 25-year-old females 1.75 m with different body weights and body mass indices, using three different methods: (□——□). Schofield *et al* (1985). ■——■. Fleish (1951). ●——●. Owen *et al* (1986) (From, Elia 1992). Reproduced with permission.

and 60+ years and both sexes separately. BMR is highly correlated with body weight and including surface area or body height in the prediction equations made no significant difference to the accuracy of prediction. The equations were subsequently adjusted by the COMA Panel (DoH 1991) on DRVs by excluding some of the data derived from studies in Third World countries. These are given in Table 2.1. Appendix 4 gives look-up tables for BMR by age, sex and body weight derived from these equations (Tables 7.40 and 7.41).

In one laboratory (Prentice *et al* personal communication), comparison of individual measured BMR values with those predicted by the Schofield equations gave a mean difference of 2% (measure: predicted values, mean 1.02, standard deviation 0.09, range 0.82–1.19). The subjects however were all healthy adults and few were at the extremes of body composition. Schofield *et al* (1985) suggest that, at any given body weight, the variance of an individual value about the predicted mean results in a CV of about 8%. This includes both the error on using a predicted rather than a measured value and the biological variation. The deviation may be greater at extremes of body composition, but there is limited data on BMR of individuals with weights greater than 80 kg.

2.1.3 Energy requirements

The principles currently used to estimate energy requirements are set out in detail in the report of the FAO/WHO/UNU Joint Expert Consultation (1985). These same principles were used by the COMA Panel on Dietary Reference Values (DoH 1991) with minor modifications appropriate to the UK situation.

> 'The energy requirement of an individual is the level of energy intake from food that will balance energy expenditure when the individual has a body size and composition, and level of physical activity, consistent with long-term good health; and that will allow for the maintenance of economically necessary and socially desirable physical activity. In children and pregnant or lactating women the energy requirement includes the energy needs associated with the deposition of tissues or the secretion of milk at rates consistent with good health.'
>
> (FAO/WHO/UNU 1985)

> 'As far as possible, energy requirements should be determined from estimates of energy expenditure.'
>
> (FAO/WHO/UNU 1985)

The major component of energy expenditure is the Basal Metabolic Rate. The FAO/WHO/UNU (1985) committee established a new principle of expressing energy expenditure as multiples of BMR. Thus the energy expenditure during sleep is 1.0 × BMR, while cycling uphill might cost 7.0 × BMR. These figures for the energy costs of specific activities are called Physical Activity Ratio or PAR. Examples of PAR are given in the COMA report, Annexe 3 (DoH 1991).

Table 2.1 Equations for predicting basal metabolic rate from body weight (DoH 1991)

	Males		Females	
Age range	kcal/day	MJ/day	kcal/day	MJ/day
10–17	17.7w + 657	0.074w + 2.754	13.4w + 692	0.056w + 2.898
18–29	15.1w + 692	0.063w + 2.896	14.8w + 487	0.062w + 2.036
30–59	11.5w + 873	0.048w + 3.653	8.3w + 846	0.034w + 3.538
60–74	11.9w + 700	0.0499w + 2.930	9.2w + 687	0.0386w + 2.875
75+	8.4w + 821	0.0350w + 3.434	9.8w + 624	0.041w + 2.610

w = body weight (kg)

Energy requirements of adults

Estimates of energy requirements in adults and teenage children have been determined from estimates of energy expenditure. To estimate the total energy requirement of an individual, the BMR is calculated from body weight (see above) and multiplied by a factor that covers the energy cost of increased muscle tone, physical activity, the thermic effect of food and, where relevant, the energy requirements for growth and lactation.

From information in the literature, the energy cost of various occupational and discretionary activities in terms of multiples of the BMR has been estimated. A factorial calculation is then used to determine the overall 24 hour energy requirement. For example, a value of 1.4 times BMR was obtained from the literature for waking hours to cover the cost of washing, dressing, and short periods of standing. If eight hours are spent in bed at 1.00 × BMR, then the overall energy requirement for 24 hours is 1.27 × BMR. This is the level of expenditure to be found only in totally inactive dependent persons. It is not compatible with long term health and makes no allowance for energy needed to earn a living or prepare food. This was termed the 'survival requirement' by the FAO/WHO/UNU (1985) committee.

The COMA (DoH 1991) panel also used this factorial approach to calculate the energy requirements for varying life styles and differing levels of occupational and discretionary activity. For adults total energy requirement is estimated as the sum of energy needed for BMR plus additional energy needed for specific activities. The additional costs of specific activities are estimated from knowledge of the time spent in each activity and the energy cost (PAR) of that activity. While the gross energy costs of certain activities may be very high while the activity is being undertaken – labouring tasks such as digging or hand sawing, or strongly athletic recreations such as rowing – these are rarely maintained for extended periods of time.

Energy costs of activity are 'diluted' by time spent merely sitting or standing around and the daily average is further reduced by hours spent asleep. Examples of the energy costs of various activities and occupations are given in the COMA Report, Annexes 3, 4 and 6 (DoH 1991).

An example of the factorial approach is given in Table 2.2.

The average daily energy requirements of adults obtained using the factorial approach are given in Table 2.3. These figures for 24-hour energy expenditure expressed as multiples of BMR have since come to be referred to as physical activity levels or PALs. In the UK it is likely that the overall energy expenditure of an individual may be influenced more by the recreational than the occupational activity. PAL values varying with both occupational and recreational activity levels are given in Table 2.3.

Energy requirements of children and adolescents aged 10–18 years

These are based on the same principles as for adults (see Table 2.3). They are best estimated on the basis of body weight rather than age, since weight may vary widely at any given age. An additional 5% allowance is added for the average daily cost of weight gain. The EARs for children and adolescents are given by the COMA Panel (DoH 1991), Annexe 7, p. 207.

Energy requirements of children aged 3–10 years

Information on the time and cost of activities of children is not available. Estimated requirements have therefore been based on data on energy intake obtained from dietary surveys. The COMA Panel based their estimates on data from UK studies. The estimated energy requirements for children aged 3–10 years are set out on page 21 of the COMA Report (DoH 1991).

Energy requirements of children aged 0–36 months

Data from recent doubly-labelled water measurements was used by the COMA panel (1991) to provide information on

Table 2.2 Example of a factorial calculation of energy expenditure

Subject: Clinical dietitian, age 28 y, weight 55 kg, BMR = 5.45 MJ

Activity	Time in activity hr	Physical Activity Ratio (PAR)	Total energy cost, MJ (5.45 × PAR × Time/24)
Bed	8.0	1.0	1.82
Getting dressed	0.5	2.8	0.32
Morning chores	0.5	2.1	0.24
Driving to work	0.5	1.6	0.18
Walking around hospital	2.0	2.8	1.27
Standing, ward round etc.	2.0	2.1	0.95
Sitting, office work, OP clinic	3.5	1.6	1.27
Sitting, meal breaks	1.0	1.2	0.27
Driving to sports club	0.5	1.6	0.18
Exercise, squash	0.5	6.9	0.78
Standing, socializing	0.5	1.6	0.18
Driving home	0.25	1.6	0.09
Evening chores	2.0	2.1	0.95
Watching TV	1.75	1.2	0.40
Preparing for bed	0.5	2.8	0.31
Total	24.0		9.21

$$\text{Physical activity level (PAL)} = \frac{\text{Energy expenditure}}{\text{BMR}} = 1.69$$

Table 2.3 Calculated Physical Activity Level (PAL) of adults at three levels of occupational and non-occupational activity. (DoH 1991). Reproduced with the permission of the Controller of Her Majesty's Stationery Office

	Occupational activity					
Non-occupational activity	Light		Moderate		Moderate/Heavy	
	Male	Female	Male	Female	Male	Female
Non-active	1.4	1.4	1.6	1.5	1.7	1.5
Moderately active	1.5	1.5	1.7	1.6	1.8	1.6
Very active	1.6	1.6	1.8	1.7	1.9	1.7

Footnote:
Physical activity ratio (PAR) = the energy cost of a specific activity e.g. 7.0 × BMR for cycling uphill
Physical activity level (PAL) = the overall energy cost of a 24-hour period encompassing varying periods of time spent in activities of varying PAR

total energy expenditure. These were on average in agreement with observed dietary energy intakes from modern infant formulas and with FAO/WHO/UNU estimates of observed intake of toddlers. The EARs for children ages 0–36 months are set out in the COMA report on page 20 (DoH 1991).

2.1.4 Prescribing energy intakes

In any dietary prescription the limiting parameter is the energy intake of the individual, whether the intention is to maintain or to change body weight. It has been customary in the past to take a dietary history from patients in order to estimate their energy requirements and obtain the baseline for the dietary prescription. It is considerably less time-consuming and probably more accurate (certainly no less) to use PAL values.

1 Weigh the subject.

2 Calculate BMR as predicted from weight by equations (Table 2.1) or use the look-up tables (Tables 7.40 and 7.41 in Appendix 4). Note that deviations of predicted BMR from true BMR may be greater at the extremes of body composition. There is limited data on the BMR of individuals with body weights greater than 80 kg, and Schofield *et al* (1985) did not consider it appropriate to include heavier weights in their own look-up table. They are included in Appendix 4 for ease of reference for those

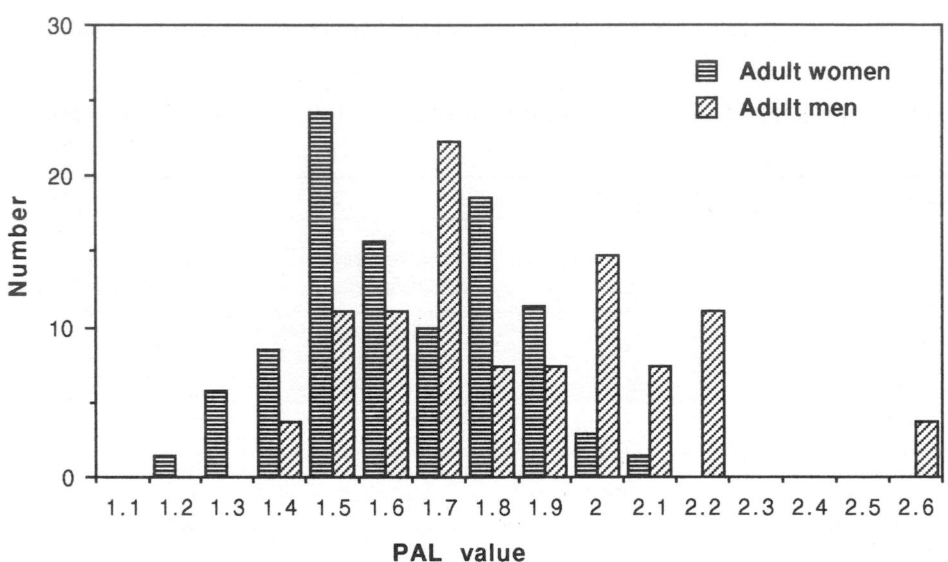

Fig. 2.3a Distribution of PAL values in adult men and women as determined from measurements of BMR by calorimetry and total energy expenditure by doubly-labelled water (Data from Dunn Nutrition Centre, Cambridge).

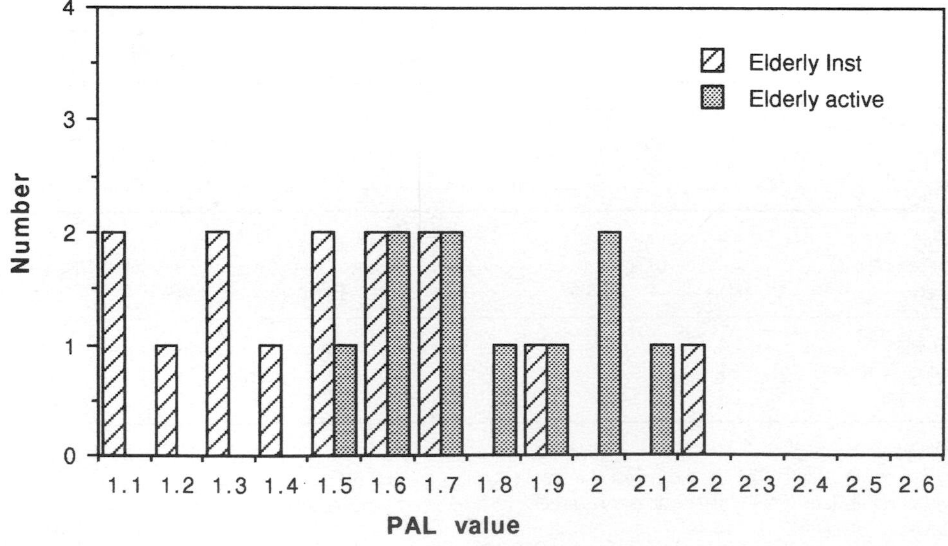

Fig. 2.3b Distribution of PAL values as determined from measurements of BMR by calorimetry and total energy expenditure by doubly-labelled water in a group of elderly institutionalized women and a group of elderly women living in their own homes (Data from Dunn Nutrition Centre, Cambridge).

working in obesity clinics, although it is probable that the equations overestimate BMR in the heaviest individuals.
3 Obtain information on the recreational and occupational activity of the subject and choose an appropriate PAL from Table 2.3 to calculate the total energy requirements. Examples of the PAR or PAL for various activities and occupations are given in the COMA Report Annexes 3 and 4 (DoH 1991).
4 Multiply BMR by the chosen PAL factor to obtain total energy requirement.

The PAL values in Table 2.3 are recommended population averages (DoH 1991). The distribution of individual PAL values for total energy expenditure in free-living conditions from studies at the Dunn Nutrition Centre are shown in Figs 2.3a and 2.3b. The range is from 1.1 × BMR in a totally sedentary Alzheimers patient to 2.6 in a building labourer working 12 hour shifts. These two figures indicate the limits of the range likely to be sustained for any length of time in day-to-day life. A value of 2.8 × BMR has been obtained in female athletes during a period of rigorous training and an extreme of 5.4 × BMR in a cyclist during the Tour de France. Guidance on typical PAL values for different activities and occupations are given in the COMA report, Annexes 3 and 4 (DoH 1991).

2.1.5 Dietary sources of energy

Principal dietary sources in the average British diet

Figure 2.4 shows the contributions made by different food groups to energy intakes from household food purchases in the UK, excluding the contribution from alcohol, chocolate and sugar confectionery and meals purchased and eaten away from the home (MAFF 1991). The national average energy intake for 1990 was 1872 kcal (7.9 MJ) per person per day. In addition, the national supplies of alcoholic drinks provided 151 kcal (0.63 MJ) and those of chocolate and sugar confectionery 137 kcal (0.57 MJ) per person per day and an average of 3.76 meals per person per week were eaten out.

Factors affecting the contribution of food to total energy intake

Energy content per 100 g (energy density)

Fat, alcohol, protein, carbohydrate and water provide 9, 7, 4, 3.75 and 0 kcal (37, 29, 17, 16, 0 kJ) per g respectively. The energy density of a food therefore depends primarily on its water and fat content. Fruits and vegetables containing 80–90% water and no fat have a large bulk for low

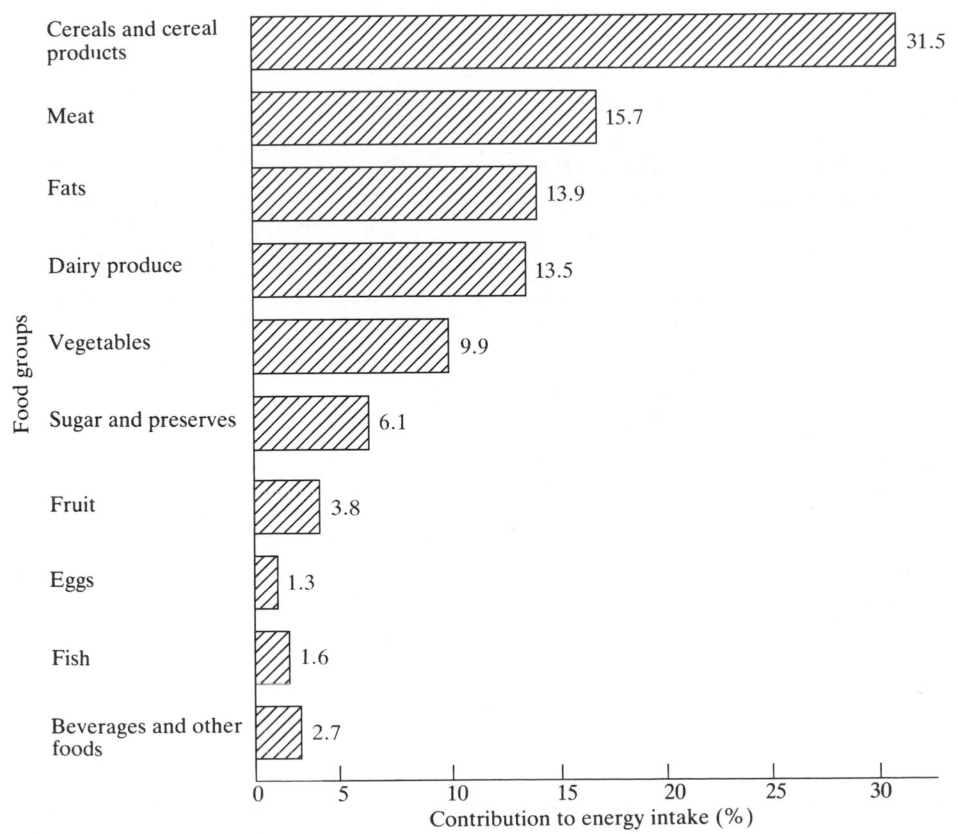

Fig. 2.4 Sources of energy in the British diet. Contribution made by groups of foods to energy intake of the average British household in 1990 (MAFF 1991).

Table 2.4 Energy contribution of different foods taking typical portion size** into account

Food group	High energy (>150 kcal/portion)	Medium energy (75–150 kcal/portion)	Low energy (<75 kcal/portion)
Cereal and cereal products	Pastry*, pies*, puddings* cakes*, scones*, doughnuts* pancakes*, sweetened breakfast cereals, chocolate and sweet biscuits*, pizza, quiches	Bread, flour, pasta, rice, semi-sweet and water biscuits*, unsweetened breakfast cereals	Crispbreads
Milk and milk products	Channel Island and full-fat milk, cream*, milk puddings, full and medium fat cheeses	Semi-skimmed milk, reduced fat cheeses, sweetened yoghurts	Low fat cheeses, natural yoghurt
Eggs	Egg yolk	Whole eggs	Egg white
Fats and oils	Butter*, margarine*, cooking and vegetable oils*, lard* suet*, dripping*, all fried foods*	Low fat spreads*	—
Meat and meat products	Fat on meat*, fatty meats* poultry skin*, sausages*, meat pies*, pasties, cold cuts e.g. luncheon meat*, salami*, spam, mortadella*, tongue, samosas*	Lean meat, poultry without skin	—
Fish and fish products	Oily fish, fish tinned in oil/tomato sauce, taramasalata	White fish, shellfish, fish tinned in brine, fish fingers	—
Vegetables	Fried and roast vegetables*, potato crisps*	Potatoes, pulses, baked beans, parsnips, sweetcorn, beetroot, yams, sweet potatoes, plantain	Green leafy vegetables, onions, leeks, swede, turnips runner/French beans, beansprouts, peppers, salad vegetables
Fruit	Avocado pears, dried fruit	Bananas, grapes, cherries mangoes, stewed dried fruit, fruit cooked with sugar, tinned fruit in syrup*, olives	All other fresh fruit, fresh fruit stewed without sugar
Nuts and seeds	All nuts except chestnuts, all seeds, peanut butter	Chestnuts	—
Sugar, preserves and confectionery	Sugar*, sweets*, chocolates*	Jam*, marmalade	Reduced sugar jams
Beverages	Chocolate and malted drinks made with whole milk	Sugar-containing fizzy drinks*, fruit squash*, fruit juice (sweetened)* fruit juice (unsweetened)	Tea, coffee, Bovril, tomato juice, low calorie drinks*
Alcoholic beverages (per measure or $\frac{1}{2}$ pint)	—	Spirits*, wine*, beer*, lager*, low alcohol beers and lager*	—
Sauces, soups and miscellaneous	Mayonnaise, salad cream*, French dressing*, crisps* and savoury snacks*, oily pickles and chutneys*	Proprietary sauce mixes*, gravy mixes*, sweetened pickles*, thickened soups	Oxo, Bovril, Marmite, low calorie and thin soups, low calorie salad dressings made without oil*, herbs and condiments, pickles in vinegar, Worcester sauce

* Foods with a relatively low nutrient density
** See Appendix 5 Table 7.42

energy intake; conversely cheese and cakes and biscuits with high fat and low water content are energy dense.

Typical portion size Energy dense foods do not necessarily contribute large amounts of energy to the diet if eaten in small portions, for example 10–15 g portions of jam or marmalade.

The frequency of consumption Milk contains less energy per 100 g than cream but is customarily consumed more frequently (and often in larger quantities) and therefore makes a larger contribution to total energy intake.

In summary

$$\text{Energy from a given food} = \text{Energy content per g} \times \text{Typical portion size} \times \text{Frequency of consumption}$$

For example

Whole milk in tea	$0.66 \times 30\,g \times 10/d$	$= 198\,kcal$
Potatoes	$0.52 \times 300\,g \times 1/d$	$= 52\,kcal$
Marmalade	$2.61 \times 10\,g \times 1/d$	$= 26\,kcal$
Sugar in tea	$3.94 \times 5\,g \times 10/d$	$= 197\,kcal$
Chips, retail	$2.39 \times 300\,g \times 1/d$	$= 717\,kcal$
Chips, retail	$2.39 \times 300\,g \times 1/w$	$= 102\,kcal$

Other considerations

Nutrient density The content of a food in vitamins and minerals may be expressed per unit of weight or per unit of energy. Since ultimately total nutrient intake is limited by the total food intake i.e. energy requirement, it makes sense when planning diets to measure nutrient density per unit of energy.

Foods that have a high nutrient density for their energy content include fruit, vegetables, whole grain cereals, dairy products and meat. Nutrient density tends to be reduced by added fat or sugar. When planning diets for people with low energy requirements, for example institutionalized elderly people, it is wise to maximize nutrient density. On the other hand this must not be at the cost of producing so bulky a diet that total energy intake will be limited by appetite to inadequate levels. A satisfactory energy intake is the paramount consideration. When planning low energy diets for weight reduction, nutrient density must be maximized; in this instance bulk is unlikely to be a limiting factor.

Satiety value It can be argued that the bulk of low energy foods will provide a higher sense of satiety than the small bulk of high energy dense foods – for example 285 g of apple has the same energy value (100 kcal) as 25 g of cheddar cheese. On the other hand anecdotal experience suggests that a high fat meal may suppress hunger for longer than a high carbohydrate meal.

2.1.6 Altering the energy content of the diet

The contribution of different food groups to the total energy intake in the UK, taking typical portion size (Crawley 1988) into account, is given in Table 2.4.

Energy reduction

The diet should be composed of foods relatively low in energy with high nutrient density per unit of energy and high satiety value (see Table 2.4).

Energy supplementation

If the aim is to increase energy intake in sick persons with defective appetite or possibly enhanced nutrient requirements, then emphasis should be on foods of high nutrient density. Proprietary energy supplements (see Appendix 6, Tables 7.44–7.46) can be used to modify recipes and supplement meals. If mineral and vitamin intake is already satisfactory, for example in healthy young persons with hearty appetites but who may require additional energy for a period of high intensity sports activity, then emphasis on foods of high nutrient density is less important than the provision of adequate calories in a small bulk.

References

Crawley H (1988) *Food portion sizes*. HMSO, London.

Department of Health (1991) *Dietary Reference Values for food energy and nutrients for the United Kingdom*. Rep Hlth Soc Subj 41. HMSO, London.

Elia M (1992) Energy expenditure in the whole body. In *Energy metabolism: Tissue determinants and cellular corollaries*. Kinney JM and Tucker HN (Eds) Raven Press, New York, pp 19–59.

Fleish PA (1951) La métabolisme basal standard et sa détermination au moyen du 'metabocalculator' *Helv Med Acta* **18**, 23–44.

FAO/WHO/UNU (1985) *Energy and protein requirements. Report of a Joint FAO/WHO/UNU Expert Consultation*. WHO Tech Rep Ser **724**. World Health Organization, Geneva.

Harris JA and Benedict FG (1919) *A biometric study of basal metabolism in man*. Carnegie Institute of Washington. Publications No 279. Washington DC.

Jequier E (1984) Energy expenditure in obesity. *Clinics in Endocrinology and Metabolism* **13**, 563–77.

Ministry of Agriculture, Fisheries and Food (1991) *Household food consumption and expenditure 1990*. Annual Report of the National Food Survey Committee. HMSO, London.

Owen OE, Karle E, Owen RS *et al* (1986) A reappraisal of the caloric requirements of healthy women. *Am J Clin Nutr* **44**, 1–19.

Passmore R and Eastwood MA (1986) *Davidson and Passmore Human Nutrition and Dietetics*. Churchill Livingstone, Edinburgh.

Prentice AM (1986) Energy expenditure in free-living people. *Nutrition and Food Science* **98**, 2–5.

Schofield WN, Schofield C and James WPT (1985) Basal metabolic rate review and prediction together with an annotated bibliography of source material. *Hum Nutr: Clin Nutr* **39C**,Suppl 1.

Spurr GB, Prentice AM, Murgatroyd PR, Goldberg GR, Reina JC and Christman NT (1988) Energy expenditure using minute-by-minute heart rate recording: comparison with indirect calorimetry. *Am J Clin Nutr* **48**, 552–9.

2.2 Dietary protein and amino acids

Information on the biochemistry and physiology of proteins, their digestion and functions in the body may be found in Passmore and Eastwood (1986). Those concerned with assessing protein requirements or evaluating the adequacy of diets are also referred to the FAO/WHO/UNU Report on Energy and Protein Requirements (1985) and the COMA report on Dietary Reference Values (DoH 1991).

2.2.1 Protein requirements

Definition

The protein requirement of an individual is defined as the amount of dietary protein needed to balance the losses of nitrogen from the body in those maintaining energy balance at modest levels of physical activity. In children this includes the requirements for growth and in pregnant and lactating women the needs for increases in maternal tissue, growth of the fetus and milk production. The requirements are set for populations and not for individuals, and represent the needs averaged over time although expressed as a daily requirement. Within any population there is a range of individual requirements.

Protein turnover

In the body protein is constantly being broken down and resynthesized. Some amino acids are lost at every stage by oxidation, but reutilization of amino acids is a major factor in the overall protein economy. This process, under hormonal and metabolic control, can be modified to take account of the status of the body. For example during catch-up growth in children or after injury or infection there is an increase in the efficiency of utilization of amino acids.

The body has some capacity for adjustment to the supply of dietary protein. Low protein intakes result in decreased protein turnover and a reduction in amino acids used for oxidation. However the extent of adaptation which can occur without a detrimental effect on health or long term survival is uncertain. There is also uncertainty as to the extent to which individuals can adapt to a high protein diet. Excessive protein intakes are known to cause some elevation of blood urea nitrogen, demineralization of bone (Garn and Kangas 1981; Orwell *et al* 1987) and a deterioration of renal function (Brenner *et al* 1982; Wiseman *et al* 1987a, 1987b; Rudman 1988). Concerns have been expressed about possible detrimental effects associated with consumption of single amino acid supplements (Belongia *et al* 1990). Purported relationships between high protein intakes and longevity and well-being are thwarted by the many confounding variables. High protein intakes tend to be associated with affluence and other health advantages and also with higher intakes of micronutrients.

Factorial estimates

Protein requirements have traditionally been assessed by the factorial method in which requirements for maintenance and growth were added to a baseline of obligatory losses. These were then adjusted for protein quality and digestibility. Losses of nitrogen from urine and faeces were taken to be 49 mg nitrogen per kg body weight, with an additional 5 mg nitrogen lost via other routes (sweat etc.). However, studies in which individuals were fed only sufficient protein to meet the calculated obligatory losses did not achieve nitrogen balance even using only high quality protein. Accordingly the FAO/WHO/UNU committee (1985) chose to use nitrogen balance studies to establish the quantity of nitrogen needed to achieve zero balance. Unfortunately there remain several drawbacks to this biological approach.

Nitrogen balances

Individuals are fed different levels of protein and the requirement is assessed by interpolating the data to give the zero balance point. The technique involves determining the difference between the intake of nitrogen and the amount excreted in urine, faeces, sweat and minor losses by other routes. However in the majority of studies only dietary nitrogen and the urinary and faecal losses have been measured directly while an estimate has been added for other losses. These are usually taken as 8 mg nitrogen per kg body weight for adults and 10 mg per kg for children up to 12 years.

Ideally subjects should be maintained on each level of protein intake for a sufficient period to allow complete adaptation to each new level. This is rarely possible and thus there is a tendency to overestimate protein requirements.

The aim of balance studies is to find the minimum amount of protein required to maintain the body protein mass. This is not ideal since there is no independent method for assessing the optimal state of protein stores.

The functional significance of increased or decreased body nitrogen pools or protein turnover is uncertain. Most biochemical markers of protein status (e.g. albumin) remain unchanged even after relatively long periods on reduced intakes and will not detect protein inadequacy before it becomes clinically apparent.

Nitrogen balance studies determine nitrogen requirements which are then converted to protein requirements by assuming that a gram of nitrogen is contained in 6.25 g of protein. This is a crude estimate; some proteins have a higher or lower percentage of nitrogen or contain non-protein nitrogen. More accurate conversion factors exist for many food proteins (Table 2.5).

Most balance studies have been performed on young adult males. The average protein requirement is calculated to be 0.6 g/kg/d. Given a between-person coefficient of variation of 12.5%, a value 25% above the mean will cover the needs of 97.5% of the population. The protein requirement is therefore set at 0.75 g/kg/day. Women are assumed to have similar needs. In the elderly protein utilization is probably less efficient and requirements may be increased, but lean body mass is proportionally reduced and therefore the intake per unit lean body mass is automatically higher. Thus an intake of 0.75 g/kg/day is also deemed appropriate for this group.

2.2.2 Dietary Reference Values for protein

The DRVs for the UK for protein are given in Table 2.6. These figures are based on the requirement of 0.75 g protein/kg/day assuming that dietary protein contains 6.25 g N per gram of protein and that the requirement will be met from high quality protein sources that are 100 per cent digested. To apply these figures to populations consuming protein from mixed sources the requirement must be adjusted to allow both for the digestibility of the diet and for the adequacy of the amino acid profile.

Table 2.5 Factors for converting total nitrogen in foods to protein (Paul and Southgate 1978)

	Factor (per gN)		Factor (per gN)
Cereals		Nuts	
Wheat		Peanuts, Brazil nuts	5.41
Wholemeal	5.83	Almonds	5.18
Flours, except wholemeal	5.70	All other nuts	5.30
Macaroni	5.70		
Bran	6.31	Milk and milk products	6.38
Rice	5.95		
Barley, oats, rye	5.83	Gelatin	5.55
Soya	5.71	All other foods	6.25

Data/information from the Composition of Foods and Supplements is reproduced with the permission of the Royal Society of Chemistry and the Controller of HMSO.

Table 2.6 Dietary Reference Values for Protein[a] (DoH 1991)

Age	Weight kg	Estimated Average Requirement EAR g/d[c]	Reference Nutrient Intake RNI g/d[c]
0–3 months	5.9	–[d]	12.5[d]
4–6 months	7.7	10.6	12.7
7–9 months	8.8	11.0	13.7
10–12 months	9.7	11.2	14.9
1–3 years	12.5	11.7	14.5
4–6 years	17.8	14.8	19.7
7–10 years	28.3	22.8	28.3
Males:			
11–14 years	43.0	33.8	42.1
15–18 years	64.5	46.1	55.2
19–50 years	74.0	44.4	55.5
50+ years	71.0	42.6	53.3
Females:			
11–14 years	43.8	33.1	41.2
15–18 years	55.5	37.1	45.4
19–50 years	60.0	36.0	45.0
50+ years	62.0	37.2	46.5
Pregnancy[b]			+6
Lactation[b]:			
0–6 months			+11
6+ months			+8

[a] Values from WHO/FAO/UNU, 1985.
[b] To be added to adult requirement through all stages of pregnancy and lactation.
[c] Milk or egg protein. These figures assume complete digestibility. For diets based on high intakes of vegetable proteins, a correction may need to be applied.
[d] No figures were given by WHO for infants aged 0–3 months[1], therefore no EAR has been derived. The RNI is calculated from the recommendations of COMA (DHSS 1980)

Reproduced with the permission of the Controller of Her Majesty's Stationery Office.

For diets based on refined cereals (i.e. the majority of UK diets at the present time), a correction of 95% for digestibility should be applied. For diets which contain considerable amounts of unrefined cereal grains and vegetables a correction of 85% for digestibility should be applied (see below). For most UK diets no allowance for protein quality need be made, but it might be necessary for vegan diets or diets of idiosyncratic or limited food choice when given to children (see below).

2.2.3 Protein digestibility

The digestibility of a protein is the comparison between the amount of protein eaten and the quantity of amino acids absorbed. Differences in protein digestibility arise from differences in the nature of the food protein (e.g.

intrinsic differences in the cell wall), or the presence of other dietary factors which alter the release of amino acids from proteins.

Protein digestibility is calculated as follows.

$$\text{Apparent protein (N) digestibility (\%)} = \frac{I - F}{I} \times 100$$

$$\text{True protein (N) digestibility (\%)} = \frac{I - (F - Fk)}{I} \times 100$$

Where I = Nitrogen intake
F = Faecal nitrogen output on the test diet
Fk = Faecal nitrogen output on a non-protein diet

Fk is frequently not measured but assumed to be 12 mg nitrogen per kg per day for individuals consuming diets without excessive quantities of fibre.

In general animal proteins are the most, and vegetable proteins the least, digestible. Values for the digestibility of food proteins and diets in man are given in Table 2.7. High fibre intakes increase nitrogen excretion in faeces and may reduce the apparent digestibility by up to 10%. Protein digestibility of whole diets have been found to range from 78% for an Indian diet of rice and beans to 96% for a North American diet (Table 2.7).

2.2.4 Protein quality

Protein quality is determined by its content of amino acids. Amino acids can be classified as follows (see Table 2.8).
1 Essential, i.e. they cannot be synthesized by the body.
2 Semi-essential, i.e. they can be supplied by the metabolism of certain amino acids provided that these are consumed in adequate amounts.
3 Non-essential, i.e. they can be synthesized from carbon and nitrogen precursors.

Proteins which contain all the essential amino acids in sufficient amounts to support growth or maintain nutritional status are termed high biological value (HBV) protein. Proteins with a relatively low concentration of one or more essential amino acids are of low biological value (LBV).

Animal foods generally contain HBV protein while plant foods supply LBV protein. The major limiting essential amino acids in vegetable proteins are
1 Lysine (cereals).

Table 2.7 Values for the digestibility of protein in man

Protein source	True digestibility (mean ± SD)	Digestibility relative to reference proteins	Reference[a]
Egg	97 ± 3		
Milk, cheese	95 ± 3 95	100	
Meat, fish	94 ± 3		
Maize	85 ± 6	89	
Rice, polished	88 ± 4	93	
Wheat, whole	86 ± 5	90	
Wheat, refined	96 ± 4	101	
Oatmeal	86 ± 7	90	
Millet	79	83	Hopkins, 1981
Peas, mature	88	93	
Peanut butter	95	100	
Soyflour	86 ± 7	90	
Beans	78	82	
Maize + beans	78	82	b
Maize + beans + milk	84	88	b
Indian rice diet	77	81	
Indian rice diet + milk	87	92	Panemangalore *et al* 1964
Chinese mixed diet	96	98[c]	Huang and Lin, 1982
Brazilian mixed diet	78	82	Vannucchi *et al* 1981
Filipino mixed diet	88[d]	93	Intengan *et al* 1976
American mixed diet	96[d]	101	McClanahan-Hunt and Schofield, 1969
Indian rice + beans diet	78[d]	82	Cergueira *et al* 1979

[a] Except as indicated all figures are from Hopkins 1981
[b] Viteri, F., unpublished data, 1971
[c] Relative to egg measured in the same study
[d] Recalculated from apparent digestibility, using $F_a = 12$ mg N/kg (see text)

Reprinted from FAO/WHO/UNU (1985) with permission

Table 2.8 Amino acids

Essential amino acids	Leucine Isoleucine Valine Lysine Threonine Methionine Phenylalanine Tryptophan Histidine
Semi-essential	Cystine (can be synthesized from methionine) Tyrosine (can be synthesized from phenylalanine)
Non-essential	Glycine Arginine Proline Glutamic acid Aspartic acid Serine Alanine

2 Tryptophan (maize).
3 Sulphur-containing amino acids i.e. methionine and cystine (peas, beans and pulses).

However, by combining plant proteins limited in certain essential amino acids with others which contain relatively high amounts of those amino acids, a plant protein mixture which is of high biological value can be produced. This is a cardinal principle of vegan diets (see Section 3.10) where pulse dishes must be eaten with rice, bread or other cereal foods.

Amino acid score

The amino acid score is used to evaluate the capacity of a given protein or mix of proteins to meet the essential amino acid requirements of the recipient. The amino acid composition of the test protein is compared with that of the requirement pattern. The score is calculated as a percentage of adequacy.

$$\text{Amino acid score} = \frac{\text{mg amino acid in 1 g test protein} \times 100}{\text{mg amino acid in requirement pattern}}$$

The amino acid score for any given food or diet is the score for the amino acid present in the lowest amount compared with the requirement pattern for the relevant age group, usually referred to as the limiting amino acids. These are normally lysine in cereals, methionine + cystine in pulses and tryptophan in maize. Table 2.9 gives the requirement pattern for different ages. These are tentative figures and more research is required.

In adults consuming mixed diets it is generally unnecessary to be concerned about the amino acid score of the diet, but in children, particularly those consuming protein from a limited number of sources, the amino acid composition may become significant in assessing the adequacy of protein supply.

Table 2.9 Suggested requirement pattern of amino acids for different age groups (mg/g protein) (FAO/WHO/UNU 1985)

	Lysine	Methionine +cystine	Threonine	Tryptophan
Pre-school child	58	25	34	11
School child	44	22	28	9
Adult	16	17	9	5

Example of adjusting the DRV for protein to take digestibility and protein quality into account

Safe level of reference protein for a pre-school child 4–6 years = 19.7 g/d
Digestibility of high fibre diets = 85%
Amino acid score for limiting amino acid (e.g. wheat based Indian diet) = 76%
Safe level of dietary protein intake $= 19.7 \times \frac{100}{85} \times \frac{100}{76}$
$= 30.5$ g/d

2.2.5 Protein requirements for vegan diets

Table 2.7 shows the digestibility of a cereal and bean diet to be about 78%. It may be more appropriate therefore to use a factor of 80% digestibility for vegan diets containing a high proportion of wholegrain cereals and pulses rather than the 85% suggested for high fibre omnivorous diets.

Information on the amino acid scores for vegan diets as eaten is scanty and there is no hard information to provide rule-of-thumb guidance on factors for adjusting DRV for protein quality. It is unlikely that adults do not obtain all their amino acid requirements, but children may be at risk. The WHO/FAO/UNU committee (1985) calculated limiting amino acid scores for pre-school children ranging from 55–91% for a variety of cereal/legume based Third World diets. Vegan children in Western societies often fail to grow as well as their omnivorous cohorts but the relative importance of energy intake, protein intake, fibre intake, dietary bulk, digestibility/absorption of energy and protein and the bioavailability of amino acids is unclear. Langley (1988) has reviewed studies of nutrition in vegan children and concludes that in committed vegans taking thought over their diets, protein requirements of even young children will be met, provided that the energy requirement is also met. However there are several studies in the literature of protein-energy malnutrition in children on fruitarian and macrobiotic diets, diets restricted for 'allergy' and bulky diets of inadequate energy density.

2.2.6 Sources of protein in the average British diet

The Household Food Consumption Survey (MAFF 1992) showed that in the UK in 1990 the average daily consumption of protein was 63 g compared to 73 g in 1979 and 74 g in 1969. Despite this downward trend in the amount of protein consumed there was an upward trend in the proportion of the energy intake derived from protein which was 11.6% in 1969, 13.0% in 1979 and 13.5% in 1990. In the average UK diet, most protein is obtained from meat and meat products (29%) and cereals and cereal products (26%); milk, cheese and other milk products together provide about 22% (MAFF 1992).

Most proteins contain about 16% nitrogen so the concentration of protein in a particular food can be obtained by multiplying its nitrogen content by 6.25. The approximate protein density (g protein/100 g food) of some common foods is listed in Table 2.10. However, as with all foods, the nutrient density alone does not necessarily reflect the importance of a food as a contributor to the daily protein intake; the likely portion size and the frequency of consumption must also be taken into account. For example, skimmed milk is one of the most concentrated sources of protein yet usually makes a minimal contribution to dietary protein content; in contrast, cereal foods contain a lower percentage of protein yet provide about one-quarter of the average person's daily protein intake.

It is important to remember that, unlike fat and carbohydrate, protein consumed in excess of immediate requirement cannot be stored by the body. In essence, only the energy component of any surplus will be retained and the excess nitrogen will be excreted.

Table 2.10 Typical protein content of some foods

Food	Protein content (g/100 g)
Dairy produce	
Dried skimmed milk	36.1
Liquid milk	3.2
Cheese (cheddar)	25.5
Yoghurt	3.5–6.4
Meat, fish and eggs	
Beef, lamb, pork, chicken (lean, raw)	20.5
Liver (raw)	20.1
Kidney (raw)	16.5
White fish (raw)	17.5
Mackerel (raw)	19.0
Pilchards (in tomato sauce)	18.8
Prawns (boiled)	22.6
Eggs	10.8
Cereals and cereal products	
Bread	
wholemeal	9.2
white	8.4
Flour	
wholemeal	12.7
white, plain	9.4
Cornflakes	7.9
Muesli	10.6
All-bran	15.1
Rice (boiled)	2.2
Pasta (boiled)	3.2
Vegetables	
Beans	
baked (canned)	4.8
broad (boiled)	5.1
butter (boiled)	7.1
haricot (boiled)	6.6
runner (boiled)	1.2
Brussels sprouts (boiled)	2.9
Cabbage (boiled)	1.7
Carrots (boiled)	0.6
Lentils (boiled)	7.6
Peas (boiled)	6.7
Potatoes (boiled)	1.8

2.2.7 Altering the protein content of the diet

Protein supplementation

A protein intake above normal requirements is indicated in cases of hypoproteinaemia. It may be useful, in conjunction with an increased energy intake, in short-bowel syndrome, intractable malabsorption, inflammatory bowel disease, bowel fistulae, for pre-operative preparation of undernourished patients and in anorexia nervosa.

In those patients able to eat a normal diet, an increase in protein intake can most easily be achieved by regular consumption of foods which are rich sources of high biological protein (see Table 2.11). For patients unable or unwilling to do this, the addition of skimmed milk powder to milk-based drinks and to some cooked foods increases protein intake with little effect on palatability or portion size.

There is a wide range of high protein proprietary products which can be used as supplementary sip feeds or to provide complete nutrition. Details of these can be found in Appendix 6. Many of the products are prescribable for certain conditions and information on this can be obtained from the manufacturers or publications such as the *British National Formulary* or the *Monthly Index of Medical Supplies* (*MIMS*).

Protein restriction

A protein restriction is frequently indicated in the management of disorders associated with liver and renal dysfunction (see Sections 4.11 and 4.13).

The degree of protein restriction required will depend on the severity of the disease state and will be a compromise between the body's requirement for protein and the clinical

Table 2.11 High biological value (HBV) protein exchanges

Food	Quantity for a 7 g protein exchange	Quantity for a 6 g protein exchange	Also high * in		
			Na[1]	K[1]	P[1]
Dairy produce					
Milk					
cows'/goats'	$\frac{1}{3}$ pt	180 ml		√	√
evaporated	3 fl.oz	70 ml		√	√
breast, modified baby milk	$\frac{3}{4}$ pt	400 ml			
Cheese (cheddar)	1 oz	25 g	√		√
Cottage cheese[2]	$1\frac{3}{4}$ oz	45 g			
Cheese curd[2]	$1\frac{1}{4}$ oz	30 g			√
Yoghurt	5 oz	120 g			√
Fromage frais	$3\frac{1}{2}$ oz	80 g			√
Eggs					
Hen's egg	One large	One small			√
Meat					
Bacon (lean, cooked)	$\frac{3}{4}$ oz	20 g	√		
Meat (lean, cooked)	1 oz	25 g			
Poultry (cooked)	1 oz	25 g			√
Liver/kidney	1 oz	25 g			
Fish					
White fish (e.g. cod), cooked	$1\frac{1}{4}$ oz	35 g			
Smoked fish (steamed)	1 oz	25 g	√		
Sardines, canned	1 oz	25 g	√		√
Fish fingers[2]	2	$1\frac{1}{2}$			
Shrimps/prawns (without shells)	1 oz	25 g	√		√
Mussels	$1\frac{1}{2}$ oz	35 g	√		√

Table 2.12 Low biological value (LBV) protein exchanges

Food	Quantity for a 7 g protein exchange	Quantity for a 6 g protein exchange	Also high * in		
			Na[1]	K[1]	P[1]
Meat products					
Sausage (cooked)	$1\frac{1}{2}$ oz	45 g	√		
Haggis	$2\frac{1}{4}$ oz	55 g	√		√
Peas and beans					
Baked beans	5 oz	120 g		√	√
Haricot beans					
raw	1 oz	25 g		√	√
cooked	$3\frac{1}{2}$ oz	90 g		√	√
Peas (fresh, frozen)	4 oz	100 g		√	√
Mung beans (raw)	1 oz	25 g		√	√
Lentils					
raw	1 oz	25 g		√	√
cooked	$3\frac{1}{4}$ oz	80 g		√	√
Nuts					
Almonds	$1\frac{1}{2}$ oz	35 g		√	√
Brazil nuts	2 oz	40 g		√	√
Chestnuts	11 oz	250 g		√	√
Hazel nuts	3 oz	75 g		√	√
Peanuts (unsalted)	1 oz	25 g		√	√

[1] Na = sodium; K = potassium; P = phosphorus
[2] Contains some sodium — usually allowed on a 'No added salt' diet

* All protein foods contain K+ and P but those which are highest are marked √

Table 2.13 2 g protein exchanges (All are low biological value (LBV) unless marked with an asterisk)

Food	Imperial	Metric	Also high (√) in Na[1]	K[1]	P[1]
Cereal products					
Bread (1 large thin slice)	1 oz	25 g			
Flour (wheat, plain)	$\frac{1}{2}$ oz	15 g			
Pastry	1 oz	25 g	√		
Pasta					
raw	$\frac{1}{2}$ oz	15 g			
boiled	$1\frac{3}{4}$ oz	50 g			
Oatmeal	$\frac{1}{2}$ oz	15 g			
Rice					
raw*	1 oz	30 g			
cooked*	$3\frac{1}{2}$ oz	100 g			
Breakfast cereals					
Cornflakes	1 oz	25 g			
Puffed Wheat	$\frac{1}{2}$ oz	15 g			√
Rice Krispies*[2]	1 oz	25 g			
Shredded Wheat	1	1			√
Sugar Puffs	1 oz	25 g			
Weetabix	1 biscuit	1		√	√
Biscuits and cakes					
Cream crackers[2]	3	3		√	
Digestive biscuits[2]	2	2			
Semi-sweet biscuits	4 small	4 small			
Sponge cake (without fat)	1 oz	25 g			
Dairy produce					
Cream cheese*	2 oz	60 g		√	
Double cream*	$4\frac{1}{2}$ oz	125 g			
Malted drink[2]	3 tsp	3 tsp		√	√
Vegetables					
Green vegetables	$2\frac{1}{2}$ oz	75 g		√	
Carrots/celery/cucumber/lettuce	11 oz	300 g		√	
Sweetcorn (boiled)	$1\frac{3}{4}$ oz	50 g		√	
Potatoes (boiled)*	5 oz	140 g		√	
Yam (raw)	$3\frac{1}{2}$ oz	100 g		√	
Miscellaneous					
Chocolate					
milk	1 oz	25 g		√	√
plain	$1\frac{3}{4}$ oz	50 g		√	√
Crisps*	1 small pkt	30 g	√	√	
Chappati	1 small	1 small			
Yorkshire pudding*	1 oz	25 g			√

[1] Na = sodium; K = potassium; P = phosphorus
[2] Contains some sodium — usually permitted on 'No added salt' diets
* High biological value protein

indications. Because protein intake is limited, the biological value of the protein which is consumed is a vital consideration.

In some instances, the intake of other nutrients such as sodium, potassium or phosphorus may also have to be controlled and this further limits the choice, as well as the amount, of protein foods which can be consumed. In such cases protein-containing foods high in sodium, potassium and phosphorus must also be identified and excluded from or limited in the patient's diet.

These potentially complicated dietary manipulations are usually achieved by means of protein exchange lists. These give the quantity of food which provides a certain amount of protein of either high or low biological value.

The dietary plan should specify the number of exchanges to be eaten at each meal but the patient, if well enough, is free to choose the food. The patient will also require guidance as to which foods may be eaten freely and which are contraindicated.

The most commonly used protein exchanges are 6 g or 7 g of HBV protein and 2 g of LBV protein. 7 g protein exchanges lend themselves to imperial measures whilst 6 g

Table 2.14 Composition of low protein diets

	Protein intake				
	20 g	30 g	40 g	50 g	60 g
Daily allowance of					
Milk	150 ml	200 ml	200 ml	200 ml	200 ml
Protein exchange	1 × 6 g protein exchange divided between two meals	2 × 6 g protein exchanges divided between two meals	3 × 6 g protein exchanges divided between three meals	5 × 6 g protein exchanges divided between three meals	7 × 6 g protein exchanges divided between three meals
Breakfast cereal[1]	—	—	1 × 2 g protein exchange	1 × 2 g protein exchange	1 × 2 g protein exchange
Bread[3]	2 × 2 g protein exchanges	2 × 2 g protein exchanges	3 × 2 g protein exchanges	4 × 2 g protein exchanges	3 × 2 g protein exchanges
Potatoes, rice or pasta[2]	2 × 2 g protein exchanges	2 × 2 g protein exchanges	2 × 2 g protein exchanges	2 × 2 g protein exchanges	2 × 2 g protein exchanges

Average portions of low protein vegetables, salad[4] or fruit[4] will increase protein intake by 2–3 g.
Average portions of sugar and butter or polyunsaturated margarine[3] may be eaten.
Extra energy from glucose polymers and/or fat emulsions may be necessary. An allowance of double cream can be given in place of a 2 g protein exchange

[1] Type of cereal not specified unless sodium intake is restricted. Muesli should be avoided due to variability of composition and protein content
[2] Potatoes should be limited or avoided if potassium restriction is necessary
[3] Salt free butter should be used if there is need for a strict sodium restriction
[4] Fruit and vegetables will need to be limited if a potassium restriction is indicated
Low protein products may be used to add variety and increase energy intake

Table 2.15 Foods not allowed on a low protein diet. Meat, fish, eggs and cheese should be eaten only in the quantities specified in the diet plan

Dairy products
Extra milk (see exchange list)
Milk powders*
Instant creams
Single cream
Yoghurt (can be exchanged for milk allowance)
Tinned milk
Sour cream
Skimmed milk powder
Buttermilk

Cereal products
Extra bread (see exchange list)
High protein breads and cereals
Biscuits (see exchange list)
Bought cakes (see exchange list)
Bought pastry (see exchange list)
Semolina
Macaroni
Barley
Breakfast cereals (see exchange list)
Muesli
Extra porridge oats (see exchange list)

Sweet foods
Lemon curd
Fruit pastilles and gums
Fancy chocolates
Extra chocolate (see exchange list)
Drinking chocolate
Cocoa
Malted drinks (see exchange list)
Marzipan
Extra nuts (see exchange list)
Dried fruit and prunes
Ice cream (see exchange list)
Ice cream mixes
Mousse
Jelly, (agar jelly allowed)
Whips and instant puddings
Virol
Advocaat

Vegetables
Extra butter beans, Baked beans, Broad beans, Haricot beans, Peas, Lentils, Spinach — see exchange list
Mushrooms (except as a garnish)

Savoury foods
Salad cream
Mayonnaise
Tinned and packet soups
Sauce mixes
Batter mixes
Packet stuffings
Meat pastes
Fish pastes
Bemax
Bovril, Oxo, Marmite

* Coffeemate and similar whiteners not made from milk can be used to extend the milk allowance

exchanges are more appropriate for metric quantities. Most adults prefer to use imperial measures but there are an increasing number of adolescents who are more familiar with metric quantities.

Tables 2.11–2.15 provide details to protein exchanges and the construction of low protein regimens. However, it should be noted that these tables are for use by dietitians and are not presented in a format which is suitable to be given directly to the patient.

Proprietary low protein products

A wide range of specially manufactured low protein items such as biscuits, bread, bread mixes, crackers, flour and pasta are prescribable under the NHS for conditions specified by the Advisory Committee on Borderline Substances (ACBS). Details can be found in the *British National Formulary* or MIMS. Some low protein products (e.g. egg replacer and egg white replacer) are not available on prescription.

In the 1980s, two major companies, Welfare Foods (using the brand name of Rite-Diet) and the GF Dietary Group (using several brand names including Juvela), had the largest share of the specially produced low protein (and gluten-free) food market. Neither of these companies now exists having been taken over by Nutricia Dietary Products Ltd, and some of the old brand names have been acquired by other companies. Numerous other products have been discontinued and some renamed, all causing immense confusion to doctors, patients, dietitians and pharmacists.

The situation is not as complicated for low protein products as for gluten-free foods. The two companies producing the majority of the low protein products are Nutricia Dietary Products Ltd and Scientific Hospital Supplies. Ultraphram Ltd also produces a number of suitable products.

It should be noted that, while most proprietary low protein foods can be used on a gluten-free diet, only some proprietary gluten-free products can be used on a low protein diet.

Manufacturers provide comprehensive details of all products, their indications for use and prescribability (addresses are given in Appendix 9, at the end of this book).

References

Belongia EA, Hedberg CW, Gleich GJ *et al* (1990) An investigation of the cause of the eosinophilia-myalgia syndrome associated with tryptophan use. *New Eng J Med* **323**, 357–65.

Brenner BM, Meyer TW and Hostetter TH (1982) Dietary protein intake and the progressive nature of kidney disease: The role of hemodynamically mediated glomerular injury in the pathogenesis of progressive glomerular sclerosis in aging, renal ablation, and intrinsic renal disease. *New Eng J Med* **307**, 652–9.

Cergueira MT, McMurry-Fry M and Connor WE (1979) The food and nutrient intakes of the Tarahumara Indians of Mexico. *Am J Clin Nutr* **32**, 905–915.

Department of Health and Social Security (1980) Artificial feeds for the young infant. *Rep Hlth Soc Subj* **18**. HMSO, London.

Department of Health (1991) Dietary reference values for food energy and nutrients for the United Kingdom. *Rep Hlth Soc Subj* **41**. HMSO, London.

FAO/WHO/UNU (1985) Energy and protein requirements. *WHO Tech Rep Ser* **724**. World Health Organization, Geneva.

Garn SM and Kangas J (1981) Protein intake, bone mass and bone loss. In Deluca H *et al* (Eds) *Osteoporosis: recent advances in pathogenesis and treatment* pp. 257–63. University Park Press, Baltimore.

Hopkins DT (1981) Effects of variations in protein digestibility. In Bodwell CE *et al* (Eds) *Protein quality in humans: assessment and in vitro estimation* pp. 178–81. AVI Publishing Co, Westport.

Huang H-C and Lin CP (1982) Protein requirements of young Chinese male adults on ordinary Chinese mixed diets and egg diet at ordinary levels of energy intake. *J Nutr* **112**, 897–907.

Intengan CL, Roxas BV, Bautista CA and Alejo LG (1976) Studies on protein requirements of Filipinos. *Philippine J Nutr* **29**, 94–8.

Langley G (1988) *Vegan nutrition. A survey of research*. Vegan Society, Oxford.

McClanahan-Hunt S and Schofield FA (1969) Magnesium balance and protein intake level in adult human female. *Am J Clin Nutr* **22**, 367–73.

Ministry of Agriculture, Fisheries and Food (1992) *Household food consumption and expenditure 1990*. Annual report of the National Food Survey Committee. HMSO, London.

Orwell ES, Weigel RM, Oviatt SK, Meier DE and McClung MR (1987) Serum protein concentrations and bone mineral content in aging normal men. *Am J Clin Nutr* **46**, 614–21.

Paul AA and Southgate DAT (1978) *McCance and Widdowson's The Composition of Food*. HMSO, London.

Panemangalore M, Parthasarathy HN, Joseph K, Sankaran AN, Narayana-Rao M and Swaminathn M (1964) The metabolism of nitrogen and the digestibility and biological value of the proteins and net protein utilization in poor rice diets supplemented with methionine-fortified soya flour or skim milk powder. *Canad J Biochem* **42**, 641–50.

Passmore R and Eastwood MA (1986) *Davidson and Passmore Human Nutrition and Dietetics* 8e. Churchill Livingstone, Edinburgh.

Rudman DK (1988) Kidney senescence: a model for aging. *Nutr Rev* **46**, 209–214.

Vannucchi H, Duarte RMF and Dutra de Oliveira JE (1981) Nutritive value of a rice and beans based diet for agricultural migrant workers in Southern Brazil. *Nutr Rep Int* **24**, 129–34.

Wiseman MJ, Bognetti E, Dodds R, Keen H and Viberti GC (1987a) Changes in renal function in response to protein restricted diet in Type 1 (insulin-dependent) diebetic patients. *Diabetologia* **30**, 154–9.

Wiseman MJ, Hunt R, Goodwin A, Gross JL, Keen H and Viberti G (1987b) Dietary composition and renal function in healthy subjects. *Nephron* **46**, 37–42.

2.3 Dietary fats and fatty acids

2.3.1 Composition of food fats

Dietary fats consist of triglycerides, cholesterol and phospholipids of which the triglycerides comprise by far the greatest component (>95%). Triglycerides consist of three long or medium chain fatty acids esterified with glycerol. Fatty acids vary according to chain length and the presence and number of double bonds. The type of fatty acids present in a triglyceride determine not only the physical characteristics of the fat, but also the stability to storage and nutritional value of foods which contain fat. A brief review of the chemistry of dietary fatty acids is given to provide a better understanding of the nutritional properties of different fatty acids. Some information on nomenclature is also included because the current use of mixed terminology, and the increasing preference for the use of notional names for fatty acids is a cause of much confusion.

Chemistry

Fatty acids are composed of a chain of carbon atoms with an acid (carboxyl) group at the end. The carbon atoms may be linked by single or double bonds. Saturated fatty acids contain carbon atoms linked only by single bonds. If one double bond is present the fatty acid is described as monounsaturated. Fatty acids with more than one double bond present are described as polyunsaturated. Fats containing mainly saturated fatty acids (SFAs) are solid at room temperature and are chemically stable, both within the body and when present in foods. Fats containing a large proportion of polyunsaturated fatty acids (PUFAs) are liquid (oils) at room temperature and are susceptible to oxidation. Double bonds in fatty acids may be in the *cis* or *trans* form; in the *cis* form the hydrogen atoms bonded to the carbon atoms at either end of the double bond are on the same side, in the *trans* form these hydrogen atoms are on opposite sides (Fig. 2.5). Most dietary fatty acids contain *cis* double bonds, a characteristic which makes the fatty acid more rigid and bulky. Although *trans* bonds are rarely found in naturally occurring fats they may be introduced during the hydrogenation of PUFAs during the manufacture of margarine. *Trans* unsaturated fatty acids appear to be metabolized in a similar fashion to saturated fatty acids so that it has been suggested that, in terms of their nutritional properties, they should be considered as equivalent to saturated fatty acids.

Nomenclature

About 21 different fatty acids are found in the diet in appreciable amounts (Table 2.16), although the most common are palmitic, stearic, oleic, linoleic and arachidonic acids. Individual fatty acids frequently have common names according to their source of origin, although there is a systematic method of naming fatty acids according to their chain length and number of double bonds. The common name is used for many of the important dietary fatty acids (e.g. linoleic acid) although, for reasons which are not clear, the systematic name is more frequently used for the fish oil fatty acids (e.g. eicosapentaenoic acid; *eicosa* = 20 carbon atoms and *penta* = 5 double bonds).

Notional systems for naming fatty acids also exist and with the increasing use of fatty acid supplements as therapeutic agents, this system of naming fatty acids is becoming more prevalent. In this system the total number of carbon atoms in the fatty acid is designated as C12, C16 etc., with numbering starting from the carboxyl end. The total number of double bonds are then shown following a colon. Thus palmitic acid is C16:0, linoleic acid as C18:2, etc. The position of the first double bond is defined in relation to the methyl end of the carbon chain, with the carbon atom at the methyl end termed the omega (or n) carbon. Thus linoleic acid has its first double bond between the sixth and seventh carbons from the methyl end and its full notional name is C18:2 omega-6, or C18:2, ω-6, or, as shown in Table 2.16, C18:2, n-6.

2.3.2 Metabolism of fatty acids in humans

Essential fatty acids

It has long been known that two 18 carbon atom PUFAs, linoleic and linolenic acids, are essential dietary constituents in man and other animals. Animals including humans can synthesize saturated fatty acids from carbohydrates and from some amino acids and can insert double bonds between the ninth and tenth carbon atoms and anywhere between that point and the carboxyl end of the fatty acid. Animals cannot insert double bonds at any point between carbon number nine and the methyl end of the fatty acid. The reason for this is that the necessary enzyme is absent in animal tissues but is present in plant systems. Consumption of plant products provides the only source of these dietary fatty acids. Although estimates of requirements vary, expert committees currently recommend that at least

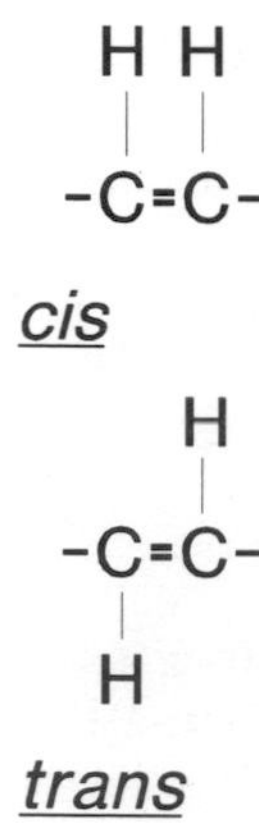

Fig. 2.5 *Cis* and *trans* forms of dietary fatty acids.

1% dietary energy should be provided by dietary linoleic acid and 0.2% by dietary linolenic acid (DoH 1991).

Omega-6 and omega-3 pathways

Although animal tissues cannot synthesize linoleic and linolenic fatty acids, under most circumstances they can readily transform these products into 20 and 22 carbon atom fatty acids with three to six double bonds (Fig. 2.6). Indeed the essentiality of linoleic and linolenic fatty acids is due to their ability to act as precursors of these functionally important fatty acids. Transformation of linoleic acid along the omega-6 pathway results in the production of two important 20 carbon atom fatty acids dihomo-γ-linolenic acid (GLA) and arachidonic acid (AA). Linolenic acid is transformed in a similar manner (omega-3 pathway) to a series of highly polyunsaturated fatty acid products, the most important of which is the 20 carbon fatty acid, eicosapentaenoic acid (EPA). This latter pathway is extremely active in marine animals so that fish provide a very rich source of EPA.

Prostaglandins

Interest in these 20 carbon fatty acids lies in the fact that each has been shown to act as a precursor for the synthesis of a separate family of prostaglandins and leukotrienes (the eicosanoids). Arachidonic acid is the precursor for the most potent family of prostaglandins, the PG2 family, whereas GLA and EPA are the precursors of the less potent

Table 2.16 Nomenclature of fatty acids commonly found in food

Carbon: double bonds	Common name	Systematic name	Common natural sources
Saturated			
4:0	Butyric	Tetranoic	Coconut oil and dairy products
6:0	Caproic	Hexanoic	
8:0	Caprylic	Octanoic	
10:0	Capric	Decanoic	
12:0	Lauric	Dodecanoic	
14:0	Myristic	Tetradecanoic	
16:0	Palmitic	Hexadecanoic	Palm oil, cottonseed oil, butter, meat fat
18:0	Stearic	Octadecanoic	Meat fat, butter, chocolate
20:0	Arachidic	Eicosanoic	Nut and seed oils
22:0	Behenic	Docosanoic	Peanut oil, peanuts
Monounsaturated			
16:ln7	Palmitoleic	9 cis-hexadecenoic	Cod liver oil, meat fat, fish
18:ln9	Oleic	9 cis-octadecenoic	Olive oil, nut and seed oils, meat fat, butter, eggs, avocado
18:ln9	Elaidic	9 trans-octadecenoic	Hydrogenated oils, fats from ruminants
20:ln9	—	11 cis-eicosaenoic	Fish, peanut oil
22:ln9	Erucic	13 cis-docosaenoic	Rapeseed if not a low erucic variety
Polyunsaturated			
18:2n6	Linoleic	9,12 cis, cis-octadecadienoic	Vegetable oils, nuts, lean meat and eggs
18:3n3	Alpha-linolenic	9,12,15 all cis-octadecatrienoic	Soyabean and rapeseed oils
18:3n6	Gamma-linolenic	5 trans, 9 cis, 12 cis-octadecatrienoic	Evening Primrose oil
20:4n6	Arachidonic	5,8,11,14 all cis-eicosatetraenoic	Offal, game, lean meat, egg
20:5n3	—	Eicosapentaenoic (EPA)	Fish
22:6n3	—	Docosahexaenoic	Fish, liver, egg yolk

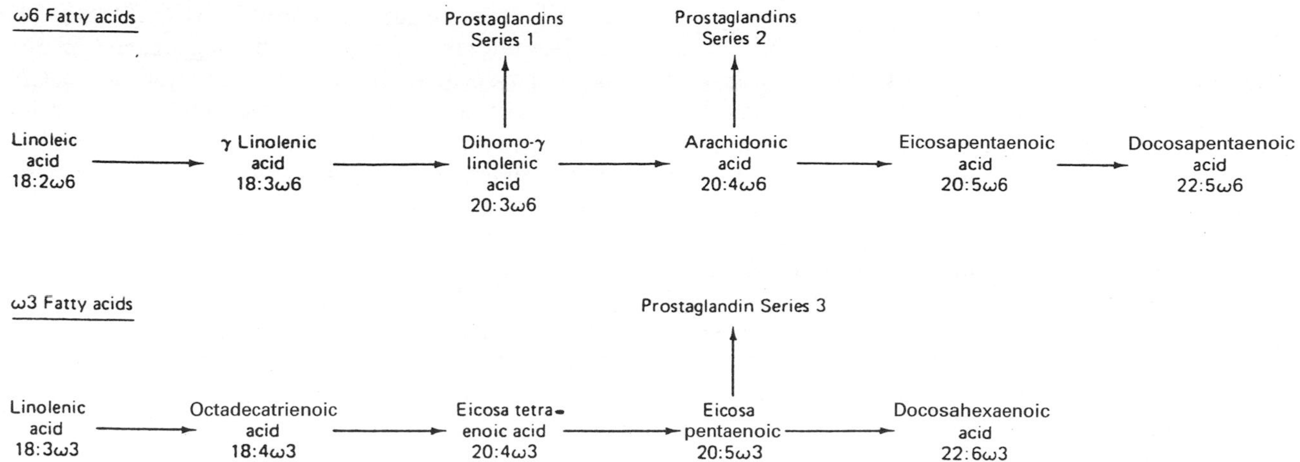

Fig. 2.6 Pathways of linoleic and linolenic acid metabolism: relationship to prostaglandin production.

PG1 and PG3 prostaglandins, respectively. Prostaglandins are involved in inflammation and platelet aggregation and disturbance in prostaglandin metabolism is thought to underlie a number of common inflammatory diseases of man, including psoriasis, asthma and rheumatoid arthritis and in the increased tendency to platelet aggregation seen in thrombotic conditions. Recent clinical trials have shown that large daily doses of evening primrose oil (rich in GLA) or fish oils (rich in EPA) are effective in ameliorating the symptoms of psoriasis and rheumatoid arthritis in a significant proportion of affected individuals (Kremer *et al* 1987; Bittiner *et al* 1988). Cyclical breast pain has also been shown to be effectively treated by the administration of large doses of evening primrose oil (Pye *et al* 1985). The efficacy of these treatments is thought to be due to increased production of PG1 and PG3 series prostaglandins at the expense of the more potent PG2 series prostaglandins but further research is required before the detailed mechanism of action of these dietary fatty acids is completely understood. At the present time it is not clear whether an inborn error of metabolism in one of the enzymes involved in the omega-6 and omega-3 pathways (delta-6-desaturase) is responsible for the susceptibility of some individuals to these conditions and whether dietary supplementation therefore acts as a form of replacement therapy.

2.3.3 Dietary fatty acids

Saturated fatty acids

In the UK, current average intakes of saturated fatty acids are 50% higher than levels recommended in the recent dietary guidelines drawn up by a government expert committee (DoH 1991) (Table 2.17). The committee considered there was strong evidence to suggest that this level of restriction in saturated fatty acid intake would result in a fall in cardiovascular disease in the population, due to beneficial effects on serum LDL concentrations.

Table 2.17 Comparison of current dietary fatty acid intakes with recommended values

	Percentage of total dietary energy	
	Recommended*	Current+
Saturated fatty acids	10	16
Cis-monounsaturated fatty acids	12	11.6
Cis-polyunsaturated fatty acids (n-6; n-3)	6	6
Trans fatty acids	<2	2 (approx)

* DoH (1991); + Gregory *et al* (1990)

Polyunsaturated fatty acids

Incorporation of increased amounts of PUFAs into the diet has been shown to be an effective method of reducing circulating LDL concentrations. Current practice is to define diets in terms of their total fat content and their P/S ratio. The P/S ratio refers to the balance of PUFA to SFA and various recommendations for optimal P/S ratios have been made ranging from 1.0 (FAO/WHO 1980) to 0.45 (BMA 1986). Although previous reports on diet and health emphasised the potential benefits of increasing intakes of PUFAs (FAO/WHO 1980; NACNE 1983), the most recent report (DoH 1991) did not recommend that the consumption of these fatty acids should be increased (Table 2.17). Greater caution in recommending higher intakes of PUFAs by the population as a whole is largely due to recognition of the potentially damaging effects of the products of PUFA oxidation. Although there is no evidence from human populations to suggest that high levels of PUFA are harmful, experimental studies have led to claims that lipid peroxidation may be involved in the pathogenesis of cancer, atherosclerosis and ageing. Until further evidence is available government guidelines suggest that PUFA intakes should be maintained at current levels and that a P/S ratio of 0.6 is one which is unlikely to be associated with harmful effects.

Balance of n-6 and n-3 polyunsaturated fatty acids

At the present time the average intake of n-6 PUFAs is 11.6 g/day whilst that of the n-3 PUFAs is 1.6 g/day. N-3 fatty acids have been shown to reduce fasting and post-prandial serum triglyceride levels but have no effect on, or even raise, serum cholesterol concentrations. However the n-3 fatty acids have beneficial effects on blood clotting since increased n-3 PUFA intake has been shown to inhibit thrombus formation, probably through inhibition of platelet aggregation. One study has shown that addition of fish to the diet reduces the risk of further myocardial infarction in men with at least one previous episode (Burr *et al* 1989). Some authorities believe current dietary habits result in an imbalance in the ratio of n-6 to n-3 fatty acids, with excessive intake of the former and inadequate intake of the latter (Kinsella *et al* 1990). At the present time the optimal balance of dietary n-6 to n-3 fatty acids required for health is not known and recommendations cannot be made with any confidence.

Monounsaturated fatty acids

Monounsaturated fatty acids (MUFA) make a significant contribution to fatty acid intake in the UK (Table 2.17). There is some evidence from studies of Mediterranean countries to suggest that additional consumption of these dietary fatty acids may be beneficial in reducing the incidence of cardiovascular disease and some types of cancer. However differences in the intake of other dietary constituents (e.g. fruit and vegetables) in Mediterranean countries may in part be responsible for these effects. At the present time no recommendation has been made that the consumption of MUFAs should be increased. Some studies have suggested that in non-insulin dependent diabetes mellitus (NIDDM), substitution of some dietary carbohydrate with MUFAs may be allowed without detrimental effects on glucose control (Garg *et al* 1988). These findings offer the possibility of allowing moderate increases in fat intake in individuals who find very low fat diets unpalatable, although further research in this area is required to establish the extent to which substitution of carbohydrates with MUFAs may be achieved without adverse effects on glucose control.

Trans fatty acids

Although *trans* fatty acids are introduced during the processing of hard margarines, ruminant bacteria also generate *trans* fatty acids so that milk and other dairy products and lamb and beef are also important sources of these fatty acids. The average consumption of *trans* fatty acids is about 5 g/day (about 2% dietary energy) but estimates of intake may be inaccurate. Although harmful effects of *trans* fatty acids have been suggested, the biological effects of *trans* fatty acids are only poorly understood. On this basis it has been recommended that intake of *trans* fatty acids should be monitored and that increased consumption should not be advised.

2.3.4 Fatty acid content of principal fat sources

Recent developments in our understanding of the roles of different dietary fatty acids in human health mean that in the future, diets are likely to be characterized in terms of their MUFA, n-6/n-3 ratios and *trans* fatty acid contents as well as their total fat and P/S ratios (Ulbricht and Southgate 1991). This will require dietitians to have a working knowledge of the fatty acid contents of principal food fat sources (Table 2.18). Additional information on the n-6/n-3 ratios of food fats is not available at the present time but is likely to be published in the near future.

Table 2.18 Fatty acid content of the principal fat sources in food

	Total fat (g/100 g)	Saturates (g/100 g)	Monoenes (g/100 g)	PUFA (g/100 g)	Trans (g/100 g)
Dairy foods					
(mean of summer and winter)					
Cheese					
cottage	3.9	2.4	1.1	0.1	0.2
cheddar	34.4	21.7	9.4	1.4	1.9
cream	47.4	29.7	13.7	1.4	2.8
Milk					
skimmed, fresh	0.1	0.1	Tr	Tr	Tr
whole, fresh	3.9	2.4	1.1	0.1	0.2
Channel Island	5.1	3.2	1.4	0.1	0.3
Cream					
single	19.1	11.9	5.5	0.5	1.2
whipping	39.3	24.6	11.4	1.1	2.1
double	48.0	30.6	13.9	1.4	2.8
Egg					
whole raw	10.8	3.1	4.7	1.2	Tr
fried in corn oil	13.9	4.0	6.0	1.5	Tr

Meat					
Chicken (roast)					
no skin	4.3	1.6	2.5	1.0	—
with skin	14.0	4.2	6.5	2.5	—
Beef topside (roast)					
lean	4.4	1.4	2.2	0.2	0.1
lean and fat	12.0	4.1	6.4	0.7	0.1
Lamb, leg (roast)					
lean	8.1	3.9	3.0	0.4	0.5
lean and fat	17.9	8.9	6.9	0.9	1.3
Pork, leg (roast)					
lean	6.9	2.4	2.7	1.0	0.02
lean and fat	19.8	7.3	8.0	3.0	0.08
Corned Beef					
Sausages (grilled)					
pork	24.6	9.5	11.0	2.7	0.1
beef	17.3	6.7	8.2	1.3	0.8
Pork pie	27.0	10.2	12.5	2.7	—
Cornish pastie	20.4	8.9	8.7	2.2	—
Fish					
Oily fish					
Herring (grilled)	13.0	3.7	5.9	2.1	0.9
Kipper (baked, net weight)	11.4	1.8	6.0	2.5	0.9
Mackerel (raw)	16.3	3.3	8.0	3.3	1.0
Pilchards in tomato sauce	5.4	1.1	1.5	2.3	1.0
Salmon (tinned)	8.2	1.5	3.5	2.4	1.0
Sardines (fish only)	13.6	2.8	4.7	4.8	1.0
White fish					
Haddock (steamed)	4.0	0.2	0.1	0.3	2.4

Note. The fat content of fish will vary with maturity of fish and time of year. Oily fish caught in British waters, e.g. herring and mackerel, are highest in fat content in the winter months

Nuts and seeds (net weights)					
Almonds	55.8	4.7	34.4	14.2	0.0
Brazil nuts	68.2	16.4	25.8	23.0	0.0
Cashew (dry roasted)	50.9	10.1	29.4	9.1	0.0
Coconut (fresh)	36.0	30.9	2.4	0.6	0.0
Hazel nuts	63.5	4.7	50.0	5.9	0.0
Peanuts	46.1	8.2	21.1	14.3	0.0
Peanut butter	53.7	11.7	21.3	18.4	0.0
Sesame seeds (dried)	58.0	8.3	21.7	25.5	0.0
Walnuts	68.5	5.6	12.4	47.5	0.0
Plant foods (net weights)					
Avocado	19.5	4.1	12.1	2.2	0.0
Olives (in brine)	11.0	1.7	5.7	1.3	0.0
Potato crisps	37.6	9.2	12.0	9.9	1.5
Cakes and Biscuits					
Biscuits					
Cream crackers	16.3	8.8	6.8	0.6	—
Digestives	20.9	8.6	9.6	1.7	—
Semi-sweet	16.6	8.0	5.9	1.7	—
Cakes					
Gateau	16.8	9.5	5.3	0.8	0.8
Fruit cake	12.9	5.8	5.2	1.1	0.7
Chocolate					
Mars bar	18.9	10.0	7.2	0.8	0.5
Chocolate (milk)	30.3	17.8	9.5	1.5	0.3
Chocolate (plain)	29.2	16.9	9.3	1.2	0.2

Data from McCance and Widdowson, 5e, (Holland *et al*, 1991)

Data/information from the Composition of Foods and Supplements is reproduced with the permission of the Royal Society of Chemistry and the Controller of HMSO

Variability in the fatty acid composition of manufactured foods

A wide range of oils and margarines is available for human consumption (Table 2.19) with P/S ratios varying from the most unsaturated, safflower oil (P/S ratio 7.1), to the most saturated, coconut oil (P/S ratio 0.02). The fatty acid composition of margarines, blended vegetable oils and foods to which fats is added (such as biscuits, cakes and pastry products) will vary from one manufacturer to another. Individual manufacturers may also change the fat used according to the market price of oils and fats. For many manufactured foods, fatty acid composition will mainly be determined by the fats added during manufacturing and cooking processes, rather than from the food itself. This means that differences in the fats used will alter the contents of saturated, polyunsaturated and *trans* fatty acids. When accurate assessments of fatty acid intake are required it is important that detailed information on fats and oils used for spreading and cooking are obtained and in the case of manufactured foods that the oils and fats used during processing are identified.

2.3.5 Reduction of dietary fat intake

The total amount of fat consumed may need to be reduced as a general health measure in response to government guidelines or for a specific therapeutic purpose. Consideration must be given to the degree and type of fat restriction required in individuals since this will influence the type of dietary changes required. If government guidelines are followed it is suggested that, on average, individuals in the UK will need to reduce their saturated fat intake by 11 g/day (women) and 13.5 g/day (men). Low fat and very low fat diets prescribed for therapeutic purposes may require reductions in total fat intake in the region of 20–60 g/day.

Table 2.20 shows the fat density of certain foods and the food portions which provide 10 g fat; when severe fat restriction is required patients may find a fat exchange list compiled from this information useful. However, it must be remembered that the fat density of a food is not necessarily a good reflector of that foods importance to the daily fat consumption. For most people meat and meat products, spreading fats and cooking oils, milk and products (including cheese) are the major sources of fat in the diet (Fig. 2.7) because these are commonly eaten on a daily basis. Cereal products also provide a considerable amount of fat in the diet in the form of biscuits, buns, cakes and puddings and their contribution to fat intake is increasing. It can be seen from Fig. 2.7 that full-fat milk and its products make a greater contribution to saturated fat intake than they do to total fat intake so that where a specific reduction in saturated fat intake is required, restriction of these products should be emphasized.

2.3.6 Dietary cholesterol

A 'cholesterol-lowering diet' is not the same as a 'low cholesterol diet'. The former might incorporate high linoleic acid foods such as sunflower oil which has the effect of lowering blood cholesterol; the latter simply aims to reduce

Table 2.19 Fatty acid content and P/S ratios of the principal edible fats and oils in order of PUFA content

Oils/fats	Total fat (g/100 g)	Saturates (excl. trans) (g/100 g)	Monoenes (g/100 g)	PUFA (g/100 g)	P/S ratio
Safflower oil	99.9	10.1	12.6	72.1	7.1
Corn oil	99.9	12.7	24.7	57.8	4.5
Soya oil	99.9	14.0	23.2	56.5	4.0
Sunflower oil	99.9	11.9	20.2	63.0	5.3
Sesame seed oil	99.9	14.2	37.3	43.9	3.1
Margarine (good quality)	81.0	16.2	20.6	41.1	2.5
Peanut/groundnut/arachis oil	99.9	18.8	47.8	28.5	1.5
Blended oil (good quality)	99.9	6.5	60.2	28.4	4.3
Blended oil (poor quality)	99.9	13.8	53.5	23.1	1.7
Lard (pork fat)	99.0	40.8	43.8	9.6	0.2
Palm oil	99.0	45.3	41.6	8.3	0.2
Olive oil	99.9	14.0	69.7	11.2	0.8
Margarine (poor quality)	81.0	34.7	32.0	3.8	0.1
Dripping	99.0	54.8	36.7	2.5	0.04
Butter	82.0	54.0	19.8	2.6	0.04
Coconut oil	99.0	85.2	6.6	1.7	0.02
Coconut cream	82.0	87.2	6.3	1.0	0.01

Data from McCance and Widdowson. 5e (Holland *et al*, 1991)

Data/information from the Composition of Foods and Supplements is reproduced with the permission of the Royal Society of Chemistry and the Controller of HMSO

Table 2.20 Food portions which contain 10 g fat

	High fat foods		Medium fat foods		Low fat foods		Very low fat foods	
Food group	Fat density ≥20 g/100 g	Portion containing 10 g fat	Fat density 10–20 g/100 g	Portion containing 10 g fat	Fat density 5–10 g/100 g	Portion containing 10 g fat	Very low fat density or fat free	Portion containing 10 g fat
Milk, cream	Butter	12 g	Full fat yoghurt	300 g	Evaporated, condensed milk	100 g	Silver top milk[a]	$\frac{1}{2}$pt
	Double cream	20 g					Semi-skimmed[a]	1 pt
	Whipping cream	30 g					Skimmed milk, fresh or dried, low fat yoghurt	
	Milk powder	40 g			Gold top milk[a]	$\frac{1}{3}$pt		
	Single or soured cream	50 g						
Oils, fats, spreads and sauces	Vegetable oils, lard, dripping	10 g					Bottled sauces and pickles, Marmite, jams, honey, Bovril, tomatoes etc. onions, herbs, spices	
	Margarine, butter	12 g						
	Mayonnaise	12 g						
	Low fat spread	25 g						
	Salad cream	35 g						
	Reduced fat Salad cream	58 g						
Eggs	Scrambled eggs	45 g	Boiled eggs (2)	100 g			Egg white	
	Fried eggs	50 g						
	Scotch egg	50 g						
Cheese	Stilton	25 g	Feta	50 g			Cottage cheese	
	Cream cheese	20 g	Tendale	70 g				
	Cheddar, Cheshire	30 g	Curd cheese	90 g				
	Danish blue, Parmesan,	35 g						
	Edam, cheese spread (e.g. Dairla)	45 g						
Cheese dishes	Quiche	35 g	Cheese souffle	55 g	Macaroni cheese	100 g		
	Welsh rarebit	40 g	Pizza	90 g	Cauliflower cheese	125 g		
			Cheese pudding	95 g				
Meats	Fried streaky bacon	20 g	Grilled lean back bacon	50 g	Home cooked lean ham	100 g	Turkey breast, White fish	
	Boiled brisket	40 g	Fried rump steak, (with fat)	70 g	Lean grilled rump steak	170 g		
			Stewed mince	70 g	Lean roast beef	110 g		
	Lamb chop (with fat)	30 g	Lean lamb chop	85 g	Lean roast leg lamb	120 g		
	Pork chop (with fat)	40 g	Lean pork chop	95 g	Lean roast leg pork	150 g		
	Roast duck, (with fat)	25 g	Roast chicken, (with skin)	70 g	Roast chicken (no skin	185 g		
	Liver paté	40 g	Fried lamb's liver	70 g	Grilled lamb's kidney	100 g		
	Luncheon meat	40 g	Corned beef	80 g	Canned lean ham	195 g		
	Pork sausages	40 g	Steaklets, beefburgers, hamburgers	60 g				
	Sausage roll	25 g	Moussaka	75 g	Lean meat in stew, hot pot, shepherd's pie, curry	150–200 g		
	Pork pie	35 g	Bolognese sauce	100 g				
	Pastie, meat pie,	50 g						
Fish	Taramasalata	20 g	Fried cod in batter	100 g	Pilchards in tomato sauce	185 g	All poached or steamed white fish and shellfish	
	Fried whitebait	20 g	Canned salmon	120 g				
			Sardines	85 g				
			Fish fingers	100 g				
			Fried scampi	55 g				

Table 2.20 *contd*

Food group	High fat foods: Fat density ≥20 g/100 g	Portion containing 10 g fat	Medium fat foods: Fat density 10–20 g/100 g	Portion containing 10 g fat	Low fat foods: Fat density 5–10 g/100 g	Portion containing 10 g fat	Very low fat foods: Very low fat density or fat free	Portion containing 10 g fat
Vegetables and *nuts* and *soups*	Crisps Low fat crisps Frozen fried chips Soya beans Avocado pears Nuts and nut butters	30 g 50 g 50 g 45 g 45 g 20 g	Thick chips Olives	100 g 90 g	Roast potatoes Oven ready chips Cream and thick soups (e.g. tomato, lentil, oxtail)	200 g 140 g 250 g	All potatoes cooked without fat. All vegetables, salad, peas, beans, lentils (except soya) with no added fat	
Sweets and chocolates	Milk chocolate	35 g	Mars bar Toffees	50 g 60 g			All plain sweets	
Breads, breakfast cereals	Fried bread	25 g	Chapatis	80 g	Muesli Readybrek Soft rolls	133 g 115 g 150 g	All other bread, pasta, rice, cereals, breakfast cereals	
Biscuits	Chocolate (orange creams, Penguins, etc.) Filled wafers Custard creams Chocolate digestive Shortbread Home made Easter Lincoln, crunch biscuits	35 g 35 g 40 g 40 g 40 g 45 g 45 g	Cream crackers Rich tea Oatcakes Ginger nuts Wafer biscuits	60 g 60 g 55 g 65 g 80 g	Starch reduced	130 g	Matzo, rye crispbread	
Cakes	Flaky pastry Short pastry Victoria sponge Chocolate eclairs Mince pies	25 g 30 g 40 g 40 g 50 g	Madeira, rock cakes Doughnuts, jam tarts Scones Plain iced cakes Fruit cake	60 g 65 g 70 g 70 g 85 g	Currant bun Sponge with no fat, (e.g. Swiss roll)	130 g 150 g	Meringues	
Puddings	Cheesecake	30 g	Custard tart Pancakes Sponge pudding Fruit pie (two crust) Lemon meringue pie, Treacle tart	60 g 60 g 60 g 65 g 70 g	Trifle Fruit tart Bread and butter pudding Ice cream Apple crumble Egg custard	165 g 130 g 130 g 140 g 150 g 170 g	Jelly, low fat yoghurt, fresh, canned or frozen fruit, custard or other milk pudding made with skimmed milk (fresh or powdered)	

[a] Milk contains the following fat per 100 g: gold top (Channel Island) 4.8 g; silver top (Friesian) and red top (homogenized) 3.8 g; silver and red top (semi-skimmed) 2.0 g; blue top (skimmed) 0.1 g.

Reproduced (with permission) from Bingham (1987).

the intake of foods containing cholesterol. It must be pointed out that the amount of cholesterol synthesized and metabolized by the body itself is far greater than the amount usually consumed in the diet, of which only 50% may be absorbed. It is also worth noting that in healthy people, little correlation has been found between the intake of cholesterol and blood cholesterol levels. However, the level of cholesterol in the blood is increased with high intakes of dietary saturated fat and it can be lowered by increasing the intake of linoleic acid. A high intake of fibre, particularly gel forming fibres (found for example in beans and pulses), also leads to a reduction in cholesterol absorption from the intestine and increased faecal excretion of dietary cholesterol (Kritchevsky and Story 1974). A list of high, medium and low sources of cholesterol is given in Table 2.21.

2.3.7 Low and reduced fat products and fat substitutes

Low and reduced fat products

The past five years have seen a vast increase in the production and marketing of low fat and reduced fat

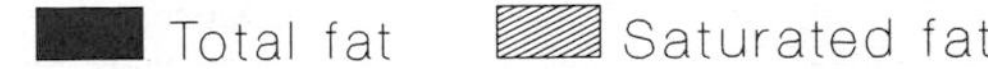

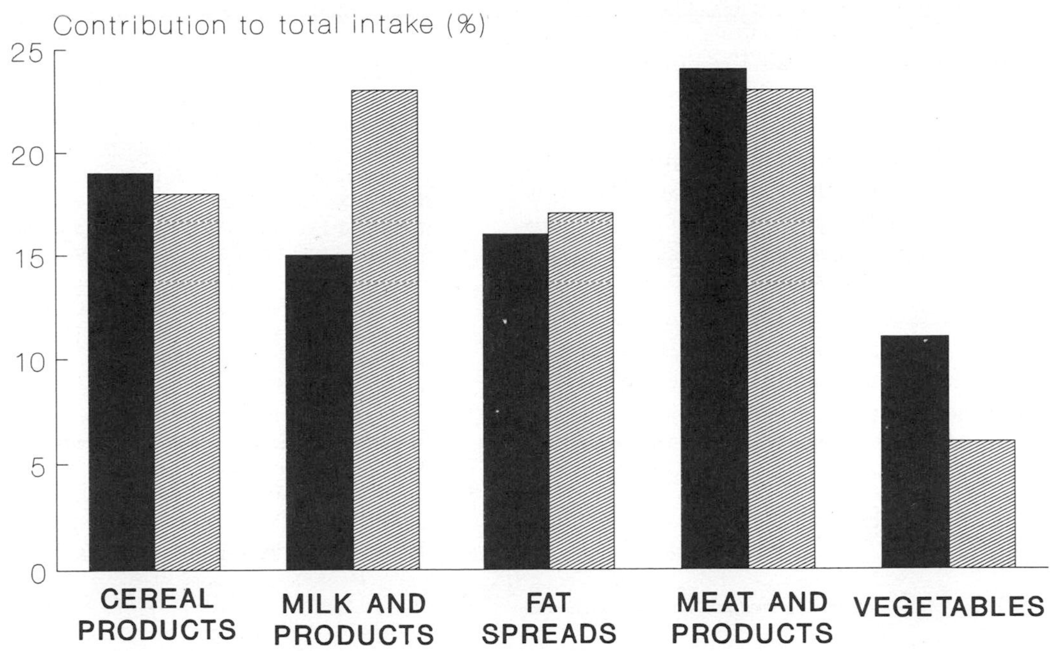

Fig. 2.7 Percentage contribution made by major food groups to total and saturated fat intakes in the British adult diet (Gregory *et al* 1990).

products and these are now available country wide in all types of food retail outlets. Legislation on the fat content of foods labelled as 'low', 'medium' or 'high' in fat is soon to be introduced and will be of great value to the consumer in selecting foods according to their fat and energy contents. Low fat and reduced fat foods currently available include:

1 Skimmed and semi-skimmed milks.

2 Low fat dairy products including yoghurts, fromage frais, reduced fat cheeses. There have been marked improvements in the texture and flavour of reduced fat cheeses which have greatly increased their uptake.

3 Low fat spreads. Low fat/high PUFA spreads have been a recent introduction and very low fat spreads (<5% fat) are also now available as a result of the use of fat substitutes in margarine manufacture (see below).

4 Low fat ready made meals. A range of products including Lean Cuisine, Waistline and supermarkets' own lines has proved to be very popular and new recipes are produced on a regular basis.

Other products such as low fat crisps, oven chips, sausages and salad dressings are also widely available.

Table 2.21 Sources of dietary cholesterol

Rich sources	All offal including paté, egg yolk, fish roes, mayonnaise, shell fish and dishes made with these ingredients
Moderately rich sources	Fat on meat, duck, goose and cold cuts (e.g. salami) whole milk, tinned milks, cream, ice cream, cheese, butter, most commercially made cakes, biscuits and pastries, homemade dishes containing any of the above ingredients. Crisps and all shop bought foods made with unspecified fat/oil
Poor sources	All fish (white and oily) and fish tinned in vegetable oil, very lean meats, poultry (no skin), skimmed milk, low fat yoghurt, cottage cheese, bread, margarines claiming to be low in cholesterol (i.e. <0.005% cholesterol)
Cholesterol-free	All vegetables and vegetable oils, fruit including avocado and olives, nuts, cereals, pasta (without added eggs), rice, popcorn (unbuttered), egg white, meringue, sugar

Fat substitutes

Despite the availability of reduced fat products, many individuals find compliance with low fat diets difficult. Part of the reason for this is that, without fat, meals lack flavour and the pleasant 'mouth feel' that is associated with fatty food. Recognition of this problem has led to the development of a number of fat substitutes, which when incorporated into manufactured foods, confer the same properties as fat and provide a creamy fat-like texture and flavour to the final product (Gillatt and Lee 1991). Some of these fat substitutes have gained 'generally regarded as safe' (GRAS) status and are incorporated into foods sold in the UK. These include Polydextrose (Pfizer) and Simplesse (Nutrasweet) which are used in confectionary, salad dressings, frozen desserts, ice creams, mayonnaise and margarines. Neither of these products can be used in foods which require heating so that their application is limited to the type of uses listed above. However the development by Procter and Gamble of the Sucrose Polyesters (Olestra), a group of compounds which are non-hydrolysable and non-digestible and which are heat stable, means that a fat substitute is now available which can be used in a wide range of baked products and also as a cooking oil. This product has not yet gained clearance from the USA Food and Drug Administration (FDA) because of concern over potential laxative effects and the possibility of malabsorption of the fat soluble vitamins. Should these problems be resolved, this fat substitute will potentially have a vast number of applications and, it has been suggested, will revolutionize the dietary approach to the treatment of conditions such as obesity and hyperlipidaemia.

References

Bingham SA (1987) *Everyman companion to food and nutrition*. Dent and Sons, London.

Bittiner SB, Tucker WFG, Cartwright I and Bleehen SS (1988) A double-blind randomised, placebo-controlled trial of fish oil in psoriasis. *Lancet* **i**, 378–80.

Burr ML, Gilbert JF, Holliday RM and Fehily A (1989) Effects of changes in fat, fish and fibre intakes on death and myocardial reinfarction; Diet and Reinfarction Trial. *Lancet* **ii**, 757–61.

British Medical Association (1986) *Diet, nutrition and health*. Report of the Board of Science and Education. BMA, London.

Department of Health (1991) *Dietary Reference Values for food energy and nutrients for the United Kingdom. Rep Hlth Soc Subj* **41**. HMSO, London.

FAO/WHO (1980) *Dietary fats and oils in human nutrition*. FAO Food and Nutrition Series No 20, Rome.

Garg A, Bonanome A, Grundy SM, Zhang Z-J and Unger RH (1988) Comparison of a high carbohydrate diet with a high monounsaturated fat diet in patients with non-insulin-dependent diabetes mellitus. *New Eng J Med* **319**, 829–34.

Gillatt PN and Lee SM (1991) Changes in dietary energy with novel proteins and fats. *Proc Nutr Soc* **50**, 391–7.

Gregory J, Foster K, Tyler H and Wiseman M (1990) *The dietary and nutritional survey of British adults*. HMSO, London.

Holland B, Welch AA, Unwin ID, Buss DH, Paul AA and Southgate DAT (1991) *McCance and Widdowson's The Composition of Foods* 5e. Royal Society of Chemistry, Cambridge.

Kinsella JE, Broughton KS and Whelan JW (1990) Dietary unsaturated fatty acids: interactions and possible needs in relation to eicosanoid synthesis. *J Nutritional Biochem* **1**, 123–41.

Kremer JM, Jubiz W, Michalik A, Rynes RI, Bartholemew LE, Bigaouette J, Timchalk M, Beeler D and Lininger L (1987) Fish-oil fatty acid supplementation in active rheumatoid arthritis. *Ann Intern Med* **106**, 497–502.

Kritchevsky D and Story JA (1974) Binding of bile salts *in vitro* by non-nutritive fibre. *J Nutr* **104**, 458.

National Advisory Committee on Nutrition Education (1983) *Proposals for nutrition education in Britain*. Health Education Council, London.

Pye JK, Mansell RE and Hughes LE (1985) Clinical experience of drug treatments for mastalgia. *Lancet* **ii**, 373–7.

Ulbricht TLV and Southgate DAT (1991) Coronary heart disease: seven dietary factors. *Lancet* **338**(ii), 985–92.

2.4 Dietary carbohydrate

2.4.1 Composition of carbohydrate

Available dietary carbohydrate is comprised of sugars and starches. Sugars are a soluble form of carbohydrate characterized by varying degrees of sweetness. Starches are a storage form of carbohydrate derived from plants.

Chemically, sugars and starches are classified according to the number of saccharide units in their structure. Sugars are either mono- or disaccharides; starches are polysaccharides.

Monosaccharides

Glucose

Most carbohydrates are ultimately digested or converted to glucose and this is the form in which they are transported in the blood.

Fructose

Fructose is found in some fruits and vegetables and honey. It is a component of sucrose.

Galactose

Galactose is not found in the free state but as a component of lactose in milk and milk products.

Disaccharides

Disaccharides are comprised of two chemically bound monosaccharide units. These are broken down in the intestine and absorbed as monosaccharides.

Sucrose

Sucrose is a combination of glucose and fructose. It occurs naturally in some fruits and root vegetables but is usually extracted from sugar beet and sugar cane.

Maltose

Maltose is comprised of two glucose units. It is formed during the breakdown of starch by digestion or fermentation.

Lactose

Lactose is a combination of glucose and galactose. It is found only in milk and products derived from milk.

Polysaccharides

Polysaccharides are comprised of large numbers of saccharide units.

Starch

Starch is comprised of glucose units linked together in either straight (amylose) or branched (amylopectin) chains. The availability of starch is influenced by its physical state. Raw starch is insoluble and in some foods unavailable for digestion. On heating, starch swells and gelatinizes and can be rapidly hydrolysed to glucose and absorbed. Some forms of cooked starch (e.g. that in potato) retrograde on cooling and becomes resistant to digestion ('resistant starch').

Non-starch polysaccharide

Many other polysaccharides exist in nature but most cannot be digested by humans and are classified as non-starch polysaccharide (NSP), i.e. 'dietary fibre' (see Section 2.5).

Glucose syrup

Glucose syrup (liquid glucose) is a manufactured mixture of glucose, maltose and some complex carbohydrates chemically derived from the partial hydrolysis of starch. Glucose syrup is less sweet than glucose but, in metabolic terms, can be considered to be similar in effect. It is used in many manufactured products such as confectionery and soft drinks and hence can make a significant contribution to carbohydrate intake. Commercial fructose syrups are also used in the manufacture of some products (e.g. jams).

2.4.2 Function of carbohydrate

Carbohydrate is an important source of energy in the human diet. All carbohydrates are ultimately converted to, and absorbed into the blood in the form of, glucose. Glucose is a vital fuel substrate for all body tissues, especially the brain, and the body attempts to maintain a constant level of glucose in the blood at all times. In normal circumstances, when blood glucose rises above a certain level (i.e. following the consumption of carbohydrate), surplus glucose is removed and stored as liver or muscle glycogen or, ultimately, body fat. In the pre-prandial state or during exercise, a minimum level of blood glucose is maintained by breakdown of glycogen or by gluconeogenesis from other fuel stores. However, the body's supply of such fuels is limited, and prolonged absence of carbohydrate from the diet will result in excessive ketone production.

2.4.3 Sources of carbohydrate

In the UK, carbohydrate consumption has declined in recent years, both in absolute terms and as a proportion of total energy intake (MAFF 1991). In the UK, adults obtain about 45% of dietary energy from carbohydrate, just over half of which is derived from starches (Gregory *et al* 1990).

In the average diet, almost half of total carbohydrate intake comes from cereal foods, especially bread which contributes about one-fifth of the total intake. Vegetables, particularly potatoes, provide a further 16%. About 13% of total carbohydrate intake comes from table sugar, confectionery and preserves (Gregory *et al* 1990).

The proportion of sugars in the diet decreases with age. Infants derive about 40% of dietary energy from sugars (primarily lactose), pre-school children obtain about 25–30% energy from sugars, and older children and adults about 17–25% (DoH 1989).

2.4.4 Recommended carbohydrate intake

In its recent report on Dietary Reference Values, the Department of Health (1991) did not set a specific requirement for carbohydrate but recommended that starch intake should be increased in order to compensate for the recommended reductions in the amount of dietary energy derived from fat, alcohol and protein.

The effects of dietary sugars on health were considered in detail by the COMA report (DoH 1989). They suggested that the health implications of dietary sugars depend on whether the sugars are present as an integral part of the cells in food (intrinsic sugars) or in a free form (extrinsic sugars). Distinction can also be made between the extrinsic sugars present in milk and non-milk extrinsic sugars (NMES) (Table 2.22). In some respects this classification is a spurious one since the body cannot ultimately distinguish between a molecule of glucose derived from a bar of chocolate, a glass of milk or a piece of fruit. It is incorrect therefore to assert that intrinsic and milk sugars have inherently different metabolic effects from those of non-milk extrinsic sugars. The value of the intrinsic/extrinsic distinction is that it is a useful pointer to the overall quality of a diet. A diet containing a high proportion of NMES is more likely to be inadequate in other nutritional respects (e.g. its content of dietary fibre or micronutrients), and its high palatability/low satiety value is more likely to lead to over-consumption of food energy and hence in turn to obesity and obesity-related disorders. The frequent consumption of NMES (which can be rapidly fermented in the mouth) will also increase the risk of dental caries. The Department of Health (1991) therefore recommended that the adult population's average intake of non-milk extrinsic sugars should not exceed 10% of total energy intake (about 60 g/day).

Table 2.22 Classification of dietary sugars

Dietary sugars		
Intrinsic sugars	Extrinsic sugars	
	Milk extrinsic sugars	Non-milk extrinsic sugars (NMES)
Whole fruit Vegetables	Milk Milk products	Packet sugars Honey Manufactured foods with added sugars or glucose/fructose syrups

2.4.5 Alteration of carbohydrate intake

Carbohydrate supplementation

An increase in carbohydrate intake may be required in order to help meet the body's requirement for energy. This may be necessary as a result of energy requirements being increased (e.g. during catabolic states) or because the existing requirement for energy is not being met (e.g. due to loss of appetite or a therapeutic diet which curtails the intake of other energy-providing nutrients). In some patients, carbohydrate supplementation is relatively easy because there are so many foods which are concentrated sources of sucrose or starch. However, when appetite is poor or solid foods cannot be eaten, proprietary drinks or supplements based on glucose or liquid glucose polymers may be required. These provide a concentrated source of readily assimilable energy and in a form which is less sweet, and hence more palatable, than an equivalent amount of sucrose. The use of proprietary carbohydrate supplements is discussed in Section 1.13.3 and the composition of these products is given in Appendix 6.

General carbohydrate restriction or regulation

Strict control of carbohydrate intake used to be a central feature of the management of diabetes and most patients were encouraged to use a carbohydrate exchange system as a way of regulating the amount of carbohydrate eaten at each meal. Nowadays, carbohydrate exchange lists are used less often. This is partly because the principles of dietary management have changed and dietary guidance needs to encompass fat restriction and control of energy intake as well as considerations of carbohydrate intake (see Section 4.16). In addition to this, the principle behind the carbohydrate exchange list – that equivalent amounts of carbohydrate have equivalent effects on blood sugar levels – is now known to be flawed; the 'glycaemic index' of a food or meal is more relevant.

Nevertheless, ensuring that people with diabetes consume sufficient carbohydrate of an appropriate type, and that those on insulin do so at appropriate times, remains important. Many patients, particularly those who are newly diagnosed and the parents of diabetic children, feel reassured by knowing roughly how much carbohydrate should be eaten at each meal and the carbohydrate content of different foods. For them, Food Values Lists giving such guidance are therefore helpful. Table 2.23 provides information from which such lists can be devised but it should be noted this table is not in a format which is appropriate for patients. The British Diabetic Association provides Food Values Lists suitable for patients from a variety of cultural groups. The carbohydrate content of many manufactured foods can be found in the publication *Countdown*, also produced by the Association.

Table 2.24 gives a low sodium carbohydrate list which is sometimes used in the management of liver disease (see Section 4.11).

Table 2.23 10 g carbohydrate exchange list

Food item	Household measure	Weight (g)	Energy content (kcal)
Bread[1]			
* Wholemeal bread	Thin slice small loaf	25	50
	¾ large slice (medium thickness)		
White bread	1 small slice (medium thickness)		
	⅔ large slice (medium thickness)	17	44
	½ large thick slice		
Breakfast cereals			
* All Bran	5 tbs	20	50
* Bran Flakes	5 tbs	20	50
* Cornflakes	5 tbs	10	40
* Muesli (unsweetened)	2 tbs	15	50
Puffed Wheat	15 tbs	15	50
Rice Krispies	6 tbs	10	40
* Shredded Wheat	⅔ of one	10	50
Special K	8 tbs	15	50
* Spoonsize Cubs	12–14	–	45
* Weetabix	1 biscuit	15	60
* Weetaflakes	4 tbs	15	50
Porridge (made with water)	4 tbs	120	55
Biscuits[2]			
Plain or semi-sweet	2	15	60
* Oatcake	1	15	55
* Digestive or wholemeal	1	15	70
Crackers (plain)	2	15	70
Crispbread	2	15	50
Flours and grains			
Flour			
white, plain or self-raising	1 tbs	10	40
* wholemeal	1½ tbs	15	50
Arrowroot, custard powder, cornflour	1 tbs	10	35
Barley (raw)	1 tbs	10	40
* Oats (uncooked)	3 tbs	15	60
Rice			
* brown (uncooked)	1 tbs	10	40
white (uncooked	1 tbs	10	45
Spaghetti			
* wholewheat	20 10″ strands	15	50
white	6 long (19″) strands	10	45
Sago, tapioca, semolina, uncooked	2 tsp	10	35

Table 2.23 *contd*

Food item	Household measure	Weight (g)	Energy content (kcal)
Vegetables[3]			
* Beans			
* baked (canned)	5 tbs	75	55
* broad (boiled)	10 tbs	150	75
* dried (all types, raw)	2 tbs	20	55
* Beetroot (cooked whole)	2 small	100	45
* Lentils dry (raw)	2 tbs	20	60
Onions (raw)	1 large	200	45
Parsnips (raw)	1 small	90	45
* Peas (marrowfat or processed)	7 tbs	75	60
* Peas (dried, all types, raw)	2 tbs	20	60
Plantain, green (raw, peeled)	Small slice	35	40
Potatoes –			
raw	1 egg sized	50	45
boiled	1 egg sized	50	40
chips (cooked weight)	4–5 average chips	25	65
* jacket (weighed with skin)	1 small	50	45
mashed	1 small scoop	50	80
roast	1 egg sized	40	65
* Sweetcorn			
canned or frozen	5 tbs	60	45
on the cob	$\frac{1}{2}$ medium cob	75	60
* Sweet potato (raw peeled)	1 small slice	50	45
Fruits[4]			
Apples –			
eating (whole)	1 medium	110	50
cooking (whole)	1 medium	125	55
stewed without sugar	6 tbs	125	40
Apricots			
fresh (whole)	4 medium	160	40
dried (raw)	4 small	25	45
Bananas with skin	1 small	90	40
Blackberries (raw)	10 tbs	150	45
Blackcurrants (raw)	10 tbs	150	45
Cherries (fresh, whole)	12	100	40
Currants (raisins, dried)	$1\frac{1}{2}$ tbs	15	35
Damsons (raw, whole)	7	120	40
Dates			
fresh, whole	3 medium	50	40
dried, without stones	3 small	15	40
Figs			
fresh whole	1	100	40
dried	1	20	40
Grapes (whole)	10 large	75	40
Grapefruit (whole)	1 very large	400	45
Greengages (fresh, whole)	5	90	40
Guavas (fresh, flesh only)	1	70	45
Mango (fresh whole)	$\frac{1}{3}$ of a large one	100	40
Melon (all types, weighed with skin)	large slice	300	40
Nectarine (fresh, whole)	1	90	40
Orange (fresh, whole)	1 large	150	40
Paw-paw (fresh, whole)	$\frac{1}{6}$ of a large one	80	50
Peach (fresh, whole)	1 large	125	40
Pear (fresh, whole)	1 large	130	40
Pineapple (fresh, no skin or core)	1 thick slice	90	40
Plums			
cooking (fresh, whole)	4 medium	180	40
dessert (fresh, whole)	2 large	110	40
Pomegranate (fresh, whole)	1 small	110	40
Prunes (dried, without stones)	2 large	25	40
Raisins (dried)	$1\frac{1}{2}$ tbs	15	35

Table 2.23 *contd*

Food item	Household measure	Weight (g)	Energy content (kcal)
Strawberries (fresh)	15 medium	160	40
Sultanas (dried)	$1\frac{1}{2}$ tbs	15	40
Tangerines (fresh, whole)	2 large	175	40
Fruit juices (unsweetened)			
Apple juice	6 tbs	85	40
Blackcurrant juice	7 tbs	100	40
Grapefruit juice	8 tbs	125	45
Orange juice	7 tbs	100	40
Pineapple juice	6 tbs	85	40
Tomato juice	1 large glass	275	50
Milk and milk products			
Milk –			
fresh, whole	$\frac{1}{3}$ pint	200 ml	130
fresh, semi-skimmed	$\frac{1}{3}$ pint	200 ml	90
fresh, skimmed	$\frac{1}{3}$ pint	200 ml	70
dried, whole	8 tsp	25	125
dried, skimmed	10 tsp	20	70
evaporated	6 tbs	90 ml	145
Yoghurt (plain)	1 small carton	150 ml	80
Manufactured foods[5]			
Beefburgers (frozen)	3 small	–	450
Fish fingers	2	–	110
Ice cream	1 scoop	–	90
Sausages	2 thick	110	400
Soup (thickened)	1 cup	200	115
Sugar-rich foods[6]			
Glucose	2 tsp	10	40
Dextrosol	3 tablets	–	40
Sugar	2 tsp	10	40
Golden syrup	1 tbs	15	40
Marmalade/jam/honey	2 tsp	15	40
Lucozade	3–4 tbs	50 ml	36
Cola	8 tbs	100 ml	40

[1] Figures of carbohydrate and energy are contained on the packaging of many sliced breads. Details are also given in *Countdown.*
[2] Details of many individual brands are given in *Countdown.*
[3] A portion of the following will not add more than 5 g of carbohydrate and 20–25 kcal to the diet and need not be counted as an exchange:
Artichokes, asparagus, aubergine, beans (runner), beansprouts, broccoli, brussels sprouts, cabbage, carrots, cauliflower, celery, courgettes, cucumber, leeks, lettuce, marrow, mushrooms, mustard and cress, okra, peas (fresh or frozen), peppers, pumpkin, radishes, spinach, spring onions, swede, tomatoes (raw and canned), turnip, watercress.
[4] Cranberries, gooseberries, lemons, loganberries and rhubarb need not be counted into the diet.
[5] Different brands of the same product vary considerably in nutrient composition. Precise figures can be obtained from *Countdown.* The figures in the table are given for guidance only.
[6] For use at times of illness or hypoglycaemia by the insulin dependent diabetic.
* Valuable source of fibre.

Specific restriction or avoidance of carbohydrate

Sucrose avoidance

Sucrose intolerance may be either primary (congenital sucrose deficiency) or secondary to some other malabsorption state (see Section 4.6).

Many sources of dietary sucrose are readily apparent (e.g. table sugar and obviously sweetened foods). However, most fruits, many vegetables and many manufactured (especially canned) products contain sucrose and must also be eliminated from the diet.

Sucrose-intolerant infants will require a milk formula in which the sucrose is replaced by glucose. Weaning presents less of a problem than it used to as many manufactured baby foods are free from added sucrose; however, fruit and

Table 2.24 Low sodium, 10 g carbohydrate exchange list

Food item	Household measure
Salt-free bread	1 small, thin slice $\frac{1}{2}$ large, thick slice
Tea Matzos	2 biscuits
Matzos (large)	$\frac{1}{2}$
Salt-free crackers	2
Pasta (macaroni, noodles, spaghetti)	
raw	1 heaped tbs
cooked	3 heaped tbs
Rice (boiled)	2 heaped tbs
Sago, semolina, rice, tapioca (raw)	1 level tbs
Puffed Wheat	5 heaped tbs
Shredded Wheat	$\frac{2}{3}$ biscuit
Porridge (cooked)	4 tbs
Flour, cornflour, custard powder (raw)	1 rounded tbs
Potato	
boiled, roast	1 egg sized
mashed	1 heaped tbs
chips	6 large
Unsalted crisps (Salt'n shake)	1 small packet

some vegetable-based weaning foods will still contain sucrose of natural origin and must be avoided. Vitamin supplementation (especially of vitamin C) is vital.

Secondary sucrose intolerance is commonly accompanied by lactose intolerance and if this is the case, products containing milk, milk solids, and lactose must also be excluded (see lactose-free foods).

Table 2.25 provides broad guidelines for a sucrose-free diet (and associated lactose intolerance). The presence or absence of *added* sucrose in a manufactured food can be determined from its label. However, 'sucrose' will not appear on the list of ingredients if it originated naturally, e.g. fruit canned in natural juice.

Lactose avoidance

Lactose intolerance may be primary (and is common in certain racial groups) or secondary as a result of acute diarrhoeal illness. In the former instance, complete avoidance of lactose is usually unnecessary; there is usually

Table 2.25 Guidelines for a sucrose-free diet

Food group	Permitted foods	Excluded foods
Cereals and cereal products	Porridge oats Sugar-free breakfast cereals* Bread* Sucrose-free biscuits* Some crispbreads* Flour, cornflour Rice, tapioca and sago* Pasta	Sugar-containing breakfast cereals Sweetened bread, biscuits, cakes, pastries and pies Manufactured desserts and puddings Canned pasta
Milk and milk products	Milk* Evaporated milk (unsweetened)* Most coffee whiteners* Unsweetened yoghurt* Cheese* Cream*	Condensed milk Sweetened yoghurt
Eggs	Egg yolk, egg white and whole egg	Meringues (unless made with a sucrose substitute)
Fats and oils	All types*	
Meat and meat products	Beef, lamb and pork Poultry Ham and bacon (unless sweet cured)	Most canned meats Meat paste Some meat products Casseroles with unsuitable vegetables (see below)
Fish and fish products	Fresh and frozen fish Most tinned fish	
Vegetables	Green leafy vegetables — broccoli, cabbage, spinach, brussels sprouts and cauliflower Salad vegetables — lettuce, cucumber, chicory, cress, celery and tomato Asparagus Marrow	Pulses — peas, beans and lentils Root vegetables — carrots, parsnips, turnips and swede Beetroot Leeks

Table 2.25 *contd*

Food group	Permitted foods	Excluded foods
	Mushrooms Potatoes Runner beans	Sweetcorn Many canned vegetables Some varieties of baked beans
Fruit	Cherries Grapes Figs	All other fruit (fresh, canned or dried) Glace cherries Fruit juice (except unsweetened tomato juice)
Nuts		All
Sugars, preserves, confectionery	Glucose, fructose Saccharine, aspartame and other sucrose-free artificial sweeteners Sugarless drinks Some brands of honey	Sugar Sugar-containing drinks and baked products Jam, marmalade Syrup, treacle Ice-cream, jelly Confectionery Drinking chocolate, Bournvita and malted milk drinks
Alcoholic drinks	Spirits Sugar-free mixers	Wines, sherries and ports Beer, lager Liqueurs
Miscellaneous	Gelatine Marmite, Bovril Oxo, stock cubes Salt, pepper, herbs and spices	Gravy browning Canned or packet soups Pickles, chutneys Salad cream Syrup-based medicines
Baby foods	Baby milks* without added sugar Sugar-free weaning foods Baby rice	Sugar-containing milks or foods Fruit-based weaning foods

* Items which contain milk, milk products or lactose and will need to be excluded if there is associated lactose intolerance.

a threshold for lactose (in the region of around 10 g/day) below which no symptoms of intolerance will occur. However, some individuals and some cases of secondary lactose intolerance will have a very low lactose tolerance.

Lactose is contained in human, cows', sheep's and goats' milk, in milk products and manufactured foods containing milk. It is also present in some medicines and artificial sweeteners.

Lactose-intolerant infants will require a low lactose milk based on soya. Lactose-intolerant children may require extra protein from meat, fish and eggs.

For practical purposes, no differentiation is generally made between cows' milk protein intolerance and lactose intolerance. The construction of milk-free diets is discussed in detail in Section 2.14. However, guidelines for a low lactose diet are summarized in Table 2.26.

Manufactured foods free from lactose are included in the list of foods free from milk and milk products printed by the British Dietetic Association (but see Section 2.14).

Table 2.26 Principal sources of dietary lactose (and suggested alternatives)

Food group	Foods containing lactose	Lactose-free alternative
Milk and milk products	Human, cows', sheep's and goats' milk Yoghurt Cream and cheese	Low lactose milk substitute (see Section 2.14)
Fats and oils	Butter Most margarines	Tomor margarine Some low fat spreads Lard Vegetable oil
Manufactured and baked products	Cakes, biscuits, bread and pastry containing milk Milk puddings Ice cream	Milk-free products (see Section 2.14)
Miscellaneous	Lactose-containing sweeteners Tablets with a lactose filler Many manufactured products	

Note: Milk-free diets are discussed in detail in Section 2.14.

Galactose avoidance

Galactosaemia, an inborn error of metabolism requires a galactose-free diet. Since galactose is a constituent of lactose, this entails *severe* restriction of lactose-containing foods as well as other sources of galactose and galactosides.

It is usually possible to replace milk with a low lactose milk substitute, but in young infants a feed based on comminuted chicken, milk-free cereal, egg and glucose may be required.

Guidelines for a galactose-free diet are given in Table 2.27. These should be used in conjuction with an up-to-

Table 2.27 Guidelines for a galactose-free diet

Food group	Permitted foods	Excluded foods
Milk and milk products	Lactose-free or low lactose milk substitute (e.g. Formula S (Cow and Gate), Prosobee (Mead Johnson) or Wysoy (Wyeth)** Some coffee whiteners	Human, sheep's, cows' and goats' milk, cheese, cheese spread, yoghurt and cream Any manufactured food containing milk, milk solids, lactose, galactose, whey, casein or caseinate
Cereals	Breakfast cereals without added milk solids Flour, cornflour Milk-free bread, biscuits, cakes and puddings Baby rice Rice, sago, tapioca and semolina (made without milk) Pasta	Some baby cereals
Eggs	Egg yolk, egg white, whole egg	Scrambled egg made with milk
Fats and oils	Tomor margarine Some low fat spreads Lard Vegetable oils	Butter Margarine
Meat and meat products	Cooked without milk	Meat products containing milk solids or lactose Offal*
Fish and fish products	Cooked without milk	Fish products containing milk solids or lactose
Vegetables	All except those listed opposite	Peas*, beans*, lentils*, soya*, legumes* and pulses*
Fruits	All	
Nuts	All	
Sugar and preserves	Boiled sweets Water ices Sugar Jam, honey, marmalade Syrup, treacle Jelly	Milk-containing confectionery (chocolate, fudge and toffees) Ice cream Milk-based desserts
Beverages	Milk or lactose-free tea, coffee, fruit juice, squash and fizzy drinks	Malted milk or chocolate drinks
Miscellaneous	Marmite, Bovril Oxo, stock cubes, salt, pepper, herbs and spices	Soups made with milk or cream Tablets with lactose filler Some artificial sweeteners Many canned or manufactured foods

* Contain galactosides

** Details of products suitable for use in milk-free diets are given in Section 2.14.

date list of manufactured foods free from milk and milk derivatives printed by the British Dietetic Association (but see Section 2.15). The construction of milk-free regimens is also discussed in detail in Section 2.14.

Starch avoidance

Primary starch intolerance is due to isomaltase deficiency and is usually associated with primary sucrose intolerance. This will require exclusion of the sucrose-containing foods listed in Table 2.25 as well as foods which contain the following:

1 Flour and foods containing flour (i.e. bread, cakes and biscuits).
2 Breakfast cereals.
3 Cornflour (and most manufactured desserts).
4 Rice.
5 Pasta.
6 Food coated in breadcrumbs or batter.
7 Potatoes
8 Many manufactured meat products (e.g. sausages, beefburgers, rissoles and meat and fish pastes).

It may be possible to use a soya-based flour as an alternative for baking.

References

Department of Health (1989) *Dietary Sugars and Human Disease.* Committee on Medical Aspects of Food Policy. Report of the Panel on Dietary Sugars. *Rep Hlth Soc Subj* **37**, HMSO, London.

Department of Health (1991) *Dietary Reference Values for foods and nutrients for the United Kingdom.* Committee on Medical Aspects of Food Policy. Report of the Panel on Dietary Reference Values. *Rep Hlth Soc Subj* **41**. HMSO, London.

Gregory J, Foster K, Tyler H and Wiseman M (1990) *The Dietary and Nutritional Survey of British Adults.* Office of Population Censuses and Surveys. HMSO, London.

Ministry of Agriculture, Fisheries and Food (1991) *Household food consumption and expenditure: 1990.* Annual Report of the National Food Survey Committee. HMSO, London.

2.5 Dietary fibre (non-starch polysaccharides)

2.5.1 Definition and principal fibre components

Dietary fibre is a class of carbohydrate; it is defined chemically as non-starch polysaccharides (NSP). The average UK diet for example contains approximately 244 g total carbohydrate, of which about 100 g is composed of sugars such as glucose, fructose and sucrose. Approximately 130 g is starch, and the remainder, approximately 12 g, is NSP (Gregory *et al* 1990). Figure 2.8 shows the range in individual intake, from 5 to 25 g per day. Most individuals consume between 7 and 15 g NSP per day.

NSP are complexes of cellulose, a polysaccharide of glucose, which comprises about 20% of total NSP in the average UK diet, and of various other polysaccharides (the non-cellulosic polysaccharides). These contain the pentose sugars, xylose and arabinose (36% of the total NSP), the hexose sugars, glucose and arabinose (27% of the total) and the uronic acids found particularly in pectin (15% of the total). Small amounts of mannose may also be found. Lignin is sometimes included in the definition of dietary fibre but it is extremely difficult to measure. Current analytical methods which attempt to measure it in human foods actually isolate various inert substances which are better referred to as 'substances analysing as lignin'. These amount in total to less than 1 g in human diets.

The term 'hemicellulose' is sometimes used together with 'pectin' to mean non-cellulosic polysaccharides, but this nomenclature is now rarely used.

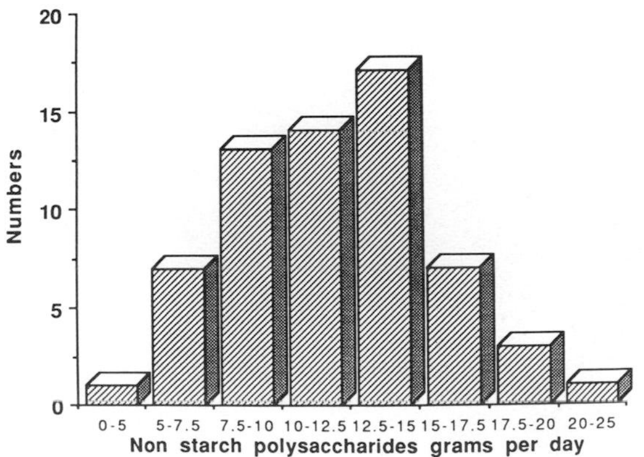

Fig. 2.8 Distribution of individual NSP intake in 63 men and women (from Bingham *et al* 1990).

2.5.2 Analysis

Dietary fibre can be difficult to measure, particularly in starch-rich foods such as potatoes and cereals. In these, starch may be inadequately removed and contaminate the analyses, giving erroneously high results. Conversely, some of the polysaccharides, particularly water soluble ones, may be lost and dietary fibre values will be underestimated. As a result of these and other problems, different methods of analysis give different results. Two methods, those of Southgate and Englyst, are used in the current set of British food tables (see Section 1.4). The Englyst technique is recommended for food labelling in the UK, and is the basis for DRV and WHO recommendations (see Section 1.2).

2.5.3 Low/high NSP foods

The current intake of NSP in Britain is 12 g per day on average and yet the Dietary Reference Value population average is 18 g (Section 1.2). About half the population are consuming less than the recommended individual minimum intake of 12 g and hardly any are consuming more than 18 g per day (Fig. 2.8). Considerable effort will be required to change food choice so that NSP increases by 50% on average.

Some suggestions for the national diet are made in Section 1.2 but there will be distinct differences in the way in which individuals increase their intake. This should be from mixed sources, especially whole grain cereals and vegetables. Table 2.28 is a guide to good, moderate and poor sources of NSP per portion. At least four portions of fruits and vegetables and two good sources of cereal NSP would be needed to achieve 18 g per day. Large quantities of unprocessed bran should be avoided because of its high phytic acid content; the enzyme phytase is present in yeast so leavened wholemeal bread contains smaller amounts of phytic acid than bran.

Low fibre foods are shown in Table 2.28. When devising diets low in residue, however, it is probably important to limit starch in addition, since if this escapes digestion in the small bowel it will act in a similar manner to NSP by acting as an energy source for bacterial growth in the large bowel, and faecal weight will be increased. Potatoes, for example, contain little NSP and the starch in these is readily digested if they are eaten freshly cooked. On cooling, the starch retrogrades or becomes 'resistant' and in cooked cooled potatoes (for instance eaten as potato

Table 2.28 Guide to good, medium and poor sources of non-starch polysaccharides

Good sources of NSP (more than 4 g per portion)	Peas, beans, brussels sprouts, parsnips, spring greens Wholemeal, rye and granary bread, wholemeal pasta All Bran, Bran Flakes, muesli
Moderate sources of NSP (1–4 g per portion)	Most fruits, vegetables and nuts Other Bread, brown rice, other pasta, wholemeal and fruit cakes Weetabix, porridge
Poor sources of NSP (less than 1 g per portion)	Lettuce, marrow, grapes, canned mandarin oranges White rice, sago, cornflour, tapioca, arrowroot, plain cakes and biscuits Cornflakes, Rice Krispies

salad) a significant quantity of the starch will enter the large bowel. In practice, low residue diets are difficult to achieve if they contain cereals, even highly refined cereals. In some cases, specially designed diets may be necessary for research purposes, consisting entirely of meat, cheese, eggs, fish and sugar; alternatively, a liquid formula diet may be necessary. For more detailed discussion of low residue diets see Bingham (1979).

2.5.4 Sources of different NSP constituents

Different constituents are identified in the analytical method, for example pentose sugars, uronic acids, soluble fibre, but the physiological significance of these constituents is not always clear. The proportion of soluble to insoluble NSP in foods depends largely on the pH at which it is measured on analysis, hence different food table data may give confusing values. Those used in Britain are based on the Englyst technique and details can be found in the supplements to *The Composition of Food* relating to vegetables and cereals (Holland *et al* 1988; 1991). Most of these data and those for fruits are also available in Englyst *et al* (1988; 1989).

In general fruit and vegetables contain more of their NSP as cellulose and uronic acids (pectin). The presence of soluble fibre (for example, gums or pectins) may be particularly important in the control of plasma glucose and cholesterol levels. Oat fibre, which is higher in soluble fibre than other cereal fibres, can also reduce elevated blood cholesterol levels. NSP from other cereals, particularly wheat, which contain a greater proportion of pentose sugars and insoluble dietary fibre, may be particularly important in increasing faecal weight and therefore valuable in the treatment of constipation and diverticular disease. Some soluble NSP such as guar and pectin, however, do not bring about an increase in faecal weight.

Although in human diets, NSP is derived mainly from the cell walls of plants, gums and mucilages used as food additives and sometimes fibre supplements, are also NSP. Ispaghula, for example, consists mainly of soluble pentose sugar-containing polysaccharides, and the polysaccharides of guar gum contain mainly the hexose sugars, galactose and mannose. Supplements may be prescribed as drugs, for certain clinical conditions, but DRV for the normal population of 18 g per day should be provided by foods.

References

Bingham S (1979) Low residue diets. *J Hum Nutr* **33**, 15–16.

Bingham S, Pett S and Day KC (1990) NSP intake of a representative sample of British adults. *J Hum Nutr* **3**, 333–7.

Englyst HN, Bingham SA, Runswick SA, Collinson E and Cummings JH (1988) Dietary fibre (non-starch polysaccharides) in fruit, vegetables and nuts. *J Hum Nutr* **1**, 247–86.

Englyst HN, Bingham SA, Runswick SA, Collinson E and Cummings JH (1989) Dietary fibre (non-starch polysaccharides) in cereal products. *J Hum Nutr* **2**, 253–71.

Gregory J, Foster K, Tyler H and Wiseman M (1990) *The dietary and nutritional survey of adults*. OPCS, London.

Holland B, Unwin ID and Buss DH (1988) *Cereals and Cereal Products, Third Supplement to The Composition of Foods*. Royal Society of Chemistry, Cambridge.

Holland B, Unwin ID and Buss DH (1991) *Vegetables, herbs and spices. Fifth Supplement to The Composition of Foods*. Royal Society of Chemistry, Cambridge.

2.6 Vitamins

2.6.1 Dietary sources of vitamins

Figure 2.9 shows the contributions of various food groups to the intake of vitamins in the UK. These figures are taken from data derived from the National Food Survey (Spring *et al* 1979; Bull and Buss 1982; MAFF 1984). For comparative purposes, the intakes from the food groups are expressed as a percentage of the total intake. It is thus possible to see at a glance which foods make the most important contribution to the intake of each vitamin.

While Fig. 2.9 indicates the relative importance of certain food groups in providing vitamins it does not indicate which individual foods are most valuable in boosting intake. The contribution which an individual food makes to nutrient intake depends on three factors: the vitamin content/100 g; the size of the portion eaten, and the frequency of consumption.

Table 2.29 lists some 130 commonly eaten foods (as the cooked form if usually eaten cooked) and their nutrient content per portion (derived from the Cambridge Survey,

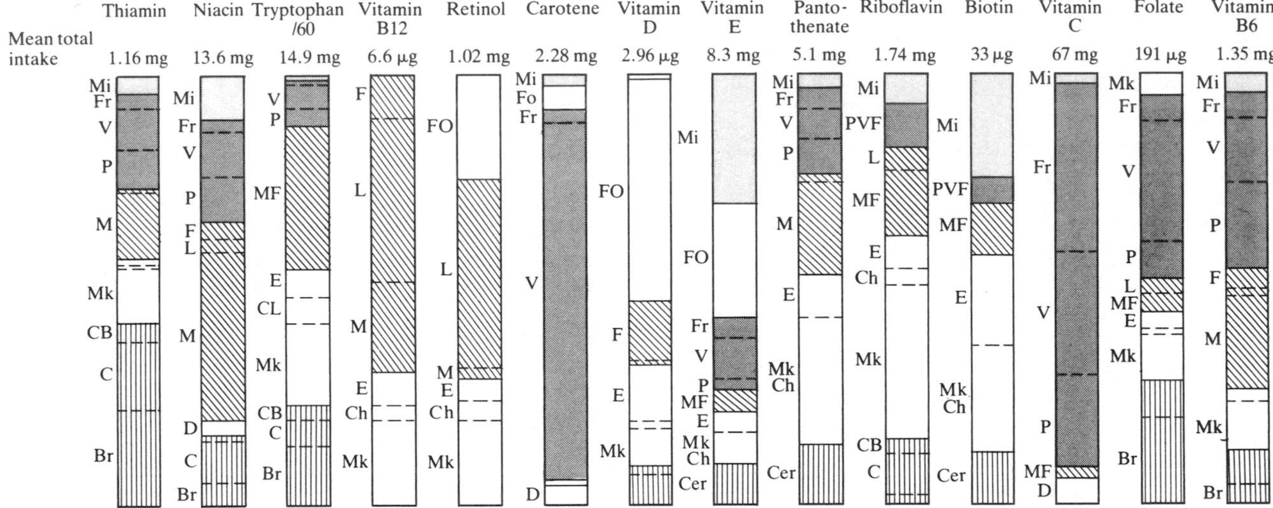

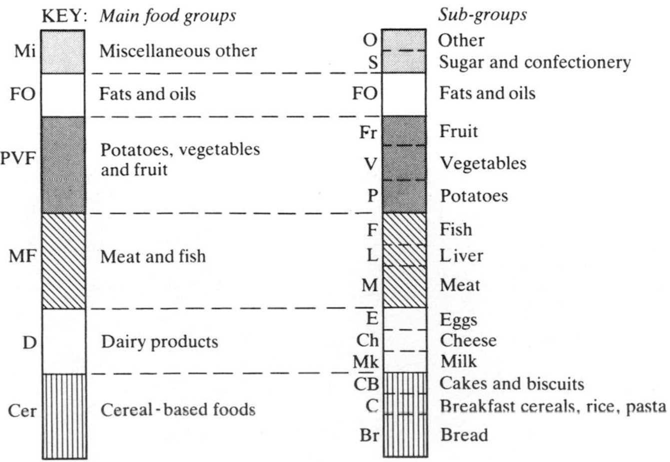

Fig. 2.9 Mean intakes of vitamins in British household diets and the proportion derived from different food groups. Drawn from Spring *et al* (1979); Bull and Buss (1982); MAFF (1984).

Table 2.29 Vitamin contents of foods in portions eaten by adult women in Cambridge, UK. (Portions eaten by men are given in brackets for comparison). (Derived from the data of M Nelson, personal communications).
Tr = trace N = No data ( ) = Estimated value

Food	MW 4[1] Code	*MW 5[2] Code*	Women's[3] Portion g	Men's[4] Portion g	Retinol μg	Carotene μg	Vit D μg	Thiamin mg	Riboflavin mg	Nicotinic Acid mg	Trytophan/60 mg	Vit C mg	Vit E mg	Vit B6 mg	Vit B12 μg	Folate μg	Pantothenic Acid mg	Biotin μg
Bran, wheat	11005	*1*	8			0	0	0.07	0.03	2.37	0.24	0	0.24	0.11	0	20.8	0.19	3.6
Porridge, made with water	11143	*76*	190	(240)		0	0	0.11	0.02	0.19	0.57	0	0	0.019	0	7.6	0.19	3.8
Rice, white, boiled	11050		140	(160)		0	0	0.01	(0.01)	0.42	0.70	0	Tr	0.070	0	(4.2)	0.28	1.4
Spaghetti, white, boiled	11062	*30*	190	(240)		0	0	0.02	0.02	0.95	1.33	0	0	0.038	(0)	7.6	0	0
Bread, wholemeal	11113	*56*	60	(65)		0	0	0.2	0.05	2.46	1.08	0	0	0.072	0	23.4	0.36	3.6
Bread, brown	11070	*33*	55	(75)		0	0	0.15	0.05	1.38	0.94	0	0	0.071	0	22	0.17	1.7
Hovis, average	11079	*40*	55	(70)		0	0	0.44	0.05	2.31	1.04	0	N	0.06	0	21.5	(0.17)	(1.1)
Bread, white	11099	*48*	55	(85)		0	0	0.12	0.03	0.94	0.94	0	0	0.038	0	16	0.17	0.6
Wheatgerm	11034	*17*	10			0	0	0.2	0.07	0.45	0.53	0	2.2	0.33	0	33.1	0.19	2.5
All Bran	11126	*65*	30	(20)		0	0.9	0.3	0.45	4.8	0.96	0	0.6	0.54	0.6	75	0.51	7.5
Corn Flakes	11130	*69*	30	(40)		0	0.9	0.3	0.45	4.8	0.27	0	0	0.54	0.6	75	0.09	0.6
Muesli, Swiss style	11137	*73*	60	(50)		0	0	0.3	0.42	3.9	1.38	0	1.8	0.96	0	(84)	0.72	9
Rice Krispies	11146	*81*	30	(35)		0	0.9	0.3	0.45	4.8	0.42	0	0.3	0.54	0.6	75	0.21	0.6
Weetabix	11154	*90*	35	(35)		0	0	0.24	0.35	3.5	0.73	0	0.35	0.077	0	17.5	0.24	2.8
Crispbread, rye	11168	*95*	20	(20)		0	0	0.06	0.03	0.22	0.36	0	0.2	0.058	0	7	(0.22)	(1.4)
Digestive biscuits, plain	11170	*97*	30	(30)		Tr	0	0.04	0.03	0.33	0.39	0	N	0.027	0	3.9	N	N
Short-sweet biscuits	11184	*105*	25	(25)		12	0	0.04	0.01	0.22	0.32	0	0.25	0.013	0	(3.2)	N	N
Fruit cake, rich	11201	*114*	70	(100)		63	0.7	0.06	0.05	0.42	0.56	0	0.7	0.077	0	5.6	0.14	3.5
Sponge cake	11211	*119*	50	(60)		75	1.5	0.05	0.06	0.25	0.8	0	1.5	0.03	0.5	5	0.25	3.5
Whole milk average	12012	*189*	30		16	6	0.009	0.01	0.05	0.02	0.23	0.3	0	0.018	0.12	1.8	0.11	0.6
Skimmed milk, average	12001	*181*	30		0	0	0	0.01	0.05	0.03	0.23	0.3	0	0.018	0.12	1.5	0.1	0.6
Whole milk average	12012	*189*	200		104	42	0.06	0.06	0.34	0.16	1.5	2	0	0.12	0.8	12	0.7	3.8
Skimmed milk, average	12001	*181*	200		2	0	0	0.08	0.34	0.18	1.56	2	0	0.12	0.8	10	0.64	3.8
Cream, fresh, single	12113	*212*	30	(45)	94	38	0.042	0.01	0.05	0.02	0.18	0.3	0	0.015	0.09	2.1	0.08	0.5
Cream, fresh, double	12116	*215*	30	(45)	180	98	0.081	0.01	0.05	0.01	0.12	0.3	0.3	0.009	0.06	2.1	0.06	0.3
Cheese, Camembert	12133	*227*	35		80	110	(0.063)	0.02	0.18	0.34	1.72	0	0.35	0.077	0.38	35.7	0.13	2.7
Cheese, Cheddar, average	12134	*228*	35	(45)	114	79	0.091	0.01	0.14	0.02	2.1	0	0.35	0.035	0.38	11.6	0.13	1
Cheese, cottage, plain	12147	*232*	70		31	7	0.021	0.02	0.18	0.09	2.27	0	0	0.056	0.49	18.9	0.28	2.1
Cheese, Edam	12154	*237*	40	(30)	70	60	(0.076)	0.01	0.14	0.03	2.45	0	0	0.036	0.34	16	0.15	0.7
Cheese, Stilton, blue	12180	*249*	30	(40)	107	56	0.081	0.01	0.13	0.15	1.6	0	0.3	0.048	0.3	23.1	0.21	1.1
Cheese spread, plain	12142	*231*	20		55	21	0.034	0.01	0.07	0.02	0.63	0	0	0.016	0.12	3.8	0.1	0.7
Low fat yogurt, plain	12188	*255*	140	(140)	11	7	0.014	0.07	0.35	0.21	1.68	1.4	0	0.126	0.28	23.8	0.63	4.1
Eggs, chicken, boiled	12806	*293*	60	(60)	114	0	1.05	0.04	0.21	0.04	2.21	0	0.6	0.072	0.66	23.4	0.78	9.6
Butter	12256	*306*	12	(16)	98	52	0.091	Tr	Tr	Tr	0.01	0	0.24	Tr	Tr	Tr	Tr	Tr
Margarine	12257	*309*	12	(16)	94	90	0.953	Tr	Tr	Tr	0	0	0.96	Tr	Tr	Tr	Tr	Tr

Table 2.29 *contd.*

Food	MW 4[1] Code	*MW 5[2] Code*	Women's[3] Portion g	Men's[4] Portion g	Retinol µg	Carotene µg	Vit D µg	Thiamin mg	Riboflavin mg	Nicotinic Acid mg	Tryptophan/60 mg	Vit C mg	Vit E mg	Vit B6 mg	Vit B12 µg	Folate µg	Pantothenic Acid mg	Biotin µg
Baked beans, canned in tomato sauce	13043	*694*	115	(160)	0	80	0	0.09	0.07	0.57	0.92	Tr	0.41	0.138	0	38	0.21	2.9
Beans, runner, boiled	13113	*720*	75	(75)	0	90	0	0.04	0.01	Tr	0.23	7.5	0.17	0.03	0	31.5	0.03	0.4
Beans, Haricot, dried, boiled	13087		90	(115)	0	Tr	0	0.09	0.04	0.54	0.99	Tr	0.06	0.108	0	N	0.15	N
Beetroot, boiled in salted water	13165	*742*	40	(40)	0	11	0	0	0	0.04	0.12	2	Tr	0.016	0	44	0.04	N
Brussels sprouts, boiled in salted water	13178	*747*	85	(100)	0	272	0	0.06	0.08	Tr	0.43	51	0.76	0.162	0	93.5	0.24	0.3
Cabbage, boiled, average	13185	*750*	90	(115)	0	189	0	0.07	0.01	0.27	0.18	18	0.18	0.072	0	26.1	0.14	Tr
Carrots, old, boiled	13202	*755*	60	(80)	0	4536	0	0.05	Tr	Tr	0.06	1.2	0.34	0.06	0	9.6	0.11	0.2
Cauliflower, boiled	13217	*760*	120	(115)	0	72	0	0.08	0.05	0.48	0.84	32.4	0.13	0.18	0	61.2	0.5	1.2
Celery, raw	13221	*761*	45	(50)	0	22	0	0.03	0	0.14	0.04	3.6	0.09	0.013	0	7.2	0.18	0
Cucumber, raw	13233	*767*	30	(40)	0	18	0	0.01	0	0.06	0.03	0.6	0.02	0.012	0	2.7	0.09	0.3
Leeks, boiled	13265	*776*	80	(80)	0	460	0	0.02	0.02	0.32	0.16	5.6	0.62	0.04	0	32	0.08	0.8
Lettuce, average, raw	13266	*777*	25	(30)	0	89	0	0.03	0	0.1	0.03	1.2	0.14	0.01	0	13.8	(0.05)	0.2
Peas, boiled	13128	*730*	60	(70)	0	150	0	0.42	0.02	1.08	0.66	9.6	0.13	0.054	0	16.2	0.09	0.2
Peas, canned, re-heated, drained	13135	*733*	60	(70)	0	270	0	0.05	0.04	0.72	0.54	0.6	0.13	0.036	0	12	(0.02)	Tr
Processed peas, canned, re-heated, drained	13140	*736*	85	(90)	0	51	0	0.09	0.03	0.34	0.94	Tr	0.26	0.085	0	9.4	(0.03)	Tr
Chick peas, whole, dried, boiled	13075	*705*	75		0	17	0	0.08	0.05	0.52	0.83	Tr	0.83	0.105	0	40.5	0.22	N
Old potatoes, boiled	13013	*668*	140	(235)	0	Tr	0	0.25	0.01	0.7	0.56	8.4	0.08	0.462	0	36.4	0.53	0.4
Old potatoes, mashed	13015	*669*	140	(235)	57	53	0.546	0.22	0.03	0.7	0.56	7	0.63	0.42	Tr	33.6	0.5	0.6
Old potatoes, baked, flesh only	13011	*666*	140	(235)	0	Tr	0	0.29	0.01	0.84	0.7	11.2	0.08	0.434	0	35	0.36	0.4
Old potatoes, roast in corn oil	13016	*672*	110	(170)	0	Tr	0	0.25	0.02	0.77	0.77	8.8	0.86	0.341	0	39.6	0.28	0.3
Chips, retail, fried in vegetable oil	13022	*679*	130	(170)	Tr	Tr	0	0.1	0.01	0.91	1.04	11.7	0.51	0.416	0	N	0.32	0.5
New potatoes, boiled in salted water	13002	*661*	140	(235)	0	Tr	0	0.18	0.03	0.56	0.56	12.6	0.08	0.462	0	26.6	0.53	0.4
Swede, boiled in unsalted water	13361	*819*	80	(125)	0	132	0	0.1	0.01	0.8	0.08	12	Tr	0.032	0	14.4	0.06	Tr
Tomatoes, raw	13384	*827*	50	(55)	0	320	0	0.05	0	0.5	0.05	8.5	0.61	0.07	0	8.5	0.12	0.8
Apples, eating, average, raw	14012	*856*	80	(80)	0	14	0	0.02	0.02	0.08	0.08	4.8	0.47	0.048	0	0.8	0	1
Apricots, canned in juice	14035	*864*	100		0	210	0	0.02	0.01	0.3	0.1	14	N	0.06	0	2	0.06	0.4
Avocado, average	14037	*865*	75		0	12	0	0.08	0.14	0.83	0.23	4.5	2.4	0.27	0	8.2	0.83	2.7
Bananas	14045	*867*	70	(70)	0	15	0	0.03	0.04	0.49	0.14	7.7	0.19	0.203	0	9.8	0.25	1.8
Blackcurrants, stewed with sugar	14054	*873*	25		0	20	0	0	0.01	0.05	0.03	28.8	0.19	0.013	0	N	0.06	0.3
Dates, dried	14085	*887*	25		0	(10)	0	0.02	0.02	0.45	0.38	0	N	0.047	0	3.2	0.19	N
Gooseberries, cooking, stewed with sugar	14101	*896*	100		0	41	0	0.01	0.02	0.2	0.1	11	0.29	0.01	0	6	0.17	0.3
Grapes, average	14109	*903*	55		0	9	0	0.03	0.01	0.11	0	1.7	0	0.055	0	1.1	0.03	0.2
Grapefruit, raw	14105	*899*	85		0	14	0	0.04	0.02	0.26	0.09	30.6	(0.16)	0.025	0	22.1	0.24	(0.9)
Mandarin oranges, canned in juice	14146	*914*	100		0	95	0	0.08	0.01	0.2	0.1	20	0	(0.03)	0	12	(0.15)	(0.8)
Melon, Canteloupe-type	14157	*920*	105		0	620	0	0.02	0.01	0.31	0	15.7	0.06	0.063	0	3.1	0.08	N
Melon, Honeydew	14162	*923*	105		0	50	0	0.03	0.01	0.31	0	9.4	0.1	0.063	0	2.1	0.22	N
Oranges	14175	*931*	105	(90)	0	29	0	0.12	0.04	0.42	0.1	56.7	0.25	0.105	0	32.5	0.39	1
Peaches, canned in juice	14188	*940*	100		0	67	0	0.01	0.01	0.6	0.1	6	N	0.02	0	2	0.06	0.2
Pears, canned in syrup	14198	*946*	100		0	0	0	0.01	0.01	0.2	0	2	0	0.03	0	3	0.04	0.2
Pineapple, canned in syrup	14212	*949*	100		0	11	0	0.07	0.01	0.2	0.1	13	0.06	0.07	0	(1)	0.07	0.1
Prunes, stewed with sugar	14233		100		0	73	0	0.04	0.07	0.5	0.2	0	N	0.09	0	0	0.16	0
Raspberries, canned in syrup	14248	*960*	100		0	3	0	0.01	0.03	0.3	0.1	7	0.15	0.04	0	(10)	0.17	(0.7)
Strawberries, raw	14260	*967*	90	(80)	0	7	0	0.03	0.03	0.54	0.09	69.3	0.18	0.054	0	18	0.31	1
Tangerines	14266	*970*	45	(30)	0	44	0	0.03	0.01	0.09	0.04	13.5	N	0.032	0	9.4	0.09	N

Table 2.29 *contd.*

Food	MW 4[1] Code	*MW 5[2] Code*	Women's[3] Portion g	Men's[4] Portion g	Retinol μg	Carotene μg	Vit D μg	Thiamin mg	Riboflavin mg	Nicotinic Acid mg	Tryptophan/60 mg	Vit C mg	Vit E mg	Vit B6 mg	Vit B12 μg	Folate μg	Pantothenic Acid mg	Biotin μg
Bacon, gammon rashers, grilled (lean only)	220	*348*	80		Tr	Tr	Tr	0.80	0.22	5.68	4.72	0.0	(0.03)	(0.296)	Tr	(1.6)	(0.56)	(2.4)
Bacon, rashers, fried, middle, (lean and fat)	227	*354*	35		Tr	Tr	Tr	0.14	0.07	1.75	1.58	0.0	0.07	0.102	Tr	0.4	0.11	0.7
Bacon, rashers, grilled, average (lean only)	230	*356*	35		Tr	Tr	Tr	0.21	0.08	2.17	1.99	0.0	0.01	0.130	Tr	0.7	0.25	1.0
Bacon, rashers, grilled middle (lean and fat)	232	*358*	35		Tr	Tr	Tr	0.14	0.06	1.54	1.61	0.0	0.04	0.091	Tr	0.4	0.18	0.7
Beef, rump steak, fried (lean and fat)	250	*372*	90	(100)	Tr	Tr	Tr	0.07	0.31	4.95	5.49	0.0	0.30	0.261	1.80	13.5	0.72	Tr
Beef, sirloin, roast (lean only)	258	*382*	90	(100)	Tr	Tr	Tr	0.06	0.28	5.40	5.31	0.0	0.26	0.297	1.80	15.3	0.81	Tr
Lamb, leg, roast (lean only)	286	*406*	80	(100)	Tr	Tr	Tr	0.11	0.30	5.28	5.04	0.0	0.08	0.176	1.60	3.2	0.56	1.6
Lamb, shoulder, roast (lean and fat)	292	*412*	80	(100)	Tr	Tr	Tr	0.06	0.16	2.48	3.36	0.0	0.10	0.128	1.60	2.4	0.40	0.8
Pork chops, grilled (lean and fat)	304	*420*	85	(125)	Tr	Tr	Tr	0.56	0.17	4.85	4.51	0.0	0.03	0.263	0.85	5.1	0.85	1.7
Pork, leg, roast (lean only)	310	*426*	85	(125)	Tr	Tr	Tr	0.72	0.30	5.61	4.85	0.0	0.00	0.349	1.70	5.9	1.11	2.6
Chicken, roast (meat only)	321	*438*	80	(130)	Tr	Tr	Tr	0.06	0.15	6.56	3.68	0.0	0.09	0.208	0.00	8.0	0.96	2.4
Chicken, roast (meat and skin)	322	*439*	85	(135)	Tr	Tr	Tr	(0.05)	(0.14)	(5.35)	3.57	0.0	—	—	Tr	—	—	—
Chicken, roast (light meat)	323	*440*	80	(130)	Tr	Tr	Tr	0.06	0.11	8.24	4.00	0.0	0.06	0.280	Tr	5.6	0.88	1.6
Chicken, roast (dark meat)	324	*441*	80	(130)	Tr	Tr	Tr	0.07	0.19	4.88	3.44	0.0	0.12	0.128	0.80	10.4	1.04	2.4
Turkey, roast (meat only)	344	*462*	100		Tr	Tr	Tr	0.07	0.21	8.50	5.40	0.0	Tr	0.320	2.00	15.0	0.80	2.0
Kidney, lamb (fried)	365	*478*	60		96	—	—	0.34	1.38	5.76	3.18	5.4	0.25	0.180	47.40	47.4	3.06	25.2
Kidney, ox (stewed)	367	*480*	60		150	—	—	0.15	1.26	2.88	3.30	6.0	0.25	0.180	18.60	45.0	1.80	29.4
Kidney, pig (stewed)	369	*482*	60		84	0	—	0.11	1.26	3.66	3.12	6.6	0.22	0.168	9.00	25.8	1.44	31.8
Liver, lamb (fried)	376	*488*	90	(135)	18540	54	0.450	0.23	3.96	13.68	4.41	10.8	0.29	0.441	72.90	216.0	6.84	36.9
Liver, ox (stewed)	378	*490*	90	(135)	18090	1386	1.017	0.16	3.24	9.27	4.77	13.5	0.40	0.468	99.00	261.0	5.13	45.0
Liver, pig (stewed)	380	*492*	90	(135)	10440	0	1.017	0.19	2.79	10.35	4.95	8.1	0.14	0.576	23.40	99.0	4.14	30.6
Beef, corned (canned)	393	*507*	50	(65)	Tr	Tr	Tr	Tr	0.11	1.25	3.25	0.0	0.39	0.030	1.00	1.0	0.20	1.0
Ham (canned)	394	*360*	40	(40)	Tr	Tr	Tr	0.21	0.10	1.56	1.20	0.0	0.03	0.088	Tr	Tr	0.24	0.4
Ham and pork chopped (canned)	395	*513*	40	(65)	Tr	Tr	Tr	0.08	0.08	1.28	1.08	0.0	0.04	0.020	0.40	0.4	0.16	0.8
Luncheon meat (canned)	396	*515*	40	(65)	Tr	Tr	Tr	0.03	0.05	0.72	1.08	0.0	0.04	0.008	0.40	0.4	0.20	Tr
Tongue (canned)	398	*537*	60		Tr	Tr	Tr	0.02	0.23	1.50	2.28	0.0	0.16	0.024	3.00	1.2	0.24	1.2
Black pudding (fried)	401	*505*	45	(75)	Tr	Tr	Tr	0.04	0.03	0.45	1.26	0.0	0.11	0.018	0.45	2.3	0.27	0.9
Liver sausage	404	*514*	35	(45)	(2905)	Tr	(0.210)	0.06	0.55	1.51	0.84	Tr	0.04	0.049	2.80	6.6	0.52	2.4
Frankfurters	405	*510*	55		Tr	Tr	Tr	0.04	0.07	0.83	0.83	0.0	0.14	0.016	0.55	0.5	0.22	1.1
Salami	407	*521*	30		Tr	Tr	Tr	0.06	0.07	1.38	1.08	0.0	0.08	0.045	0.30	0.9	0.24	0.9
Sausages, pork (grilled)	413	*529*	70	(90)	Tr	Tr	Tr	0.01	0.11	2.80	1.96	0.0	0.15	0.042	0.70	2.1	0.42	2.1
Cod (fried in batter)	442	*570*	125	(135)	Tr	Tr	Tr	(0.09)	(0.09)	(2.13)	4.63	Tr	—	(0.475)	(2.50)	(15.0)	(0.25)	(3.8)
Cod (steamed)	446		100	(150)	Tr	Tr	Tr	(0.09)	(0.09)	(2.10)	3.50	Tr	(0.54)	(0.370)	(3.00)	(12.0)	(0.20)	(3.0)
Kipper (baked)	489	*615*	105	(145)	(51)	Tr	(26.250)	Tr	(0.19)	(4.20)	5.04	Tr	(0.31)	(0.599)	(11.55)	(10.5)	(0.92)	(10.5)
Mackerel (fried)	492	*618*	95		(49)	Tr	(20.045)	(0.09)	(0.36)	(8.26)	3.80	Tr	—	(0.798)	(11.40)	—	(0.91)	(7.6)
Pilchards (canned in tomato sauce)	494	*621*	75		Tr	Tr	6.000	0.02	0.22	5.70	2.63	Tr	0.52	—	9.00	—	—	—
Salmon (canned)	498	*625*	30	(45)	27	Tr	3.750	0.01	0.05	2.10	1.14	Tr	0.45	0.135	1.20	3.6	0.15	(1.5)
Sardines, canned in oil (fish only)	500	*628*	70	(85)	Tr	Tr	5.250	0.03	0.25	5.74	3.08	Tr	0.21	0.336	19.60	5.6	0.35	3.5
Tuna (canned in oil)	508	*631*	70	(85)	Tr	Tr	4.060	0.03	0.08	9.03	3.01	Tr	4.41	0.308	3.50	10.5	0.29	2.1
Prawns (boiled)	523	*639*	40	(40)	Tr	Tr	Tr	—	—	—	1.68	Tr	—	—	—	—	—	—

Table 2.29 cont'd

Food	MW 4[1] Code	*MW 5[2] Code*	Women's[3] Portion g	Men's[4] Portion g	Retinol µg	Carotene µg	Vit D µg	Thiamin mg	Riboflavin mg	Nicotinic Acid mg	Tryptophan/60 mg	Vit C mg	Vit E mg	Vit B6 mg	Vit B12 µg	Folate µg	Pantothenic Acid mg	Biotin µg
Bournvita powder	12072	*1043*	7		0	0	0	N	N	N	0.14	0	Tr	0	N	N	N	0
Cocoa powder	12082	*1050*	4		0	(2)	0	0.01	0	0.07	0.16	0	0.04	0.003	0	1.5	N	N
Drinking chocolate powder	12093	*1064*	7		0	1	0	0	0	0.04	0.08	0	0.01	0.001	0	1.7	N	N
Horlicks powder	12097	*1069*	10		62	0	0.208	0.1	0.13	1.5	0.3	0	N	N	N	N	N	N
Ovaltine powder	12108	*1076*	7		44	0	0.147	0.07	0.09	1.05	0.15	0	N	0.12	N	N	N	N
Honey (in jars)	848	*1001*	15		0	0	0.000	Tr	0.01	0.03	Tr	Tr	—	—	0.00	—	—	—
Jam (fruit with edible seeds)	849	*1004*	25		0	Tr	0.000	Tr	Tr	Tr	Tr	2.5	Tr	Tr	0.00	Tr	Tr	Tr
Marmalade	853	*1008*	20		0	10	0.000	Tr	Tr	Tr	Tr	2.0	Tr	Tr	Tr	1.0	Tr	Tr
Chocolate (milk)	857	*1015*	25	(35)	0	(10)	Tr	0.02	0.06	0.05	0.35	0.0	0.13	(0.005)	Tr	(2.5)	(0.15)	(0.8)
Keg bitter beer[5]	895	*1096*	283	(334 868)	0	Tr	0.000	Tr	0.08	0.91	0.37	0.0	—	0.054	0.42	13.0	(0.28)	(1.4)
Lager (bottled beer)[5]	896	*1099*	283	(331 669)	0	Tr	0.000	Tr	0.06	0.93	0.59	0.0	—	0.059	0.40	12.2	(0.28)	(1.4)
Stout (bottled)[5]	898	*1101*	283	(307 567)	0	Tr	0.000	Tr	0.08	0.74	0.48	0.0	—	0.040	0.31	12.5	(0.28)	(1.4)
Cider (sweet)[5]	902	*1105*	283	(252 —)	0	Tr	0.000	Tr	Tr	0.03	Tr	0.0	—	0.014	—	—	0.08	1.7
Wine (red)[5]	904	*1107*	116	(163 256)	0	Tr	0.000	Tr	0.02	0.10	Tr	0.0	—	0.017	Tr	0.2	(0.05)	—
Wine white (medium)[5]	907	*1110*	116	(163 256)	0	Tr	0.000	Tr	0.01	0.09	Tr	0.0	—	0.016	Tr	0.2	(0.03)	—
Sherry (medium)[5]	912	*1115*	60	(71 182)	0	Tr	0.000	Tr	0.01	0.05	Tr	0.0	0.00	0.005	Tr	0.1	—	—
Vermouth (dry)[5]	914	*1117*	60	(68 122)	0	0	0.000	Tr	Tr	0.02	0.00	0.0	0.00	0.005	Tr	Tr	—	—
Vermouth (sweet)[5]	915	*1118*	60	(68 122)	0	0	0.000	Tr	Tr	0.02	0.00	0.0	0.00	0.002	Tr	Tr	—	—

[1] MW4 Code = the number of the food in McCance and Widdowson's *The Composition of Foods* 4e (Paul and Southgate 1978) and supplements (Holland, Unwin and Buss 1988; 1989; 1991; 1992)

[2] MW5 Code = the number of the food in McCance and Widdowson's *The Composition of Food*, 5e (Holland *et al*) 1991

[3] Womens' portion: see text for definition in Appendix 5

[4] Men's portion: see text for definition. Where no weight is given, either men did not eat this food or data for both sexes was combined

[5] For alcoholic beverages, the nutrient content is given per typical glass. The actual average portion weights for each sex are given in brackets

see Appendix 5). It is left to the dietitian to consider how frequently the food might be eaten by the group or individual under consideration. Lack of space makes it impossible to provide lists of foods ranked for content per portion for each separate nutrient. However, it is relatively easy to run the eye down this table and pick out the foods of high or low content.

References

Holland B, Unwin ID and Buss DH (1988) Cereals and cereal products. The third supplement to McCance & Widdowson's The Composition of Foods (4th edition). Nottingham: The Royal Society of Chemistry and Ministry of Agriculture, Fisheries and Food.

Holland B, Unwin ID and Buss DH (1989) Milk products and eggs. The fourth supplement to McCance & Widdowson's The Composition of Foods (4th edition). Cambridge: The Royal Society of Chemistry and Ministry of Agriculture, Fisheries and Food.

Holland B, Unwin ID and Buss D (1991) Vegetables, herbs and spices. The fifth supplement to McCance & Widdowson's The Composition of Foods (4th edition). Cambridge: The Royal Society of Chemistry and Ministry of Agriculture, Fisheries and Food.

Holland B, Unwin ID and Buss DH (1992) Fruit and nuts. The first supplement to McCance & Widdowson's The Composition of Food (5th Edition). Cambridge: Royal Society of Chemistry and Ministry of Agriculture, Fisheries and Food.

Holland B, Welch AA, Unwin ID, Buss DH, Paul AA and Southgate DAT (1991) McCance and Widdowson's The Composition of Foods. Fifth revised and extended edition. Cambridge: Royal Society of Chemistry and Ministry of Agriculture, Fisheries and Food.

2.6.2 Vitamin requirements

For information on the biochemistry of the vitamins and for accounts of the classical deficiency diseases the reader is referred to the standard textbooks of nutrition (e.g. Passmore and Eastwood 1986).

For summaries of the body of work on which the Reference Nutrient Intakes (RNI) are based, the relevant reports should be studied (NRC 1989; Truswell 1990; DoH 1991). This section notes some of the most recent work with implications for the vitamin requirements of normal populations.

Free radicals and antioxidant nutrients

Free radicals are generated during the normal oxidative processes which occur in living cells. A free radical is an atom or molecule capable of existing independently, which contains one or more unpaired electrons. Free radicals are very reactive chemically and carry the potential for extensive damage to the organism which, therefore, must there be equipped with potent defence mechanisms.

The important oxygen species are superoxide ($O_2^{\bullet -}$), hydrogen peroxide (H_2O_2), and the hydroxyl radical ($OH^{\bullet}$). Both superoxide and the hydroxyl radical are free radicals. The reduction of molecular oxygen to water involves the production initially of the free radical superoxide. This then gains a further electron forming the peroxyl anion which, with two protons from solution, will form hydrogen peroxide. Both superoxide and hydrogen peroxide must be removed from the system as soon as they are formed, because divalent cations such as iron may cause a catalysed interaction with formation of a further free radical, the hydroxyl radical. This is highly reactive and potentially severely damaging in living systems because it can pluck an electron from almost any organic molecule in its vicinity initiating further processes that may lead to tissue damage and eventually disease. Prevention of the hydroxyl radical formation depends on the immediate removal of the superoxide and hydrogen peroxide. The superoxide anion is efficiently removed by superoxide dismutase (SOD) and hydrogen peroxide by glutathione peroxidase. These enzmes are dependent on zinc, copper, manganese and selenium (Zn, Cu, Mn, Se).

A further reactive metabolite of oxygen (but not a free radical), is singlet oxygen ($^1O_2$) in which a peripheral electron is excited to an orbital above that which it normally occupies. Singlet oxygen may be 'quenched' by retinoids or carotenoids, which absorb energy without chemical change so that the excited singlet oxygen is returned to the O_2 ground state.

Since free radical reactions involve the donation or acquisition of a single electron, they tend to create another radical, whereupon the process may be repeated. It is the nature of free radical reactions that they can initiate chain reactions and it is the function of the defence systems to prevent and stop propagation.

Defence mechanisms included the following.

1 *Water* This supplies hydroxyl ions which can donate electrons to complete a pair in an electron shell.

2 *Enzymic systems* particularly glutathione peroxidase (GPX), a Se dependent enzyme; catalase, an Fe dependent enzyme that deals with hydrogen peroxide; superoxide dismutase (SOD) which is Zn, Cu or Mn dependent.

3 *Antioxidant vitamins with a chain breaking role* Vitamin E, Vitamin C, β-carotene, and probably also other carotenoids.

4 *Preventive antioxidant vitamins* which maintain tissue integrity, such as retinol and riboflavin.

5 *Antioxidant minerals* that form part of the enzyme systems (see 2 above).

The antioxidants interact with each other and it is probable that the optimum requirement of one will depend on the intake of others. Vitamin E exerts a sparing effect on vitamin A, raising the liver stores and decreasing turnover rate of vitamin A.

Free radicals are believed to play a role in the aetiology of cardiovascular disease, cancer and ageing.

For further information see Thurnham (1990a; 1990b) BNF (1991), Slater and Block (1991).

Retinol (pre-formed vitamin A)

Retinol functions in the eye in the transmission of light stimuli to the brain; defective dark adaptation and night blindness are usually the first indicators of deficiency. The most general morphological change occurring in vitamin A deficiency is the replacement of the mucus lining of epithelial tissues by a squamous metaplastic epithelium which eventually produces large amounts of keratin. Changes in the integrity of epithelia may affect the resistance of animals to bacterial infection; this is an important factor in developing countries. The reproductive apparatus in both males and females is sensitive to vitamin A deficiency, and this can be explained in part by changes in the epithelia involved. Excess vitamin A is teratogenic (see the section below on Vitamins and toxicity). Vitamin A affects both cellular proliferation and differentiation, and in deficiency, growth is affected.

Retinol is a preventive antioxidant necessary for tissue integrity, but it possesses little if any radical-quenching properties since *in vivo* it is tightly bound to retinol-binding protein. Several epidemiological studies have shown significant negative correlations between vitamin A intake and occurrence of cancer in humans. This may be linked to its essentiality for growth and differentiation of tissues, or to its role in maintaining the integrity of epithelial tissues. However, many of these studies failed to distinguish between retinol and β-carotene and their relative importance is still uncertain.

Vitamin A toxicity

See Section 2.6.3 below on Megadoses of vitamins and toxicity.

β-carotene

β-carotene has been best known as the precursor of vitamin A. However, it is now apparent that it has an antioxidant role in its own right. It is the single most effective, naturally occurring quencher of singlet oxygen. Five prospective studies have shown that low plasma concentrations of β-carotene are associated with an elevated risk of lung cancer.

Vitamin E

Vitamin E has been known for decades as the vitamin in search of a function. In recent years it has become clear that it is nature's most effective lipid-soluble, chain-breaking antioxidant, protecting cell membranes from peroxidative damage (Packer 1991).

Vitamin E may be protective against cancer through its functions as a free-radical scavenger, by enhancing the body's immune responses, and by inhibiting the conversion of nitrites to nitrosamines in the stomach. Vitamin E inhibits platelet aggregation, a significant factor in the development of atherosclerosis and other vascular diseases, and production of prostaglandins, which further stimulate platelet aggregation.

Vitamin E has been shown to inhibit the elevation of free-radical concentrations associated with arthritis and also to provide some relief of pain and improvement of mobility.

Lipids and lipid vitamins are poorly absorbed by neonates weighing less than 1500 g at birth. Low serum levels of vitamin E are commonly seen and are associated with haemolytic anaemia, bronchopulmonary dysplasia and retrolental fibroplasia.

Vitamin E deficiency also occurs in patients with abetalipoproteinaemia and in malabsorption syndromes such as cystic fibrosis, massive ileal resection, blind loop syndrome and congenital cholestatic jaundice. It is associated with neuropathological syndromes (*Lancet* 1986). In these cases, pharmacological doses of vitamin E are required for treatment.

Vitamin C

There is more debate over the optimum intake of vitamin C than any other vitamin. An adult requires 10 mg/d to prevent scurvy. The UK RNI is 40 mg/d and the US RDA is 60 mg/d. However tissue saturation appears to require an ascorbic acid intake above 100 mg/d, which is also the amount estimated to be necessary to maintain a body pool of 20 mg/kg body weight. Megadosing with intakes in excess of 1 g/d remains popular.

Vitamin C and the common cold

The role of vitamin C in the common cold has been reviewed by Hemilä (1992). The results of 18 studies from 1972 to 1988 in which subjects regularly received at least 1 g of vitamin C per day over periods of 1–9 months are summarized. These do not support the hypothesis that megadoses of vitamin C have a prophylactic effect. However, vitamin C consistently decreased the duration and severity of symptoms. No conclusion could be drawn as to the effective dose or duration of treatment. Benefits appear to have been greater when the background level of intake was lowest. In one study, urinary excretion before supplementation was 300 mg/d indicating normal intakes even higher than this. The benefits may be due to the antioxidant property of vitamin C. In an infection, phagocytic leucocytes become activated and produce oxidizing compounds which are released from the cell. By reacting with these oxidants, vitamin C may decrease their inflammatory effects.

Vitamin C may be protective against cardiovascular disease or cancer. A substantial body of evidence suggests that the incidence is lower in populations that have an abundant intake of leafy green vegetables or fruit. Several prospective epidemiological studies have shown a correlation between a low dietary level or blood concentration of vitamin C and ischaemic heart disease or cancer. The strongest case is for protection against gastric and oesophageal cancers, possibly because of a role in preventing the reaction of secondary and higher amines with nitrite to form nitrosamines in the stomach.

Vitamin D

Dietary vitamin D is listed in the both UK food tables and UK RNIs, and nutritionists still continue to measure dietary intake. However, it is clearly established that in people regularly exposed to sunlight, dietary vitamin D (about 2.5 μg; 100 iu/day) makes an insignificant contribution to plasma 25(OH)D levels. In only a minority of the population does it play a significant role in maintaining vitamin D status. Fraser (1983; 1990) provides important reviews of recent advances.

Elderly people

In people deprived of sunshine, dietary vitamin D does make a valuable contribution to vitamin D status even though it has been calculated that an intake of about 12.5 μg (500 iu) is necessary to maintain plasma 25(OH)D at satisfactory levels. For the elderly therefore, particularly the housebound and those in institutions, supplements of 10 μg (400 iu) are to be recommended (Fraser 1983; Holdsworth *et al* 1984; Dattani *et al* 1984; Sheltawy *et al* 1984; Morris *et al* 1984).

Infants

It has been shown in animals (Clements and Fraser 1984) that there is active transport of vitamin D from the mother to the fetus. The newborn therefore, even in the absence of sunlight and dietary vitamin D, do not develop rickets if maternal vitamin D status is adequate. Therefore, the vitamin D status of the infant is best determined by ensuring an adequate prenatal status in the mother rather than by giving oral vitamin D_2 supplements to the infant. There is also a suspicion from experience with animals that giving oral vitamin D to infants promotes arteriosclerosis, and may therefore be harmful (Peng *et al* 1978).

Milk, it must be noted, contains very little vitamin D. The suggestion by Lakdawala and Widdowson (1977) that it contains considerable amounts of water soluble vitamin D sulphate has not been confirmed by other workers (Leerbeck and Sondergaard 1980; Hollis *et al* 1981; Reeve *et al* 1982).

Asians

Asian mothers have a low vitamin D status and many Asian infants show signs of vitamin D deficiency (e.g. neonatal tetany). Attempts to get Asians to increase dietary vitamin D have not been very successful and concerned people would like to see fortification of chapati flour. However, this action has been rejected by the Committee on Medical Aspects of Food Policy (COMA). Arguments for and against fortification are set out in DHSS (1980) and Sheiham and Quick (1982).

The incidence of neonatal tetany has a seasonal variation, indicating that sunlight does make an important contribution to vitamin D status, and that it is not a total absence of exposure to sunlight which causes low vitamin D status in Asian women. Recent work (Clements *et al* 1987) suggests that deficiency is precipitated by the low Ca:P ratio and the low availability of calcium in the Asian diet. It is thought that this leads to enhanced destruction of vitamin D in the liver. Thus strategies for preventing vitamin D deficiency other than supplementation with pills or fortification of foods with vitamin D may emerge.

Vitamin B_6

The various forms of pyridoxine, pyridoxal, pyridoxamine and their phosphates and some other conjugated forms all contribute to the vitamin B_6 activity in foods. Bioavailability has been found to vary widely (Gregory and Kirk 1981), and uncertainty exists over how well this is reflected by the current forms of assay. The figures given in food tables must be regarded as tentative (Paul and Southgate 1978; Cooke 1983).

Ten years ago the UK had not established an RNI for vitamin B_6, but other countries had put it at 0.2 mg per gram of protein (NRC 1980; Rutishauser 1982). However recent reports (NRC 1989; DoH 1991) have accepted a figure of 0.15 and 0.1 mg per gram of protein for adults. This figure has also been used by the Department of Health for other age groups, but in the absence of new information the NRC (1989) report upheld the earlier figure of 0.2 mg/g protein in pregnancy, lactation and for children. It has been suggested that oral contraceptive use increases the requirement for vitamin B_6; the COMA panel on DRVs (DoH 1991) rejected this conclusion.

Vitamin B_6 and premenstrual tension

Vitamin B_6 is claimed to alleviate the symptoms of premenstrual tension. Two mechanisms have been proposed, but neither has received firm support from research. Vitamin B_6 may help in alleviating some symptoms in some women but the literature is contradictory, and the scientific case must be regarded as not proven. Studies achieving the best response have used doses of 50–500 mg/d, suggesting a pharmacological response rather than a correction of nutritional deficiency (Mira *et al* 1988). A major concern is that preparations containing 25, 50 and 100 mg per tablet are readily available over the counter and that self-prescribing might achieve toxic intakes (see below).

Folate

The primary biochemical function of folate co-enzymes is in the transfer and utilization of one-carbon units in a variety of essential reactions involved in amino acid interconversions, biosynthesis of the nucleic acids, purines and pyrimidines and certain methylation reactions. The major clinical sign of deficiency (macrocytic anaemia) is the result of blockage of synthesis of DNA. Rapidly dividing cells (e.g. mucosal epithelium) are most affected by deficiency.

In pregnancy, folate needs are increased by the demand from increased cell turnover. That these needs cannot always be met from an individual's normal diet is shown by the significant number of women who developed megaloblastic anaemia of pregnancy before antenatal supplementation became routine (Chanarin 1973). The amount necessary to prevent a fall in red cell folate is an additional 100 μg/day in women who start pregnancy with adequate stores.

Until recently there was a discrepancy between reported folate intakes ranging from 120–300 μg/d and RDAs of 400–800 μg (NRC 1980), while there was apparently no widespread deficiency of folate except in pregnancy. Reasons for the discrepancy were reviewed by Bates *et al* (1982) and Truswell (1984). They included uncertainties in methods for assaying folate in foods, possible underestimation of bioavailability, and the addition of large 'safety' factors. Recent committees have placed the RDA (NRC 1989) or RNI (DoH 1991) at a figure which is generally achievable in real diets.

Folate and neural tube defects

The association between poor nutrition during pregnancy and neural tube defects (NTD) has been documented since the 1970s. Many studies suggested that vitamin supplementation, particularly with folate, in the periconceptual period would reduce the prevalence and recurrence rate. Unfortunately these studies, reviewed by Schorah and Smithells (1991), did not resolve the role of multivitamins versus folate. However, the UK Medical Research Council's study (MRC 1991) has finally done so. In a randomized multicentre study, a significant reduction (72%) in NTD recurrence was achieved by periconceptual supplementation with folate, but not with multivitamins. A number of questions remain unanswered and were raised in the *Lancet* (1991) editorial that accompanied the research report. The dose of folate used, 4 mg/d (10 times the RNI for pregnancy) was much higher than can be achieved in normal diets. Is it necessary? Smithells *et al* (1989) obtained a reduction in occurrence with a multivitamin supplement containing 0.36 mg folate/d. Would the lower amount be effective if used alone or was its action potentiated by the presence of other vitamins? The ongoing study of Lenehan *et al* (1988) should resolve this, as it includes a low dose of folate with and without other vitamins. It is also uncertain whether the occurrence of NTD is a straight dietary deficiency or whether an inborn error of metabolism is overcome by folate supplementation. At 4 mg/d, potential adverse effects include potentiation of neurological damage from vitamin B_{12} deficiency and deleterious effects on zinc metabolism (Simmer *et al* 1987).

Folate and cancer

It has been hypothesized that localized folic acid deficiency may play a role in the development of metaplasia. Krumdieck has suggested that exposure to cigarette smoke results in a folate deficiency affecting principally the bronchial epithelium and rendering it more susceptible to neoplastic transformation by the carcinogenic hydrocarbons of tobacco smoke. In clinical studies, Krumdieck and colleagues (Heimberger *et al* 1987) have demonstrated lower levels of plasma and erythrocyte folate in smokers than in non-smokers. There have also been suggestions that folate may play a role in cervical cancer (see Potischman *et al* 1991; Butterworth *et al* 1992). These associations have yet to be confirmed.

Niacin and tryptophan

The term niacin is used generically to cover nicotinic acid and nicotinamide. It has a central role in intermediary metabolism and the requirement is related to energy expenditure. Nicotinamide can be synthesized from dietary tryptophan. The equivalence of preformed niacin and dietary tryptophan varies between individuals and from day to day. The widely used convention that 60 mg tryptophan are equivalent to 1 mg niacin contains an allowance for variation. Oestrogens reduce the rate of tryptophan metabolism such that, in areas of the world where the deficiency disease pellagra is seen, women are more likely than men to suffer. This is of no practical importance in the UK and the normal diet contains approaching twice the RNI in niacin equivalents.

Tryptophan supplements

L-tryptophan is among the single amino acid supplements promoted by the health food industry. In this context it acts not as a niacin supplement but as an amino acid. Because of substantial safety queries, the US Food and Drug Administration declared all single amino acids as non-GRAS (not Generally Recognized As Safe) in 1974. There are several potential harmful effects.

- L-tryptophan supplements have caused the eosinophilia-myalgia syndrome (EMS) in the US and several deaths have been reported (CDC 1991; Kamb 1992). It is believed this was caused by a contaminant produced during manufacture of the drug but this has yet to be confirmed (Roufs 1992).

- L-tryptophan in large amounts (e.g. 2 g) produces a relatively high blood level compared to other neutral amino acids, thereby increasing its ability to compete with them for transport across the blood-brain barrier to form serotonin which induces sleep. This could be a dangerous effect if taken during the day while driving a car for instance.
- Eating purified amino acids promotes osteoporosis, probably by chelating dietary calcium so that it is not only readily absorbed but also readily excreted. A similar effect is obtained with 'chelated' mineral supplements that are promoted as 'easily absorbed'.

Niacin and hyperlipidaemia

Nicotinic acid, but not nicotinamide, in pharmacological doses (1.5–6 g per day) has been used to treat hyperlipidaemia (Naito 1987). Doses greater than 75 mg stimulate histamine release and produce a temporary vasodilation and unpleasant flushing. If levels are increased gradually, patients can increase their tolerance.

Thiamin

Thiamin requirement is related to energy, and particularly to carbohydrate intake. High carbohydrate diets require more thiamin than high fat diets. A number of naturally occurring compounds have antithiamin activity, including fermented tea leaves, tea leaf extracts, betel nuts and coffee. Thiaminases are present in raw fish and shell fish and ferns, but are destroyed by cooking.

In developing countries, thiamin deficiency (beri-beri) is usually due to diets of milled rice or to consumption of thiaminase containing foods such as raw fish. Physical exertion and high calorie intake are common precipitants of acute beri beri. In developed countries, alcoholism is the major cause of thiamin deficiency. It manifests itself as Wernicke's encephalopathy and/or Korsakoff's psychosis state. However these conditions are not cured by thiamin alone indicating a multiple deficiency (Reuler *et al* 1985). Acute deficiency has been precipitated by glucose loading in a deficient individual. Food faddism and iatrogenic causes such as parenteral nutrition or dialysis account for some cases. Wernicke's encephalopathy has been reported in situations associated with vomiting and malnutrition including Hodgkin's lymphoma, carcinoma of the stomach, chronic gastritis and gastric partitioning. Patients are usually chronically malnourished and receive carbohydrate without adequate thiamin (Butters 1981; Watson *et al* 1981; Fawcett *et al* 1984).

Riboflavin

Riboflavin functions primarily as a component of two flavin coenzymes that catalyse many oxidation-reduction reactions. Deficiency symptoms are non-specific, and clinically obvious deficiency is rarely reported in Western countries, but is common in countries with low intakes of meat and dairy products. Those most likely to be at risk in the UK are vegans. Riboflavin has a role as a preventive antioxidant; it is associated with epithelial cell lesions and with potential control of the regeneration of reduced glutathione.

Vitamin B_{12}

Vitamin B_{12} deficiency is most likely in elderly with gastrointestinal problems (Carethers 1988; Nilsson-Ehle *et al* 1989) and in vegans. The label declaration on some vegan products supposedly high in vitamin B_{12} may be misleading, since the compounds measured as vitamin B_{12} by microbiological assay probably do not have biological activity in the human (Herbert 1988). (See also Veganism, Section 3.10).

Pantothenic acid

Food table values are derived from microbiological assays after enzyme treatment to release bound forms. Data is lacking for many foods. Calculated intakes must be regarded as tentative. Deficiency has been produced only by use of semi-synthetic diets (Fry *et al* 1976) or by giving an antagonist (Hodges *et al* 1959). Indications of deficiency take several weeks to appear, and studies of intake and excretion (Fry *et al* 1976) suggest the body has considerable stores. The COMA Panel (DoH 1991) concluded that reported intakes of 3–7 mg must be adequate.

Biotin

Biotin occurs in bound and unbound forms and the biological availability in foods varies enormously. Food table values are based on 'values obtained by microbiological assay. . . after acid hydrolysis to release the bound form. Recent improvements have resulted in lower amounts. . . and these are believed to be more correct than the older ones' (Paul and Southgate 1978). Data is lacking for many foods. Calculated food intakes must be regarded as tentative. Biochemical evidence on which to assess the daily requirement is virtually non-existent. Deficiency has been reported as a complication of total parenteral nutrition (Mock *et al* 1981; Gillis *et al* 1982) and in individuals who have consumed large amounts of egg white. It is thought that synthesis by intestinal microorganisms may contribute significantly to intake. The COMA Panel (DoH 1991) agreed that intakes between 10 and 220 μg/day were both adequate and safe.

2.6.3 Megadoses of vitamins and toxicity

The use of vitamins in doses far exceeding the RDA has grown in recent years. They are claimed to cure or prevent a variety of conditions including the common cold, schizophrenia, cancer, hyperactivity, to increase ability to deal with stress and to delay ageing. Megadosing is promoted primarily by food faddists and 'ortho-molecular' physicians. It can also arise through injudicious medical prescribing or by unwitting self-administration of high content vitamin preparations from health food shops. The best controlled studies have found no benefits from megadosing and significant toxic effects have emerged.

The toxic effects of the fat soluble vitamins are well recognized, but the water soluble vitamins are generally regarded as safe on the grounds that excess is eliminated in the urine. This is not so. All biologically active substances have a toxic level. The toxic effects of water soluble vitamins have been reviewed by Miller and Hayes (1982), Flodin (1990) and the Department of Health (1991). Adverse effects are of four kinds

1 Direct toxicity.
2 Induced dependency.
3 The masking of other diseases.
4 Interactions with other drugs.

The reported adverse effects are summarized in Table 2.30 together with an indication of the doses at which adverse effects have been reported.

The vitamins most likely to have toxic effects are vitamin A, vitamin D and vitamin B_6. Toxic levels of these vitamins can be achieved by injudicious dosing with readily available products. The toxic effects of other vitamins listed in Table 2.30 occur rarely.

Vitamin D toxicity

Infants are most at risk from vitamin D toxicity. It is characterized by hypercalcaemia and failure to thrive of sudden onset between three and nine months of age. There is evidence that infantile hypercalcaemia is the result of a comparatively rare degree of sensitivity to moderately excessive intakes of vitamin D. In 1953 and 1954 around 100 new cases were recorded annually. At that time infants might easily have received 100 μg per day of vitamin D in fortified milks, vitamin drops and baby cereals. In 1957, the levels of fortification were reduced such that vitamin D intake from these sources was halved. Infantile hypercalcaemia is now rare, but the risk of excessive intakes remains real. Maternal hypercalcaemia may contribute to supravalvular aortic stenosis in the fetus and to suppression of parathyroid function in the newborn. Administration of vitamin D above RNI levels to pregnant women is contraindicated.

Vitamin A toxicity

Toxicity is caused by retinol, retinol esters and retinoic acid but not by β-carotene. Most cases of toxicity are due to self-medication. The toxicity of vitamin A has been reviewed by Hathcock *et al* (1990). They conclude that an intake of 10 000 iu/d (3000 μg/d) is adequate to provide for good nutrition but low enough to avoid toxicity in most people, that an intake of 25 000 iu/d (7500 μg/g) is nutritionally excessive and carries some risk of toxicity, and that the effects between these boundaries cannot be anticipated.

Chronic vitamin A toxicity in children may produce permanent long bone deformities by premature closure of epiphyses. Excessive maternal intake has teratogenic potential in experimental animals and possibly in humans. Administration of vitamin A in greater than RNI amounts is contraindicated in pregnant women or those planning pregnancy. In October 1990 the Chief Medical Officer of Health issued the Vitamin A and Pregnancy Hazard Notice HC (Hazard) (90) 41 stating 'The vitamin supplements currently prescribed as part of ante-natal care for pregnant and nursing mothers contain a safe amount of vitamin A and should continue to be taken, [but] I must caution women who are or who may become, pregnant against taking dietary supplements containing vitamin A except on the advice of a doctor. . . . as a matter of prudence [pregnant women] are advised not to eat liver or products made from it such as liver paté and liver sausage.' This hazard notice was issued as a result of some case reports from abroad and concern over elevated levels of vitamin A in liver possibly due to changes in agricultural practice in the UK.

Vitamin B_6 toxicity

Chronic dosing with high levels of vitamin B_6 produces sensory neuropathy with unsteady gait, numb feet and numbness and clumsiness of hands. There may be irreversible residual neuropathy after withdrawal of the vitamin. Toxicity has been reported at a dose of 200 mg/d for three years, although most reports are of higher doses. Since vitamin B_6 has been promoted as alleviating pre-menstrual tension, and preparations containing 25, 50 and 100 mg are readily available over the counter in health food shops, self-prescribing could achieve a toxic dose.

2.6.4 Vitamin supplementation

Vitamins and work capacity or sporting performance

The idea that vitamin supplementation can improve stamina and increase muscular strength is attractive to many adults. The supposed rationale is the premise that there must be increased demand for the B-complex vitamins because of their biochemical reactions that make energy available for muscular work. There is also a mistaken belief that there are large losses of vitamins in sweat. Studies that have examined the effect of vitamin supplementation on work performance have been summarized by Consolazio (1983). A majority agree that a healthy person on a normal diet will not benefit from further nutrient supplementation.

Table 2.30 Toxicity of vitamins

Vitamin	Toxic effects	Toxic intakes	Reference
Vitamin A	Liver and bone damage, hair loss, double vision, vomiting, headaches	Daily doses should not exceed — Infants 900 μg 1–3 yrs 1800 μg 4–6 yrs 3000 μg 7–12 yrs 4500 μg — Adolescents 6000 μg — Adult females 7500 μg — Adult males 9000 μg	DoH (1991)
Vitamin D	Infants are most at risk. Hypercalcaemia, calcification of soft tissues, damage to kidneys and cardiovascular system	50 μg/d 15 mg every 3 to 5 m	DHSS (1980) Markestad *et al* (1987)
Vitamin B_6	Peripheral sensory neuropathy	2–7 g/d 50–500 mg/d	Schaumberg *et al* (1983) Dalton and Dalton (1987)
Nicotinic acid	Changes in liver structure and function, in carbohydrate tolerance; in uric acid metabolism	3–6 g/d	McCreanor and Bender (1986)
Folic acid	Masking of B_{12} deficiency	The risks are small except in vegans	
Vitamin C	Diarrhoea at intakes of g/d; increased production of oxalate and kidney stones in a small group of individuals with a high propensity for oxalate production	The risks are small	Balcke *et al* (1984)
Thiamin	Headache, irritability, insomnia, rapid pulse, weakness, contact dermatitis, pruritis	The risks are small 50 mg/kg; 3 g/d	Iber *et al* (1982)
Riboflavin	None		
Vitamin B_{12}	None		
Vitamin E	None reported consistently		Bendich and Machlin 1988
Vitamin K	Synthetic vitamin K has been linked to liver damage in the newborn. Natural vitamin K is of low toxicity		

Vitamins and IQ

In 1988 a paper by Benton and Roberts was given national press coverage. It purported to show that in 12–13 year old children with apparently normal growth and no nutritional deficiency, additional vitamins and minerals had a positive effect on performance in tests of non-verbal intelligence. This finding was not confirmed by a subsequent double-blind study by Nelson *et al* (1990). It seems unlikely that marginal deficiencies would affect brain function. Vitamins and minerals are transported from the blood to the brain by specific active mechanisms that are saturable (Bradbury 1979). Thus nutrient homeostasis occurs in the central nervous system. Further, the levels of nutrient intake in British schoolchildren are, in the majority of cases, well above the RDA (DoH 1989).

Vitamins in vegetarian and vegan diets (see Section 3.10)

Welfare foods scheme supplements

COMA (DHSS 1980) recommended that vitamin tablets (vitamins A and D) continue to be made available to expectant and nursing mothers up to 30 weeks after parturition, and children's vitamin drops (vitamins A, D and C) for children up to the age of 5 years.

Further reading

Bender DA (1992) *Nutritional biochemistry of the vitamins.* Cambridge University Press, Cambridge.

Bendich A and Butterworth CE (Eds) (1991) *Micronutrients in health and in disease prevention.* Marcel Dekker, New York.

Block G (1991) Epidemiologic evidence regarding vitamin C and cancer. *Am J Clin Nutr* **54**, 1310S–14S.

Combs GF (Ed) (1992) *The vitamins: fundamental aspects in nutrition and health.* Academic Press, San Diego.

Diplock AT (1991) Antioxidant nutrients and disease prevention: an overview. *Am J Clin Nutr* **53**, 189S–93S.

Gaby SK, Bendich A, Singh VN and Machlin LJ (1991) *Vitamin intake and health. A scientific review.* Marcel Dekker, New York.

Machlin LJ (1984) *Handbook of the vitamins: nutritional, biochemical and clinical aspects.* Marcel Dekker, New York.

Slater TF and Block G (eds) (1991) Antioxidant vitamins and β-carotene in disease prevention. *Am J Clin Nutr* **53**(1 — Supplement), 189S–396S.

Trout DL (1991) Vitamin C and cardiovascular risk factors. *Am J Clin Nutr* **53**, 322S–25S.

Weisburger JH (1991) Nutritional approach to cancer prevention with emphasis on vitamins, antioxidants, and carotenoids. *Am J Clin Nutr* **53**, 226S–37S.

Zeigler RG (1991) Vegetables, fruits and carotenoids and the risk of cancer. *Am J Clin Nutr* **53**, 251S–59S.

References

Balcke P, Schmidt P, Zazgarnik J, Kopsa H and Haubenstock A (1984) Ascorbic acid aggravates secondary hyper-oxalaemia in patients on chronic hemodialysis. *Ann Intern Med* **100**, 344–5.

Bates CJ, Black AE, Phillips DR, Wright AJA and Southgate DAT (1982) The discrepancy between normal folate intakes and the folate RDA. *Hum Nutr: Appl Nutr* **36A**, 422–9.

Bendich A and Machlin LJ (1988) Safety of oral intake of vitamin E. *Am J Clin Nutr* **48**, 612–19.

Benton D and Roberts G (1988) Effects of vitamin and mineral supplementation on intelligence of a sample of schoolchildren. *Lancet* **i**, 140–3.

Bradbury M (1979) *The concept of a blood brain barrier.* John Wiley, Chichester.

British Nutrition Foundation (1991) *Antioxidant nutrients in health and disease.* Briefing paper 25. British Nutrition Foundation, London.

Bull NL and Buss DH (1982) Biotin, pantothenic acid and vitamin E in the British household food supply. *Hum Nutr: Appl Nutr* **36A**, 190–6.

Butters N (1981) The Wernicke-Korsakoff syndrome: a review of psychological, neuropathological and etiological factors. *Curr Alcohol* **8**, 205–32.

Butterworth CE, Hatch KD, Macaluso M, Colel P, Sauberlich HE, Soong S, Borst M and Baker VV (1992) Folate deficiency and cervical dysplasia. *J Am Med Ass* **267**, 528–33.

Carethers M (1988) Diagnosing vitamin B_{12} deficiency, a common geriatric disorder. *Geriatrics* **43**, 89–112.

Centers for Disease Control (1991) Eosinophilia myalgia syndrome: follow-up survey of patients, New York, 1990–91. *J Am Med Ass* **226**, 195–6.

Chanarin I (1973) Dietary deficiency of vitamin B_{12} and folic acid. In *Nutritional deficiencies in modern society* Howard AN and McLean Baird I (Eds) Newman Books, London.

Clements MR and Fraser DR (1984) Quantitative aspects of vitamin D supply to the rat foetus and neonate. *Calcif Tissue Int* **36**[Suppl 2], S31.

Clements MR, Johnson L and Fraser DR (1987) A new mechanism for induced vitamin D deficiency in calcium deprivation. *Nature* **324**, 62–5.

Consolazio CF (1983) Nutrition and performance. *Prog Fd Nutr Sci* **7**, 1–210.

Cooke JR (1983) Food composition tables – analytical problems in the collection of data. *Hum Nutr: Appl Nutr* **37A**, 441–7.

Dalton K and Dalton MJT (1987) Characteristics of pyridoxine overdose neuropathy syndrome. *Acta Neurol Scand* **76**, 8–11.

Dattani JT, Exton-Smith AN and Stephen JML (1984) Vitamin D status of the elderly in relation to age and exposure to sunlight. *Hum Nutr: Clin Nutr* **38C**, 131–8.

Department of Health (1989) *The diets of British schoolchildren.* Rep Hlth Soc Subj **36**, HMSO, London.

Department of Health (1991) *Dietary Reference Values for food energy and nutrients for the United Kingdom.* Rep Hlth Soc Subj **41**, HMSO, London.

Department of Health and Social Security (1979) *Recommended daily amounts of food energy and nutrients for groups of people in the United Kingdom.* Rep Hlth Soc Subj **15**, HMSO, London.

Department of Health and Social Security (1980) *Rickets and osteomalacia.* Rep Hlth Soc Subj **19**, HMSO, London.

Fawcett S, Young PK and Holliday RL (1984) Wernicke's encephalopathy after gastric partitioning for morbid obesity. *Can J Surg* **27**, 169–70.

Flodin NW (1990) Micronutrient supplements: toxicity and drug interactions. *Prog Fd Nutr Sci* **14**, 277–331.

Fraser DR (1983) The physiological economy of vitamin D. *Lancet* **i**, 969–72.

Fraser DR (1990) Vitamin D. In *Recommended Nutrient Intakes: Australian Papers.* Truswell AS (Ed) Australian Professional Publications, Sydney.

Fry PC, Fox HM and Tas HG (1976) Metabolic response to a pantothenic acid deficient diet in humans. *J Nutr Sci Vitaminol* **22**, 339–46.

Gillis J, Murphy FR, Boxall LBHG and Pencharz PB (1982) Biotin deficiency in a child on long term TPN. *J Parent Ent Nutr* **6**, 308–310.

Gregory JF and Kirk JR (1981) The bioavailability of vitamin B_6 in foods. *Nutr Rev* **39**, 1–8.

Hathcock JN, Hattan DG, Jenkins MY, McDonald JT, Sundaresan PR and Wilkening VL (1990) Evaluation of vitamin A toxicity. *Am J Clin Nutr* **52**, 183–202.

Heimberger DC, Krumdieck CL, Alexander B, Birch R, Dill R and Bailey WC (1987) Localised folic acid deficiency and bronchial metaplasia in smokers: hypothesis and preliminary report. *Nutrition International* **3**, 54–60.

Hemilä H (1992) Vitamin C and the common cold. *Br J Nutr* **62**, 3–16.

Herbert V (1988) Vitamin B_{12}: plant sources, requirements, and assay. *Am J Clin Nutr* **48**, 852–8.

Hodges RE, Bean WB, Ohlson MA and Bleiler B (1959) Human pantothenic acid deficiency produced by omega-methyl panthothenic acid. *J Clin Invest* **38**, 1421–5.

Holdsworth MD, Dattani JT, Davies L and Macfarlane D (1984) Factors contributing to vitamin D status near retirement age. *Hum Nutr: Clin Nutr* **38C**, 139–50.

Hollis BW, Roos BA, Draper HH and Lambert PW (1981) Occurrence of vitamin D in human milk whey. *J Nutr* **109**, 384–90.

Iber FL, Blass JP, Brin M and Leevy CM (1982) Thiamin in the elderly – relation to alcoholism and to neurological degenerative disease. *Am J Clin Nutr* **36**, 1067–82.

Kamb MLE (1992) Eosinophilia-myalgia syndrome in L-tryptophan exposed patients. *J Am Med Ass* **267**, 77–82.

Lakdawala DR and Widdowson EM (1977) Vitamin D in human milk. *Lancet* **i**, 167–8.

Lancet (1986) Vitamin E deficiency. *Lancet* **i**, 423–4.

Lancet (1991) Folic acid and neural tube defects. *Lancet* **338**, 153–4.

Leerbeck E and Sondergaard H (1980) The total content of vitamin D in human milk and cows' milk. *Br J Nutr* **44**, 7–12.

Lenehan P, MacDonald D and Kirke P (1988) Neural tube defects and vitamin prophylaxis. In *Vitamins and minerals in pregnancy and* lactation. Berger H (Ed) Nestle Nutrition Workshop Series 16. Raven Press, New York.

Markestad T, Hesse V, Siebenhuner M *et al* (1987) Intermittent high dose vitamin D prophylaxis during infancy: effect on vitamin D metabolites, calcium and phosphorus. *Am J Clin Nutr* **46**, 652–8.

McCreanor GM and Bender DA (1986) The metabolism of high intakes of tryptophan, nicotinamide and nicotinic acid in the rat. *Br J Nutr* **56**, 577–86.

Miller DR and Hayes KC (1982) Vitamin excess and toxicity. In *Nutritional toxicology* Vol 1. Darby WJ (Ed) pp. 81–133. Academic Press, New York.

Ministry of Agriculture, Fisheries and Food (1984) *Household food consumption and expenditure: 1982*. Annual report of the National Food Survey Committee. HMSO, London.

Mira M, Stewart PM and Abraham SF (1988) Vitamin and trace element status in premenstrual syndrome. *Am J Clin Nutr* **47**, 636–41.

Mock DM, De Lorimer AA, Liebman W, Sweetman L and Baker H (1981) Biotin deficiency: an unusual complication of parenteral alimentation. *New Engl J Med* **304**, 820–3.

Morris HA, Morrison GW, Burr M, Thomas DW and Nordin BEL (1984) Vitamin D and femoral neck fractures in elderly South Australian women. *Med J Aust* **140**, 519–21.

MRC Vitamin Study Research Group (1991) Prevention of neural tube defects: results of the Medical Research Council vitamin study. *Lancet* **338**, 131–7.

Naito HK (1987) Reducing cardiac deaths with hypolipidaemia drugs. *Postgrad Med* **82**, 102–112.

National Research Council (1980) *Recommended dietary allowances*. 9e. National Academy of Sciences, Washington DC.

National Research Council (1989) *Recommended dietary allowances*. 10e. National Academy of Sciences, Washington DC.

Nelson M, Naismith DJ, Burley V, Gatenby S and Geddes N (1990) Nutrient intakes, vitamin-mineral supplementation, and intelligence in Britith schoolchildren. *Br J Nutr* **64**, 13–22.

Nilsson-Ehle H, Landahl S, Lindstedt G, Netterblad L, Stockbruegger R, Westin J and Ahren C (1989) Low serum cobalamin levels in a population study of 70- and 75-year-old subjects: gastrointestinal causes and hematological effects. *Dig Dis Sci* **34**, 716–23.

Packer L (1991) Protective role of vitamin E in biological systems. *Am J Clin Nutr* **53**(4), 1051S–1055S.

Palmer N *et al* (1982) Recommended dietary intakes for use in Australia. *J Food Nutr* **39**, 157–93.

Palmer N *et al* (1984) Recommended dietary intakes for use in Australia. *J Food Nutr* **41**, 109–54.

Passmore R and Eastwood M (1986) *Human nutrition and dietetics*, 8e. Churchill Livingstone, Edinburgh.

Paul AA and Southgate DAT (1978) McCance and Widdowson's *The Composition of Foods*. HMSO, London.

Peng SK, Taylor CB, Tham P and Mikkelson B (1978) Role of mild excesses of vitamin D_3 in arteriosclerosis. A study in squirrel monkeys. *Paroi Arterielle* **4**, 229–43.

Potischman N, Brinton LA, Laiming VA, Reeves WC, Brenes MM, Herrero R, Tenorio F, de Britton RC and Gaitan E (1991) A case-control study of serum folate levels and invasive cervical cancer. *Cancer Research* **51**, 4785–9.

Reeve LE, Jorgensen NA and DeLuca HF (1982) Vitamin D compounds in cows' milk. *J Nutr* **112**, 667–72.

Reuler JB, Girard DE and Coonay TG (1985) Current concepts: Wernicke's encephalopathy. *New Eng J Med* **312**, 1035–9.

Roufs JB, (1992) Review of L-tryptophan and eosinophilia-myalgia syndrome. *J Am Dietet Assoc* **50**, 844–50.

Rutishauser IHE (1982) Vitamin B_6. *J Food Nutr* **39**, 158–67.

Schaumberg H, Kaplan J, Windebank A *et al* (1983) Sensory neuropathy from pyridoxine abuse: a new megavitamin syndrome. *New Eng J Med* **309**, 445–8.

Schorah CJ and Smithells RW (1991) Maternal vitamin nutrition and malformations of the neural tube. *Nutr Res Rev* **4**, 33–49.

Sheiham H and Quick A (1982) *The rickets report: 'Why do British Asians get rickets?* Haringey CHC London.

Sheltawy M, Newton H, Hay A, Morgan DB and Hullin RP (1984) The contribution of dietary vitamin D and sunlight to the plasma 25-hydroxyvitamin D in the elderly. *Hum Nutr: Clin Nutr* **38C**, 191–4.

Simmer K, Iles CA, James C and Thompson RPH (1987) Are iron-folate supplements harmful? *Am J Clin Nutr* **45**, 122–5.

Slater TF and Block G (Eds) (1991) Antioxidant vitamins and β-carotene in disease prevention. *Am J Clin Nutr* **53**(Supplement to Issue 1), 198S–369S.

Smithells RW, Sheppard S, Wild J and Schorah CJ (1989) Prevention of neural tube defect recurrence in Yorkshire: final report. *Lancet* **ii**, 498–9.

Spring JA, Robertson J and Buss DH (1979) Trace nutrients 3. Magnesium, copper, zinc, vitamin B_6, vitamin B_{12} and folic acid in the British household food supply. *Br J Nutr* **41**, 487–93.

Thurnham DI (1990a) Anti-oxidant vitamins and cancer prevention. *J Micronut Anal* **7**, 279–99.

Thurnham DI (1990b) Antioxidants and pro-oxidants in malnourished populations. *Proc Nutr Soc* **49**, 247–59.

Truswell AS (1984) Folate. *J Food Nutr* **41**, 143–54.

Truswell AS (Ed) (1990) *Recommended Nutrient Intakes. Australian papers*. Australian Professional Publications, Sydney.

Watson AJS, Walker JF, Tomkin GHF and Keogh JAB (1981) Acute Wernicke's encephalopathy precipitated by glucose loading. *Ir Med J* **150**, 301–303.

2.7 Minerals

2.7.1 Sodium and potassium

Requirements

Sodium and potassium are of major importance in the body as they maintain fluid volume and pressure both intracellularly and extracellularly. They are both essential minerals and it is possible to find signs of deficiency if the dietary intake is reduced (Whitney and Boyle 1984).

The body normally has a good homeostatic mechanism for control of the body content of these two minerals. The major excretory route is urine. Losses in the stools amount to only 2% of ingested sodium (Sanchez-Castillo and James 1984) and about 11% of potassium (Caggiula *et al* 1985). Loss of sodium in sweat is very small (2%/day) and individuals can become acclimatized, thereby reducing the loss. This does not appear to be the case with potassium and large losses can occur with profuse sweating (Lane and Cerda 1978, cited by Whitney and Boyle 1984).

The requirements for sodium and potassium are not easy to establish but 500 mg (22 mmol)/day has been quoted for sodium (BNF 1981) and 1560 mg (40 mmol)/day for potassium (Lee 1974) in adults. The requirement for potassium is higher because there is an obligatory loss of potassium in the urine and stools which amounts to about 590 mg (15 mmol)/day.

Sodium

Dietary sources and intake

The dietary intake of sodium may be divided into discretionary (i.e. added to the food by the individual) and non-discretionary (the sodium which is added to food during manufacture or present naturally in foods).

It has been estimated, that 84–88% of sodium intake in the UK is non-discretionary (Shepherd *et al* 1984; Sanchez-Castillo *et al* 1984). Bull and Buss (1980a) estimated from National Food Survey data that the intake of sodium in the British diet was between 2.9 and 3.7 g/day from non-discretionary sources, 86% being from processed foods.

Foods which make a significant contribution to the non-discretionary intake are the staples in the diet such as cereal products (bread and breakfast cereals in particular) and margarine or butter. A study in Australia (Greenfield *et al* 1984) demonstrated that this group of staples provided 36% of the total sodium intake and that if cakes were also added, nearly 50% of sodium intake came from this group which would not be classified as 'highly salted foods'. In fact, 'highly salted foods' were shown to contribute 33% to the total. The remaining 17% of the total came from milk, beer and meat. Similar percentages have been shown for British diets although cereals provided 40% of the total (Bull and Buss 1980a). A diet relying heavily on processed foods could supply up to 6.5 g of sodium/day (282 mmol sodium or 16.6 g of salt) while one relying on take-away foods could contain about 5.1 g of sodium (Greenfield *et al* 1984). The same authors estimated that a diet which included very few processed foods and no take-away foods may supply as little as 1.6 g of sodium (70 mmol sodium or 4.1 g of salt).

Discretionary addition of sodium includes salting of food at the table and during cooking, although Sanchez-Castillo *et al* (1984) estimated that 29% of the sodium added when cooking was discarded with the cooking water. In a large observational study of over 2000 people, 64% were observed to add salt to their food, 16% of them without prior tasting (Greenfield *et al* 1984). The amount added to the meal was largely dependent on the total diameter of the holes in the shaker but could be as much as 1.2 g of salt or 20.4 mmol (469 mg) of sodium. The use of a single-holed shaker of hole area 3 mm resulted in the smallest addition of salt. The amount added to foods has been shown to correlate with preference for salty foods (Shepherd *et al* 1984) but not with total sodium intake nor sensitivity to the salt taste (Pangborn and Pecore 1982). However, it was of interest to find that in a controlled experiment, those men and women who added salt to their food did so in an amount proportional to the energy content of the diet, 0.4–0.6 g/1000 kcal (Kumanyika and Jones 1983). The amount added per day by individuals showed little intraindividual variability.

Clearly there is much more that needs to be done to establish just how individuals perceive the need for adding salt to food and to estimate the real contribution that this discretionary addition of sodium makes to total intake. What, perhaps, is clear is that the processed/manufactured foods in the diet make a larger contribution to sodium intake than does individual salting. Therefore, salt taken in processed foods needs to be reduced in order to reduce the sodium intake of the population. Furthermore, if sodium intake is reduced then the preference for salty foods also decreases (Bertino *et al* 1982), i.e. the sensitivity to salt taste increases. Since a preference for salt in food and sensitivity to salty taste has been recognized in infants of only two years of age (BNF 1981), the sodium content of food offered to this age group could conceivably affect their preference for salt in later life.

Estimation of sodium consumption is notoriously difficult (Pangborn and Pecore 1982). The 24-hour excretion of sodium provides a more realistic estimate of sodium intake. Caggiula *et al* (1985) found the urinary excretion of sodium in salt users to be 157 mmol (estimated intake was 119 mmol) and 119 mmol excretion in non-salt users (estimated intake was 104 mmol). This study demonstrates that the error in estimating sodium intake is likely to increase where individuals add salt to their food; the percentage underestimate of sodium intake (as judged from excretion) was 24% for salt users and 13% for non-salt users.

One other source of sodium which must be considered when estimating intake of sodium, especially where the individual has been advised to reduce sodium, is in laxative and other drug usage (BNF 1981).

Sodium restriction

Three categories of sodium restriction are used in clinical practice, depending on the degree of restriction required

1 No added salt: 80–100 mmol sodium/day (1.8–2.3 g sodium/day).
2 Low salt: 40 mmol sodium/day (1 g sodium/day).
3 Low sodium: 22 mmol sodium/day (0.5 g sodium/day).

A 'no added salt' (NAS) diet requires that the patient does not use salt in cooking or at the table. In addition, the consumption of salt-rich foods (Table 2.31) may need to be limited if the usual intake of these is particularly frequent or excessive.

Guidance for the construction of low salt or low sodium regimens is given in Tables 2.32 a and b. In some disorders, additional constraints on protein or fluid intake may have to be taken into account.

Table 2.31 Foods high in sodium

Food group	High sodium foods
Meat and meat products	All meat and poultry which is either tinned, smoked, cured or pickled, e.g. bacon, ham, sausages, salt beef, salt tongue, corned beef, luncheon meat and haslet. Meat paste and paté. Made-up, frozen, ready prepared meat stews, casseroles and other dishes
Fish and fish products	Smoked or tinned fish, shellfish, kippers, sardines, etc. Fish paste and paté, made-up fish dishes
Dairy products	Cheese (cottage cheese is lower in sodium)
Vegetables	All tinned vegetables
Miscellaneous	Dehydrated prepacked meals. Tinned, packet and bottled sauces and soups. Marmite, Oxo, Bovril, yeast extracts, stock cubes and gravy powders. Crisps and other snacks. Instant puddings and cake mixes

Because sodium restricted diets tend to be bland in flavour, alternative ways of flavouring foods using freely allowed herbs and spices should be suggested to patients. Some suggestions are given in Table 2.33. The formulation of a low sodium baking powder is given in Table 2.34. Retail pharmacists are often unwilling to make this up in small quantities and patients may therefore experience difficulty in getting the baking powder. If a number of patients at any centre are going to need this baking powder, the hospital pharmacist should be asked to prepare it. The powder can then be used within the hospital for low sodium diets, and patients be given a supply when they leave and on subsequent visits.

Potassium

Dietary sources and intake

Potassium is found widely distributed in foods. Bull and Buss (1980b) have calculated the contributions which various food groups made to the supply of potassium in the UK diet. Out of a total intake of 2.99 g (76.6 mmol/day), root vegetables supplied the greatest percentage (27%), and significant amounts were also provided by milk (19%), meats and eggs (13%), cereal products (11%) and other vegetables (10%). From analysis of diet samples, Bull and Buss (1980b) found the total intake of potassium to be slightly less at 2.51 g/day and the proportion supplied by cereals higher (16%) and that from root vegetables lower (23%).

Dietary potassium is not completely absorbed and 24-hour urinary potassium excretion is a more accurate way of measuring potassium intake (Caggiula *et al* 1985).

Potassium restriction

Potassium is present in nearly all foods. Foods which are particularly high in potassium are summarized in Table 2.35. Low potassium foods are listed in Table 2.36. In some instances (for example, certain renal disorders), dietary potassium intake may need to be regulated by means of a system of potassium exchanges. A 4 mmol potassium exchange list is given in Table 2.37.

2.7.2 Calcium, phosphorus and magnesium

Calcium

The British Nutrition Foundation have published a review of calcium and nutrition (BNF 1991).

The major role of calcium in the body is as a constituent of hydroxyapatite ($Ca_{10}(PO_4)_6(OH)_2$), which comprises the mineralized part of bone. In addition calcium has a number of other functions including enzyme activation, nerve transmission, membrane transport and stability, smooth muscle tone and blood clotting. About 1% of the

Table 2.32(a) and **(b)** Sodium restricted regimens

a) Daily allowances

Food	22 mmol sodium (Low sodium)	40 mmol sodium (Low salt)
Milk	200 ml	300 ml
Ordinary bread	None	2 thin slices

NO SALT to be used in cooking or added to food at the table

b) Guidelines for sodium restricted regimens

Foods allowed	Foods to avoid
† *Meat*	
Fresh or frozen meat, poultry, game, sweetbreads, tripe or liver	Bacon, ham, sausages, kidney, tongue tinned meat, meat pastes, and spreads; any salted and/or smoked meats or sausages. Manufactured meat products, e.g. meat pies and beefburgers
† *Fish*	
Fresh or frozen fish or fish roe	Tinned or smoked fish, shellfish molluscs, fish pastes and spreads Manufactured fish products, e.g. fish fingers and fish in sauce
Dairy products	
Milk and eggs as an allowance. Unsalted butter, double cream and unsalted cream cheese. Yoghurt may be used in exchange for milk (but has a slightly higher sodium content)	Milk in excess of allowance. Cheese, evaporated or condensed milk and single cream
Cereals	
Plain flour, wholemeal flour, salt-free bread, salt-free cakes and salt-free biscuits. Matzos and kosher crackers. Shredded Wheat, Puffed Wheat, Sugar Puffs and porridge. Rice, spaghetti, macaroni, semolina, tapioca, arrowroot and sago	Self-raising flour, ordinary bread, cakes and biscuits (unless otherwise directed). Breakfast cereals other than those listed opposite
Vegetables	
All fresh or frozen vegetables except those listed opposite. Unsalted potato crisps	Baked beans, instant mashed potato and tinned vegetables. Salted potato crisps. *Use sparingly* carrots, spinach, celery and beetroot
Fruits and nuts	
All fresh, tinned or stewed fruit, fruit juices, dates and unsalted nuts	Dried fruit (except dates). Pickled olives, salted nuts and peanut butter
Sugar products	
All sugars, glucose, jam, marmalade, honey, jelly, plain chocolate, boiled sweets, peppermints, marshmallows and marzipan	Toffee, fudge, milk chocolate and filled chocolates. *Use sparingly* golden syrup and treacle

Table 2.32(b) *contd.*

Foods allowed	Foods to avoid
Soups, sauces and gravies	
Home made salt-free soups and sauces. Salt-free meat or vegetable stock. Salt-free stock cubes, salt-free gravy browning (made from pure caramel). Salt-free tomato puree (check label)	Tinned and packet soups, gravy mixes and brownings. Stock cubes (unless salt-free). Salted yeast and meat extracts (e.g. Marmite, Bovril and Oxo). Commercial sauces, ketchups, salad creams, pickles, chutneys and tomato puree, unless labelled unsalted
Beverages	
Tea, coffee and fresh fruit juices. Suitable low sodium fruit squashes, minerals and fizzy drinks, (manufacturers will usually provide information)	Soda water, mineral waters (unless permitted brand). Lucozade, tomato juice, cocoa powder, drinking chocolate, Bournvita, Horlicks and rosehip syrup
Miscellaneous	
Herbs (see Table 2.33). Spices e.g. turmeric, ginger, nutmeg, curry powder, cloves, chilli, pepper, paprika, garlic and powdered mustard. Lemon juice, vinegar (check label for salt). Cooking oils, lard, suet and yeast. Salt substitute (based on potassium chloride§). Salt-free baking powder, custard powder and blancmange powder (check label)	Salt, celery salt or other flavoured salt. Bicarbonate of soda, baking powder, ready-mixed mustard and any products containing salt, soda or sodium

* In cases of renal and liver disease, a sodium restriction may need to be accompanied by a fluid restriction

† In cases of renal and liver disease, a protein restriction may also be indicated

§ Not allowed in renal disease

Table 2.33 Flavouring food on low sodium diets

Food	Suggested flavourings
Fish	Allspice, bay leaf, dill, red cayenne pepper
Roast meat	Allspice. Pork — cloves, apples. Lamb — marjoram, rosemary, apricot. Veal — tarragon. Chicken — tarragon, dill, grapes. Liver — oranges
Grills and roasts	Fresh lemon juice
Stews	Basil, bay leaf, dill, garlic, bouquet garni, marjoram, oregano, chilli, sage, thyme, orange or lemon peel, red cayenne pepper
Tomatoes	Basil, marjoram, oregano
Potatoes	Bay leaf, nutmeg, dill, garlic, mint
Rice	Bay leaf, nutmeg, coriander, cardamom, peppercorns, turmeric
Scrambled egg	Chilli, chives red paprika pepper
Omelette	Chives, chervil, tarragon, garlic, red paprika pepper
Courgettes	Coriander, garlic
Carrots	Thyme
Cauliflower, cabbage	Dill, caraway
All dishes	Freshly ground black and white pepper

Table 2.34 Low sodium baking powder (makes 100 g)

21 g starch
30 g potassium bicarbonate
6 g tartaric acid
43 g potassium acid tartrate

The powder should be stored in a cool, dry place

Table 2.35 Foods high in potassium

Food group	Foods high in potassium
Wholegrain cereals*	It may be possible to incorporate these into potassium restricted diets. The absorption of K^+ varies between subjects and therefore blood biochemistry needs careful monitoring
Meat and meat products	All meat*
Fish and fish products	All fish*
Dairy products	Milk*, eggs*, yoghurt*, cheese*
Fruit	All fruit, especially dried and crystallized fruit, bananas, apricots, rhubarb and blackcurrants. Fruit juices, tomato juice
Nuts	All nuts
Vegetables	Dried pulses, baked beans, beetroot, sweetcorn, mushrooms, spinach. Instant potatoes*, chips*, jacket potatoes*, potato waffles*, crisps and other manufactured potato snacks. Vegetable juice, tomato juice
Beverages	Build Up, drinking chocolate, Horlicks, Ovaltine, other malted milk drinks. Coffee and cocoa. Wine and sherry, beer, cider
Sugar and confectionery	Chocolate and all foods containing it, toffees, liquorice. Molasses, black treacle, syrup, mincemeat and dried fruit
Miscellaneous	Marmite and all yeast extracts, Oxo, Bovril, gravy powders, stock cubes, bottled sauces and ketchups, pastes, pickles and chutneys. Packet sauces, tinned and packet soups. Instant puddings, Gram flour, Cream of Tartar
Herbs and spices	Salt substitutes, e.g. Ruthmol, Selera. Reduced sodium salts. Curry powder, chilli and ginger

* These foods may be incorporated into the diet using an exchange list.
Note that some foods may be unsuitable in renal or liver failure due to their high sodium and/or protein content

total body calcium is in the soft tissues and plasma; 45% of plasma calcium exists as free ions (ionized calcium), the remainder is complexed with citrate or bicarbonate. Three hormones control the level of ionized calcium, which in health is maintained within narrow limits by using bone as a 'reservoir'. Parathyroid hormone (PTH) raises levels by increasing renal tubule resorption and by stimulating the formation of 1,25 dihydroxycholecalciferol – $1,25(OH)_2D$. This hormonal form of vitamin D also raises levels by increasing gut absorption and renal tubule resorption. Calcitonin decreases plasma calcium levels by inhibiting the release of calcium from bone and by increasing urinary excretion.

Table 2.36 Low potassium foods

Food group	Low potassium foods
Bread and cereals	Arrowroot, cornflour, custard powder, flour, oatmeal porridge, rice, sago, tapioca, white bread
Fats and oils	Butter, dripping, margarine, oils, suet, fats
Sugar and confectionery	Boiled sweets, barley sugars, glucose, honey, glace cherries, jam, marshmallows, Opal fruits, Opal mints, pastilles, peppermints, marmalade*
Beverages	Tea, weak ground coffee, spirits e.g. whisky, ginger ale, lemonade, orangeade, Lucozade, soda water, Hycal, lime juice cordial, Tizer, Pepsi-cola, water, Schweppes: American sweet ginger, bitter lemon, dry ginger, sparkling grapefruit, lemonade, sparkling golden orange, sugar-free tonic and tonic water

Note that some items will not be suitable if a sodium and/or protein restriction is necessary
* Reduced sugar jams and marmalades have a higher potassium content

The Dietary Reference Values for calcium (DoH 1991) are given in Table 2.38. Requirements depend upon growth rate and the rate at which calcium is incorporated into bone; they are therefore highest during infancy and adolescence and fall after peak bone mass is achieved at about 25 years (Fig. 2.10). Premature infants are particularly at risk from calcium depletion since their bones are less mineralised than term infants. It is expected that the additional requirements of pregnancy (with the exception of adolescent pregnancy) will be met by increased absorption and no additional calcium is recommended. A higher intake is recommended for lactation to cover the amount secreted in milk.

The current RNI is higher than intakes seen in many countries, where there is no evidence of calcium deficiency. The apparently high requirement of Western populations may be spurious and may reflect an adaptation to high dietary calcium intakes seen in dairy/wheat-eating areas; alternatively it may be that other constituents of the diet such as phosphorous, protein and sodium increase the dietary requirement for calcium.

The normal dietary intake of calcium is given in Table 2.39 and the calcium content of some foods in Table 2.40. Calcium intakes in the UK have decreased over the last few decades, largely due to a reduction in the amount of dairy products consumed. There is now anxiety that some groups, particularly teenage girls, may not be consuming sufficient calcium to achieve maximum bone density and may be at increased risk of developing osteoporosis in later life. The major dietary sources of calcium in the UK are given in Table 2.39. These are mainly milk and dairy products, but 22% of dietary calcium comes from cereals while water is a significant source of calcium in hard water areas.

Table 2.37 Potassium exchange list. Each exchange provides approximately 4 mmol potassium

Food group	Foods	Exchange
High biological value protein foods	Milk	100 ml
	Soya milk	300 ml
	Yoghurt	60 g
	Cheddar cheese	130 g
	Eggs, hens	2 eggs
	Meat, average, lean (cooked)	50 g
	Fish (cooked)	50 g
	Tofu	200 g
Cereals	White wheat flour	120 g
	Wholemeal flour	45 g
	Wheat bran	13 g
	Wholemeal bread	70 g
	White bread	160 g
	Rye crispbread	30 g
	Digestive biscuits	100 g
	All Bran	15 g
	Cornflakes	160 g
	Rice Krispies	100 g
	Weetabix	3 biscuits
	Noodles (raw)	60 g
	Spaghetti (raw)	60 g
	Rice, brown (raw)	60 g
	Millet flour	40 g
	Poppadums	15 g
Fruit	Apple	125 g
	Bilberries	
	Pineapple, canned (with syrup)	
	Strawberries, canned (with syrup)	
	Cranberries	
	Pear	
	Tangerine (weighed with skin)	
	Watermelon (weighed with skin)	
	Peaches, canned (with syrup)	100 g
	Strawberries, fresh	
	Lemon (whole or juice)	
	Orange (weighed with skin)	
	Passion fruit (weighed with skin)	
	Tangerine (weighed without skin)	
	Blackberries	
	Gooseberries	75 g
	Lychees	
	Mango	
	Melon (weighed with skin)	
	Plums	
	Quince	
	Raspberries	
	Apricots (fresh)	50 g
	Cherries	
	Damsons	
	Figs, fresh (raw)	
	Grapes	
	Loganberries	
	Melon (weighed without skin)	
	Mulberries	
	Nectarines	
	Orange (weighed without skin)	
	Peach	
	Pineapple	
	Pomegranate	
	Redcurrants	
	Whitecurrants	
Fruit *contd.*	Apricots (dried)	<25 g
	Avocado pear	
	Banana	
	Blackcurrants	
	Currants (dried)	
	Figs (dried)	
	Prunes (dried)	
	Raisins (dried)	
	Rhubarb	
	Sultanas (dried)	
Vegetables	Carrots, old (boiled)	125 g
	Chayote	
	Marrow (boiled)	
	Onions	
	Swede (boiled)	
	Cabbage	100 g
	Cucumber	
	Runner beans (boiled)	
	Turnip (boiled)	
	Water chestnuts	
	Cauliflower	75 g
	Chicory (raw)	
	Courgettes	
	Green pepper	
	Marrow (raw)	
	Okra	
	Radish	
	Ackee	50 g
	Artichokes, globe (edible portion)	
	Aubergine	
	Beans	
	broad (boiled)	
	baked	
	Beetroot (raw)	
	Broccoli (boiled)	
	Brussels sprouts (boiled)	
	Cabbage (raw)	
	Carrots (raw)	
	Leeks	
	Lettuce	
	Cress	
	Parsnips	
	Peas	
	Potato (boiled)	
	Pumpkin	
	Sweetcorn	
	Sweet potato	
	Tomato	
	Ginger root	
	Beans	<25 g
	mung	
	haricot	
	Cassava	
	Gourd (dried)	
	Lentils (dried)	
	Mushrooms	
	Peas	
	chick	
	dried	
	Pigeon peas (dried)	
	Plantain	

Table 2.37 *contd.*

Food group	Foods	Exchange	Food group	Foods	Exchange
Vegetables *contd.*	Potato	<25 g		Sherry	
	jacket			dry	175 ml
	chips			sweet	140 ml
	roast			Vermouth	400 ml
	crisps		Miscellaneous	Golden syrup	60 g
	Spinach			Black treacle	10 g
	Yam			Jam (not low sugar)	150 g
Beverages*	Milk	100 ml		Marmalade (not low sugar)	350 g
	Soya milk	300 ml		Chocolate	
	Pure orange juice			plain	50 g
	canned	120 ml		milk	35 g
	fresh	90 ml		Toffee	75 g
	Pure grapefruit juice (canned)	140 ml		Marzipan	40 g
	Pineapple juice	110 ml		Indian sweets (average)	25 g
	Tomato juice	60 ml	Spices†	Anise seeds	10 g
	Coffee			Allspice	1 g
	instant	4 g		Caraway seeds	10 g
	ground, infusion	240 ml		Cardamom powder	10 g
	Tea (infusion)	920 ml		Chilli powder	5 g
	Bournvita	40 g		Cinnamon powder	30 g
	Cocoa	10 g		Coriander seeds	10 g
	Drinking chocolate	40 g		Cumin seeds	5 g
	Horlicks	20 g		Dill seeds	10 g
	Ovaltine	20 g		Fennel seeds	5 g
	Beer			Fenugreek seeds	20 g
	keg bitter	1 pint		Ginger (ground)	15 g
	pale ale	350 ml		Mustard powder	15 g
	stout	350 ml		Nutmeg	40 g
	stout extra	180 ml		Paprika	5 g
	strong ale	140 ml		Saffron	5 g
	Cider	200 ml		Sesame seeds	35 g
	Wine			Turmeric	5 g
	red	120 ml			
	white, average	200 ml			

* Spirits, carbonated drinks, fruit-flavourd drinks and fruit squashes contain negligible amounts of potassium

† White pepper has a negligible potassium content

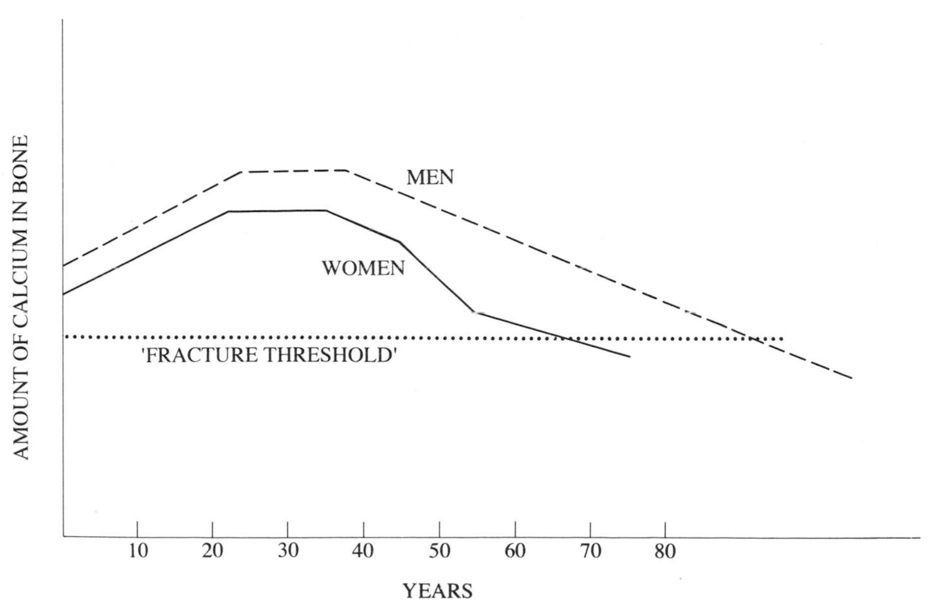

Fig. 2.10 Bone density in men and women.

Table 2.38 Dietary Reference values for calcium, phosphorus and magnesium (mmol/day)* (DoH 1991)

Age	Calcium and phosphorus		Magnesium	
	LNRI	RNI	LNRI	RNI
0–3 mnths	6.0	13.1	1.2	2.2
4–6 mnths	6.0	13.1	1.7	2.5
7–9 mnths	6.0	13.1	1.9	3.2
10–12 mnths	6.0	13.1	1.9	3.3
1–3 yrs	5.0	8.8	2.1	3.5
4–6 yrs	6.9	11.3	2.9	4.8
7–10 yrs	8.1	13.8	4.7	8.0
Males				
11–14 yrs	11.3	25.0	7.4	11.5
15–18 yrs	11.3	25.0	7.8	12.3
19–50 yrs	10.0	17.5	7.8	12.3
50+ yrs	10.0	17.5	7.8	12.3
Females				
11–14 yrs	12.0	20.0	7.4	11.5
15–18 yrs	12.0	20.0	7.8	12.3
19–50 yrs	10.0	17.5	6.2	10.9
50+ yrs	10.0	17.5	6.2	10.9
Pregnancy	10.0	17.5	6.2	10.9
Lactation	10.0	31.8	6.2	13.0

1 mmol calcium = 40 mg
1 mmol phosphorus = 30.9 mg
1 mmol magnesium = 24.3 mg

Table 2.39 Daily intakes and dietary sources of calcium, magnesium and phosphorus

Element	Molecular Weight	Quantity in adult man	Adult daily intakes in the UK*(mmol)	Major dietary sources
Calcium	1 mmol = 40 mg	1200 g	*Males* 23.5 *Females* 18.3	Milk and milk products, flour**, cereals, some vegetables
Magnesium	1 mmol = 24.3 mg	25.0 g	*Males* 13.3 *Females* 9.8	Cereals, green vegetables
Phosphorus	1 mmol = 30.9mg	900 g	*Males* 47.0 *Females* 34.6	Milk and milk products, bread and cereals, meat and fish

* Gregory *et al* (1990)
** White flour is fortified with calcium in the UK

Calcium bioavailability depends on a number of factors. Vitamin D status is a major determinant of calcium absorption. Absorption is highest in infants and decreases with age, and in adults on mixed diets comprises about 30% of the intake (Bullamore *et al* 1970). Absorption is higher during pregnancy and lactation in response to increased requirements.

The percentage of the dietary calcium that is absorbed is inversely related to the intake. Calcium from milk is well absorbed, particularly that from breast milk (80% of calcium from this source is absorbed, compared with 10–20% from infant formulae); there is evidence to suggest that lactose and casein increase the bioavailability of calcium.

Several studies have described a decrease in calcium absorption with an increase in NSP intake; however these studies have mainly used test diets. Phytate, oxalate and non-fermentable NSP such as cellulose may decrease the percentage absorption but, in practice, diets rich in these substances also contain fairly high levels of calcium. Fermentable NSP such as pectins are thought to release bound calcium for absorption in the large bowel. It would appear that a moderate intake of NSP does not significantly decrease calcium absorption in the long term (Allen 1982).

Table 2.40 Calcium, magnesium and phosphorus content of foods (mg/100 g)*

Food	Calcium	Magnesium	Phosphorus
Cereals			
Rice, boiled – white	1	4	34
– brown	4	43	120
Spaghetti, boiled – white	7	15	44
– brown	11	42	110
Bread – white	110	24	91
– wholemeal	54	76	200
Chapati	60	37	120
Flour, plain – white	140	20	110
self-raising – white	350	20	450
wholemeal	38	120	320
All Bran	69	370	620
Corn Flakes	15	14	38
Porridge (with water)	7	18	47
Rice Krispies	20	50	130
Weetabix	35	120	290
Milk/dairy			
Cow's milk – whole	115	11	92
– skimmed	120	12	94
Soya milk	13	15	47
Human milk, mature	34	3	15
Infant milk (whey based)	51	7	32
Cheese, Cheddar	720	25	490
Cream – single	91	9	76
– double	50	6	50
Cottage cheese	73	9	160
Fromage frais	89	8	110
Ice cream, dairy	130	13	110
Yogurt, plain low fat	190	19	160
Butter	15	2	24
Whole egg, raw	57	12	200
Meat/fish			
Beef, roast	15	21	160
Lamb, roast	8	25	220
Pork, roast	10	22	200
Chicken, roast	9	24	210
Sausage, pork – grilled	53	15	220
Cod, baked	29	26	180
Herring, grilled	39	35	340
Sardines, canned in oil	550	52	520
Vegetables and fruit			
Potatoes, old – boiled	5	17	37
Baked beans	48	31	95
Peas, boiled	19	29	130
Cabbage, boiled	33	4	25
Carrots, boiled	24	3	17
Spinach, boiled	160	34	28
Apples, eating	4	5	11
Oranges	47	10	21
Mixed nuts	78	200	430
Miscellaneous			
Chocolate – milk	220	55	240
– plain	38	100	140
Baking powder	1130	9	8430
Marmite	95	180	1700

* Holland *et al* (1991; 1992)

Data/information from the *Composition of Foods and Supplements* is reproduced with the permission of the Royal Society of Chemistry and the Controller of HMSO

The dietary calcium:phosphorus ratio was formerly thought to be important in determining calcium absorption, but this is no longer thought to be the case in adults unless phosphate intake is excessive. However, it is still important in small infants and there is a recommendation (EEC 1991) for the calcium:phosphorus ratio to be 2.0 in milks for infant feeding.

High sodium intakes may decrease calcium retention (Shortt *et al* 1989).

Because of the large reservoir of calcium in bone, deficiency symptoms are rarely seen except as a result of a metabolic disorder (e.g. hypoparathyroidism, pancreatitis). There is no satisfactory biochemical method for assessing calcium status; serum levels of calcium do not reflect dietary adequacy, since these parameters are maintained at the expense of bone mineral. Newer measurements of bone density and total body calcium, such as photon absorptiometry and neutron activation analysis, are used only as research tools at present (Gibson 1990). Other disorders in which calcium deficiency may be implicated are discussed in Disorders of bone minerals later in this section.

Phosphorus

A review of phosphorus metabolism was published in 1988 (Berner and Shike 1988).

Phosphorus is present in all cells of the body and is closely linked to calcium and protein metabolism. The majority (85%) of the body phosphorus is in bone in the form of hydroxyapatite. The remaining 15% is a constituent of substances such as phospholipids and nucleic acids or is concerned with the release of oxygen and energy to the cells and the mediation of the intracellular effects of hormones. Phosphate excretion through the kidney is one of the mechanisms for regulating acid-base balance in the body.

Phosphorus shares similar homeostatic mechanisms with calcium (i.e. PTH, 1,25(OH)D). Calcium metabolism indirectly affects phosphorus by stimulating hormones such as 1,25(OH)D. Phosphate balance is maintained largely by the renal tubules.

Although phosphorus in the form of dairy food or cereals does not appear to affect calcium balance, some authors have noted that phosphorus in the form of food additives, such as phosphoric acid in carbonated drinks, may behave differently and increase bone resorption (Spencer and Kramer 1986).

Phosphorus and calcium exist in the body in equimolar amounts and requirements for phosphorus parallel those of calcium (Table 2.38).

Current UK intakes of phosphorus are shown in Table 2.39 and the phosphorus content of foods in Table 2.40.

Milk and dairy products are the richest sources of phosphorus in the UK, although meat, fish, egg, nuts, fruit, cereals and vegetables provide useful amounts. Inorganic phosphorus is added to processed foods, particularly baked goods and carbonated drinks, and intakes from these have risen to about 10% of the total phosphorus intake over the last 20 years.

Approximately 60% of the dietary intake of phosphorus is absorbed. A decrease in phosphate absorption has been described with increasing NSP intakes; however, high NSP diets are generally higher in phosphate, so the quantitative absorption is not reduced. Phytic acid phosphorus from wholegrain cereals and pulses is not absorbed in the small intestine because mammals do not produce phytase; however this enzyme is naturally present in some wholegrain cereals and renders the phosphorus more available. In addition, some absorption may take place in the large bowel following bacterial fermentation.

Serum phosphate is the usual method of determining phosphorus status; normal values vary with age and sex. High levels may be seen during bone remodelling after a fracture.

Although a dietary phosphorus deficiency is unlikely, phosphate depletion in blood and soft tissue may occur in any metabolic disorder where body pH is altered or where there is excessive loss of phosphate through urine or stools. Deficiencies have been described where there has been inadequate provision in intravenous regimens, in elderly persons receiving diuretic drugs, with excessive use of magnesium and aluminium antacids, in diabetic acidosis, alcoholism and malabsorption. Symptoms include myopathy, respiratory and cardiac failure, neuropathy and tissue hypoxia. Low birth weight infants require more phosphorus than is supplied by human milk, and a rachitic-like disease may develop if supplements are not given (Chan *et al* 1986).

Magnesium

A review of magnesium in health and disease was published in 1988 (Shils 1988).

Magnesium functions in many enzyme systems, including decarboxylation and those concerned with phosphate group transfer and energy release. It is also involved in protein synthesis and neuromuscular transmission. There appear to be no major hormonal factors controlling magnesium balance and homeostasis is largely controlled by the kidney.

Dietary Reference Values for magnesium (DoH 1991) are shown in Table 2.38, intake data for the UK are shown in Table 2.39 and the magnesium content of some foods in Table 2.40. Magnesium is a component of chlorophyll, so green vegetables are a rich source. Meats, pulses and cereals (particularly wholegrain) also provide useful amounts. Hard drinking water may make a significant contribution to intake.

About 20–30% of the dietary intake of magnesium is absorbed, mainly from the small intestine; absorption is an active process partly dependent on 1,25(OH)D. High

NSP diets have been described as inducing magnesium deficiency (Mills 1985) although other studies using cellulose or soluble gums were not able to reproduce this (Behall *et al* 1987). When a normal diet is eaten, any decrease in the percentage of magnesium absorbed is likely to be masked by an increase in dietary magnesium in the high NSP foods. Dietary deficiency of magnesium is unlikely. A number of disorders may cause depletion of body stores and these include alcohol abuse, protein-energy malnutrition, malabsorption, poorly controlled diabetes and diuretic therapy. The elderly sick have been described as having low serum and erythrocyte levels (Touitou *et al* 1987). Hypomagnesaemia results in hypocalcaemia, muscular weakness, neuromuscular dysfunction and cardiac muscle fibrillation.

Some 40% of the body magnesium is in the soft tissues; about 0.3% is present in the serum. Serum magnesium is the most commonly used parameter for assessing status, although serum levels may not accurately reflect those present in other tissues and normal values do not preclude deficiency. Serum magnesium concentrations vary with age and sex, exercise and protein status.

The concentrations of magnesium in erythrocytes and leukocytes have also been used as a measure of magnesium status and may be more representative of tissue values (Gibson 1990). Urinary magnesium excretion after a magnesium load is a useful test for magnesium depletion (Holm *et al* 1987).

Disorders of bone minerals

Osteoporosis

The incidence of osteoporosis in the UK and in other Western countries has doubled in the last 30 years. About 20% of orthopaedic beds in the UK are occupied by patients with a fractured neck of femur (Smith 1990), although there are signs that the rate of increase is slowing (Spector *et al* 1990). The incidence in elderly men also appears to have increased. The reasons for this increase are not clear but race, reproductive hormones, smoking, exercise and dietary intakes of protein, sodium, fluoride as well as calcium, phosphorus and magnesium may play a part. These factors are discussed in detail in Section 4.28, Osteoporosis.

The COMA Panel has suggested that, because the evidence relating to the place of high calcium intakes in the prevention of osteoporosis is equivocal and the risk of toxicity due to over-consumption is low, those considered to be at risk of developing osteoporosis may benefit from intakes higher than the DRV (DoH 1991).

The place of phosphorus is even less clear. Although an increased phosphorus intake has been shown to improve calcium balance (Munro *et al* 1987), diets in the UK contain more phosphorus than calcium so, unless there is an increased loss of phosphorus from the gut, phosphorus deficiency is unlikely to play a part. High intakes of inorganic phosphate in the form of food additives may increase calcium losses from bone.

The magnesium content of trabecular bone has been shown to be low in post-menopausal women (Cohen and Kitches 1982). The elderly are less able to mobilize magnesium from bone in response to low serum levels (Thomas 1984). However primary magnesium deficiency is unlikely to be a factor in the aetiology of osteoporosis.

Hypertension and coronary heart disease (CHD)

An inverse relationship between dietary calcium intake and the incidence of hypertension has been described, though some studies have disagreed with these findings (Karanja and McCarron 1986). Similar evidence has been provided for the implication of magnesium in hypertension (Altura and Altura 1985). The dietary Ca:Mg ratio may be more important than actual dietary intake, a reduced ratio with more Mg relative to Ca being advantageous (Wester and Dyckner 1987).

Decreased deaths from CHD have been described in hard water areas and this has been attributed to the higher mineral content of the water. However a large study in the UK produced negative results (Elwood *et al* 1980). At present there is no consensus on the place of calcium and magnesium in the aetiology of CHD.

References

Allen LH (1982) Calcium bioavailability and absorption: a review. *Am J Clin Nutr* **35**, 783–808.

Altura BM and Altura BT (1985) New perspectives on the role of magnesium in the pathophysiology of the cardiovascular system. I Clinical aspects. *Magnesium* **4**, 226–44.

Behall K, Scholfield B, Lee K, Powell A and Moser P (1987) Mineral balance in adult men: effect of four refined fibers. *Am J Clin Nutr* **46**, 307–14.

Berner YN and Shike M (1988) Consequences of phosphate imbalance. *Ann Rev Nutr* **8**, 121–48.

Bertino M, Beauchamp GK and Engleman K (1982) Long term reduction in dietary sodium alters taste of salt. *Am J Clin Nutr* **36**, 1113–44.

British Nutrition Foundation (1981) *Salt in the diet*. BNF Briefing Paper (2). BNF, London.

British Nutrition Foundation (1991) *Calcium*. BNF Briefing Paper (24). BNF, London.

Bull NL and Buss DH (1980a) Contributions of foods to sodium intakes. *Proc Nutr Soc* **39**, 30A.

Bull NL and Buss DH (1980b) Contributions of foods to potassium intakes. *Proc Nutr Soc* **39**, 31A.

Bullamore J, Gallagher J, Wilkinson R and Nordin B (1970) Effect of age on calcium absorption. *Lancet* **II**, 535–7.

Caggiula AW, Wing RR, Nowalk MP, Milas NC, Lee S and Langford H (1985) The measurement of sodium and potassium intake. *Am J Clin Nutr* **42**, 391–8.

Chan GM, Mileur L and Hansen JW (1986) Effects of increased calcium and phosphorus formulas and human milk on bone mineralisation in preterm infants. *J Paediatr Gastroenterol Nutr* **5**, 383–8.

Cohen L and Kitzes R (1982) Relationship of bone and plasma magnesium in magnesium deficient cirrhosis patients. *Isr J Med Sci* **18**, 679–82.

Department of Health (1991) Dietary Reference Values for food energy and nutrients for the United Kingdom. *Rep Hlth Soc Subj* No **41** HMSO, London.

EC Commission (1991) Directive on infant formulae and follow-up formulae (91/321/EEC). *Official Journal of the European Communities* **L/175** 35–49.

Elwood P, Sweetman P, Beasley W, Jones D and France R (1980) Magnesium and calcium in the myocardium: cause of death and area difference. *Lancet* **II**, 720–2.

Gibson RS (1990) *Principles of nutritional assessment.* Oxford University Press, Oxford.

Greenfield H, Smith AM, Maples J and Wills RBH (1984) Contributions of foods to sodium in the Australian food supply. *Hum Nutr: Appl Nutr* **38A**, 203–210.

Gregory J, Foster K, Tyler H and Wiseman M (1990) *The dietary and nutritional survey of British adults.* HMSO, London.

Holland B, Unwin ID and Buss DH (1991; 1992) *McCance and Widdowson's* The composition of foods *5e and Supplement 1. Fruit and nuts.* HMSO, London.

Holm CN, Jepsen JM, Sjogaard G and Hessov I (1987) A magnesium load test in the diagnosis of magnesium deficiency. *Human Nutr: Clin Nutr.* 41C, 301–306.

Karanja N and McCarron DA (1986) Calcium and hypertension. *Ann Rev Nutr* **6**, 475–94.

Kumanyika SK and Jones DY (1983) Patterns of week to week table salt use by men and women consuming constant diets. *Hum Nutr: Appl Nutr* **37A**, 348–56.

Lee HA (1974) Normal fluid and electrolyte requirements. In *Parenteral nutrition in acute metabolic illness* pp. 97–112. Academic Press, London and New York.

Mills CF (1985) Dietary interactions involving the trace elements. *Ann Rev Nutr* **5**, 173–93.

Munro HN, Suter PM and Russell RM (1987) Nutritional requirements of the elderly. *Ann Rev Nutr* **7**, 23–49.

Pangborn RM and Pecore SD (1982) Taste perception of sodium chloride in relation to dietary intake of salt. *Am J Clin Nutr* **35**, 510–20.

Sanchez-Castillo CP and James WPT (1984) Estimating dietary sources of sodium with lithium tagged salt. *Proc Nutr Soc* **43**, 154A.

Sanchez-Castillo CP, Warrender S, Whitehead T and James WP (1984) Epidemiological assessment of sodium sources in the diet by the use of the lithium-marker technique. *Proc Nutr Soc* **43**, 153A.

Shepherd RE, Farleigh CA and Land DG (1984) Effects of taste sensitivity and preference on salt intake. *Proc Nutr Soc* **43**, 87A.

Shils ME (1988) Magnesium in Health and Disease. *Ann Rev Nutr* **8**, 429–60.

Shortt C, Madded A, Flynn A and Morrissey P (1989) Influence of dietary sodium intakes on urinary calcium excretion in selected Irish individuals. *Europ J Clin Nutr* **42**, 595–604.

Smith R (Ed) (1990) *Osteoporosis*. Royal College of Physicians, London.

Spector TD, Cooper C and Fenton Lewis A (1990) Trends in admissions for hip fracture in England and Wales. *Brit Med J* **300**, 1173–4.

Spencer H and Kramer L (1986) NIH Consensus Conference: Osteoporosis. *J Nutr* **116**, 316–19.

Thomas AJ (1984) Magnesium. In *Clinical Biochemistry of the elderly* Ed. Hodkinson M. Churchill Livingstone, Edinburgh.

Touitou Y, Godard J-P, Ferment O *et al* (1987) Prevalence of magnesium and potassium deficiencies in the elderly. *Clin Chem* **33**(4), 518–23.

Wester P-O and Dyckner T (1987) Magnesium and hypertension. *J Amer Coll Nutr* **6**, 321–8.

Whitney EN and Boyle MA (1984) *Understanding nutrition* 3e. West Publishing Co, Minnesota.

2.8 Trace elements

2.8.1 General aspects

Definition

Twenty-six of the 90 naturally occurring elements are considered to be essential for animal life; eleven are classified as major elements and the remainder as trace elements. Of the fifteen trace elements, nine are known to be essential for humans and these are shown in Table 2.41. Fluoride is considered to be semi-essential. A further 6 elements are essential for some species of animals but not for man (Table 2.42). Trace elements were originally so described because early workers were unable to make precise measurements of the small quantities usually present in biological materials; concentrations are usually lower than 100 μg/100 g tissue. The sub classification of 'ultra trace elements' for substances present in concentrations of less than 0.01 μg/100 g tissue has not gained general acceptance. A trace element is generally regarded as one where the average daily requirement is 1 mg or less. Iron is usually classified as a major element, although requirements are small.

Functions and requirements

Trace elements usually form part of an enzyme system, functioning as a co-enzyme or catalyst. Their action may depend upon ionic effects or upon the formation of a metalloenzyme where the element is bound to the protein. Some trace elements function as part of a molecular structure rather than as part of an enzyme system. It has been suggested that some trace elements are involved in protection against free radicals, which have numerous implications in disease states (Diplock 1991).

Dietary Reference Values for trace elements are given in Tables 2.43 and 2.44. Requirements for patients receiving intravenous nutrition are much smaller and are given in Table 2.45.

Bioavailability

Absorption of trace elements is regulated at the mucosa of the small intestine and the mechanism appears to involve ion-specific low molecular weight proteins.

A number of factors affect the bioavailability of elements

Table 2.41 Trace elements essential for humans

Element	Molecular weight	Quantity in adult man	Adult daily intakes in the UK	Major dietary sources*
Chromium	1 μmol = 52 μg	<6 mg	13.6–47.7 μg[1]	Brewers' yeast, meat, cheese, wholegrain cereals, nuts, prunes mushrooms, wine, beer
Copper	1 μmol = 63.5 μg	70–80 mg	1.23–1.63 mg[2]	Liver, oysters, shellfish, nuts, chocolate, green vegetables, dried fruit
Iodine	1 μmol = 127 μg	15–20 mg	176–243 μg[2]	Milk, seafood, eggs vegetables
Iron	1 μmol = 55.9 μg	4.0 g	12.3–14.0 mg[2]	Liver, red meat, bread**, wholegrain cereals, pulses, chocolate
Manganese	1 μmol = 55 μg	12–20 mg	4.6–5.4 mg[3,6]	Tea, nuts, wholegrain cereals, dried fruit, vegetables
Molybdenum	1 μmol = 95.9 μg	0.7–7.0 mg	120–140 μg[5] (USA)	Cereals, legumes, leafy vegetables, milk, liver, kidney
Selenium	1 μmol = 79 μg	15 mg	25–129 μg[4]	Cereals, meat, seafood, nuts, mushrooms, garlic
Zinc	1 μmol = 65.4 μg	1.5–2.0 g	8.4–11.4 mg[2]	Oysters, seafood, meat, nuts, wholegrain cereals
Cobalt	Only essential as part of vitamin B_{12}			
Fluoride	No essential function apparent			

* The trace element content of vegetables may vary according to soil levels
** White bread is supplemented with additional iron in the UK

[1] Bunker *et al* (1984)
[2] Gregory *et al* (1990)
[3] Wenlock *et al* (1979)
[4] Bunker *et al* (1988a)
[5] Tsongas *et al* (1980)
[6] Bunker *et al* (1988b)

Table 2.42 Other trace elements

Essential for some species	No known function
Arsenic	Aluminium
Boron	Antimony
Bromine	Caesium
Cadmium	Germanium
Lead	Gold
Lithium	Mercury
Nickel	Silver
Silicon	Strontium
Tin	Titanium
Vanadium	

from the diet. These include interactions between ions themselves, or between ions and other dietary components such as dietary fibre. For some elements the valency state plays a key role in determining the mechanism of absorption and bioavailability. Generally trace elements are poorly absorbed from the diet and once absorbed are only excreted in very small quantities through the urine or bile, though a few (e.g. iodine) are readily absorbed and excreted in the urine.

Assessment of intake and status

In the plasma, trace elements are bound by specific proteins such as transferrin and caeruloplasmin, or by albumins and globulins, although some are transported in association

Table 2.43 Dietary Reference Values for trace elements (μmol/day) (DoH 1991)

Age	Copper		Iodine		Iron		Selenium		Zinc	
	LNRI	RNI	LNRI	RNI	LNRI	RNI	LNRI	RNI	LNRI	RNI
0–3 mnths	—	5	0.3	0.4	15	30	0.05	0.12	40	60
4–6 mnths	—	5	0.3	0.5	40	80	0.06	0.16	40	60
7–9 mnths	—	5	0.3	0.5	75	140	0.06	0.12	45	75
10–12 mnths	—	5	0.3	0.5	75	140	0.05	0.12	45	75
1–3 yrs	—	6	0.3	0.6	65	120	0.09	0.19	45	75
4–6 yrs	—	9	0.4	0.8	60	110	0.12	0.25	60	100
7–10 yrs	—	11	0.4	0.9	80	160	0.20	0.38	60	110
Males										
11–14 yrs	—	13	0.5	1.0	110	200	0.32	0.57	80	140
15–18 yrs	—	16	0.6	1.1	110	200	0.51	0.89	85	145
19–50 yrs	—	19	0.6	1.1	80	160	0.51	0.95	85	145
50+ yrs	—	19	0.6	1.1	80	160	0.51	0.95	85	145
Females										
11–14 yrs	—	13	0.5	1.0	140*	260	0.32	0.57	80	140
15–18 yrs	—	16	0.6	1.1	140*	260	0.51	0.76	60	110
19–50 yrs	—	19	0.6	1.1	140*	260	0.51	0.76	60	110
50+ years	—	19	0.6	1.1	80*	160	0.51	0.76	60	110
Pregnancy	—	19	0.6	1.1	*		0.51	0.76	60	110
Lactation										
0–4 mnths	—	24	0.6	1.1	*		0.70	0.95	60	200
4+ mnths	—	24	0.6	1.1	*		0.70	0.95	60	150

Factors for converting μmol to μg can be found in Table 2.41
LNR — Lower Reference Nutrient Intake
RNI — Reference Nutrient Intake
* See text

Table 2.44 Safe intakes for trace elements (per day) (DoH 1991)

Age	Chromium	Manganese	Molybdenum	Fluoride
Infants	*	0.3 μmol/kg/d	5–16 nmol/kg/d	3 μmol/kg/d
Children and Adolescents	2–20 μmol/kg/d	0.3 μmol/kg/d	5–16 nmol/kg/d	*
Adults	0.5 μmol/d	26 μmol/d	0.52–4.17 μmol/d	*

* No recommendation

Table 2.45 Recommended daily trace element intakes for parenteral nutrition

Element	ADULTS (1) umol/day	CHILDREN >10 kg per kg	max daily total[2]	INFANTS <10 kg per kg
Chromium	0.2	4 nmol[2]	96 nmol	4 nmol[2]
Copper	20	0.2 μmol[3]	4.7 μmol	0.375 μmol[3]
Iodine	1.0	8 nmol[2]	8 μmol	8 nmol[2]
Iron	20	1.0 μmol[3]	nr	2.5 μmol[2]
Manganese	5.0	18 nmol[2]	90 nmol	18 nmol[2]
Molybdenum	0.2	2.6 nmol[2]	52 nmol	2.6 nmol[2]
Selenium	0.4	25 nmol[2]	380 nmol	25 nmol[2]
Zinc	100	2.0 μmol[3]	76 μmol[2]	2.0 μmol[3]

[1] Shenkin (1986)
[2] Greene *et al* (1988)
[3] Booth and Shaw (1988)

with amino acids or small peptide complexes. Atomic absorption spectrophotometry is the most widely used method for the analysis of trace metals in biological samples. In order to obtain accurate results, careful precautions need to be taken to avoid contamination during the collection and preparation of samples for analysis. The methodology has developed rapidly in the last decade, but prior to 1980 many analyses are an overestimation due to low sensitivity of the method and sample contamination, and data from before this period should be viewed with caution (Gibson 1990).

Normal adult blood levels of trace elements are given in Table 2.46. Because of the low concentrations and small quantities involved the analysis of trace elements in food, the diagnosis of deficiency disorders and assessment of requirements is difficult.

Table 2.46 Normal adult biochemical values for trace elements (per litre) (Gibson 1990)

Element	Normal value per l plasma or serum	
Chromium	serum	2.5 nmol
Copper	serum plasma	19 μmol 17 μmol
Iodine	serum T3 serum T4	1.0–3.4 nmol 58–154 nmol
Manganese*	serum	5.9 nmol
Molybdenum*	serum	14.5 nmol
Selenium	serum plasma	0.9 μmol 0.8 μmol
Zinc	serum	0.14 μmol

* Versiek and Cornelius (1989)

Table 2.47 lists the trace element content of some foods. A number of factors will affect the trace element content of a food, including the soil in which vegetables are grown and animals grazed, seasonal variation and the species and maturity of the animal or plant. Processing will also have a major effect on trace metal content: it may be decreased where foods are refined, or increased by contamination from external sources during manufacture. Food tables do not yield an accurate indication of intake, but can be used in conjunction with information on local variations and foods that are rich or poor sources of a particular element. Disorders resulting from trace element deficiency are rare, and are usually seen only in patients on a grossly inadequate diet or who are receiving inadequate nutritional support.

Assessment of trace element status is usually biochemical and involves measurement of trace element content in body fluids such as blood or plasma, in other tissues such as hair or fingernails or a functional test examining the activity of trace element-dependent enzymes. More recently the use of stable isotopes has enabled the study of trace element homeostasis to advance (Turnlund 1989). The most useful body fluid in which to measure trace element status remains to be determined; plasma or whole blood may not accurately reflect body stores of an element such as zinc, where considerable stores are present in bone. In addition a large number of factors affect blood concentration including age, sex, time of day, posture, exercise, pregnancy and a number of disease states.

Analyses of hair, saliva and nails are subject to influence of cosmetics and shampoos and may not be an accurate reflection of internal status.

Other physiological or behavioural tests such as taste acuity in zinc depletion are subjective and open to misinterpretation.

Table 2.47 Essential trace element content of foods per 100 g

Food	Chromium µg[1]	Copper mg	Iodine µg	Iron mg	Manganese mg	Molybdenum µg[2]	Selenium µg	Zinc mg
Cereals								
Rice, boiled — white	0.6	0.06	5	0.20	0.3	10	4	0.7
— brown	1.0	0.33	N	0.50	0.9	N	tr	0.7
Spaghetti, boiled — white	1.0	0.10	tr	0.50	0.3	11	tr	0.5
— brown	N	0.18	N	1.40	0.9	N	N	1.1
Bread — white	0.3	0.19	6	1.60	0.5	21	28	0.6
— wholemeal	0.2	0.26	tr	2.70	1.9	N	35	1.8
All Bran	N	0.44	N	12.00	N	N	N	8.4
Cornflakes	0.7	0.03	10	6.70	0.1	N	2	0.3
Rice Krispies	0.5	0.10	N	6.70	1.0	N	N	1.1
Weetabix	N	0.54	N	6.00	N	N	N	2.0
Milk & dairy								
Cows' milk	1.0	tr	15	0.06	tr	5	1	0.4
Soya milk	N	0.06	N	0.40	0.1	N	N	0.2
Human milk, mature	0.03	0.04	7	0.07	tr	N	1	0.3
Infant formula	N	0.40	7	0.60	0.07	N	15*	0.4
Cheese, cheddar	1.0	0.03	39	0.30	tr	11	12	2.3
Whole egg, raw	0.5	0.08	53	1.90	tr	9	11	1.3
Butter (and margarine)	6.0	0.03	38	0.20	tr	<1	tr	0.1
Meat and fish								
Beef, roast	2.0	0.14	6	2.80	0.04	4	3	5.5
Lamb, roast	4.0	0.31	5	2.70	0.02	N	1	5.3
Pork, roast	4.0	0.29	3	1.3	0.04	4	14	3.5
Chicken, roast	4.0	0.12	5	0.8	0.03	5	7	1.5
Kidney, fried — lamb	2.0	0.65	N	12.0	0.13	70[3]	N	4.1
Liver, fried — lamb	1.0	8.70	5	9.4	0.32	150[3]	20	3.9
Cod, baked	1.0	0.07	110	0.4	0.01	N	34	0.5
Herring, grilled	N	0.11	32	1.0	0.05	N	41	0.5
Prawn, boiled	N	0.70	28	1.1	0.01	1	18	1.6
Vegetables and fruit								
Potato, boiled — old	0.5	0.07	3	0.4	0.10	7.0	1	0.3
Baked beans	N	0.04	3	1.4	0.30	N	2	0.5
Lentils, boiled — whole	N	0.33	N	3.5	0.50	N	40	1.4
Peas, boiled	1.0	0.03	2	1.5	0.40	130	1	1.0
Cabbage, boiled	0.5	0.01	2	0.3	0.20	6	2	0.1
Carrots, boiled	1.0	0.01	2	0.4	0.10	8[1]	1	0.1
Apple, eating	0.5	0.02	tr	0.1	tr	3	tr	0.1
Banana	3.0	0.10	8	0.3	0.4	8	1	0.2
Orange	1.0	0.05	2	0.1	tr	1	1	0.1
Sultanas	10.0	0.40	N	2.2	0.3	N	N	0.3
Mixed nuts	10.0	0.79	12	2.1	2.1	N	5	3.1
Miscellaneous								
Chilli powder	N	0.43	N	14.3	2.2	N	N	2.7
Curry powder	N	1.04	N	58.3	4.7	N	N	4.1
Chocolate — milk	6.0	0.30	N	1.6	0.5	N	4	0.2
— plain	N	0.7	N	2.4	0.5	N	2	0.2
Coffee, infusion	tr	tr	tr	tr	tr	N	tr	N
Tea, infusion	0.5	tr	tr	tr	0.14	N	tr	tr
Beer, bitter	0.9	0.08	8	0.01	tr	N	tr	0.05
Wine — red	1.0	0.12	N	0.9	0.1	2[1]	tr	0.05
— white	12.0	0.01	N	0.5	0.1	2[1]	tr	0.02

N no data available
* data from single manufacturer
Figures (except molybdenum and chromium) from Holland *et al* (1991; 1992)

[1] Koivistoinen *et al* (1980)
[2] Tsongas *et al* (1980)
[3] Schroeder *et al* (1970)

Data/information from the *Composition of Foods and Supplements* is reproduced with the permission of the Royal Society of Chemistry and the Controller of HMSO

2.8.2 Specific aspects

Chromium

A review of chromium in human nutrition was published in 1988 (Offenbacher and Pi-Sunyer 1988). The physiologically active form of chromium appears to be an organic molecule which may contain nicotinic acid and glutathione. This molecule appears to potentiate the action of insulin in cellular glucose uptake. It may also have a role in lipid and amino acid metabolism, in maintaining the structure of nucleic acids and in gene expression. Chromium does not appear to form part of any enzyme system.

There is little recent data on the chromium content of foods and published values are likely to be falsely high. Refined foods are generally low in chromium. Because of the paucity of reliable recent data on intakes and indices of chromium status it was not possible for the COMA Panel (DoH 1991) to make precise recommendations and a safe and adequate intake was suggested. Requirements may be affected by nutritional or physiological stress which alter glucose metabolism. Because chromium excretion is increased by exercise (Anderson *et al* 1982) and possibly by high sugar intakes (Schroeder *et al* 1970), requirements may be increased in physically active people and those who eat large quantities of refined sugar. It is recommended that chromium is added to long term intravenous feeding regimens, although it has been suggested that because of outside contamination of fluids this may not be necessary (Moukarzel *et al* 1991).

Chromium is usually present in food as trivalent chromium (Cr^{3+}) and the absorption of this is 0.5–2% of intake. Factors in the diet such as phytate decrease chromium absorption, but oxalate increases it (Chen *et al* 1973).

Chromium in serum exists mainly as Cr^{3+}, and is largely bound to transferrin which acts as a transport protein. The very low levels of chromium found in plasma, serum and urine make accurate measurement very difficult; some anticoagulants contaminate plasma samples. The usefulness of serum or plasma levels as an index of total body content of chromium is uncertain as tissue concentrations are much higher than blood levels.

Urine is the main excretory route for absorbed chromium; urinary chromium levels of 0.2–0.4 μg per day are considered to be normal (Anderson and Kozlovsky 1985). Improvement in glucose tolerance after supplementation with physiological doses of chromium can be used as an indicator of marginal chromium deficiency.

The essential role of chromium in human nutrition was first demonstrated in a patient receiving a chromium-free intravenous regime (Jeejeebhoy *et al* 1977). Other reports have described long term parenteral nutrition without adequate chromium leading to weight loss, glucose intolerance refractory to insulin and a peripheral neuropathy. Frank chromium deficiency has never been reported in humans except during parenteral nutrition. Marginal chromium deficiency has been described in malnourished children and in diabetics. In those patients with abnormal glucose tolerance tests, improvements were seen after chromium supplementation. There is a possible link between a long term marginally deficient chromium intake, type II diabetes and atherosclerosis (Schroeder 1974). It has been suggested that ageing in Western societies is accompanied by a gradual depletion in chromium body stores. The ability to convert Cr^{3+} to a biologically active form has been shown to be defective in elderly subjects with an impaired glucose tolerance (Mertz 1982).

Cobalt

The only known function of cobalt in man is as part of vitamin B12; as this cannot be synthesized in the human body, dietary intake of inorganic cobalt is only important because it impinges on the absorption of other trace metals.

Copper

Copper is a component of a number of oxidative enzymes; cytochrome c oxidase is active at the terminal end of the mitochondrial electron transport chain; uricase is involved in the renal and hepatic metabolism of uric acid; in connective tissue, amine oxidases contribute to the elasticity and tensile strength of elastin and collagen, particularly in blood vessels.

Caeruloplasmin is a copper-containing glycoprotein which appears to be important not only in copper transport but also as an enzyme (ferroxidase) in the control of free radicals, in defences against infection and in the intracellular oxidation of Fe^{2+} to Fe^{3+}.

There is very little data available on human requirements and the COMA Panel were not able to derive EARs or LNRIs. Table 2.43 shows the RNIs for copper (DoH 1991).

The full-term infant has relatively large copper stores and is not dependent on dietary intake for the first few weeks of life. Since homeostasis for copper is mainly achieved by adjustment of biliary excretion, requirements are increased if there is a jejunostomy or other loss of bile such as chronic diarrhoea. Care should be taken when administering copper to intravenously fed patients with impaired biliary excretion, since copper overload is likely to occur if intake is high (Greene *et al* 1988).

In addition to the food sources listed, the copper content of drinking water can be high if copper plumbing is used and can provide up to 0.8 mg (12 μmol) per day (Delves 1988). Milk and dairy products are poor sources of copper. Intakes are higher in vegetarians than in those consuming a mixed diet.

About 35–70% of dietary copper is absorbed; absorption seems to be lower in the elderly (Bunker *et al* 1988b). Soluble phytate in the diet may affect availability but other fibres seem to have little effect on absorption. Copper absorption is inhibited by large excesses of dietary zinc, iron and calcium and may be increased by protein (Forbes and Erdman 1983).

Most of the circulating copper is bound to caeruloplasmin; a small amount is associated with albumin. Serum copper levels are useful to detect frank deficiency but are not a sensitive indicator of poor status generally. Levels may vary according to age, sex and recent exercise experience. They are elevated in pregnancy and in a number of clinical conditions. Caeruloplasmin levels suffer similar drawbacks and are also affected by factors which affect plasma protein concentrations. In mild deficiency states, a rise in serum caeruloplasmin levels occur after a few days of supplementation with physiological (1 – 2 mg) quantities of copper and this can be used as an indicator of status. Urine copper levels are too low to be of value in assessing possible deficiency. Although hair changes are a feature of copper deficiency, hair copper levels do not appear to correlate with blood values (Gibson 1990).

Copper deficiency produces a wide variety of clinical and metabolic defects. The processes which are most sensitive to deficiency are those concerned with melanin pigment formation, particularly in the hair, and hair changes usually accompany depletion. Copper deficiency during pregnancy has severe effects on early fetal development and survival. Later manifestations of deficiency include defects in elastin formation, myelin and noradrenaline synthesis, myocardial lesions and coronary artery aneurysms. In childhood, copper deficiency results in poor growth and delay in sexual maturation.

Low copper intakes have been associated with raised cholesterol levels and altered lipid metabolism, although the significance of this is not certain (Fischer *et al* 1980). Anaemia is a late consequence of copper deficiency and is difficult to separate from iron deficiency anaemia. Low copper levels have been described in premature infants, infants fed on unsupplemented cows milk, in kwashiorkor and a number of malabsorptive states (Danks 1988), and in patients on parenteral nutrition (Fujita *et al* 1989).

Fluoride

Fluorine forms calcium fluorapatite in tooth and bone. It assists remineralization of bone in pathological demineralizing conditions; the presence of 1 mg/kg (1 ppm) in drinking water protects against tooth decay in children (Schamschula and Barmes 1981). However an intake of 0.1 mg/kg body weight in children has been associated with tooth enamel changes indicative of mild fluorosis (Leverett 1982).

The major source of fluoride in most diets is water which provided 1.3 mg/day in British adolescents; 0.6 mg from fluoridated drinking water (Rugg-Gunn *et al* 1987). Tea and some mineral waters provide appreciable amounts (Meunier *et al* 1989). Most plant foods are low. Mechanically deboned meat products (sausages, burgers etc. and particularly chicken), fish canned with bones and gelatin products are all high in fluorine. The quantity of fluorine ingested from toothpastes and mouthwashes is not known, and it has been suggested that young children should be discouraged from swallowing large quantities of fluoridated toothpastes because of the danger of fluorosis (Murray 1986).

The declining prevalence of dental caries in non-fluoridated areas may reflect increased amounts of fluoride in the food chain, including fluoridated water used by manufacturers (Subba Rao 1984).

There is insufficient evidence to suggest that fluoride is an essential element. However its beneficial effects on dental caries means that it is important that children are exposed to fluoride. The COMA Panel endorsed the recommendation that water supplies are fluoridated at a level of 1 ppm (DoH 1991). For children on long term nutritional support the fluorine content of the feed used should be checked; there is no requirement to add it to enteral feeds and levels will be low if deionized water is used during preparation. Where the diet necessarily contains a high quantity of simple sugars (high energy density regimens or some therapeutic diets) fluorine should be supplemented from the age of six months. For children with delayed oro-motor development it may be beneficial for topical fluoride to be applied.

Fluoride is rapidly and efficiently absorbed from the gut; unbound fluoride in water is more bioavailable than protein-bound forms, such as in milk. Excretion of fluorine is mainly by the kidney. A deficiency of fluorine has never been demonstrated in man, hence it is not considered to be an essential element.

Fluoride increases osteoblast and osteoclast activity and has been used in the treatment of osteoporosis. However, large doses impair bone mineralization and lead to osteomalacia; fluoride therefore needs to be given with a calcium supplement to prevent this. There is also a suggestion that a lower incidence of cardiovascular disease is found in areas with a high water fluoride level (Schamschula and Barmes 1981).

Iodine

Iodine functions as part of the thyroid hormones thyroxine (T^4) and triiodothyronine (T^3). These are necessary for the maintenance of metabolic processes, thermoregulation, protein synthesis and the integrity of connective tissue. In the fetus and the neonate, protein synthesis in the brain and central nervous system is dependent on iodine or an iodine-containing compound.

There is little data on iodine intakes in populations and the COMA Panel were unable to derive an EAR (DoH 1991). For patients on short term intravenous nutrition it may not be necessary to add iodine as sufficient may be absorbed through the skin from topical applications, although a recommendation is made for long term nutritional support (Greene *et al* 1988).

Seawater is rich in iodine (5 mg/l) and seafoods are good sources. Iodine in drinking water is low (1–5 μg/litre) in the UK. In Western countries, milk is the major source and the iodine content of milk has risen in recent years due to use of iodine supplemented animal feedstuffs and contamination from iodophors as sterilizing agents. Vegetables are low in iodine, although the levels depend on soil content. In some countries, all table salt is fortified with iodine.

Large areas of the world have low iodine intakes due to low soil levels. This is most commonly seen in isolated inland mountainous regions and iodine deficiency is common in these areas (Hetzel and Dunn 1989). In areas of the UK which had a previously low iodine intake, some of the older members of the population have become sensitive to high iodine intakes and have developed autoimmune thyroid disease (Braverman 1987).

The element is readily absorbed from the gut as inorganic iodide. Excretion is via the urine. Some minerals such as calcium, fluoride, magnesium and manganese which may be present in hard water make iodine less available from the gut.

A number of foods such as turnips, cabbage, cassava, millet, maize, bamboo shoots, lima beans and sweet potato contain goitrogens (mainly thiocyanates) which interfere with iodine metabolism. These substances are usually destroyed in cooking and, although goitrogens are a problem in areas where cassava is a staple, they are rarely important in Western countries unless large quantities of uncooked brassicas are eaten as part of a low iodine diet (Hetzel and Dunn 1989).

Urinary iodine excretion closely matches intake since urine is the major route for excretion. A 24-hour urinary iodine measurement is useful in the assessment of iodine deficiency. Concentrations of serum T^3 and T^4 are also routinely used and a low T^4 with normal or raised T^3 level is indicative of iodine deficiency. Thyroid function can be measured by determining the uptake of radioactive iodine by the thyroid gland (Gibson 1990).

Iodine deficiency disorders constitute a major public health problem in many areas of the world with an estimated 800 million people at risk. Prior to the middle of this century iodine deficiency was common in some central areas of the UK, but the disorder is now rare in Europe.

Deficiency in adults causes a fall in the blood level of T^4 which in turn stimulates thyroid stimulating hormone (TSH). TSH causes hyperplasia of the thyroid gland and the development of a goitre. Decreased fertility has been reported in women in deficient areas; there is also an increase in the rate of stillbirths, spontaneous abortions, perinatal deaths and congenital abnormalities. Iodine is essential for neonatal brain development and mental retardation is common in iodine deficient regions; endemic cretinism, prevalent in very low iodine areas, is characterized by mental deficiency, hypothyroidism and dwarfism (Hetzel and Dunn 1989).

Iron

A review of iron metabolism with particular reference to children was published in 1989 (Aggett and Wharton 1989).

The major role of iron is as an oxygen carrier in haemoglobin and myoglobin and as part of the cytochrome system involved in electron transfer. Haem-containing enzymes include catalase and peroxidases (peroxide and superoxide metabolism); non-haem iron containing proteins include flavoproteins and prolyl hyroxylase (nucleotide and collagen synthesis); in addition iron acts as a cofactor for enzymes in the citric acid cycle and amino acid metabolism. Iron is stored as ferritin or haemosiderin predominantly in the liver, spleen and bone marrow. It is transported to receptors on cell membranes by the plasma protein transferrin.

Homeostasis is maintained by regulating absorption. Some iron is excreted via bile; very little is lost via the urine, skin or sweat. Menstrual losses are variable and usually range from 13–56 ml per month but may be as high as 118 ml (Cole *et al* 1971). In women with high menstrual losses it may not be possible to meet requirements from the diet and iron supplements will be necessary. During pregnancy (providing iron stores are adequate) and during lactation increased iron needs may be offset by amenorrhoea. Dietary requirement depends upon the bioavailability of iron from the diet. An adult male needs to absorb approximately 0.9 mg daily to remain in balance.

Iron absorption is low and bioavailability is affected by many dietary factors. Breast fed infants absorb about 50% of the iron in breast milk, but absorption from milk formulae is only about 10% (Flanagan 1989). Approximately 20–40% of haem iron is available; iron from vegetable sources, egg and milk is about 5–20% available. For adults eating a mixed diet including meat and fish, absorption is assumed to be about 15%. Those eating a vegetarian diet may have higher dietary requirements. Dietary factors acting as enhancers or inhibitors of iron absorption are given in Table 2.48. Iron is absorbed as part of a meal and in a mixed diet there are a large number of

Table 2.48 Dietary factors affecting iron absorption

Enhancers	Inhibitors
Tissue protein – meat and fish	Vegetable polyphenols – spinach
Organic acids – ascorbic acid	Tannins – tea, coffee
Amino acids – cysteine, lysine, histidine	Vegetable proteins – soy protein
	Oxalate – chocolate
Peptides – glutathione	NSP – phytate
Sugars – fructose	Metals – zinc, manganese
Alcohol	

complex factors interacting together. One of the most potent enhancers, particularly of low-bioavailable or non-haem iron is ascorbic acid eaten at the same meal as the iron (Monsen 1988).

Different pathways exist for the absorption of haem and non-haem iron although the exact mechanism is not known. Absorption is increased by low iron stores and in response to increased erythropoeisis; intestinal factors such as pH and motility will also affect absorption.

Parameters for the diagnosis of iron deficiency have been suggested and are shown in Table 2.49. Serum ferritin provides a useful indicator of iron stores; levels decrease with reduction of stores. Reduced ferritin levels are the earliest sign of iron depletion (Johnson 1990), although levels of transport iron and haemoglobin may be normal. Serum ferritin levels rise during infection and liver disease and vary during pregnancy. Decreased serum levels of transferrin and iron and increased total iron-binding capacity (TIBC) indicate a decrease in iron availability for erythropoiesis and iron-dependent reactions. Transferrin saturation (the ratio of serum iron to TIBC) is decreased in iron deficiency. Erythrocyte protoporphyrin (a precursor of haem) levels rise at this stage of deficiency. The third stage of iron deficiency is microcytic hypochromic anaemia as haemoglobin production falls and levels decrease. The haematocrit, mean corpuscular volume (MCV), mean cell haemoglobin concentration (MCHC) and mean cell haemoglobin (MCH) are all decreased in iron deficiency anaemia.

Iron deficiency is the most common nutritional deficiency in the world (Expert Scientific Working Group 1985). Sectors of the population most affected are pregnant women, infants and pre-school age children (Dallman *et al* 1980). In children, deficiency is particularly associated with the use of cows' milk as a main drink before the age of one year, and it is common in Asian families where weaning is delayed (Ederhardt 1986).

Systems affected by iron deprivation include heart, skeletal muscle, liver and gastrointestinal system. Iron deprivation can affect brain function, psychomotor development and mood. Low iron intakes have also been linked to an increased incidence of cancer and infections (Dallman *et al* 1980).

Manganese

Manganese functions as a structural element in bone and cartilage; a large number of enzymes include manganese as part of the molecule or as a cofactor, including glycosyl transferases (glycoprotein synthesis), pyruvate carboxylase (carbohydrate synthesis) and superoxide dismutase (protection from free radical damage).

There is limited data available on body composition, manganese turnover and metabolism. For this reason in

Table 2.49 Indicators of iron status (Adapted from Gibson 1990)

Index	Normal adult value	Iron depletion	Iron deficiency	Iron deficiency anaemia
Haemoglobin g/l	*Males* 150 *Females* 140	Normal	Normal	Low *Males* <130 *Females* <120
Haematocrit %	*Males* 47 *Females* 41	Normal	Normal	Low *Males* <41 *Females* <36
Mean corpuscular volume (fl)	90	Normal	Normal	Low <80
Serum iron μmol/l	20	Normal	Low <10	<7
Transferrin saturation %	35	Normal	Low <15	<15
Erythrocyte protoporphyrin μmol/l RBC	*Males* 0.8 *Females* 0.9	Raised >1.0	>1.24	>1.47
Total iron-binding capacity μmol/l	60	Raised >64	>70	>74
Serum ferritin μg/l	*Males* 100 *Females* 50	Low <12	<12	<12

the UK the COMA Panel were unable to make precise recommendations (DoH 1991). Since deficiencies have never been described in free-living populations, current ranges of intake are presumed to meet requirements. The Panel have suggested safe intakes (Table 2.44). Because of analytical difficulties, few studies of intakes have been carried out. In the UK, approximately 50% of the manganese intake is derived from tea.

Absorption from the diet is normally about 5%. Excretion appears to be mainly via the bile. Little is known about the absorption of manganese or the factors which affect it, although it appears to increase in iron deficiency (Valberg and Flanagan 1983). There are conflicting views on the effect of dietary fibre on manganese absorption: natural fibre as part of a mixed diet appears to have little or no effect on absorption (Lawson *et al* 1987), whilst purified fibre preparations may increase absorption (Behall *et al* 1987). Other studies have shown reduced absorption in vegetarians consuming a high fibre diet (Kelsay *et al* 1988).

Measurement of manganese in plasma and blood is difficult as levels are close to the detection limits of most currently available techniques. It is also a common contaminant introduced during blood collection.

Much of the cofactor activity of manganese can be replaced by other divalent cations. Possible manganese deficiency in a human subject fed on a purified experimental diet was characterized by weight loss, slow hair growth, dermatitis, low plasma levels of cholesterol, phospholipids and triglycerides (Doisy 1972). Low plasma manganese levels have been found in children and adults with convulsive disorders (Papavasiliou *et al* 1979) although the significance of this is not clear.

Molybdenum

A review of molybdenum metabolism was published in 1988 (Rajagopolan 1988).

Molybdenum is part of three enzyme systems, xanthine oxidase, aldehyde oxidase and sulphite oxidase, all of which are involved in oxidation-reduction reactions and which may also be involved with detoxification processes in the liver. Molybdenum appears to be particularly important in the early stages of brain development.

There have been few studies of intakes (food levels are affected by local soil concentration); requirements and deficiency in free-living humans have never been clearly documented. The COMA Panel was unable to set a RNI; safe intakes are given in Table 2.44 (DoH 1991). About 50–70% dietary molybdenum appears to be absorbed from most diets. The addition of molybdenum to parenteral nutrition solutions is recommended only if treatment is prolonged (Greene *et al* 1988).

There appears to be wide variation in molybdenum levels in plasma between high and low molybdenum areas. However few surveys have been carried out on whole blood or serum molybdenum levels in normal populations and there are no generally accepted parameters for diagnosing molybdenum deficiency.

Deficiency of molybdenum in animals causes neuropathology due to inability to oxidize sulphite to sulphate, resulting in low levels of available sulphate for DNA synthesis.

A report of molybdenum deficiency in a patient receiving parenteral nutrition described general symptoms and biochemical abnormalities including raised plasma methionine and low serum uric acid levels which responded to molybdenum supplementation (Abumrad *et al* 1981). There is some epidemiological evidence linking molybdenum deficiency with oesophageal cancer in some areas (Nielsen 1988).

Selenium

Two useful reviews of selenium nutrition have been published (Neve *et al* 1985; Levander 1987). Selenium forms part of the peroxide-destroying enzyme glutathione peroxidase, which protects tissues from oxidative breakdown. It is also thought to have a role as modifier of enzymes involved in the metabolism of cancer-promoting and chemotherapeutic agents. A link between selenium deficient diets and cancer has been postulated. There is considerable interaction between selenium and vitamin E in the body and the effects of selenium deficiency may be decreased by high doses of vitamin E.

In the absence of data, the RNI for selenium has been set at the current daily intake in the UK, which is sufficient for the population; these values may be higher than true requirements. Adaptive changes in selenium metabolism occur during pregnancy, so extra selenium appears not to be necessary, although there is a higher requirement during lactation. There appears to be no need to add selenium for short term parenteral regimens, but it should be added if treatment lasts for more than 10–14 days. Care should be taken in supplementing selenium where there is renal insufficiency, since the kidney is the major route of excretion. The margin between selenium requirements and toxicity is narrower than for many trace elements and it should not be over supplemented.

Selenium is widely distributed in the environment but consumption by humans depends upon its concentration in soils and availability. High protein foods generally contain the greatest amounts of selenium. Absorption from food is high: 85–100% is available from brewers yeast; 20–50% is absorbed from animal foods (Forbes and Erdman 1983).

The best index of selenium status is not clear. Selenium concentrations in plasma or serum are sensitive to short term changes in intake; whole blood values are more indicative of long term status. Twenty-four hour urinary excretion is an indication of the dietary intake and low concentrations can indicate deficiency. Glutathione peroxidase activity in erythrocytes, plasma or whole blood is a fairly insensitive measure of deficiency; it is difficult to use these to compare populations since there is no standard method for measurement.

Two selenium deficiency disorders have been described: in parts of China where soil selenium levels are very low Keshan disease, a fatal congestive cardiomyopathy mainly affecting young women and children, is widespread. Kashin-Beck disease, an endemic polyarticular degenerative joint disease occurring in the Far East is also thought to be a result of selenium deficiency. There is some epidemiological evidence in support of the role of low selenium status in pathogenesis of cardiovascular disease and cancers. Muscle pain and tenderness after use of parenteral nutrition solutions devoid of selenium (Van Rij *et al* 1979), and a fatal congestive cardiomyopathy after prolonged parenteral feeding (Fleming *et al* 1982) have been described.

Pre-term infants have low selenium stores and may be prone to deficiency, although their requirement is not precisely known. Children receiving artificial therapeutic diets for inborn errors of metabolism have been shown to have a lower selenium status than controls (Lloyd *et al* 1989).

Zinc

Zinc is a component of more than 70 mammalian enzymes. It participates in carbohydrate, lipid, protein and nucleic acid synthesis and degradation. Zinc also appears to play a structural role in maintaining the stability of presecretory insulin granules and the configuration of gene transcription proteins.

The recommendations of the COMA Panel are given in Table 2.43 (DoH 1991). Additional zinc appears to be necessary during pregnancy and lactation although some intestinal adaptation may take place in response to increased needs and a greater proportion of dietary zinc may be absorbed. Requirements are likely to be increased during severe stress such as injury or surgery due to increased urinary losses.

The amount of dietary zinc absorbed appears to range from 14–41%, and a number of factors are thought to affect bioavailability. Zinc in foods of plant origin is generally less available than that from animal sources. The ratio of phytate: zinc in diets has been shown to affect bioavailability (Oberleas and Harland 1981). The presence of high calcium concentrations further depresses absorption. Dietary iron competes with zinc and high iron concentrations in the gut will also decrease availability (Forbes and Erdman 1983).

Muscle, bone, skin and hair contain 90% of the body zinc content. The plasma zinc pool comprises less than 1% of the total body content; about 80% of plasma zinc is associated with albumin. Serum or plasma zinc is the most commonly used index of status, although factors other than nutrition affect levels. Zinc levels fall during infection, stress and myocardial infarction. Chronic disease in which the plasma albumin alters will affect zinc levels. Leucocyte zinc levels have been suggested as a better index of status than plasma, as it reflects body tissue more closely, although there are technical problems which compromise its usefulness. Diminished taste acuity has been reported in zinc deficiency and has been used as a functional index of zinc status, but this is a somewhat subjective assessment and is only suitable for co-operative subjects.

A full review of zinc deficiency disorders is given by Prasad (1985).

Zinc deficiency was first described in humans in the Middle East; features included growth stunting, hypogonadism, anorexia and cognitive dysfunction. Delayed wound healing has been reported to respond to zinc supplementation; zinc deficiency has been implicated in the aetiology of Alzheimer's disease (Burnett 1981) and in type II diabetes. Impairment of the immune response also appears to be related to zinc deficiency. Zinc deficiency has also been noted in patients on parenteral nutrition, in gastrointestinal disorders, cystic fibrosis, sickle cell disease, burns, renal and hepatic disease and alcoholism. Groups who may be at risk of marginal or sub clinical zinc deficiency (characterized by slow growth, anorexia and decreased taste acuity) are infants and children (Gibson *et al* 1990), pregnant women and the elderly.

References

Aggett PJ and Wharton B (Eds) (1989) Iron nutrition in childhood. *Acta Paed Scand* Suppl **361**, 1–112.

Abumrad NN, Schneider AJ, Steel D and Rogers LS (1981) Amino acid intolerance during prolonged total parenteral nutrition reversed by molybdate therapy. *Am J Clin Nutr* **34**, 2551–9.

Anderson RA, Polansky MM, Bryden NA, Roginsky EE, Patterson KY and Deamer DC (1982) Effect of exercise on serum glucose, insulin, glucagon and chromium excretion. *Diabetes* **31**, 213–16.

Anderson RA and Kozlovsky AS (1985) Chromium intake, absorption and excretion of subjects consuming self-selected diets. *Am J Clin Nutr* **41**, 1177–83.

Behall KM, Schofield BS, Lee K, Powell AS and Moser MB (1987) Mineral balance in adult men: effect of four fibers. *Amer J Clin Nutr* **46**, 307–314.

Booth IW and Shaw V (1988) Parenteral Nutrition. In *Harries Paediatric Gastroenterology and Nutrition* 2e. Milla PJ, Muller DP (Eds) pp. 558–83. Churchill Livingstone, Edinburgh.

Braverman LE (1987) Iodine excess and thyroid function. In *Dietary iodine and other aetiological factors in Hyperthyroidism*. Conference Report MRC Environmental Epidemiology Unit. (MRC Scientific Report No 9) pp. 29–37.

Bunker VW, Lawson MS, Delves HT and Clayton BE (1984) The uptake and excretion of chromium by the elderly. *Amer J Clin Nutr* **39**, 797–802.

Bunker VW, Lawson MS, Stansfield MF and Clayton BE (1988a) Selenium balance studies in apparently healthy and housebound people eating self-selected diets. *Brit J Nutr* **59**, 171–80.

Bunker VW, Lawson MS, Stansfield MF and Clayton BE (1988b) Trace element nutrition in the elderly – a review of zinc, copper, manganese and chromium. *Internat Clin Nutr Rev* **8**, 111–27.

Burnett FM (1981) A possible role of zinc in the pathology of dementia. *Lancet* **I**, 186–8.

Chen NS, Tsai A and Dyer IA (1973) Effect of chelating agents on chromium absorption in rats. *Brit J Nutr* **103**, 1182–6.

Cole SK, Billewicz WZ and Thomson AM (1971) Sources of variation in menstrual blood loss. *J Obstet Gynaecol Brit Commonwealth* **78**, 933–9.

Dallman PR, Siimes MA and Stekel A (1980) Iron deficiency in infancy and childhood. *Am J Clin Nutr* **33**, 1354–8.

Danks DM (1988) Copper deficiency in humans. *Ann Rev Nutr* **8**, 235–57.

Delves HT (1988) Dietary sources of copper. *Ciba Foundation Symposium 79. The biological roles of copper*. pp. 5–22.

Department of Health (1991) *Dietary Reference Values for food energy and nutrients for the United Kingdom*. Rep Hlth Soc Subj **41** HMSO, London.

Diplock AT (1991) Antioxidant nutrients and disease prevention: an overview. *Am J Clin Nutr* **53**(Suppl 1), 189s–193s.

Doisy EA (1972) Micronutrient controls on biosynthesis of clotting proteins and cholesterol. In *Trace substances in environmental health* Vol VI, Hemphill DD (Ed) pp. 193–9. University of Missouri Press, Columbia.

Ederhardt P (1986) Iron deficiency in young Bradford children from different ethnic groups. *Brit Med J* **292**, 90–93.

Expert Scientific Working Group (1985) Summary of a report on assessment of the iron nutritional status of the United States population. *Am J Clin Nutr* **42**, 1318–30.

Fischer PW, Giroux A, Belonje B and Shah BG (1980) The effect of dietary copper and zinc on cholesterol metabolism. *Am J Clin Nutr* **33**, 1019–25.

Flanagan PR (1989) Mechanisms and regulation of intestinal uptake and transfer of iron. *Acta Paed Scand* **361**(Suppl), 21–30.

Fleming CR, Lie JT and McCall JT (1982) Selenium deficiency and fatal cardiomyopathy in a patient on home parenteral nutrition. *Gastroenterology*. **83** 682–93.

Forbes RM and Erdman JW (1983) Bioavailability of trace mineral elements. *Ann Rev Nutr* **3**, 213–31.

Fujita M, Itakura T, Tagaki Y and Okada A (1989) Copper deficiency during total parenteral nutrition: clinical analysis of three cases. *J Parent Ent Nutr* **13**, 421–5.

Gibson RS (1990) *Principles of Nutritional Assessment*. Oxford University Press. New York, Oxford.

Greene HL, Hambidge KM, Schanler R and Tsang RC (1988) Guidelines for the use of vitamins, trace elements, calcium, magnesium, and phosphorus in infants and children receiving total parenteral nutrition. *Am J Clin Nutr* **48**, 1324–42.

Gregory J, Foster K, Tyler H and Wiseman M (1990) *The dietary and nutritional survey of British adults*. HMSO, London.

Hetzel BS and Dunn JT (1989) Iodine deficiency disorders. *Ann Rev Nutr* **9**, 21–108.

Holland B, Unwin ID, Buss DH (1991/1992) *McCance and Widdowson's The Composition of Foods* 5e and supplement 1. *Fruit and nuts*. HMSO, London.

Hurley LS (1982) Clinical and experimental aspects of manganese in nutrition. In *Clinical, Biochemical and Nutritional aspects of trace elements*. Prasad AS (Ed) pp. 369–78. AR Liss Inc, New York.

Jeejeebhoy KN, Chu RC, Marliss EB, Greenbury GR and Bruce-Robertson A (1977) Chromium deficiency, glucose intolerance and neuropathy reversed by chromium supplements in a patient on long-term parenteral nutrition. *Am J Clin Nutr* **30**, 531–8.

Johnson MA (1990) Iron: nutrition monitoring and nutrition status assessment. *J Nutr* **120**, 1486–91.

Kelsay JL, Frazier CW, Prather ES, Canary JJ, Clark WM and Powell BS (1988) Impact of variation in carbohydrate intakes on mineral utilisation by vegetarians. *Am J Clin Nutr* **48**, 875–9.

Koivistoinen P (Ed) (1980) Mineral content of Finnish foods. *Acta Agric Scand* **22**(Suppl).

Kumpulainen J, Vuori E, Makinen S and Kara R (1980) Dietary chromium intake of lactating Finnish mothers: effects on the Cr content of their breast milk. *Brit J Nutr* **4**, 257–63.

Lawson MS, Bunker VW and Clayton BE (1987) The effect of dietary fibre on apparent absorption of zinc, copper, iron and manganese in the elderly. *Proc Nut Soc* **46**, 53A.

Levander OA (1987) A global view of human selenium nutrition. *Ann Rev Nutr* **7**, 227–50.

Leverett DH (1982) Fluorides and the changing prevalence of dental caries. *Science* **217**, 26–30.

Lloyd B, Robson E, Smith I and Clayton BE (1989) Blood selenium concentrations and glutathione activity. *Arch Dis Childh* **64**, 352–6.

Mertz W (1982) The clinical and public health significance of chromium. In *Clinical, biochemical and nutritional aspects of trace elements*. Prasad A (Ed) pp. 315–23. AR Liss Inc, New York.

Meunier PJ, Femenias M, Diboeuf F, Chapuy MC and Delmas PD (1989) Increased vertebral bone density in heavy drinkers of mineral water rich in fluoride. *Lancet* **I**, 152.

Monsen ER (1988) Iron nutrition and absorption: dietary factors which impact iron bioavailability. *J Am Diet Assoc* **88**, 786–90.

Moukarzel A, Vargas J, Buchman A and Ament ME (1991) Chromium requirements of patients on long term parenteral nutrition are not the recommended chromium intake. *Amer J Clin Nutr* **53**(Suppl), 25.

Murray JJ (Ed) (1986) *Appropriate use of fluorides for human health*. WHO, Geneva.

Neve J, Vertongen F and Molle L (1985) Selenium deficiency. *Clin Endoc Metab* **14**, 629–56.

Nielsen FH (1988) Nutritional significance of the ultratrace elements. *Nutr Rev* **46**, 337–42.

Oberleas D and Harland B (1981) Phytate content of foods: effect on dietary zinc bioavailability. *J Amer Dietet Assoc* **79**, 433–7.

Offenbacher EG and Pi-Sunyer FX (1988) Chromium in human nutrition. *Ann Rev Nutr* **8**, 543–63.

Papavasiliou PS, Kutt H, Miller ST, Rosal V, Wang YY and Aronson RB (1979) Seizure disorders and trace metals. *Neurology* **29**, 1466–73.

Prasad AS (1985) Clinical, endocrinological and biochemical effects of zinc deficiency. *Clin Endoc Metab* **14**, 567–89.

Rajagopolan KV (1988) Molybdenum: an essential trace element in human nutrition. *Ann Rev Nutr* **8**, 410–27.

Rugg-Gunn AJ, Hackett AF, Appleton DR, Easoe JE, Dowthwaite L and Wright WG (1987) The water intake of 405 Northumbrian adolescents aged 12–14 years. *Brit Dent J* **162**, 335–40.

Schamschula RG and Barmes WD (1981) Fluoride and health: dental caries, osteoporosis and cardiovascular disease. *Ann Rev Nutr* **1**, 427–35.

Schroeder HA, Nason AP and Tipton HI (1970) Chromium deficiency as a factor in atherosclerosis. *J Chron Dis* **23**, 123–42.

Schroeder HA (1974) The role of trace elements in cardiovascular disease. *Med Clin North Amer* **58**, 381–96.

Shenkin A (1986) Vitamin and essential trace element recommendations during intravenous nutrition: theory and practice. *Proc Nut Soc* **45**, 383–90.

Subba Rao G (1984) Dietary intake and bioavailability of fluoride. *Ann Rev Nutr* **4**, 115–35.

Tsongas TA, Meglen RR, Walravens PA and Chappel WR (1980) Molybdenum in the diet: an estimate of average daily intakes in the United States. *Amer J Clin Nutr* **33**, 1103–107.

Turnlund J (1989) The use of stable isotopes in mineral nutrition research. *J Nutr* **119**, 7–14.

Valberg LS and Flanagan PR (1983) Intestinal absorption of iron and chemically related compounds. In *Biological aspects of metals and metal-related diseases*. Sakar B (Ed) pp. 41–66. Raven Press, New York.

Van Rij AM, Thomson CD, McKenzie JM and Robinson MF (1979) Selenium deficiency in total parenteral nutrition. *Amer J Clin Nutr* **32**, 2076–85.

Versiek J and Cornelius R (1989) *Trace elements in human plasma or serum*. CRC Press Inc, Florida.

Wenlock RW, Buss DH and Dixon EJ (1979) Trace nutrients 2. Manganese in British diets. *Brit J Nutr* **41**, 253–61.

2.9 Fluid

In adults water comprises 50−70% of total body weight. The percentage varies according to age (being higher in infants than in adults) and sex (women have larger stores of adipose tissue and therefore less body water than men). Body water is divided between the intracellular and extracellular compartments, the latter being composed of the interstitial fluid and the plasma volume (Table 2.50). These compartments are separated by semi-permeable barriers which permit the free passage of salt and water but only limited movement of other solutes such as proteins. All three compartments are interdependent and movement of fluid between them is regulated largely by pressure gradients and osmosis. Since it is difficult to gain access to the intracellular fluid compartment, extracellular fluid volume is the most important consideration when providing clinical care for a patient, particularly in the acute stages of an illness.

2.9.1 Regulation of body fluid

Regulation of the body fluid is called homeostasis. This is a dynamic function governed by biochemical and physiological processes. Normally the total fluid volume fluctuates by less than 1% per day, despite variations in intake. Changes of as little as 1−2% can lead to illness and sometimes death. An understanding of the functions of fluid within the body helps to clarify the factors affecting its regulation. Fluid is needed

1 To act as a solvent for ions and molecules.

2 To act as a transport medium especially for the excretion of osmotically active solutes such as urea and salts.

3 As a lubricant.

4 To regulate body temperature.

2.9.2 Fluid requirement and fluid balance

Fluid intake

Fluid intake is normally controlled by the sensation of thirst which is regulated by the hypothalamus. Fluid is present in food as well as in oral liquids. Small quantities of water are also produced by the metabolic processes of the body.

Fluid output

Fluid output is primarily controlled by the kidneys, although there are also insensible losses via the skin, lungs and gastrointestinal tract. The amount of insensible loss depends on factors such as climate, activity, state of health and dietary intake.

Management of the patient should always be influenced by the need to maintain a state of balance between fluid intake and output (Table 2.51). Assessment of current fluid status requires meticulous completion of daily fluid balance charts and careful monitoring of blood and urine results with particular emphasis on sodium and osmolality.

Individual requirements for additional fluids vary considerably. The *minimum* intake should be sufficient to replace losses from all sources and provide adequate dilution for the excretion of solutes via the kidney. The *maximum* intake from oral liquids (or enteral or parenteral fluids) should be that which the kidney can excrete. In normal circumstances this is approximately 30−35 ml/kg body weight *or* 1 ml/kcal in adults and 1.5 ml/kcal in children.

Renal solute load

This refers to solutes which have to be excreted in the urine. These consist mainly of electrolytes and nitrogenous materials. Fats and carbohydrates are not involved in this process because they are usually metabolized to carbon dioxide and water. It is essential to make sure that enough fluid is available to enable the solute load to be excreted and this is particularly important in infants or patients with fluid restrictions — for example those with renal failure (Zeigler and Fomon 1971; Francis 1987). The calculation is performed as follows:

1 Analyse the diet or feed for protein, sodium, potassium, chloride and any other attendant anions.

2a Each mmol of sodium, potassium, chloride or other anion contributes 1 mmol to the renal solute load.

(*Note*: If details of attendant anion intake are not available, double the content contributed by sodium and potassium.)

2b Each gram of protein contributes 4 mmol to the renal solute load.

3 Add the above figures together and then divide by the urine osmolality. This gives a figure which is the number of litres needed to excrete the renal solute load generated by the diet or feed.

4 Remember to make an additional allowance for *insensible losses* (approximately 1000 ml); and *increased temperature* (approximately 500 ml per 1°C).

Table 2.50 Body fluids – location, percentage and composition

Compartment	Location	% Body weight	Principal cation	Principal anion
Extracellular				
Interstitial	Fluid surrounding the cells	16%	Na^+	Cl^-
Vascular	Fluids within the blood vessels (6.5% solids-mainly protein)	4%		
Intracellular	Fluids within the cells (Protein content higher than plasma)	30–40%	K^+	PO_4^- (+ protein)

The only common feature between these three compartments is the osmolality which is 290 mosmol/kg water

Table 2.51 Fluid balance

Input/24 hrs		Output/24 hrs	
Source	Typical volume (ml)	Source	Typical volume (ml)
Oral liquids	1500	Urine	1500
Water contained in food*	1000	Faeces	150
Metabolism†	300	Lungs	400
		Insensible losses	750
Total	2800	Total	2800

* The water content of food can be ascertained by looking up the appropriate item in McCance and Widdowson's *The Composition of Foods*. It may not always be necessary to calculate this figure accurately, but an estimate of the fluid derived from food should be included in the daily input. If the patient is not eating, the fluid usually derived from food should be replaced by another source

† Metabolism of 1 g starch yields 0.6 g water; 1 g protein yields 0.4 g water and 1 g fat yields 1.1 g water

2.9.3 Factors affecting fluid movement

Movement of water

Fluid shifts between the three compartments are controlled by a variety of sensitive and highly complex mechanisms which include osmosis and the effect of hydrostatic pressure gradients. Particles within the body fluid are electrically charged; the main extracellular cation is sodium and the main intracellular cation is potassium (Table 2.50). In normal circumstances the osmolalities of the plasma and interstitial fluid are equal. Plasma osmolality usually reflects the serum sodium which, in turn, reflects the total extracellular volume. It may be useful to note that, provided water is distributed normally between the three compartments, a high serum sodium level may indicate dehydration while a low level could point to over hydration.

Plasma osmolality

This is a key factor in the determination of fluid movement and slight alterations in plasma osmolality are usually corrected by the movement of fluid between the interstitial compartment and the plasma. This may be accompanied by variations in oral intake. If the plasma osmolality increases then the hypothalamus is stimulated by a sensation of thirst and increased amounts of antidiuretic hormone (ADH) are released. This leads to the reabsorption of water from the distal renal tubules and correction of the plasma osmolality. Decreased plasma volume can also lead to a raised osmolality; aldosterone is then released which results in increased sodium and water retention.

Renal function is therefore an important factor in the regulation of fluid balance and any impairment is often characterized by oedema.

'*Pitting oedema*' is the most common clinical symptom of an expanded interstitial volume. Fluid balance is normally maintained within the extracellular compartment but can be upset for a number of reasons. It is important to remember that the location of pitting oedema is affected by gravity and that a bedridden patient may show signs of sacral oedema in the absence of ankle oedema. Correction of oedema should never be attempted without a precise knowledge of its cause. It is also important to remember that severe cases of disturbed osmolality or volume depletion can lead to the movement of water between the intracellular and extracellular compartments; this is more difficult to diagnose and can have fatal consequences if not treated promptly.

Hydrostatic pressure

Plasma volume is also maintained by the effects of hydrostatic pressure. Essentially, a higher pressure is exerted within the arterial end of the capillary. At the same time there is the lesser effect of osmotic pressure exerted by the plasma proteins (oncotic pressure) resulting in the movement of fluid into the interstitial space. The process is reversed at the venous end of the capillary with a consequent movement of fluid back into the plasma (Starling's Hypothesis, summarized in Fig. 2.11). The plasma proteins therefore play an important role in the movement of fluid between the vascular and interstitial compartments.

2.9.4 Correction of fluid balance

This is sometimes managed by the administration of Plasma Protein Fraction (PPF) or additional nutritional support. The fluid level in the intracellular compartment is maintained by a water shift from the extracellular space.

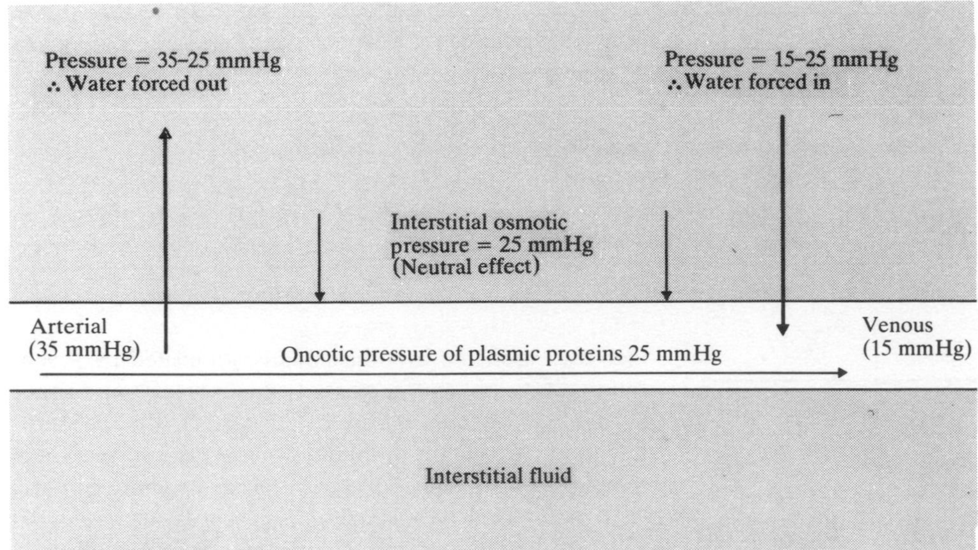

Fig. 2.11 Starling's hypothesis

Administration of extra protein as PPF will lead to the retention of water and consequent expansion of the plasma volume. However, it is important to note that serum albumin levels are maintained by a balance between albumin synthesis, breakdown and redistribution. Giving a bolus of additional protein may help to restore fluid balance but it is unlikely to confer any long term benefit on the serum albumin level. Approximately one third of the albumin pool is in the plasma and the remaining two thirds are distributed throughout the extracellular compartment. The plasma pool is maintained by the movement of albumin from the extracellular space. PPF administration will result in albumin diffusing back to the extracellular compartment rather than remaining in the plasma pool and thus the serum albumin level should not be used in isolation when considering the nutritional status of patients.

Intestinal control of fluid balance

This is chiefly related to any losses incurred during bouts of diarrhoea and/or vomiting. Normally, the large quantities of digestive juices which are secreted into the gastrointestinal tract are reabsorbed. If there is abnormal gastrointestinal function leading to excessive fluid loss this is replaced by extracellular fluid which crosses the mucosa into the gut. This may be caused by a variety of conditions including short bowel syndrome and ileostomy losses. The average composition of various intestinal fluids is shown in Table 2.52.

Insensible losses

The *respiratory system* is involved to a lesser degree in the maintenance of fluid volume. Normally, a constant amount of water (approximately 400 ml) is lost daily from the lungs. This loss can increase dramatically in hyperventilation, whatever the cause.

Fluid is also lost by evaporation from the skin. Losses amount to approximately 500–750 ml daily but will increase as a result of a hot climate, fever, burns or any other situation which increases the metabolic rate.

Summary

Fluid is essential to life and, although man can survive for remarkably long periods without food, he cannot withstand

Table 2.52 Volume and composition of gastrointestinal secretions and sweat (Adapted from Harper 1971; Caldwell and Kennedy-Caldwell 1981)

Fluid	Average adult volume (ml/24 hours)	Electrolyte concentration (mEq/l)			
		Na^+	K^+	Cl^-	HCO_3^-
Gastric juice	2500	31–90	4.3–12	52–124	0
Bile	700–1000	134–156	3.9–6.3	83–110	38
Pancreatic juice	700–1000	113–153	2.6–7.4	54–95	110
Small bowel (Miller-Abbott Section)	3000	72–120	3.5–6.8	69–127	30
Ileostomy					
Recent	100–4000	112–142	4.5–14	93–122	30
Adapted	100–500	50	3	20	15–30
Caecostomy	100–3000	48–116	11.1–28.3	35–70	15
Faeces	100	<10	<10	<15	<15
Sweat	500–1000	30–70	0–5	30–70	0

Table 2.53 Patients at particular risk of inadequate fluid intake and consequent depletion

Increased requirements for fluid	Patients with tracheostomies or on ventilators; diarrhoea and/or vomiting; increased fluid losses e.g. sepsis, any other conditions associated with pyrexia, diabetes insipidus Patients receiving high protein/high osmolar diets (e.g. tube feeding regimens; patients with nephrotic syndrome) Infants — particularly with any of the above conditions
Lack of awareness of, or inability to express, the need for fluid	Patients who are unable to communicate — those who are unconscious; those who have suffered a stroke Patients who are unable to eat normally — those with dysphagia (e.g. cancer of the oesophagus); those with diminished food intake (e.g. anorexia nervosa); those with a poor appetite (e.g. the elderly or chronically ill); those on 'nil by mouth' regimens who are receiving inadequate fluids intravenously

Patients on long term diuretic therapy should have their fluid balance monitored closely to avoid any risk of dehydration.

Some patients may require a *reduced* fluid intake. These could include patients in various stages of renal failure; congestive cardiac failure; respiratory failure; or post-operative recovery — especially chest surgery

a prolonged deprivation of fluid. It is unlikely that the majority of patients will suffer from severe fluid imbalance. However, there are certain groups of patients in whom the possibility of fluid imbalance should be considered carefully and these are listed in Table 2.53. Awareness of the problems created by fluid imbalance will help to ensure successful management of these patients.

Further reading

Bunton GL (1976) *Fluid balance without tears*. Lloyd-Luke, London.

Martin DW (1983) Water and minerals. In *Harpers review of biochemistry* 17e. Martin DW, Mays PA and Rodwell VW (Eds). Lange, Los Altos.

Moghissi K and Boore J (1983) *Parenteral and enteral nutrition for nurses*. p. 18. Heinemann Medical, London.

Morgan DB and Grant A (1980) Water, electrolytes and acid base. In *Biochemistry of hospital nutrition* Woolfson A (Ed). Blackwell Scientific Publications, Oxford.

Richards P and Truniger B (1983) *Understanding water, electrolyte and acid-base balance*. Heinemann Medical, London.

Smith K (1980) *Fluids and electrolytes — a conceptual approach*. Churchill Livingstone, Edinburgh.

Tweedle DEF (1982) *Metabolic care*. Churchill Livingstone, Edinburgh.

Willats M (1982) *Lecture notes on fluid and electrolyte balance*. Blackwell Scientific Publications, Oxford.

References

Caldwell MD and Kennedy-Caldwell C (1981) Normal nutritional requirements. *Surg Clin North Am* **61**(3), 489–507.

Francis D (1987) *Diets for sick children* 4e pp. 198–9. Blackwell Scientific Publications, Oxford.

Harper HA (1971) *Physiological chemistry* 13e. Lange, Los Altos.

Zeigler EE and Fomon SJ (1971) Fluid intake, renal solute load and water balance in infancy. *J Paed* **78**(4), 561–8.

2.10 Drug-nutrient interactions

The relationship between nutrition and drug metabolism is an important but poorly documented subject. Diet can affect drug action and metabolism in a number of ways and conversely, drugs themselves may affect nutrient intake and metabolism.

2.10.1 Effects of nutrition on drug action and metabolism

The metabolism of a drug usually involves the following stages:

1 Absorption from the gastrointestinal tract (if the drug is orally administered).

2 Transport in the blood, usually bound to plasma proteins.

3 Deactivation by a two-stage metabolic process, i.e.

- Oxidation by microsomal enzyme systems involving reduced nicotinamide adenine dinucleotide (NADPH) and cytochrome P450, predominantly in the liver but also in the lung and small intestine;
- Conjugation with glucuronic acid, sulphate or glycine.

4 Excretion of the conjugate in urine or bile.

Nutrient intake and drug absorption

The pharmacological response to a drug depends on the rate at which it is absorbed from the gastrointestinal tract.

The presence of food in the stomach and proximal intestine may delay the absorption of drugs from the gut. Food will alter the rate of gastric emptying and will therefore delay the rate of drug absorption (although not necessarily the quantity of drug absorbed). For this reason, some drugs (e.g. oral hypoglycaemics or antibiotics) must be taken on an empty stomach.

Cations in foods can chelate with some drugs and reduce their intestinal absorption. For example, tetracyclines and ferrous sulphate both chelate with Ca^{2+}, therefore milk or milk products should not be consumed within two hours of ingesting these drugs. Drugs that are partly ionized (e.g. amiloride) will have reduced absorption due to the presence of food.

Other dietary constituents such as fat may impede the absorption of drugs that are hydrophilic. Foods that alter the pH of the gut may also affect drug absorption. Some antihypertensives (atenolol and captopril) and antituberculous compounds (rifampicin and isoniazid) also have impaired absorption in the presence of food.

There are some drugs that have an increased rate of absorption in the presence of food (e.g. nitrofurantoin and hydrochlorothiazide), and in some cases the bioavailability of drugs (e.g. propranolol, metoprolol and hydralazine) can be increased when administered with food (Melander and McLean 1983).

Plasma binding protein

Plasma protein transports the drug from the gastrointestinal tract. Therefore in cases of malnutrition where tissue protein is used as a source of energy, transportation of the drug will be impaired. Thus the effectiveness of drugs such as chloramphenicol, digoxin, phenylbutazone, salicylates and tetracyclines will be decreased.

Rate of deactivation and conjugation

In some cases the metabolic derivative of a drug is its active constituent. Abnormalities in the deactivation or conjugation of a drug may affect the pharmacological or toxic effect of the drug. Periods of short term starvation or prolonged periods of nutritional inadequacy can affect microsomal drug metabolizing enzymes (Dickerson 1978; Cusack and Denham 1984). These states are likely to occur in cases of severe illness where correct drug metabolism is of greatest importance.

2.10.2 Effects of drugs on nutrition

Absorption of nutrients

Laxatives can interfere with the biological availability of nutrients by decreasing intestinal absorption. The chronic use of peristaltic stimulants (such as senna or phenolphthalein) can reduce nutrient absorption. Absorption of fat-soluble vitamins is impaired by the use of intestinal lubricants (such as liquid paraffin).

Colonic flora are altered by the use of antibiotics, and diarrhoea can often result. Prolonged use, therefore, of antibiotics can lead to a malnourished state. One antibiotic, neomycin, decreases the absorption of carotene, glucose, fat and iron. Tetracycline increases the urinary excretion of vitamin C. Drugs such as sulphasalazine cause folate malabsorption, while cholestyramine impairs the absorption of fat soluble vitamins. The gut mucosa may be affected by cytotoxic drugs, producing villous atrophy resulting in malabsorption.

Malabsorption of vitamin C occurs with consumption of large doses of aspirin.

Appetite

Appetite may be either increased or decreased by drug administration. Indomethacin and cytotoxic drugs have a directly anorectic effect while others such as theophylline, amphetamines and sulphonamides can cause nausea. Some drugs, notably drugs used in psychiatry, give an altered taste sensation (anticholinergics, tricyclics and lithium carbonate) which can affect the quantity and type of food eaten.

Drugs such as insulin, sulphonylureas, phenothiazines, benzodiazepines, alcohol and newer agents such as mianserin, can increase appetite. The effect of some drugs on nutrient intake are shown in Table 2.54.

Increased nutrient requirement

Anticonvulsants, phenothiazines and tricyclics induce the synthesis of cytochrome P 450 and therefore increase the requirement for folic acid. Labadarios *et al* (1978) suggest that these drugs cause low blood levels of folate if they are given to patients over a long period of time. This, they suggest is especially true for those patients where the intake of folate is particularly low, (e.g. elderly and mentally ill patients).

Penicillamine, used occasionally in the treatment of rheumatoid arthritis, chelates zinc and prolonged administration could lead to a deficiency, especially when the intake of the mineral is also reduced.

Table 2.54 Effects of drugs on nutritional intake

Drugs	Action affecting nutritional intake
Diethylpropion	Anorexia/decreased appetite
Mazindol	
Biguanides	
Fenfluramine	
Cytotoxic drugs	
Neomycin sulphate	
Cyclophosphamide	
Digitalis	
Glucagon	
Amphetamines	Nausea
Indomethacin	
Digoxin	
Theophylline	
Clomipramine	
Diphenylhydantoin	
Sulphonamides	
Anticholinergic drugs – all members	Altered taste sensation
Tricyclic drugs	
Lithium carbonate	
Zopiclone	
L-Dopa	
Androgens	Increased appetite
Sulphonylureas	
Corticosteroids	
Phenothiazines	
Benzodiazepines	
Insulin	
Alcohol	
Mianserin	

Table 2.55 Effects of drugs on carbohydrate and lipid metabolism

Drugs	Disturbance
Thiazides	Carbohydrate metabolism
Corticosteroids	
Oral contraceptives	
Diphenylhydantoin	
Sulphonylureas	
Aspirin	
Monoamine oxidase inhibitors	
Alcohol	
Aspirin	Lipid metabolism
Chlortetracycline	
Colchicine	
Phenindione	
Indomethacin	
Oral contraceptives	
Alcohol	
Adrenal corticosteroids	
Growth hormone	
Chlorpromazine	
Phenobarbitone	

Table 2.56 Effects of drugs on electrolytes and minerals

Drug	Effect
Thiazide diuretics	Depletion of body potassium
Purgatives	
Adrenal steroids	
Corticosteroids	Retention of water and salt
Phenylbutazone	
Oxyphenbutazone	
Carbenolone	
Oral contraceptives	
Phosphates	Decreased iron absorption
Antacids	
Tetracyline	
Sulphonylureas	Decreased iodine uptake by the thyroid gland
Phenylbutazone	
Cobalt	
Lithium	
Oral contraceptives	Reduction in plasma zinc Increase in plasma copper
Thiazide diuretics	Increased reabsorption of calcium from the kidney

Table 2.57 Effects of drugs on vitamin absorption and metabolism

Drug	Vitamin	Effect
Alcohol Antacids	Thiamin	Malabsorption
Isoniazid Hydralazine Penicillamine Oral contraceptives	Pyridoxine	Antagonist of the vitamin
Alcohol Aspirin Biguanides Metformin Oral contraceptives Sulphasalazine	Folate	Malabsorption
Anticonvulsants Phenothiazines Tricyclics Methotrexate	Folate	Interaction between drugs and co-enzymes
Para amino salicylate Colchicine Metformin Phenformin Cholestyramine Oral contraceptives Trifluoperazine	B_{12}	Malabsorption
Tetracycline Aspirin Corticosteroids Barbiturates Oral contraceptives	C	Increase excretion and decrease storage levels
Anticonvulsants	D	Induce enzymes that convert the vitamin to its active form
Warfarin	K	Inhibit bacterial synthesis of the vitamin
Liquid paraffin Cholestyramine	A, D, E, K	Malabsorption

Alterations in nutrient metabolism

Tyramine

Tyramine is an indirectly sympathomimetic amine which releases noradrenaline from adrenergic neurones causing a rise in blood pressure. Normally tyramine is metabolized by the enzyme monoamine oxidase before any significant hypertension can occur. If the enzyme's activity is blocked by a monoamine oxidase inhibitor (MAOI) drug, a severe and possibly fatal rise in blood pressure can result from the ingestion of tyramine rich foods. These foods listed elsewhere (Section 2.11, Table 2.59) must therefore be avoided by patients taking MAOI drugs.

Carbohydrate metabolism

Antidiabetic agents such as sulphonylureas are prescribed precisely because of their effect on carbohydrate metabolism. Drugs such as oral contraceptives or corticosteroids can produce adverse effects on carbohydrate metabolism and provoke glucose intolerance. Tricyclic drugs are known to cause carbohydrate craving, but do not affect metabolism.

Lipid metabolism

Some drugs are used to correct lipid metabolism, whilst others such as chlorpromazine and phenobarbitone induce hyperlipidaemia (Table 2.55).

Vitamin and mineral metabolism

Anticonvulsants (phenytoin, phenobarbitone and primidone) affect vitamin D metabolism resulting in impaired calcium absorption and, with prolonged treatment, osteomalacia or rickets. These drugs also decrease folate levels leading to megaloblastic anaemia.

Antimetabolite drugs such as methotrexate (used in the treatment of some cancers) directly antagonize folic acid metabolism by inhibiting the activity of the enzyme dehydrofolate reductase. Anti-cancer drugs can also affect vitamin status.

The mood stabilizer lithium carbonate is affected by salt intake. A high salt intake will decrease the lithium level whilst the converse is also true. This is an important fact in the use of lithium therapy. This is discussed in more detail in Section 4.23.

Tables 2.56 and 2.57 show the effects of some drugs on electrolytes, minerals and vitamins. Interactions between nutrition and drugs used in psychiatric disorders are discussed in Section 4.23.

Further reading

Awad AG (1984) Diet and drug interactions. The treatment of mental illness — a review. *Can J Psychiat* **29**, 609–613.

Basu TK (1977) Interactions of drugs and nutrition. *J Hum Nutr* **31**, 449–58.

References

Cusack B and Denham MJ (1984) Nutritional status and drug disposition in the elderly. In *Drugs and nutrition in the geriatric patient* Roe DA (Ed) pp. 71–91. Churchill Livingstone, Edinburgh.

Dickerson JWT (1978) The interrelationships of nutrition and drugs. In *Nutrition and the clinical management of disease* Dickerson JWT and Lee HA (Eds) pp. 308–31. Edward Arnold, London.

Labadarios D, Obuwa G, Lucas EG, Dickerson JWT and Parke DV (1978) The effects of chronic drug administration on hepatic enzyme induction and folate metabolism. *Br J Clin Pharmacol* **5**, 167–73.

Melander A and McLean A (1983) Influence of food intake on presystemic clearance of drugs. *Clin Pharmacokinet* **8**, 286–96.

2.11 Miscellaneous substances

2.11.1 Caffeine, theophylline and theobromine

Caffeine, theophylline and theobromine are all methyl derivatives of xanthine. They are pharmacologically active substances. Caffeine is the most potent and acts as a stimulant to the heart and central nervous system. It also increases gastric acid secretion and is known to cause vasodilatation. Effects are most likely when excessive quantities are taken or in highly sensitive people.

A retrospective survey of caffeine consumption in the UK (Scott *et al* 1989) showed that most dietary caffeine was obtained from tea and coffee. The mean daily intake was found to be 259 mg/day (sd 189). However this population included those who deliberately avoided caffeine, so the mean intake of habitual caffeine consumers is likely to be higher. Some people consume in excess of 1 g caffeine/day (Heaney and Recker 1982); this is equivalent to the consumption of about 10 cups of percolated coffee or 15 cups of instant coffee per day, although this does vary with the brand and preparation method used (Bunker and McWilliams 1979). Caffeine intake has been shown to be higher in smokers than non-smokers and tends to increase with age (Scott *et al* 1989).

The principal dietary sources of caffeine are summarized in Table 2.58. Caffeine may also be present in some foods for flavouring purposes but such foods are difficult to identify because added flavours are not usually identified by name on a food label, only as 'flavouring'. Proprietary cold relief, pain relief or caffeine stimulant tablets can be additional sources of caffeine (Graham 1978).

Table 2.58 Principal dietary sources of caffeine (Nagy 1974; Bunker and McWilliams 1979)

Food	Caffeine content
Coffee (mg/cup)	
Instant	61–70
Percolated ground	97–125
Tea (mg/cup)	15–75
Cocoa (mg/cup)	10–17*
Chocolate bar	60–70*
Cola drinks (mg/12 oz can) e.g. Pepsi Cola, Coca Cola, Diet Coke	43–65
Lucozade (mg/100 g)	18

* Main stimulant is theobromine

2.11.2 Monoamines

Monoamine oxidase inhibitors (MAOIs) are drugs used in the treatment of depression. Current MAOI drugs in use include:

- Tranylcypromine (trade names Parnate, Parstelin);
- Phenelzine (trade name Nardil);
- Isocarboxazid (trade name Marplan).

Additionally, procarbazine (Natulan), an antineoplastic drug, is a mild MAOI. The data sheet advises that interaction with diet should be borne in mind when it is prescribed to patients.

Monoamine oxidase is required for the metabolism of catecholamines. There are biologically active amines (e.g. tyramine, histamine and dopamine) in certain foods which, if taken during a course of MAOI, can result in unpleasant and even life-threatening reactions. The most commonly reported reactions are headaches, but substantial rises in blood pressure leading to subarachnoid haemorrhage and death have also been documented.

The Pharmaceutical Society and the British Medical Association produce up-to-date dietary guidelines for patients on MAOIs in the form of a card which is normally issued to the patient by the pharmacist. Foods to be avoided when MAOI drugs are taken are listed in Table 2.59.

This area of food and drug interaction has been comprehensively reviewed by McCabe and Tsung (1982) and McCabe (1986) who conclude that some dangers of MAOI drugs and food have been poorly documented and the need for complete exclusion of certain foods exaggerated. These include avocado, chocolate, yogurt, soya sauce, tea, coffee and cola beverages. The main problem is the presence of tyramine (produced by the decarboxylation of tyrosine). There is a wide variation in the tyramine content of different samples of the same type of food and there is also a variation in patient tolerance to tyramine.

Eating fresh foods, or meals freshly prepared from tinned and frozen ingredients, reduces the risk of consuming protein which has undergone degradation and possibly resulted in the production of tyramine.

2.11.3 Oxalates

Oxalates are found mainly in foods of plant origin. The actual content varies considerably with season, species, variety, age, maturity and part of the plant.

Table 2.59 Foods to be avoided on MAOI drugs (and for 14 days after the end of treatment)*

Alcoholic drinks and low alcohol beers, lagers and wines
Broad bean pods
Cheese, especially that which is fermented (e.g. blue cheeses), matured or processed and cheese spreads
Game
Meat extracts and yeast extracts (e.g. Oxo and other stock cubes, Marmite and Bovril)
Manufactured foods containing meat or yeast extracts (check label)
Pickled herrings
Flavoured textured vegetable protein
Any food which has been kept for a long time
Any food which has previously produced unpleasant symptoms

* Information derived from the Pharmaceutical Society, British Medical Association and MIMS

Table 2.60 Principal dietary sources of oxalate (Kasidas and Rose 1980 and Kasidas, personal communication)

Food	Oxalic acid content (mg/100 g)
Beetroot	500
Carob powder	73
Chocolate (and other products containing cocoa)	117
Parsley (can be used in small amounts)	100
Peanuts*	187
Rhubarb	600
Spinach	600
Tea infusion (mg/100 ml)	55–78

* All nuts should be considered to be high in oxalates

Foods which contain moderate amounts of oxalates and which should be taken in controlled amounts are strawberries, celery and instant coffee

The oxalate content of the diet may need to be modified as part of the treatment of some renal stones (see Section 4.14).

A typical UK diet contains approximately 70–150 mg oxalic acid per day (Zarembski and Hodgkinson 1962). A low oxalate diet should provide no more than 60–70 mg oxalic acid per day. Principal sources of dietary oxalate are summarized in Table 2.60. Note that herbal teas are low in oxalate so make a good alternative to ordinary tea. However, carob, sometimes used as a substitute for chocolate, is not suitable for those on a low oxalate diet. For a more comprehensive list of the oxalate content of foods, see Kasidas and Rose (1980).

2.11.4 Purines

Drug therapy has largely replaced dietary restriction in the treatment of gout (hyperuricaemia). However, it is still reasonable to advise patients with recurrent gout to eliminate the principal sources of purines from their diet because this is not difficult and dietary nucleoproteins contribute about 5% of urate present in blood. Purine restriction is not necessary for the treatment of uric acid stones (see Section 4.14).

Principal dietary sources of purines are summarized in Table 2.61.

Table 2.61 Principal dietary sources of purines (Clifford *et al* 1976; Wyngaarden and Kelly 1976)

Meat sources	Fish sources
Liver	Anchovies
Heart	Crab
Kidney	Fish roes
Sweetbreads	Herring
Meat extracts (e.g. Oxo)	Mackerel
	Sardines
	Shrimps
	Sprats
	Whitebait

2.11.5 Salicylates

Much of the interest in the salicylate content of foods arose from the demonstration that urticaria, asthma, angioedema or rhinitis may follow the ingestion of aspirin (acetylsalicylic acid) (James and Warin 1970; McDonald *et al* 1972; Juhlin 1980). This led some to believe that all food and drug sources of salicylates should be avoided by patients who show a positive response to oral aspirin challenge (Lockey 1971). Some practitioners have also excluded 'structurally related compounds' such as azo dyes and benzoates (Noid *et al* 1974; Ros *et al* 1976).

However, from a dietetic viewpoint, a request for advice on salicylate avoidance is highly problematical owing to the lack of accurate information on the salicylate content of foods consumed in the UK. Available analytical data are not only limited in scope but also contain many inconsistencies, partly as a result of variation in analytical methods but also because the salicylate content of a food appears to vary with factors such as its country of origin, variety, degree of ripeness and degree of processing. As a consequence, there is a wide discrepancy in the types of foods recommended for exclusion on low salicylate diets. It is difficult therefore to construct low salicylate diets with any degree of confidence and hence to investigate their efficacy.

Apart from the practical difficulties, the rationale for placing someone on a low salicylate diet has also been questioned. The most comprehensive study of the salicylate content of foods is that of Swain *et al* (1985) on foods consumed in Australia. Based on their data, these authors suggest that Western diets contain between 10–200 mg

Table 2.62 Possible sources of yeast in the diet (Warin 1976; Workman *et al* 1984)

Bread	Bread made with yeast or yoghurt (soda breads are yeast-free) Buns and cakes made with yeast (e.g. crumpets, doughnuts, teacakes, bath buns) Foods made with bread (e.g. bread sauce, stuffing, bread and butter pudding, apple charlotte, summer pudding) Foods containing bread as a 'filler' (e.g. sausages, beefburgers, rissoles, meat loaf) Foods coated in breadcrumbs (e.g. fish fingers, fish cakes, breaded fish, potato cakes, scotch eggs) Pizza
Fermented foods	Cheese, yoghurt, buttermilk, soured cream, some synthetic creams Wine, fortified wines (e.g. vermouth), beer, cider Fruit juices (unless freshly prepared and consumed) Grapes, plums and any over-ripe fruit Dried fruit such as sultanas, raisins, currants, dates, figs or prunes and foods containing dried fruit (e.g. fruit cake, mincemeat, muesli, eccles cakes) Soy sauce Pickles (e.g. pickled onions, pickled beetroot) Vinegar and vinegar-containing products (e.g. tomato sauce, salad dressing, mayonnaise)
Yeast and meat extracts	Marmite, Bovril Oxo and similar beef, chicken or vegetable stock cubes Gravy mixes Many tinned and packet savoury foods (e.g. soups, sauces)
Vitamin tablets	Brewers yeast tablets B vitamins, either as multivitamin or single preparations, are often produced from yeast
Miscellaneous	Malted milk drinks Cream crackers Twiglets Any manufactured food with yeast as an ingredient on the label

salicylate/day. Since the usual adult pharmacological dose of aspirin is 600 mg (two tablets), which may be taken several times per day, Swain *et al* suggest that it is unlikely that foods could trigger similar effects to salicylate medication. Others have also challenged the assumption that aspirin intolerance represents a broad intolerance to salicylates (Oliver 1974; Dahl 1980; Warner 1987). The value of dietary salicylate avoidance therefore remains to be demonstrated.

2.11.6 Benzoates

Benzoates occur naturally in a wide range of foods but, as with salicylates, analytical information on this subject is limited and subject to wide discrepancies. The benzoate content of a food appears to vary according to factors such as its variety and the soil and conditions in which it is grown. Juhlin (1980) suggests that the amounts of benzoates present naturally in foods are small compared with the amounts added as preservatives, and would only be sufficient to produce urticaria in extremely sensitive patients.

2.11.7 Yeast

Yeast has been implicated in certain food allergy conditions although this remains contentious (see Section 4.31). Yeast can be an ingredient in foods or occur as a microbiological contaminant. Possible sources of yeast are listed in Table 2.62.

References

Bunker ML and McWilliams M (1979) Caffeine content of common beverages. *J Am Dietet Assoc* **74**, 28–32.

Clifford AJ, Riumullo JA, Young VR and Scrimshaw NS (1976) Effect of oral purines on serum and urinary uric acid of normal and gouty humans. *J Nutr* **106**, 428.

Dahl R (1980) Sodium salicylate and aspirin disease. *Allergy* **35**, 155–6.

Graham DM (1978) Caffeine – its identity, dietary sources, intake and biological effects. *Nutr Rev* **36**, 97–102.

Heaney RP and Recker RR (1982) Effects of nitrogen, phosphorus and caffeine on calcium balance in women. *J Lab Clin Med* **99**, 46–55.

James J and Warin RP (1970) Chronic urticaria: the effect of aspirin. *Br J Dermatol* **82**, 204.

Juhlin L (1980) Incidence of intolerance to food additives. *Int J Dermatol* **19**, 548–51.

Kasidas GP and Rose GA (1980) Oxalate content of some common foods: Determination by an enzymatic method. *J Hum Nutr* **34**, 255–66.

Lockey SD (1971) Reactions to hidden agents in foods, beverages and drugs. *Ann Allergy* **29**, 461–6.

McCabe BJ (1986) Dietary tyramine and other pressor amines in MAOI regimens: a review. *J Am Dietet Assoc* **86**(8), 1059–64.

McCabe BJ and Tsung MT (1982) Dietary considerations in MAO Inhibitor regimens. *J Clin Psych* **43**(5), 178–81.

McDonald JR, Mathieson DA and Stevenson PD (1972) Aspirin intolerance in asthma. Detection by oral challenge. *J Allergy* **50**, 198.

Nagy M (1974) Caffeine content of beverages and chocolate. *J Am Med Assoc* **229**, 337.

Noid HE, Schulze TW and Winkelmann RK (1974) Diet plan for patients with salicylate-induced urticaria. *Arch Dermatol* **109**, 866–9.

Oliver NE (1974) Diet plan for patients with salicylate induced urticaria. *Arch Dermatol* **110**, 957.

Ros AM, Juhlin L and Michaelsson G (1976) A follow-up study of patients with recurrent urticaria and hypersensitivity to aspirin, benzoates and azo dyes. *Br J Dermatol* **95**, 19.

Scott NR, Chakraborty J and Marks V (1989) Caffeine consumption in the United Kingdom: a restrospective survey. *Food Sciences and Nutrition* **42F**, 181–91.

Swain AR, Dutton SP and Truswell AS (1985) Salicylates in foods. *J Am Dietet Assoc* **85**, 950–60.

Warin RP (1976) Food factors in urticaria. *J Hum Nutr* **30**(3), 181–2.

Warner JO (1987) Artificial food additive intolerance – Fact or fiction? In *Food intolerance* Dobbing J (Ed) pp. 133–47. Baillière Tindall, London.

Workman E, Hunter J and Alun Jones V (1984) *The allergy diet* (Positive Health Guide). Optima, London.

Wyngaarden JB and Kelly WN (1976) *Gout and hyperuricaemia* pp. 453–5. Grune and Stratton, New York.

Zarembski PM and Hodgkinson A (1962) The oxalic acid content of English diets. *Br J Nutr* **16**, 627–34.

2.12 Food additives

There are some 3500 additives used in food manufacturing processes today.

Before any additive is permitted for use it undergoes a lengthy and detailed process of approval, with most of the research funded by the food manufacturer who wishes to use the new additive.

2.12.1 Approval process

The manufacturer has first to demonstrate to the Food Advisory Committee (FAC) that the benefits to the consumer of the proposed additive cannot be achieved by an already approved additive.

There are six factors to consider:

1 The need to keep food safe and wholesome until eaten.
2 The extension of choice in the diet.
3 The convenience of purchasing, packaging, storage, preparation and use.
4 The need for it to be attractively presented.
5 Economic advantage such as increasing shelf life or reducing cost.
6 The need for nutritional supplementation.

Once the need has been justified, the results of the safety testing are examined by the Committee on Toxicity of Chemicals in Food Consumer Products and the Environment (COT). Judgement is based on evidence supplied by the manufacturer and from other published work in the field. The COT can recommend to the FAC that:

1 An additive can be permitted.
2 An additive can be permitted for use only if more information is made available.
3 An additive should not be used until further research is undertaken.
4 An additive not be approved for use at all.

Based on these safety recommendations the FAC makes its own recommendations to the Ministry of Agriculture, Fisheries and Food.

If the additive is one of the categories considered by the European Community, the EC must also approve it.

Once the additive is approved by one or both of the groups, regulations concerning its use are drawn up and details are circulated to interested individuals and organizations for comment. If no new evidence of significance is received, regulations are signed jointly by ministers and laid before Parliament for approval.

2.12.2 The E number system for food additives

The E numbers code a list of permitted food additives, generally regarded as safe, for use within the European Community. Since January 1 1986, all food labels have to give the E numbers or the actual name of the additives in the ingredients list. At the moment flavourings are exempt from this ruling and have no E number. However at the time of publication, an EC discussion document has been circulated to interested parties proposing control on various categories of flavourings.

The E number classification is summarized in Table 2.63.

2.12.3 Food additives and their uses

Colours

Food is coloured:

1 To restore losses occurring during processing and storage.
2 To reinforce colour to meet consumer expectations.
3 To give colour to otherwise colourless foods in the development of new foods.
4 To ensure similar products look the same.

By weight, 98% of all food colour is caramel (E150) (Denner 1984).

Natural versus man-made colours

Natural and man-made additives, including colours, come under the same rigorous approval testing procedures. In recent years some man-made colours have virtually disappeared from food due to consumers indicating their preference for either natural colours or removal of additives altogether. However, some natural colours may fade in some food products or may cost more than the man-made alternative. Examples of natural and man-made colours and their uses are given in Tables 2.64 and 2.65.

Preservatives

Preservatives are substances added to food to prevent food poisoning and spoilage of food in shops and at home. Their use enables the consumer to have a wider choice of safely imported foods, which stay available out of season.

Table 2.63 Summary of E numbers

E number	Type of additive	Example
E100–180	Colours	E163 Anthocyanins
E200–290	Preservatives	E210 Benzoic acid
E300–322	Antioxidants	E320 BHA
E400–495	Emulsifiers/stabilizers	E322 Lecithin
E420–421	Sweeteners	E420 Sorbitol
E170–927	Miscellaneous additives	E170 Calcium carbonate

Some additives are under consideration by the EEC and have a number but no E prefix, e.g. 621 Monosodium glutamate

Table 2.64 Examples of natural colours

Name	E number	Typical food uses
Riboflavin (yellow)	E101	Processed cheese
Chlorophyll (green)	E140	Fats, oils, canned and dried vegetables
Carbon (black)	E153	Jams and jellies
Alpha carotene (yellow/orange)	E160(a)	Margarine and cakes

Table 2.65 Examples of man-made colours

Name	E number	Specific food use
Tartrazine (yellow)*	E102	Soft drinks
Quinoline Yellow	E104	Scotch eggs and smoked fish
Yellow 2G*	107[a]	
Sunset Yellow*	E110	Orange squash
Carmoisine (red)*	E122	Swiss roll
Amaranth (red)*	E123	Blackcurrant products
Ponceau 4R (red)*	E124	Tinned red fruits
Erythrosine (red)	E127	Glace cherries
Red 2G*	128[a]	Sausages
Patent Blue V	131[a]	Tinned vegetables
Indigo Carmine (blue)	E132	Savoury food mixes
Brilliant Blue FCF	133[a]	Canned vegetables
Green S	E142	Tinned peas, mint jelly and sauce
Black PN*	E151	Brown sauce and blackcurrant products
Brown FK*	154[a]	Kippers and smoked fish
Brown HT*	155[a]	Chocolate flavoured products

[a] Waiting consideration for E prefix by EC
* Contain azo group in their chemical structure

Traditional preservatives include salt, vinegar, saltpetre, alcohol and spices.

The Preservatives in Food Regulations 1979 (amended 1989) (MAFF) give detailed information on the use of preservatives including:

1 The current permitted preservatives.
2 The foods in which a preservative may be used.
3 The maximum permitted level of preservative in parts per million (ppm).

Some commonly used preservatives are given in Table 2.66. Those of particular interest to dietitians include benzoic acid and its derivatives, sulphur dioxide and nitrates/nitrites.

Benzoic acid and derivatives

Benzoic acid and benzoates are widely used by the food industry as preservatives. Benzoates occur widely in fresh foods, such as peas, bananas and berry fruit (see Section 2.11.6). Some fruits, such as cloudberries, may contain as much as 2% by weight of benzoic acid (but note analytical discrepancies mentioned in Section 2.11.6).

Adverse reactions have been seen in some people to benzoic acid but this is rare. For those who are sensitive, check food labels of products such as soft drinks, fruit products, jams, pickles and sauces for E210–E219.

Sulphur dioxide

This chemical is known to destroy thiamin. It is not permitted in any food which is considered to be a significant source of this vitamin.

Sulphur dioxide and sulphites are used extensively to kill yeasts that can cause fermentation in food and drink products.

Nitrates and nitrites

These preservatives act against the potentially lethal

Table 2.66 Commonly used preservatives

Name	E number	Specific food use
Sorbic acid and its derivatives	E200–E203	Cheese, yoghurt and soft drinks
Acetic acid	E260	Pickles and sauces
Lactic acid	E270	Margarine, confectionery and sauces
Propionic acid and its derivatives	E280–E283	Bread, cakes and flour confectionery
Carbon dioxide	E290	Fizzy drinks
Benzoic acid and its derivatives	E210–E219	Soft drinks, pickles, sauces, fruit products and jams
Sulphur dioxide	E220	Widely used in soft drinks, fruit products, beer, cider and wine
Nitrites	E249, E250	Cured meats, cooked meats and meat products
Nitrates	E251, E252	Bacon, ham and cheese (not Cheddar or Cheshire)

bacterium *Clostridium botulinum*. They also preserve the red colour of meats by reacting with myoglobin. They are used in a whole range of meat products and in some cheeses (not Cheddar, Cheshire or soft cheese).

Food is not the only source of nitrates and nitrites. These chemicals are used in fertilizers and the consequent leaching from the soil into the water supply has increased the levels available to the body.

Nitrites may react with secondary amines in the gastrointestinal tract to produce nitrosamines which have been shown to be carcinogenic in experimental animals. There is no evidence, as yet, in man to substantiate the role of these preservatives in the causation of cancer.

Antioxidants

As with preservatives, our current methods of food production would not produce goods with satisfactory shelf life without the use of antioxidants. The most important use of antioxidants is to prevent the unpleasant taste and smell which occur if fats or oils go rancid. Table 2.67 lists permitted antioxidants.

BHA and BHT (butylated hydroxyanisole and butylated hydroxytoluene)

These are two of the most used antioxidants. They are used in a wide variety of foods from dried soup mixes to cheese spreads. In certain circumstances high doses of BHA and BHT have been shown to give cancerous tumours in rats. Some diets also restrict their use in treatment of urticaria.

Emulsifiers and stabilizers

These additives are used to affect the texture and consistency of food. They are often needed because of the long shelf life of some manufactured foods. They constitute the largest group of additives and many are natural substances. The most controversial additives in this group are the polyphosphates, whose use as a meat tenderizer also enables water to be retained, so increasing product weight, e.g. frozen poultry, cured meats.

Some examples of emulsifiers and stabilizers are given in Table 2.68.

Table 2.67 Permitted antioxidants

Name	E number	Specific food use
Ascorbic acid and its derivatives	E300–E305	Beer, soft drinks, powdered milks, fruit products, (e.g. jams) and meat products (e.g. sausages)
Tocopherols (vitamin E and its derivatives)	E306–E309	Vegetable oils
Gallates	E310–E312	Vegetable oils and fat, margarine
Butylated hydroxyanisole (BHA)	E320	Margarine, fat in baked products, e.g. pies, sweets and convenience foods
Butylated hydroxytoluene (BHT)	E321	Crisps, margarine, vegetable oils and fats and convenience foods

Table 2.68 Examples of emulsifiers and stabilizers

Name	E number	Specific food use
Lecithins*	E322	Chocolate and chocolate products, powdered milk, margarine and potato snacks
Citric acid and its derivatives	E472a–c	Pickles, bottled sauces, dairy and baked products
Tartaric acid and its derivatives	E472d–f	Baking powder
Alginic acid and its derivatives	E400–E401	Ice cream, instant desserts and puddings
Agar	E406	Tinned ham (jelly), meat glazes and ice cream
Carrageenan	E407	Ice cream
Gums		
locust bean gum	E410	Ice cream, soups, bottled sauces and confectionery
guar gum	E412	
tragacanth	E413	
gum arabic	E414	
xanthan gum	E415	
Pectin	E440	Preserves, jellies and mint jelly
Sodium and potassium phosphate salts (polyphosphates)	E450	Frozen poultry and meat products, e.g. sausages

* Also used as an antioxidant

Sweeteners (See also Section 2.13)

These are a class of food additives that fall into two categories:

1 Caloric sweeteners, e.g. mannitol, sorbitol, xylitol, hydrogenated glucose syrup.

2 Non-caloric sweeteners, e.g. acesulpame K, aspartame, saccharin and thaumatin.

Some, such as saccharin, have been used for many years. Others, such as aspartame, probably one of the most extensively tested food additives, have been in use since the mid eighties.

Sucrose, glucose, fructose and lactose are all classified as foods rather than as sweeteners.

Solvents

Alcohol is the most common solvent use to enable the incorporation of a substance into a food product.

Miscellaneous additives

These include

1 Anti-foaming agents, to prevent frothing during processing.

2 Propellant gases, e.g. in aerosol cream.

3 Flavour modifiers, e.g. monosodium glutamate.

Many of these additives have a number but no E prefix as they are under consideration by the EEC.

Further reading

Amos HE and Drake JJP (1965) Problems posed by food additives. *J Hum Nutr* **30**(3), 165–78.

British Dietetic Association manufactured foods lists (but see Section 2.15 in this Manual):

1 *Additive free*. Excludes all E numbers and all foods with added vitamins but does not exclude natural sources of salicylates and benzoates.

2 *Added preservative free*. Excludes E200–299 inclusive but does not exclude natural sources of salicylates and benzoates or preservatives carried over into a product in one of the ingredients.

3 *Colour free*. Excludes E100–199 inclusive, but riboflavin and carotene are included.

4 *Colour and preservative free*. A combination of 2 and 3.

Food and Agriculture Committee (1972) *Interim report on the review of preservatives in food regulations*. HMSO, London.

Food and Agriculture Committee (1979) *Interim report on the review of colouring matter in food regulations*. HMSO, London.

Hanssen M (1984) *E for additives – the complete E number guide*. Thorsons, Wellingborough.

Joint Report of the Royal College of Physicians and the British Nutrition Foundation (1984) Food intolerance and food aversion. Reprinted from the *J Roy Coll Phys* **18**(2), 3–41.

Ministry of Agriculture, Fisheries and Food (1973) *Colouring matter in food regulations*. HMSO, London.

Ministry of Agriculture, Fisheries and Food (1979) *Preservatives in food regulations*. HMSO, London.

Ministry of Agriculture, Fisheries and Food (1983) *Look at the label*. HMSO, London.

Ministry of Agriculture, Fisheries and Food (1991) *About food additives – a guide from the Food Safety Directorate*. HMSO, London.

Reference

Denner WHB (1984) Colourings and preservatives in foods. *Hum Nutr: Appl Nutr* **38A**(6), 435–50.

2.13 Artificial and substitute sweeteners

Alternative sweeteners are used both in the home and in industry as a replacement for simple sugars – sucrose and glucose. They are generally categorized as either intense (non-nutritive) or nutritive (caloric) sweeteners.

2.13.1 Intense sweeteners

Intense sweeteners are used widely in the dietary management of diabetes and obesity, and are also used by the general population as a low calorie substitute for sugar (Table 2.69). They are food additives which have the unique property of imparting an intensely sweet flavour in minute amounts. Although some do have an energy value, their caloric contribution to a food is negligible, since they are used in such small quantities. Hence, their incorporation into manufactured foods has led to the development of a wide range of reduced calorie and sugar-free products. They are used extensively in diabetic or low-calorie versions of soft drinks, desserts, made-up salads and processed foods, but are not permitted in foods specifically prepared for babies and young children. Since they do not add bulk in the same way as sucrose, their use cannot be extended to baking and preserving unless an alternative bulking aid is also added. However, they are currently used in some preserves and may in future be incorporated into baked goods. They are non-cariogenic.

Since all sugar substitutes are food additives, they are required by law to undergo rigorous evaluation procedures before being approved for use. In the UK, the use of intense sweeteners is subject to *The Sweeteners in Food Regulations 1983* (Statutory Instruments 1983 No 1211) as subsequently amended in 1988 (Statutory Instruments 1988 No 2112).

Currently permitted intense sweeteners

Four intense sweeteners are currently permitted for use in food in the UK. They are:

1 Saccharin
2 Aspartame.
3 Acesulfame potassium (acesulfame K).
4 Thaumatin.

Saccharin

Saccharin was the first available artificial sweetener and it has been used in food for more than 80 years (Atkins 1990). It is approximately 300 times as sweet as sucrose at common levels of use (sweetening intensity can vary according to technical application). Concern regarding the safety of saccharin arose in the late 1970s because it had been shown to cause bladder cancer in male rats. Its use was temporarily banned. Public demand then led to a moratorium on the ban, and it is now approved for use in the UK, Canada and USA as a tabletop sweetener. In Italy, it is only available on prescription, and products containing saccharin in the USA must carry a health warning. Numerous studies to date have shown that there is no evidence that saccharin consumption increases the risk of bladder cancer in humans (Armstrong *et al* 1976; Kessler and Clark 1978; Morrison and Buring 1980).

Two surveys by the Ministry of Agriculture, Fisheries and Food (MAFF 1990) suggested that some people may be exceeding the Acceptable Daily Intake (ADI) for saccharin. (The ADI is the amount of a food additive, expressed on a bodyweight basis, which can be ingested daily over a lifetime without appreciable health risk.) It appears that the high intakes are derived largely from the consumption of tabletop sweeteners based on saccharin, and that people with diabetes may be particularly at risk. The British Diabetic Association consequently advises diabetics to vary their choice of tabletop sweeteners and products which contain them so that they do not rely exclusively on saccharin-based foods (BDA 1989; Govindji 1990).

One saccharin tablet contains around 15 mg of saccharin. The ADI for saccharin is 0–5 mg/kg body weight/day, which for a 60 kg adult is equivalent to 0–20 saccharin tablets daily. The Food Advisory Committee (FAC) recommended that the Food Minister considers placing a maximum recommended dose on food labels of saccharin-based tabletop sweeteners.

Ministers decided to accept a voluntary system of labelling table-top sweeteners, specifically to alert diabetics who consume large quantities of saccharin-based sweeteners to the possibility that they may have a high dietary intake of saccharin. In addition, a leaflet has been produced and widely circulated by industry, in consultation with MAFF and the British Diabetic Association, to inform diabetics about appropriate dietary use of saccharin (International Sweeteners Association 1992).

Saccharin-aspartame blends in diet drinks have been very popular, although manufacturers are now reformulating products to replace the saccharin with acesulfame K or aspartame. As a consequence, intakes of saccharin from diet soft drinks may decline in the future. Con-

Table 2.69 Intense non-nutritive sweeteners available in the UK in 1991

Brand name	Manufacturer	Sweetener used	Calorie values	Uses
Canderel (tablets)	Searle	Aspartame	0.3 kcal/tablet	Hot drinks
Flix (tablets)	Searle	Aspartame	0.3 kcal/tablet	Hot drinks
Hermesetas (liquid)	Hermes Sweeteners	Saccharin	4 kcal/tsp (5 ml)	Cold drinks stewed fruit, custard etc.
Hermesetas (tablets)	Hermes Sweeteners	Saccharin	negligible	Hot drinks
Hermesetas (Gold) (tablets)	Hermes Sweeteners	Acesulfame K	negligible	Hot drinks
Hermesetas Light	Hermes Sweeteners	Aspartame/ Acesulfame K	0.2 kcal per tablet	Hot drinks
Natrena (tablets)	Scholl Consumer Products Ltd	Saccharin	negligible	Hot drinks
Saxin (tablets)	Nicholas Laboratories Ltd	Saccharin	negligible	Hot drinks
Shapers (tablets)	Boots	Aspartame	0.2 kcal per tablet	Hot drinks
Sweetex (liquid)	Crookes Healthcare Ltd	Saccharin	4 drops = 1 kcal	Drinks, stewed fruit, custard
Sweetex (tablets)	Crookes Healthcare Ltd	Aspartame/Saccharin/ Lactose	0.16 kcal/tablet	Hot drinks
Natriblend (tablets)	Crookes Healthcare Ltd	Aspartame/Saccharin/ Lactose	0.16 kcal/tablet	Hot drinks

sumption of aspartame and acesulfame K is likely to increase.

The advantages and disadvantages of saccharin and other non-nutritive sweeteners are summarized in Table 2.70.

Aspartame

Aspartame was approved for use in the UK in 1983. It is approximately 200 times sweeter than sucrose. Aspartame is marketed world-wide, most frequently under the brand name Nutrasweet, and is essentially a combination of two amino acids – phenylalanine and aspartic acid – both of which occur naturally in foods. Therefore, like all proteins, aspartame has an energy value of 4 kcal per gram.

Aspartame is widely used in soft drinks and manufactured foods, and also as a tabletop sweetener. It is currently the most commercially successful intense sweetener. It has been largely responsible for the great surge in the market for 'diet' soft drinks and yoghurts. Although originally used in combination with saccharin, a number of higher quality drinks are now sweetened with aspartame alone.

Because of the presence of phenylalanine, products containing aspartame are not suitable for those on low or controlled phenylalanine diets. Therefore, all food and drink which incorporates aspartame should carry a warning to this respect (this is not a statutory requirement in the UK).

There have been concerns regarding the safety of aspartame (Centers for Disease Control 1984). Symptoms of dizziness, headaches, mood swings and impaired vision have been linked to aspartame although no scientific evidence to date suggests that these claims are justified. The safety of aspartame has recently been confirmed following review by the Committee on Toxicity of Chemicals in food (COT) and the FAC (MAFF 1992).

The advantages and disadvantages of aspartame are summarized in Table 2.70.

Acesulfame potassium (acesulfame K)

Acesulfame K is approximately 150 times sweeter than sucrose. Although approved for use in the UK in 1983, (SI 1983, No 1211) the development of its market has been slow. However, within the last few years a growing number of 'diet' and 'low-calorie' products have been reformulated using acesulfame K.

It is synergistic with other intense sweeteners such as aspartame which has both quantitative and qualitative advantages. Its ability to enhance sweetness means that smaller quantities of a sweetener are required than when it

Table 2.70 Advantages and disadvantages of permitted non-nutritive sweeteners

Non-nutritive sweetener	Advantages	Disadvantages
Saccharin	1 Very stable to food processing and storage 2 High intensity of sweetness 3 Cost-effective tabletop sweetener	1 Very apparent aftertaste reported by some people (Crapo 1988). Saccharin therefore tends to be used only as a partial replacement for sugar or in combination with other sweeteners in order to mask the bitter aftertaste 2 High temperatures may provoke a more pronounced bitter, metallic aftertaste. It is hence usually necessary to add saccharin at the end of any cooking or baking process
Aspartame	1 No aftertaste 2 Sweetness profile very close to that of sucrose	1 Unstable to prolonged heating, when it breaks down into its constituent amino acids with resulting loss of sweetness 2 Expensive, although the growing market may help reduce costs 3 Poor stability in liquid form (Horwitz and Bauer-Nehrling 1983)
Acesulfame-K	1 Stable to heat, and thus can be used in cooking and in manufactured products 2 Clean, sweet taste 3 Water-soluble 4 Maintains sweetness over a long shelf life 5 It is synergistic with other sweeteners	1 Expensive
Thaumatin	1 Intensely sweet	1 Provokes a delayed perception of sweetness 2 Has a liquorice flavour which can persist for 30 minutes 3 Not stable to processing 4 Problem of equal dispersion in the product because it is used in such small quantities

is used in isolation and this reduces costs for manufacturers.

The advantages and disadvantages of acesulfame K are summarized in Table 2.70.

Thaumatin

Thaumatin is approximately 2000 to 2500 times as sweet as sucrose. It is a protein which is extracted from the seeds of a West African plant. It is not suitable for use as a tabletop sweetener on its own, but can be combined with other sweeteners or is incorporated into foods as a flavour enhancer.

Its advantages and disadvantages are summarized in Table 2.70.

Intense sweeteners under consideration for approval

The European Commission has proposed a sweeteners directive which has already progressed through most of the discussion stage, but there have been a number of delays to its agreement. This proposal currently includes two sweeteners which are not approved in the UK.

Cyclamate

Cyclamate was originally prohibited in the UK because of concerns about carcinogenicity. However, the COT have now proposed a temporary ADI of 0–1.5 mg cyclamate/kg body weight/day.

Cyclamate is currently permitted in a number of European countries, and the EC will be reviewing the safety of cyclamate before its directive on the use of sweeteners throughout the EC is finalised. This legislation is likely to come into force in 1994 or 1995 and will supersede the existing UK regulations.

Neohesperidine dihydrochalcone

A draft proposal for the EC directive on sweeteners for use in foodstuffs has suggested that neohesperidine dihydrochalcone (NHDC) should be permitted for use. In February 1991 Agriculture and Health ministers in the UK stated that they would not oppose the inclusion of NHDC on the EC permitted list. However, the UK industry has expressed little interest in using it.

2.13.2 Nutritive sweeteners

These are sugar substitutes which make some contribution to energy and/or carbohydrate intakes. Currently, nutritive sweeteners fall into two categories

1 Compound mixtures of an intense sweetener and either:
   - a sugar (e.g. sucrose, lactose);
   - a bulk sugar substitute (e.g. sorbitol); or
   - an inert starch (e.g. maltodextrin).

2 Pure bulk sugar substitutes.

Compound mixtures

Products in this category need to be used with care since

their nutritional contribution varies. The nutritional analysis per 100 g and the likely quantities of the product to be used by the consumer must both be considered.

Products available

The two most common formulations are
1 Intense sweetener plus a sugar (sucrose or lactose).
2 Intense sweetener plus bulk sugar substitute.

The most widely available combination of intense sweetener plus a sugar is saccharin and sucrose, resulting in a product which is about four times as sweet as sucrose alone. Thus one teaspoon of this mixture replaces four teaspoons of sucrose, resulting in a 75% saving in energy intake.

Currently the most widely available combinations of an intense sweetener with a bulk sugar substitute are a mixture of aspartame and maltodextrin (see Table 2.71). However, in the near future, saccharin with fructose, acesulfame K with fructose, and aspartame with fructose are all likely to become commercially available. Care must be taken in selecting the products used since equivalent sweetness (which affects the quantity consumed and thus nutritional intake) varies considerably.

Advantages of compound mixtures

1 Some may help reduce total energy intake.
2 They can be useful to reduce consumption of simple sugars (e.g. to help prevent dental caries).

Disadvantages of compound mixtures

1 Products which contain sucrose must be used with care by some individuals (e.g. people with diabetes).
2 Not all products are suitable for use in cooking. They cannot be used to replace sugar in recipes where bulk or the reaction of sugar with fat and flour is important in the final product, i.e. in sponge cakes and some biscuits.

Bulk sugar substitutes

The bulk sweeteners currently available in the UK are fructose and the sugar alcohols or polyols: sorbitol, lactitol, mannitol, xylitol, isomalt and hydrogenated glucose syrup. Hydrogenated glucose syrup is a mixture of sugar alcohols and contains between 50% and 90% maltitol.

Table 2.71 Compound nutritive sweeteners (mixture of intense sweeteners and bulking agents) available in the UK in 1991

Brand name	Sweetener formulation	Suitability for Use in Baking	Sweetening Power Compared with Sucrose	Energy Saving
Canderel Spoonful (Searle)	Maltodextrin, aspartame	Limited	10 times as sweet	Yes
Diamin Powder (Vitalia Ltd)	Acesulfame K/cellulose	Limited	11 times as sweet	Yes
Flix Granules (Searle)	Maltodextrin, aspartame	Limited	10 times as sweet	Yes
Hermesetas Sprinkle Sweet (Hermes Sweeteners)	Maltodextrin, saccharin, thaumatin	Limited	10 times as sweet	Yes
Natrena Granules (Scholl Consumer Products)	Maltodextrin, saccharin	Limited	Equal	Yes
Shapers Granulated (Boots)	Maltodextrin, aspartame	Limited	Equal	Yes
Sionon (Boots)	Sorbitol/saccharin	Suitable	Equal	No
Sweet 'n' Low (Dietary Foods Ltd)	Saccharin, lactose	Limited	10 times as sweet	Yes
Sweet 'n' Low (2) (Dietary Foods Ltd)	Acesulfame K, lactose	Limited	10 times as sweet	Yes
Sweet 'n' Low Minicubes (Dietary Foods Ltd)	Acesulfame K	Unsuitable	10 times as sweet	Yes
Sweetex Granulated (Crookes Healthcare)	Maltodextrin, aspartame, saccharin	Limited	10 times as sweet	Yes
Trim Spoon (Whitworths)	Maltodextrin, aspartame	Unsuitable	Equal	Yes

Products available

Fructose Fructose or fruit sugar is probably the sweetest of the naturally occurring sugars. It is around 1.5 times as sweet as sucrose, although this is dependent on the prevailing physical and chemical conditions.

Sorbitol This occurs naturally in plants and is about half as sweet as sucrose. It is more slowly absorbed and is metabolized in the liver. Ingestion of around 30 g per day can cause osmotic diarrhoea, although some people may be sensitive to even less (BDA 1990). All of the sugar alcohols have a similar laxative potential.

Xylitol Found naturally in virtually all plants, xylitol is a palatable sweetener, the sweetness intensity being dependent on existing physical and chemical conditions. Some polyols, especially sorbitol and xylitol, can be used in products which require their particular properties of mild sweetness and mouth cooling (e.g. chewing gum, toothpaste, pastilles and mints).

Isomalt Isomalt has a sweetness of around 0.5 relative to sucrose. Since 1989, sugar-free confectionery based on isomalt has been marketed in the UK by several manufacturers. The products are more widely available in the rest of Europe, where they are promoted as being non-cariogenic or 'tooth-friendly'. These countries also have ice cream, biscuits and marzipan products containing isomalt although they are not yet available in the UK.

Hydrogenated glucose syrup (Lycasin®) This has a sweetness of around 0.75 relative to sucrose, and a calorific value of 3.75 kcal/g. It is used mainly in the manufacture of sucrose-free confectionery and pharmaceutical syrups where its low cariogenic properties can be useful.

Advantages of bulk sugar substitutes

Dental caries With the exception of fructose (for which only weak data exist) all the other bulk substitutes have been shown to be less cariogenic than sucrose.

Food processing The polyols do not crystallize at high temperatures so they can be used very successfully to replace sucrose in confectionery such as boiled sweets. Fructose tends to be hygroscopic so is advantageous in baking processes where staling or drying can be a problem.

Disadvantages of bulk sugar substitutes

Costs All are substantially more expensive than sucrose or glucose. This limits their use in industry and in the home.

Low relative sweetness With the exception of fructose and xylitol, all are less sweet than sugar. So, unless they are combined with intense sweeteners, greater quantities will be needed to obtain equivalent sweetness.

Gastrointestinal side effects All the polyols have pronounced effects on the gastrointestinal tract. Individual tolerance varies and, to a certain extent, depends on dosage and previous exposure. However, diarrhoea, flatulence and unpleasant stomach cramps can all be experienced on relatively low intakes of less than 25–50 g/day (BDA 1992). Some individuals, particularly children, may experience pronounced symptoms following the ingestion of very small amounts.

Browning effect Fructose-sweetened products tend to brown more quickly, so care must be taken in any baking process where fructose has been used.

Dietary application

Sorbitol and fructose are the main sugar substitutes used in the manufacture of special diabetic products. These foods have been on the market since the 1960s, when the traditional very restricted low carbohydrate diet was recommended for people with diabetes. Diabetic products had a use at that time, since some of the carbohydrate and all of the sucrose was replaced by substances with little or no glycaemic effect. The possibility of osmotic diarrhoea lead to a preferential use of fructose. However, modern dietary management of diabetes encourages a high complex carbohydrate intake within a mix of healthy low fat, low sugar foods (BDA 1991). Specialist diabetic products are of little value in such a regimen and their use is now actively discouraged (BDA 1992).

Fructose was traditionally recommended as a suitable alternative to sucrose, since initial steps of its metabolism do not require insulin. However, on review of the evidence on the use of fructose compared to sucrose, fructose is no longer advocated for people with diabetes (BDA 1990). In poorly controlled diabetes, fructose and the sugar alcohols can be converted to glucose (Akgun and Ertel 1985).

Being a monosaccharide, fructose contains 3.75 kcal/g, and it would appear that the provision of a sweet taste at a relatively lower calorie cost would be an advantage. However, there is no conclusive scientific evidence to support the use of fructose as an aid to weight reduction.

The sugar alcohols (or polyols) contain on average 2.4 kcal/g, according to the EC Proposals for Directives on Compulsory Nutrition Labelling and on Nutrition Labelling Rules for Foodstuffs (1989). However, they are unlikely to offer significant calorie savings in made-up foods. The polyols have low cariogenic properties and have been used in the preparation of a wide range of specialist products.

Table 2.72 Properties of bulk and intense sweeteners

	Sweetener	Kcal/g	Approx sweetening intensity compared to sucrose	Acceptable daily intake (ADI)	Heat tolerant	Properties	Uses	Commercial application
INTENSE	Saccharin	0	300	0–5 mg/kg[b] body weight	Yes			
	Aspartame	4.0	200	40 mg/kg[b] body weight	No	Intense sweetening power; virtually calorie and carbohydrate free	Drinks Cereals Milk puddings; Stewed fruit etc.	Soft drinks Table-top sweeteners Yogurts Sugar-free chewing gum and medicines
	Acesulfame Potassium	0	150	2.0 mg/kg[b] body weight	Yes			Not permitted for use in foods specially prepared for babies and young children
	Thaumatin	4.0	2000–2500	Not specified	Yes	Delayed and prolonged sweetness	Flavour modifier	Chewing gum and products requiring flavour enhancement
BULK	Fructose	3.75	1.5	25 g total bulk sweeteners daily (BDA* Recommendation)	Yes	Provide bulk and sweetness	Creaming mixtures and preserving	Diabetic products
	Sorbitol	2.40[a]	0.5		Yes			Tooth-friendly products;
	Lactitol		0.4		Yes			
	Mannitol		0.6		Yes			Boiled sweets (Bulk sweeteners may also not be added to soft drinks or baby foods)
	Xylitol		1.0		Yes			
	Isomalt		0.5		Yes			
					Yes			
	Hydrogenated glucose syrup	3.75	0.75		Yes			

[a] Values as outlined in the EC Proposals for Directives on Compulsory Nutrition Labelling and on Nutrition Labelling Rules for Foodstuffs (1989)
[b] Set by International Advisory Bodies
* British Diabetic Association

2.13.3 Comparative use of intense and bulk sweeteners

Table 2.72 summarizes the main properties of intense and bulk sweeteners. The intense sweeteners are marketed widely as tabletop sweeteners and in manufactured food and drink. They continue to be successful low-calorie, non-cariogenic alternatives to simple sugars and are likely to maintain their existing popularity well into the future.

Although many bulk sugar substitutes are currently available, their use at present is limited. At the moment their most effective and proven role appears to be as a substitute for sugar as part of the campaign to prevent dental caries. Even so, until they can be successfully combined with an intense sweetener, their applications will be limited both by their cost and by their gastrointestinal effects.

References

Akgun S and Ertel NH (1985) The effects of sucrose, fructose, and high-fructose corn syrup on plasma glucose and insulin in non-insulin dependent diabetic subjects. *Diabetes Care* **8**, 279–83.

Armstrong B, Lea AJ, Adelstein AM, Donovan JW, White GG and Ruttle S (1976) Cancer mortality and saccharin consumption in diabetics. *Br J Prev Soc Med* **301**, 151–7.

Atkins D (1990) Intensely sweet. *Nutrition and Food Science* **122**, 2–4.

British Diabetic Association (1989) Consumption of saccharin. *Balance* **114**, 5.

British Diabetic Association, Nutrition Sub-Committee (1990) Sucrose and fructose in the diabetic diet. *Diabetic Med* **7**, 764–69.

British Diabetic Association, Nutrition Sub-Committee (1991) Dietary recommendations for people with diabetes: an update for the 1990s. *J Hum Nutr Dietet* **4**, 393–412.

British Diabetic Association, Nutrition Sub-Committee (1992) Diebetic foods and the diabetic diet. *Diabetic Med* **9**, 300–306.

Centers for Disease Control, Division of Nutrition, Center for Health Promotion and Education (1984) Evaluation of consumer complaints related to aspartame use. *Morbid Mortal Weekly* **Rep 33**, 605–607.

Crapo PA (1988) Use of alternative sweeteners in diabetic diets. *Diabetic Care* **11**, 174–82.

Govindji A (1990) Not sugar – but Sweet! *Balance* **116**, 56–60.

Horwitz DL and Bauer-Nehrling JK (1983) Can aspartame meet our expectations? *J Am Diet Assoc* **83**, 142–6.

International Sweeteners Association (1992) *Saccharin – an information leaflet: Diabetics and sweeteners*. Available from the Saccharin Table Top Group, c/o Boswell House, 37/38 Long Acre, Covent Garden, London WC2E 9RJ.

Kessler II and Clark JP (1978) Saccharin, cyclamate and human bladder cancer. *J Am Med Assoc* **240**, 349–55.

Ministry of Agriculture, Fisheries and Food (1990) Intakes of Intense and Bulk Sweeteners in the UK 1987–88. HMSO, London.

Ministry of Agriculture, Fisheries and Food (1992) *Sweetener intake within safe limits*. MAFF Food Safety Directorate News Release. FSD 44/92, 30 July 1992.

Morrison AS and Buring JE (1980) Artificial sweeteners and cancer of the lower urinary tract. *N Eng J Med* **302**, 537–41.

Statutory Instruments (SI) (1983) No 1211. The Sweeteners in Food Regulations. HMSO, London.

Statutory Instruments (SI) (1988) No 2112. The Sweeteners in Food (Amendment) Regulations. HMSO, London.

2.14 Sources of specific foods and food components

2.14.1 Sources of gluten

Gluten-free foods

Gluten-free foods are required by those with coeliac disease (Section 4.7) and dermatitis herpetiformis (Section 4.30.4). It is generally accepted that a gluten-free diet involves the complete avoidance of all foods made from, or containing, wheat, rye, barley and usually oats (Table 2.73). Oats may be permitted, this will be decided by the consultant, however the Coeliac Society advise *against* their inclusion in the gluten-free diet.

Some manufactured products bear the gluten-free symbol on their label

indicating their suitability for inclusion in gluten-free diets. However, not all manufacturers have adopted this policy and it is not satisfactory to attempt to deduce suitability of a given product by looking at the ingredients listed on the label.

The Coeliac Society publishes a list of gluten-free manufactured products in booklet form which is up-dated every year. Where the column of permitted foods states 'certain brands', these should be sought in the Coeliac Society's list. Where necessary, categories of products are prefaced by an informative, explanatory paragraph.

It is essential that the *current* edition of the list should be referred to in order to complement the basic diet sheet and that this list is regularly updated. Patients should be strongly recommended to enrol as members of the Coeliac Society, not only in order that they be in receipt of the list but also for the other benefits which membership affords.

The address of the Society is The Coeliac Society, PO Box 220, High Wycombe, Bucks HP11 2HY, Tel: 0494 437278.

Communion wafers

Ordinary Communion wafers do contain gluten, however gluten-free wafers can be obtained at a small cost from The Poor Clares, Monastery of St Joseph, Lawrence Street, York YO1 3EB. The Coeliac Society's list of gluten-free manufactured products may list alternative sources.

New methods of analysis

Recent advances in technology using enzyme linked immunosorbant assays (ELISAs) have now made it possible to detect the presence of very small but measurable amounts of gliadin and similar proteins toxic to coeliacs such as hordein in barley and certain fruits and vegetables. Obviously these substances have always been present but previously undetectable analytically. Hordein has been found in most beers, lagers, ales and stouts which in the past have been considered suitable for inclusion in a gluten-free diet, and attention is now being drawn to malt extract and specially manufactured wheat starch. There is no clinical evidence currently available to indicate that these minute quantities are harmful to coeliacs and such evidence is unlikely to be forthcoming in the near future. Patients who have doubts about products such as beer should leave it out of their diet or consult their own medical advisers.

Gluten-testing kits

Gluten-testing kits for use by laboratories have been available in the UK for a few years and are used by public analysts. A simple 'home-test' kit, based on monoclonal antibodies to heat-stable gluten proteins has been developed and used in Australia (Skerritt and Hill 1991) and this may become available in the UK.

Prescribable items

A wide range of specially manufactured gluten-free items, e.g. biscuits, bread, bread mix, cakes, crispbread, flour, flour mix, pastas and rusks are prescribable under the NHS for gluten-sensitive enteropathies.

Full use of these products should be encouraged. Their inclusion in the diet not only adds variety, palatability and bulk but also aids compliance. Dietary indiscretions are much more likely to occur in a hungry patient.

Gluten-free bread is now available vacuum-packed, sliced and unsliced, in sealed plastic/polythene packs for longer shelf life, as well as in tins. Bread can also be made easily from a variety of mixes. Gluten-free bread can be frozen and will keep for a long time in a freezer – individual slices can be frozen to allow economical use of small amounts.

Gluten-free flours and flour mixes are available to make cakes, biscuits and other baked goods and now give

Table 2.73 Gluten-free and gluten-containing foods

Food group	Gluten-free foods	Gluten-containing foods
Cereals and flours	Arrowroot, buckwheat, corn or maize, cornflour or maize flour, gluten-free flour, potato flour (or fecule or farina), rice and rice flour, sago, soya, soya flour, tapioca. Oats* (if permitted)	Wheat, wholemeal, wholewheat and wheatmeal flours, bran, barley, rye, rye flour, pasta (macaroni, noodles, spaghetti, etc.), semolina
Prepared cereals	Made from corn or rice e.g. Cornflakes, Rice Krispies, baby rice. Porridge oats* (if permitted)	Cereals made from wheat, barley or rye, e.g. muesli, Shredded Wheat, Sugar Puffs, Weetabix
Baked goods	*Gluten-free* biscuits, bread, bread mix, cakes, crispbread, flour, flour mix, pasta, rusks. *Certain brands* of oatcakes* (if permitted)	*All ordinary baked goods* made from wheat, barley, rye flour, suet and semolina. Crispbreads and starch reduced bread and rolls. Ice cream wafers and cones. Communion wafers (see above)
Milk	Fresh, condensed, dried, evaporated, skimmed, sterilized. Fresh or tinned cream. Most brands of yoghurt. Coffee creamers and whiteners	Artificial cream containing flour. Yoghurt containing muesli
Cheese	Plain, e.g. Cheddar, cottage cheese, cream cheese, curd cheese. *Certain brands* of cheese spreads	Cheese spreads containing flour
Eggs	Prepared and cooked without flour and breadcrumbs	Prepared and cooked with flour or breadcrumbs e.g. Scotch eggs
Fats and oils	Butter, margarine, oil, lard, dripping	Suet
Meat and fish	All varieties prepared and cooked without flour and breadcrumbs. *Certain brands* of canned meat and canned fish in sauce. *Certain brands* of meat and fish pastes. *Certain brands* of continental sausages. *Certain brands* of burgers	Savoury pies and puddings containing flour, breadcrumbs, stuffing and suet. Sausages and burgers containing breadcrumbs. Battered or crumbed fish, fish fingers, fish cakes
Vegetables	Fresh, cooked, canned, dried, frozen, pulses, soya. *Certain brands* of baked beans. *Certain brands* of potato crisps	Vegetables canned in sauce e.g. creamed mushrooms. Potato croquettes. Textured vegetable protein containing wheat
Fruit	Fresh, cooked, canned, dried, frozen	
Nuts	Fresh and plain, salted. *Certain brands* of dry roasted nuts	
Preserves and confectionery	Sugar, glucose, jam, honey, malt, malt extract, marmalade, molasses, treacle, *certain brands* of mincemeat. *Certain brands* of sweets and chocolate. Plain ice lollies	Sweets containing or rolled in flour, e.g. liquorice, unwrapped sweets, Smarties, Twix
Puddings and desserts	Jelly, milk puddings made from permitted cereals **NOT** semolina. Home-made puddings using gluten-free ingredients. *Certain brands* of instant desserts. *Certain brands* of ice cream	Puddings and desserts containing flour, breadcrumbs and suet. Ice cream cones and wafers
Beverages	Tea, pure instant or fresh ground coffee, cocoa, fizzy drinks, squashes and cordials, fresh fruit juices, wines, spirits, beers[1] lagers[1]	Barley-based instant coffee, barley flavoured fruit drinks. Bengers, malted drinks e.g. Horlicks. Home brewed beer, cloudy real ale, hot drinks from vending machines
Soups, sauces and gravies	Soup, sauce and gravy if thickened with suitable cereal. *Certain brands* of tinned and dried soups. *Certain brands* of stock concentrates, gravy brownings and gravy salts	Soup, sauce and gravy thickened with or containing wheat, barley, rye or pasta. Bisto

Table 2.73 *contd.*

Food group	Gluten-free foods	Gluten-containing foods
Seasonings	Salt, fresh ground or pure pepper. Herbs, pure spices, vinegar. *Certain brands* of ready-to-eat mustard. *Certain brands* of ready mixed spices, seasonings and curry powders. Monosodium glutamate	Pepper compound, ready-mixed spices, seasonings and curry powders containing flour as a 'filler'
Miscellaneous	Bicarbonate of soda, cream of tartar, tartaric acid. *Certain brands* of baking powder, fresh and dried yeast, colourings and essences, gelatine	Medication containing gluten

The foregoing lists are intended only as a basic guide to the suitability of 'everyday' foods
[1] See preceding text on 'New Methods of Analysis'

results which look and taste exactly like items cooked with ordinary flour. To obtain the best results, the recipes given by individual manufacturers for their own products *must* be followed; it is no longer satisfactory to substitute gluten-free flour for ordinary flour in ordinary recipes, or to interchange one gluten-free flour for another.

A list of prescribable items appears in the current editions of *Monthly Index of Medical Specialities* (MIMS) and the *British National Formulary* under the Borderline Substances Appendix, and in Appendix 1 of the current Coeliac Society food list. Prescriptions should be marked 'ACBS' (Advisory Committee for Borderline Substances). Prescribable items (at the time of going to press) are listed in Table 2.74.

Children under 16 years, pregnant women, men aged 65 years or over and women aged 60 years or over are exempt from prescription charges. Other adults may find it economical to buy a 'season ticket', (prepayment of charges) for their prescriptions. Form FP 95 (EC 95 in Scotland) is available from Post Offices, local social security offices and chemists. Further information may be found in leaflet P11 – *NHS prescriptions, how to get them free.*

Certain other gluten-free products are considered non-essential luxuries rather than staple items, and therefore must be purchased – they are *not* available on prescription. These products can be ordered from a chemist. Alternatively, certain products may be available by mail order direct from the manufacturers or distributors. Before recommending 'over the counter' products to their patients, dietitians should be aware that most of these products are inordinately expensive and often represent poor value for money.

Table 2.74 Gluten-free foods available on prescription (as at April 1992)

The following food preparations are listed as prescribable under the NHS Service for Coeliac and Dermatitis Herpetiformis patients. It is necessary for such prescriptions to be marked 'as per ACBS'

Bread	Ener-G brown rice bread (sliced) Ener-G white rice bread (sliced) Ener-G tapioca bread (sliced)	GD[1]
	Glutafin gluten-free loaf (sliced or unsliced) Glutafin gluten-free fibre loaf (sliced or unsliced)	NUT
	Juvela gluten-free loaf (sliced and whole) Juvela gluten-free fibre loaf (sliced and whole) Juvela low protein loaf (sliced and whole)	SHS
	Loprofin low protein loaf (sliced or unsliced) Rite-Diet gluten-free white bread Rite-Diet high fibre bread Rite-Diet low protein white bread with added fibre Rite-Diet gluten-free low protein canned white bread Rite-Diet gluten-free low protein canned bread with added soya bran Rite-Diet gluten-free low protein canned white bread with no added salt	NUT
	Schär bread Schär bread rolls Schär pizza bases Ultra high fibre bread Ultra low protein and gluten-free canned brown bread Ultra low protein and gluten-free canned white bread	ULT

Table 2.74 *contd.*

The following food preparations are listed as prescribable under the NHS Service for Coeliac and Dermatitis Herpetiformis patients. It is necessary for such prescriptions to be marked 'as per ACBS'

Category	Product	Manufacturer[1]
Biscuits	Aproten biscuits	ULT
	Arnott's Rice Cookies	ULT
	Bi-Aglut gluten-free biscuits	ULT
	Farley's gluten-free biscuits	FAR
	G.F. Dietary gluten-free biscuits	NUT
	Glutafin gluten-free biscuits	NUT
	Glutafin gluten-free tea biscuits	NUT
	Glutafin gluten-free sweet biscuits	NUT
	Glutafin gluten-free digestive biscuits	NUT
	Glutafin gluten-free savoury biscuits	NUT
	Liga gluten-free rusks	JAC
	Polial gluten-free biscuits	ULT
	Schär Savoy biscuits	ULT
Flours and mixes	Aproten bread mix	ULT
	Aproten cake mix	ULT
	Aproten flour	ULT
	Glutafin gluten-free mix	NUT
	Glutafin gluten-free fibre mix	NUT
	Juvela corn mix	SHS
	Juvela gluten-free mix	SHS
	Juvela gluten-free fibre mix	SHS
	Juvela low protein mix	SHS
	Kallo brown flour alternative	KAL
	Kallo white flour alternative	KAL
	Kallo low protein flour alternative	KAL
	Loprofin low protein mix	NUT
	Rite-Diet white bread mix	NUT
	Rite-Diet brown bread mix	NUT
	Rite-Diet gluten-free flour mix	NUT
	Rite-Diet low protein flour mix	NUT
	Rite-Diet baking mix	NUT
	Schär bread mix	ULT
	Tritamyl gluten-free flour	PROC
	Trufree flours Nos 1–7	CANT
Crackers	Aproten crispbread	ULT
	Bi-Aglut cracker toast	ULT
	Glutafin gluten-free crackers	NUT
	Glutafin high fibre crackers	NUT
	Loprofin low protein crackers	NUT
	Schär crackers	ULT
	Schär crispbread	ULT
	Ultra crackerbread	ULT
Pasta	Aproten – low protein anellini, ditalini, rigatini, tagliatelle, spaghetti	ULT
	Ener-G – shells, small shells, spaghetti, lasagna, tagliatelle, vermicelli, cannelloni	GD
	Glutafin – macaroni, pasta spirals, short cut spaghetti	NUT
	Loprofin – low protein macaroni, short cut spaghetti, pasta spirals	NUT
	Pastariso – spaghetti, elbow macaroni, fettucini, fusilli, mini elbows, spirals, twists	GD
	Schär – fusilli, rigatoni, tagliatelle, penne, spaghetti	ULT

All of these products are available through chemists' shops, but may have to be specially ordered

See the subsection on 'Prescribable items – the changing scene'

[1] Manufacturers:
CANT Cantassium Co
FAR Farley Health Products
GD General Designs Ltd
JAC Jacob's Bakery Ltd
KAL Kallo Foods Ltd
NUT Nutricia Dietary Products Ltd
PROC Procea
SHS Scientific Hospital Supplies Ltd
ULT Ultrapharm Ltd

Manufacturers' addresses are given in Appendix 9

Prescribable items — the changing scene

In the 1980s, two major companies, Welfare Foods (using the brand name of Rite-Diet) and the GF Dietary Group (using several brand names including Juvela), had the largest share of the specially produced gluten-free food market. Neither of these companies now exist having been taken over by Nutricia Dietary Products Ltd, and some of the old brand names have been acquired by other companies. Coincidentally, several other companies have increased their market share or come into the market, resulting in the introduction of many new products. Numerous other products have been discontinued, and some renamed, all causing immense confusion to the doctor, patient, dietitian and pharmacist.

In April 1992, 105 different items were available to coeliacs on prescription and it has become impossible to keep up with the changes in non-prescribable items. There are now nine manufacturers who produce product information and technical handouts of varying quality — not all companies have medical or dietetic advisers to provide input of a suitable standard.

The Coeliac Society publishes an up-to-date list of prescribable items six-monthly in each issue of their magazine *The Crossed Grain* and the current list is always available on receipt of a stamped addressed envelope. Accompanying the list is an index of manufacturers and the latter should be contacted directly for their own lists of non-prescribable items.

Due to these changes and the recent proliferation of gluten-free items on prescription, considerable difficulties have been experienced by dietitians in knowing what to suggest to patients, and by newly diagnosed coeliacs in particular in knowing what to select. Tastes vary and some products are of a better quality and more acceptable than others. For example, gluten-free products made specifically for coeliacs are usually more palatable than those which are also suitable for low protein diets. The situation is further complicated by the computerized systems which most general practitioners are now, very sensibly, using for repeat prescriptions. If patients do not like a product, or if they wish to try something new or different, it can be difficult to change a prescription once on the computer.

Dietitians are the best people to advise GPs what is available for coeliacs and how much an individual patient may require. In order not to appear biased towards one company or a particular product, dietitians require sufficient information about all products to advise both patients and their doctors. Talking to coeliac patients and listening to their experiences and preferences as well as contacting the manufacturers to request samples and full information would seem to be the best way of acquiring this information.

Gluten-free, soya-free foods

Reference should be made to the foregoing section covering 'everyday' gluten-free foods. In addition to the forbidden foods listed, the following should also be avoided

1 Soya beans.
2 Soya grits.
3 Soya flour.
4 Hydrolysed, 'spun' or 'textured' vegetable protein of soya origin.
5 Soya milk.
6 Soya-based flavouring.
7 Soya oil.
8 Soya protein isolate.

Using the Coeliac Society food list, the ingredients of those foods listed should be checked for the presence or absence of soya.

Up to 2% soya (usually as soya isolate) fulfils such purposes as water binding, emulsification and whippability in a wide range of foods including baby foods, hams, sausages, pastes and other meat products, fish products, dessert toppings, yoghurt, coffee whiteners, dairy products and ice cream, snack foods and sugar confectionery.

Soya products may be the major component of products intended for use as meat 'extenders' usually in textured forms such as extruded defatted soya flour or spun soya isolate. These textured products may be present in some meat products in addition to the legally required minimum meat content. Soya flour is often present in sausages as a binder at levels of 2–3%.

Prescribable items

Many gluten-free prescribable items contain soya to improve protein content, palatability and texture, and are therefore contraindicated. Details of foods which are both gluten-free and soya-free should be obtained from manufacturers.

Gluten-free low lactose foods

A gluten-free, low lactose diet involves the complete avoidance of several cereals (see 'gluten-free foods'; Table 2.73) and of milk, most milk products and milk derivatives (see 'milk-free foods'; Table 2.76).

Combining these two sections will provide comprehensive lists of everyday foods which are permitted and forbidden on a gluten-free, milk-free diet. However, the percentage of lactose in butter is so small (approximately 0.4–1% maximum) as to render it suitable for use in most cases of simple lactose intolerance. Similarly, most types of pure cheese contain only traces of lactose. Norwegian Mysost does contain significant quantities of lactose, as does cottage cheese and processed cheeses such as cheese spreads and cheese portions. Hence apart from allowing butter and pure cheese, the permitted and forbidden foods are the same for a low lactose regimen as for a milk-free regimen.

A list of 'wheat-free, milk-free manufactured foods' is

available to dietitians at a small cost from The British Dietetic Association (but see Section 2.15). This may be used as a basis for ascertaining suitable gluten-free, low lactose proprietary items.

Details of products which may be prescribed for gluten-sensitive enteropathies with associated lactose intolerance should be obtained from manufacturers.

2.14.2 Sources of wheat

Wheat is present in a wide variety of foods (including flour, pasta, many breakfast cereals, cakes, biscuits) and in many manufactured foods in the form of, for example, gluten, wheat starch, rusk and hydrolysed vegetable protein of wheat origin. It is important that all sources of wheat (including wheat protein and starch) are excluded from a patient's diet. Many special gluten-free products (e.g. bread and biscuits) contain wheat starch and are not suitable for use in wheat intolerance. This, in fact, reduces the variety of special foods available, which ultimately increases the difficulties of adhering to the diet. In practice, patients may react not only to wheat but also to other grains such as oats, rye, corn and barley. These as well may need to be excluded initially and reintroduced at a later stage.

Table 2.75 lists foods to be included and excluded on a wheat free diet. A list of wheat-free manufactured foods is available to dietitians from the British Dietetic Association (see Section 2.15).

2.14.3 Sources of egg

Egg is one of the foods to which sensitivity is more common. An egg-free diet involves the complete avoidance of eggs and foods containing whole egg, dried egg, egg yolk, egg albumin or egg lecithin. Such foods include egg pasta, most biscuits and cakes, meringues and mayonnaise. The British Dietetic Association produces a list of manufactured egg-free foods for use by dietitians (see Section 2.15).

Substitutes for egg

Rite-diet egg replacer (Nutricia Dietary Products Ltd) This is a low protein, low phenylalanine, low fat and cholesterol-free product which can be used as a substitute for egg. It is composed of potato starch, modified maize starch, thickener, cellulose gum, calcium polyphosphate, carotene and potassium carbonate. One teaspoon of egg replacer mixed with two tablespoons of water is equivalent to one egg.

Rite-diet egg white replacer (Nutricia Dietary Products Ltd) This is comprised of purified methyl ethyl cellulose which, when made up into a solution, provides an excellent meringue substitute.

Ener-G low protein egg replacer (General Designs Ltd) This is a low protein and cholesterol-free culinary replacement for egg. It comprises potato starch, tapioca flour, methylcellulose, calcium carbonate, citric acid and calcium lactate. It is available in a 510 g carton which is equivalent to 180 eggs.

2.14.4 Sources of milk

Milk is particularly difficult to exclude from a patient's diet. In addition to the fact that milk and products based on milk are important components of the average diet, many popular manufactured foods contain milk or milk derivatives. A dietitian's help is essential if a patient (or parent) is to remove milk completely from a diet without adverse nutritional consequences.

A milk-free diet involves the complete avoidance of cows' milk, goats' and sheep's milk, milk products such as butter, cheese, cream and yoghurt and milk derivatives such as casein, whey, skimmed milk, non-fat milk solids and hydrolysed whey. Lactose is also found in many foods and in retail brands of monosodium glutamate (MSG),

Table 2.75 Foods suitable or unsuitable for a wheatfree diet

	Wheat-free foods	Foods containing wheat or wheat products
Cereal foods	Rice, oats, corn, (maize), barley, millet, arrowroot, banana flour, barley flour and barley flakes, buckwheat and buckwheat flour, buckwheat flakes, chestnut flour, chickpea flour, cornflour, maize flour, potato flour, popping corn, oats and oatmeal, rice, rice flour, rye flour and rye flakes, sago and sago flour, tapioca and tapioca flour	
	Certain brands of crispbreads e.g. Ryvita Light and Dark Rye, Finn Crisp Original Rye and Light Rye Rice cakes without added wheat bran Bread, cake, pastry and biscuits made from permitted ingredients	Batter, bread, breadcrumbs, biscuits, buns, cakes, chapatis, crackers, croissants, crumpets, doughnuts, dumplings, fritters, muffins, noodles, oatcakes, pancakes, pasta (including buckwheat spaghetti), pastry, pies, pizza, rusks,

Table 2.75 *contd.*

	Wheat-free foods	Foods containing wheat or wheat products
	Certain brands of gluten-free products	scones, semolina, shortbread, starch-reduced rolls, stuffings, wheatgerm, wheat bran, wheat crispbreads, e.g. high fibre Ryvita
	Cornflakes, Rice Krispies, Porridge, Crunchy Nut Cornflakes, Homemade Muesli, Frosties, Ricicles Soya, oat and rice bran	Wheat or bran-containing breakfast cereals such as All-Bran, Weetaflakes, Shredded wheat, Bran Flakes, Muesli, Special K, Sugar Puffs
Meat and meat products	Fresh or plainly frozen beef, chicken, duck, goose, lamb, offal, pork, rabbit, turkey, venison Bacon	Any meat cooked in batter, breadcrumbs, gravy, pastry, flour or sauce (unless known to be suitable)
	Plain soya protein and mince	Certain brands of beefburgers, croquettes, tinned meats, forcemeat, frankfurters, haggis, ham, salami, sausages. Dehydrated and ready prepared meat dishes Vegeburger mixes and soya protein mixes and dishes Meat paste, paté and spread
Fish and fish products	All fresh and plainly frozen fish Shellfish Fish canned in oil or brine Smoked fish	Any fish cooked in batter, breadcrumbs, pastry, flour or sauce (unless known to be suitable) Fish fingers, fish cakes Taramasalata Certain brands of ready prepared fish dishes, tinned fish in sauce, fish paste, paté and spread
Eggs	Egg — boiled, fried, poached, scrambled, omelette Meringue nests	Scotch egg, quiche and other egg dishes made with flour
Dairy and soya milk products	Fresh, dried, evaporated and condensed milk Fresh cream, sour cream Plain unsweetened yoghurt Smetana, buttermilk	Certain brands of sweetened yoghurts
	Cheese, plain cottage cheese, cottage cheese and pineapple	Certain brands of cheese spread and processed cheese Some flavoured cottage cheese
Fats and oils	Butter, most margarines and low-fat spread Sunflower, safflower, olive, peanut, grapeseed, rapeseed, sesame and soya oils Lard, suet coated in rice flour	Wheatgerm oil, vegetable oil of unspecified origin Suet coated in wheat flour Margarines containing wheatgerm oil e.g. Vitaquell
Vegetables	All fresh or plainly frozen varieties or those canned in salt and water only Certain brands of dehydrated vegetable dishes. Dried pulses e.g. butter beans, kidney beans, lentils, chickpeas Tofu Certain brands of baked beans e.g. Heinz	Tinned vegetables in sauce, ready prepared salads in dressing, mayonnaise or salad cream Potato waffles, potato croquettes

Table 2.75 *contd.*

	Wheat-free foods	Foods containing wheat or wheat products
Fruit	Fresh fruit or plainly frozen fruit of all kinds Tinned fruit in natural juice, syrup or water Dried and stewed fruit Certain brands of fruit pie filling Fruit juices	Fruit pies
Desserts	Homemade puddings from permitted ingredients e.g. rice pudding, custard, egg custard Jelly and jelly crystals Sorbet and water ice	Blancmanges, bread puddings, cakes, creme caramel, Christmas pudding, custards, gateaux, flans, icing, pancakes, pies, instant mixes, steamed puddings, semolina, souffles, tarts, trifles. Ice cream cones and wafers
Soups, sauces and gravy	Homemade, from permitted ingredients Heinz Tomato Ketchup	Most tinned, packet, powdered and creamed varieties Bottled sauces Gravy granules and mix
Beverages and fruit drinks	Tea, teabags, freshly ground coffee 100% instant coffee powder, coffee essence, cocoa, drinking chocolate Most coffee whiteners — check label Fruit squashes, fizzy drinks, barley cup, Caro Fruit juice, V8 juice, tomato juice	Malted milks e.g. Horlicks Ovaltine, Bournvita Instant drinking chocolate Herbal teas Cereal based beverages such as Bambu
Alcoholic beverages	Wine, champagne, sherry, brandy, slivowitz, calvados, tequila, vodka, rum, cider	Ale, beer, lager, stout, whisky, gin, liqueurs, vermouth
Sugar spreads and preserves	Sugar brown or white, icing sugar, jam, marmalade and fruit spread Sunflower and sesame spread Golden syrup, treacle, molasses Marmite and Vecon	Orange or lemon curd Commercial spreads including sandwich spread, chocolate spread honey spread. Mincemeat, Bovril
Condiments	Table salt, peppercorns, fresh herbs and spices, homemade curry powder Check that no flour has been added to spices e.g. chilli compound Vinegar, tomato puree Clear pickles e.g. onions, gherkins	Celery salt, garlic salt, ready-mixed curry powder, mustard, pepper compounds, stock cubes e.g. OXO Meat tenderizer, thickened pickles and chutney
Raising agents	Yeast, sodium bicarbonate, tartaric acid, cream of tartar, grain-free baking powder, e.g. salt-free Baking Powder. Homemade baking powder	Commercial baking powder
Confectionery	Boiled sweets, fruit gums and pastilles, milk and plain chocolate. Hard mints Plain Ice lollies Dried fruit bars	Liquorice, filled chocolates, and chocolate bars e.g. KitKat, Mars Bar Fancy ice lollies
Nuts and savoury snacks	Nuts in shells, e.g. almonds, cashews, brazils Peanut butter Ready-salted crisps	Dry roasted peanuts, marzipan, praline Twiglets, Cheeselets and similar savoury snacks. Flavoured crisps

Note. Where reference is made to 'certain brands', these should be sought in the wheat-free manufactured products list which may be purchased by dietitians from the British Dietetic Association certain low calorie sweeteners and as a constituent of some crisps, stock cubes and dried soups. Lactose is also used by the pharmaceutical industry as a filler in some tablets.

For practical purposes, no differentiation is usually made between cows' milk protein intolerance and lactose intolerance. However, goats' and sheep's milk may be tolerated in the diet of some cases of cows' milk protein intolerance but, since goats' and sheep's milk contain lactose, they are unsuitable for those with lactose intolerance.

Foods which are either suitable or unsuitable for inclusion in a milk-free diet are listed in Table 2.76. However, these are only guidelines and it must be stressed to patients that the ingredient list of manufactured brands of items should be checked for the presence of milk or a milk derivative. The British Dietetic Association regularly prints a list of milk-free manufactured foods for use by dietitians, but it must be remembered that this rapidly becomes out of date owing to the changes in formulation of foods or the introduction of new products (see Section 2.15).

Fortunately, many recipes can be adapted by using milk-free margarines to replace butter or ordinary margarine and by using a milk substitute to replace milk, Since milk normally provides a major source of protein, energy, calcium, riboflavin and vitamin A in the diet of infants and young children, it is vitally important that a nutritionally complete milk substitute is given to those who are milk intolerant. Nutritionally complete milk substitutes are prescribable in cases of milk or lactose intolerance and galactosaemia. A list of prescribable soya-based milk substitutes can be found in MIMS or the *British National Formulary* and those available as in 1991 are listed in Table 2.77.

Casein hydrolysate milks (i.e. Nutramigen and Pregestimil) show virtually no antigenic cross-reactivity with cows' milk (McLaughlan *et al* 1981) and because of their

Table 2.76 Foods suitable or unsuitable for a milk-free diet

Milk-free foods		Foods containing milk or milk derivatives
Complete milk substitutes		*All milk*
Infasoy	Cow and Gate Nutricia	Fresh, condensed, dried, evaporated, skimmed
Wysoy	Wyeth Laboratories	
Isomil	Abbott	
Ostersoy	Farleys	
Prosobee	Mead Johnson	
Pregestimil	Mead Johnson	
Nutramigen	Mead Johnson	
Milk-free margarines		*Milk products*
DP Pure, Rakusens, Tomor, Telma, Vitaquel, Suma, Vitasieg		Butter, all types of cheese Fresh and tinned cream
Certain brands of low fat spread, Suma, Outline, Granose diet half-fat spread, Tomor sunflower low-fat spread		Margarines and spreads containing milk
Vegetable oil, lard, suet, dripping		
Soya yoghurt, soya 'ice cream', soya desserts		Yoghurt, ice cream, dairy desserts, mousse
Prepared cereals		
Certain brands of baby cereals e.g. Farley's Farex, Boot's baby rice		Baby cereal containing milk e.g. Robinson's baby rice, Boot's strawberry baby rice
Certain brands of rusks e.g. Farley's original, banana and orange rusks		Rusks containing milk e.g. Farley's low sugar and granulated rusks, Jacob's Liga rusks
Certain brands of breakfast cereals e.g. Cornflakes, Rice Krispies		Breakfast cereals containing milk e.g. Special K, Coco pops, Weetos chocolate flavour, some brands of muesli
Cereals and flour		
Cornflour, all varieties of flour, *certain brands* of blancmange powder, oats, rice, sago, semolina, tapioca, spaghetti, macaroni		Instant desserts, instant porridge, milk puddings
Baked goods and puddings		*Baked goods and puddings*
Bread (standard white, brown and wholemeal). Home-made cakes, biscuits and puddings using milk-free ingredients. *Certain brands* of cakes, biscuits and puddings.		Milk bread, fancy bread and buns, cakes, biscuits and puddings made with milk or milk products
Meat and fish		*Meat/fish products*
All varieties prepared and cooked without milk and milk products		Meat products containing milk derivatives
Certain brands of sausages, fish fingers etc.		
Eggs		

Table 2.76 *contd.*

Milk-free foods	Foods containing milk or milk derivatives
Vegetables Fresh, cooked, canned, dried, frozen, pulses, soya beans *Certain brands* of baked beans *Certain brands* of instant potato *Certain brands* of potato crisps	*Vegetables* Vegetables canned in sauce containing milk or milk products Instant potato containing milk or milk products
Fruit Fresh, cooked, canned, dried, frozen, fruit pie filling Fresh fruit juice	
Nuts Fresh and plain salted Peanut butter	*Nuts* Dry roasted nuts with a lactose-containing flavouring
Preserves and confectionary Sugar, glucose, jam, honey, syrup, marmalade, molasses, treacle, mincemeat. *Certain brands* of lemon curd, *certain brands* of sweets and plain chocolate. Plain ice lollies, sorbet, jelly. *Certain brands* of carob bars and carob coated items	*Preserves and confectionary* Toffee, fudge, caramels, butterscotch, milk chocolate, filled chocolates, milk gums, milk lollies
Beverages Soya milks, e.g. Granose, Sunrise, Provamel, Plamil, Soyagen. Tea, coffee, cocoa. *Certain brands* of 'drinking chocolate' Bovril, Marmite, squashes and cordials, fizzy drinks, wines, spirits and beers etc.	*Beverages* Malted milks e.g. Bournvita, Horlicks, Ovaltine Instant and vending machine tea Cream based liquers and cocktails
Soups, sauces, gravies and salad cream Home-made using milk free ingredients. *Certain brands* of convenience soups, sauces and gravies. *Certain brands* of mayonnaise and salad cream, seasoning. Salt, pepper, herbs, spices, vinegar, mustard	*Soups, sauces, gravies and salad cream* Soups, sauces, gravies and salad cream containing milk products or milk derivatives Monosodium glutamate with a lactose filler
Miscellaneous Bicarbonate of soda, cream of tartar, tartaric acid, baking powder, fresh and dried yeast, colourings and essences. Canderel Spoonful	*Miscellaneous* Tablets containing a lactose filler. Low calorie sweeteners containing lactose e.g. 'Sweet 'n' Low'. Canderel tablets

Note: Where reference is made to *certain brands*, these should be sought in the milk-free manufactured products list, which may be purchased by dietitians from the British Dietetic Association

Table 2.77 Nutritionally complete milk substitutes (soya) available for infants and children

Milk	Protein source	Fat source	Carbohydrate source	Suitable for	
				Vegetarian	Vegan
Infasoy (Cow and Gate)	Soya protein isolate L methionine, taurine, carnitine	Palm, coconut, maize safflower oils	Glucose syrup	Yes	No
Prosobee Powder (Mead Johnson)	Soya protein isolate L methionine	Corn, coconut oils	Glucose syrup solids	Yes	No
Prosobee Liquid (Mead Johnson)	Soya protein isolate L methionine	Soya, coconut oils	Glucose syrup solids	Yes	No
Wysoy Powder (Wyeth)	Soya protein isolate L methionine, taurine, carnitine	Palm, coconut, oleic oil, soya or corn, lecithin	Glucose syrup solids	Yes	No
Wysoy Liquid (Wyeth)	Soya protein isolate L methionine, taurine, carnitine	Palm, coconut, oleic oil, soya or corn, lecithin	Glucose syrup solids	Yes	No
Isomil (Abbott)	Soya protein isolate L methionine, taurine, carnitine	Corn, coconut oils	Glucose syrup solids Sucrose	Yes	Yes
Ostersoy (Farleys)	Soya protein isolate L methionine, taurine, carnitine	Groundnut, palm kernel, palm oils	Glucose syrup solids	Yes	Yes

low allergenic properties they are preferable to soya, goats' and sheep's milks, especially for children under one year. However, the choice of milk substitute will depend on the age of the patient, the range of foods included in the diet and the quantity consumed. Casein hydrolysate milks, for example, have a strong taste and smell and may be unacceptable to a young child drinking from an open feeding cup. Nutritionally adequate soya protein-isolate formula such as Infasoy, Wysoy, Isomil, Prosobee and Ostersoy may be more acceptable to a child over the age of one year. Many other available soya milk preparations, containing soya and sugar only, are nutritionally incomplete and therefore unsuitable for infants and young children.

Nutritionally incomplete milk replacements are available from health food shops and some supermarkets. These do not provide the same nutrients as cows' milk and should never be regarded as an adequate nutritional supplement. Such 'social' milk replacements may be a useful adjunct to the diet of older children and adults.

Further reading

Ambasna C, Brostoff J and Scadding G (1987) *Cooking and eating for allergies*. Details available from the Good Housekeeping Institute, National Magazine House, 72 Broadwick Street, London W1V 2BP.

Armstrong D and Cant A (1986) *The Allergy Free Cookbook*. Octopus, London.

Dowell P and Bailey A (1988) *The book of ingredients*. Michael Joseph, London.

Francis D (1987) Food Intolerance and Allergy. In *Diets for Sick Children* 4e pp. 77–127. Blackwell Scientific Publications, Oxford.

Hanssen M (1987) *The new E for additives*. Thorsons, Wellingborough, Northants.

Igoe RS (1989) *Dictionary of Food Ingredients* 2e. Van Nostrand Reinhold, London.

Workman E, Hunter J and Alun Jones V (1984) *The allergy diet*. Martin Dunitz, London.

Workman E, Alun Jones V and Hunter J (1986) *The food intolerance diet book*. Martin Dunitz, London.

References

McLaughlan P, Anderson KJ and Coombs RRA (1981) An oral screening procedure to determine the sensitizing capacity of infant feeding formulae. *Clin Allergy* **11**, 311–18.

Skerritt JH and Hill AS (1991) Self management of dietary compliance in Coeliac Disease by means of ELISA 'home-test' to detect gluten. *Lancet* **337**, 379–82.

2.15 Manufactured food products free from specified ingredients

Lists of manufactured foods free from specified ingredients are available to State Registered Dietitians for use as part of the dietary advice given to patients requiring a medically prescribed diet.

In 1965 the dietitian at the Hospital for Sick Children, Great Ormond Street, London, compiled a list of gluten-free foods to help coeliac patients. Over the years other dietitians collected information for their own patients on other types of products, e.g. lactose-free. In 1976 this was systematized when specific dietetic departments undertook responsibility for compiling specific food lists, e.g. lactose-free, wheat-free, etc. These were then made available to all from the British Dietetic Association (BDA). In 1984 the BDA took this a stage further when it centralized the collection of information and put it on computer.

However, in April 1984, a Joint Royal College of Physicians/British Nutrition Foundation (RCP-BNF) Report on Food Intolerance and Food Aversion recommended that food manufacturers consider the possibility of setting up a central databank where products free of ingredients known to be responsible for intolerance could be registered. As a result of this recommendation, the Scientific and Technical Committee of the Food and Drink Federation set up a working party to examine the feasibility of setting up such a databank. The working party included representatives from the Food and Drink Federation, Leatherhead Food Research Association, the Food Research Institute, Norwich, the British Nutrition Foundation, the Royal College of Physicians and the British Dietetic Association.

The databank was set up, and was in operation by the end of 1986. At the time of writing, lists of foods 'free' from any combination of wheat, milk, egg, soya, cocoa, sulphur dioxide, benzoate, glutamate, azo colour and the antioxidants BHA and BHT can be produced, and used in the diagnosis and management of food intolerances.

The more frequently used lists are published by, and may be purchased from, the British Dietetic Association. Other lists may be obtained by State Registered Dietitians on application to the Leatherhead Food Research Association.

The definition of 'free from' caused the Working Party great problems, there being virtually no evidence in the medical literature on the levels of ingredients or additives in foods which can provoke reactions in a susceptible individual. The definitions finally adopted in September 1986 are given in Table 2.78.

The RCP/BNF Joint Report also concluded that:

'The dietary approach to the management of food intolerance is particularly complex and may lead to nutritional difficulties and social disruption. There are considerable

Table 2.78 Definitions of 'free from' adopted by the Food Intolerance Working Party of the FDF in 1986

Food/food additive	Derivatives/additives covered	Notes
Milk and milk derivatives	Butter, caseinates, cheese, cream, lactose, margarine or shortening containing whey, whey, whey syrup sweetener, yoghurt	'Free from' is to be interpreted as contains no added milk or milk derivative
Egg and egg derivatives	Dried egg, egg albumen, egg lecithin, egg yolk, fresh egg	'Free from' is to be interpreted as contains no added egg or egg derivative
Wheat and wheat derivatives	Breadcrumbs, hydrolysed wheat protein, rusk, wheat bran, wheat binder, wheatflour, wheat germ, wheat germ oil, wheat gluten, raising agent containing wheat starch, wheat starch, wheat thickener, wholewheat	'Free from' is to be interpreted as contains no wheat or wheat derivative. NB the wheat-free list will be for actual wheat intolerance and not for gluten intolerance; gluten-free lists are already available from The Coeliac Society
Soya and soya derivatives	Flavouring (soya), hydrolysed vegetable protein (soya), lecithin (soya) (E322), soya protein products	'Free from' is to be interpreted as contains no added soya or soya derivatives. NB a product declared as 'free from soya and soya derivatives' may contain soya oil and/or shortening. Such products will be separately identified in a manner similar to that undertaken in the current BDA list of soya-free manufactured foods, from products declared as free from soya and soya derivatives **and** free from soya oil and soya shortening

Table 2.78 contd.

Food/food additive	Derivatives/additives covered	Notes
Cocoa	Cocoa powder, cocoa butter	
BHA and BHT		These are the permitted antioxidants butylated hydroxyanisole (E320) and butylated hydroxytoluene (E321) 'Free from' is to be interpreted as contains less than 1 mg/kg BHA and/or BHT calculated from the level of addition to the food but having due regard to the presence of these compounds in ingredients and thereby carried over into the food
Sulphur dioxide	Sulphur dioxide (220), sodium sulphite (E221), sodium hydrogen sulphite (sodium bisulphite) (E222), sodium metabisulphite (E223), potassium metabisulphite (E224), calcium sulphite (E226), calcium hydrogen sulphite (calcium bisulphite) (E227)	'Free from' is to be interpreted as contains less than 1 mg/kg free sulphur dioxide as determined by the Tanner* method or an equivalent technique
Benzoate	Benzoic acid (E210), sodium benzoate (E211), potassium benzoate (E212), calcium benzoate (E213), ethyl 4-hydroxybenzoate (ethyl para-hydroxybenzoate) (E214), ethyl 4-hydroxybenzoate, Na salt (sodium ethyl para-hydroxybenzoate) (E215), propyl 4-hydroxybenzoate (propyl para-hydroxybenzoate) (E216), propyl 4-hydroxybenzoate, Na salt (sodium propyl para-hydroxybenzoate) (E217), methyl 4-hydroxybenzoate (methyl para-hydroxybenzoate) (E218), methyl 4-hydroxybenzoate, Na salt (sodium methyl para-hydroxybenzoate) (E219)	'Free from' is interpreted as contains less than 1 mg/kg benzoate as calculated from the level of addition to the food having due regard to the presence of these compounds in ingredients and thereby carried over into the final food
Glutamate	L-glutamic acid (620), sodium hydrogen L-glutamate (mono sodium glutamate or MSG) (621), potassium hydrogen L-glutamate (mono potassium glutamate) (622), calcium dihydrogen di-L-glutamate (calcium glutamate) (623)	'Free from' is to be interpreted as contains no added glutamate either in one of these forms or in the form of a protein hydrolysed before addition
Azo colour	Amaranth (E123), Black PH (E151), Brown FK (154), Brown HT (155), Carmoisine (122), Pigment Rubine (E180), Ponceau 4R (E124), Red 2G (128), Sunset Yellow (E110), Tartrazine (E102), Yellow 2G (107)	'Free from', is to be interpreted as contains no added azo colour

* Tanner H (1963) *Mitt Geb Lebensmitt u Hyg* **54**, 158. An English text of a suitable procedure based upon the Tanner method, is included in the LFRA *Analytical Methods Manual*

dangers in the unsupervised use of diets, especially for infants and young children'.

The working party accepted this conclusion. The information on the databank is therefore only available to State Registered Dietitians, and the lists can only be obtained from dietitians as part of a medically prescribed diet. They include a warning against the risks of self-diagnosis and self-treatment.

Reference

RCP/BNF (1984) Food intolerance and food aversion. A Joint Report of the Royal College of Physicians and the British Nutrition Foundation. *J Roy Coll Physicians London* **18**, No 2.

2.16 Health foods and alternative diets

In recent years there has been growing interest in the relationship between food and health. As a result, an increasing proportion of people buy 'health foods' or follow an alternative way of eating in the hope of attaining better health, despite the fact that there is little scientific evidence to justify their use. Nevertheless, since it is important that dietitians are aware of what some of their patients or clients may be eating, some of these products and dietary regimens are described below.

2.16.1 Health foods

A fundamental problem with 'health foods' is their name. The term implies something which is necessary for, or improves, health. A more realistic view is the one offered by Bender (1985) that there is no such thing as a health food, only a health food industry.

These foods are available in a number of retail outlets including specialist shops and, increasingly, supermarkets. Herbert (1980) argues that the purveyor of health foods attempts to con the public by trying to create a need for the product: 'To those in pain, he promises relief. To the incurable he offers hope. To the nutrition conscious, he says "make sure you have enough". To one and all he promises better health and a longer life'.

To an extent this strategy seems to have been successful. In 1988 a Key Note Report on Health Foods noted that the industry was worth over £220 million per annum. It is likely that this figure has increased since then.

The report also found that the predominate users of health foods are female, in socioeconomic groups A, B and C1 and living in the south of England. This group of the population has been termed 'healthy bandwaggoners' as they tend to 'read all food labels, consume vitamin pills, read articles and watch television programmes about health and dietary issues'. While only a small proportion of the population can be categorized in this way, everyone wants to feel fit and healthy and the idea that this can be achieved quickly and easily via pills and potions has considerable appeal. People want health foods to work and are ready to believe the apparently scientific claims made for them. They are also perhaps impressed by the price – if something costs that much it *must* be beneficial.

Not all products sold in health food shops are undesirable. 'Wholefoods' such as brown rice, dried fruit, dried pulses, wholewheat pasta and cereals have a valuable place in a healthy eating regimen. However specialist outlets are no longer the only source of such foods and it can be argued that the sale of foods of genuine value to health alongside others of more uncertain value may bestow a certain amount of 'health credibility' to the latter.

Organically grown fruit, vegetables and cereals are becoming increasingly available. Although there is little evidence to show that they are nutritionally superior to conventionally grown produce, sales of these foods do have a significant market share. There is of course no reason why people should not use such produce if they wish to and are prepared to pay the extra cost. The main drawback to organic foods is that they can exploit people's fears about 'chemicals in their food' – and such people are often the most vulnerable members of society who can least afford them.

It is the use of dietary aids and supplements available at increasing numbers of outlets which is the area of greatest concern. There is a vast array of substances available for a variety of different purposes (Table 2.79). Some of the products may even appear to work owing to the power of the placebo effect; if you expect that product 'x' will make you feel better, then it probably will. But these supplements must not be dismissed as placebos in the sense of being inert pieces of chalk. These substances are what they say they are, and many of them have powerful pharmacological effects (though not necessarily those claimed for them). The danger from hypervitaminosis is an obvious example. The effects of excess quantities of other substances have never been fully explored and may be no less hazardous.

Even if consumed at a level which is not harmful, use of these supplements is still undesirable. In most instances they are unnecessary, either providing nutrients which are surplus to requirements or supposed nutrients which may not be needed at all. Their use as remedies for various ailments may have little scientific justification and may lead to a delay in seeking, or even abandonment of, medical advice.

Of fundamental concern is the fact that their use depends on dietary ignorance and tends to reinforce such ignorance. This also hampers efforts to explain the genuine issues of healthy eating.

2.16.2 Alternative diets

From time to time, a new alternative diet which is supposed to improve health, aid slimming or cure illness receives publicity via books, magazines, television or radio. As with health foods, the use of these regimens largely depends on people's hopes, fears and ignorance.

Table 2.79 Health food supplements and remedies

Reasons for use	Products used	Comments
To correct dietary deficiencies	Vitamins, Minerals, Amino acids } in isolated form or in combination Kelp (a source of minerals) Spirulina (vitamins and minerals) Aloe vera (sugars, vitamins and minerals)	Probably surplus to requirements in most cases. Considerable dangers from over-use A nutritionally inadequate diet is not transformed into an adequate one merely by taking vitamin and mineral tablets
To supply 'nutrients' deficient in a normal diet	Vitamin B_{15} (Panganic acid) — found naturally in brewer's yeast, brown rice and whole grains	This is a B complex factor but *not* a vitamin. Claims that it cleanses the body, extends cell life, lowers cholesterol and increases immunity have little scientific support
	Vitamin B_{17} (laetrile or amygdalin) is extracted from apricot kernels	This is a B complex factor but *not* a vitamin. It has been used in the USA as an alternative cancer cure. It is now banned as a result of deaths due to the cyanide content
	Inositol	Also a B complex factor, not a vitamin as it can be synthesized by the body. There is little evidence to substantiate claims that it lowers cholesterol, reduces oestrogen levels, prevents hair loss and high blood pressure
	Selenium (RNI 60–75 μg/day for adults)	Evidence that it may have a role in the prevention of cancer and heart disease. Can be toxic at levels of just 1 mg/day. US National Cancer Institute recommends 200 μg/day as a prophylactic measure
To aid digestion	Enzymes	Cannot possibly act in this way. Are denatured on reaching the stomach and then treated as any other protein
Rejuvenation/to retard ageing	DNA and RNA	The body makes all the DNA and RNA it needs. Dietary excess can cause hyperuricaemia
	Amino acids	Selective deficiency of amino acids is rare. Large amounts of isolated amino acids can be toxic
	Gingko (extract of a tree, used by Buddhist monks)	Reported to reverse ageing of the brain, insufficient evidence to substantiate this
	Coenzyme Q (key component in the release of energy from food)	Reported to reverse degenerative diseases; little scientific evidence for this
To 'cleanse' the body of toxins	Cider vinegar Garlic Panganic acid (B_{15}) Herbs (e.g. Shepherd's purse, yarrow, lemon balm, parsley)	In the absence of severe liver or renal disease, the body is quite capable of doing this for itself
As a slimming aid	Spirulina Cider vinegar Honey Lecithin Evening primrose oil Fennel, Chickweed, Kelp } supposedly appetite suppressants	Claims that substances can burn up fat or stimulate metabolism are nonsense; if true, obesity would be a thing of the past. Honey and lecithin are significant sources of energy
	Pantothenic acid (said to speed up transit time)	If true, the absorption of valuable nutrients would be jeopardized

Table 2.79 *contd.*

Reasons for use	Products used	Comments
To restore vigour/induce feelings of well-being	Ginseng (herb obtained from the root of a plant grown in Korea and China)	Ginseng has certain pharmacological effects although these are variable and unpredictable, perhaps because ginseng itself is of variable composition. Extremely expensive. Contradictions over its use; some suggest it helps normalize blood pressure, others that it shouldn't be used in those with high blood pressure. Problems with over-use have been reported (Dukes 1978; Palmer *et al* 1978; Bender 1985)
	Bees Royal Jelly (substance which transforms a worker bee into a Queen bee)	Reported benefits include relieving fatigue, reducing stress, fighting infection, promoting fertility and longevity. Rich in pantothenic acid but little evidence that this is deficient in UK diets
	Honey	Provides energy but little else. No evidence of health benefits
	Pollen (a mixture of bee saliva, plant nectar and plant (or flower) male gametes)	Anecdotal claims of increased longevity, improved athletic performance, relief of fatigue, improved resistance to infection, relief of hay fever
	Kelp Spirulina	These may provide traces of vitamins and minerals (at a price) but little in the way of magic
To reduce cholesterol/heart disease	Lecithin B_{15} Inositol Selenium Garlic Evening primrose oil	None of these substances is likely to be successful in isolation i.e. without attention to dietary and other risk factors. The effects of garlic are well-documented although the recommended level varies between 3–50 g/day (1–12 large cloves)
As a cure	Aloe vera (arthritis) Green lipped mussel (rheumatism)	It should be borne in mind that chronic disorders such as arthritis and rheumatism tend to have periods of partial remission in any case.
	Salt bush (diabetes) Kelp (healing) Laetrile (cancer) Various herbs	A skilled herbalist may well be able to relieve minor ailments via the pharmacological effects of some plants. But these effects can be powerful, and sometimes toxic (e.g. hemlock, strychnine) and indiscriminate use of these remedies by the uninformed can be dangerous
	Germanium (said to protect against cancer, leukaemia, asthma, diabetes, senility and a range of other disorders)	Has potentially lethal side effects and has been banned from sale in the UK
Because they are 'natural'	'Natural' as distinct from 'synthetic' vitamins Sea salt	By definition, a synthetic vitamin must be identical to a natural one or it wouldn't be a vitamin Sea salt is, in effect, dirty salt. People often assume that anything 'natural' is automatically superior to anything manufactured. They should be reminded that some of the most toxic substances known to man (e.g. certain plant alkaloids or botulinus toxin) are 'natural'

Alternative diets tend to develop in societies where food is plentiful and people have sufficient disposable income to be able to follow them. In less affluent countries, the main priority is simply to obtain sufficient food in order to survive; factors such as optimum health or longevity are somewhat irrelevant.

People may follow an alternative eating regimen for a variety of reasons:

- Concern about their health;
- Fear of additives;
- Influence of family, friends or the media;
- Strongly formed beliefs;
- In response to diagnosis of a particular illness;
- Wanting a quick result in terms of health or improved appearance.

Some alternative diets quickly fade into obscurity, others persist for longer, most are useless. Some of the regimens which dietitians may encounter among their clients are summarized below. The use of alternative diets by people with cancer is discussed in Section 4.34.3, by those with AIDS/HIV disease in Section 4.32.13 and by those with rheumatoid arthritis in Section 4.29.4.

Elimination and cleansing diets

Elimination diets carried out under qualified medical and dietetic supervision have a proper place in the diagnosis and management of food intolerance (Section 4.31). But alongside this has grown the belief among the general public that 'elimination' or 'cleansing' diets can remove 'toxins' from the modern day diet and can relieve ailments such as catarrh or arthritis. In some instances, genuine food intolerance may indeed be responsible for some of these symptoms, but this possibility should be explored with qualified dietetic help and not on a do-it-yourself basis. The latter course of action may well:

1 Be expensive.
2 Be ineffective.
3 Result in nutritional deficiencies as a result of prolonged dietary imbalance.
4 Offer false hope.

Food combining diets

Food combining diets have been reported to cure stomach acidity, heartburn, bloating, dyspepsia, headaches, allergies and nervousness. In addition they 'almost invariably result in weight loss' (Sharon 1989).

The principle behind the regimen is that some digestive processes are chemically opposed and hence foods should not be eaten in combinations which interfere with the digestion of each other. It is suggested that proteins and fat may be eaten together, also carbohydrates and fat; however, protein and carbohydrate should not be combined together or this will 'stress' the system. The scientific basis for this presumption is dubious at best. Furthermore, listed examples of 'suitable' food combinations often ignore single food sources of carbohydrate and protein such as pulses. Diets based on a food combining system can be unbalanced in nutritional terms and contrary to the principles of healthy eating.

Anti-candida diets

Crook (1984), Chaitow (1985) and others claim that yeasts (*Candida Albicans*) can make you feel 'ill all over'. They suggest that yeasts present in the body under 'normal circumstances' do no harm. There are however triggers such as diets rich in sugar and yeasts, oral contraceptives, pregnancy and – more especially – treatment with broad spectrum antibiotics which cause yeasts to multiply resulting in an 'overgrowth'. This results in toxin production which is a contributing factor along with nutritional deficiencies, environmental moulds and chemicals in weakening the immune system.

There are no fewer than 40 symptoms which Crook attributes to intestinal candidiasis, two of which are food sensitivity and myalgic encephalomylitis.

Non-dietary suggestions for treatment include various antifungal drugs such as nystatin, amphotericin, ketaconazole, evening primrose oil, garlic capsules, *lactobacillus acidophilus*, vitamin and mineral supplements 'to boost the immume system', stopping smoking and 'avoiding chemicals'. Dietary treatments centre on avoiding yeasts and all foods containing them, sugar including milk, and some also include advice for restricting total carbohydrate to 60–80 g/day. Foods to avoid include bread, vinegar, pickles, alcohol, cheese, yeast extracts, sweets, chocolates, cakes, biscuits, honey, syrups etc. To date, this treatment can only be considered experimental and there have been no reported clinically controlled trials supporting the relevance of anticandida therapy in the treatment of food allergy. In a study on the use of nystatin therapy for the candidiasis hypersensitivity syndrome, the authors conclude that, in the treatment regimens employed, nystatin did not significantly alter the systemic symptoms attributed to the condition. They did not, however, address the issues of special diets or measures to control the environment (Dismukes *et al* 1990).

Feingold Diet/diet and hyperactivity

Feingold (1975) made the assertion that hyperactivity and learning disorders are frequently caused by an intolerance to additives and salicylates found in foods. The Feingold Diet therefore excludes all artificial flavourings, colours, preservatives and foods containing salicylates. It has been popularized through the media and promoted by a number of self-help groups for the dietary treatment of hyperactivity.

Cant (1985) after reviewing double-blind studies testing the validity of Feingold's dietary views, has suggested that his hypothesis has been largely disproved. However some recent studies have reported improved behaviour in some hyperkinetic children after periods of elimination of some dietary components, particularly tartrazine and benzoic acid (Egger *et al* 1989) and foods such as soya and cows' milk, grapes, wheat, oranges, eggs and peanuts (Graham 1987; Kaplan *et al* 1989). Graham suggests that adverse behavioural responsiveness to food does exist in a number of hyperkinetic children, particularly those with an allergic condition such as asthma or eczema. However it also seems likely that genuine diet-linked hyperkinesis only affects a small proportion of those diagnosed as 'hyperactive'; the remainder are probably just badly behaved children!

'Fad' reducing diets

There is a multiplicity of diets which are claimed to be of benefit in achieving weight reduction. Most fall into two categories.

Distorted nutrient composition

Diets such as the 'Mayo Clinic' diet, the 'Chicago' diet or 'Beverly Hills' diet are based on a marked distortion in the nutrient composition of the diet, e.g. a severe carbohydrate restriction sometimes in association with a high protein intake. Many of these diets claim to have discovered the secret of 'speeding up metabolism' or 'burning up fat' more effectively than any other type of diet. In reality, whether they achieve weight loss will depend solely on whether an individual's energy intake is less than his requirement. Their effectiveness depends on the length of time the diet can be tolerated (which is not usually very long).

Restricted food group diets

Women's magazines are particularly fond of recommending diets based on a few foods, e.g. the 'grapefruit' diet. While these diets may achieve short term weight loss (much of which is due to the loss of body water), they are obviously nutritionally unsound and of no value whatsoever in the long term treatment of obesity.

Further reading

Bender AE (1985) *Health or hoax?* Elvendon Press, Reading.
Mayes A (1991) *The A–Z of nutritional health*. Thorsons, London.
Werback MR (1989) *Nutritional influences on illness*. Thorsons, London.

References

Bender AE (1985) *Health or hoax?* Elvendon Press, Reading.

Cant AJ (1985) Food allergy in childhood. *Hum Nutr: Appl Nutr* **39A**, 277–93.

Chaitow L (1985) *Candida Albicans: Could yeast be your problem?* Thorsons, Wellingborough.

Crook WG (1984) *The yeast connection. A medical breakthrough* 2e. Professional Books, Tennessee.

Dismukes WE, Scott Wade J, Lee JY, Dockery BK, Hain RN and Hain JD (1990) A randomised, double-blind trial of Nystatin therapy for the candidiasis hypersensitivity syndrome. *New Eng J Med* **323**, 25.

Dukes MN (1978) Ginseng and mastalgia (letter). *Br Med J* **1**, 1621.

Egger J, Carter CM, Soothill JF and Wilson J (1989) Oligoantigenic diet treatment of children with epilepsy and migraine. *J Paediat* **114**, 51–8.

Feingold BF (1975) Hyperkinesis and learning disabilities linked with artificial food flavours and colours. *Am J Nurs* **75**, 797–803.

Graham P (1987) Dietary aspects of management in childhood hyperactivity. In *Food intolerance* Dobbing J (Ed) pp. 59–67. Baillière Tindall, London.

Herbert V (1980) *Nutrition cultism – facts and fiction*. GF Stickly.

Kaplan BJ, McNicol J, Conte RA and Moghadam HK (1989) Dietary replacement in pre-school aged hyperactive boys. *Paediat* **83**, 7–17.

Key Note Publications (1988) *Health foods – an industry sector overview*. Details available from 22/42 Banner Street, London EC1Y 8QB.

Palmer BV, Montgomery ACV and Monteiro JCMP (1978) Ginseng and mastalgia (letter). *Br Med J* **1**, 1284.

Sharon M (1989) *Complete nutrition – how to live in total health*. Prion, London.

2.17 Food legislation

2.17.1 Background and current regulations

The earliest record of food legislation in this country was an Act passed in 1266 which protected the purchaser against sale of unsound meat and short weight in bread. Whilst apparently far sighted, the enforcement of the Act left a lot to be desired and was largely ineffective. However, Guilds, which played a very important role at that time, helped to ensure that the commodities were as pure as possible. This meant checking the pepper to ensure there was no added gravel, leaves or twigs, checking the coffee to ensure there was no added grass, acorns or lard and checking bread to ensure that no mashed potato, sand or ashes had been added.

As the population grew, the industrial revolution caused a massive shift from country to town; more people needed to be fed and a larger proportion of them were no longer able to grow their own food and became dependent on others for its supply.

By the middle of the 19th century the abuses were appalling. Increased publicity was now being given to the problem of food adulteration in both the scientific journals and popular press of the day and as a result public pressures led to the establishment of a Select Committee on Food Adulteration. After much dissatisfaction concerning its effectiveness, another Committee was set up, the result of which was the 1875 Sale of Food and Drugs Act. This Act is the basis of present UK law and includes the statement fundamental to current practice.

> 'No person shall sell to the prejudice of the purchaser any article of food or any food thing which is not of the nature, substance or quality demanded by such purchasers.'

By the turn of the century, significant improvements had been made to the purity of basic commodities – bread, flour and coffee were no longer adulterated. The 1875 Act remained in force until 1928 when it was replaced by the consolidated Food and Drugs (Adulteration) Act. It was at this time that regulations pertaining to composition and labelling were first introduced.

In 1943 the Food and Drugs Act combined *all* legislation concerning the retailing of foodstuffs. This Act was the basis of Government control during the war years.

In 1955 the Food and Drug Act came into being and was to remain the basis of food legislation until general legislation covering the composition, labelling, hygiene and safety of food in the UK was introduced in 1984 by the Food Act. (The 'drug' aspect was superseded by the Medicines Act in 1968 and from 1974 has no longer been included in this schedule).

In view of the considerable changes which have occurred in both food production and eating habits in the past 40 years, legislation was increasingly criticized for being out of date and in need of amendment. As a result the Government proposed a number of major amendments which were the subject of wide consideration among interested parties. These changes were welcomed by both the consumer and the food industry and the result was the Food Safety Act 1990.

Whilst the Food Act provides the basic legislation, the making of new regulations is divided between the Ministry of Agriculture, Fisheries and Food in matters dealing with composition and labelling and the Secretary of State for Social Services in matters relating to hygiene. Figure 2.12 shows how a substance, e.g. a food additive, is dealt with by MAFF when referred for approval.

2.17.2 Food Safety Act

The Food Safety Act, which came into force on January 1, 1991, results from the first major review of food legislation since the 1940s. With the harmonization of Europe in 1992 in sight, the need to remain flexible was recognized and the Act concentrates on the principal issues of legislation, leaving the details to be completed through subsidiary orders, regulations and codes of practice.

Content of the Food Safety Act

The act is divided into four parts: Preliminary; Main Provisions; Administration and Enforcement; Miscellaneous and Supplemental.

Part I: Preliminary

In this section, the full scope of the Act is detailed, also the responsibilities for those involved in enforcing it. As the new Act now covers the whole of Great Britain, its scope is much wider than that of previous Food Acts. Its definitions of food and premises are wider, with the former now including slimming aids and dietary supplements as well as tap water, and the latter including, from 1 April 1992, most Crown properties as well as ships and aircraft. There are regulations covering all aspects of food production, processing and selling, from the farm to the retailer. It also

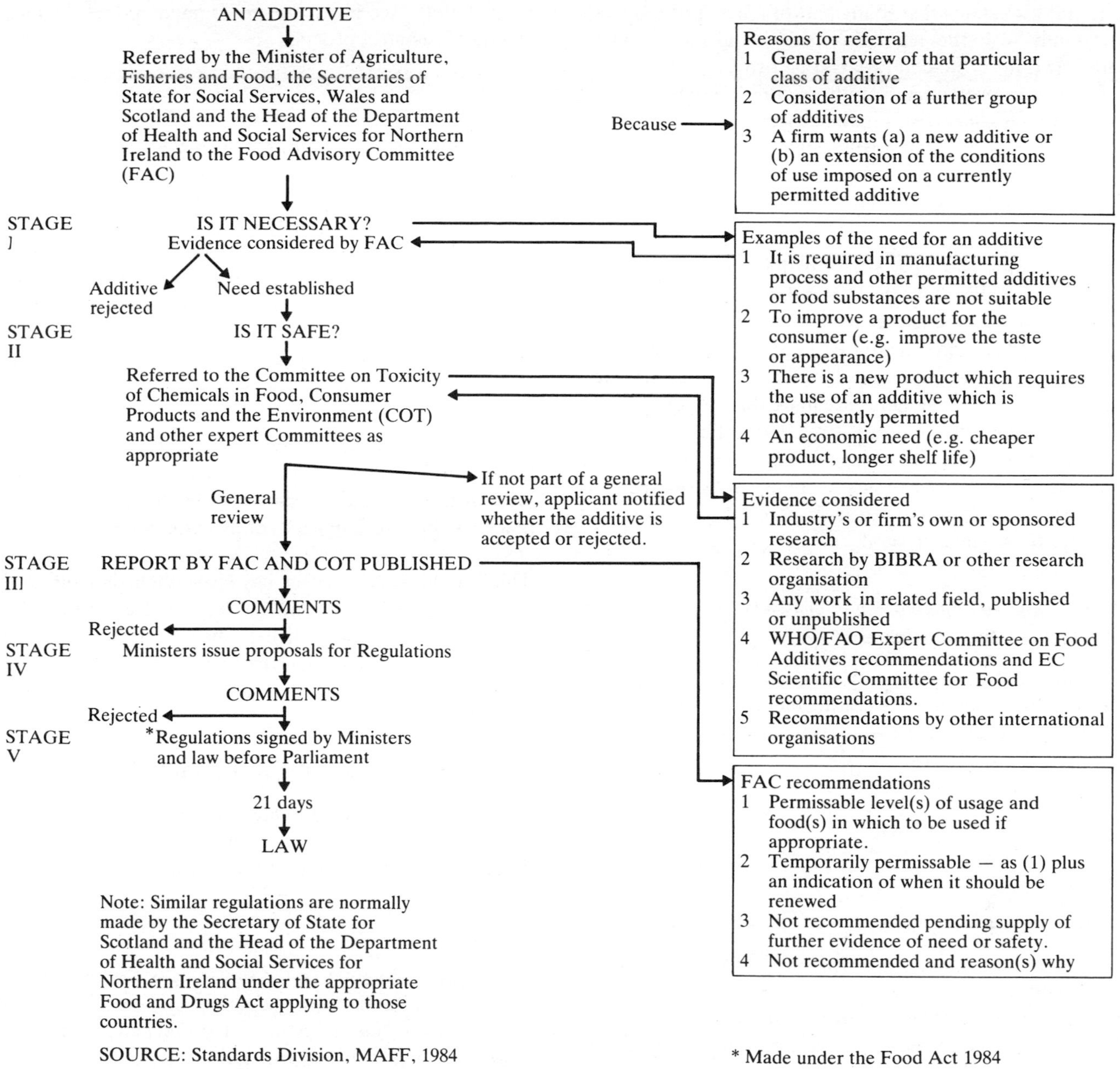

Fig. 2.12 The process of evaluating food additives

covers growing crops and live animals destined to become food.

Under the new Food Safety Act responsibility for enforcement is not set out in detail. Instead the Act makes it clear that all local authorities are responsible for enforcing the food law that is within their remit and not specifically given to somebody else. It also gives ministers powers to specify in an order or code of practice which type of local authority is to enforce each aspect of the food law.

Part II: Main Provisions

Offences The main provisions of the Act, namely food safety, consumer protection, regulation making powers and defences are covered in this part of the Act.

Food safety is dealt with under three sections of the Act. In Section 7 it is made clear that it is an offence to render food injurious to health by any process or treatment. It is no longer necessary for there to be an intention that the food will be consumed in that state, i.e. it is an offence as soon as the food has been rendered injurious to health.

In another section under the Act it is now also an offence to sell food that does not comply with food safety requirements. These requirements are based on the two existing criteria, i.e. being injurious to health and unfit for human consumption, and a new criterion — contamination.

The Act also states that if any part of a batch of food fails to comply with the regulation, the whole batch will be withdrawn until the contrary can be proved.

Consumer protection is addressed in Section 14 of the Act in two familiar ways. Firstly, it is an offence to sell food which is not of the nature, substance or quality demanded and secondly, it is an offence to give misleading information about food in an advertisement or label.

Defences This is a new aspect of food legislation introduced under this Act. If a defendant can show that he exercised due diligence to avoid committing the offence, then he is likely to be acquitted. The onus is clearly with manufacturers and importers therefore to ensure that their quality control arrangements are more than adequate. To a lesser extent it also applies to retailers selling both their own brand and other brand goods. This is considered to be one of the most far reaching and comprehensive aspects of the new Act and puts a clear responsibility on the food industry to supply safe food.

Parts III and IV: Administration and Enforcement; Miscellaneous and Supplemental

Procedures for sampling and analysis of products, powers of entry, obstruction and enforcement, are laid down in this section. It also deals with legal aspects of prosecution and appeal procedures.

Enforcement of the Act

Enforcement officers

Under the Act local authority staff may, by right:

- Enter any food premises to investigate possible offences;
- Take away samples for investigation;
- Detain suspect food or ask for it to be destroyed through local court procedures;
- Require food hygiene to be improved or, in an extreme case, close down a premises if considered to be a public health risk.

Trading standards officers deal with the labelling of food, its composition and most cases of chemical contamination; environmental health officers deal with hygiene, with cases of microbiological contamination of foods and with food which is unfit for human consumption.

Throughout the UK, public analysts are responsible for carrying out chemical analysis of food and food examiners are responsible for microbiological examination of food. They both form an integral part of the enforcement team.

At the extreme end of such control, when for example shutting down a food premises is insufficient to limit further contaminated food reaching the consumer, the Food Safety Act gives the government power to make emergency control orders.

Regulations

Apart from enabling ministers to make regulations on a wide range of food matters such as composition, additives, hygiene, labelling and packaging materials, two new sets of regulations have been introduced.

1 *Registration* Premises used for food business now have to be registered with their local authority. This will also include premises, vehicles, market stalls, etc. used by charities and those where catering is provided over several consecutive days (e.g. at conference or sports events).

2 *Training for food handlers* The Act requires that all those handling food should be trained to an appropriate level in hygiene and be shown to be competent in such practices through independent assessment.

The new Food Safety Act has strengthened significantly pre-existing legislation and has provided a stronger and more streamlined legislative framework to address food safety issues at all stages of the food chain and to enhance consumer protection on such matters.

2.17.3 International food legislation

Food is both imported into and exported from the UK, so legislation on standards of composition and on labelling should attempt to comply with international standards.

Codex

The Codex Alimentarius Commission is the main international food standards organization. It is the joint body of the two United Nation bodies – the Food and Agriculture Organization (FAO) and the World Health Organization (WHO). Codex sets out to establish procedures and principles which are acceptable to member countries in relation to meeting agreed standards for food in international trade and to help lower trade barriers.

European Community

Membership of the EC requires the Government to take into account regulations and directives of the EC. Two major objectives underlie the legislation in member countries

1 To protect the health of the consumer.
2 The prevention of fraud.

Harmonization of legislation is therefore essential if goods such as foodstuffs are to be able to move freely in a single market. The original aim of the EC therefore was to introduce common standards for those products currently controlled by food regulations.

Harmonization can be achieved by either Regulations or Directives.

Regulations

These are applicable directly to all market countries and, whilst they may need additional measures to help in enforcement, no national exactment is required.

Directives

This is the more usual method used for harmonization of food laws. The directive, once adopted by the EC Council of Ministers, lays down the ultimate objective for a particular food law, but leaves each member country free to decide how it will be implemented.

In regulatory terms, the major effect of the achievement of a single market in the EC will be that much food regulatory work will be done at Community level in Brussels rather than at the national level in the 12 capitals of member states. Problems which require regulations will then have to be negotiated among the 12 member states rather than by an individual country drawing up its own conclusions and taking its own actions. Community food law will then concentrate on issues concerned with food safety and public health, proper information for consumers and rules to ensure fair trading. It will move away from qualitative issues such as food composition and recipe laws.

Useful addresses

EC Commission (London Office), EC Commission, 8 Storey's Gate, London SW1P 3AT.

Enforcement

1 Trading standards – Local Authorities Co-ordinating Body on Trading Standards (LACOTS), PO Box 6, Fell Road, Croydon CR9 1LG.

2 Weights and measures – National Metrological Co-ordination Unit (NMCU), PO Box 6, Fell Road, Croydon CR9 1LG.

(LACOTS and NMCU were established after the 1979 Trading Standards Act.)

Government departments

Food standards (England and Wales)

Ministry of Agriculture, Fisheries and Food, (Standards Division), Horseferry Road, London SW1P 2AE.

Milk (England and Wales)

Ministry of Agriculture, Fisheries and Food, (Milk and Milk Products Division), 10 Whitehall Place (East block), London SW1A 2HH.

Food Standards (Scotland)

Scottish Home and Health Department, St Andrew's House, Edinburgh EH1 3DE.

Milk, imported meat, etc. (Scotland)

Department of Agriculture and Fisheries for Scotland, Chesser House, 500 Gorgie Road, Edinburgh EH11 3AW.

Food and milk (Northern Ireland)

Department of Health and Social Services (Medicines and Food Control Branch), Annexe A, Dundonald House, Upper Newtonards Road, Belfast BT4 3SF.

Trade descriptions (UK)

Department of Trade, (Consumer Affairs Division), Millbank Tower, Millbank, London SW1P 4QU.

Hygiene (England and Wales)

Contact local authority or
Department of Social Security, (Health Services Division), Alexander Fleming House, Elephant and Castle, London SE1 6BY.

Imported Food (England and Wales)

Ministry of Agriculture, Fisheries and Food, (Meat Hygiene Division), Tolworth Tower, Surbiton, Surrey KT6 7DX.

Weights and Measures (UK)

Department of Trade, (Consumer Affairs Division), 26 Chapter Street, London SW1 4NS.

Further reading

The Food Safety Act 1990 and You:

A guide for the food industry (PB0351). HMSO, London.
A guide for caterers and their employees (PB0370). HMSO, London.
A guide for farmers and growers (PB0371). HMSO, London.

Copies of all three leaflets are available from Food Sense, London SE99 7TT.

Copies of the Act, Statutory Instruments and Codes of Practice may be obtained from HMSO Publications Centre, PO Box 276, London SW8 5DT.

2.18 Food labelling

The Food Act 1984 (and the regulations made under it) is the main legislation governing the labelling of food in the UK.

The most important *regulations* are The Food Labelling Regulations 1984 which became fully operative in September of that year. In addition, there are regulations which are specific to certain foods, for example, the Meat Regulations which came into force in July 1986. Two Weights and Measures Acts and the Trade Descriptions Act also have an impact on what information is given on a food label.

Because the UK is a member of the EC, Community Regulations and Directives have to be adopted. EC Regulations are effective in all member states as soon as they are adopted by the EC Council. Directives, on the other hand, do not become effective until they are written into a country's legislation.

2.18.1 The Food Labelling Regulations

Almost all food sold to the 'ultimate consumer' or to a catering establishment has to comply with these regulations. Exemptions include certain sugar products, cocoa and chocolate products, honey, condensed and dried milk and cheese. These, and some other foods, have their own special regulations.

Almost all the foods covered by The Food Labelling Regulations must be marked with the following information:

1 The name of the food.
2 A list of ingredients.
3 An indication of minimum durability.
4 Any special storage conditions or conditions of use.
5 Its weight, volume or number in pack.
6 The name and address of the manufacturer or packer or seller.
7 The place of origin (if omitting this information would mislead the purchaser).
8 Instructions for use (if omitting them would make it difficult to use the product properly).

Ingredients

Nearly all foods which come within the scope of the Food Labelling Regulations must carry a list of ingredients. The few exceptions include fresh fruits and vegetables which are not cut in pieces, carbonated water to which nothing except carbon dioxide has been added, vinegar to which nothing has been added, most cheeses, butters and fermented milks, flavourings, alcoholic drinks with an alcohol content of less than 1.2% by volume and foods which consist of a single ingredient.

When ingredients are listed they must appear in descending order of weight. With the exception of added water, the weight of each ingredient is the amount used during preparation of the food. Water is now generally considered to be an ingredient (in the same way as flour, sugar or beef) but its position in the ingredients list depends on the amount in the final product. Water need not be declared if it is used solely to reconstitute a dried or concentrated ingredient, nor if it is part of a medium not normally consumed, such as the brine in canned vegetables. Water need not be listed if it is 5% or less of the finished product. There are specific EC regulations governing water in frozen poultry.

If a compound ingredient is used, such as pasta in lasagne, the ingredients may be listed in one of two ways. Either all the constituents of the pasta, meat sauce and cheese sauce are given in one list or the compound ingredient may appear in the appropriate position followed by a list of its ingredients. Thus, in lasagne the ingredients panel may be: water, beef, tomato, semolina, skimmed milk powder, cheese, pork, etc. *or* pasta (semolina, water, egg white), skimmed milk, beef, tomato, vegetable stock, etc.

Additives

All categories of additives must be listed in the ingredients. In every case except flavours the additive must be described by its generic name, for example, acidity regulator and either the specific name, e.g. 'sodium citrate', or the EC code number or other serial number, e.g. 'E331'. All flavours are covered by the single word 'flavouring(s)'.

Although the current Food Labelling Regulations require more information on the food label than any of the preceding labelling regulations, there may still be ingredients in foods which do not appear on the label.

If an additive is present in an ingredient rather than being added as such to the food it may not need to be listed. For example, sulphite is often added to fruit to preserve it, and if the fruit is made into jam some sulphite may remain in the finished product. If, however, the amount carried over is too small to have any preservative effect on the jam, it need not be declared. Additives used solely as processing aids, for example, tin-greasing agents, do not have to be listed, neither do solvents or carriers of flavours.

If a compound ingredient constitutes less than 25% of the finished product, only its additives, not the main ingredients, need be listed. The other exemption which may be important to dietitians is bread and bread flour. Flour is considered to be a single ingredient food and, provided only the additives stipulated in the Bread and Flour Regulations (1984a) are used, they need not appear on the label.

Special emphasis

If one ingredient in a product is given special emphasis, for example, 'with extra fresh cream', the minimum amount of that ingredient (as a percentage of the total product weight) must appear close to the name or in the list of ingredients. Just using the word 'cream' in the name of the food does not constitute special emphasis. Similarly, if particular attention is drawn to the *small* amount of an ingredient, the maximum amount of that ingredient which could be present must be stated.

Minimum durability

Nearly all foods have to be marked with a date up to and including that which the food can reasonably be expected to 'retain its specific properties' if properly stored. The time that any food will keep in good condition depends very much on the storage temperature. This is especially true of frozen and chilled/fresh foods. If a manufacturer is not too sure about the temperatures his food will encounter during distribution and retail display he is going to be very cautious about the 'life' he claims for the food. So, the vast majority of foods are likely to be perfectly edible after the date marked on the packet.

Foods which are currently exempt from date marking include: foods which are not pre-packed, foods with a shelf life of more than 18 months, eggs, very long life foods such as vinegar and sugar, cheese intended to ripen after it is packed, most alcoholic drinks, fresh fruit and vegetables which are not peeled or cut, frozen foods and ice cream which carry star marking, flour confectionery and bread intended to be eaten within 24 hours.

The date which appears on the packet depends on the expected 'life' of the food. Current regulations (effective since 1 January 1991) require that, if this is less than six weeks, the label must show either 'use by' followed by a day and month *or* 'best before' followed by a day and month. 'Use by' dates have been introduced to provide a clear and final date for use of microbiologically highly perishable food while 'best before' remains the principal system for the majority of foods. The 'sell by' date marking system is no longer permitted.

Foods with an expected life of six weeks to three months must show 'best before' followed by a day and month. Those with a life of three months to 18 months must state either 'best before' followed by a day, month and year *or* 'best before end' followed by a month and year. Foods with an expected shelf life of more than 18 months do not *have* to carry any date but they *may* show a 'best before' or 'best before end' date. In all cases, if any special storage conditions such as refrigeration are necessary, these must be shown close to the date.

Weight

Nearly all packaged foods have to show the net weight in g, the volume in ml or some other approved measure. The imperial measure may also be given. Where a weight is given, it must be the average contents of packs provided that no pack has an unreasonable deficiency. 'Unreasonable deficiency' is defined and the tolerances allowed are so tight that far more than half the packs have to contain more than the declared weight if the regulations are to be met. So the move from declaration of minimum weight to average weight which might appear to be against the consumer's interest has not had any detrimental effect.

Claims

The Food Labelling Regulations make provision for certain claims on labels and elsewhere. They do not state precisely what constitutes a claim, but many enforcement authorities regard any statement as a claim and, therefore, subject to the provisions of the regulations. But the regulations do say that a statement of the energy content of a food is not a claim.

A special schedule in the regulations specifies the criteria which must be met if certain words or descriptions are to be used. Of special interest to dietitians are the criteria for use of the words 'dietary' and 'dietetic'. They may be applied to food which

> 'has been specially made for a class of person whose digestive process or metabolism is disturbed or who, by reason of their special physiological condition, obtain special benefit from a controlled consumption of certain substances'.

Also, the food has to be

> 'suitable for fulfilling the particular nutritional requirements of the class of person'.

A food may be described as 'starch reduced' if less than 50% of the dry food is anhydrous carbohydrate and the starch content is substantially less than that of the same weight of similar food to which the description is *not* applied.

A drink may be described as 'tonic wine' only if the words 'the name tonic wine does not imply health-giving or medicinal properties' appear close by.

Diabetic claims

Diabetic claims may be made only if a number of conditions are met. Among them are that the food must not normally be higher in fat or energy than a similar food not carrying a diabetic claim, and it must not contain more mono- or disaccharide (other than fructose) than is necessary.

A diabetic food must state that it is not suitable for overweight diabetics unless the energy value is 50% or less than that of an equivalent food for which no diabetic claim is made.

If a diabetic food contains fructose, sorbitol, mannitol, xylitol, isomalt or hydrogenated glucose syrup, the label must make the recommendation that a total of no more than 25 g of these substances should be eaten daily. It must also show the amounts of these carbohydrates, total carbohydrate content and 'other' carbohydrates present.

Slimming claims

Slimming claims may be made only if the food is 'capable of contributing to weight loss'. The claim must be accompanied by the words 'Can help slimming or weight control only as part of a calorie (or joule or energy) controlled diet'.

If a food is claimed to be reduced energy it must have an energy value of no more than 75% that of the same weight of an equivalent food which does not carry a reduced energy claim.

To qualify for a *low* energy claim a food must contain no more than 167 kJ (40 kcal)/100 g or 100 ml and the energy value of a normal portion must be no more than 167 kJ (40 kcal).

2.18.2 Nutrition labelling

Discussions on the whole subject of nutrition labelling were prompted by the publication of the report of the Committee on Medical Aspects of Food Policy (COMA) on Diet and Cardiovascular Disease in 1984 which recommended more on-pack information to help consumers select a nutritionally better diet. The Ministry of Agriculture, Fisheries and Food (MAFF) responded to this by developing regulations on fat content labelling and later by producing guidelines for fat nutritional labelling.

Fat labelling

The COMA Panel, in making its recommendations on reducing fat consumption, asked that more informative labelling be given for all foods with a fat content above 10% or for those foods which were major contributors to fat intake. Proposals were issued by MAFF in 1986 outlining the Government's intention of introducing statutory fat labelling for foods which made a significant contribution to total fat intake. Such foods were to be labelled with total fat and their saturated fat content. These proposals were not considered acceptable because:

- Such selective labelling perpetuated the myth of 'good' and 'bad' foods;
- Labelling of fat alone did not fully implement the COMA Panel's advice;
- Labelling of fat was considered to be a barrier to European trade.

MAFF was advised by the Commission of the European Community that this was an area of food law which was being harmonized within the Community and MAFF has therefore not proceeded any further with its plans for mandatory fat labelling.

Full nutritional labelling

Shortly after the draft Fat Labelling Regulations were published, guidelines for fuller nutrition information were issued by MAFF. It was not intended that these should be mandatory but it was recommended that, if manufacturers did give fuller information, they should follow the proposed format. This, it was hoped, would enable shoppers to compare products and reduce the confusion which might result if many different formats were used.

Views about how much information should be given on labels vary. Some authorities believe that, unless people have the complete nutrition picture including vitamins and minerals, they will be misled. Others believe that such a large amount of information is both unnecessary and confusing and will detract from the main issues which, they argue, are to prevent or correct obesity and reduce total and saturated fat intake.

After much debate and some consumer research, draft guidelines have been produced suggesting formats for three levels of nutrition labelling:

- I – Energy, protein, carbohydrate, fat (The Big Four); *or*
- II – Energy, protein, carbohydrate, fat with a breakdown to show saturates; *or*
- III – Energy, protein, carbohydrate with a breakdown to show sugars, fat with a breakdown to show saturates, sodium, and 'fibre' (the Big Four plus the Little Four).

Optional additions to Category III were:

1 Starch in addition to sugars in the breakdown of carbohydrates and trans and/or polyunsaturates in the breakdown of fat. Monounsaturates could only be shown if polyunsaturates were shown too.

2 Energy was to be expressed in kilojoules or kilocalories and other nutrients in grams.

3 The amounts to be given per 100 g or per 100 ml or, if smaller, per portion or per serving.

4 No other information including visual information was to be given under the heading of nutritional information.

The Food Advisory Committee, concerned about the

frequency of additional nutritional claims and the misleading effect they may have on consumers, also made some recommendations on the need to standardize such claims. The FAC recommended that nutritional claims should be controlled through legislation in a similar way to those existing regulatory controls on slimming, energy and protein.

European Community (EC) Nutrition Labelling Rules Directive

Common rules on such matters as nutrition labels on food are needed so that trade within the Community is not impaired. Two proposals were issued in 1988, one dealing with the introduction of selective compulsory nutrition labelling and the other laying down rules to be followed whenever nutrition labelling is provided.

The first proposal was not popular other than with the UK and has not progressed further as yet.

The Directive for the second proposal was adopted by the EC members in September 1990. In summary it states that whenever nutrition labelling is given, the information must consist of either Group I or Group II:

- Group I – Energy values and the amounts of protein, carbohydrate and fat;
- Group II – Energy values and the amounts of protein, carbohydrate, sugars, fat, saturates, 'fibre' and sodium.

Nutrition labelling may also list amounts of starch, polyols, monounsaturates, polyunsaturates and cholesterol. It may also indicate the levels of a number of vitamins and minerals where these are present in significant amounts. Nutrition labelling will remain voluntary unless a claim is made for any of the items in Group II in which case full nutritional labelling of Group I is required.

Whilst the EC Directive is broadly similar to the MAFF guidelines, there are some differences but it has brought a reasonable consistency at national and European level for the time being.

There are still some outstanding issues, for example whether there should be compulsory labelling of all eight nutrients – a concept much supported by organizations such as the Health Education Authority and the Consumers' Association, and the format that nutrition information should take (e.g. whether the weight basis is the best option – some would prefer to see the information on a percentage of energy basis or in a graphical format). There are also analytical considerations, in particular the need to clarify the position of dietary 'fibre'.

References and further reading

British Nutrition Foundation (1990) *Nutrition Labelling.* Briefing Paper No 21. BNF, London.

Committee on Medical Aspects of Food Policy (1984) *Diet and Cardiovascular Disease.* HMSO, London.

The Food Labelling Regulations (1984) SI 1305. HMSO, London.

Weights and Measures Acts (1985; 1985(a)). HMSO, London.

The Food Act (1984). HMSO, London.

Section 3 **Nutritional needs of population sub-groups**

3.1 Pregnancy

3.1.1 Preconceptional and periconceptional nutrition

Preconceptional nutrition in men

The preconceptional effects of diet in men are poorly researched. Most studies relating to the subject have been carried out on animals and the relevance to humans is unclear. It is known however that gross dietary inadequacies or excesses in men can affect either the likelihood of and/or the outcome of conception. For example, undernutrition delays puberty and in adults reduces sex drive and performance, while both undernutrition and gross obesity alter sex hormone production (Calloway 1983). Zinc deficiency can reduce sperm numbers while iodine deficiency lessens libido and androsterone production (Calloway 1983). Cadmium, boron, titanium and excess molybdenum can all injure the gonads (Calloway 1983). Alcohol increases zinc loss and may interfere with vitamin A metabolism (Calloway 1983). The effects of lesser degrees of dietary imbalance are unknown. The most prudent preconceptional nutritional advice for men at the present time (at least in relation to infertility) would therefore appear to be to consume an adequate and varied diet, to correct grossly abnormal body weight, and to moderate alcohol intake. Any such changes should probably be made at least two to three months before the intended time of conception.

Pre- and periconceptional nutrition in women

Nutrition and fertility

When energy stores are low, menarche may be delayed and if energy stores are diminished after menarche the menses are likely to become irregular, infrequent and possibly stop (Frisch and MacArthur 1974). Amenorrhoea has been well described in excessive weight loss and anorexia nervosa (Fries 1974).

Conception can occur in women who are well below average or ideal weight (for height) and it has been reported in women with a BMI as low as 14.9 (Treasure and Russell 1988). However, women who are thin at conception do have a higher frequency of intra-uterine growth retardation leading to smaller and possibly disadvantaged babies. Very thin women can produce healthy offspring provided a healthy and varied diet is available and weight is gained adequately throughout the pregnancy (Rosso 1985).

Thus, pre-pregnancy counselling should be available for the very thin woman aiming at weight gain before conception and certainly throughout pregnancy. Overweight women are also commonly infertile and there are data to suggest that the overweight have reduced sexual activity (Crisp 1967).

Nutrition and early fetal development

The fetus is most susceptible to nutritional imbalance during the first trimester of pregnancy, since this is the time of most rapid cell differentiation and establishment of embryonic systems and organs (Basu 1981). The time of greatest nutritional vulnerability is possibly before a woman even suspects she is pregnant, and certainly before the first antenatal appointment. Much of pre-pregnancy care then (including nutrition) should form part of health education for living which should be started in schools and continued into the pre-pregnancy zone of life (Chamberlain 1986).

Much remains to be learned about the intricacies of nutrition and early fetal development. However several areas can be highlighted as being of particular relevance.

Undernutrition During the 'Dutch Hunger Winter' of October 1944 to May 1945 there were significant famine effects on fetal growth but these were limited in that they occurred mainly with exposure in late pregnancy and not with exposure in the first two trimesters (Susser 1980). The size of the effects of various growth indices were concomitant with the time order in which they became apparent. First maternal weight was affected, then birth weight, then placental weight, then length and then head size. Thus women exposed to starvation in the early stages of pregnancy did not have smaller babies although other developmental problems such as neural tube defects were more frequent (Stein *et al* 1975).

Although overt food shortage is rare in the UK the consequences of undernutrition are seen in anorexia nervosa patients. Pregnancy is, of course, unlikely to occur during the anorexic state, but fertility will return during the recovery phase and pregnancy at this time is perhaps unwise. Extremely poor eating habits (due to factors such as ignorance or low income) may also lead to a diminished food intake but slimming is perhaps the greatest hazard.

Large numbers of women spend periods of time following reducing 'diets' of dubious nutritional quality which may result in very low energy intakes. Additionally, overweight women trying to start a family are often encouraged to lose weight because of the increased risk of late pregnancy complications and perinatal mortality in overweight mothers (Naeye 1979; Edwards *et al* 1979). It is preferable for weight to be reduced well in advance of conception in order to lessen the likelihood of nutritional inadequacy. If this is not practicable then efforts should be made to ensure that the diet is adequate in terms of quality for at least three to four months prior to the intended time of conception.

Vitamin deficiency There is now considerable evidence that low periconceptional vitamin intake may be linked with the development of neural tube defect (NTD) (Smithells *et al* 1980, 1981a, 1981b; Laurence *et al* 1981; Smithells 1983). However, it is likely that most cases of NTD arise from a combination of unknown genetic and environmental components, both of which must be triggered for the defects to occur (Seller 1987).

Several environmental agents have been studied in the aetiology of NTD including tea drinking (Frederick 1974) and blighted potatoes (Renwick 1972). However, studies of vitamin supplementation have provided the strongest evidence for a dietary link so far. In supplementation studies (Smithells *et al* 1980; Smithells 1983) observed lower rates of recurrent NTD in the offspring of women who complied with a regimen of multivitamin supplements compared to women who were pregnant prior to study or who had not complied with the prescribed regimen. However, Smithells' studies have been heavily criticized for using self-selected subjects (i.e. compliers) (Rush 1986). Laurence *et al* (1980) reported decreased recurrence in Wales where women with previous NTD births had received dietary counselling. All recurrences were in women judged to have a 'poor diet'. The interpretation of these studies is however complicated because of social and environmental factors associated with a poor dietary intake.

The results of the Medical Research Council Vitamin Study (MRC 1991) on the prevention of neural tube defects clearly demonstrate a link between folic acid and the development of NTDs. In this study, a daily 4 mg folic acid supplement given around the time of conception to women at high risk (i.e. those who already had one or more NTD pregnancies) was shown to prevent neural tube defects (anencephaly, spina bifida, encephalocele). The effects of multivitamins were also assessed but there was no indication that these conferred any preventative effect or that they enhanced folic acid.

The conclusions from the study group are that folic acid supplementations can now be recommended for all women who have had a previously affected pregnancy and that public health measures (e.g. fortification of staple foods) should be taken to ensure that all women of childbearing age receive adequate dietary folic acid. It is unclear whether all women planning a pregnancy should take folic acid supplementation. In dietetic practice it would be appropriate to provide dietary counselling for all women with a previous NTD pregnancy although some women will have dietary intakes close to or greater than the estimated average requirement (250 μg/day) and Reference Nutrient Intake (300 μg/day) (DoH 1991). This suggests that the mechanism of vitamin action may be related to a metabolic block, defect in embryonic uptake from maternal blood or other disorder (i.e. genetically controlled disturbance of folic acid metabolism) rather than a simple dietary deficiency.

Alcohol The affects of alcohol taking during the preconceptual period on the outcome of pregnancy are unknown. However animal work by Keiffer and Ketchel (1970) suggests that a single administration of alcohol may reduce the likelihood of conception. However, it is considered rare that a woman will be anovulatory on the basis of alcohol alone, although it has been reported during the acute phase of alcoholism (Ryback 1977) with return of ovulation after cessation of alcoholic episode.

The term 'fetal alcohol syndrome' (FAS) is used to describe the congenital malformations associated with alcohol intake. These include growth retardation, abnormal craniofacial features, plus developmental problems (Beattie 1988). FAS is seen in the children of heavy drinking mothers (more than 80 g pure alcohol per day) and abstinence during pregnancy protects the infant. Some women drinking at this alcoholic level produce children with full FAS; other infants from such pregnancies may exhibit only partial FAS features and are considered to have 'fetal alcohol effect' (FAE). The incidence of FAS is around one case per thousand live births (Beattie *et al* 1983), with 3–4 cases of FAE per thousand in the general population. However, incidence varies from region to region and in the UK cases have mainly been seen in the West of Scotland, Liverpool and Belfast (Beattie 1988).

It has been suggested that the regular consumption of 1–2 drinks a day during the first trimester of pregnancy is associated with an increased relative risk of mid-trimester abortion (Harlap and Shiono 1980). It would appear at present that moderate drinking does not increase neonatal mortality (Newman 1986). There may however be a small influence on birth weight if more than 5 drinks weekly are taken (Wright *et al* 1983) but the biological significance of this is unknown.

In summary, it is clear that alcohol intoxication should be avoided at any stage of pregnancy and especially in the early weeks where it is associated with teratogenesis (Beattie 1988). Regular excessive drinking is linked with FAS and FAE and has an adverse effect on perinatal mortality and brain development.

Occasional social drinking is thought to be fairly innocuous (Beattie 1988) but it would be advisable to consume fewer than five drinks per week. It is appropriate to remember that tolerance to alcohol may be affected by nutritional status, body weight, body fat and other factors.

The recommendation by the US Surgeon General for pregnant women to abstain totally from alcohol has been

Table 3.1 Nutritional aspects of preconceptional counselling for women

1	Make dietary changes at least 3–4 months before attempting conception
2	Achieve acceptable body weight for height
3	Eat a diet with adequate energy
4	Eat a varied diet to ensure intake of all nutrients
5	Restrict, or preferably exclude, alcohol
6	Seek advice from a doctor before taking any dietary supplements

criticized because of lack of evidence (Wright *et al* 1983; Beattie 1988).

Nutritional aspects of preconceptional advice for women are summarized in Table 3.1.

3.1.2 Nutritional considerations during pregnancy

Nutritional requirements

During the second and third trimesters of pregnancy rapid growth of the fetus inevitably imposes increased nutritional demands on the mother. However, it is worth remembering that there are a number of ways in which the nutrient supply to the fetus may be regulated:

1 Changes in food and diet.
2 Altered maternal absorption.
3 Fetal uptake (i.e. maternal loss).
4 Varying placental transfer.

The extent to which increased nutritional needs must be met by dietary adjustment is unclear. Although Recommended Dietary Allowances (RDAs) or Dietary Reference Values (DRVs) can be calculated which take the nutritional cost of pregnancy into account, these figures cannot be applied indiscriminately to all pregnant women, for two reasons.

- RDAs are set at a level which should prevent nutritional deficiencies in the vast majority of the population. The actual requirement of many individuals will be considerably less than the RDA.
- As a physiological response to pregnancy there is considerable adaptation to meet increased nutritional needs. The absorption of many nutrients is increased and their excretion decreased and metabolism is generally more efficient. In general, RDAs do not take these factors into account and thus may be unnecessarily high, although the current UK DRVs have considered the adaptive processes which occur at this time.

Nevertheless there will be some pregnant women in whom the nutritional needs will not be met. If these women can be identified at the appropriate time then they need to be selected for specific dietetic counselling. However, because of the difficulty in identifying 'at risk' individuals, it may be more appropriate to advise all women on a healthy varied diet as part of health education initiated by schools.

Dietary advice in pregnancy must be aimed not only at ensuring a satisfactory outcome of pregnancy but also should be aimed at promoting family health and preventing disease.

The healthy varied diet

The majority of pregnant women can meet their nutrient needs by consuming a diet in fibre-rich carbohydrate and low in fat, as recommended for the general population. The advantages of this type of diet for pregnant women are described by James (1986) who expresses the view that if women are to meet the nutrient requirements of themselves and their children they should eat a low-fat, low-sugar diet. The suitability of this type of diet for pregnancy is also commented on by Johnstone (1983). He concludes in his review of dietary advice during pregnancy that a healthy active woman who has maintained her optimal body weight for some years prior to pregnancy on a NACNE style diet will eat slightly more during pregnancy, but there is no good evidence that any other quantitative or qualitative changes need to be made. A study in Aberdeen (Lean and Anderson 1990) of a sample of randomly selected women attending routine antenatal clinics in the first trimester of pregnancy indicated that women in the lowest quartile of energy from fat (mean fat intake 35% energy) had a good overall nutrient intake (Table 3.2). This suggests that a NACNE style diet can be associated with adequate nutrient intake (including energy).

Energy

The total energy costs of pregnancy were estimated by Hytten and Leitch (1964) to be about 80 000 kcal (336 MJ). This includes the cost of the increase in maternal tissues, the growth of the product of conception, an assumed 3–4 kg gain in lipid reserves and the increased basal metabolic rate resulting from the increased body weight.

If the whole of this cost were to be met from increased food intake, an additional 150 kcal per day would be required during the first trimester and 350 kcal per day in the second and third trimesters. However dietary surveys show increases of only around 200 kcal in the third trimester. The remainder of the energy cost was assumed to be met from energy savings from reduced activity.

Recent work in Scotland has shown that the average gain in adipose tissue is only about 2.3 kg, and this does not seem to be detrimental to the fetus (Durnin *et al* 1985; 1987). The total cost of pregnancy is therefore calculated as 40 000 kcal for the tissue deposition and 30 000 kcal for increased BMR, giving a total of 70 000 kcal. However, in view of the disparity between calculated costs and the dietary findings, the panel on Dietary Reference Values took a cautious view and set the Estimated Average Requirement (EAR) for pregnancy at 200 kcal per day in the third trimester only (DH 1991).

The above calculations are based on the average costs of

Table 3.2 Nutrient intake in a random sample of Aberdeen women in the first trimester of pregnancy (Lean and Anderson 1990).

Daily nutrient intake (mean ± sd) of 34 pregnant women

Nutrient	Unit	All ($n = 34$)	Low fat group ($n = 8$)
Energy	kcal	1909 ± 363	2017 ± 485
Protein	g	68.9 ± 13.8	72.5 ± 15.1
Protein	% energy	14.5 ± 1.7	14.8 ± 1.9
Fat	g	88.4 ± 19.6	78.6 ± 22.5
Fat	% energy	41.7 ± 5.1	34.6 ± 3.5
Carbohydrate	g	221 ± 50.1	247 ± 82.5
Carbohydrate	% energy	43.4 ± 5.1	50.0 ± 3.8
Alcohol	g	0.9 ± 2.2	0.6 ± 1.2
Alcohol	% energy	0.3 ± 0.8	0.2 ± 0.4
Dietary fibre	g	17.6 ± 5.8	22.3 ± 3.9
Thiamin	mg	1.5 ± 1.6	1.4 ± 0.3
Riboflavin	mg	1.6 ± 0.6	1.9 ± 0.6
Nicotinic acid equivalents	mg	19.7 ± 5.8	21.2 ± 7.3
Total folate	μg	144 ± 51	176 ± 31.5
Ascorbic acid	mg	89.3 ± 49	115 ± 43.7
Calcium	mg	881 ± 255	990 ± 320
Iron	mg	12.4 ± 5.2	16.0 ± 5.5

a pregnancy. Goldberg *et al* (1993) have shown that there are wide variations between individuals in the energy economy of pregnancy. Some women may show a reduction in BMR during the early months, while others show an increase almost from conception. The amount of fat laid down also varies enormously. The total cost of pregnancy in only 12 individuals ranged from 34 MJ to 1192 MJ. Probably the best practical advice for pregnant women is to eat to appetite. Some women with weight problems who normally keep slim by restrained eating may suffer 'motivational collapse' during pregnancy when their body shape and lifestyle are radically altered (Prentice *et al* 1987). These women may need help and guidance during pregnancy and afterwards. In general, dieting for weight loss during pregnancy is to be discouraged and may result in a low birth weight incidence (Campbell 1983).

Protein

The optimal protein requirements for pregnancy are unknown. Calculations based on foetal maternal growth suggest that 900 grams are needed for the entire pregnancy or approximately 5 g/day during the last two trimesters (Hytten and Leitch 1971). The current UK DRV (DoH 1991) is an additional 6 g per day throughout pregnancy, making the RNI approx 51 g/day. However, recent studies of dietary intake have shown that women consume much greater quantities (Anderson and Lean 1986; Black *et al* 1986; Schofield *et al* 1987; Thompson *et al* 1989), and up to 16% of dietary energy as protein. Schofield *et al* (1987) found no significant difference in protein intake among different social class groups in Edinburgh and London which they thought to be due to the widespread belief 'that protein foods are less fattening than starch or fat'.

Caution needs to be exerted in over-zealous recommendation of protein-rich foods during pregnancy. Rush *et al* (1980) demonstrated that high protein supplementation (40 g protein/470 kcal) was associated with an excess of very early premature births, associated neonatal deaths and significant growth retardation up to 37 weeks of gestation.

Minerals and trace elements

Iron Typical iron losses incurred as a result of pregnancy comprise

Iron transferred to the fetus	300 mg
Placenta and cord iron	50 mg
Postpartum blood loss	200 mg
Total	550 mg

Offset against this is the saving of 200 mg due to the absence of menstruation, making a net iron cost to the body of 350 mg. This represents a theoretical extra requirement over the non-pregnant state of 1.8 mg iron/day during the second and third trimesters.

In addition to this, the body requires approximately 500 mg iron for the expansion in red cell mass which occurs after 12 weeks. Normally this is met from internal reserves and creates no extra requirement. However, if iron stores are depleted at the start of pregnancy then, theoretically, an additional 2.6 mg/day will be required from dietary sources throughout the last two trimesters.

While these estimates of additional daily needs are convenient, they are not totally realistic. They assume that the requirement for iron remains constant throughout the last two trimesters whereas, in fact, proportionally less is needed at 12 weeks and correspondingly more as term approaches.

Nevertheless, provided that habitual iron intake is adequate, it seems likely that the extra requirement to cover iron losses can be met through physiological adaptation and without the need for a dietary increase. The current DRV (DoH 1991) for iron in adult women is 14.8 mg/day with no recommended increase during pregnancy. This is based on the assumption that all women of childbearing age should have sufficient stores to cope with the metabolic demands of pregnancy and diminished losses because of the absence of menstrual bleeding. Iron absorption increases during pregnancy, and increases progressively as pregnancy advances, therefore meeting the rising demand (Bowering *et al* 1979). Furthermore, a greater percentage increase in absorption will occur in anaemic than in non-anaemic women. Apte and Iyenger (1970) showed that iron absorption rose from 7.4% at the 16th week of pregnancy to 25.7% in the third trimester; in those who were anaemic, iron absorption rose to 37.9%. Even a lower than average dietary iron intake is not necessarily an indication for supplementation since this too will tend to be offset by an increased absorption (Bowering *et al* 1979).

However, in women who start pregnancy without adequate iron stores, the situation may be rather different. Low reserves in conjunction with a low iron intake will inevitably result in iron deficiency. It is this group of women who require dietary intervention and, probably, iron supplementation. The problem is that this sub-group is not easy to identify. Some indication of iron stores can be derived from the serum ferritin level but this is rarely carried out as a routine measure. Conversely, regular measurements are usually made of the blood haemoglobin level, although this is not a sensitive reflector of iron status. A fall in haemoglobin during pregnancy does not necessarily indicate iron insufficiency; more usually it is simply a dilution effect caused by the expansion in plasma volume. On the other hand, if iron deficiency is present, few clinicians would wish to wait until frank anaemia (a low haemoglobin coupled with reduced red cell size) appears before instituting corrective therapy. It is for this reason that routine iron supplementation to all pregnant women is so common even though for the majority it is unnecessary.

However, some antenatal clinics do now adopt a more discriminatory approach to iron supplementation. Iron supplements are not always well tolerated and significant numbers of women suffer from nausea, diarrhoea or constipation (Bennett 1982; Lind 1983). There is also some evidence to suggest that unnecessary supplementation may do more harm than good. Lind (1983) showed that iron supplements resulted in an increased mean cell volume (MCV) compared with that in unsupplemented pregnant women. This increased red cell size may be highly undesirable since it could affect blood flow in small capillaries and impair oxygen and/or nutrient supply to the placenta.

It has also been suggested that the level of iron supplement commonly used may adversely affect maternal zinc status (Solomons and Jacob, 1981; Hambidge *et al* 1983). Iron supplementation is known to affect the bioavailability of zinc. An American study has shown an inverse association between circulating levels of zinc and the amount of iron consumed as part of the prenatal vitamin-mineral supplementation (Hambidge *et al* 1983).

Ideally, rather than routine supplementation, iron insufficiency should be diagnosed and corrected preconceptionally or at an early stage of pregnancy before physiological changes make the usual laboratory indices difficult to interpret. If women are not seen until pregnancy is more advanced, efforts should be made to identify those who appear to have a habitually low iron intake. If subsequent screening then reveals either a haemoglobin of 10.0 g/dl in association with a MCV of 82 fl or less, or a progressive fall in MCV, dietary intervention or supplementation is indicated.

In women who have neither evidence of, nor a history of, anaemia, the advice to include some lean meat in the diet every day is probably sufficient (haem iron from animal sources is better absorbed than inorganic iron from vegetable sources). In non-meat eaters, care should be taken to ensure that the diet is high in vitamin C (which improves the absorption of inorganic iron).

Calcium The metabolism of calcium in pregnancy has been summarized by Reeve (1980). A baby at birth contains 25–30 g calcium, most of which is laid down in the last ten weeks of pregnancy. The requirement specific to pregnancy is for approximately 260 mg/day at this time. There is a consensus (Misra and Anderson 1990) that the concentration of maternal free (biologically active) 1,25 dihydroxyvitamin D3 is raised during pregnancy thus increasing net calcium absorption. Thus the increased requirement for calcium during pregnancy may be met entirely from increased absorption. There is no evidence to suggest that the UK intakes of 0.8–1.0 g/day (Doyle *et al* 1982; Anderson and Lean 1986; Thompson *et al* 1989) are inadequate, and current DRVs (DoH 1991) suggest an RNI of 800 mg (for women aged 15–18 years) and 700 mg (for women aged 19–50 years) per day with no increment for pregnancy.

There is also evidence that even in populations with habitual intake as low as 400 mg/day, increased absorption can compensate for the increased requirements of pregnancy (Shenolikar 1970; Walker *et al* 1972). The well nourished woman will be in slight calcium imbalance during pregnancy but this may be reversed in breast feeding. There is concern that repeated pregnancies and prolonged lactation (without adequate replenishment) may lead to osteomalacia in women and neonatal rickets, although this is likely to be confined only to economically deprived communities and Asian immigrants in Northern parts of Europe (Misra and Anderson 1990).

Special attention may be needed for Asian mothers because not only do they have a low vitamin D status but they have high fibre intakes which may impair calcium absorption.

Where increases in calcium intake are indicated the following foods will provide approximately an additional 300 mg calcium to the usual diet.

1 Half a pint of milk.
2 One small piece (30–40 g) Cheddar cheese.
3 One 90 g serving of sardines.
4 A small carton of yoghurt.
5 A 200 g serving of milk pudding.

Zinc Animal studies have shown that deficiency of zinc is associated with abnormal pregnancy but this has not been clearly demonstrated in humans. With respect to retarded fetal growth, some studies have shown an increase in plasma zinc concentration (Patrick *et al* 1982), some a decreased plasma zinc concentration (Mukkerjee *et al* 1984), and some unchanged levels (Tuttle *et al* 1985). Studies of dietary intake (Abraham 1983; Hunt *et al* 1983) suggest that zinc intake is less than the previous recommended daily allowance for pregnant women of 20 mg/day (US National Research Council 1980) although the UK RNI (DoH 1991) of 7 mg/day (with no increment during pregnancy) has been met. Zinc intakes tend to parallel protein intake. In the majority of these studies the outcome of the pregnancy was entirely satisfactory with normal healthy babies.

Plasma zinc levels decrease in early pregnancy (Campbell 1988) but return to normal by 6 weeks post-partum. This observation is probably due to an expansion in plasma volume and increase in intravascular zinc mass (Tuttle *et al* 1985). Altered zinc status in pregnancy has been linked with neural tube defects (Soltan and Jenkins 1982; Hinks *et al* 1989).

Vitamins

Although routine multivitamin supplementation is common, it is probably unnecessary other than in those in high risk groups (see below) or where there is evidence of dietary inadequacy. The majority of pregnant women can meet their vitamin needs by consuming a healthy varied diet, high in fibre-rich carbohydrates and low in fat, as recommended for the general population. Vitamins which may be particularly important in pregnancy are as follows.

Folate (see also *vitamin deficiency* on p 236) Requirement for folate is increased during pregnancy to prevent megaloblastic anaemia (Chanarin *et al* 1968). The current UK DRV (DoH 1991) for folic acid in pregnancy is for 100 μg/day extra to the RNI of 200 μg/day for non-pregnant adults. The folate content of the diet has been reported to vary from 30 to 2681 μg/day in different studies (Rogozinski *et al* 1983) and there is some debate regarding the analytical techniques used to measure folic acid.

Vitamin C Vitamin C-rich fruit and vegetable consumption should be encouraged as part of a healthy varied diet. Vitamin C requirement is increased by 10 mg during pregnancy (and thus increases from 40 mg/day to 50 mg/day). The anti-oxidant properties of vitamin C may be beneficial for general health (WHO 1990). In women who have problems eating fruit (e.g. edentulous women), appropriate vitamin C rich fruit juices should be encouraged. Vitamin C intakes have also been found to be lower amongst women who smoke during pregnancy (Haste *et al* 1990), thus appropriate advicė should be provided for this group.

Vitamin D Vitamin D is important in order to sustain the heightened calcium absorption and utilization during pregnancy. Normally, the body's requirements of vitamin D are supplied through exposure to sunlight, but whether the increased needs during pregnancy can be met via this route is unclear. In France (where food is not supplemented with vitamin D) vitamin D deficiency has been described in mothers and neonates, especially during winter and spring in areas where sunlight is scarce (Salle *et al* 1982). Brooke (1983) showed that vitamin D supplemented Asian women gained more weight than unsupplemented controls and had fewer small infants. All pregnant women should be encouraged to get out of doors as much as possible to get some sunlight.

For most women, diets which regularly contain vitamin D enriched margarine, cheese, fatty fish and eggs are probably adequate in vitamin D. Supplements may be necessary for 'at risk' individuals, especially Asian women, and should be accompanied by clear written instructions in the appropriate language to avoid any possibility of vitamin D overdose. Current DRVs (DoH 1991) recommend that pregnant women should receive supplementary vitamin D to achieve an intake of 10 μg/day.

Vitamin A In 1990 the Department of Health cautioned women who were (or who intended to become) pregnant to avoid excessive intake of vitamin A, either in the form of supplements or as liver products (such as paté or liver sausage) (DoH 1990). This advice related to recent analysis of the vitamin A content of liver, which showed that an average portion (i.e. 3–5 oz or 100 g), could contain 4–12 times the maximum RDA for pregnancy (2700–3300 μg). These excessively high levels were thought to result from the vitamin A content of animal foodstuffs.

Vitamin supplements containing 400–1250 μg of vitamin A given under medical supervision are still considered safe although pregnant women are currently advised not to eat liver. The effects of vitamin A intake in pregnancy are reviewed by Hathcock *et al* (1990) who conclude that the maternal dose threshold for birth defects could not be identified from present data. Current DRVs (DoH 1991) for vitamin A recommend an increment of 100 μg/day throughout pregnancy (raising the maternal RNI to 700 μg/day).

Globally, vitamin A deficiency is a much more frequent problem.

Non-nutritional considerations

Smoking

Smoking is associated with a decrease in birth weight of around 175–200 g (Lumley and Astbury 1989). Smokers tend to have an increased risk of a delivery between 24 and 34 weeks gestation, particularly those smoking 20 or more cigarettes a day (Meyer *et al* 1976). Placenta praevia, abruptio placenta and premature rupture of the membranes are all more common in smoking mothers.

The relationship between smoking and maternal nutrition is summarized by Sexton (1986) who reported that smokers tend to weigh less and gain less weight during pregnancy than non-smokers, although both of these observations may be linked more closely to social class than dietary intake. Haste *et al* (1990) reported that women who smoked had a poorer quality of diet (other than energy intake) than did non-smokers and this was independent of social background. Non-smokers were found to have persistently higher mean intakes of all nutrients (except energy) analysed in all social class groups.

How smoking relates to nutrition is complex and incompletely understood. Metabolic rate is elevated, taste is altered, nutrient metabolism may be affected.

Factors implicated in a poor outcome to pregnancy

Parents who fall into one or more of the following categories should be monitored closely and the fetus considered at risk. Dietary counselling is particularly important for the following groups:

1 Adolescent mothers. If pregnancy follows soon after menarche, those with a late menarche are likely to be more developed and therefore less at risk than those with an early menarche (Beal 1981). Thomas (1984) recommends a pregnancy weight gain of around 14 kg for the normal weight teenager.

2 Women more than 20% above or 10% below ideal body weight (Pitkin 1981).

3 Immigrant women who may be consuming an inadequate diet in this country.

4 Vegans or vegetarians who follow an inadequate diet.

5 Women with bizarre eating habits such as those suffering with bulimia nervosa.

6 Families with a limited food budget or food management problems.

7 Women with closely spaced pregnancies.

8 Parents with pre-existing medical complications, such as diabetes mellitus or gastrointestinal disease.

9 Women with a poor obstetric history including low birth weight babies (less than 2500 g), spontaneous abortion, prolonged labour, and abruptio placenta.

10 Exposure of either parent to high levels of cadmium or lead via water supplies, food, occupation or place of residence (Stephens 1981).

11 Parents with alcohol or drug problems.

12 Parents who smoke or are exposed to cigarette smoke (Grant 1981).

However, it is important to remember that antenatal care is one situation which is unique in providing the opportunity to reach large numbers of healthy women with the potential to influence the health of the next generation. There is a case for providing all pregnant women with information on a healthy varied diet, because it is not always obvious which individuals are 'at risk' and many women with poor birth outcome cannot be identified.

Weight gain during pregnancy

Desirable weight gain during pregnancy

It seems reasonable to avoid massive weight gain during pregnancy and the amount to be gained should be related to the pre-pregnant weight (Fig. 3.1). However, assessing desirable weight gain in pregnancy is complicated by the fact that it is difficult to distinguish between weight gain caused by fat deposition and weight gain due to fluid retention. Hytten and Leitch (1971) found that overweight women tended to gain more water and less fat than thin women. Campbell (1983) found that primigravidae who

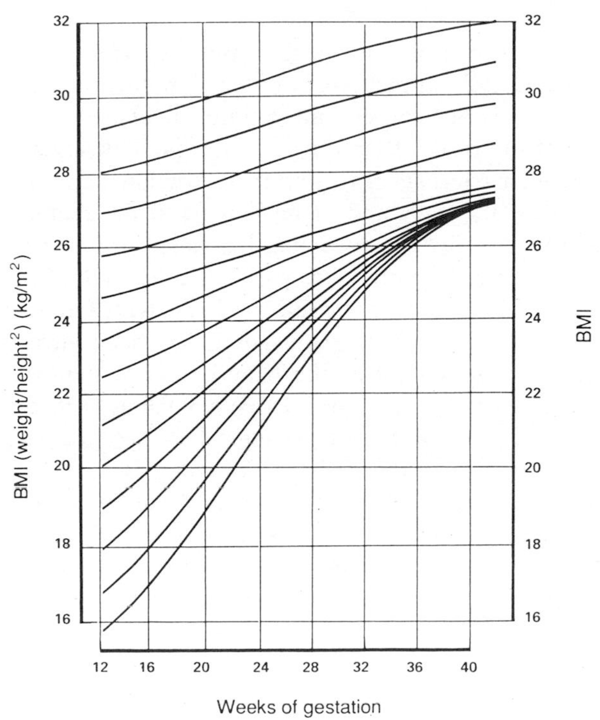

Fig. 3.1 Recommended weight gain during pregnancy.

restricted their food intake gained less weight than those who ate to appetite. However the difference was mainly due to reduced water retention and less expansion of plasma volume rather than a large reduction in body fat stores. Young teenage mothers may have high weight gains but these have been attributed to increased fluid volume and fluid retention rather than addition to body mass (Garn *et al* 1984).

Inadequate weight gain

Poor weight gain may be due to low food intake although pre-pregnant weight should be taken into consideration. Some women may fear excessive body weight and find it difficult to cope with changing body shape. These women should be encouraged towards a realistic weight gain and reassured that they will lose weight post-partum. Dugdale and Eaton Evans (1989) found that women who wanted to lose weight after pregnancy are more likely to do so and that changes in weight and skinfold thicknesses are independent of breast feeding. They also reported that most women had returned to their pre-pregnant weight by six months post-partum. There is some variation in how breast feeding affects mothers' weight, but current consensus is that it has a rather small effect. Certainly it doesn't cause weight gain, and should always be recommended as the perfect diet for the healthy newborn child. Advice on slimming after pregnancy (Anderson and Lean 1989) should be provided for women who are anxious about weight gain during pregnancy.

Excessive weight gain

In obese pregnant women, limitation of weight gain has been and still is practised in order to reduce high blood pressure, pre-eclampsia and gestational diabetes, and to prevent the birth of large babies, to ease delivery and to prevent long-term obesity. Dietary restriction may be detrimental to the baby and of no benefit to the mother. In some studies dietary restriction has failed to lower blood pressure or reduce pre-eclampsia, but it has reduced birth weight (Campbell and McGillivray 1975; Kerr Grieve *et al* 1979; Campbell 1983). Although it has been suggested that this is important as the baby is merely deprived of optional fat reserves (Hytten 1983) any fall in birth weight is undesirable since neonatal mortality rates increase at birth weights less than 3400 g (Van den Berg 1981). In addition Campbell (1983) found that gestation was longer in a diet restricted group of women, i.e. 32% delivered later than 40 weeks compared with 15% of control. The reasons for these observations were complex.

3.1.3 Nutrition-related problems in pregnancy

Nausea and vomiting

Nausea and vomiting are generally accepted as a common occurrence which accompany half of all pregnancies (Fairweather 1968). Estimates of incidence vary from 50–86% (Taggart 1961; Pickard 1982; Wiegel and Wiegel 1989). Wiegel and Wiegel (1989) reported that 46% of women experienced both nausea and vomiting, whilst 23% reported nausea with no vomiting. They noted that symptoms started as early as 4–6 weeks gestation, peaked at 8–12 weeks, and diminished thereafter. They found that only vomiting was associated with decreased risk of miscarriage.

Taggart (1961), in her study of pregnant Aberdeen women, reported that it was usual for appetite to be normal or even increased in spite of nausea and vomiting, whilst Wiegel and Wiegel (1989) showed that women with vomiting gained less weight in the first 20 weeks than those with nausea only or no symptoms.

Anecdotal reports suggest that nausea may become worse when the stomach is empty and may be relieved by eating. Other factors which might induce nausea include long journeys and smells (particularly those of cigarettes, coffee and toothpaste). Many cures for morning sickness have been described in folklore, but none have been scientifically validated. These treatments include consuming liquids between meals instead of with the food (Worthington Roberts *et al* 1981), consumption of ginger, peppermint tea, wheatgerm milk mixture, and stopping iron tablets (Kitzinger 1988).

There is a general impression that small carbohydrate-rich snacks given at frequent (e.g. two-hourly) intervals may provide some relief from nausea although the reason is not clear (Table 3.3). Snacks which involve little preparation and/or cooking smells may be preferable. Women should be reassured that snacks can be as nourishing as full meals and that this type of regimen will not necessarily lead to excessive weight gain. This approach provides an

Table 3.3 Snacks which may alleviate nausea and vomiting during pregnancy

Breakfast cereals with low-fat milk
Toast and jam, no butter
Plain biscuits, e.g. oatcakes
Hot or cold low-fat milky drinks
Sandwiches with low-fat filling
Boiled egg and toast
Baked beans on toast
Soup and toast/bread
Jacket potatoes with a low-fat filling
Lean cold meat or poultry with potato or roll
Yogurt or fromage frais, low-fat varieties
Milk puddings with low-fat milk
Fruit salad and cottage cheese

opportunity to discuss healthful snacks suitable for the entire family. As with the general population it is important to point out that high fat, high sugar snacks may reduce appetite for more nutrient-dense foods generally.

Anti-emetics are not considered appropriate for use in pregnancy.

Hyperemesis gravidarum

In a superb review of nausea and vomiting in pregnancy, Fairweather (1968) defined hyperemesis gravidarum as 'vomiting occurring in pregnancy appearing for the first time before the twentieth week of gestation and as of such severity as to require the patient's admission to hospital'. The aetiology is unknown although factors such as multiple pregnancy, parity, race, social circumstances may contribute. Incidence appears to vary across the UK and figures range from 0.1 to 1% (Fairweather 1968).

Early intervention is important in hyperemesis gravidarum to avoid severe dehydration and associated problems. Once hospitalized, initial attention must focus on intravenous rehydration, correction of electrolyte imbalance and energy provision. Vitamins, minerals and trace elements should also be supplied as these may be severely depleted. Reports of total parenteral nutrition given during the first trimester suggest that this is a safe and effective method of nutritional support (Levine and Esser 1988) but this is rarely necessary. Small frequent feeds of clear fluids should be introduced initially and continued for at least 24 hours. Once these are well tolerated, small quantities of liquid energy or preferably a complete food supplement should be taken at frequent intervals. As tolerance improves the amounts can be increased gradually until intake approaches the daily requirement, weaning onto three small meals a day. Small supplemental drinks should still be given between meals but phased out gradually as the meals increase in size. Body weight, electrolytes, urinary ketones, fluid balance and food consumption should be monitored throughout.

Discharge can be planned once the women is tolerating her oral regimen and progressively gaining weight. She should be instructed to have at least three meals a day at home, perhaps with more frequent snacks. There should be early follow up with immediate re-admission and initiation of supplementary feed if there is any decrease in weight. Advice on suitable snacks should be given prior to discharge.

Cravings, aversions and pica

Women may seek dietary advice following symptoms such as cravings, aversions and pica. In general, these symptoms cause much amusement for those individuals who do not experience them. They are popularly believed to be related to the nutritional needs of the mother, to have symbolic value, or to be related to sensory or physiological causes (Schwab and Axelson 1984).

Food cravings and aversions have been the centre of folk beliefs concerning pregnancy for many years (Murphree 1968; Snow and Johnson 1978) to explain infants' physical attributes, personality traits, birth marks and congenital malformations. For example, red spots on a baby may be attributed to excessive consumption of strawberries or cherries (Snow and Johnson 1978).

Food aversions have been defined as 'a definite revulsion against food and drink not previously disliked' (Dickens and Trethalum 1971). In Aberdeen, Taggart (1961) reported aversions to tea and coffee, fried food and eggs in early pregnancy, and to sweet foods in later pregnancy. Similar food findings were described by Hook (1978) in the US who also reported aversions to alcohol.

Food cravings have been defined by Dickens and Trethalum (1971) as 'a compulsive urge for a food for which there was no previous excessive desire'. Harries and Hughes (1957) described 991 cravings reported by 509 women in the UK. Most were for fruit and vegetables. Confectionery and cereal products were also mentioned. Taggart (1961) reported that about two thirds of Aberdeen women experienced cravings during pregnancy, the most common being for fruit. She also described some women who spontaneously developed a craving for milk. In the US, Hook (1978) describes common cravings as ice cream, sweets, candy, fruit and fish. Tierson *et al* (1985) were able to demonstrate that women who reported cravings generally increased their consumption of food items craved, and women reporting aversions decreased their consumption of those food items.

The explanation for these cravings and aversions are incomplete. Hytten and Leitch (1964) suggest that food cravings may be due to dulling of the sense of taste in pregnancy, and Tierson *et al* (1985) suggests that they may relate to changes in olfactory and taste sensitivity during pregnancy. Taste changes may be difficult to detect, but they are widely discussed in pregnancy health guides and are often said to result in foods developing a 'metallic' taste (SHEG 1979). Brewin (1980) has found similar taste changes in patients with tumours. There is a rapid return to normal taste perception with delivery of the baby or removal of the tumour.

Pica is the craving for, and ingestion of, substances usually considered inedible for human consumption. A wide variety of items have been described including laundry starch, ice (Schwab and Axelson 1984), rocks, match boxes and clay (Snow and Johnson 1977). The importance of pica is probably overstated in the lay literature. Taggart (1961) found only one case out of 900 women in Aberdeen. This woman ate coal and spent match heads during the last six weeks of pregnancy. Apparently she preferred 'good quality coal which crunched in a satisfying manner'. There is no convincing evidence that pica has any physiological significance, or indicates any mineral deficiency.

Heartburn

Gastro-oesophageal reflux, the basis of heartburn in pregnancy, can start as early as the third month but is generally worst in the third trimester and occurs in 30–50% of women (Taggart 1961; Seymour and Chadwick 1979). It is the result of increased abdominal pressure, combined with altered gastrointestinal motility. Davison *et al* (1970) found that women with heartburn had slower gastric emptying times than those without. There is widespread opinion that small frequent meals or snacks are usually tolerated better than infrequent large ones in the management of heartburn. Milk and yogurt may help to relieve the symptoms in some people but antacids tend to be widely used. The discomfort can be severe, and sustained – particularly when the woman is lying down. Certain foods such as spicy and fatty foods, fizzy drinks, citrus fruit and fruit juices, and alcohol may exacerbate the problem.

Constipation

In the UK, 38% of women report having been constipated some time during pregnancy, and 20% in the third trimester (Anderson 1984). Its aetiology is complex and includes depressed gut mobility in pregnancy (Hytten and Chamberlain 1980), increased fluid absorption from the large intestine (Parry *et al* 1970), decreased physical activity and dietary changes (Burgess 1972).

Reported treatments include dietary manoeuvres, drug therapy and changes in iron supplementation. Anderson (1985) has shown that many women attempt to relieve the symptoms of constipation by increasing the fibre content of the diet, but they often fail to achieve this. However, if a genuine increase in fibre is achieved, from an average intake of about 18 g to 27 g per day, then it is effective in treating constipation (Anderson and Whichelow 1985). Advice to follow a high fibre diet must include specific recommendations to increase complex carbohydrate intake with complementary reduction in fat intake. Simple advice to change to wholemeal bread, etc will only be effective if a substantially greater proportion of energy comes from carbohydrate.

Increasing fluid intake, while not supported by scientific evidence, is very widely recommended to treat constipation in pregnancy. Fluid intake may be intentionally reduced in pregnancy if frequency of micturition is a problem, and additionally colonic absorption of water is increased in pregnancy (Parry *et al* 1970). Tea drinking is only likely to be a problem at levels well above the amounts generally taken, but increasing fluid intake could be counter productive if tea intake is allowed to approach the 2 litres per day found by Hojgaard *et al* (1981) to produce constipation in non-pregnant subjects.

Pre-eclampsia

The cause of pre-eclampsia is unknown but various dietary links have been postulated. A frequent problem in assessing the relationship between diet and pre-eclampsia is the variable and often imprecise nature of the criteria which are used to diagnose the condition. In a review of diet and the prevention of pre-eclampsia, Green (1989) defines true pre-eclampsia as the presence of hypertension (diastolic pressure of 90 mmHg or more) and significant proteinuria (above 0.2 g/l) arising in the second half of pregnancy, with the obvious proviso that other causes of these signs (essential hypertension, renal disease, urinary tract infection) have been ruled out (MacGillivray 1983).

Obesity is widely regarded as a risk factor for the development of pre-eclampsia (Ruge and Anderson 1985) although the situation is complicated by evidence that the overall increase in incidence of pre-eclampsia among obese women is accompanied by a fall in the incidence of severe pre-eclampsia (Thomson and Billewicz 1957). However, none of the controlled studies (Campbell and MacGillivray 1975; Campbell 1983) on limiting weight gain in pre-eclampsia have been able to demonstrate a decreased incidence of pre-eclampsia with restricted weight gain. Indeed energy restriction may exacerbate the situation by further reducing cardiac output (Rosso 1983) which is already decreased in pre-eclampsia (Llewellyn-Jones 1982). Reduced cardiac output may reduce uterine blood flow and so compromise fetal development. Dietary restriction may also result in a reduction of birth weight (Campbell Brown 1983).

Attempts to use dietary manipulation to prevent pre-eclampsia have included protein supplements (Strauss 1935), zinc supplements (Hunt *et al* 1983), folic acid (Hemminki and Starfield 1978), B vitamins (Hillman *et al* 1963), vitamin mineral supplementation (People's League of Health 1946). Salt supplementation was examined with an apparently beneficial response, by Robinson (1958). More recently, salt restriction has been studied with inconclusive results.

A preventive effect of dietary marine n-3 fatty acids on early delivery (Olsen *et al* 1986) and toxaemia has recently been hypothesized, largely based (Olsen and Secher 1990) on the dietary supplementation trial conducted by the People's League of Health (1946). The role of fish oil supplements on pre-eclampsia is currently being assessed.

In summary, there is no conclusive evidence that dietary restriction or supplementation can reduce pre-eclampsia.

Listeriosis

Listeriosis is a disease caused by a bacterium, *Listeria monocytogenes*. Listeriosis is a rare illness but has a high mortality rate (Gellin and Broome 1989). Two hundred and fifty-one cases were reported in the general population of England and Wales in 1989 although only 59 were reported in the first half of 1990 (Cooke 1990).

Infection of the fetus can lead to abortion, stillbirth or delivery of an acutely ill infant. It is considered prudent for pregnant women to avoid foods known to be sometimes heavily contaminated with *L. monocytogenes*. Some obstetricians feel that information on food implicated in the transmission of listeria should be detailed in all antenatal clinics throughout the UK (Buchdahl *et al* 1990).

The main foods to be avoided are soft ripened cheeses including Camembert, Brie, goats' and sheep milk cheeses. It is thought that 5–15% of these cheeses for sale in European countries might be contaminated (usually in low numbers), irrespective of the heat treatment of the original milk (Roberts 1990). Care must also be taken with mould ripened cheeses which have a higher pH and permit growth of *L. monocytogenes*. Hard cheeses, yoghurt and butter can be regarded as safe because of a low pH and lack of moisture. Processed cheese spread and cottage cheese are also likely to be free from contamination.

Sufficient heat will eliminate the organism. Raw milk (cow, sheep, goat) should be avoided or boiled before consumption. Purchased ready-made salad/ingredients (including coleslaw) are best avoided. Other foods to avoid include paté, raw or under-cooked meat, non-canned meat products (pies, sausage rolls, unless they are cooked first). Pre-cooked foods and cook-chill meals should not be eaten cold, but cooked till very hot once only, and the leftovers discarded.

Good kitchen hygiene is essential. The Listeria Support Group recommends the following measures:

1 Cook food thoroughly (heat food through to 70°C and maintain for at least two minutes).
2 Buy chilled and frozen foods last; take home and store them quickly.
3 Check fridge and freezer temperatures.
4 Avoid mixing raw and cooked food.
5 Don't re-heat any food more than once.
6 Check dates on packets etc.

Useful addresses

A large stamped addressed envelope should accompany all requests for information.

Foresight (The Association for the Promotion of Preconceptual Care) The Old Vicarage, Church Lane, Witley, Godalming, Surrey GU8 5PN
Booklets include *Environmental factors and foetal health – the case for preconceptual care* and *Guidelines for future parents and other information*.

National Childbirth Trust, Alexandra House, Oldham Terrace, London W3 6NH
General information about pregnancy, breast feeding and local groups.

Maternity Alliance, 59–61 Camden High Street, London NW1 7JL
Regular bulletin and leaflets.

The Alfawap Trust Fund Ltd, 4 Woodchurch Road, London NW6
Leaflets and information on the effects of alcohol preconceptually and during pregnancy.

Foundation for Education and Research in Childbearing, 27 Walpole Street, London SW3

The Listeria Support Group, c/o Mark Horvath, Worlingworth, Woodbridge, Suffolk IP13 7NZ

References

Abraham R (1983) Ethnic and religious aspects of diet. In *Nutrition in pregnancy*. Campbell DM and Gillmer MDG (Eds) pp. 243–50. Royal College of Obstetricians and Gynaecologists, London.

Anderson AS (1984) Constipation during pregnancy: Incidence and methods used in its treatment in a group of Cambridgeshire women. *Health Visitor* **57**, 363–4.

Anderson AS (1985) Dietary factors in the aetiology and treatment of constipation during pregnancy. *Br J Obstet Gyn* **83**(3), 202–207.

Anderson AS and Lean MEJ (1986) Dietary intake in pregnancy: A comparison between 49 Cambridgeshire women and current recommended intakes. *Hum Nutr: Appl Nutr* **40A**, 40–48.

Anderson AS and Lean MEJ (1989) Dieting after pregnancy. *Midwife, Health Visitor and Community Nurse* **25**(11), 475–7.

Anderson AS and Whichelow M (1985) Constipation during pregnancy: Dietary fibre intake and the effect of fibre supplementation. *Hum Nutr: Appl Nutr* **39A**, 202–207.

Apte SV and Iyenger L (1970) Absorption of dietary iron in pregnancy. *Am J Clin Nutr* **23**, 73–7.

Basu TK (1981) The significance of vitamins in pre-natal life. *Int J Environ Stud* **17**, 31–5.

Beal VA (1981) Assessment of nutritional status. *Am J Clin Nutr* **34**, 691–6.

Beattie JO (1988) Alcohol and the child. *Proc Nutr Soc* **47**(2), 121–7.

Beattie JO, Day RE, Cockburn F and Garg RA (1983) Alcohol and the fetus in the West of Scotland. *Br Med J* **287**, 17–20.

Bennett CA (1982) *Health awareness and practices among pregnant women in Glasgow*. Department of Child Health and Obstetrics, University of Glasgow.

Black AE, Wiles SJ and Paul AA (1986) The nutrient intakes of pregnant and lactating mothers of good socioeconomic status in Cambridge, UK: some implications for recommended daily allowances of minor nutrients. *Br J Nutr* **56**, 59–72.

Bowering J, Sanchez AM and Irwin MI (1979) A conspectus of research on iron requirements of man. *J Nutr* **106**, 985–1074.

Brewin TB (1980) Can a tumour cause the same appetite perversion or taste change as a pregnancy? *Lancet* **ii**, 907–908.

Brooke OG (1983) Vitamin D supplementation and pregnancy outcome. In *Nutrition in pregnancy*. Campbell DM and Gillmer MDG (Eds) pp. 167–170. Royal College of Obstetricians and Gynaecologists, London.

Buchdahl R, Hird M, Gamsu H, Tapp A, Gibb D and Tzannotos L (1990) Listeriosis revisited: the role of the obstetrician. *Br J Obstet Gyn* **97**, 186–9.

Burgess DE (1972) Constipation in obstetrics. In *Management of constipation*. Avery Jones F and Godding E (Eds) pp. 177–8. Blackwell Scientific Publications, Oxford.

Calloway DM (1983) Nutrition and reproductive function of men. *Nutr Abst Rev* **53**(5), 361–77.

Campbell DM and MacGillivray I (1975) The effect of a low calorie diet or a thiazide diuretic on the incidence of pre-eclampsia and birth weight. *Br J Obstet Gynaecol* **82**, 572–7.

Campbell DM (1983) Dietary restriction in obesity and its effect on neonatal outcome. In *Nutrition in pregnancy*. Campbell DM and Gillmer MDG (Eds) pp. 243–50, Royal College of Obstetricians and Gynaecologists, London.

Campbell DM (1988) Trace element needs in human pregnancy. *Proc Nutr Soc* **47**(1), 45–53.

Campbell-Brown M (1983) Protein energy supplements in primigravid women at risk of low birthweight. In *Nutrition in pregnancy*. Campbell

DM and Gillmer MDG (Eds) pp. 85–99. Royal College of Obstetricians and Gynaecologists, London.

Chamberlain G (1986) Prepregnancy care. In *Prepregnancy care.* Chamberlain G and Lumley J (Eds) John Wiley, Chichester.

Chanarin I, Rothman D, Ward A and Perry J (1968) Folate status and requirement in pregnancy. *Br Med J* **2**, 390–94.

Cooke ME (1990) Epidemiology of foodborne illness: UK. *Lancet* **336**, 790–93.

Crisp AH (1967) The possible significance of some behavioural correlates of weight and carbohydrate intake. *J Psychomatic Res* **11**, 117–31.

Davison JS, Davison MC and Hay DM (1970) Gastric emptying time in late pregnancy and labour. *J Obstet Gynaecol Brit Commonw* **77**, 37.

Department of Health (1990) Press Release 90/507. Women Cautioned. HMSO, London.

Department of Health (1991) *Dietary Reference Values for food energy and nutrients for the United Kingdom.* Report on Health and Social Subjects, No 41. HMSO, London.

Dickens G and Trethalum WH (1971) Cravings and aversions during pregnancy. *J Psychosom Res* **15**, 259–68.

Doyle W, Crawford MA, Laurance BM and Drury P (1982) Dietary survey during pregnancy in a low socioeconomic group. *Hum Nutr: Appl Nutr* **36A**, 95–106.

Dugdale AE and Eaton-Evans J (1989) The effect of lactation and other factors on postpartum changes in body-weight and skin fold thickness. *Br J Nutr* **61**, 149–53.

Durnin JVGA, McKillop FM, Grant S and Fitzgerald G (1985) Is nutritional status endangered by virtually no extra intake during pregnancy? *Lancet* **ii**, 823–25.

Durnin JVGA, McKillop FM, Grant S and Fitzgerald G (1987) Energy requirements of pregnancy in Scotland. *Lancet* **ii**, 897–900.

Edwards LE, Alton IR, Barrada MI and Hakanson EY (1979) Pregnancy in the underweight woman. *Am J Obstet Gynecol* **135**, 297.

Fairweather DV (1968) Nausea and vomiting in pregnancy. *Am J Obstet Gynecol* **102**(2), 135–75.

Frederick J (1974) Anencephalus and maternal tea drinking: evidence for a possible association. *Proc Roy Soc Med* **67**, 356–60.

Fries H (1974) Secondary amenorrhoea, self-induced weight reduction and anorexia nervosa. *Acta Psychiatr Scand* **248**(Suppl), 1–70.

Frisch RE and McArthur JW (1974) Menstrual cycles: fatness as a determinant of minimum weight for height necessary for their maintenance or onset. *Science* **185**, 949–51.

Garn SM, Lavelle N, Pesick SD and Ridella SA (1984) Are pregnant teenagers still in rapid growth? *Am J Dis Childh* **138**, 32–4.

Gellin BG and Bromme CV (1989) Listeriosis. *J Am Med Assoc* **261**, 1313–20.

Goldberg GR, Prentice AM, Coward WA, Davies HL, Murgatroyd PR, Wensing C, Black AE, Ashford J and Sawyer M (1993) Longitudinal assessment of energy expenditure in pregnancy by the doubly labelled water method. *Am J Clin Nutr* **57**, 494–505.

Grant ECG (1981) The harmful effects of common social habits, especially smoking and using oral contraceptive steroids, on pregnancy. *Int J Environ Stud* **17**, 57–66.

Green J (1989) Diet and the prevention of pre-eclampsia. In *Effective care in pregnancy and childbirth.* Chalmers I and Enkin M (Eds) pp. 281–300. Oxford University Press, Oxford.

Hambidge KM, Krebs NF, Jacobs MA, Favier A, Guyette L and Ilke DN (1983) Zinc nutritional status during pregnancy: a longitudinal study. *Am J Clin Nutr* **37**, 429–42.

Harlap S and Shiono PH (1980) Alcohol, Smoking and incidence of spontaneous abortions in the first trimester of pregnancy. *Lancet* **ii**, 173–176.

Harries JM and Hughes TG (1957) An enumeration of the 'cravings' of some pregnant women. *Proc Nutr Soc* **16**.

Haste FM, Brooke OG, Anderson HR, Bland JM, Shaw A, Griffin J and Peacock JL (1990) Nutrient intakes during pregnancy: observations on the influence of smoking and social class. *Am J Cin Nutr* **51**, 29–36.

Hathcock JN, Hattan DG, Jenkins MJ, McDonald JT, Sundaresan PR and Wilkening VL (1990) Evaluation of vitamin A toxicity. *Am J Clin Nutr* **52**(2), 183–202.

Hemminki E and Starfield B (1978) Routine administration of iron and vitamins during pregnancy – a review of controlled clinical trials. *Br J Obstet Gynaecol* **85**, 404–410.

Hillman RW, Caband PG, Nilsson DE, Arpin PD and Tufano R (1963) Pyridoxine supplementation during pregnancy. *Am J Clin Nutr* **12**, 427–30.

Hinks LJ, Ogilvy-Stuart A, Hambidge KM and Walker V (1989) Maternal zinc and Fe status in pregnancies with a neural tube defect or elevated plasma and feta-proteins. *Br J Obstet Gynaecol* **96**, 61–6.

Hojgaard L, Artmann S, Jorgensen M and Krag E (1981) Tea consumption: a cause of constipation? *Br Med J* **282**, 864.

Hook EB (1978) Dietary cravings and aversions during pregnancy. *Am J Clin Nutr* **31**, 1355–62.

Hunt IF, Murphy NJ, Cleaver AE, Faraji B, Swendseid ME, Louken AH, Clark VA, Laine N, Davis CA and Smith JC (1983) Zinc supplementation during pregnancy: zinc concentration of serum and hair from low-income women of Mexican descent. *Am J Clin Nutr* **37**, 572–582.

Hytten FE, (1983) Nutritional physiology during pregnancy. In *Nutrition in pregnancy.* Campbell DM and Gillmer MDG (Eds) pp. 1–8. Royal College of Obstetricians and Gynaecologists, London.

Hytten FE and Chamberlain G (1980) *Clinical physiology in obstetrics.* Blackwell Scientific Publications, Oxford.

Hytten FE and Leitch I (1964) *The physiology of human pregnancy.* Blackwell Scientific Publications, Oxford.

Hytten FE and Leitch I (1971) *The physiology of human pregnancy* 2e. Blackwell Scientific Publications, Oxford.

James WPT (1986) *Nutrition in pregnancy and early childhood.* Coronary Prevention Group, London.

Johnstone FD (1983) Assessment of dietary intake and dietary advice in pregnancy. In *Nutrition in pregnancy,* Campbell DM and Gillmer MDG (Eds). Royal College of Obstetricians and Gynaecologists, London.

Keiffer JD and Ketchel MM (1970) Blockade of ovulation in the rat by ethanol. *Acta Endocrinologica* **65**, 117–24.

Kerr-Grieve JF, Campbell Brown M and Johnstone FD (1979) Dieting in pregnancy: a study of the effect of a high protein low carbohydrate diet on birthweight in an obstetric population. In *Carbohydrate metabolism in pregnancy and the newborn.* Sutherland HW and Stowers JM (Eds) pp. 518–33. Springer Verlag, Berlin.

Kitzinger S (1988) *Freedom and choice in childbirth.* Penguin Books, London.

Laurence KM, James N, Miller H *et al* (1980) Increased risk of recurrence of pregnancies complicated by fetal neural tube defects in mothers receiving poor diet and possible benefits of dietary counselling. *Br Med J* **281**, 1592.

Laurence KM, James N, Miller MH, Tennant GB and Campbell H (1981) Double-blind randomized controlled trial of folate treatment before conception to prevent recurrence of neural tube defects. *Br Med J* **282**, 1509–511.

Lean MEJ and Anderson AS (1990) How much to eat? In *Perspectives in pre-pregnancy care.* Sutherland HW and Smith NC (Eds) pp. 19–31. Smith-Gordon, London.

Levine MG and Esser DE (1988) Hyperemesis gravidarum: Maternal nutritional effects on fetal outcome. *Obstet Gynaecol* **72**(102), 102–107.

Lind T (1983) Iron supplementation during pregnancy. In *Nutrition in pregnancy.* Campbell DM and Gillmer DG (Eds) pp. 181–91. Royal College of Obstetricians and Gynaecologists, London.

Llewellyn-Jones D (1982) *Fundamentals of obstetrics and gynaecology* Vol 1, 3e. Faber and Faber, London.

Lumley J and Astbury J (1989) Advice for pregnancy. In *Effective care in pregnancy and childbirth.* Chalmers I and Enkin M (Eds) Oxford University Press, Oxford.

MacGillivray I (1983) *Pre-eclampsia: the hypertensive disease of pregnancy.* WB Saunders, London.

MRC Vitamin Study Research Group (1991) Prevention of neural tube defects: Results of the Medical Research Council Vitamin Study. *Lancet* **338**, 131–7.

Meyer MB, Jones BS and Tonascia JA (1976) Perinatal events associated with maternal smoking during pregnancy. *Am J Epidem* **103**, 464–76.

Misra R and Anderson DC (1990) Providing the fetus with calcium. *Br Med J* **30**, 1220–21.

Mukkerjee MP, Sandstead HH, Ratuaparki MV, Johnson LK, Milne DG and Stelling HP (1984) Maternal zinc, iron, folic acid and protein nurtiture and outcome of human pregnancy. *Am J Clin Nutr* **40**, 496–507.

Murphree AH (1968) A functional analysis of Southern folk beliefs concerning birth. *Am J Obstet Gynecol* **102**(1), 125–34.

Naeye RL (1979) Weight gain and the outcome of pregnancy. *Am J Obstet Gynecol* **135**, 3–9.

Newman N (1986) Alcohol. In *Prepregnancy care: A manual for practice.* Chamberlain G and Lumley J (Eds) John Wiley, Chichester.

Olsen SF, Hansen HS, Sorensen TI, Jensen B, Secher NJ, Sommer S and Knudsen LP (1986) Intake of marine fat rich in n-3-polyunsaturated fatty acids may increase birth-weight by prolonging gestation. *Lancet* **ii**, 367–9.

Olsen SF and Secher NJ (1990) A possible preventive effect of low-dose fish oil on early delivery and pre-eclampsia: indicators from a 50-year old controlled trial. *Br J Nutr* **64**, 599–609.

Parry E, Shields R and Turnbull AC (1970) The effect of pregnancy on the colonic absorption of sodium, potassium and water. *J Obstet Gynaecol Br Commonw* **77**, 616–19.

Patrick J, Dervish C and Gillison M (1982) Zinc and small babies. *Lancet* **i**, 169–170.

Peoples League of Health (1946) The nutrition of expectant and nursing mothers in relation to maternal and infant mortality and morbidity. *J Obstet Gynaecol Br Emp* **53**, 498–509.

Pickard B (1982) Vitamin B_6 during pregnancy – a review. *Nutr Health* **1**, 78–84,

Pitkin RM (1981) Assessment of nutritional status of mother, fetus and newborn. *Am J Clin Nutr* **34**, 658–68.

Prentice A, Coward A, Murgatroyd P, Goldberg G, Black A and Davies H (1987) Energy expenditure during pregnancy. In *Recent advances in obesity research.* Berry EM, Blondheim SH, Eliahou HE and Shafrir E (Eds) pp. 251–6. John Libbey, London.

Reeve J (1980) Calcium metabolism. In *Clinical physiology in obstetrics.* Hytten FE and Chamberlain G (Eds) pp. 257–69. Blackwell Scientific Publications, Oxford.

Renwick JM (1972) Hypothesis: anencephaly and spina bifida are usually preventable by avoidance of a specific but identifiable substance present in certain potato tubers. *Br J Prev and Soc Med* **26**, 67–88.

Roberts D (1990) Sources of infection: Food. *Lancet* **336**, 859–61.

Robinson M (1958) Salt in pregnancy. *Lancet* **1**, 178–181.

Rogozinski C, Finkers L, Lennen D, Wild J, Schorah C, Sheppard S and Smithells RW (1983) Folate nutrition in early pregnancy. *Hum Nutr: Appl Nutr* **37A**, 357–64.

Rosso P (1983) Nutrition and maternal-fetal exchange. *Am J Clin Nutr* **34**, 744–55.

Rosso P (1985) A new chart to monitor weight gain during pregnancy. *Am J Obstet Gynecol* **41**, 644–52.

Ruge S and Anderson T (1985) Obstetric norms in obesity — an analysis of the literature. *Obstet Gynecol Surv* **40**, 57–60.

Rush D (1986) Nutrition in the preparation for pregnancy. In *Prepregnancy care: a manual for practice.* Chamberlain G and Lumley J (Eds) pp. 113–41. John Wiley, Chichester.

Rush D, Stein Z and Susser M (1980) A randomized controlled trial of prenatal nutritional supplementation in New York City. *Pediatrics* **65**(4), 683–97.

Ryback RS (1977) Chronic alcohol consumption and menstruation. *J Am Med Assoc* **238**, 21–43.

Salle BL, David L, Glorieux FH, Delvin E, Senterre J and Renaud H (1982) Early oral administration of vitamin D and its metabolites in premature neonates. Effect on mineral homeostasis. *Paediatr Res* **16**, 75–8.

Schofield C, Wheeler E and Stewart J (1987) The diets of pregnant and post-pregnant women in different social groups in London and Edinburgh: energy, protein, fat and fibre. *Br J Nutr* **58**, 369–81.

Schwab EB and Axelson ML (1984) Dietary changes of pregnant women: compulsions and modifications. *Ecol Food Nutr* **14**, 143–153.

Scottish Health Education Group (1979) *The book of the child.* SHEG, Edinburgh.

Seller MJ (1987) Nutritionally induced congenital defects. *Proc Nutr Soc* **46/2**, 227–35.

Sexton M (1986) Smoking. In *Prepregnancy care: a manual for practice.* Chamberlain G and Lumley J (Eds) pp. 41–64. John Wiley, Chichester.

Seymour CA and Chadwick VS (1979) Liver and gastrointestinal function in pregnancy. *Postgrad Med J* **55**, 343–52.

Shenolikar IS (1970) Absorption of dietary calcium in pregnancy. *Am J Clin Nutr* **23**, 63–7.

Smithells RW (1983) Diet and congenital malformation. In *Nutrition in pregnancy.* Campbell DM and Gillmer MDG (Eds) pp. 155–65. Royal College of Obstetricians and Gynaecologists, London.

Smithells RW, Sheppard S, Schorah LJ, Seller MJ, Nevin NC, Harris R, Read AP and Fielding DW (1980) Possible prevention of neural tube defects by periconceptual vitamin supplementation. *Lancet* **ii**, 339–40.

Smithells RW, Sheppard S, Schorah LJ, Sellar MJ, Nevin NC, Harris R, Reach AP and Fielding DW (1981a) Apparent prevention of neural tube defects by periconceptual vitamin supplementation. *Arch Dis Childh* **56**, 911–18.

Smithells RW, Sheppard S, Schorah LJ, Seller MJ, Nevin NL, Harris R, Read AD, Fielding DW and Walker S (1981b) Vitamin supplementation and neural tube defects. *Lancet* **ii**, 1425.

Snow LF and Johnson SM (1978) Folklore, food, female reproductive cycle. *Ecology of Food and Nutrition* **7**, 41–9.

Solomons NW and Jacob RA (1981) Studies on the bioavailability of zinc in humans: effects of haem and non-haem iron on the absorption of zinc. *Am J Clin Nutr* **34**, 475–82.

Soltan MH and Jenkins DM (1982) Maternal and fetal plasma zinc concentrations and fetal abnormality. *Br J Obstet Gynaecol* **89**, 56–8.

Stein Z, Susser M, Saenger G and March F (1975) *Famine and human development. The Dutch Winter of 1944–45.* Oxford University Press, Oxford.

Stephens R (1981) Human exposure to lead from motor vehicle emissions. *Int J Environ Stud* **17**, 7–12.

Strauss MB (1935) Observations on the etiology of the toxaemias of pregnancy. *Am J Med Sci* **190**, 811–24.

Susser M (1980) Prenatal nutrition, birthweight and psychological development: an overview of experiments, quasi-experiments and natural experimentations in the past decade. *Am J Clin Nutr* **34**, 784–803.

Taggart N (1961) Food habits in pregnancy. *Proc Nutr Soc* **20**, 35.

Thomas MR (1984) Nutritional recommendations for pregnant and lactating teens. In *Proceedings of the 9th International Congress of Dietetics*, Toronto.

Thomson AM and Billiewicz WZ (1957) Clinical significance of weight trends during pregnancy. *Br Med J* **i**, 243–7.

Thompson B, Skipper D, Fraser C, Hewett A and Hunter D (1989) Dietary intake of Aberdeen primigravidae in 1950/51 and 1984/85. *J Hum Nutr Dietet* **2**, 345–59.

Tierson FD, Olsen C and Hook EB (1985) Influence of cravings and aversions on diet in pregnancy. *Ecology of Food and Nutrition* **17**, 117–29.

Treasure JL and Russell GFM (1988) Intrauterine growth and neonatal weight gain in babies of women with anorexia nervosa. *Br Med J* **296**, 1038.

Tuttle S, Aggett PJ, Campbell DM and MacGillivray I (1985) *Am J Clin Nutr* **41**, 1032–41.

US National Research Council (1980) Recommended Dietary Allowances 9e. National Academy of Sciences, Washington DC.

Van den Berg BJ (1981) Maternal variables affecting fetal growth. *Am J Clin Nutr* **34**, 722–6.

Walker ARP, Richardson B and Walker F (1972) The influences of numerous pregnancies and lactations on bone dimensions in South African Bantu and Caucasian mothers. *Clin Sci* **42**, 189–96.

Wiegel M and Wiegel R (1989) Nausea and vomiting of early pregnancy and pregnancy outcome. *Br J Obstet and Gynaecol* **96**, 1304–11.

World Health Organization (1990) *Diet, nutrition and the prevention of chronic diseases*. WHO Tech Rep Ser No 797. WHO, Geneva.

Worthington-Roberts BS, Vermeersch J and Rodwell-Williams S (1981) *Nutrition in pregnancy and lactation*. CV Mosby, London.

Wright JT, Toplis PJ and Barrison IG (1983) Alcohol and coffee consumption during pregnancy. In *Nutrition in pregnancy*. Campbell DM and Gillmer MDG (Eds) pp. 195–205. Royal College of Obstetricians and Gynaecologists, London.

3.2 Low birth weight infants

Low birth weight (LBW) infants are defined as weighing less than 2500 g at birth, and those of very low birth weight (VLBW) less than 1500 g. About one third of LBW infants are small for gestational age (SGA) or small for dates (SFD) and show intrauterine growth retardation (IUGR). About two thirds of LBW infants have a size which is appropriate for gestational age (AGA), but are born before 37 weeks gestation and are considered to be 'pre-term'.

The clinical management and nutritional requirements of the immature or pre-term infant will be different from a mature IUGR infant born after 37 weeks. Pre-term infants experience renal, hepatic, gastrointestinal and respiratory problems due to immaturity of organ systems. They are more likely to need assistance with breathing and are less likely to tolerate oral feeds.

3.2.1 Nutritional requirements

The optimum growth rate for small infants has yet to be defined. Although growth rates similar to those seen *in utero* might appear to be desirable, there are practical difficulties in achieving this and there may be some disadvantages in increasing growth velocity above that of a normal weight infant, particularly in immature pre-term infants, because of the extra stresses imposed by extra-uterine life (Stern 1982). It is important to ensure that adequate nutrition is achieved as early as possible: there is now considerable evidence that nutrient deprivation in early life has a considerable effect on long-term outcome (Lucas *et al* 1990). Since these infants have very small reserves of fat or glycogen they are extremely susceptible to even short periods without nutrition. Many of the nutritional recommendations for the LBW infant have been derived from those for normal term infants; relatively little is known about requirements for many nutrients.

The European Society for Paediatric Gastroenterology (ESPGAN) has compiled a report summarizing current knowledge (Wharton *et al* 1987) and the recommendations are given in Table 3.4. The American Academy of Paediatrics has also reported on the subject (Mauer *et al* 1985). A more recent comprehensive review of requirements has been published by Neu *et al* (1990).

Table 3.4 Nutrient requirements of low birth weight infants

Nutrient	Requirement per kg body weight per day
Fluid	150–200 ml
Energy	130 kcal
Protein	3.0–4.0 g
Sodium	1.3 mmol
Calcium	2.0–4.5 mmol
Phosphorus	Ca : P 1.4–2.0 : 1
Iron	35–45 μmol (max 270 μmol)
Copper	1.8–2.5 μmol
Vitamin B_6	45 μg
Vitamin K	2–3 μg
	Suggested total daily intake
Vitamin A	200–1000 μg
Vitamin D	20–40 μg
Folic acid	65 μg
Vitamin C	20 mg

Source: *ESPGAN Nutrition and feeding of pre-term infants.* (Wharton *et al* 1987)

3.2.2 Milks for low birthweight infants

Human milk

Several studies show that LBW infants fed on human milk alone show a reduced growth velocity compared with those fed a more nutrient-dense formula (Lucas *et al* 1984); neurological development is also impaired when infants fed standard formula are compared at age nine months with those receiving an energy-dense formula (Lucas *et al* 1989) and this difference persists at the age of 18 months (Lucas *et al* 1990).

It would appear from the above studies that human milk (particularly pooled human milk from a milk bank) does not provide the optimum amount of protein and energy for growth in LBW infants. However, human milk feeding appears to prevent infection (Narayan *et al* 1981) and the use of even small quantities significantly reduces the incidence of the bowel disease necrotizing enterocolitis (Lucas and Cole 1990). More recently (Lucas *et al* 1992), it has been demonstrated that infants fed human milk (particularly their own mother's milk) had a significant advantage in terms of intelligence quotient at 7–8 years over infants who received only formula.

The milk of mothers who deliver pre-term has a different composition from that of mature human milk. It has a higher content of protein, sodium and iron; the energy content of mature and pre-term milk appears to be similar. Table 3.5 lists the differences between mature and pre-term milk.

If human milk is used then it may need to be sup-

Table 3.5 Composition of mature and pre-term human milk

Nutrient	Mature milk per 100 ml*	Colostrum per 100 ml*	Pre-term milk per 100 ml** (8–18 days)
Energy (kcal/kJ)	69/289	56/236	71/298
Protein (g)	1.3	2.0	1.8
Fat (g)	4.1	2.6	4.2
Carbohydrate (g)	7.2	6.6	5.6
Sodium (mmol)	0.65	2.04	1.08
Calcium (mmol)	0.85	0.70	1.45
Phosphorus (mmol)	0.48	0.45	0.48
Iron (μmol)	1.25	1.25	1.72
Zinc (μmol)	4.59	9.17	6.93

Sources:
* Holland *et al* (1991) *McCance and Widdowson's The Composition of Foods* 5e.
** Anderson *et al* (1981)

plemented with sodium and phosphate and possibly with protein and calcium. A complete vitamin supplement should be used and iron should be introduced from about eight weeks of age.

One method of increasing the nutrient content of human milk is to supplement it with a small amount (5 g/100 ml) of a whey-based infant milk or a hydrolysed infant formula such as Prejomin (Milupa). A commercially produced enhancer for human milk is also available in the USA, and some European countries. Since the protein content of mature breast milk is low, additional energy should not be added without protein, as it may result in a low protein-energy ratio.

Standard formulae

The use of standard infant formulae containing 65–70 kcal/270–295 KJ per 100 ml has been shown to provide a less than adequate range of nutrients for the growth and development of LBW infants in the studies described above (Lucas *et al* 1984, 1989, 1990). In order to achieve their energy requirement, infants need to be fed very large quantities of milk, and this is often not possible. Fluid intakes above 180 ml/kg, whether orally or intravenously, have been shown to be associated with a higher incidence of patent ductus arteriosis and necrotizing enterocolitis (Bell and Oh 1983).

Low birthweight formulae

A number of ready-to-feed formulae designed for the low birth weight infant are available in the UK. They have a higher nutrient density than standard milks and contain all necessary vitamin, mineral and trace elements, although some infants may need an additional iron supplement. Guidelines for the composition of these formulae have been published by the European Society for Paediatric Gastroenterology (Wharton *et al* 1987). As yet there are no EC compositional guidelines for these milks.

The milks available in the UK conform to the ESPGAN guidelines. Table 3.6 sets out the ESPGAN recommendations. Table 3.7 gives the composition of LBW milks available in the UK.

Other formulae

A small minority of infants will not be able to tolerate a cows' milk based formula, and they should be treated according to their clinical symptoms and should receive a lactose-free or milk protein-free formula. The use of medium chain triglycerides, while in theory enabling improved fat absorption, has not shown to be beneficial (Bustamente *et al* 1989). Soya formulae are not recommended for long-term use in LBW infants because of the possibility of altered calcium and iron availability from these milks (Mauer *et al* 1983).

3.2.3 Feeding low birthweight infants

In very immature infants with poor gut development, enteral feeding is usually not possible and parenteral feeding must be initiated. The American Academy of Paediatrics discusses the requirements of the parenterally fed LBW infant (Mauer *et al* 1985).

Enteral feeding should be possible from about 25–28 weeks gestation. Suckling will not be established at this time and feeding by tube will be necessary. Intermittent feeding via a gastric tube is recommended by ESPGAN (Wharton *et al* 1987), although improved weight gain has been demonstrated in VLBW infants fed by continuous infusion (Toce *et al* 1987).

Mothers can express their milk and can either put it straight down a feeding tube or the milk can be suitably stored (refrigerated for up to four hours or microbiologically tested and frozen for longer than four hours) and fed when required.

It appears that the most satisfactory regimen for LBW infants may be a combination of human milk to supply

Table 3.6 Guidelines for the composition of pre-term formulae

Nutrient	Recommendation per 100 kcal	Recommendation per 100 ml (assuming 80 kcal/100 ml)	Comments
Energy (kcal/kJ)	65–85/273–357		
Protein (g)	2.25–3.1	1.8–2.5	Amino acid content should not be below that of breast milk
Fat (g)	3.6–7.0	2.9–5.6	Not more than 40% MCT
Linoleic acid (g)	0.5–1.4	0.4–1.1	Not more than 20% of total fatty acids
Linolenic acid (mg)	55	44	No maximum recommended
Carbohydrate (g)	7.0–14.0	5.6–11.2	Lactose not more than 8 g/100 ml; glucose, sucrose, starch hydrolysates acceptable
Calcium (mmol)	1.75–3.5	1.4–2.8	Ca:P ratio 1.4–2.0:1
Sodium (mmol)	1.0–2.3	0.6–1.5	Intake not less than 1.3 mmol/kg
Iron (μmol)	approx 27	21	Intake should be 35–45 μmol/kg/day (max. 270 μmol total)
Zinc (μmol)	8.4	6.7	No upper guide; no reason to exceed current levels of 17 μmol/100 kcal
Vitamin C (mg)	7.0	5.6	No upper guide; no reason to exceed current levels of 40 mg/100 kcal
Folic acid (μg)	60	48	No upper guide
Selenium Chromium Taurine Carnitine	No recommendation		

* Source: *ESPGAN Nutrition and feeding of pre-term infants.* (Wharton *et al* 1987)

Table 3.7 Low birthweight milks available in the UK

Milk	Composition per 100 ml*: Energy kcal/kJ	Protein g	Fat g	CHO g	Sodium mmol	Iron μmol
Cow and Gate LBW (Cow and Gate)	80/330	2.2	4.4	8.5	1.34	15.7
Osterprem (Farleys)	80/330	2.0	4.9	7.0	1.83	7.0
Prematil (Milupa)	68/286	2.0	3.5	7.7	1.00	13.4
SMA LBW (Wyeth)	80/336	2.0	4.4	8.6	0.94	11.7

* Source: Manufacturers' data

approximately 50% of the energy requirements and a LBW formula supplying the remainder. It is customary to continue a supplemented breast milk or LBW formula until the infant is 2.0 kg and growth velocity is normal; a standard infant formula or unsupplemented breast milk can be used from this time.

3.2.4 Weaning the low birthweight infant

Factors to be taken into consideration when deciding on the time of weaning for a LBW infant are

1 The degree of prematurity.
2 The chronological age.
3 The developmental level.

It is suggested that weaning does not take place prior to 16 weeks post delivery (as with a term infant), and not before the infant is 5.0 kg in weight. One formula used is to add half the number of weeks of prematurity to 16 weeks – for example, if a baby is 10 weeks pre-term, wean at 16 weeks + 10/2 (i.e. 16 + 5 = 21) weeks post-delivery, providing the infant is 5.0 kg by this time and appears to be able to eat from a spoon.

References

Anderson GH, Atkinson SA and Bryan MH (1981) Energy and macronutrient content of human milk during early lactation from mothers giving birth prematurely and at term. *Am J Clin Nutr* **34**, 258–65.

Bell EF and Oh W (1983) Water requirements of premature newborn infants. *Acta Paediatr Scand* **305**(Suppl), 21–6.

Bustamente SA, Fiello A and Pollack PF (1987) Growth of premature infants fed formulas with 10%, 30% or 50% medium-chain triglycerides. *Am J Dis Childh* **141**, 516–19.

Holland B, Welch AA, Unwin ID, Buss DH, Paul AA and Southgate DAT (1991) *McCance and Widdowson's The Composition of Foods* 5e. Royal Society of Chemistry/Ministry of Agriculture, Fisheries and Food. HMSO, London.

Lucas A, Gore SM, Cole TJ, Bamford MF, Dossetor JFB, Barr I, Dicarlo L, Cork S and Lucas PJ (1984) Multicentre trial on feeding low birthweight infants: effects of diet on early growth. *Arch Dis Childh* **59**, 722–30.

Lucas A, Morley R, Cole TJ, Gore SM, Davis JA, Bamford MFM and Dossetor JFB (1989) Early diet in preterm babies and developmental status in infancy. *Arch Dish Childh* **64**, 1570–78.

Lucas A, Morley R, Cole TJ, Gore SM, Lucas PJ, Crowle P, Boon AJ and Powell R (1990) Early diet in preterm babies and developmental status at 18 months. *Lancet* **335**, 1477–81.

Lucas A and Cole TJ (1990) Breast milk and necrotising enterocolitis. *Lancet* **336**, 1519–21.

Lucas A, Morley R, Cole TJ, Lister G and Leeson-Payne C (1992) Breast milk and subsequent intelligence quotient in children born preterm. *Lancet* **339**, 261–4.

Mauer AM, Dweck HS, Holmes I, Reynolds JW, Suskind RM, Walker WA and Woodruff CW (1983) Soy-protein formulas: recommendations for use in infant feeding. *Paediatrics* **72**, 359–63.

Mauer AM, Dweck HS, Finberg L, Holmes I, Reynolds JW, Suskind RM and Woodruff CW (1985) Nutritional needs of low-birth-weight infants. *Paediatrics* **75**, 976–86.

Narayan I, Prakash K and Gujral VV (1981) The value of human milk in the prevention of infection in the high risk infant. *J Pediatr* **99**, 496–8.

Neu J, Valentine C and Meetze W (1990) Scientifically-based strategies for nutrition of the high-risk low birth weight infant. *Eur J Pediatr* **150**, 2–13.

Stern L (1982) Early postnatal growth of low birthweight infants: what is optimal? *Acta Paediatr Scand* **296**(Suppl), 6–11.

Toce SS, Keenan WJ and Homan SM (1987) Enteral feeding in very-low-birth-weight infants. *Amer J Dis Childh* **14**, 439–44.

Wharton BA, Bremer HJ, Brooke OG, Orzalesi M, Putet G, Raiha NCR, Senterre J and Shaw JCL (1987) Nutrition and feeding of preterm infants. *Acta Paed Scand* **336**(Suppl).

3.3 Infants

The feeding of infants is subject to old wives' tales and unsound advice based on neither careful observation nor scientific fact. Well-informed advice before and after the birth is important. In this country, mothers can exercise considerable choice over how to feed their infants. However, many are ill-informed about the implications and practicalities of the feeding method chosen.

3.3.1 Breast feeding

To some mothers, breast feeding is a natural progression of pregnancy, but others find the idea less attractive. Around 65% of mothers in the UK start to breast feed their babies but by six weeks post-partum only 40% are still doing so (Martin and White 1988). This 'lost' 25% is of great concern to all those involved in the care and support of the breast feeding mother.

Advantages and disadvantages of breast feeding

Advantages of breast feeding

A complete food Breast milk provides complete nutrition when feeding is successfully established. Additional vitamins may be necessary after six months (DHSS 1988).

Protection against infection Breast milk provides protection against infection, both bacterial and viral. Human milk contains macrophages (which produce lysozymes and lactoferrin), lymphocytes (which secrete interferon and secretory immunoglobulin A), bifidus factor (which enhances growth of *Lactobacillis bifidus*) and antibodies (Downham *et al* 1976; Ogra and Ogra 1978; Adinolfi and Glynn 1979; Pittard 1979; Welsh and May 1979; Yap *et al* 1979; Brock 1980). Significantly less gastrointestinal disease is found in babies breast fed for at least 13 weeks, the effect persisting beyond the period of breast feeding (Howie *et al* 1990). This protective effect had previously only been shown in developing countries (Plank and Milanesi 1973; Victoria *et al* 1987). There is a small but less clearly defined reduction in rates of respiratory illness in breast fed infants (Wright *et al* 1989; Howie *et al* 1990).

Breast feeding may afford partial protection against atopic disease. However, there are conflicting views on this subject (Kramer 1988). Sensitization to food antigens may occur *in utero* and from breast milk (Warner 1980; Jakobsson *et al* 1985; Chandra *et al* 1986).

No risk of solute overload Unlike powdered milks, breast milk cannot be reconstituted incorrectly.

Availability Breast milk is immediately available. No kitchen preparation is required.

Effect on mother-baby relationship It helps emotional bonding between mother and baby. This is important for the emotional and physical development of the child (Klaus and Kennell 1976). Suckling ensures frequent contact between mother and infant.

Maternal benefits Breast feeding assists uterine involution and utilizes surplus body fat deposited in pregnancy thus aiding a return to previous body weight. Breast feeding also has a limited contraceptive effect. Although this should not be relied upon as a method of contraception, the reduction in fertility may be advantageous in developing countries.

Cost Breast feeding is cheaper than bottle feeding, even when the 'hidden' cost of the additional nutritional needs of the lactating mother are taken into account.

Disadvantages of breast feeding

Demands on the mother's time The mother has to be available day and night to feed the baby, especially in the early weeks while breast feeding is being established.

Physical problems Establishing a successful lactation is not always straighforward. Physical discomfort in the early days from engorged breasts and sore nipples discourages some mothers.

Difficulty in measuring supply The mother cannot see the volume of milk taken. Many mothers need continual reassurance that their milk supply is adequate and are unhappy that they do not know how much the baby consumes. They need to be taught that the infant itself provides the best guide; a baby who is contented and is gaining weight is adequately fed.

The milk supply may be inadequate Poor weight gain and an unsettled baby may be due to an inadequate supply of breast milk. There are ways in which the milk supply can be increased (see the section below on 'Establishing and maintaining breast feeding'). Sometimes, however, supplementary bottle feeding may be advised instead and, once this is started, breast feeding is frequently abandoned altogether.

Embarrassment Some mothers are embarrassed to breast feed even within the home, particularly those in lower socioeconomic groups (Martin and White 1988). Many women find that the attitude of other people to breast feeding in public, coupled with the frequent lack of facilities to feed in private, make prolonged excursions outside the home very difficult.

Breast feeding can create jealousy Husbands, relatives and siblings may, in different ways, resent the exclusive role of the mother in breast feeding. These problems can be helped by involving everyone in all other aspects of caring for the infant.

Incompatible with work Owing to the lack of suitable child-care facilities in most places of work, returning to work shortly after giving birth makes continuing with full breast feeding almost impossible. However, partial breast feeding (e.g. in the mornings and evenings) should be encouraged.

Contraindications to breast feeding

Serious chronic maternal illness necessitating drug therapy Many drugs are passed into the breast milk which consequently may have adverse effects on the baby. These effects have been reviewed by Wilson *et al* (1980) and White and White (1980). Maternal diabetes mellitus does not preclude lactation.

Human immunodeficiency virus Mothers in the UK who are HIV positive are at present advised against breast feeding their babies (DHSS 1988).

Severe physical problems These can occur in either the baby (e.g. cleft palate) or the mother (e.g. inverted nipples).

Low birth weight Breast milk may not always be suitable for low birth weight infants (see Section 3.2).

Impending adoption If the baby is to be adopted, breast feeding may be discouraged on psychological grounds.

Illness in the baby Small or sick babies may require intravenous or tube feeding although it may be possible to tube feed expressed breast milk. Some chronic illnesses such as galactosaemia necessitate milk exclusion.

Maternal nutritional needs for lactation

Energy

The amounts of food energy and nutrients required for lactation have been summarized by the Department of Health (1991) (see Section 1.2). Energy requirements take account of the age of the baby and whether weaning foods have been introduced. As with all recommended intakes, however, these figures are designed to cover the needs of all lactating women and the inbuilt safety factor inevitably means that they will be too high for some individuals.

For most lactating women, increased quantities of a normal and varied diet, based on 'healthy eating' principles, will provide adequate nutrition. The mother's appetite is the best guide to energy requirements. Sensations of hunger and thirst are often particularly intense during the lactating period. Mothers should be encouraged to respond to these signals and increase their food and liquid consumption accordingly (Table 3.8).

Many women lactate successfully on apparently low-energy intakes; enhanced metabolic efficiency probably reducing the true energy cost of lactation (Illingworth *et al* 1986). The milk output by Gambian mothers with an energy intake of 1500–1800 kcal/day was very similar to that of Cambridge mothers with an energy intake of 2330 kcal/day (Whitehead *et al* 1980). Giving the Gambian mothers a dietary supplement of 1000 kcal daily, thus bringing their intake to the Cambridge level, had no effect on the amount of milk taken by their babies (Prentice *et al*

Table 3.8 General dietary guidelines for lactation

Food	Fluids
Eat regularly Let your appetite dictate how much you eat. If you are hungry, eat more Do not attempt to slim Eat a variety of foods. Try to include the following in your diet every day: Milk, cheese or yoghurt Meat, fish or eggs Yellow or green leafy vegetables Fruit or fruit juice Wholemeal bread or high fibre breakfast cereals Potatoes, rice or pasta If you think some foods in your diet are upsetting your baby, try avoiding them for a few days to see if it helps Only take vitamin supplements on medical advice	Drink plenty of fluids If you are thirsty, drink more Do not drink much alcohol, strong coffee, strong tea

1983). The results of these and other studies have been comprehensively reviewed by Prentice *et al* (1986).

Deliberately attempting to limit food intake in order to lose weight is inadvisable, however. This will only exacerbate any feelings of stress or tiredness being experienced by the mother and may in turn lead to a decrease in milk production.

Minerals

Current recommendations (see Section 2.7, Table 2.38) (DoH 1991) suggest an additional daily intake of 550 mg calcium for breast feeding mothers. Adaptation of calcium metabolism resulting in increased absorption of dietary calcium may occur but this has yet to be proved. Higher calcium intakes are likely to be particularly important for adolescent mothers (Chan *et al* 1987).

Increased intakes of phosphorus, magnesium, zinc, copper and selenium are suggested.

Additional iron is not recommended. Requirements are decreased through lactational amenorrhoea (DoH 1991).

Vitamins

Vitamin D supplements are recommended to achieve a daily intake of 10 μg/day (DoH 1991). This is in part to ensure an adequate vitamin D content of breast milk throughout the year. However it is particularly important that women of immigrant communities achieve this level of intake in order to minimize the risk from osteomalacia and rickets (Park *et al* 1987).

Possible dietary exclusions

The maternal diet influences the composition of breast milk (Craig-Schmidt *et al* 1984), and breast milk may contain a number of non-nutritive substances (DHSS 1988). Alcohol is excreted in breast milk (Binkiewicz *et al* 1978), and is ideally avoided, or at least restricted, during breast feeding. Other substances which can pass into breast milk include caffeine, nicotine, senna and other amines and alkaloids. High intakes of coffee and other caffeine-containing beverages may promote sleeplessness in some babies (Clement 1989). Drugs, including oral contraceptives, should only be taken on medical advice. Details of the suitability of drugs for use during breast feeding are given in the *British National Formulary*.

The hypothesis that maternal avoidance of cows' milk products will benefit the breast fed baby with colic remains controversial. However, it has recently been suggested that bovine IgG may be present in sufficiently high concentrations to support this theory (Clyne and Kulczycki 1991). Occasionally eczema in breast fed infants can result from cows' milk protein present in the breast milk (Jakobssen *et al* 1985; Cant *et al* 1986).

If cows' milk and milk products are excluded from the mother's diet, dietary advice should be given to ensure that calcium intake is adequate. A calcium supplement may be required.

The vast majority of breast feeding mothers need not exclude any food items from their diet. In particular they should be reassured that the very loose stools produced by the baby during the early days of breast feeding are not related to the mother's diet.

Establishing and maintaining breast feeding

The decision to breast feed

Virtually all women decide before the birth how they will feed their baby and carry out this intention. The most common reason given is that breast feeding is best for baby. Convenience is also important to many mothers (Martin and White 1988).

Breast feeding is most common amongst mothers:

- Of first babies;
- Aged 25 years or more;
- Of higher social class;
- Educated beyond 18 years;
- Living in London and the South East.

Initiation of breast feeding

Consistent and rational advice from midwives and other staff is essential for the optimal care of the breast feeding mother and her baby. Conflicting advice is common, but is unhelpful and confusing for the new mother.

A good understanding of the physiology of lactation is essential for all who are involved in the care of breast feeding mothers. The book *Successful Breast Feeding* published by the Royal College of Midwives (1991) is an excellent practical guide on the management of breastfeeding.

The composition of breast milk is not homogenous. It alters between feeds, within feeds and during a lactation. The hind-milk has a higher fat and thus greater energy content than the fore-milk obtained at the beginning of a feed. Incomplete emptying of the breasts may lead to a baby receiving an inadequate energy intake (Woolridge and Fisher 1988).

Putting the baby to the breast immediately after birth assists in developing the suckling reflex which is particularly strong for a short while after delivery (Righard and Alade 1990).

The supply of breast milk is determined largely by demand and is stimulated by frequent (rather than prolonged) suckling. Therefore feeding 2–3 hourly (or even more frequently) for a few minutes at each breast will help the milk supply to become established by the third or fourth day post-partum. Complementary feeds are not necessary and will hinder the establishment of breast feeding. The changes in the composition of breast milk in the early post-partum period are summarized in Table 3.9.

It takes 3–6 weeks for lactation to become fully established; it is during this period that feeding 'on demand' round the clock (at least every 3–4 hours) is most valuable. Once lactation is well established, feeds can be spaced further apart without diminishing the milk supply.

If the baby is unable to suckle at birth, the mother can use an electric or hand pump to simulate suckling and the baby can be fed expressed breast milk until normal breast feeding can commence.

Milk supply can be reduced by tiredness and tension, so practical and emotional support is very important at this time. Establishing lactation is more difficult to achieve in some babies than in others. Some infants seem to fight at the breast or may be irritable and scream or cry. This is often a result of the very rapid initial flow of milk which overwhelms and frustrates the baby. Expressing a little milk before the feed often resolves the problem.

Mothers should be reminded that crying in a baby does not always signal a demand for food. It may be because the baby is uncomfortable, overtired, or just bored and lonely.

Maintaining lactation

Support for the lactating mother from family, friends, midwife, health visitor, National Childbirth Trust breast feeding counsellors or local mother-child support groups is important if breast feeding is to continue. Martin and White (1988) found one third of mothers in their study stopped breast feeding within six weeks. The most common reason given was 'insufficient milk'. Few had been offered or received any guidance as to whether this was really the case.

The breast feeding mother needs to feed on demand, day and night, and may find herself feeding every 3–4 hours for several weeks. Practical help in the house with other children will help the mother get as much rest as possible. Regular meals are needed during this busy and demanding period.

Once the milk supply is established, the mother may get a break from her responsibilities by expressing breast milk for someone else to feed to the baby from a bottle. Not all babies co-operate with this occasional bottle feed. Expressed breast milk can be stored in a refrigerator for 24 hours or it can be frozen. Careful attention to hygiene is important. Bottles, containers for storage and other utensils must be sterilized.

Table 3.9 Changes in breast milk composition

Day	Milk	Description
1–3	Colostrum	Thick, yellowy milk, high in protein, antibodies and some vitamins and minerals
3–7+	Transitional	Thinner, white appearance. Composition approaching mature milk
7–10+	Mature	More watery appearance, almost blue in colour as the feed begins and becoming white by the end of a feed as the fat content increases

Complementary bottle needs

Some mothers complement breast feeds with milk formula from a bottle. This may be for reasons of convenience, illness in the mother or an inadequate supply of breast milk. If done for the latter reason it is likely that the mother's own milk supply will diminish further, making a return to complete breast feeding impossible. If a mother is keen to persevere with breast feeding, other measures to improve her lactation should be tried before starting complementary feeds (see below). If complementary feeds are used, they should be given after the breast feed.

Additional nutritional requirements of the infant

Vitamins

Provided that the maternal diet is adequate, breast milk will meet the vitamin requirements of the baby. In practice, the following vitamin supplements may be given:

1 Vitamin K (1 mg) administered at delivery to prevent haemolytic disease of the newborn.

2 Children's vitamin drops (available from baby clinics) are recommended for breast fed infants over the age of six months until the age of two or preferably five years of age. Five drops daily provide 200 μg vitamin A, 20 mg vitamin C and 7 μg vitamin D. Vitamin supplements are particularly important when the child is being weaned.

Fluoride

A daily intake of 0.25 mg fluoride is recommended by the British Dental Association for infants and young children. This amount cannot be obtained from breast or infant milk formulae. However, the level of fluoride in water supplies varies greatly and local levels, together with the infant's water consumption, must be taken into account when deciding whether or not to use fluoride supplements (Dowell and Joyston-Bechal 1981). As a general guide, fluoride drops providing 0.25 mg fluoride daily should be given (see Section 4.1.1) if the water supply contains less than 0.3 ppm fluoride.

Fluid

Additional fluid is not necessary for exclusively breast fed babies (Goldberg and Adams 1983). A thirsty baby will demand more breast milk. Additional fluids in the early days of breast feeding should be actively discouraged as they interfere with the establishment of lactation. Older babies may be offered cooled, boiled water from a feeding cup or by cup and spoon, as part of the weaning process.

Monitoring the progress of a breast fed baby

Weight gain

Most breast fed babies gain weight and thrive. Weight loss during the first few days of life should not exceed 10% of birth weight. This loss of weight usually ceases by days 4–7 and birth weight has been regained by 7–10 days. Over the first three months, weight gain averages approximately 200 g per week, then 150 g per week for the 3–6 month period. A healthy full-term baby of average birth-weight doubles its weight by about five months and trebles it by the end of the first year of life. A meaningful assessment of a baby's growth can only really be made by the regular use of centile growth charts. Typically a successfully breast fed baby gains weight more rapidly than a bottle fed baby in the first 2–3 months. The rate of weight gain slows from around 4 months and may be less than that of a bottle fed baby from 6–12 months. Energy intakes of 0.40 MJ (95 kcal)/kg/day at five weeks falling to 0.39 MJ (93 kcal)/kg/day at eleven weeks have been reported by investigators using the doubly-labelled water technique (Lucas *et al* 1987). These energy intakes are lower than current recommended intakes and this reduced energy intake of breast fed infants may persist into childhood (Paul *et al* 1990).

In summary, weight gain is not always consistent and over frequent weighing can cause unnecessary anxiety.

General observation of the baby

A thriving breast fed baby will:

- Have a good skin colour;
- Be alert, responsive and mostly contented;
- Have frequent wet nappies;
- Produce bright yellow soft stools (frequency is unimportant).

Test weighing

Test weighing the infant (recording weight before and after several feeds) can provide an indication of the volume of feed being taken. However, by itself, this is not a particularly meaningful figure and, since obtaining it is traumatic for the mother, may even result in a reduced milk supply. The disadvantages of test weighing strongly outweigh any advantages.

Failure to thrive at the breast

Poor weight gain and growth and an unsettled or over-quiet, listless baby are clear indications of an inadequate milk intake. However there are a number of possible reasons for this and the factors responsible – in either the mother and/or the child – must be identified before they can be remedied.

Inadequate milk supply

Illness, tension or fatigue in the mother can interfere with her lactation. However, the most common cause is a lactation which has never been properly established.

Inadequate milk intake

Feeding frequency The baby may not be being fed frequently enough. Some babies need to be fed more frequently than others. Rigid feeding schedules should be discouraged; babies should be fed on demand and allowed to feed for an unrestricted length of time. More frequent feeding will increase the milk supply.

Fixing difficulties Breast engorgement, inverted nipples or a poor suckling position can prevent the correct fixing or attachment of a baby to the nipple. This is essential if the baby is to obtain the complete volume and nutrient content of the feed.

Solving problems

Advice should be sought from an experienced midwife, health visitor or breast feeding support counsellor.

Occasionally it is impossible to improve a lactation sufficiently to allow the baby to thrive. However, a change to bottle feeding may be the right decision for the baby's health and the mother's physical and mental well-being.

Problems associated with breast feeding

'Posseting' or vomiting

Many babies regurgitate small amounts of milk at the end of a feed. This is of no consequence. Projectile vomiting or vomiting both after and between feeds, or blood or bile stained vomit must be reported immediately to a doctor. Traces of blood may come from cracked and bleeding nipples.

Irregular bowel habits

The baby's stools will normally be bright yellow and loose or soft. A breast fed baby may pass several stools on one day and then several days may elapse before another one. Even after 4–5 days without a bowel movement, the breast fed baby is not constipated if the stool, when passed, is soft.

Illness of the baby

Temporary nasal obstruction due to an upper respiratory tract infection commonly interferes with feeding. A medically prescribed short course of decongestant nose drops may be helpful.

It is unusual for a breast fed baby to develop gastroenteritis, but if this does occur breast feeding should continue supplemented with an oral rehydration solution (Walker-Smith 1990).

Occasionally serious illness (e.g. congenital heart disease) may present with feeding difficulties and failure to thrive.

3.3.2 Bottle feeding

At the age of one month, the majority of babies in the UK are having some bottle feeds and by four months three quarters of babies are fully bottle fed (Martin and White 1988).

Infant formulae

Modified milk formulae

These formulae are designed as nutritionally complete feeds to replace breast milk. They are based on cows' milk modified to mimic the composition of mature breast milk (Tables 3.10 and 3.11). However no formula can provide the anti-infective properties of breast milk.

DHSS (1980) guidelines on the composition of infant formulae based on the composition of pooled samples of human milk. However, recent estimations of the energy content of mature breast milk suggest that the energy density of infant formulae may now exceed that of breast milk (Lucas *et al* 1987).

Modified milks available in the UK can be divided into two groups, whey dominant and casein dominant.

Whey dominant These are the most highly modified milks available (Table 3.10). They have a ratio of whey to casein of about 60:40 similar to that found in breast milk. Whey dominant formulae are generally considered the most suitable for babies under three months.

Casein dominant These formulae have a whey:casein ratio of about 20:80, as found in cows' milk (Table 3.11). Casein dominant feeds are marketed as suitable for the 'hungry bottle fed baby'. There is *no* scientific basis to this commonly held belief (Taitz and Scholey 1989). A whey dominant milk may be continued until the change to cows' milk is made.

Other milk formulae

Low birth weight milks Milk formulae adapted to meet the special nutritional needs of low birth weight infants are available (see Section 3.2).

Soya milks Formulae based on soya protein isolates (Table 3.12) should only be used for infants thought to be intolerant to lactose or cows' milk protein. They are prescribable for milk or lactose intolerance and can also be purchased over the counter.

Follow-up formulae

Follow-up (or follow-on) formulae are an alternative to modified milks or whole cows' milk for infants over six months. They contain more iron and vitamin D and less saturated fatty acids, sodium and protein than whole cows' milk. Four follow-up milks are marketed in the UK: Progress (Wyeth), Step-up (Cow & Gate), Junior Milk (Farley) and Junior Milk Drink (Boots). They are intended to be used as part of a mixed weaning diet. They have no advantage over modified milks but provide an equally valuable source of iron and vitamin D. It is increasingly suggested that the introduction of ordinary cows' milk should be delayed until one year of age (Wharton 1990).

Changing milk formulae

Martin and White (1988) report that 44% of mothers changed formulae by 6–10 weeks of age. The most common change (64%) was from whey dominant to casein dominant. Reasons given were that babies were 'hungry' or 'not satisfied' with their milk feed. Many mothers and some health professionals wrongly believe casein dominant milks contain more energy.

It seems likely that a variety of problems are wrongly attributed to the choice of milk feed. Frequent changes should be discouraged particularly in an attempt to treat minor symptoms of wind, posseting or colic.

International code of marketing of breast milk substitutes (WHO 1981)

This resolution, adopted by the World Health Organization in 1981, aims to promote breast feeding and ensure the correct use of infant formulae. In the UK the Food Manufacturers' Federation (FMF) has drawn up a voluntary Code of Practice covering the marketing of infant formulae. Thus can be summarized as follows:

1 The advertizing of infant formulae should be restricted to professional journals.

2 Maternity hospitals should not use promotional material such as posters or cot tags.

3 Breast feeding mothers should not be given free samples of formula.

Table 3.10 Whey dominant infant formulae

All values per 100 ml reconstituted feed		Mature Breastmilk	DHSS Guidelines (1980)	Cow & Gate Premium	Wyeth SMA Gold	Farleys Oster-Milk	Milupa Aptamil
Major nutrients							
Protein	g	1.2–1.4	1.2–2.0	1.4	1.5	1.45	1.5
Casein:Whey ratio		40:60	As for human milk	40:60	40:60	40:60	40:60
Fat	g	3.7–4.8	2.3–5.0	3.6	3.6	3.8	3.6
Essential fatty acid ratio Linoleic:α-Linolenic (ω6):(ω3)		5:1	5–15:1	5:1	14:1	Trace of α-linolenic acid	9:1
Carbohydrate	g	7.1–7.8	4.8–10.0	7.1	7.2	7.0	7.3
Minerals							
Calcium	mg	32–36	30–120	54	42	39	59
Phosphorus	mg	14–15	15–60	27	28	27	35
Calcium:phosphorus ratio		2.3:1	1.2:1–2.2:1	2:1	1.5:1	1.4:1	1.7:1
Sodium	mg	11–20	15–35	18	15	17	18
Potassium	mg	57–62	50–100	65	56	57	85
Chloride	mg	35–55	40–80	40	40	45	38
Magnesium	mg	2.6–3.0	2.8–12	5	4.5	5.2	6.5
Iron	μg	62–93	70–700	500	600	650	700
Zinc	μg	260–330	200–600*	400	450	340	400
Iodine	μg	2–12	ns	7	6.0	4.5	4
Manganese	μg	0.7–1.5	ns	7	15	3.4	4.2
Copper	μg	37–43	10–60*	40	47	42	46
Potential Renal Solute Load	mosmol/l	86	79–143	92	92	93.5	100
Vitamins							
A Retinol	μg	40–76	40–150	80	60	100	61
D_3 Cholecalciferol	μg	na	0.7–1.3	1.1	1.0	1.0	1.0
E dl-α-Tocopherol	mg	0.29–0.39	0.3–ns	0.8	0.64	0.48	0.7
K_1 Phytomenadione	μg	na	1.5–ns	5	5.5	2.7	4.0
B_1 Thiamin	μg	13–21	13–ns	40	67	42	40
B_2 Riboflavin	μg	31	30–ns	100	100	55	51
B_6 Pyridoxine	μg	5.1–7.2	5–ns	40	42	35	30
B_{12} Cyanocobalamin	μg	0.01	0.01–ns	0.2	0.13	0.14	0.16
Nicotinic acid	μg	210–270	230–ns	800	500	1200	400
Pantothenic acid	μg	220–330	200–ns	300	210	230	400
Biotin	μg	0.52–1.13	0.5–ns	1.5	1.5	1.0	1.1
Folic acid	μg	3.1–6.2	3–ns	10	5.0	3.4	10
C Ascorbic acid	mg	3.1–4.5	3–ns	8	5.5	6.9	6
Choline	mg	na	ns	7	4.7	4.8	nd
Energy							
	kJ	270–315	270–315	277	274	284	281
	kcal	65–75	65–75	66	65	68	67

na = not available   nd = not declared
ns = not specified   * = tentative guideline
Reproduced with the permission of Cow & Gate Nutricia Ltd

4 All packaging should state that breast feeding is best for babies.

Aluminium

Cows' milk formulae contain 10–20 times, and soya formulae 100 times, the aluminium found in breast milk (Weintraub *et al* 1986).

Aluminium is the third most abundant element on earth. It is found in many foods particularly those of vegetable origin such as soya. It is poorly absorbed by the gut and readily excreted by the kidney (MAFF 1989). Aluminium toxicity in patients undergoing treatment for chronic renal failure is well documented. Some links between aluminium and Alzheimer's disease have been postulated.

There is no evidence that the levels of aluminium found in infant soya formulae pose any risk to healthy infants. However, pre-term infants may be at risk of absorbing and

Table 3.11 Casein dominant infant formulae

All values per 100 ml reconstituted feed		Mature Breastmilk	DHSS Guidelines (1980)	Cow & Gate Plus	Wyeth SMA White	Farley's Oster-Milk Two	Milupa Milumil	Cows' Milk
Major nutrients								
Protein	g	1.2–1.4	1.5–2.0	1.7	1.5	1.7	1.9	3.4
Casein : Whey ratio		40 : 60	As for Cows' milk	80 : 20	80 : 20	77 : 23	80 : 20	80 : 20
Fat	g	3.7–4.8	2.3–5.0	3.4	3.6	2.6	3.1	3.9
Essential fatty acid ratio Linoleic : α-Linolenic (ω6) : (ω3)		5 : 1	5–15 : 1	5 : 1	14 : 1	Trace of α-linolenic acid	15 : 1	1 : 1
Carbohydrate	g	7.1–7.8	4.8–10.0	7.2	7.2	8.6	8.4	4.6
Minerals								
Calcium	mg	32–36	30–120	80	46	61	71	124
Phosphorus	mg	14–15	15–60	47	36	49	55	98
Calcium : Phosphorus ratio		2.3 : 1	1.2 : 1–2.2 : 1	1.7 : 1	1.3 : 1	1.2 : 1	1.3 : 1	1.3 : 1
Sodium	mg	11–20	15–35	25	18	25	24	52
Potassium	mg	57–62	50–100	90	62	86	86	15
Chloride	mg	35–55	40–80	56	42	56	44	98
Magnesium	mg	2.6–3.0	2.8–12	5.4	4.0	6.0	6.2	12
Iron	μg	62–93	70–700	500	600	650	400	50
Zinc	μg	260–330	200–600*	400	450	330	400	360
Iodine	μg	2–12	ns	10	10	10	2.1	nd
Manganese	μg	0.7–1.5	ns	7	7	3.3	13	nd
Copper	μg	37–43	10–60*	40	47	39	27	20
Potential Renal Solute load	mosmol/l	86	79–143	118	96	117	121	223
Vitamins								
A Retinol	μg	40–76	40–150	80	79	97	57	40
D_3 Cholecalciferol	μg	na	0.7–1.3	1.1	1.0	1.0	1.0	0.02
E dl-α-tocopherol	mg	0.29–0.39	0.3–ns	0.8	0.64	0.46	0.8	0.09
K_1 Phytomenadione	μg	ns	1.5–ns	5	5.5	2.6	4.1	nd
B_1 Thiamin	μg	13–21	13–ns	40	67	39	32	40
B_2 Riboflavin	μg	31	30–ns	100	100	53	49	200
B_6 Pyridoxine	μg	5.1–7.2	5–ns	40	42	33	42	40
B_{12} Cyanocobalamin	μg	0.01	0.01–ns	0.2	0.13	0.13	0.2	0.3
Nicotinic acid	μg	210–270	230–ns	800	500	1100	400	80
Pantothenic acid	μg	220–330	200–ns	300	210	220	240	360
Biotin	μg	0.52–1.13	0.5–ns	1.5	1.5	0.97	1.1	2.1
Folic acid	μg	3.1–6.2	3–ns	10	5.0	3.2	5	5
C Ascorbic acid	mg	3.1–4.5	3–ns	8	5.5	6.4	7.6	1.5
Choline	mg	na	ns	7	4.7	4.6	nd	nd
Energy								
	kJ	270–315	270–315	277	273	273	290	272
	kcal	65–75	65–75	66	65	65	69	65

na = not available nd = not declared
ns = not specified * = tentative guideline
Reproduced with the permission of Cow & Gate Nutricia Ltd

retaining aluminium (Weaver *et al* 1984). At present, soya based formulae should not be advised for pre-term infants or babies with renal impairment.

Establishing bottle feeding

Most maternity hospitals use 'ready to feed' sterilized bottles of infant formulae. Most offer a choice of product. A range of infant formulae is available from baby clinics and recipients of Family Credit may obtain these at reduced prices.

Bottle feeding techniques

Few babies seem to refuse the feed from a bottle. Occasionally a baby will show frustration by crying, refusing the teat

Table 3.12 Nutritional comparison of soya based infant formulae
Approximate composition per 100 ml

All values per 100 ml reconstituted feed		Cow & Gate Infasoy	Wyeth Wysoy	Abbott Isomil	Mead Johnson Prosobee	Farley Ostersoy	Mature Breast milk	DHSS Guidelines (1980)
Major nutrients								
Protein	g	1.8	1.8	1.8	2.05	1.95	1.2–1.4	1.5–2.0*
Fat	g	3.6	3.6	3.69	3.6	3.8	3.7–4.8	2.3–5.0
Carbohydrate†	g	7.1	6.9	7.36	6.85	7.0	7.1–7.8	4.8–10.0
Minerals								
Calcium	mg	54	60	70	63.3	56	32–36	30–120
Phosphorus	mg	27	42	50	50.1	37	14–15	15–60
Calcium:Phosphorus ratio		2.1	1.4:1	1.4:1	1.3:1	1.5:1	2.3:1	1.2:1–2.2:1
Sodium	mg	18	18	32	24.3	25	11–20	15–35
Potassium	mg	65	70	77	82.3	75	57–62	50–100
Chloride	mg	40	40	59	55.9	50	35–55	40–80
Magnesium	mg	5	6.7	5	7.38	5.7	2.6–3.0	2.8–12
Iron	μg	800	670	1200	1270	650	62–93	70–700
Zinc	μg	600	500	500	527	450	260–330	200–600*
Iodine	μg	13	6	10	6.86	8.4	2–12	ns
Manganese	μg	33	20	20	17	34	0.7–1.5	ns
Copper	μg	40	47	50	63	42	37–43	10–60*
Vitamins								
A Retinol	μg	80	60	60	63.3	100	40–76	40–150
D_3 Cholecalciferol	μg	1.1	1.0	1.0	1.05	D_2 1.1	na	0.7–1.3
E dl-α-tocopherol	mg	1.3	0.64	1.7	2.1	0.5	0.29–0.39	0.3–ns
K_1 Phytomenadione	μg	5	10	10	10.5	2.8	na	1.5–ns
B_1 Thiamin	μg	40	67	40	52.7	42	13–21	13–ns
B_2 Riboflavin	μg	100	100	60	63.3	56	31	30–ns
B_6 Pyridoxine	μg	40	42	40	42.2	36	5.1–7.2	5–ns
B_{12} Cyanocobalamin	μg	0.2	0.2	0.3	0.211	0.15	0.01	0.01–ns
Niacin	μg	400	500	900	844	700	210–270	230–ns
Pantothenic acid	μg	300	300	500	316	240	220–230	200–ns
Biotin	μg	1.5	3.5	3	5.27	1.1	0.52–1.13	0.5–ns
Folic acid	μg	10	5.0	10	10.5	3.5	3.1–6.2	3–ns
C Ascorbic acid	mg	8	5.5	5.5	5.49	7.0	3.1–4.5	3–ns
Choline	mg	7	8.5	7	5.27	na	na	ns
Energy								
	kJ	280	274	286	277.6	293	270–315	270–315
	kcal	66	65	68	66.3	70	65–75	65–75
Osmolality	mosmol/kg water	200	229	250	160	na	300	ns

na = Not available ns = Not specified * = Protein with a casein:whey ratio of 80:20 † = Expressed as monsaccharide
Reproduced with the permission of Cow & Gate Nutricia Ltd

or feeding reluctantly and this is usually due to an inappropriate flow rate of milk from the bottle. This can be altered by changing to a larger or smaller-holed teat. A teat which resembles the human nipple in size and shape may be more successful than the traditional bottle teat. Some teats have an automatic vacuum release which ensures a continuous flow of milk from the bottle.

The correct feeding technique is also important. The bottle should always be angled so that the teat is full of milk thus minimizing the amount of air consumed.

It is usual to 'wind' bottle fed babies half way through a feed and after a feed.

Calculating the bottle feed

The average milk intake from one week of age until weaning is 150 ml/kg/day. Some babies will take more milk. A baby regularly taking significantly less is being underfed.

As with breast feeding, mothers should be encouraged to feed on demand. However most young babies will feed 3–4 hourly, for example, a two-week old, 4 kg baby might take 100 ml × 6 feeds every four hours. As the volume of feed taken increases, the interval between feeds increases and a typical three-month old baby weighing 6 kg might take 180 ml × 5 feeds every four hours (missing one feed overnight).

Preparation of infant milk formulae

It is essential to encourage high standards of hygiene in feed preparation and storage. Feed preparation demonstrations are commonly given at antenatal and parentcraft classes.

Sterilizing equipment Bottles, teats and bottle caps must be rinsed after use, washed in hot water with detergent, rinsed and then sterilized in a commercial cold sterilizing solution. A variety of the latter preparations in tablet or liquid forms are produced. Bottles must be submerged for the recommended time and rinsed in previously boiled water before use. Dummies, spoons and other non-metallic items can also be sterilized in this way. Sterilizing solutions must be changed daily.

Alternatively, equipment may be boiled for three minutes. Steam sterilizers are also available.

Microwave ovens Baby feeding equipment cannot be sterilized effectively in a microwave oven. In addition, milk feeds should never be warmed in a microwave. The milk may heat unevenly and readily overheats risking scalds to the baby's mouth (DHSS 1988).

Preparing a bottle feed Powdered infant milks are reconstituted by adding one level scoop of milk powder to every 30 ml/1 fluid oz previously boiled water. Feeds are usually prepared in the feeding bottle with the milk powder being added to the measured water. A water temperature of 70°C will ensure a final pasteurization in the bottle (DHSS 1988). Bottle feeds may be prepared in advance and stored in a refrigerator for up to 24 hours.

Feeds are warmed by standing the bottle in hot water or using an electric bottle warmer. The temperature of the feed should be checked on the back of the hand before feeding the baby. Any milk remaining after a feed should be discarded.

Ready-to-use feeds are now available to the general public; Wyeth produce SMA Gold and White in cartons and Cow & Gate produce bottles of Plus and Premium.

Bottled waters Some parents wish to use mineral or spring waters for their babies as they perceive them to contain fewer chemicals and other contaminants. Bottled waters are not sterile and must be boiled for infants under six months (Paediatric Group 1990a).

The mineral content must be considered. The sodium content of reconstituted feeds must be less than 35 mg/100 ml (DHSS 1988). Waters containing less than 20 mg sodium per litre are suitable. Most bottled waters sold in the UK (e.g. Highland Spring, Evian) can be used. When travelling abroad, parents should check labels and be aware that sodium may appear under its chemical symbol (Na).

Filtered and softened waters The use of a water filter to remove organic and inorganic contaminants present in tap water has become popular in recent years. However, water filters are breeding grounds for bacteria and filtered water used for infants under six months of age must be boiled. Freshly filtered water can be given to older babies (Paediatric Group 1990b).

Softened water produced by an ion exchange system contains high levels of sodium and must not be used to prepare infant formulae (Paediatric Group 1990b).

Additional nutritional requirements of the bottle-fed infant

Vitamins and minerals

All the infant milk formulae are supplemented with vitamins and minerals during production to meet DHSS guidelines (DHSS 1980). With the exception of fluoride (see the relevant paragraph under the subsection 'Additional nutritional requirements of the infant' in Section 3.3.1 above) additional supplements are not therefore required for babies under six months fed a modified infant formula. In some areas vitamin drops may be recommended from one month.

Additional fluids

By the age of six weeks, virtually all bottle fed babies have been given drinks other than formula milk (Martin and White 1988). For a healthy baby this is an unnecessary but harmless practice. Cooled boiled water is the best choice. It is important to give additional fluid to a baby with a fever, diarrhoea or vomiting in order to replace fluid losses. Medical advice should also be sought.

Monitoring the progress of a bottle fed infant

Monitoring the progress of the baby in general terms has been discussed above. The most important factors to consider in the bottle fed infant are the growth rate (weight gain in relation to length) and the contentment of the baby.

Because the volume of feed consumed is known, it is easier to assess the nutrient intake of the bottle fed than the breast fed infant. However, this assumes that the feed is being made up correctly, and this factor must be borne in mind when either an inadequate or excessive weight gain is being investigated. Lucas *et al* (1991) measured the energy content of infant formulae as made up by a group of bottle feeding mothers. The energy content ranged from

41 kcal (209 kJ) to 91 kcal (380 kJ) per 100 ml whereas the manufacturer's intended energy content was 68 kcal (284 kJ) per 100 ml. One third of feeds contained less than 50 kcal per 100 ml and around half the feeds over 80 kcal per 100 ml.

Inadequate weight gain

This may be due to:

- Feeds being either too few or too small;
- Feed being over-diluted;
- Undercurrent illness;
- Intolerance to a component of the feed (usually evidenced by gastrointestinal symptoms).

Medical staff commonly request that energy intake be increased. However, it is clearly important that the cause for poor weight gain should be investigated. Suggested strategies include:
1 Increasing the volume of feed offered. Many babies will take up to 200 ml/kg/day.
2 Increasing the frequency of feeds.
3 In a baby over three months of age, consider introducing solids.
4 The energy density of a feed can be increased by adding 2–5% of a glucose polymer. It is important the baby is taking at least 150 ml/kg/day of milk to ensure an adequate intake of protein and other nutrients. (100 ml formula + 5% glucose polymer will provide 85 kcal/360 kJ.)

Excessive weight gain

This may be due to:

- Feeds being either too frequent or too large;
- Feeds being over-concentrated;
- Rusk or cereal being added to the bottle. Athough this practice, once common, is now discouraged by health professionals, it still occurs, mainly because it is often recommended by well-meaning relatives.

Suggested strategies:
1 Parents may need support and guidance in handling their baby.
2 A smaller-holed teat may be worth trying.
3 Additional water after a feed may help the crying baby who feeds for comfort rather than hunger. Some parents find a dummy helpful.

Problems associated with bottle feeding

Wind, posseting and vomiting

Bottle fed babies tend to take in more air with their feed than breast fed infants and are therefore more likely to suffer discomfort. For the same reason, regurgitation during or after a feed is also more common. Both can be minimized by allowing the baby to rest from feeding at intervals in a vertical position so that the swallowed air can escape. Reducing the flow rate of the milk may also help.

If a considerable proportion of the feed is being persistently regurgitated, or if the vomit contains blood or bile, medical advice should be sought. A thickening agent to add to the feed (e.g. Instant Carobel – Cow & Gate) can be prescribed and is usually very effective. A large holed or cross-cut teat must be used with thickened feeds.

Stool appearance

Artificial feeding results in stools which are often greenish in colour and these are not always easily distinguished from the green stools seen when a gut infection is present. Loose stools may be normal for a particular baby but can occasionally indicate dietary intolerance. The sudden appearance of loose stools associated with vomiting and an unwell child suggest the presence of infection.

Constipation

This is more likely to occur in bottle than breast fed infants and may reflect an inadequate fluid intake. Bottle fed infants should be offered cooled boiled water at intervals, particularly in hot weather. Diluted fresh orange juice (1 in 4) can be given to babies over one month.

Incorrect reconstitution of the milk formula

Over-concentrated feeds can be prepared either by tight packing of powder in the measuring scoop or by deliberately adding more powder or less water than recommended. This will clearly exacerbate the risk of obesity and, in addition, may lead to life-threatening problems of hyperosmolar dehydration and hypernatraemia (see below).

Hyperosmolar dehydration and hypernatraemia

The immature kidneys of the young infant can only produce a maximum osmolarity of 700 mmol/l. A high solute load may therefore result in hyperosmolar dehydration and hypernatraemia. Fortunately these conditions are much more rare than they used to be owing to modifications in infant milk formulae. However, they can still arise from a combination of factors such as over-concentrated feeds, high extra-renal fluid losses (e.g. due to diarrhoea or excessive sweating), a reduced renal output and no additional fluid.

Hypercalcaemia and hyperphosphataemia

As with the above, modern milk formulae are less likely to cause these problems. The ratio of calcium : phosphorus in breast milk is 2.3 : 1 and this is now copied in the artificial formulae. Hypercalcaemia/hyperphosphataemia can still be a problem in low birth weight infants.

Intolerances

Cows' milk protein (see Section 2.14.4);
Disaccharide intolerance (see Section 2.4.5).

3.3.3 Weaning

'Weaning begins when semi-solid food starts to be given in addition to milk' (DHSS 1988). The introduction of solids to a baby's diet is a gradual process taking several months. Weaning does not need to start at a given age or weight. Current recommendations (DHSS 1988) suggest that very few babies need solid food before three months but that the majority should have started solids by six months. Infants are weaned for two reasons:

1 *Nutritional*
The volume of milk required to meet energy needs becomes too great and the baby requires a more energy-dense diet. Stores of, for example, iron are depleted by about six months of age and additional sources of iron need to be introduced. This is particularly true for breast fed babies and those who have been changed to cows' milk.

2 *Developmental*
Feeding behaviour progresses from immature sucking and swallowing to biting and chewing. To encourage this phase of development it is important to introduce a variety of tastes and to include thicker and then lumpy foods from 6–7 months. Pridham (1990) reviews the development of feeding behaviour at weaning.

Introducing solids

Martin and White (1988) report that 62% of mothers have given their babies solid food by the age of three months. Many mothers are still introducing solids earlier than generally thought desirable or necessary.
The age at which mothers choose to start weaning is affected by both social factors and medical factors.

Social factors

- Social class and cultural differences in the age of weaning.
- Bottle fed infants tend to be weaned earlier than breast fed infants.
- Influence of family and friends.

Medical factors

- Professional advice.
- Growth rate.
- Medical conditions.

Suitable early weaning foods

Nutrient content This is relatively unimportant at this stage because of the small quantity of food involved. Commercial baby cereal is a popular first food. The baby is then gradually introduced to a range of foods. New foods should be introduced one at a time to make it easier to identify any adverse reaction.

Flavour Bland foods with a milky or neutral flavour are preferred to strongly flavoured or spiced foods. No salt or sugar should be added during food preparation, nor added to a manufactured baby food. The food is designed to suit a baby's palate not an adult's.

Consistency A thin smooth consistency is necessary initially so that the baby can use the sucking reflex to take food from the spoon. At about the age of 4–6 months, the baby develops a swallowing ability, transferring food from the spoon to the back of the mouth, and can progress to food in the form of a thicker lump-free paste (Table 3.15).

Manufactured 'first stage' weaning foods are either ready made or can be reconstituted to a smooth texture. Home-made weaning foods need liquidizing or sieving to achieve a suitable texture and consistency.

Preparation Dried manufactured weaning foods are particularly useful in the early stages as very small quantities can be made up. Manufactured baby foods in tins and jars are also useful but once opened must be refrigerated and consumed within 48 hours and there may be wastage.

Home-made baby food can be prepared and frozen, initially in ice cube trays and later in small pots (e.g. empty yoghurt cartons). A large freezer is not necessary; the small freezer compartment in a fridge is adequate for storing several days' meals.

Many mothers appreciate ideas for weaning meals. A range of leaflets and books is available (see 'Further reading' at the end of this chapter). Suitable early weaning foods are listed in Table 3.13. Practical guidelines for starting weaning are given in Table 3.14.

Introducing gluten

For several years it has been recommended that gluten should be avoided until a baby was six months old. This was because of the relationship between early introduction of gluten-containing cereals and the development of coeliac disease in susceptible infants. The incidence of coeliac disease in children has been decreasing for many years and continues to fall (Stevens *et al* 1987). It is questionable whether the relatively recent trend towards gluten-free baby foods has contributed to this decline. Current advice (DHSS 1988) is that wheat-based foods present little risk in terms of coeliac disease for the majority of infants.

Table 3.13 Suitable early weaning foods

Food	Comments
Baby cereal	Mix to a smooth runny consistency with baby milk or water according to instructions on the packet
Fruit purées	Cook fruit without sugar or use fruit canned in natural juice. Suitable fruits are dessert apples, pears, peaches or apricots
Vegetable purée	Cook vegetables without salt. Suitable vegetables include carrots, swede, potato, parsnip, cauliflower or courgettes
Commercial baby food dried, cans or jars	Choose first stage or strained varieties. Offer savoury as well as sweet products

Table 3.14 Practical guidelines for early weaning

1 Decide which foods are to be offered
2 Obtain the equipment needed;
   (a) Protective clothing for both mother and baby (weaning is a messy process)
   (b) Shallow plastic spoon — avoid large, deep or metal teaspoons
   (c) Plastic dish — initially the top of a feeding bottle or small plastic container is large enough
   (d) Liquidizer, blender or sieve if fresh foods are to be prepared
3 Choose a quiet time of day to start weaning when the baby is not tired and other members of the family are not demanding meals
4 Offer the weaning food either after or during a milk feed so that the baby is not frustrated by hunger. As the baby becomes proficient at spoon feeding give solids before the milk feed. This allows the volume of milk taken to decrease automatically
5 Stay relaxed and be patient. It can take time — days or weeks — for the baby to accept food from a spoon. All babies are different. If a young baby is very reluctant to spoon feed, try again a week or two later

Food intolerances

The DHSS (1988) recommend that, in infants with a strong family history of atopy, it is reasonable to avoid early introduction of foods most commonly implicated in adverse reactions (e.g. cows' milk, eggs, wheat, nuts and citrus fruits). Health visitors and others professionally involved with babies should be encouraged to seek help from a dietitian when advising mothers on exclusion diets.

Progression of weaning

The main steps in the progression of an infant's diet from milk to family meals are outlined in Table 3.15. However the time-scale over which they are achieved will vary considerably.

Suitable foods for later stages of weaning

At about the age of six months the baby will welcome food of a more interesting texture. A mincer or baby food mill is a useful piece of equipment. Vegetables may be mashed instead of puréed, and meats can be minced instead of liquidized. By the age of 10–12 months, the child will be able to chew chopped foods.

As soon as children can sit up unsupported, they should be fed in a high chair and given a spoon so that they can learn, gradually, to feed themselves.

Finger foods should be introduced. Suitable foods at this stage are listed in Table 3.16.

Table 3.15 Progression of weaning

Approximate age	Timescale from starting weaning	Stage of feeding
3–4 months	Weeks 1 and 2	One teaspoon of different single foods of a thin, smooth consistency at one meal
	Weeks 3 and 4	1–2 teaspoons at two meals increase consistency to a smooth paste
5 months	1 month	Gradual increase in quantity and variety of foods offered. Maintain milk intake (breast or bottle). Additional fluid from bottle or feeder cup
6–8 months	2–4 months	Food at three meals, gradually changed to minced mashed consistency. Suitable finger foods offered. Number and quantity of milk feeds may be reduced. Additional fluid from feeding cup
8–10 months	4–6 months	Diversification into minced/mashed foods at family meal times. Milk minimum 1 pint daily. Additional fluid from feeding cup. Baby uses hands to self feed
1 year	6–8 months	Chopped family meals. Milk 1 pint daily (or suitable alternatives). Feeding cup for fluids. Learning to feed self with a spoon

Table 3.16 Suitable weaning foods for later stages of weaning (over six months)

Food	Comments
Cereals	Breakfast cereals without added sugar, e.g. porridge, Weetabix, baby mixed cereals. Cereals to make milk puddings or custard, e.g. rice, custard powder. Pasta, e.g. spaghetti, macaroni
Meats, poultry, offal	Cooked without spices, salt or additional fat and minced
Fish	Grilled, steamed or baked white fish, carefully checked for bones and then flaked. Later canned fish such as sardines or tuna can be used. Fish fingers
Eggs	Eggs must be thoroughly cooked e.g. chopped hard-boiled egg
Milk	If required as a drink, infant formula should be used as an alternative to breast milk in infants under the age of one year. Cows' milk may be used in cooked dishes (e.g. milk puddings or custard)
Yoghurt/fromage frais	
Cheese	Cottage cheese or mild hard cheese
Vegetables	All except those with a stringy texture (e.g. celery) or which are spicy (e.g. chillis or peppers)
Fruits	All should be grated or chopped (with skins) until whole pieces of fruit can be eaten
Nuts	Babies must NEVER be given whole nuts but ground nuts and nut butters can be useful especially for vegetarians
Fluid	Diluted natural juice and baby fruit juices add variety of flavours. Encourage water
Finger foods	Never leave a baby alone with finger food (or indeed any food). Try cooked pasta shapes, fingers of toast/bread, biscuits, pieces of banana, pear, cooked carrot and potato, chips, peas, diced or grated cheese, small shaped breakfast cereals (e.g. Raisin Splitz, Shreddies), cold cooked meats

General considerations

Nutritional adequacy

Although a satisfactory growth rate is the most obvious sign of an adequate diet, the baby's general contentment, sleeping pattern and bowel habits are also valuable indicators. Some mothers worry over the apparently minute quantities of food eaten by their child. They should be discouraged from trying to force the child to eat more and be reassured that a healthy baby will not go hungry.

Additional vitamins The DHSS recommends the use of children's vitamin drops for all children between the ages of six months and two years (and preferably until the age of five) (DHSS 1988). Vitamin drops are strongly advised for children of Asian families to prevent the risk of rickets.

The recommended dose of five drops daily provides 200/mg Vitamin A, 20 mg Vitamin C and 7/mg Vitamin D. Childrens' vitamin drops are sold at low cost through baby clinics. They are free to mothers on Income Support.

Fluoride A daily fluoride supplement of 0.25 mg is recommended for children under two years who live in areas with low fluoride levels in the drinking water. (For more information see the paragraph on 'Fluoride' in Section 4.1.1.)

Home-made versus manufactured baby foods

Mothers often ask whether they should use home-made or manufactured baby foods. Either type is suitable. It is simply a matter of personal preference. Today convenience foods feature largely in most people's diets. Tins and jars of baby food are merely the baby equivalent.

Martin and White (1988) found that home-prepared foods were given by a minority of mothers of four month old babies – 82% used commercial baby food. However by nine months, most babies were having a wide range of home prepared and convenience baby foods.

Some mothers like to prepare all their infant's food and have the satisfaction of knowing exactly what their baby is eating. Others find it frustrating to take time and trouble preparing a suitable purée only for it to be rejected after one spoonful. In theory, home-made baby foods are more economical than manufactured ones although this is not always the case in practice if they are prepared separately from the family meals (e.g. to avoid the use of excess salt or sugar) thus incurring extra fuel costs, or if the baby then dislikes what has been produced. In the early stages, many mothers opt for the convenience of dried manufactured foods which can be made up in small quantities and gradually introduce suitably modified items from the family meals. Ready made baby foods are also useful when travelling or eating away from home.

From 6–7 months it is reasonable to offer the baby suitable food from family meals. Prolonged use of commercial baby food can make some babies reluctant to enjoy the varied textures and tastes of family food.

Salt

Commercial baby food contains no added salt. When preparing savoury meals, especially for a baby, no salt should be added.

For an older baby sharing family food, it is unrealistic to suggest that no salt is added on cooking. However it is a time when a family may become more aware of the amount of salt they consume unnecessarily. In particular, adding extra salt at the table is a habit which many children copy and a practice which can be beneficially avoided by the entire family.

Introducing cows' milk

The DHSS (1988) recommends that milks suitable for infants over six months are breast milk, modified infant formulae, follow-up milks and whole pasteurized cows' milk.

Semi-skimmed milk may be introduced from the age of two, provided that the rest of the diet is adequate in energy. Fully skimmed milk should not be used before the age of five years (DHSS 1988).

There is much to commend the use of infant formula (or breast milk) in babies throughout their first year. Follow-up milks are an alternative in babies over six months whose mothers wish to change the milk feed (Wharton 1990).

When advising individual mothers it is important to consider the rest of the baby's diet. A seven month old baby who is slow to accept solid food and is taking just a few teaspoons of cereal and fruit should clearly remain on a modified milk.

These recommendations refer to milk drinks given by bottle or cup. There is no reason why cows' milk in the form of milk puddings, sauces, yoghurt etc. should not be included in the baby's diet from around six months. Cows' milk used for babies and children should be pasteurized (or UHT). Untreated milk, such as might be available to children who live on a farm for example, must be boiled.

Goats' milk

Goats' milk is unsuitable for babies under six months of age for the same reasons as cows' milk. In addition it is deficient in folic acid. Goats' milk for older babies and children must be boiled if it has not been pasteurized. Vitamin drops should be given (DHSS 1988).

Infant drinks

A wide range of fruit and herbal flavoured drinks are sold for babies. Many contain added Vitamin C. Thirsty babies will drink water and mothers should be encouraged to offer water in preference to juices.

Drinks produced for babies contain no added sucrose but have high levels of naturally occurring sugars or added glucose syrup, which are also cariogenic (DoH 1989). Fruit drinks, even when well diluted, are acidic enough to cause erosion of dental enamel (Duggal and Curzon 1989). From a dental health point of view, the only harmless drinks are milk and water.

Realistic advice is to give juice by cup as soon as possible, ideally only at mealtimes rather than between meals. Prolonged sipping of fruit juice (e.g. from a bottle) should be discouraged.

Problems associated with weaning

Risk of choking

It is important that a baby is never left alone while feeding. Initially, finger foods should be those which soften easily in the mouth (e.g. rusk, bread or banana). Harder foods such as apple or carrot should only be given when the child has learnt to chew well.

Rejection of solids

It takes time for a baby to become accustomed to feeding from a spoon and to each new taste. There will inevitably be some rejections, but provided that weaning coincides with the baby's development, solids will be taken.

Late weaning (e.g. after nine months) may present more problems. Babies with developmental delay may be slow to wean. Pre-term babies, particularly if they experienced long periods of tube or parenteral feeding may display problems at the weaning stage. A reluctance to accept lumpy food is a common problem; this is often the result of smooth purées being offered for too long. Exclusive use of commercial baby foods also exacerbates the problem. All normal babies should be offered lumpy, mashed foods and finger foods from no later than 6–7 months.

Babies should never be force-fed. Prolonged feeding difficulties may benefit from a team approach involving a speech therapist experienced in assessing feeding development. Parents need consistent help and support over what is a most distressing problem.

Poor weaning practices

Common causes include ignorance, child neglect, economic and social problems. Some ethnic groups delay weaning, and allow the child to remain almost exclusively on cows' milk until 2–3 years of age. This problem requires tactful handling.

Over-zealous application of NACNE recommendation to infants (especially high fibre diets) can cause a number of nutritional problems, particularly too low an energy intake and impairment of trace element status (Francis 1986). Some mothers are slow to introduce foods other than fruit and vegetables into the weaning diet and the inclusion of some foods with a higher energy density is essential (Table 3.17). Self-diagnosis of food allergy and the use of goats' milk or plant-based milk, and over-restriction of foods offered at weaning can also result in nutritional inadequacies.

Restrictive diets may also be followed for religious, social or cultural reasons. More details about particular ethnic groups can be found in Section 3.9. Vegetarian and vegan diets are discussed in Section 3.10.

Table 3.17 Energy content of common weaning foods

	average per 100 g	
	kJ	kcal
Carrot purée	84	20
Unsweetened fruit purée	210	50
Jar/can savoury baby food	275–335	65–80
Baby rice mixed with milk	380	90
Rusk mixed with milk	420	100
Lentil soup	420	100
Custard (made with whole milk)	525	125
Powdered baby food (mixed with water)	525	125
Minced meat ($\frac{1}{3}$) and potato ($\frac{2}{3}$)	630	150

Failure to thrive

Poor weaning practices can, if left, result in the baby failing to thrive. Medical attention is essential to eliminate a functional cause such as coeliac disease or cystic fibrosis.

Constipation and diarrhoea

Some babies are more prone to constipation than others. Constipation can occur if the fluid or fibre intake is inadequate. Consumption of these should be increased and high fibre cereals (e.g. Weetabix) and wholemeal bread can be introduced at around 6–7 months.

Diarrhoea can be due to:

- Infection;
- Excessive fibre intake;
- Food intolerance.

Prolonged diarrhoea should receive medical advice.

Obesity (see also Section 4.17)

Infants are at greater risk of becoming obese if:

- One or both parents is obese;
- Weaning is started early, before the age of three months;
- They have certain mental or physical disabilities.

If both the weight and length of babies are regularly recorded, height-weight centile charts will show any deviations from desirable weight gain. Strict reducing diets must never be imposed at this age. General measures such as minimizing the use of added sugar and sweet drinks, increasing the content of fruit and vegetables in the diet and reducing milk intake once weaning is established are usually sufficient to restore appropriate weight for height.

Food allergy and intolerance (see Section 4.31)

Eczema (see Section 4.30.1)

Rickets (see Section 4.27 and DHHS 1980)

Inconsistent advice

The new mother is usually bombarded with advice – from professionals, the mass media, baby food manufacturers and lay groups – some of which may be contradictory (Clark and Laing 1990). Further confusion may arise with the healthy eating guidelines recommended in the NACNE (1983) and COMA (1984) reports and, for example, mothers may give their children skimmed milk in the belief that its low fat content is beneficial.

The implementation of a local child nutrition policy which endeavours to introduce some degree of uniformity to the advice given by health professionals within a particular area may help to reduce these problems. Dietitians should be available not only to give advice directly to mothers but also to advise the advisers.

Useful addresses

Association of Breastfeeding Mothers, 26 Hearnshaw Close, London SE26 4TH. Tel 081–778 4769.

Joint Breastfeeding Initiative, Department of Health, Skipton House, 80 London Road, London SE1 6LW. Tel 071–972 2000.

La Lèche League, Breastfeeding Help and Information, PO Box BM 3424, London WC1N 3XX. Tel 071–242 1278.

National Childbirth Trust, Breastfeeding Promotion Group, Alexander House, Oldham Terrace, Acton London W3 6NH. Tel 081–992 8637.

Further reading

Francis DEM (1986) *Nutrition for children*. Blackwell Scientific Publications, Oxford.

Karmel A (1991) *The complete baby and toddler meal planner*. Ebury Press, London.

Kinman J (1987) *Going on to solids*. Paperfronts, London.

La Lèche League International (1990) *The art of breast feeding*. Angus and Robertson, London.

Royal College of Midwives (1991) *Successful breastfeeding* 2e. Churchill Livingstone, Edinburgh.

Smale M (1992) *The NCT book of breastfeeding*. Vermilion, London.

Stanway P and Stanway A (Revised 1983) *Breast is best*. Pan Books, London.

References

Adinolfi M and Glynn A (1979) The interaction of antibacterial factors in breast milk. *Devel Med Child Neurol* **21**, 808–10.

Binkiewicz A, Robinson MJ and Senior B (1978) Pseudo-Cushing syndrome caused by alcohol in breast milk. *J Paediatr* **93**, 965–7.

Brock JH (1980) Lactoferrin in human milk: its role in iron absorption and protection against enteric infection in the newborn infant. *Arch Dis Childh* **55**, 417–22.

Cant AJ, Bailes JA, Marsden RA and Hewitt D (1986) Effect of maternal dietary exclusion on breastfed infants with eczema. *Br Med J* **293**, 231–3.

Chan GM, McMurray M, Estorer K, Engelbert-Fenton K and Thomas MR (1987) Effects of increased dietary calcium intake upon calcium and bone mineral status in lactating adolescent and adult women. *Am J Clin Nutr* **46**, 319–23.

Chandra RK, Puri S, Suraiya C and Cheema PS (1986) Influence of maternal food antigen avoidance during pregnancy and lactation on incidence of atopic eczema in infants. *Clin Allergy* **16**, 565–9.

Clark BJ and Laing SC (1990) Infant feeding: a review of weaning. *J Hum Nutr Diet* **3**, 11–18.

Clement MI (1989) Personal view – Caffeine and babies. *Br Med J* **298**, 1461.

Clyne P and Kulczycki A (1991) Human breast milk contains bovine IgG. Relationship to infant colic? *Paediatrics* **87**(4), 439–44.

Craig-Schmidt M, Weete JD, Faircloth SA, Wickwire MA and Livant EJ (1984) The effect of hydrogenated fat in the diet of nursing mothers on lipid composition and prostaglandin content of human milk. *Am J Clin Nutr* **39**, 778–86.

Department of Health and Social Security (1980) Artificial feeds for the young infant. *Rep Hlth Soc Subj 18.* HMSO, London.

Department of Health and Social Security (1984) Committee on Medical Aspects of Food Policy. Diet and cardiovascular disease (The COMA Report). *Rep Health Soc Subj 28.* HMSO, London.

Department of Health and Social Security (1988) Present day practice in infant feeding. *Rep Hlth Soc Subj 32*, HMSO, London.

Department of Health (1989) Dietary sugars and human disease. Report of the Panel on Dietary Sugars. *Rep Hlth Soc Subj 37*, HMSO, London.

Department of Health (1991) Dietary Reference Values for food energy and nutrients in the United Kingdom. *Rep Hlth Soc Subj 41*, HMSO, London.

Dowell TB and Joyston-Bechal S (1981) Fluoride supplements, age related doses. *Br Dental J* **150**, 283–5.

Downham MAPS, Scott R and Sims DE (1976) Does breast feeding protect against respiratory syncytial virus? *Br Med J* **2**, 274–6.

Duggal MS and Curzon MEJ (1989) An evaluation of the cariogenic potential of baby and infant fruit drinks. *Br Dent J* **166**, 327–30.

Francis D (1986) *Diets for sick children*. Blackwell Scientific Publications, Oxford.

Goldberg NM and Adams E (1983) Supplementary water for breastfed babies in a hot dry climate – not really a necessity. *Arch Dis Childh* **58**, 73–4.

Howie PW, Forsyth JS, Ogston SA, Clark A and Florey C du V (1990) Protective effect of breast feeding against infection. *Br Med J* **300**, 11–16.

Illingworth PJ, Jung RT, Howie PW, Leslie P and Isles TE (1986) Diminution in energy expenditure during lactation. *Br Med J* **292**, 437–41.

Jakobsson I, Lindberg T, Benediktsson B and Hansson BG (1985) Dietary bovine betaglobulin is transferred to human milk. *Acta Paed Scan* **74**, 342–5.

Klaus MH and Kennell JH (1976) Maternal infant bonding. CV Mosby, St Louis.

Kramer MS (1988) Does breast feeding help protect against atopic disease? *J Paediatr* **112**, 181–90.

Lucas A, Ewing G, Roberts SB and Coward WA (1987) How much energy does the breast fed infant consume and expend? *Br Med J* **295**, 75–7.

Lucas A, Lockton S and Davies PSW (1991) Milk for babies and children (letter). *Br Med J* **302**, 350–1.

Martin J and White A (1988) *Infant feeding 1985*. Office of Population Censuses and Surveys, Social Survey Division, HMSO. London.

Ministry of Agriculture, Fisheries and Food (1989) *Food Facts 20*, April 1989. HMSO, London.

NACNE (1983) *A discussion paper on proposals for nutritional guidelines for health education in Britain*. Health Education Council, London.

Ogra SS and Ogra PL (1978) Immunological aspects of human colostrum and milk. *J Paediatr* **92**, 550–55.

Paediatric Group, British Dietetic Association (1990a) The use of bottled water in the preparation of infant formulae (Policy Statement). BDA, Birmingham.

Paediatric Group, British Dietetic Association (1990b) The use of filtered water and softened water for infants under six months of age. (Policy Statement). BDA, Birmingham.

Park W, Paust H, Kauffman HJ, Offermann G (1987) Osteomalacia of the mother – rickets of the newborn. *Eur J Paediatr* **146**, 292–3.

Paul AA, Whitehead RG and Black AE (1990) Energy intakes and growth from two months to three years in initially breast fed infants. *J Hum Nutr Diet* **3**, 141–4.

Pittard WB (1979) Breast milk immunology. *Am J Dis Child* **133**, 83–7.

Plank SJ and Milanesi ML (1973) Infant feeding and infant mortality in rural Chile. *Bull WHO* **48**, 203–10.

Prentice AM, Paul AA, Prentice A, Black AE, Cole TJ and Whitehead RG (1986) Cross-cultural differences in lactational performance. In *Human Lactation 2: Maternal and environmental factors*. Proceedings of an international workshop held at Oaxacu, Mexico 1986. Plenum Publishing, New York.

Prentice AM, Roberts SB, Prentice A, Paul AA, Watkinson M, Watkinson AA and Whitehead RG (1983) Dietary supplementation of lactating Gambian women. Effect on breast milk quality and volume. *Hum Nutr: Clin Nutr* **37c**, 53–64.

Pridham KF (1990) Feeding behaviour of six to twelve month old infants. Assessment and sources of parental information. *J Paed* (Supplement to Vol 117), S174–90.

Righard L and Alade M (1990) Effect of delivery room routines on success of first breast feed. *Lancet* **336**, 1105–7.

Stevens FM, Egan-Mitchell B, Cryan E, McCarthy CF and McNichol B (1987) Decreasing incidence of coeliac disease. *Arch Dis Childh* **62**, 465–8.

Taitz LS and Scholey E (1989) Are babies more satisfied by casein based formulas? *Arch Dis Childh* **64**, 619–21.

Victoria CG, Smith PG, Vaughan PJ, Nobre LC, Lombardi C and Teixeira HB (1987) Evidence for protection by breast feeding against deaths from infectious diseases in Brazil. *Lancet* **ii**, 319–22.

Walker-Smith JA (1990) Management of infantile gastroenteritis. *Arch Dis Childh* **65**, 917–8.

Warner JO (1980) Food allergy in fully breast fed infants. *Clin Allergy* **10**, 133–6.

Weaver LT, Laker MF and Nelson R (1984) Intestinal permeability in the newborn. *Arch Dis Childh* **59**, 236–41.

Weintraub R, Hams G, Meerkin M and Rosenberg AR (1986) High aluminium content of infant milk formulae. *Arch Dis Child* **61**, 914–16.

Welsh JK and May JT (1979) Anti-infective properties of breast milk. *J Paediatr* **94**, 1–9.

Wharton B (1990) Milk for babies and children. *Br Med J* **301**, 774–5.

White CJ and White MK (1980) Breast feeding and drugs in human milk. *Vet Human Toxicol* **22**(Suppl 1), 1–43.

Whitehead RG, Paul AA and Rowland MGM (1980) Lactation in Cambridge and the Gambia. *Br Med Bull* **37**, 77–82.

World Health Organization (1981) International code of marketing of breast milk substitutes. WHO, Geneva.

Wilson JT, Brown RD, Cherek DR, Dailey JW, Hillman B, Jobe PC, Manno BR, Manno JE, Redetz HM and Stewart JJ (1980) Drug excretion in human breast milk. *Clin Pharmokinetics* **5**, 1–66.

Woolridge MW and Fisher C (1988) Colic, 'overfeeding', and symptoms of lactose malabsorption in the breast fed baby. A possible artifact of feed management. *Lancet* **ii**, 382–4.

Wright AL, Holburg CJ, Martinez FD, Morgan NNNJ and Tanssig LM (1989) Breast feeding and lower respiratory tract illness in the first year of life. *Br Med J* **299**, 946–9.

Yap PL, Pryde A, Latham PJ and McLelland DB (1979) Serum IgA in the neonate. Concentration and effect of breast feeding. *Acta Paediatr Scand* **68**, 695–700.

3.4 Pre-school children

The pre-school child is a changing individual. The developments which take place between one and five years of age are numerous and, directly or indirectly, affect eating habits.

The pre-school child is almost totally dependent on others for his or her food. Parents, and other carers, should realize that their own eating habits, likes and dislikes, will be the ones that the child imitates.

Food and eating are wonderful sources of learning for children (e.g. cooking, shopping and eating out). Food can also be a source of frustration and a cause of arguments between parents and child. Food fads are so common in young children that they can be considered a part of normal child development.

There is little published work on what pre-school age British children are currently eating and much of what has been done has been confined to a specific area such as iron deficiency.

3.4.1 Healthy eating and the pre-school child

Current guidelines on healthy eating, as given in the COMA report (DHSS 1984) or NACNE (1983) reports, are not intended to be applied to this age group. However the food intakes of young children cannot be considered in isolation from that of their families. Many people believe that early food experiences have an important effect on eating patterns in adult life although there is little evidence to support this (Rozin 1990).

Healthy eating advice can be directed at the whole family but the special nutritional needs of the young child must be borne in mind.

Energy

Recent work suggests that young children require lower energy intakes than previously thought. Intakes of 80–90 kcal/kg/day for children aged 1–5 years have been reported (Prentice *et al* 1988; Paul *et al* 1990). Energy intakes of young children in other industrialized societies are reviewed by Paul *et al* (1990).

Many young children show chaotic eating patterns, consuming very little at one meal but 'making up' later. Sometimes days of poor eating are followed by a period of improved intake. Some children have one meal a day when they eat particularly well – commonly breakfast.

This variability in eating patterns has been shown in a study of 2–5 year old American children (Birch *et al* 1991). They found that, while food consumption from meal to meal was highly erratic, total daily energy intakes were relatively constant.

Minor illness is common in this age group and inevitably interferes with feeding.

Fat

Eating less fat poses no nutritional problems for adults but, in the small child, such a measure can result in a diet of insufficient energy content. This is because the carbohydrate foods needed to replace the energy from fat are more bulky and a young child may not be able to cope with this volume, especially if the carbohydrate is high in fibre (Burkitt *et al* 1980). However Payne (1991) found no correlation between energy derived from fat and total energy intake in her study of over 200 pre-school children, suggesting that young children may adapt to reduced fat intakes.

It is widely accepted that atherosclerosis can start in early life (Strong and McGill 1962). Whilst diet is not the only determining factor, limiting total and saturated fat as part of a healthy family lifestyle can be encouraged. A breast fed (or formula fed) baby obtains 50% of its dietary energy from fat. Adults in this country are being encouraged to achieve an energy intake from fat of 30%. Debate continues on at what age this becomes a realistic target for children. Tarlow (1989) suggests a target of 35% energy from fat by the age of five years.

Young children with familial hypercholesterolaemia are special cases who require early and intensive management to improve their prognosis (Tarlow *et al* 1988).

Fibre

There are no recommendations for the amount of fibre appropriate for small children. An Australian study reported daily intakes of 2.8 g–28 g with a mean of 12 g in a group of four year old children (Magarey and Boulton 1984).

High fibre foods are bulky and young children with small appetites offered a diet high in dietary fibre may not ingest adequate energy. However Payne (1991) in her study of urban Scottish pre-school children found no evidence that children eating a high fibre diet had a reduced energy or nutrient intake. Nevertheless, encouraging the consumption of these foods as between-meal snacks rather than with main meals may be a more satisfactory alternative, particularly in children with small appetites.

The possibility exists that diets high in phytate will adversely affect mineral absorption. This risk is increased for children following vegetarian diets.

Some young children appear sensitive to a relatively modest amount of fibre in their diet. The result is symptoms of wind, colic and loose frequent stools (see 'toddlers' diarrhoea').

Sugar

Compared to adults and school-aged children, sugar in the pre-school child's diet typically provides a much higher proportion of dietary energy (27–30%), with non-milk extrinsic sugar accounting for about half of this (DoH 1989). In the diets of children taking an exceptionally high sugar intake, Payne (1991) found the main source of sugar to be pure fruit juices and blackcurrant syrups. Such drinks appear to have an exaggerated 'healthy' image, contributing to their liberal use in the diet of young children.

There are strong links between sugar intake and the development of dental caries and dental caries is also particularly prevalent in pre-school children (DoH 1989). In order to minimize the risk, frequent consumption of sugary drinks, sweets and snacks should be discouraged.

3.4.2 Nutritional problems in pre-school children

Iron deficiency (see also Section 2.8.2, 'Iron', and 4.26.1, 'Anaemia')

Iron deficiency is common in pre-school children particularly in socially disadvantaged groups and in the immigrant population. Incidence figures for iron deficiency anaemia of around 25% in the second year of life have been reported in studies from Birmingham and Nottingham (Aukett *et al* 1986; James *et al* 1989).

Iron deficiency is associated with frequent infections, poor weight gain, developmental delay and behaviour disorders (Aukett *et al* 1986) and is an important treatable condition of early childhood. The scale of the problem may merit screening programmes to detect and treat iron deficiency (Hall 1989; Marder *et al* 1990).

Iron deficiency in young children is usually of dietary origin. It is associated with late weaning, inappropriate weaning foods and the early introduction of cows' milk which is not only deficient in iron but may cause intestinal blood loss in some young children (Ziegler *et al* 1990).

Prevention of iron deficiency

Dietary advice around the time of weaning is particularly important. Extended use of iron-fortified infant formulae or of a follow-on milk should be encouraged.

Treatment

In proven iron deficiency anaemia, (for example Hb $<$ 11 g/dl; MCV below the normal range of 76–100 fl; serum ferritin $<$ 10 μg/l, but NB these criteria may vary between laboratories), a course of supplementary iron will be prescribed.

Dietary advice centres around explanation of the role of diet in anaemia and correction of dietary imbalance. Excessive milk consumption (more than a pint daily), a high intake of sweets, biscuits, crisps and little or no meat in the diet are common findings. Mothers also frequently describe 'lazy eaters' who are unwilling to chew meat and vegetables.

Acceptable sources of iron should be encouraged, for example iron fortified cereals, minced meat dishes, bread.

Ascorbic acid enhances iron absorption and a food or drink rich in vitamin C should be encouraged at mealtimes. This is particularly important for children on non-meat diets.

Obesity

Because pre-school children are totally dependent on other people for their food, obesity in this age group is entirely the fault of the parents (or carers) rather than the child. It is easy for high energy foods such as sweets, biscuits, crisps to figure to excess in the diet of a fussy eater, but it is the parents who have allowed this situation to develop. Treatment of childhood obesity is discussed in Section 4.17.2.

Poor eating

'He hardly eats a thing' is a common reason for referral to a GP, health visitor, paediatrician or dietitian. Food refusal by a toddler is a powerful weapon and causes much parental anxiety.

If a child is growing normally it is unlikely that there is significant illness. Height and weight centiles should be plotted together with previous measurements if available. Measurements falling below the 3rd centile indicate referral to a paediatrician for investigation of possible failure to thrive.

Dietary management

In a healthy child, this revolves around explanation and reassurance.

1 Many parents have unrealistic expectations of their child's weight gain and requirements for food and are worrying unnecessarily. They should be reminded that from birth to one year a child gains about 6 kg (15 lbs) but during the second, third and fourth years, the average

weight gain is only 2 kg (5 lbs). The rapid growth and constant increases in food intake of a baby do not continue.
2 It is important to discover what the child is actually eating. Taking a detailed dietary history or asking the parents to keep a three-day food diary can be very revealing.

Common findings include the following.

Frequent drinks of milk or juice Many young children prefer drinking to eating and readily fill themselves up with drinks. Useful advice is that drinks are avoided for an hour before meals and only offered at the end of a meal, not along with food. If a toddler still drinks from a bottle, a cup should be encouraged instead; this always decreases fluid intake. Large milk drinkers pose particular problems; it can be suggested that three cups a day plus milk on cereal is ample.

Eating between meals Small children may need to eat between meals but some end up eating most of their food between meals. A cup of milk and a packet of crisps mid morning will stop most toddlers eating lunch. More appropriate snacks should be suggested, for example one cup of juice and one plain biscuit or half a banana.

Some families feel that they have to offer snacks if meals are uneaten. They should be reassured that no healthy child will starve if appropriate food is offered at mealtimes. A consistent approach is essential and all those involved in the care of the child, including relatives and childminders, must co-operate.

There is never a place for force feeding which can only make the situation worse. Tactics such as eating at friends' homes, picnics and meals out can all employed to help the fussy eater. Food and mealtimes should, after all, be an enjoyable part of a child's day.

Toddler's diarrhoea

This is a common problem in children who are otherwise healthy. Frequent, loose stools containing recognizable food matter (e.g. peas, carrots, sweetcorn) may be passed up to eight or more times daily. The stools often become looser later in the day but are not passed at night. Typically the first stool of the day is passed soon after the child first eats or drinks. The condition is thought to be due to a degree of immaturity of gut function and often improves spontaneously around the age of 3–4 years. Parents often present for advice when they hope to start toilet training or when the child is due to attend nursery school.

Dietary management

Toddler's diarrhoea is a harmless condition and careful explanation reassures many parents. Dietary manipulations which have been tried include reducing fibre, increasing fat (to prolong transit times) and reducing sugar intake. Reducing fibre intake (e.g. a change to white bread, refined breakfast cereal and one helping of fruit and vegetable daily) is particularly likely to help children whose families have adopted a high fibre healthy diet. Tolerance to fibre undoubtedly improves with age.

Constipation

Young children may become constipated particularly following an anal fissure or after an intercurrent infection. There may also be a behavioural element to the problem. The child should be encouraged to consume foods with a higher fibre content and which are also enjoyed (e.g. wholegrain breakfast cereal, fruit, lentil soup, baked beans, high fibre white bread). There is no place for battles over vegetables. Young children should not be given unprocessed bran.

It is important to ensure that the child has a good fluid intake.

Food and poverty

Families on low incomes face major problems in feeding their children (NCH 1991). This subject is discussed in more detail in Section 3.8 'Low Income Groups'.

Further reading

British Dietetic Association (1987) *Children's diets and change*. Report of the child health and nutrition working party. BDA, Birmingham.

Morse E (1988) *My child won't eat*. Penguin, Harmondsworth.

References

Aukett MA, Parks YS, Scott PH and Wharton BA (1986) Treatment with iron increases weight gain and psychomotor development. *Arch Dis Child* **61**, 849–57.

Birch LL, Johnson SL, Andresen G and Peters JC (1991) The variability of young children's energy intake. *N Engl J Med* **324**, 232–5.

Burkitt D, Morley D and Walker A (1980) Dietary fibre in under and over nutrition in children. *Arch Dis Childh* **55**, 803–7.

DHSS (1984) Committee on Medical Aspects of Food Policy. *Diet and cardiovascular disease* (The COMA Report). Rep Health Soc Subj 28. HMSO, London.

Department of Health (1989) *Dietary sugars and human disease*. Rep Health Soc Subj 37. HMSO, London.

Hall MB (Ed) (1989) *Health for all children*. Report of the Joint Working Party on Child Health Surveillance, pp. 34–6. Oxford Medical Publications, Oxford.

James T, Lawson P, Male P and Oakhill A (1989) Preventing iron deficiency in pre-school children by implementing an educational and screening programme in an inner city practice. *Br Med J* **299**, 838–40.

Magarey A and Boulton TJC (1984) Nutritional studies during childhood. IV Energy and nutrient intakes at age four. *Aust Paediatr J* **20**, 187–94.

Marder E, Nicoll A, Polnay L and Shulman CE (1990) Discovering anaemia at child health clinics. *Arch Dis Childh* **65**, 892–4.

National Advisory Committee on Nutrition Education (1983) *Proposals for nutritional guidelines for health education in Britain* (The NACNE Report). Health Education Council, London.

National Children's Home (1991) *NHC Poverty and Nutrition Survey 1991*. NCH, London.

Paul AA, Whitehead RG and Black AE (1990) Energy intakes and growth from two months to three years in initially breast fed children. *J Hum Nutr Diet* **3**, 79–92.

Payne A (1991) Nutrient intake and growth in pre-school children. PhD thesis, University of Edinburgh.

Prentice AM, Lucas A, Vasquez-Valasquez L, Davies PSW and Whitehead RG (1988) Are current dietary guidelines for young children a prescription for overfeeding? *Lancet* **ii**, 1066–9.

Rozin P (1990) Acquisition of stable food preferences. *Nutrition Reviews* **48**, 106–113.

Strong JP and McGill HC Jr (1962) The natural history of coronary atherosclerosis. *Am J Pathol* **40**, 37–49.

Tarlow M, Green A, Worthington D and Buchanan E (1988) The paediatric lipid clinic in Birmingham. *J Inherited Metab Dis* **11**(Suppl 1), 91–3.

Tarlow MJ (1989) Cholesterol and diet. *Arch Dis Childh* **64**, 647–8.

Ziegler EE, Fomon SJ and Nelson SE (1990) Cow milk feeding in infancy: further observations on blood loss from the gastrointestinal tract. *J Pediatr* **116**, 11–8.

3.5 School-age children

3.5.1 Nutritional requirements

Dietary reference values (DRVs) have been discussed in detail in Section 1.2. Table 3.18 summarizes the requirements for four important dietary components for children of school age.

Young children have relatively high requirements in relation to their size. It is well documented that young children have small appetites and frequently exhibit food faddiness to whole groups of foods for long periods of time (National Dairy Council 1991).

Young children need a high quality diet to achieve appropriate nutrient intakes in accordance with DRVs. However it is important to remember if using EAR (Estimated Average Requirement) for energy, many children will require more than this average and also many children will require less. Therefore other parameters, such as anthropometric measurements, should be used when considering dietary adequacy. It should also be borne in mind that the RNI (Reference Nutrient Intake), which is used for most nutrients, is higher than most people need since the RNI is the amount that is enough for almost every individual, including those with high needs. Therefore consideration of dietary adequacy should include referral to other measures such as biochemical indices.

A Working Party of the British Dietetic Association published a document *Children's diets and change* (BDA 1987) Table 3.19 summarizes the recommendations made to ensure good feeding practices in the under-fives.

Table 3.19 Summary of Recommendations from *Children's diets and change* (BDA 1987).

1. The recommendations outlined in *Present day practice in infant feeding* (DHSS 1988 revision) and *Artificial feeds for young infants* (DHSS 1980) should be used as the basis of nutrition during the first year
2. Energy requirements which depend on age, sex and physical activity must be met for each individual child in order to obtain optimal growth
3. Once solids have been introduced and the child is on a mixed diet, milk, lean meat, poultry, fish, eggs, cheese, fruit, vegetables, bread and cereals (preferably of the wholegrain types) should form the major dietary sources of nutrients and energy
4. Changes should not be made in a young child's (i.e. age 1–5) diet which might compromise energy intake and optimal growth
5. A diet emphasizing basic whole foods, such as in Recommendation 3, is bulkier than a diet high in refined foods. Thus young children frequently need between-meal snacks in order to obtain sufficient energy intake
6. Overweight should be avoided by controlling weight gain, if excessive after the first six months of life, especially in children at greatest risk of overweight
7. The needs of each individual, the psychosocial aspects of eating and the effects of income must be considered
8. Extremes of dietary practices of any kind should be avoided

3.5.2 Dietary habits of children of school-age

In 1983, the DHSS commissioned a survey to look at the diets of British schoolchildren, partly to assess the nutritional effects of changes in schools meals provision

Table 3.18 A summary of Dietary Reference Values for children of school-age (DoH 1991)

	Energy Estimated Average Requirement (EAR)		Protein	Calcium Reference Nutrient Intake (RNI)	Iron
	MJ/day	kcal/day	g/day	mg/day	mg/day
4–6 years					
Males	7.16	(1715)	19.7	450	6.1
Females	6.46	(1545)	19.7	450	6.1
7–10 years					
Males	8.24	(1970)	28.3	550	8.7
Females	7.28	(1740)	28.3	550	8.7
11–14 years					
Males	9.27	(2200)	42.1	1000	11.3
Females	7.92	(1845)	41.2	800	14.8

engendered by the 1980 Education Act. The heights, weights and seven-day weighed dietary intakes of 3296 children were recorded along with other relevant information such as age, sex, socioeconomic status, cultural group and family size (DoH 1989). The intake of some foods and nutrients in relation to the 1979 RDAs are shown in Table 3.20. Although average intakes of many nutrients were above the RDAs, a high percentage of children did not achieve the targets set for nutrients such as iron, calcium and vitamin A. Since the DRVs (published since the completion of this survey) have set higher recommended intakes for some nutrients, as even greater proportion of children may be considered to be at risk.

Of greatest concern was the dietary composition of girls aged between 14–15 years. Mean intakes of calcium and iron were well below the RDA; 60% of the girls did not achieve the recent RNIs of 800 mg calcium and 14.8 mg iron.

Average intakes of ascorbic acid in all groups were above the new DRVs of 30–35 mg. However it is worth noting that chips provided 25% of this total.

Bread and breakfast cereals were major contributors to iron intake providing up 26% of the total intake; meat and meat products contributed a maximum of 13% of iron intake. Again, chips provided a significant amount (8%).

These unlikely sources of nutrients should be considered when designing healthy eating advice for school-aged children. If chips form a substantial part of the daily diet, then advice that they should be eaten less often should also be accompanied by suggested alternative sources of nutrients such as ascorbic acid and iron which may otherwise be lost from the diet.

3.5.3 Healthy eating and the school-age child

The general principles of a healthy diet (see Section 1.1) apply to healthy school-age children. However, the child's eating patterns and taste preferences will have been established by the family eating habits in the pre-school years. Any poor eating patterns acquired during these years will be changed only with difficulty. The child likes familiar foods and concepts of long-term health carry no weight at all.

Table 3.20 Summary of findings from *The diets of british schoolchildren* (DoH 1989)

Nutrient	Major sources of nutrients	% Nutrient provided	% Children below RDA		Average daily intakes	RDA (DHSS 1979)	DRV (DoH 1991)
Energy (kcal)	Bread	9–11%	Boys 10–11 y	10% all ages	1510	2270	1970
	Chips	8–11%	Boys 14–15 y	(but heights and	2300	2748	2220+
	Biscuits, cakes, puddings	14–17%	Girls 10–11 y	weights were	1610	2031	1740
	Milk	6–8%	Girls 14–15 y	acceptable)	1740	2151	1845+
Fat (g)	Milk	9–12%	Boys 10–11 y	22%[1]	37	Below 35% fat	
	Chips	8–11%	Boys 14–15 y	24%[1]	37	calories	
	Butter	5–7%	Girls 10–11 y	20%[1]	37		
	Crisps	4–7%	Girls 14–15 y	18%[1]	38		
	Meat products	7–9%					
	Carcase meat	6–7%					
Vitamin C (mg)	All potatoes	31–35%	Boys 10–11 y	26%	49	25	30
	Chips	16–25%	Boys 14–15 y	22%	42	25	30
	All fruit and vegetables	35–46%	Girls 10–11 y	31%	49	25	35
	Fruit juice	8–15%	Girls 14–15 y	24%	48	25	35
Iron (mg)	Bread and Cereals	21–26%	Boys 10–11 y	81%	10	12	8.7
	Chips	6–8%	Boys 14–15 y	43%	12.2	12	11.3
	Total meat	12–13%	Girls 10–11 y	95%	8.6	12	8.7
	Carcase meat	6%	Girls 14–15 y	87%	9.3	12	14.8
Calcium (mg)	Milk	30–37%	Boys 10–11 y	33%	833	600–700	550
	Bread	11–14%	Boys 14–15 y	25%	925	600–700	1000
	Cheese	8–10%	Girls 10–11 y	33%	702	600–700	550
			Girls 14–15 y	53%	692	600–700	800
Vitamin A (μg)	Carrots	16–19%	Boys 10–11 y	54%	854	575	500
	Milk	10–12%	Boys 14–15 y	46%	653	725	600
	Cheese	5–7%	Girls 10–11 y	64%	482	575	500
	Butter/margarine	11–14%	Girls 14–15 y	61%	496	725	600
	Vegetables	6–8%					

[1] Unlike other nutrients, a high percentage of people with a consumption level below the RDA is to be welcomed

Data reproduced with the permission of the Controller of Her Majesty's Stationery Office

Because of children's ability to forage for themselves, the possible freedom to choose food at school solely according to their own preferences and, in some households where both parents work, the necessity of getting their own food after school, some children may end up with particularly poor eating habits.

At school, education in healthy eating will be built in to the curriculum. However, children may not see this education as relevant to themselves if home eating patterns are very different, and if school meals run counter to the teaching. Programmes to improve the diet of school children need to be directed at the school meals and tuck shop provision, and to the parent (perhaps through parent/teacher associations) as well as to the child. Messages will be reinforced if nutrition topics can also be included in the general curriculum – for example, study of food plants in biology, trade in food in geography or economics.

3.5.4 Food and nutrition and the National Curriculum

The National Curriculum, which is being introduced progressively into schools in England and Wales for all pupils aged 5–16 years, has ten statutory foundation subjects, three of which are described as core subjects (Table 3.21). All pupils are at school for eleven years and these years are divided into four key stages. At each key stage in each subject pupils are expected to attain a certain educational level (Table 3.22). Each subject is divided into attainment targets with associated programmes of study. These describe different aspects of the subject. The attainment targets for science and technology are described in Table 3.23.

Food and nutrition were traditionally taught in home economics but this is not a foundation subject. However there are opportunities for food and nutrition education in the National Curriculum, especially in science and technology (Table 3.24); (DES/Welsh Office 1990; 1991).

Health education is identified as one of the cross-curricular themes which are considered essential parts of the whole curriculum. One of the components of a health education curriculum is food and nutrition. Appropriate areas of study in food and nutrition have been described for the four key stages. A policy encompassing the whole school is recommended to avoid conflicting messages from the classroom, school meals and tuck shops (National Curriculum Council 1990a; 1990b). However, because health education is non-statutory, there is a very real danger in a crowded school timetable that the subject will be marginalized.

The aim of food and nutrition education is to help pupils acquire the ability to make informed choices about food in line with current recommendations. In order to do this they need to:

1 Understand the relationship between diet and health and the nutritional quality of different foods.
2 Develop skills in terms of food preparation including food safety.
3 Understand the factors affecting food choice.
4 Develop decision-making skills.

There is then a need to 'marry' the non-statutory opportunities for food and nutrition education in health education with the statutory opportunities in the National Curriculum subjects science and technology.

Combining these opportunities needs careful planning to ensure that all pupils have equality of access to a syllabus which achieves coherence, continuity and progression, avoids omission and eliminates unnecessary duplication – especially as pupils progress from primary to secondary schools. In this context, school health education co-ordinators and home economics teachers have a key role to play. Dietitians have a responsibility to translate their expertise in a way which is user-friendly for teachers.

Table 3.21 National Curriculum foundation subjects

Core subjects	English Mathematics Science
Other foundation subjects	Art Geography History Modern foreign language Music Physical education Technology (including design)

Table 3.22 National Curriculum key stages

Key stage 1	5–7 year olds Years 1 and 2 Levels 1–3
Key stage 2	7–11 year olds Years 3, 4, 5, 6 Levels 2–5
Key stage 3	11–14 year olds Years 7, 8, 9 Levels 3–7
Key stage 4	14–16 year olds Years 10, 11 Levels 4–10

Table 3.23 National Curriculum attainment targets (ATs)

Science		Technology	
AT 1	Scientific investigation	AT 1	Identifying needs and opportunities
AT 2	Life and living processes	AT 2	Generating a design
AT 3	Materials and their properties	AT 3	Planning and making
AT 4	Physical processes	AT 4	Evaluating

Table 3.24 National Curriculum: examples of opportunities for food and nutrition education

Science	*Statements of attainment*
	AT 2 LIFE AND LIVING PROCESSES
	Level 2 Know that plants and animals need certain conditions to sustain life
	Level 3 Know the basic life processes common to humans and other animals
	Level 4 Understand food chains as a way of representing feeding relationships in an ecosystem
	Level 7 Understand the life processes of nutrition in animals
Technology	At each key stage pupils should be given opportunities to work with a range of materials including food
	Examples of statements of attainment
	AT 1 IDENTIFYING NEEDS AND OPPORTUNITIES
	Level 2 Find out how the school cook chooses the menus for school dinners
	Level 5 Use information from questionnaires and books to compile a database on adults' eating habits to consider ways of encouraging healthy eating
	AT 2 GENERATING A DESIGN
	Level 3 Gather information on different types of ethnic food and people's preferences when planning a party
	AT 3 PLANNING AND MAKING
	Level 5 Use knowledge and understanding of the properties of e.g. a bread dough which determine how it is cut and manipulated
	AT 4 EVALUATING
	Level 4 Understand how convenience foods have allowed altered lifestyles

This must take account of the requirements of the National Curriculum and the constraints and pressures which teachers face in their working situations.

A well-planned food and nutrition project may fulfil the requirements of not only parts of science and technology but also other National Curriculum subjects. Food and nutrition teaching packs are increasingly available with examples of how to do this (for example Wessex RHA 1990; BNF/MAFF 1991).

3.5.5 School meals

The 1980 Education Act which became law in April 1980 made major changes in the laws governing the provision of school meals. It removed the statutory obligations of local education authorities to provide meals of a certain nutritional standard at a fixed price in maintained schools. Prior to 1980, a school meal was expected to provide one-third of the child's daily requirements of protein, energy and some vitamins and minerals. The 1980 Act simply requires local education authorities to provide a meal for children in receipt of free school meals and to provide a place for children to eat sandwiches brought to school. Local education authorities therefore do not have to provide meals at all (except for free school meal recipients) and can charge whatever price they feel appropriate.

These changes were introduced by the government in an attempt to curtail the growth in public expenditure. This was to be achieved by a reduction in the working hours of the catering staff. Hours are worked out on the basis of the number of meals to be provided and divided between cooks and kitchen assistants. This in turn led to the need to make savings in preparation and cooking time which resulted in more convenience foods being used. It was also believed that, by offering foods popular with children, a good cash return could be guaranteed.

The rules governing the provision of free school meals have also been altered so that local education authorities need only provide free meals to children from families in receipt of family income supplement and supplementary benefit – it has been suggested that this has resulted in up to 30% of children losing their entitlement. Changes in the system of benefits made in April 1988 resulted in some children's entitlement to free school meals being replaced by direct cash payments to the family (which may or may not be spent on food.)

There are several nutritional consequences of these changes:

1 There is potential for a greater variety of foods to be offered thereby increasing the acceptability of school meals. However it is important that

- A wide choice of food is offered;
- 'Healthy' alternatives are included;
- Children are guided in their choice of food.

2 Now that local education authorities are released from their statutory duties to provide a meal of certain nutritional standard there is no guarantee that children will receive an adequate meal.
3 School meals were always seen in the past as being good tools for nutrition education; in many cases they are now in direct conflict with current nutritional recommendations.
4 The new menus can result in high intakes of fat and sugar and low intakes of fibre and vitamins.
5 Children may choose to spend dinner money on items other than food.
6 A number of children may now be nutritionally at risk, in particular:

- Those who used to receive free school meals but no longer do so;
- Those who receive free school meals and who make inappropriate choices;
- Those whose parents rely on school meals to provide the main meal of the day;
- Those who spend dinner money out of school on sweets or other items;
- Those who opt to take a packed lunch of an inappropriate content.

It must be remembered that school meals only provide five out of 21 meals per week in term time – parents are responsible for the rest. The midday meal is not just a stop-gap between breakfast and the evening meal. For many children, lunch is their first meal of the day as breakfast is often omitted. It is vital therefore that the midday meal is nutritionally adequate and, if it is not, this factor must be considered when other meals are being planned.

Types of school meals

These vary according to the type of school and the local education authority (Table 3.25). Prices also vary depending on the system and the local education authority.

Table 3.25 School meal services in common use

Primary schools cafeteria service	No choice or sometimes a choice from two items. Price fixed for meal; there is an upper limit of what the child can spend. Choice may be guided by a 'unit choice' system which gives a limited amount of guidance.
Middle schools cash-cafeteria system	A wider choice of foods is available. Items are individually priced. There may be some guidance in choice.
Secondary schools cash-cafeteria system	Many foods are available. The variety in nutritional terms depends on the caterer. Items are individually priced. Children may spend as much as they wish. Choice generally not guided

Guidance with food choice

'Unit choice' system

This is designed to help children choose a balanced meal and is often used in primary schools. Pupils are allowed to choose a maximum of five units for each meal in the following way: protein part of meal = 0 units and *must* be included; other items of the meal carry either 1 or 2 units depending on the nutritional desirability of the food, e.g.

Chips	2 units
Jacket potato	1 unit
Steamed jam pudding	2 units
Fresh fruit	1 unit

By allotting the least units to the most healthy foods, children are, in theory, tempted to choose these items because they can have more of them. The system does not guarantee a healthy choice but it does at least encourage healthy eating.

Colour-coded menus

This is another system which can guide food choice. It is based on one of two ideas:

Food groups Each of the four basic food groups (milk, meat, fruit and bread) is assigned a colour and items on the menu are colour-coded according to which group they belong to. Pupils are encouraged to choose at least three different colours. An example of this system is shown in Table 3.26.

Traffic light system The NACNE recommendations can be reflected by a system using traffic light colours or similar symbols. No food is labelled as 'bad', instead:
1 Foods high in fat, sugar and salt are coded as RED 'Stop and think' foods, i.e. items in the diet which should be reduced.
2 Foods high in fibre are coded GREEN 'go' foods, i.e. foods which should be encouraged and which should be eaten to replace foods for the red group.
3 All other foods are coded AMBER 'go carefully' foods, i.e. items which should be eaten in moderation.

Pupils are encouraged to choose their lunch mainly from the green and amber groups, and to limit the number of items chosen from the red group. On the menu board and/or the service counter, foods are coded with red, amber or green labels to help pupils select their lunch wisely.

Table 3.26 Example of a colour-coded menu system to guide food choice

Food groups used	Dairy = Blue Meat/fish/pulses = Red Fruit/vegetables = Green Cereal/potato = Orange
Food choice	Pupils are encouraged to choose a meal comprised of at least three different colours
Menu available	Soup and roll = Orange Beefburger = Red Fish finger = Red Peas = Green/red Salad = Green Jacket potato = Orange Bread roll = Orange Fresh fruit = Green Apple pie = Orange/green Yoghurt = Blue Fruit juice = Green Milk = Blue
Possible meal chosen	Beefburger = Red Jacket potato = Orange Salad = Green Yoghurt = Blue

Problems remaining with the school meals service

Lack of suitable foods

The composition of a protein dish may result in the child selecting a nutritionally inadequate meal.

Lack of guidance in food choice

More help needs to be given to pupils to help them identify the content of a meal. School meals supervisors need to be better informed on nutritional matters so that they can also offer guidance on food choice.

Lack of parental awareness

Parents should know:
1 The types of food offered to their children.
2 Which nutrients are lacking in the school meals.
3 Which foods should be included at home.
4 Which foods to provide for packed lunches.

Inadequate time and choice available

This is a particular problem for young children, especially those who are slow eaters. Also, if a child has to queue for a long time to obtain his or her meal, there may be little time left in which to eat it. The choice may also be limited for the children who are last in the queue.

Lack of suitable meals for minority groups

Minority groups, such as Asian children, may not be well catered for. Many authorities are, however, reviewing their policies in order to provide more suitable foods for these groups. More liaison is also required with the Asian community to remove suspicion of the meals.

3.5.6 Nutritional problems in the school-age child

Undernutrition

This is generally characterized by poor growth rates which can be demonstrated by plotting a child's height and weight on percentile charts (see Appendix 3). However it should not be assumed that maximal growth rates can be equated with optimal nutritional status; other factors besides nutritional intake (e.g. genetics) affect weight.

In order to obtain an adequate nutritional intake, children need to consume a wide variety of foods. This is not always easy to achieve in practice since children are naturally conservative. However, they are also imitators and will tend to adopt the family's eating patterns and likes or dislikes. It is therefore important that the whole family has sensible eating habits; for example, one cannot expect children to eat breakfast if their parents do not.

Various tactics can be employed to encourage the poor eater:

1 Anticipating trouble before a meal is served; new or unfamiliar foods should be produced without comment.

2 Serving food in different and novel ways may help a child to eat and enjoy otherwide unpopular food – for example:

- Vegetables can be served raw and attractively arranged rather than always cooked, e.g. a cartwheel presentation of raw sticks of carrot, celery and cucumber with nuts, fruit and raisins;
- Meat can be minced and formed into sausage or beefburgers;
- Liver can be made into liver paté or sausage.

3 Allowing children to serve themselves often encourages them to try different foods.

4 Not allowing children in a 'bad mood' to get the better of a parent – an untouched plate should simply be removed and no other food (especially not biscuits or sweets) offered until the next meal time.

5 Unfamiliar foods which are rejected when first offered can be left for a few weeks and then offered again, maybe in a different form, but without comment.

6 Eating out or with friends at home often helps a fussy child to eat better.

Obesity (see Section 4.17.2)

The prevalence of obesity in childhood is hard to assess but it somewhere between 5–15%. Obesity in children is usually obvious but can be confirmed by measurement of skinfold thickness and by plotting height and weight on percentile charts.

Overweight children, in contrast to overweight adults, tend to be taller than average due to advanced bone ages and this reflects their generally increased growth rates, both upwards and outwards. The aetiology and treatment of obesity in children is discussed in Section 4.17.2.

Rickets (see Section 4.27)

Nowadays, rickets tends to be found mainly in Asian families, but can also occur following growth spurts in borderline vitamin D deficient white British children.

Anaemia (see Section 2.8.2 'Iron' and Section 4.26.1 'Anaemia')

This may be a problem amongst children from low income families or where a poor diet is eaten. Furthermore, iron-rich foods (e.g. liver and red meats) are not always popular with children, and some children eat few green vegetables or fresh fruit, resulting in low vitamin C intakes and poor iron absorption.

Anaemia may also be due to low folic acid intakes as a result of low intakes of liver, fruit and vegetables or wholegrain cereals.

With a little ingenuity, alternative ways of providing these nutrients can usually be found. Unpopular foods can sometimes be disguised or presented in a way which is more acceptable, for example liver turned into a paté or red meat transformed into a hamburger.

Poor meal habits

Omission of meals, notably breakfast, is likely to result in reduced nutrient intakes.

Lunch among many school children may be inadequate due to poor choice of foods or a lack of guidance and supervision. Sometimes, money for school lunches is spent on non-food items. Packed lunches may be inadequate in nutritional composition. These problems are compounded if parents are unaware that the child's lunch is inadequate and that a nutritionally adequate meal is required later at home.

Frequent consumption of snacks may also result in a reduced appetite at meal times with a consequent poor nutrient intake.

Dental disease

Causation, treatment and prevention of dental disease are discussed in Section 4.1.1.

Diet-linked behavioural problems

Hyperkinesis

Many different terms are used in the literature for this condition. Hyperkinesis or the 'hyperactive child syndrome' has also been referred to as hypersensitivity, overactivity, hyperactive change syndrome, attention deficit disorder, minimal brain damage, minimal brain dysfunction and learning disorders.

The symptoms as described in the *British Medical Journal* (1975) are 'a chronic sustained level of motor activity relative to the age of the child, occurring mainly in boys between one and 16 years, but characteristically around six years, accompanied by short attention span, impulsive behaviour or explosive outbursts and causing substantial complaints at home or in school'.

Other symptoms include social, learning and behavioural problems, thirst, anxiety, aggression, poor eating and sleeping habits and temper tantrums.

Some hyperactive children may suffer from headaches, catarrh, asthma and hayfever. A few have a low IQ, but this is not a general feature. The causes of hyperactivity are unknown but several factors are suggested to have an influence, (e.g. food allergies, parental attitudes, smoking in pregnancy and genetic factors).

The incidence of hyperactivity has been suggested to range from 1–5% but the most suitable diagnostic criteria for this condition have yet to be established (MacGibbon 1983). Nevertheless, 'hyperactivity' is, unfortunately, an increasingly popular 'diagnosis' among the lay public. Often the problem is simply one of difficult family relationships which express themselves in a child's antisocial behaviour. The problem can also be exacerbated by parental worry over dietary habits or by children themselves, exploiting the situation to their own advantage.

Treatment of the condition where a true diagnosis is made is by drugs, diet or behaviour therapy and very often a combination of all three.

The use of the Feingold (1975) diet has been extensively encouraged by many lay organizations. The basis of Feingold's dietary modification is the avoidance of naturally occurring salicylates and the avoidance of food and drink containing additives and colouring. Scientists and nutritionists have remained equivocal about the benefits of this diet as it has little hard evidence to support it. However, a number of studies have lent support to the theory that some children are sensitive to some food additives and, in these cases, removal of the offending substances can produce dramatic improvements in behaviour and other symptoms, particularly asthma and severe headaches (Freedman 1977; Weiss *et al* 1980; Egger *et al* 1985) (see also Section 2.16.2).

In many cases of hyperactivity it may be beneficial to give the child a diet free from food additives and colourings for one month to see whether any improvement occurs. If it does, further tests can then be carried out to identify the additive components responsible. However, it should not be forgotten that the extra attention given to the child as a result of the effort involved in providing an additive-free diet may in itself cause an improvement in behaviour. If no improvement occurs, the parents can then be assured that the problem is not a dietary one and thereby one element of worry is removed. This may help to improve relations with the child leading to a general improvement.

In addition to the possible effects of food additives, other causative theories put forward in recent years include a link with essential fatty acid metabolism, abnormality of carbohydrate metabolism and effects of other food allergies. However, as with any behavioural disorder where the benefits of treatment can only be evaluated subjectively, and therefore carry an inherent risk of bias, proof is difficult to obtain.

Some parents with a disruptive or 'difficult' child may be tempted to try out Feingold-type diets as a result of reading a popular newspaper or magazine article or seeing a television programme, and without any medical or dietary supervision. As such diets can be very restricted, there is a real danger of nutritional inadequacy in growing children, particularly among children from families who use large amounts of processed and packaged foods or if the dietary measures are imposed for a long period of time.

Advice from a qualified dietitian is essential before any child is placed on a diet of this type. Unfortunately, dietitians are not allowed, at present, to give advice of this nature unless it is accompanied by a medical referral and this may well not be forthcoming. Liaison with the family's health visitor can sometimes resolve this very difficult problem. If parents are determined to embark on dietary experimentation in their children without medical approval, then perhaps they can be persuaded to keep it of short duration so that nutritional damage is kept to a minimum.

Vitamins supplements and IQ

See Section 2.6.4.

References

British Dietetic Association (1987) *Children's diets and change.* Report of the Child Health and Nutrition Working Party. BDA, Birmingham.

British Medical Journal (1975) Hyperactivity in children (Editorial). *Br Med J* **4**, 123–4.

British Nutrition Foundation/Ministry of Agriculture, Fisheries and Food (1991) *Food – a fact of life. The Food and Nutrition Programme.* BNF, Birmingham.

Department of Education and Science/Welsh Office (1990) *Technology in the National Curriculum.* HMSO, London.

Department of Education and Science/Welsh Office (1991) *Science in the National Curriculum.* HMSO, London.

Department of Health (1989) *The Diets of British Schoolchildren.* Rep Hlth Soc Subj 36. HMSO, London.

Department of Health (1991) *Dietary Reference Values for food energy and nutrients for the United Kingdom.* Rep Hlth Soc Subj 41. HMSO, London.

Department of Health and Social Security (1979) *Recommended Daily Amounts of food, energy and nutrients for groups of people in the United Kingdom.* Rep Hlth Soc Subj 15. HMSO, London.

Department of Health and Social Security (1980) *Artificial feeds for young infants.* Rep Hlth Soc Subj 18. HMSO, London.

Department of Health and Social Security (1988) *Present day practice in infant feeding.* Rep Hlth Soc Subj 32. HMSO, London.

Education Act (1980) Section 22. School Meals: England and Wales.

Education Act (1980) Section 23. School Meals: Scotland.

Egger J, Carter CM, Graham PJ, Gumley D and Soothill JF (1985) Controlled trial of oligoantigenic treatment in the hyperkinetic syndrome. *Lancet* **i**, 540–45.

Feingold B (1975) *Why your child is hyperactive.* Random House Inc, New York.

Freedman BJ (1977) Asthma induced by sulphur dioxide, benzoate and tartrazine contained in orange drinks. *Clin Allergy* **7**, 407–15.

MacGibbon B (1983) Adverse reactions to food additives. *Proc Nutr Soc* **42**, 223–40.

National Curriculum Council (1990a) *Curriculum Guidance 3. The whole curriculum.* National Curriculum Council, York.

National Curriculum Council (1990b) *Curriculum Guidance 5. Health education.* National Curriculum Council, York.

National Dairy Council (1991) *How do mothers feed their children?* Nutrition Services, NDC.

Weiss B, Williams JH, Margen S, Abrams B, Caan B, Citron LJ, Cox C, McKiben J, Ogar D and Schultz S (1980) Behavioural response to artificial food colours. *Science* **207**, 1487–9.

Wessex Regional Health Authority (1990) *Hampshire's nutrition activity pack for primary schools.* Wessex RHA, Winchester.

3.6 Adolescents

Adolescence is a time of change to adult behaviour. It is therefore an important time for health and nutrition education. However, as part of this process of change, some or even all advice is likely to be ignored, at least on a temporary basis, and experimentation with new foods, new drinks, including alcohol, new tastes and new eating patterns generally will be the norm.

Teenagers have a profound wish to exert their independence and make their own decisions and food choice is likely to be one of the first targets. There is also a need to conform within the peer group. Smoking, which is at a significant level in this age group, also affects nutritional status. Tact, patience and understanding are required in large measures both by parents and by professional advisers to steer the adolescent towards sensible healthy eating and away from extreme diets with potentially harmful consequences.

3.6.1 Nutritional requirements of adolescents

Table 3.27 details requirements for major nutrients in this age group. The demands for nutrients are relatively high, and differ between boys and girls, boys having a greater need because of their greater adolescent growth spurt. Many boys become very thin during this period, prior to muscular development later in their teens. Eating disorders, predominantly but not exclusively in females, have many impacts, for example on weight, general health and iron status.

Energy

Estimated Average Requirements (EAR) for energy are given in Table 3.27. The limited data on energy expenditure as measured by doubly-labelled water are higher than these figures (Bandini *et al* 1990; Davies *et al* 1991). High energy expenditures are also found in young adult men (Roberts *et al* 1991). While there is concern over the increasing number of overweight children – presumably due to excessive energy intakes, it must not be forgotten that many have genuinely high energy requirements. Adolescent boys may be consuming 3000–4000 kcal (14.2–16.8 MJ) per day and are often described by mothers as having 'hollow legs'. The frequent consumption of snack foods in addition to substantial meals is not necessarily of nutritional concern; for some it is the only way to obtain sufficient energy. Strict adherence to low-fat, high-fibre foods may lead to a diet which is both excessively bulky and unacceptable to adolescent lifestyle.

Table 3.27 Dietary Reference Values for Adolescents (DoH 1991)

	Males		Females	
	11–14 yrs	15–18 yrs	11–14 yrs	15–18 yrs
EAR Energy kcal/d	2200	2755	1845	2110
RNI Protein g/d	42.1	55.2	41.2	45.4
RNI Calcium mg/d	1000	1000	800	800
RNI Iron mg/d	11.3	11.3	14.8	14.8

Iron

Iron requirements are increased in girls with the onset of menstruation. Iron deficiency anaemia is not uncommon in girls in this age group and is quite likely in teenagers who become pregnant. Good dietary sources of iron (e.g. haem iron in red meat) may be disliked or avoided and achieving adequate iron intake can be difficult.

Calcium

The rapid increase in bone mass during the adolescent growth spurt creates a great demand for calcium. Work on osteoporosis in later life has indicated that peak bone mass is the best predictor of bone status in later life (Wolfe and Dixon 1988).

Meeting calcium requirements is relatively easy in adolescents who like and take milk and dairy products daily, but is much harder to achieve in those who avoid or dislike these foods. Absorption of calcium is more efficient during adolescence, rising to 40–45% (compared with about 30% in normal adults) and this may partly compensate for a low calcium content of the diet.

Other minerals and vitamins

Evidence on actual requirements by adolescents for many micronutrients is not available. Use of vitamin and mineral supplements may be common and some companies target this age group in their marketing.

3.6.2 Eating habits of adolescents

Much concern is shown over the possible poor eating habits of adolescents. There is a common belief that they exist solely on junk foods. However, dietary studies show that this is not so. Surveys by the Department of Health (1989) on 14–15 year olds, Bull (1985) on 15–25 year olds and Barker *et al* (1988) show that a wide variety of foods is eaten. Robson *et al* (1992), using a diet history technique, and Cresswell *et al* (1983), using 24-hour recall, both report that children do eat three meals a day. Food eaten in the morning, midday and in the evening is perceived and described as breakfast, lunch and tea or dinner, whether a cooked meal or not a cooked meal. Approximately one third of energy comes from each of the two main meals and one third from snacks or from breakfast plus snacks (Nelson 1983; Robson *et al* 1992).

Nevertheless, it is clear that snack foods are eaten frequently. Individuals in the age group 16–25 years' are more likely to have an eating pattern based on convenience foods such as chips, sauces, soft drinks, nuts, cheese, rice and pasta, savoury pies and cooked meat dishes' than are older adults (Barker *et al* 1990), while 58% of 15–25 year olds eat breakfast daily, 18% never eat breakfast, 33% eat a cooked lunch and 78% a cooked evening meal (Bull 1985). Some favoured snack foods, defined as foods eaten on occasions other than breakfast, lunch and the evening meal, are identified in Tables 3.28 and 3.29.

Snack foods are not necessarily 'junk' foods. While Robson *et al* (1992) reported 31 and 33% of energy derived from snacks, these also contributed between 23 and 33% of iron, calcium, vitamin C, thiamin and riboflavin.

There is no data on the actual frequency of snacking among adolescents. In 11–12 year olds, Rugg-Gunn *et al* (1984) found a mean frequency of 6.8 eating occasions per day, with 95% confidence limits of 4.3–11.7.

Concern is sometimes also expressed over the 'increase' in consumption of junk food and snacking. Comparison of the 1983 survey of British 14–15 years olds (DoH 1989) with the DHSS survey of 14–15 year olds in Birmingham in 1970–71 (Darke *et al* 1980), provides no evidence for a general decline in nutritional quality of the diet of this age group. Reported energy intakes are virtually identical – 10.16 and 7.88 MJ in 1970 and 10.23 and 7.88 MJ in 1983 for boys and girls respectively. Micronutrient intakes per MJ in 1983 were identical or slightly higher than in 1970.

Table 3.28 Snack foods reported by 270 14–16 year old Scottish school girls in a 24-hour recall (Cresswell *et al* 1983)

Snacks	% reporting
Crisps or similar savoury snack	56
Soft drinks	50
Chocolate confectionery	39
Sweets or lollies	31
Chewing gum	15
Ice cream	7
Cakes	6
Biscuits	2
Fresh fruit	<1

Table 3.29 Total number of portions of snack foods eaten by 84 children aged 3–18 years in a 7-day survey, Belfast, 1989 (Livingstone, personal communication)

Snack food	Number of portions
Fruit	205
Confectionery	191
All biscuits	173
Soft drinks	120
Milk	98
Crisps	71
Cakes	45
Bread	45
Butter/margarine	59
Jam/honey	33
Cheese	27
Meat	26
Vegetables	21
Ice cream	26
Breakfast cereals	24
Pudding	11
Tea/coffee	37
Sugar	14
Powder drinks	9

3.6.3 Nutrient intakes of adolescents

There have been four major dietary surveys in the UK and Ireland which have included adolescents (Barker *et al* 1988; Bull 1988; DoH 1989; Lee and Cunningham 1990). All four surveys provide much detailed information on the nutrient intakes, foods consumed and eating habits according to a variety of social and demographic variables.

Figures for nutrient intakes must be interpreted with caution, since Livingstone *et al* (1991; 1992) found that adolescents may under-report their food intake by weighed record, while intakes estimated by diet history appear to provide a better measure of mean intake although poor measures of individual intakes. Under-estimation of energy intake (i.e. total food intake), is likely to carry also under-estimation of micronutrient intakes. The reported energy intakes (EI) are shown in Table 3.30. This shows the higher intakes as obtained by diet history whether expressed as absolute amounts or multiples of the estimated BMR for the group studied. An EI/BMR of 1.7 is in line with the values for total energy expenditure found by Davies *et al* (1991).

Low energy and nutrient intakes have been found in girls who perceived themselves as overweight or claimed to be dieting or claimed to always watch their diet (Bull 1988); 35% of girls considered themselves to be overweight. Overall, 5% claimed to be on a diet to lose weight,

Table 3.30 Reported energy intakes in four surveys of adolescents and young adults (MJ per day, mean ± sd)

Survey	Age, yrs	Males	EI/BMR	Females	EI/BMR	Method
(Lee and Cunningham 1990)	12–15	11.3 (3.3)	1.77	9.1 (3.0)	1.57	DH
(Lee and Cunningham 1990)	15–18	14.0 (4.5)	1.87	8.9 (2.5)	1.46	DH
(Lee and Cunningham 1990)	18–25	13.7 (4.5)	1.85	8.6 (3.7)	1.47	DH
Department of Health 1989)	14–15	10.4 (2.3)	—	7.9 (1.7)	—	7d WR
(Bull 1988)	15–18	10.1	—	7.8	—	14d Diary
(Bull 1988)	19–21	10.1	—	7.0	—	14d Diary
(Bull 1988)	22–25	10.3	—	7.7	—	14d Diary
(Barker *et al* 1988)	16–29	10.7 (2.53)	1.32	7.6 (1.85)	1.32	7d WR

WR = Weighed Record; DH = diet history; Diary = daily record using pre-printed lists of foods with quantities in household measures. EI = Energy intake; BMR = Basal Metabolic Rate

and 15 percent claimed to 'always watch what they eat'. In these groups, reported intakes of iron, energy, thiamin and riboflavin were below the RDA (DHSS 1979). The low reported intakes (6–7 MJ per day for energy) do not necessarily represent the long term 'habitual' intake of these individuals but must give cause for concern if they indicate actual or potential eating disorders.

The study by the Department of Health (1989) identified iron, riboflavin and calcium intakes as low in the girls. The poorest nutritional quality was found among girls who avoided school meals and ate out of school at places such as cafes, take-away or 'fast food' outlets. Scottish children were identified as having lower intakes of vitamin C, β-carotene and retinol equivalents than English children.

While the average nutrient intake of adolescents is satisfactory, individual children can have eating patterns which result in poor quality diets.

3.6.4 Nutritional problems in adolescents

Vegetarianism (see Section 3.10)

This is not in itself a problem and can be a healthy way of eating, but its adoption by teenagers frequently causes problems. Many try to follow vegetarian practices without any guidance and, while they are usually successful at omitting animal products, teenagers are usually not very adept at replacing them with appropriate vegetable ones. Deficiencies of iron, vitamin B_{12} and protein often result.

An additional problem is that parents may review their child's vegetarianism as an indication of juvenile delinquency or a desire to 'drop out'. They therefore exert parental pressure which inevitably causes friction and may lead to even more restrictive eating. If instead, parents offer the child support and help them obtain reliable information, the problem – if it is a problem – usually just fades away.

Slimming regimens

About half of the adolescent girls in Western society attempt at some time to lose weight. Some of the slimming methods adopted are very restrictive. The diet may be comprised of only two or three items (e.g. fruit and black coffee) which will obviously lead to nutrient deficiencies. Sometimes inappropriate foods are eaten in large quantities due to mistaken beliefs about their food value; cheese is a common example. Teenagers are also tempted to buy various slimming aids and gimmicks. Apart from being very expensive, many of these are undesirable in nutritional terms and are of no help in achieving long-term weight loss.

Sound advice on appropriate slimming methods is essential together with encouragement to take adequate exercise. When teenagers leave school, their activity level frequently decreases dramatically and consequently their weight may increase. Dietary advice must be practical to fit in with normal adolescent lifestyle otherwise it is only counter productive. Guidance is more appropriate than rigid rules.

Eating disorders (anorexia nervosa, bulimia nervosa) (see Section 4.24)

In this age group there is a particular risk that attempts to slim will lead to anorexia nervosa. If the slimming appears to be becoming an obsession and weight is falling rapidly, professional help should be sought quickly. This age group can also develop bulimia with a very different pattern of food abuse. Dietitians in some areas have become involved with these problems, usually as part of a multidisciplinary team.

Athletic training (see Section 3.13)

Many teenagers involved in extensive training schedules adopt bizarre eating patterns. Some consume high protein diets in a mistaken belief that this is essential for stamina. Others take high doses of vitamin and mineral supplements, a practice which should be strongly discouraged. Eating times are often limited due to training schedules and there is a temptation to use products such as complete-liquid diets; however these are expensive and inappropriate. Alternatively, quick snacks may replace proper meals and provide inadequate nutrition.

Advice needs to be given about healthy eating for these circumstances — large quantities of protein are not necessary and adequate minerals and vitamins can be obtained from dietary sources. A relatively high level of carbohydrate is essential to boost muscle glycogen stores, particularly before endurance tests. Adequate fluid intake is very important, both prior to and during sporting events. Rest days should be part of a training schedule in order to allow time to eat and replenish body stores.

Skin disorders

Acne vulgaris is common in teenagers and is often attributed to eating excess sweets, chocolates and fried foods but there is no evidence to support the view that dietary factors are responsible. However, since it is of general health benefit to consume less fat and sugar and more fibre rich foods and fluid, it is still valuable to encourage teenagers to modify their diet along these lines. The skin problem may be of sufficient concern to act as a motivating factor for dietary change.

Teenage pregnancy (see Section 3.1)

The number of teenage pregnancies is increasing and exists at a higher level in girls in care settings compared with girls in their own homes.

It is obvious that pregnancy makes considerable additional demands on a body which itself is not fully developed. Pregnant teenagers can be a difficult group to reach to provide relevant diet advice. Many may have considerable financial problems and the amount available for food may be limited. Knowledge of both food and food preparation may be poor and group sessions looking at practical aspects of food choice and use may be more useful than fact sheets on a healthy diet. Good food on a low income may be vital to the health of the teenage mother and the growing child in the months ahead.

3.6.5 Encouraging healthy eating in adolescents

Health professionals are concerned about the effects of diet in adolescents on longer term health (e.g. coronary heart disease). The concern also extends to other lifestyle factors such as smoking, alcohol, exercise. However, teenagers rarely take a long-term view and the use of threats of future poor health is unlikely to act as a motivator to diet or lifestyle change.

The National Curriculum (Key stages 3 and 4) offers opportunities to encourage this age group to learn about and become involved in choosing a healthy diet: Attainment Targets are listed in Table 3.31.

These targets can be explored in many curriculum areas, for example education for citizenship, environmental education, science and technology. Teachers will need up-to-date and relevant sources to support their teaching and community dietitians can be a valuable part of the expert resource.

Many youth groups have leaders who welcome support and visitors to the sessions they organize, especially prior to a camp or holiday when food is a topic of interest to everybody. These groups can be used successfully by community dietitians to look at food and health issues.

Table 3.31 National Curriculum food and nutrition attainment targets (ATs)

Key Stage 3	Know that individual health requires a varied diet Understand malnutrition and the relationships between diet, health, fitness and circulatory disorders Understand basic food microbiology, food production and processing techniques
Key Stage 4	To be able to analyse and evaluate diet and recognize suitable adjustments which take account of a range of factors such as the availability of food and social, cultural and financial influences Know that various types of diet promote health for different groups, acknowledging cultural and ethnic variations Understand consumer aspects of food hygiene, shopping for food, legislation, including the current food labelling system Understand the relationships between food, body image and self-esteem Have accurate information to enable them to distinguish between fact, propaganda and folklore in dietary matters

Further reading

Books

Winick M (1982) *Adolescent nutrition*. John Wiley, Chichester.

Williams SR, Worthington-Roberts BS (1988) *Nutrition throughout the life cycle*. Times Mirror/Mosby, London and St Louis.

Dietary studies

Bull NL (1988) Studies of the dietary habits, food consumption and nutrient intakes of adolescents and young adults. *Wld Rev Nutr Diet* **57**, 24–74.

Hackett AF, Rugg-Gunn AJ, Allinson M, Robinson CJ, Appleton DR and Eastoe JE (1984) The importance of fortification of flour with calcium and the sources of Ca in the diet of 375 English adolescents. *Br J Nutr* **51**, 193–7.

Hackett AF, Rugg-Gunn AJ, Appleton DR and Coombs A (1986) Dietary sources of energy, protein, fat and fibre in 375 English adolescents. *Hum Nutr: Appl Nutr* **40A**, 176–84.

Hackett AF, Rugg-Gunn AJ, Appleton DR, Eastoe JE and Jenkins GN (1984) A 2-year longitudinal nutritional survey of 405 Northumberland children initially aged 11.5 years. *Br J Nutr* **51**, 67–75.

Nelson M (1986) The distribution of nutrient intakes within families. *Br J Nutr* **55**, 267–77.

Nelson M, Barker DJP and Winter PD (1984) Dietary fibre and acute appendicitis: a case-controlled study. *Hum Nutr: Appl Nutr* **38A**, 126–131.

Nelson M and Paul AA (1983) The nutritive contribution of school dinners and other mid-day meals to the diets of schoolchildren. *Hum Nutr: Appl Nutr* **37A**, 128–35.

Rugg-Gunn AJ, Hackett AF, Appleton DR, Jenkins GN and Eastoe JE (1984) Relationship between dietary habits and caries increment assessed over two years in 405 English adolescent school children. *Arch Oral Biol* **29**, 983–92.

Rugg-Gunn AJ, Hackett AF, Appleton DR and Moynihan PJ (1986) The dietary intake of added and natural sugars in 405 English adolescents. *Hum Nutr: Appl Nutr* **40A**, 115–24.

Rugg-Gunn AJ, Hackett AF, Jenkins GN and Appleton DR (1990) Empty calories? Nutrient intake in relation to sugar intake in English adolescents. *J Hum Nutr Diet* **4**, 101–11.

Woodward DR (1984) Major influences on median energy and nutrient intakes among teenagers: a Tasmanian Survey. *Br J Nutr* **52**, 21–32.

Woodward DR (1985) What sort of teenager has high intakes of energy and nutrients? *Br J Nutr* **54**, 325–33.

Woodward DR (1985) What sort of teenager has low intakes of energy and nutrients? *Br J Nutr* **53**, 241–9.

Woodward DR, Lynch PP, Waters MJ, Maclean AR, Ruddock WE, Rataj JW and Lemoh JN (1981) Dietary studies on Tasmanian High School children: intakes of energy and nutrients. *Austral Paed J* **17**, 196–201.

References

Bandini LG, Schoeller DA, Cyr H and Dietz WH (1990) A validation of reported energy intake in obese and non-obese adolescents. *Am J Clin Nutr* **52**, 421–5.

Barker ME, McClean SI, McKenna PG, Reid NG, Strain JJ, Thompson KA, Williamson AP and Wright ME (1988) *Diet, lifestyle and health in Northern Ireland.* Centre for Applied Health Studies, University of Coleraine, Coleraine.

Barker ME, McClean SI, Thompson KA and Reid NG (1990) Dietary behaviours and sociological demographics in Northern Ireland. *Br J Nutr* **64**, 319–29.

Bull NL (1985) Dietary habits of 15 to 25-year-olds. *Hum Nutr: Appl Nutr* **39A**, (Suppl 1) 1–68.

Bull NL (1988) Studies of the dietary habits, food consumption and nutrient intakes of adolescents and young adults. *Wld Rev Nutr Diet* **57**, 24–74.

Cresswell J, Busby A, Young H and Inglis V (1983) Dietary patterns of third-year secondary schoolgirls in Glasgow. *Hum Nutr: Appl Nutr* **37A**, 301–306.

Darke SJ, Disselduff MM and Try GP (1980) Frequency distribution of mean daily intakes of food energy and selected nutrients obtained during nutrition surveys of different groups of people in Great Britain between 1968 and 1971. *Br J Nutr* **44**, 243–52.

Davies PSW, Prentice AM, Coward WA, Jagger SE, Stewart C, Strain JJ and Whitehead RG (1991) Total energy expenditure during childhood and adolescence. *Proc Nutr Soc* **50**, 14A.

Department of Health (1989) *The Diets of British Schoolchildren.* Rep Hlth Soc Subj 36. HMSO, London.

Department of Health (1991) *Dietary References Values for food energy and nutrients for the United Kingdom.* Rep Hlth Soc Subj 41. HMSO, London.

Department of Health and Social Security (1979) *Recommended Daily Amounts of food energy and nutrients for groups of people in the United Kingdom.* Rep Hlth Soc Subj 15. HMSO, London.

Lee P and Cunningham K (1990) *Irish National Nutrition Survey 1990.* Irish Nutrition and Dietetic Institute, Dublin.

Livingstone MBE, Davies PSW, Prentice AM, Coward WA, Black AE, Strain J and McKenna P (1991) Comparison of simultaneous measures of energy intake and expenditure in children and adolescents. *Proc Nutr Soc* **50**, 15A.

Livingstone MBE, Prentice AM, Coward WA, Strain JJ, Black AE, Davies PSW, Stewart CM, McKenna PG and Whitehead RG (1992) Validation of estimates of energy intake by weighed dietary record and diet history in children and adolescents. *Am J Clin Nutr* **56**, 29–35.

Nelson M (1983) A dietary survey method for measuring family food purchases and individual nutrient intakes concurrently, and its use in dietary surveillance. PhD Thesis, University of London.

Roberts SB, Heyman MB, Evans WJ, Fuss P, Tsay R and Young VR (1991) Dietary energy requirements of young adult men, determined by using the doubly labelled water method. *Am J Clin Nutr* **54**, 499–505.

Robson PG, Strain JJ, Cran GW, Savage JM, Primrose ED and Boreham CAG (1992) Snack energy and nutrient intakes of Northern Ireland adolescents. *Proc Nutr Soc* **50**, 180A.

Rugg-Gunn AJ, Hackett AF, Appleton DR, Jenkins GN and Eastoe JE (1984) Relationship between dietary habits and caries increment assessed over two years in 405 English adolescent school children. *Arch Oral Biol* **29**, 983–92.

Wolfe AD and Dixon ASJ (1988) *Osteoporosis: A clinical guide.* Martin Dunitz, London.

3.7 Elderly people

In the UK the term 'elderly' generally refers to persons of pensionable age, i.e. men of 65 years and over, women of 60 years and over. Life expectancy has continued to rise throughout this century and the newly retired can now look forward to some 20 years or more of life, a time when all will be keen to maintain their health and independence. One of the cornerstones for their future health will be the attention which is paid to diet.

In 1989 there were 10.5 million elderly in the UK, nearly 19% of the total population. During the last decade the number of pensioners below 75 decreased slightly, reflecting the casualties of the second world war and the small number of men born in the first world war who reached retirement. The population over 75 increased. The over 85s alone increased by 18% between 1986 and 1989. The projected increase for this upper age range is 63% by the turn of the century. At 85 years the ratio of women to men is 3:1 and at 80 years 2:1, at present (OPCS 1990).

There is evidence of a growing divide in health status and expectations between people in their 60s and 70s and the very elderly. GPs are giving an increasing amount of their time to elderly patients and now make a statutory annual health check on those over 75. The private nursing and residential home industry was one of Britain's most rapidly expanding industries in the 1980s. The number of residential places for over 75s increased from 88 to 112 per thousand between 1980 and 1988 (Bosanquet and Gray 1989).

It is the so-called 'frail elderly', those no longer active, who are most in need of carers to support them. The processes of biological ageing are incompletely understood but the consequences and effects of ageing are better documented. Geriatric medicine departments seek to maintain or restore functional abilities. Clinical standards are based upon maintenance of function, and changes in biochemistry are a better indicator of disease process than absolute standards which are set for a lower age range.

The closure of large residential hospitals consequent upon government policy to transfer funding for long-term care to local community services has resulted in a widely scattered population of frail elderly needing support in their own homes. This changing pattern of care is a challenge to geriatric nutrition and social workers who must develop wide ranging methods of monitoring and advice systems. It remains to be seen whether society can evolve ways to support further increases in the frail elderly population. If good nutrition can only be delivered to a limited number, the pace of increase will slow down below the projected rate. Community support and practical guidance are needed for all elderly persons to retain their independence for as long as possible.

It should be noted that, in European terms, 'elderly' is considered to be the 50-plus age bracket, so published research on 'elderly' populations should be interpreted with caution. The inter-group or intra-group variations may be so wide that it is inadvisable to make comparisons or draw conclusions. Research projects carried out on elderly people can also be impaired by the problem of finding suitably matched controls.

3.7.1 Principles of healthy eating for the elderly

Sound nutritional principles apply to all age groups but an over zealous attempt to apply present healthy eating guidelines to the elderly can result in a backlash of other problems – increased anxiety among elderly people over issues concerning diet, disinterest in food and inappropriate dietary restrictions.

Therefore, before expounding on the virtues of dietary change for older individuals several important points should be considered:

1 Dietary change is often equated to dietary restriction. For the elderly one of the greatest risks to health is to lose interest in food – neglect your diet: neglect your health. Imposing unrealistic rules or grading foods as 'good', 'bad' or 'forbidden' is counter-productive and not based on sound scientific principles. For the older person 'a little of what you fancy' really is beneficial if it stimulates an interest and pleasure in eating.

2 Some individuals may have seemingly small or poor intakes yet often there is adaptation to this level of nutrient intake. If such people are managing adequately, maintaining weight, retaining independence and unwilling to change, why should they? A 94 year old who enjoys a sugary cup of tea is, after all, 94.

3 Some changes may inadvertently be for the worst. For example, encouraging a reduction in total fat consumption unless carefully explained, may result in the omission of valuable foods from diet such as cheese or fatty fish. The former decision could affect total calcium intake, the latter omitting an excellent dietary source of vitamin D. Furthermore, trying to retard the development of atherosclerosis in the over-80s by reducing fat intake is inappropriate as any arterial damage will have already been done.

Care should therefore be taken not to discourage foods unless there is a special reason. Wherever possible, the *positive* aspects of nutrition should be stressed. It has been demonstrated that the elderly are not necessarily set in their ways (Bilderbeck *et al* 1981) and will try new foods. Dietary changes, when they occur, are often motivated by taste preference, ease of preparation or for purported 'health' reasons. It is this latter factor which can make elderly people vulnerable to cranky health messages and can tempt them to turn to expensive 'wonder' foods or supplements.

The overall message should be to keep up an interest in and enjoyment of food and be aware that nourishing foods are of prime importance to health. This can be a strong motivating force to encourage the preparation and cooking of simple, tasty, nutritious meals and snacks. A monotonous menu or a dependence on dried instant foods of the 'just-add-boiling-water' type should be discouraged. Pureed or liquid meals are a textural travesty to the palate and should be used only for short-term exceptional circumstances. Such regimens can lead rapidly to disinterest in food and the slippery slope to malnutrition.

Appropriate nutrition guidelines for the elderly are urgently needed. Some of the suggestions made in the COMA (DHSS 1984) and NACNE (1983) Reports are too restricting. These guidelines concentrate mainly on the excesses in the diet, whereas most of the problems confronting a dietitian dealing with the elderly will be related to loss of appetite. Deficiency states are more common than 'excess states' among the elderly.

3.7.2 General nutritional considerations

Nutrient intakes and Dietary Reference Values

Nutritional studies on different groups of elderly people in the UK have revealed that intakes of vitamin C, folate, riboflavin and other water soluble vitamins, vitamin D, iron, potassium and other trace elements and fibre are almost certainly lower than is desirable (DHSS 1972, 1979; Exton-Smith *et al* 1972, 1978; Vir and Love 1979; Davies 1981; Bunker and Clayton 1989).

The elderly, as a group, can therefore be considered to be especially at risk from deficiencies of these nutrients. However, caution must be exercised when comparing the intake of an individual or small group to a parameter such as the Reference Nutrient Intake (RNI) or Lower Reference Nutrient Intake (LRNI). There is a lack of data for deriving DRVs which are specific to elderly people. Because of the great diversity of this population group, it is wrong to assume that the distribution of nutrient requirements is symmetrical (as is assumed to be the case in the calculation of DRVs). In an elderly population the distribution may well be skewed. A low intake will not always be a deficient one owing to variations in individual requirements or adaptation. Conversely, some nutrient intakes may seem adequate when compared with RNIs but may, in fact, be inadequate for those individuals with extra requirements due to short-term trauma (e.g. following burns or surgery) or as a result of long-term changes (e.g. bone loss).

Individual intakes must therefore be considered in conjunction with other factors such as the general eating habits, health and activity of the person concerned.

Energy

The consumption of sufficient energy to maintain satisfactory body weight is important. It has been suggested that low weight may be a biological marker for persons more likely to end up in institutions (Morgan and Hullin 1982). A diet low in energy is also more likely to be deficient in other nutrients.

Vitamin D

Where sunlight exposure is poor, for example in the housebound or institutionalized, vitamin D status is also likely to be poor (Corless *et al* 1979; Sheltawy *et al* 1984; Dattani *et al* 1984). Elderly people should be encouraged to venture out of doors even if only to make use of a balcony. In the UK, the best time of day for sunlight exposure is between 11 AM and 4 PM during the months May–September. Those at retirement age have been found to have an excellent mean vitamin D status (Holdsworth *et al* 1984) and this needs to be maintained following retirement by encouraging sunlight exposure.

In addition, the COMA panel on DRVs has recommended that the population over 65 years should consume 10 μg vitamin D daily. Dietary sources of vitamin D are often those which the elderly find difficult to eat; fatty fish, for example, is often ignored because of the bones. More suitable alternatives such as fish patés or softer canned fatty fish should therefore be suggested. The new recommendation to consume 10 μg daily has led to debate on the need for vitamin drops or for a new formula food for this population group.

Minerals

Potassium As most foods contain moderate amounts of potassium there should be no shortage of this essential mineral. However, diets based on highly refined foods, with an excess of sugar, may be potassium deficient. Depletion of potassium has been associated with depression, muscle weakness and mental confusion (Judge and Cowan 1971; Dall and Gardiner 1971). Conversely, depression may cause some individuals to lose their appetite and to turn to a convenient but high sugar diet (Davies 1981).

Sodium In order to avoid the risk of sodium depletion, salt restrictions recommended for the general population are inappropriate for most elderly persons, especially those over 85 years of age (Brown *et al* 1984).

Calcium Milk is an important source of calcium for the elderly and if nutritional supplementation is to be given, milk-based food has been demonstrated to improve nutritional status (Katakity *et al* 1983).

Zinc Some features of old age such as delayed wound healing, decreased taste acuity and anorexia are also findings associated with zinc deficiency (Hsu 1979). However, healthy elderly subjects have been shown to be in zinc balance despite an apparent low dietary intake (Bunker *et al* 1982), suggesting that there is at least some degree of adaptation.

Fibre

Transit time in elderly people is no different from that in younger people but constipation is a common complaint, particularly in immobile patients.

There is great enthusiasm to encourage the consumption of fibre-containing foods but any increase should be gradual otherwise bowel discomfort, distention and flatulence will result. An excess of fibre may compromise the absorption of iron and certain trace elements. Adequate fluid intake should be encouraged simultaneously.

Fluid

Some elderly individuals may have a fading sense of thirst and may go for long periods without fluid. Others avoid liquid for fear of incontinence or to prevent urgency when away from home.

Dehydration can result in mental confusion, headaches and irritability. If a normally alert elderly person complains of phases of confusion, the fluid intake should be checked. Extra fluids can be taken earlier in the day and bedtime drinks can be avoided by those concerned about nocturnal incontinence. Elderly persons should be advised to consume some fluid at regular intervals even if they are not thirsty.

Physical activity

It has been suggested that, for the elderly, maintenance of physical activity should be the principal objective of nutrition education (NACNE 1983). Where there is reduced physical activity this may be a key factor leading to muscular atrophy. Physical activity and the prevention of immobilization are also important in the prevention of osteoporosis.

Deterioration in physiological function

Changes in physiological function with age must not be ignored. Deterioration in renal function may have profound implications for drug therapy (see below). Changes in digestive function may have several nutritional consequences, including malabsorption. The subject of digestive function and ageing has been comprehensively reviewed by Bowman and Rosenberg (1983). However, these authors (Rosenberg and Bowman 1984) also state that 'although changes in swallowing, gastric secretion, fat digestion or calcium absorption may have a significant influence on the nutritional status of certain elderly people, the impact of these functional alterations is modest relating to the far more pervasive influence of social and economic factors on food intake and dietary habits in the elderly population'.

Illness

Illness, which is generally more common among the elderly than the young, may affect nutritional intake (via effects on appetite and access to food), nutritional requirement and nutrient absorption. Protein turnover has been shown to be significantly increased in ill geriatric patients as a response to tissue trauma, inflammation or sepsis and further influenced by factors such as nutrition or physical activity (Phillips 1983).

Adapting therapeutic diets for elderly people

Where therapeutic diets are essential for the older person, they can tax the skills of even the most experienced dietitian. As well as knowledge of the appropriate therapies for different disease states, there are invariably other conditions which need to be considered. There may be evidence of multiple diseases, including stroke, Parkinson's disease, arthritis and the physical disabilities which may accompany ageing, e.g. hearing defects, poor sight or poor dentition. Mental states need to be considered; there may be confusion, depression, loneliness, apathy, a recent bereavement or recent loss of will to live. Social factors such as isolation or poverty also need to be recognized. When planning menus for elderly hospital inpatients, the majority of dishes should be familiar recipes, easy to handle for those with stiff fingers who cannot grip cutlery firmly or open packets. Attractive presentation with variety in condiments and colour is important. A healthy, high fibre menu planned by younger people with different tastes, will defeat its own ends if the patients cannot chew it or will not eat it. Taste alters with age so new recipes and supplements should be tested by the consumers rather than the cooks.

Drug-nutrient interaction in elderly people

Special attention needs to be paid to drug-nutrient interaction (see Section 2.10). The likely behaviour of a drug in an elderly recipient cannot be assumed from a consideration of that drug's behaviour in younger people. The Committee on Safety of Medicines now requires that drug data sheets provide details of suitable dosages for elderly people.

Many studies show that there is an increased liability to adverse drug reactions with ageing. Older people often have significant reduction in renal clearance. Multiple drugs are more often used and many elderly individuals, whether institutionalized or not, regularly take medicines – either prescribed or as self-medication. Poor compliance with complex dose regimens may be exacerbated by failing memory, poor hearing and vision, and difficulty with opening containers. Diminished salivation may make it more difficult to swallow tablets, and oesophageal motility disorders lead to bulky drugs sticking in the oesophageal mucosa. Dietary histories should include details of the usage of drugs which may be relevant to nutrition, with both the quantity and the timing being recorded. Alcohol is often taken as a medicine by elderly people.

When dealing with elderly people, dietitians need to be aware that poor nutritional status can impair drug metabolism, and that drug treatment can have a detrimental effect on nutritional status. This subject has been reviewed by Roe (1976), Dickerson (1978), Hyams (1981) and Denham and George (1990).

General considerations

General points which are relevant to the use of drugs in elderly people include the following:

Changes in body composition in old age (Denham and George 1990) These comprise:
1 Decline in total body size.
2 Increase in body fat stores.
3 Decline in total body water.
4 Decline in liver mass.
5 Decline in kidney mass.

Highly water-soluble drugs such as digoxin require a smaller loading dose as the total body water declines. Stores of lipid-soluble drugs may increase as the body fat stores increase with a resultant enhanced drug effect and toxicity.

In general drug doses are reduced to avoid toxicity. The aim is to find the lowest appropriate dose for therapeutic effect.

Changes in metabolism and excretion With ageing, there is a diminished ability to metabolize and to excrete drugs. Renal function in particular may be impaired. The mean glomerular filtration rate and tubular function have been shown to be reduced by 30% in otherwise healthy people over the age of 65 years when compared with normal young adults. There is an increased inter-individual variability consequent upon the effects of ageing *per se*, and the prevalence of disease (which may be occult). Social factors such as smoking and alcohol intake may play a part in this variability. The optimal dose for each individual is decided by clinical observation.

Percentage of body water A lower percentage of body water results in greater alcohol effects per unit of body weight.

Energy and protein intakes When energy and protein intakes are low, there is often a reduced capacity to metabolise drugs.

Timing The timing of drug intake and food consumption is important. Some drugs are more rapidly absorbed in the fasting state (e.g. ethanol, aspirin, barbiturates, penicillin and tetracycline) and should be taken on an empty stomach either to attain an effective concentrations in the blood (e.g. some antibiotics) or to avoid drug-food interactions (e.g. tetracycline should not be taken simultaneously with milk, or with antacids or mineral supplements containing salts of calcium, magnesium or iron, because of the formation of non-absorbed complexes). Other drugs *should* be taken with food in order to increase bioavailability or to minimize side effects.

Length of regimen The longer period of time a drug is administered, the greater will be the effect on nutritional status and a poor nutrient status will alter drug requirements.

Confusion Drug side effects can cause confusion states. Patients may therefore forget whether they have recently eaten or been without food. They may also forget whether they have taken medication or even exchange drugs with other people.

Specific considerations

Drugs which may be particularly relevant to the nutritional status of the elderly are:
1 Cytotoxic drugs and antibiotics which impair absorption.
2 Cimetidine and other gastric acid blockers.
3 Drugs which alter gastric emptying time. Anticholinergic drugs delay emptying. Anti-emetics such as metoclopramide and domperidone speed gastric emptying.
4 The prokinetic drug cisapride, used for symptomatic relief of gastric reflux, increases the motility of the whole gut.
5 Alcohol, cathartics, cholestyramine, clofibrate and liquid paraffin can be implicated in malabsorption in geriatric patients.

6 The theophyllines (oral bronchodilators) are commonly associated with anorexia, nausea and vomiting.
7 Drugs which alter mineral and vitamin metabolism. These include.

- *Anticonvulsants* such as phenytoin which affect vitamin D metabolism and folate absorption;
- *Biguanides* which reduce B_2 and folate status;
- *Tetracyline* which depresses leucocyte levels of ascorbic acid and increases urinary excretion of ascorbic acid;
- *Anti-cancer drugs* which can affect thiamin status;
- *Prolonged aspirin treatment* which produces tissue depletion of ascorbic acid and can also induce chronic bleeding in the gastrointestinal tract, resulting in iron deficiency anaemia.
- *Thiazide and loop diuretics* which can cause potassium depletion and magnesium and zinc deficiency. These diuretics may be used in reduced dose with a potassium sparing diuretic such as spironolactone.
- *Potassium sparing diuretics* can cause hyperkalaemia; Vasodilator angiotensin converting enzyme (ACE) inhibitors and the non-steroidal anti-inflammatory drugs (NSAIDs) also carry this risk;
- *Potassium supplements* can cause oesophageal, gastric and bowel ulceration. In elderly patients, a substantial supplement of potassium may be indicated in those with a combination of a reduced dietary intake, low body stores and less effective renal conservation of potassium. Since potassium tablets are difficult to swallow, high potassium foods should be encouraged as an additional supplement, particularly when the required dose is not met.

8 Drugs which decrease appetite include anti-cancer drugs such as cyclophosphamide; NSAIDs such as indomethacin; biguanides; glucagon; morphine and the digitalis group.
9 Drugs which increase appetite include alcohol, insulin, thyroid hormone, steroids, some antihistamines, sulphonylureas and psychotropic drugs.

Carers who are involved with the provision of food should be advised on the importance and relevance of related drug therapy. Two drugs of particular relevance to dietary therapy in old age are tolbutamide and levadopa.

Tolbutamide This drug can have a profound hypoglycaemic effect in some older people. The decline in plasma albumin levels with age may result in more tolbutamide remaining free, rather than bound, in plasma. Liver mass, and hence the rate at which this drug is metabolized, may also be reduced. An alternative hypoglycaemic agent with a shorter half-life such as glipizide may be preferred for older diabetics. If tolbutamide is used, it should be given with, or immediately after, food to lessen the risk of hypoglycaemia.

Levodopa The level of levodopa in the plasma is critical for clinical status in the later stages of Parkinson's disease. Levodopa is a precursor of dopamine. All factors which delay gastric emptying of levodopa – both food and drugs such as anti-cholinergics – result in delayed and reduced peak plasma concentration. This is turn reduces the effective conversion to dopamine.

Levodopa is absorbed rapidly in the fasting state. Maximum absorption takes place in the upper small intestine; the stomach can metabolize levodopa but has limited absorptive capacity. Animal studies have shown that levodopa absorption is by an active transport mechanism in which the levodopa has to compete with neutral amino acids. A similar transport mechanism is involved in the transport of levodopa across the blood-brain barrier. Meals containing protein will alter levodopa absorption by their effect on the gastric emptying time and on the transport mechanism.

Severe Parkinson's disease, with tremor and reduced swallowing ability, can markedly reduce food intake. Patients eat slowly and with great effort. The likely undernutrition usually indicates a need for a high protein, high energy diet with modified texture, either soft or purées. (If the tremor is marked, sip feeds boxed with a straw are easier to handle.) However, this nutritional need for protein conflicts with the pharmacological need for a reduced protein intake to maximize the effect of the levodopa. It is therefore important that an agreed meal pattern should be maintained while dosage of levodopa is adjusted to find the optimum treatment. The timing and content of meals should be decided on the basis of a home assessment (taking account of factors such as habitual eating habits and the times at which meals may be provided by carers) and the clinical state. When a suitable pattern of meals and drug administration has been established, variability in eating habits should then be avoided as this may reduce the effect of the levodopa and result in clinical deterioration.

3.7.3 **Malnutrition in the elderly**

Although it may be relatively easy to diagnose overt malnutrition, the identification of marginal or subclinical malnutrition is beset with difficulties. The condition can be disguised by disease states, biochemical results can be influenced by factors other than nutritional status (such as dehydration), or there may be low stores but no clinical indication of disturbed form or function until the full manifestation of nutritional crisis occurs.

The prime objective of nutrition policies and practices concerning the elderly should be directed towards the *prevention* of malnutrition. This calls for a wider definition to our concept of malnutrition so that risk factors can be identified in order that appropriate policies, both for groups and for individuals, can be established and appropriate action taken.

Recognizing different types of malnutrition in the elderly

Davies (1989) has defined four main types of malnutrition which are distinct, yet which may be interrelated.

Type 1 – 'long-standing' For some people there can be a long latent period between nutritional deficiency and its clinical appearance. For these people there needs to be recognition of warning signs so that early preventive action can be taken.

Type 2 – 'sudden' For some elderly men or women a medical or social stress (e.g. a bereavement) can tip marginal, or even perfectly adequate, nutrition swiftly over into poor nutrition. For these people prompt action needs to be taken at that critical stage.

Type 3 – 'specific' This is defined as the occurrence of a deficiency disease, such as scurvy, or nutrition-related diseases such as diabetes, arthritis, osteoporosis and atherosclerosis. These call for diagnosis, followed by treatment which may include medication and/or dietary manipulation.

Type 4 – 'recurrent' In some cases there is a repeated return of malnutrition accompanied by a weakening resistance to disease. For these people, monitoring and support must follow the previous episode of acute malnutrition.

Lehmann (1989) has reviewed undernutrition in elderly people.

Risk factors to identify those at risk of malnutrition

Exton-Smith (1971) recognized primary and secondary causes of malnutrition in the elderly (see Table 3.32) which call for improved social and public health measures or appropriate medical/dietetic treatment.

Table 3.32 Causes of malnutrition in the elderly

Primary causes	Secondary causes
Ignorance	Impaired appetite
Social isolation	Masticatory inefficiency
Physical disability	Malabsorption
Mental disturbance	Alcoholism
Iatrogenic disorder	Drugs
Poverty	Increased requirements

The DHSS Report (1979) associated the incidence of undernutrition with the following social and medical 'at risk' factors:

Living alone	Chronic bronchitis
Housebound	Emphysema
No regular cooked meals	Gastrectomy
Supplementary benefit (i.e. poverty bracket)	Poor dentition
Social classes IV and V	Difficulty in swallowing
Low mental test score	Smoking
Depression	Alcoholism

Active measures for those at risk

Elderly people living in the community

Although the majority of our elderly UK population is community based, many are in need of nutritional support in order to prevent Type 1 (long-standing) or Type 2 (sudden) malnutrition and unnecessary institutionalization. To identify those in need of nutritional support, such as meals-on-wheels or other services, ten main risk factors have been highlighted (Davies 1981).

1 Fewer than eight main meals, hot or cold, eaten in a week.
2 Very little milk consumed.
3 Virtual abstention from fruits and vegetables.
4 Wastage of food – even that supplied hot and ready to eat.
5 Long periods in the day without food or beverages.
6 Depression or loneliness.
7 Unexpected weight change, either a significant gain or loss (this is a more valuable index of risk than either obesity or underweight).
8 Shopping difficulties.
9 Poverty.
10 Indication in medical record of disabilities, including alcoholism.

Elderly individuals vary widely in their ability to cope with difficulties; a risk factor in isolation does not therefore necessarily indicate the need for intervention. Each risk is only a potential danger sign and must be considered in relation to the others. Thus depression or loneliness in themselves may not affect nutrition, but when found in combination with wastage of food and weight loss, the danger is apparent. Almost without exception it was found in the DHSS survey that when *four or more* risk factors were evident, an individual was likely to be malnourished (DHSS 1979).

Elderly people living in residential homes

Research on nutrition and catering in old people's homes has led to the identification of 26 risk factors, any of which may affect nutritional intake. Many of these are social factors known to influence food intake (Davies and Holdsworth 1979) and are listed in Table 3.33.

Table 3.33 An A–Z checklist of potential risk factors in residential homes

A	Weekly cyclic menu *or* monotony of menu
B	Difficulties with tea/supper meal menus. (This highlights lack of experience in menu planning and recipe ideas, and may affect costing)
C	Tea/supper meal at or before 5 pm. (This frequently occurs in the UK, mainly because of staffing difficulties. Biscuits often have to be supplied later in the evening because some residents become hungry before bedtime)
D	Lack or rapport between head of home and cook, or the cook resists and resents suggestions
E	Residents' suggestions (e.g. for recipes) unheeded. Residents' needs for special diets ignored. Inadequate contact between the residents and the home's decision-making committee or board
F	Residents not allowed choice of portion size *or* poor portion control *or* no second helpings available
G	No heed taken of food wastage
H	Very little home-style cooking. (Residents frequently express a desire for familiar foods they have been used to eating, rather than institutional type catering)
I	No special provision for food treats from the local community or from the home, apart from Christmas dinner
J	For active residents: poor or no facilities for independence in providing food and drink (e.g. tea making)
K	Hot foods served lukewarm or poorly flavoured
L	Poor presentation of food, including table setting and appearance of the dining room
M	Unfriendly or undignified waitress service. Meal too rushed
N	No observation of weight changes of the residents. (Significant changes in weight can be used as an early diagnostic tool for illness, depression or other conditions which can affect nutritional status)
O	No help in feeding very frail residents. No measures taken to protect other residents from offensive eating habits
P	Head of home and cook lacking basic nutritional or catering knowledge. Isolation from possible help
Q	Lengthy period between preparation, cooking and serving. Time lag between staff meals and resident meals
R	Lack of vitamin C-containing foods or risk of destruction of vitamin C due to poor cooking procedures
S	Few vitamin D-containing foods used, combined with lack of exposure of residents to sunlight
T	Low fibre diet and complaints of constipation
U	Possible low intake of other nutrients, e.g. iron, folate and vitamin B_{12},
V	Preponderance of convenience foods of poor nutritional content
W	Disproportionate expenditure between animal protein/fruit and vegetables/high energy foods may lead to a nutritionally imbalanced menu
X	Obvious food perks to staff to detriment of residents' meals. High proportion of food served to others
Y	Conditions conductive to food poisoning. Lack of cleanliness
Z	Recommendations may not be implemented

Elderly people in hospital

It is pitiful to see an elderly, ill, frail patient struggling to reach a tray of food placed insensitively out of reach. Such events should not occur. In busy wards, however, unless there is close supervision, problems like this do arise. Constant attention must therefore be paid to meal service. It is especially in geriatic wards that Type 3 (specific) and Type 4 (recurrent) malnutrition may be evident.

Evaluating the meal service and identifying the problems

A dietitian confronting the problems in a geriatric ward firstly needs to know what happens at meal times. This may necessitate several visits to each ward before action is taken and the ward sister should be consulted beforehand. The following points should be observed:

1 At meal times, are the patients in bed, in chairs by their beds, or communally dining at small tables?
2 Are patients sitting in positions where they can eat comfortably?
3 Who serves the meals?
4 Who delivers the food and beverages to the patients?
5 What do the meals look like?
6 Is the food appetizing?
7 Are portion sizes appropriate for individual appetites?
8 Are needs for special diets met and are the appropriate diets being given to the right people?
9 What is the reaction of the patients to the food?
10 Can patients handle crockery and cutlery?
11 Is there help with feeding when necessary? If so, how is this done?
12 Is there much food wastage? If so, which food or dish is it?
13 Are meal times rushed or is there adequate time to eat?
14 Is the food kept appetizing if the patient is interrupted by a visit?
15 Are dentures available – or are they hidden away in a drawer?
16 Are sufficient staff around at meal times to cope with the patients' extra needs?
17 Is there an over-emphasis on puréed foods?
18 How would you react to being served this food on a long-term basis?
19 Other general comments or complaints.

Diplomatic enquiries should be made regarding:
1 Whether the patients have any suggestions concerning the food.
2 What the staff on the ward think of the food.
3 Whether weight checks are made at least monthly and what action is taken if there is a loss or gain of 2 kg or more.
4 Whether staff are getting patients into the sunlight in summer.

Taking action

An important use of a dietitian's time is to educate those already involved in food preparation and service. Suggestions are given below.

Discussion Arrange meetings for nursing, ancillary and catering staff to discuss the service of beverages and food and to inspire enthusiasm regarding the importance of their work. Remind them that patients need to be able to help themselves; if patients are unable to reach the meals the frustration may lead to anorexia or depression. Suggest ways of motivating those disinterested in food or who have lost the will to live – perhaps a change in menu is required, some home-style cooking or even a series of small treats. Where appetites are small, a large meal can be off-putting. Watch out for monotony of the menu and inflexibility of meal size due to standardized servings. Discuss the observations made over the previous weeks and discuss ways to correct poor practices.

Discuss what the staff would most like to eat or drink if they were destined to be a patient in a long stay ward. Try some practical exercises: get a staff member to volunteer to be a patient, then immobilize in a chair and feed an unidentified puree at a brisk pace. Try getting them to drink out of a feeding beaker. Note the reaction.

Liaison Keep up good liaison with the catering manager and make sure that he accompanies you to the wards from time to time and discusses any problems with you and the nursing staff. Do likewise with a member of the diet kitchen staff, keeping these visits short but informative.

Refresher courses With the catering manager, arrange refresher courses in dietetic practices for chefs and cooks. These need be for only an hour each week for, say, a six week period. Subjects could include theoretical topics and practical sessions related to the elderly.

Updating medical staff Medical staff also need updating in dietetic practice. This is often best conducted informally in quieter moments on the ward.

Teamwork Contribute as part of the team in ward rounds and in case conferences where appropriate.

A multidisciplinary feeding team can give co-ordinated support to the patient with feeding difficulties. At different times, the dietitian will want to liaise with the speech therapist advising on swallowing problems, the physiotherapist concerned with positioning at table and movements related to independent feeding, the occupational therapist devising eating aids and the pharmacist for pharmaceutical nutritional support. A mental test score, usually obtained by the occupational therapist, is a background pointer to whether the patient can give a constructive and relevant dietary history as well as indicating the most appropriate approach for nutritional advice.

Health care assistants There are opportunities for a nutrition input in the new vocational training guidelines for health care assistants.

Client input Set up a 'clients' food group' for permanent residents. This enables people to contribute ideas to the menu and encourages valuable comments on the total meal service.

Special diets Where special diets are required for the elderly, much the same principles apply as for pathological conditions at younger ages, but see the paragraphs an 'Adapting therapeutic diets for elderly people' in Section 3.7.2. above. The aim of dietary treatment is likely to be symptom control and avoidance of complications. Clinical standards for the elderly must be written with this in mind.

New admissions undernourished through self-neglect

When an elderly man or woman is admitted to hospital with undernourishment through self-neglect, the stay in hospital should be used to teach the patient the importance of diet. Discuss with the doctor whether the patient's condition is caused primarily through self-neglect or a disease state. If the former, encourage the patient to regard *food*, not just vitamin or mineral supplements, as the main treatment. Monitor the diet carefully checking that extra food supplements including fresh fruit juices are provided when necessary.

In order to prevent recurrence of the malnutrition, the cause of the pre-existing condition, i.e. a poor diet, must also be tackled. When alcohol has tended to replace meals, emphasizing the importance of food in relation to health is of particular importance.

The anorexic patient will need encouragement to eat especially if loss of appetite is due to drug administration. The patient's food preferences should be considered and meals should be small, dainty and served frequently. Such individual care can motivate the patient to eat. Lowered intakes are not inevitable with ageing (Davies 1984).

Rehabilitation

The main aim in rehabilitation is to enable the individual to retain sufficient independence to prevent constant readmissions to hospital. Where there is risk of Type 4 (recurrent) malnutrition, special support outside the hospital environment will need to be arranged.

Support services

The social worker will be able to suggest local support services which may assist the patient. These may include:

Meals-on-wheels	Community centres
Home helps	Social clubs
Luncheon clubs	Cookery classes
Visits to a day hospital	Local church facilities
Day visits to a residential home	Street wardens
	Good neighbour schemes
Day centres	Shops with delivery services

Most elderly people living at home will not be totally dependent on these services for their meals. Most will still need to cook a few times a week and to prepare breakfasts. They may therefore need advice on meal planning and preparation, together will recipe suggestions which are easy to prepare, economical, tasty and nourishing. Ideally suitable are two paperback books by Louise Davies: *Easy cooking for one or two* (1972) and *More easy cooking for one or two* (1979). These books contain chapters on 'Nutrition on your own', 'Recipes for non-cooks', 'Store-cupboard cookery' and 'Cooking for companionship'. The print is large and clear for fading eyesight and the recipes are tested and approved by the elderly themselves.

If recommending other books, consider the size of the print. If designing leaflets, make sure the print is large and clear (see Section 3.11.4, concerning the visually handicapped).

Nutrition education

With the changing nutrition scene there is an increased need for updating other health professionals regarding the nutritional needs of elderly people. These professionals include doctors, medical students, nurses, occupational therapists and other hospital staff, especially ancillary staff who can influence a patient's food intake. Those outside the hospital setting, e.g. home helps, health visitors, officers in charge of old people's homes, meals-on-wheels organizers and wardens of 'sheltered housing' will also benefit from nutrition education.

Teaching sessions should be conducted informally in small groups or on a one to one basis. Alternatively, they can be in the form of one day seminars where 20–30 people with a common interest (e.g. officers in charge or cooks/chefs of old people's homes, cooks in luncheon clubs or hospital based staff) can gather to hear a series of short talks on relevant topics, followed by a discussion or questions and answers session. Topics could include menu planning, how to improve the diet, getting the elderly out of doors, fibre in the diet, costing and budgeting, nutritional risk factors in residential homes, use of freezers, prevention of food poisoning, or special diets (where relevant). Such seminars can also involve discussion groups, demonstrations (especially on cookery techniques and recipes for supper ideas), recipe exchanges or slide or film sessions.

For the elderly themselves, ideal venues for teaching 'eating for health and pleasure' are luncheon clubs, day hospitals, Darby and Joan clubs and cookery classes for the over 60s.

For those approaching retirement, talks and demonstrations can be given to groups within pre-retirement courses. Here the overall message should be 'keep interested in food and if you can't be bothered to cook at any time, turn to the nourishing easy-to-prepare foods rather than neglecting your diet'. Appropriate topics have been reported elsewhere (Davies *et al* 1985). A nutrition survey on a pre-retirement sample has indicated the need for nutrition education at this age (Holdsworth and Davies 1984).

Teaching aids and assessment kits

An updated list of leaflets is available for dietitians from the British Dietetic Association's Nutrition Advisory Group for Elderly People (NAGE), contactable through the BDA in Birmingham. Details of some NAGE publications are given below. Prices are given for guidance but are obviously subject is alteration. All enquiries should be accompanied by a stamped self-addressed envelope.

NAGE Publications

1 Position Paper 'Eating through the 90s' (1992 price, £2.50)

This booklet provides information on nutrition and dietetics for those involved in catering for any group of elderly people. It aims to maintain and/or improve the quality of care for an ever increasing sector of our community.

Details from Mrs E Haughton, Dietetic Dept, Gloucestershire Royal Hospital, Great Western Road, Gloucester GL1 3NN.

2 Nutrition assessment checklist and guidance notes (1992 price, 80p)

A screening tool for use by health professionals when interviewing older people. Its purpose is to help health professionals identify clients who are 'at risk' of nutritional inadequacy and implement appropriate intervention.

Details from Mrs H White, 30 Winford Terrace, West Park, Leeds LS16 6HY.

3 Food and health policies for elderly people (1992 price, £1)

This booklet shows how healthy eating guidelines can be adapted to the needs of elderly people. It is primarily aimed at providers of meals for elderly people.

Details from Mrs E Haughton, Dietetic Dept, Gloucestershire Royal Hospital, Great Western Road, Gloucester GL1 3NN.

4 Video 'Aspects of nutrition awareness among the elderly' (1992 price, £20)

This video is the first of a series of short trigger training videos produced by NAGE. 'Supermarket shopping' and 'The store cupboard' are the themes on this cassette. Each sequence lasts ten minutes and is intended to stimulate discussion.

Details from Mrs B Hayton, Senior Dietitian for the Elderly, Chapel Allerton Hospital, Harehills Road, Leeds LS7 4RB.

ALL CHEQUES SHOULD BE MADE PAYABLE TO THE NUTRITION ADVISORY GROUP FOR THE ELDERLY (NAGE)

Open University Publications

Training packs available from The Open University, Department of Health and Social Welfare include:

P577 Mental health problems in old age
P650 Caring for old people
P654 Working with older people
(1992 Cost – £14.50 per pack)

Details and order forms are available from The Information Officer, Department of Health and Social Welfare, The Open University, Walton Hall, Milton Keynes, MK7 6AA.

Gerontology Nutrition Unit Publications

Slide Lecture Kits

Set A An emergency food store for the elderly
Set B What is a balanced diet?
Set C Vitamin D and calcium

Assessment kits

A Meals-on-wheels assessment kit
B For dietitians: Nutrition and Catering in old peoples' homes assessment kit
C Information pack for officers in charge of residential homes

For details current prices and availability please write, enclosing a stamped, addressed envelope to Dr Louise Davies, Consultant in Gerontology Nutrition, 85a Redington Road, Hampstead, London NW3 7RR.

Useful addresses

Age Concern England, Astral House, 1268 London Road, Norbury, London SW16 4ER. Tel. 081–679 8000.
Local branches of Age Concern can advise on local services.

Alcohol Concern, 275 Gray's Inn Road, London WC1X 8QF. Tel. 071–833 3471.

Alzheimer's Disease Society, 158–160 Balham High Road, London SW12 9BN. Tel. 081–675 6557.

British Geriatric Society, 1 St Andrew's Place, Regents Park, London NW1 4LB.

Carers National Association, 29 Chilworth Mews, London W2 3RG. Tel. 071–724 7776.
The local social service department will also give up-to-date local information on carers' support groups.

Centre for Policy on Ageing, 25–31 Ironmonger Row, London EC1V 3QP. Tel. 071–253 1787.
An independent policy unit with a library and information service. Publications include *Residential case notes no. 6 on Catering and Nutrition* and *Home Work: meeting the needs of older people in residential homes* a set of nine booklets including one on nutrition and catering.

CRUSE Bereavement Care,Cruse House, 126 Sheen Road, Richmond, Surrey TW9 1UR. Tel. 081–940 4818.

Disabled Living Foundation, 380–384 Harrow Road, London W9 2HU. Tel. 071–289 6111.

Meals on Wheels, Information on local provision comes from the Social Services Department.

Motor Neurone Disease Association, PO Box 256, Northampton NN1 2PR. Tel. 0604 22269.

Parkinson's Disease Society, 36 Portland Place, London W1N 3DG. Tel. 071–323 1174.

Research into Ageing, 49 Queen Victoria Street, London ECAN 4SA.

Standing Conference of Ethnic Minority Senior Citizens, 5 Westminster Bridge Road, London SE1 7XW. Tel. 071–928 0095.

The Stroke Association, CHSA House, 123–127 Whitecross Street, London EC1Y 8JJ. Tel. 071–490 7999.

Further reading

Albanese AA (1980) Nutrition for the elderly. In *Current topics in nutrition and disease* Vol 3. Alan Liss, New York.

Andrews J and von Hahn HP (Eds) (1981) *Geriatrics for everyday practice.* S Karger, London.

Davies L (1981) *Three score years. . .and then? A study of the nutrition and well-being of elderly people at home.* Heinemann Medical, London.

Department of Health and Social Security (1972) *A nutrition survey of the Elderly* Rep Hlth Soc Subj 3. HMSO, London.

Department of Health and Social Security (1979) *Nutrition and health in old age.* Rep Hlth Soc Subj 16. HMSO, London.

Exton-Smith AN and Caird FI (Eds) (1980) *Metabolic and nutritional disorders in the elderly.* John Wright, Bristol.

Isaacs B (1985) *Understanding stroke illness.* A CHSA Publication, Tavistock House North, London WC1H 9JE.

Parliamentary White Paper (1989) *Working for patients*, CM 555, HMSO, London.

Parliamentary White Paper (1989) *Caring for people. Community care in the next decade and beyond.* CM 849, HMSO, London.

Addendum

The following report was published too late for its findings to be incorporated in this edition of the *Manual of Dietetic Practice.* The report is essential reading for any dietitian working with elderly people.

Department of Health (1992) *The Nutrition of elderly people.* Report of the Working Group on the Nutrition of Elderly People of the Committee on Medical Aspects of Food Policy. Rep Hlth Soc Subj 43. HMSO, London.

References

Bilderbeck N, Holdsworth MD, Purves R and Davies L (1981) Changing food habits among 100 elderly men and women in the UK. *J Hum Nutr* **35**, 448–55.

Bowman BB and Rosenberg IH (1983) Digestive function and ageing. *Hum Nutr: Clin Nutr* **37C**, 75–89.

Brown JJ, Lever AF, Robertson JIS, Semple PF, Bing RF, Heagerty AM, Swales JD, Thurston H, Ledingham JGG, Laragh JH, Hansson L, Nicholls MG and Espiner EA (1984) Salt and hypertension. *Lancet* **ii**, 1333–4.

Bosanquet N and Gray A (1989) *Will you still love me? New opportunities for elderly people in the 1990s and beyond.* National Association of Health Authorities Research Paper 2. NAHA, Birmingham.

Bunker VW and Clayton BE (1989) Research review: Studies in the nutrition of elderly people with particular reference to essential trace elements. *Age and Ageing* **18**, 422–9.

Bunker VW, Lawson MS, Delves HT and Clayton BE (1982) Metabolic balance studies for zinc and nitrogen in healthy elderly subjects. *Hum Nutr: Clin Nutr* **36C**, 213–21.

Corless D, Gupta SP, Salter DA, Switala S and Boucher BJ (1979) Vitamin D status of residents of an old people's home and long stay patients. *Gerontology* **25**, 350–5.

Dall JLC and Gardiner HS (1971) Dietary intake of potassium by geriatic patients. *Geront Clin* **13**, 119–24.

Dattani J, Exton-Smith AN and Stephen JML (1984) Vitamin D status of the elderly in relation to age and exposure to sunlight. *Hum Nutr: Clin Nutr* **38C**, 131–7.

Davies L (1972) *Easy cooking for one or two*. Penguin Handbooks, London.

Davies L (1979) *More easy cooking for one or two*. Penguin Handbooks, London.

Davies L (1981) *Three score years...and then*? Heinemann Medical Books Ltd, London.

Davies L (1984) Nutrition and the elderly: identifying those at risk. *Proc Nutr Soc* **43**, 295–302.

Davies L (1989) Nutritional risk factors for disease in the elderly. In *Malnutrition in the elderly*. WHO Publication, USA.

Davies L, Anderson JP and Holdsworth MD (1985) Nutrition education at the age of retirement from work. *Health Education* **44**(4), 187–92.

Davies L and Holdsworth MD (1979) A technique for assessing nutritional 'at risk' factors in residential homes for the elderly. *J Hum Nutr* **33**, 165–9.

Denham MJ and George CF (1990) Drugs in old age. New perspectives. *Br Med Bull* **46**, No 1.

Department of Health and Social Security (1972) *A nutrition survey of the elderly*. Rep Hlth Soc Subj 3. HMSO, London.

Department of Health and Social Security (1979) *Nutrition and health in old age*. Rep Hlth Soc Subj 16. HMSO, London.

Department of Health and Social Security (1984) Committee on Medical Aspects of Food Policy. *Diet and cardiovascular disease* (The COMA Report) Rep Hlth Soc Subj 28. HMSO, London.

Dickerson JWT (1978) The interrelationships of nutrition and drugs. In *Nutrition in the clinical management of disease*. Dickerson JWT and Lee HA (Eds) pp. 308–31. Edward Arnold, London.

Exton-Smith AN (1971) Nutrition of the elderly. *Br J Hosp Med* **5**, 639–45.

Exton-Smith AN (1978) Nutrition in the elderly. In *Nutrition in the clinical management of disease*. Dickerson JWT and Lee HA (Eds) pp. 72–104. Edward Arnold, London.

Exton-Smith AN, Stanton BR and Windsor ACM (1972) *Nutrition of housebound old people*. King's Fund, London.

Holdsworth MD, Dattani J, Davies L and Macfarlane D (1984) Factors contributing to vitamin D status near retirement age. *Hum Nutr: Clin Nutr* **38C**, 139–49.

Holdsworth MD and Davies L (1984) Nutrition at retirement age. *Proc Nutr Soc* **43**, 303–13.

Hsu JM (1979) Current knowledge on zinc, copper and chromium in ageing. *World Rev Nutr Diet* **33**, 42.

Hyams DE (1981) Drugs in the elderly. In *Geriatrics for everyday practice*. von Hahn and Andrews (Eds). Karger, Basel.

Judge TG and Cowan NR (1971) Dietary potassium intake and grip strength in older people. *Gerontol Clin* **13**, 221–6.

Katakity M, Webb JF and Dickerson JWT (1983) Some effects of a food supplement in elderly hospital patients: a longitudinal study. *Hum Nutr: Appl Nutr* **37A**, 85–93.

Lehmann AB (1989) Review: undernutrition in elderly people, *Age and Ageing* **18**, 339–53.

Morgan DB and Hullin RP (1982) The body composition of the chronic mentally ill. *Hum Nutr: Clin Nutr* **36C**, 439–48.

National Advisory Committee on Nutrition Education (1983) *Proposals for nutritional guidelines for health education in Britain*. (The NACNE Report) Health Education Council, London.

Office of Population, Censuses and Surveys (1990) *Population Trends* No 62. Winter 1990. OPCS, London.

Phillips P (1983) Protein turnover in the elderly: a comparison between ill patients and normal controls. *Hum Nutr: Clin Nutr* **37C**, 339–44.

Roe DA (1976) *Drug-induced nutritional deficiencies* pp. 272. AVI Publishing Co Inc, Westport, Connecticut.

Rosenberg IH and Bowman BB (1984) Gastrointestinal function and ageing. In *The role of the gastrointestinal tract in nutrient delivery*. Bristol-Myers Nutrition Symposia Vol 3, Green M, Greene HL (Eds). Academic Press, London.

Sheltawy M, Newton H, Hay A, Morgan DB and Hullin RP (1984) The contribution of dietary vitamin D and sunlight to the plasma 25-hydroxyvitamin D in the elderly. *Hum Nutr: Clin Nutr* **38C**, 191–4.

Vir SC and Love AHG (1979) Nutritional status of institutionalized aged in Belfast, Northern Ireland. *Am J Clin Nutr* **32**, 193–207.

3.8 Low income groups

3.8.1 The size and nature of the problem

Is there a problem?

> 'Children of Poor Going Hungry – A political dispute was sparked yesterday by research indicating that children of families on low incomes regularly go hungry even though their parents put them first as the cupboard becomes bare'.
>
> (Horsnell 1991)

This article followed the publication of a report by NCH, a national children's charity, which showed major cause for concern about the diets of women and children in families with low incomes in Britain (NCH 1991). In a questionnaire survey of 350 families living on benefits in different parts of the country, 55% of those on income support said that their children had not had enough to eat at some time during the month before the survey. Of these families, 23% said cited the cost of food as the main reason for this; 42% said the child didn't like what they could offer and in many cases no alternative was available to provide the child with a choice. Nearly half of the families felt that they were not giving their child a good enough diet, and food cost was the most common reason given for this. More than half of the parents had gone without food themselves to ensure that their child had had enough to eat and, as a result, over 40% had been hungry themselves in the previous month.

The NCH survey also found that families were having other financial problems apart from not being able to afford to feed themselves. Nearly three quarters of the families were behind in paying their bills or other payments, and this compounded the problem of finding enough money for food. When the quality of the families' diets were assessed by means of a food frequency questionnaire, none conformed with a pattern of healthy eating.

Other studies carried out in recent years have made similar findings. Lang *et al* (1984) interviewed 1000 people in the North of England living on low incomes (two thirds of whom were living on less than £50 a week) and reported that a third of the participants were eating inadequate diets; 37% of those who were unemployed had gone without food at some time in the previous year because they could not afford it, and 10% of all participants said that they did not usually have enough money for food all week. Food was one of the first items they cut back on when short of cash, despite the fact that the main budget priorities were housing, fuel and food.

In 1989 the Health Education Authority published its own study on the eating habits of low income families based on interviews with 47 households in South London, Sheffield and Liverpool (HEA 1989). Families with children were shown to be planning their spending very carefully and consistently in order to meet their household's basic needs. Because they were aware that money could easily be spent on non-essentials, there was a tendency to buy a week's or a fortnight's food soon after receiving the benefit. This often used up about 50% of their income. To minimize the frustration of shopping on a low budget, the families tended to use a 'tunnel vision' approach to buying food, shopping quickly and looking only for familiar items. As a result choices tended to be habitual and it was rare for the families to experiment. When choosing food the most important factors tended to be price, ease and speed of preparation and family acceptability. Most of the families ate relatively large amounts of convenience foods such as burgers and fish fingers because they were popular with the children, easy to budget for, relatively cheap, and simple to prepare. Most of the families were cooking from raw food only once or twice a week, the main problems of cooking from basics being the difficulty of budgeting, the cost of the food, the fear of waste and lack of confidence in their cooking skills. For single people, price was the most important factor to influence their choice of food. Most of the people involved in the survey were bored with their diet and felt frustrated by the lack of choice. Almost all would have liked to eat a wider variety of foods and to have been able to afford better quality lean, tender meat. More fruit, salad and cheese would also have been desirable for reasons of both enjoyability and health. As a general rule, the less money the lower the morale and the shorter the perspective on health for the family. Lack of money appeared to be the main barrier to further change towards a low-fat, high-fibre diet.

Similar findings to those of the HEA were reported by Malseed (1990) in a survey conducted in the North of England.

In recent years, many families in Britain have found themselves on a reduced income as a result of the rise in unemployment and the effects of economic recession. Most of the findings in the above studies relate to people living on Income Support; in 1991, approximately 8 million people in Britain were dependent on this benefit. Income Support is given to people who are not working and for whom unemployment benefit is not available or insufficient to live on. The 1992 level of Income Support for a family of two adults and two children is £105.00 which has to cover their poll tax contribution, water rates, bills and loan repayments as well as all households needs. Young adults not living at home are no longer entitled to any benefits at all and increased numbers of such people live on the streets in big cities.

What is the problem?

Ill-health and premature mortality are significantly increased among the unemployed and those on low incomes compared with those who are better-off (Davey-Smith *et al* 1990; Cole-Hamilton 1991). Many of the health problems experienced are diet-related. Low birth weight, perinatal mortality and morbidity rates and birth anomalies are relatively high amongst disadvantaged groups and all can be influenced by diet, particularly in the pre-conceptual period and during early pregnancy (Doyle *et al* 1989). Children from low income families tend to be shorter (DoH 1989), more obese (Garman *et al* 1982; RCP 1983) and to have poorer dental health (Schou *et al* 1991) than their more advantaged peers.

An analysis of National Food Survey data from the late 1980s (MAFF 1989) shows that food intake is closely related to both income level and the number of children in the household. Households on low incomes eat considerably less cheese, carcase meat, meat in total, butter, cooking oils, fresh and frozen vegetables, fresh fruit and wholemeal bread than higher income groups. This effect is sometimes compounded by the presence of children. For example, households with three or more children in the lowest income group eat less than half the amount of fruit consumed by similar households in the highest income group. In households with adults only, the lower income groups eat significantly less fruit but the difference is not as great.

Low income households also tend to eat more of the relatively cheap foods with a high sugar and fat content and which are energy dense (Table 3.34). This suggests that the diet of people with low incomes are likely to be lower in dietary fibre, vitamin C, beta carotene, folic acid, vitamin E, and possibly zinc, and higher in sugar than the diet of people from higher income groups. A recent Government survey on the diets of British adults (Gregory *et al* 1990) found similar differences in diet according to income and employment status. Analysis of national food survey data over the 1980s shows that all groups of people have made some changes to their eating patterns but those in the lowest income groups have made the smallest changes towards healthier eating patterns.

The problems of availability and price

The potential problems of poor nutrition amongst people from disadvantaged households are likely to be primarily connected with the relative price and availability of healthy food; people can only eat the food available in accessible shops and at a price they can afford. These problems will be compounded by other needs and priorities as well as lack of access to relevant useful information. On average the highest income groups recorded in the 1990 Family Expenditure Survey (CSO 1991) spent over one and a half times as much on food as the low income households.

In some large cities there is rapid expansion by major retailing chains of 'Superstores' (London Food Commission 1985). These are increasingly situated away from local shopping centres and in areas of relative affluence. At the same time smaller supermarkets owned by these retailing chains are being run down. The result is that in deprived inner city areas the main food shops are the smaller, relatively expensive supermarkets and grocers' shops. Some of the retailing chains actually have pricing policies which result in prices for some products being higher in small, local shops than in large superstores (London Food Commission 1985).

At the same time the type of foods currently encouraged for a healthy diet are often relatively expensive. For example wholemeal bread can be 25% more expensive than white; reduced fat cheese, wholewheat pasta, brown rice, fresh fruit and many fresh vegetables are all comparatively expensive. Table 3.34 shows that these are the types of food lacking in the diets of people on low incomes. The availability of these foods in many small shops is also often limited.

Cheaper foods are not necessarily better value for money. For example, cheap cuts of meat tend to be fattier than more expensive cuts and use more fuel in cooking. Similarly, even though many beans and pulses are considerably cheaper than meat, and have the added advantages of being low in fat and high in fibre, the fuel costs involved in cooking them must be taken into consideration. Chips cook more quickly than boiled potatoes and take considerably less fuel than jacket potatoes, while crisps present no fuel costs at all.

Table 3.34 Relative amounts of different foods eaten by low income households compared with high income households (MAFF 1989)

Relative consumption		
More	Less	No consistent difference*
Meat products	Cheese	Milk
Margarine	Carcass meat	Poultry
Lard	Total meat	Fish
Sugar	Butter	Total fat
Jam	Cooking oils	Cakes and biscuits
Potatoes	Fresh and frozen vegetables	
Canned vegetables (including baked beans)	Fresh fruit	
White bread	Wholemeal bread	
Total bread		

* Although there were differences, in some sized households they were higher, and in others lower

A study which examined individual diet histories from people on low incomes in the North of England, revealed diets which could well lead to nutritional problems (Lang *et al* 1984). Blaxter and Paterson (1982) when discussing their work into social class, poverty and nutrition concluded:

> 'Thus cultural, commercial and practical pressures dictated dietary habits. . . . This study suggested that poverty can be defined in terms of constraints upon choice, and powerlessness over the environment. In the circumstances of deprived lives, certain behaviours – from early childbearing to patterns of eating – are inevitable. The 'culture of poverty' is a concept now largely discredited, if it implies simply persisting subcultural beliefs and behaviours. However, the very practical constraints of poverty remain.'

3.8.2 Practical advice from dietitians

Often the main items of expenditure in the household food budget of low income groups are processed foods such as meat pies, fish fingers, sausages, bacon, breakfast cereals, biscuits, cakes and other convenience and canned foods. The price of foods such as these varies widely, but the cheaper ones are usually high in fat, sugar or salt and low in dietary fibre.

With very careful shopping and the use of relatively cheap foods such as dried pulses and larger amounts of potatoes instead of bought pies, etc. it is possible for a healthy diet to cost no more, and sometimes less, than an unhealthy one (Leverkus *et al* 1985). But this may not be the case if food expenditure is already low, however carefully menus are planned or budgeted. A NACNE diet costed by the London Food Commission cost 50% more than the average diet consumed by households with low incomes (Cole-Hamilton and Lang 1986). The NCH survey showed that the cost of a healthy diet is more expensive than a less healthy one in all parts of the country and especially in rural areas (NCH 1991). Since people on low incomes have little or no means of increasing their expenditure on food, consuming a healthier diet necessitates drastic changes in eating patterns, cooking techniques and the type of food consumed. Such changes may be neither acceptable nor practicable. If people are asking for this type of advice then it should, of course, be given. For some people, however, these concepts are totally inappropriate and of little interest. Like many people, they do not want to spend time shopping round, preparing cheap foods which take longer to cook, and eating the sort of diet which has long been associated with poverty. There is no justifiable reason why poverty should force a person to eat differently from anyone else.

Social Security benefits

Dietitians can greatly assist those on low incomes by helping them find out if they are receiving all the welfare benefits to which they are entitled. Millions of pounds of benefits go unclaimed every year. Dietitians cannot be expected to investigate in detail whether every individual is receiving their full entitlement of benefits but they should have some knowledge of benefits currently available should and be able to tell people where they can get advice.

Since 1988, when the benefit system changed, most people who are either unemployed or in low paid jobs are entitled to one of two benefits. Income Support is available to people who are not in work whether or not they have families. Unemployment Benefit at a flat rate is available to people who are unemployed, available for work and who have paid enough National Insurance contributions to qualify for it. In 1992, both Unemployment Benefit and Income Support for a single adult were around £40 a week. Housing costs are paid separately and in addition to this.

Family Credit is available to families with children whose income from work is below a certain level. The calculation for working out Family Credit is very complicated and only about half those families entitled to receive it actually claim. There are some advantages to being on Income Support in that any children in the family are entitled to free school meals, milk and vitamins. These are not available to those on Family Credit or Unemployment Benefit. However, all families on Income Support, Unemployment Benefit and Family Credit are entitled to free prescriptions, dental and eye checks.

Before 1988 it was possible to get additional payments for special needs, for example for food for special diets. Since 1988 these have no longer been available and if a family or person living on Income Support needs extra money, for example to replace a worn-out cooker, they have to apply for a loan from the Social Fund. This has to be repaid and the money is deducted over a period of time from their Income Support. In exceptional circumstances (for example, a person returning to the community from prison) a person may be entitled to a Community Care Grant which does not have to be repaid. However, Community Care Grants are difficult to get. Neither the Community Care Grant nor Social Fund Loan is a statutory entitlement; their provision is at the personal discretion of the local Social Security Officer. Furthermore, the budgets for Community Care Grants and Social Fund Loans are cash limited which means that if they run out before the end of the financial year, then subsequent applicants will be unable to receive anything.

There are a wide range of benefits available to people with disabilities whether or not they are in work.

More information about the benefit system can be obtained from the Citizen's Advice Bureaux and local law centres, where these exist. The Child Poverty Action Group (CPAG) annually produces two inexpensive publications giving details of all benefits available, eligibility and how to apply for them (CPAG 1992a; 1992b). These are available from bookshops or direct from CPAG. The Department of Social Security also produces a number of leaflets which give information about different types of benefits.

Dietary advice

The type of dietary advice given to individuals and groups will depend very much on their own needs and interests.

Dietitians must be aware of what foods are available in the local shops and their relative prices. They must also assess the individual's cooking skills and interest in food preparation.

Ideally, *everyone* should be able to afford healthy, convenience foods. This unfortunately is not the case at present and, until it is, dietary advice has to be realistic and sensitive. As stated previously, fuel costs are an important consideration and both the gas and electricity boards provide leaflets and information about economizing on fuel during cooking. Supplies of these leaflets could be held in dietetic departments. Some foods being recommended may be unfamiliar and involve new cooking practices. Demonstrations and tasting sessions are useful if the facilities exist.

Lang *et al* (1984) showed that parents, newspapers and magazines were important for the role they played in teaching people 'how to manage' and 'what was good for them'. Dietitians should use these media when possible. Interesting, quick, easy, cheap recipes and meals in a regular column in a local free newspaper could reach thousands of people. Lang *et al* (1984) also found that when people were really short of money they tended to eat, firstly, sandwiches, toast or bread (white bread); then eggs; then beans and chips. Dietitians could provide information about inexpensive sandwich fillings and spreads.

Lean meat is considerably more expensive than fatty meat and in the past dietitians have often advised that cheap meat is 'just as good for you' as expensive meat. This advice should now be turned on its head and people advised that a small amount of lean meat is 'much better for you, and more economical to cook, than a larger amount of fatty meat costing the same.

Ways of increasing the nutritional quality of the diet, which may save money as well, include:

1 Using less meat and more vegetables in stews and casseroles.
2 Using as little fat or oil in cooking as possible.
3 Using natural yoghurt instead of cream.
4 Using skimmed or semi-skimmed milk instead of whole milk.
5 Using lentils, peas and dried beans to replace some of the meat in mince dishes.
6 Having larger portions of potatoes, rice or starchy vegetables with smaller portions of meat or meat products.
7 Spreading butter or margarine thinly on thick slices of bread (rather than the other way round).
8 Making stale bread into breadcrumbs which can be used for meat loaves, rissoles and stuffings.
9 Grating cheese for salads and sandwiches. Grated cheese goes much further than sliced.
10 Using a small amount of a very strong cheese in a cheese sauce rather than a larger amount of a mild cheese.
11 Buying fruit and vegetables in small quantities to avoid storing them.
12 Being careful not to buy too many sweets, cakes and biscuits.
13 Avoiding convenience foods with little nutritional value such as instant meals in pots, sweet dessert mixes and sweet drinks.

These need to be offset against increased costs such as wholegrain products, reduced fat cheeses, extra fresh fruit and more vegetables.

Shopping advice

When giving advice about shopping it is important to remember that people with low incomes not only have a limited amount to spend on food each week, but also that this problem is compounded by the fact that small quantities are often relatively more expensive, local shops are usually dearer than superstores, transport facilities are often poor in deprived areas and there is insufficient money to buy in the quantities needed to justify a trip to a big, cheaper shop. These problems are not easily resolved but a few tips which may be useful are:

1 Make a list of all the most important items and buy those first.
2 Try to think ahead to avoid wastage and to make sure there is no need to go to more expensive shops outside normal opening times.
3 Share shopping trips with friends and neighbours to make better use of transport.
4 If it is cheaper to buy in larger quantities, share products with friends and neighbours and split the costs between you. Setting up small buying co-operatives can be a useful form of social contact as well as making food cheaper.
5 Be careful not to buy bruised or damaged fruit or vegetables as, although these may be cheaper, they deteriorate more quickly and the vitamin content is lower.
6 Shopping last thing in the afternoon (especially on a Saturday) often means the price of perishable goods is reduced.

Food preparation

Time and fuel costs are as important to most people as maintaining the nutritional quality of the food. Cost can be kept down by:

1 Eating more raw fruit and vegetables.
2 Cooking vegetables very rapidly in a small amount of water.
3 Stir frying vegetables in a small amount of oil.
4 Grilling tender lean meat rather than stewing tough fatty meats.

5 Sharing meals with friends and neighbours. This cuts costs and increases social contact.

Summary

Dietitians cannot alleviate poverty directly but they can, by means of sensitive and appropriate advice, help to minimize some of its likely nutritional consequences. In addition, dietitians have a general responsibility to highlight the nutritional problems which can result from a low income to the policy makers and planners.

Useful addresses

Child Poverty Action Group, 4th Floor, 1–5 Bath Street, London EC1V 9PY, Tel. 071–253 3406.

The Food Commission, 102 Gloucester Place, London WC1, Tel. 071–935 9078.

NCH, Highbury Grove, London N1.

References

Blaxter M and Paterson E (1982) Social class, poverty and nutrition. In *Food and people.* Turner M (Ed) John Libbey, London.

Central Statistical Office (1991) *Family Spending: a report on the 1990 Family Expenditure Survey.* HMSO, London.

Child Poverty Action Group (1992a) *National welfare benefits handbook.* Unwins, London.

Child Poverty Action Group (1992b) *Rights guide to non-means-tested benefits.* Unwins, London.

Cole-Hamilton I (1991) *Poverty can seriously damage your health – a response to the green paper 'The Health of the Nation'.* Child Poverty Action Group, London.

Cole-Hamilton I and Lang TML (1986) *Low income and food.* The Food Commission, London.

Davey-Smith G, Bartley M and Blane D (1990) The Black Report on socio-inequalities in health, 10 years on. *Br Med J* **301**, 373–7.

Department of Health (1989) *The Diet of British School Children.* Rep Hlth Soc Subj 36. HMSO, London.

Doyle W, Crawford MA, Wynn HA and Wynn SW (1989) Maternal nutrient intake and birth weight. *J Hum Nutr Dietet* **2**, 415–22.

Garman AR, Chinn S and Rona RJ (1982) Comparative growth of primary school-children from one and two parent families. *Arch Dis Childh* **57**, 453–8.

Gregory J, Foster K, Tyler H and Wiseman M (1990) *The Dietary and Nutritional Survey of British Adults.* Office of Population Census and Survey – Social Survey Division HMSO, London.

Health Education Authority (1989) *Diet, nutrition and healthy eating in low income groups.* HEA, London.

Horsnell M (1991) Children of poor going hungry. *The Times*, Tuesday 4 June, 1991.

Lang *et al* (1984) *Jam Tomorrow.* Food Policy Unit, Hollings Faculty, Manchester Polytechnic, Manchester 14.

Leverkus C, Cole-Hamilton I, Gunner K, Starr J and Stanway A (1985) *The Great British Diet.* British Dietetic Association, Birmingham.

London Food Commission (1985) *Access to food stores in London: a pilot study of three large retailers.* A report commissioned from CES Ltd. LFC, London.

Malseed J (1990) *Bread without dough: understanding food poverty.* Horton Publishing, Bradford.

Ministry of Agriculture, Fisheries and Food (1989) *Household food consumption and expenditure.* Annual Report of the National Food Survey Committee. HMSO, London.

NCH (1991) Poverty and Nutrition Survey. NCH, London.

Royal College of Physicians (1983) Obesity. *J Roy Coll Physcns Lond* **17**, 3–58.

Schou L *et al* (1991). Deprivation and dental health. The benefits of a child's dental health campaign in relation to deprivation as estimated by the uptake of free meals at school. *Community Dental Health* **8**, 147–54.

3.9 Black and minority ethnic communities

Britain today is referred to as a multiracial and multicultural society. Over 2 million citizens in the UK belong to ethnic minority groups (Goodwin *et al* 1987). The largest group – over one and a quarter million – comprises people from the Indian sub-continent, South Asians, who are often loosely referred to as *Asians*. About 600 000 Afro-Caribbeans are currently resident in Britain.

The group has brought with it diverse cultures and habits. This necessitates the provision of medical care which takes the different practices into account. Tailoring of dietary advice is always an integral part of the dietitian's work and this is especially important when advising patients from different ethnic backgrounds.

Eating patterns may be influenced by a number of factors, namely:

1 Religious beliefs or other strongly held principles.
2 Cultural background and ethnic origins.
3 Availability of traditional foods.
4 Time constraints.
5 The belief that the Western way of life (and hence diet) is superior.

Health professionals need to acquire sound knowledge and understanding of the diet, religious beliefs, cultural habits, lifestyle and attitudes in order to ensure that dietary instruction fits in with traditional customs and eating habits. The use of visual aids such as photographs, video cassettes, audio-cassettes and model foods can provide more effective dietary education than leaflets and diet sheets. Health flash cards have been used in the Third World, and this may be an area worth exploring.

It is important to ask patients about their food choices rather than to make assumptions. For example, it should not be assumed that all Hindus are vegetarians nor that all Muslims do not drink alcohol. Similarly, not all Asians will observe the traditional fasts.

3.9.1 Asian diets

General features

This is a heterogeneous group. There is great cultural diversity between the different Asian groups, and even within the same group. There is also variation within the same household.

The middle aged and elderly Asians are usually first-generation immigrants. They are held in great respect and are generally more resistant to change and tend to be more orthodox. The younger population and working adults have adapted to a fast and convenient way of life. Exposure to Western foods has resulted in younger members of the family demanding such foods at home in preference to traditional meals. English is the main language spoken by the younger Asian population.

The extended family is the centre of all Asian cultures. In the UK, living together is less practical; however, family members may join each other for an evening meal several times a week.

The prevalence of diabetes has been shown to be some four times higher in Asians than in Europeans (Mather and Keen 1985). Ischaemic heart disease is common and HDL cholesterol levels have been shown to be lower in the Asian population (McKeigue *et al* 1989). The high prevalence of diabetes and coronary heart disease may be related to central obesity in this population. As waist-to-hip ratio increases, the prevalence of diabetes and coronary heart disease appears to be higher (McKeigue *et al* 1991). Thus distribution of obesity may be significant in this group.

Being overweight is often considered to be a sign of affluence and good health in Asian societies. The cultural ideal of body weight favours a rounder shape than that desired by Europeans. Thus, there is no great social pressure to lose weight.

Rickets and osteomalacia may be common among Asian immigrants (see Section 4.27).

Religious beliefs

Religion is considered to be a way of life. The three main religions of Asians living in the UK are Hinduism, Islam (the religion of Muslims) and Sikhism. Each has its specific dietary restrictions but there are some points in common.

Hindus

Hinduism is founded on reverence for life, non-violence and a belief in reincarnation. Because they will not kill, many Hindus are strict vegetarians. They believe in many Gods and Goddesses. Most Hindus in Britain have come from Gujarat on the North-West coast of India; some come from the Indian Punjab and East Africa. Their first language is likely to be Gujarati.

Naming system The Hindu naming system consists of: a first name, used by family and friends; a complementary name, used only with the first name and never on its own; and a subcaste name which is used like a British surname.

It is the subcaste name which indicates the religion. The most frequently used Hindu subcaste name in Britain is 'Patel'.

Food restrictions

1 Most Hindus will not eat meat or fish of any kind. Less strict Hindus (particularly men) may eat lamb, chicken or white fish.
2 Very strict Hindus may not eat eggs since they are potentially a source of life.
3 Fats such as dripping or lard are not acceptable. Ghee (clarified butter) and vegetable oil are used in cooking.
4 Strict Hindus will be unwilling to eat food unless they are certain that the utensils used in preparation and service have not been in contact with meat or fish.

Festivals and fasting Three festivals in the Hindu calendar are observed as fast days:

1 Mahashivrati – the birthday of Lord Shiva (March).
2 Ram Naumi – the birthday of Lord Rama (April).
3 Jan Mash Tami – the birthday of Lord Krishna (late August).

Additionally, some devout Hindus will fast on one or two days a week. The fast is observed from dawn to sunset. During this time some Hindus will eat 'pure' foods such as yoghurt and fruit, whilst others forego all food and may take fluids only. It is a matter of individual preference.

Two important festivals where an abundance of rich food is available are *Holi* and *Diwali*.

Muslims

The religion of Muslims is Islam. Muslims believe in one God, *Allah*. There are five main principles, known as the 'pillars of Islam', one of which is to fast during the month of Ramadan. The Muslim community in Britain comes mainly from Pakistan, Bangladesh and East Africa, with a smaller number from the Middle East, Malaysia and Indonesia. Many Muslims of Indian origin will speak Punjabi, Mirpuri or Bengali, but some speak Urdu and Gujarati.

Naming system This is complex and needs detailed study for a full understanding (see the *Asian names and records* training pack, details of which are given in the Further Reading list). The personal name, which has its origin in religion, is not usually the first name listed. Each person also has a Muslim title which is never a personal name. The principal Muslim titles are Abdul, Allah, Mohammed, Shah, Syed and Ullah (spellings may vary). Khan and Chaudry are frequently used titles amongst Muslims from Pakistan. It is quite usual to use the title followed by the personal name when addressing someone. Bibi, Begum and Khatoon occur in some female names and signify the sex of the bearer. Members of the same family may not share a common family name, nor does a woman always take her husband's name on marriage (Thomas 1988).

Food restrictions In the Islamic tradition all wholesome things may be used for food and the general rule is that every food is lawful (*Halal*) unless it is declared unlawful (*Haram*).

Unlawful foods are:

1 Foods and food products from the pig. Manufactured foods which contain animal fat or gelatine may be rejected.
2 All meat which has not been ritually slaughtered (Kosher meat is acceptable).
3 Alcohol, including that used in cooking.

It should be noted that a Muslim may refuse a food if he cannot be sure that it does not contain an unlawful ingredient. Similarly, a devout Muslim will be concerned that the dishes used for cooking have not been in contact with unlawful foods.

Festivals and fasting There are two major festivals in the Muslim calendar:

1 Id-al Fitr marks the end of the month of Ramadan, and celebrations are held both in the community and at home.
2 Id-al Adha commemorates the pilgrimage to Mecca and is celebrated, by those who can afford it, by the sacrifice of a lamb and sharing the meat amongst family, friends and the poor.

Muslims are required to fast from dawn to sunset during the month of Ramadan, which is the ninth month of the Muslim calendar. Fasting involves abstinence from all food and drink. Feelings of weakness and lethargy often occur as a result of this abstinence and, to help overcome this, most Muslims rise early and eat a substantial high carbohydrate meal before dawn. Another heavy meal is taken after sunset. Old people and children under 12 are exempt from fasting. Women who are pregnant, breast feeding or menstruating and people who are ill or travelling during Ramadan are exempt from fasting, but are expected to compensate by fasting at some other time. Special exemption can be granted for chronically ill people for whom fasting would by physically harmful. Ramadan fasting did not have a deleterious effect on a group of non-insulin dependent diabetics studied in Bombay (Chandalia *et al* 1987).

Sikhs

Sikhism began as an offshoot of Hinduism and Islam and has developed into a religion in its own right. Sikhs believe in one personal God, with whom each Sikh must make his own relationship and through that lead a virtuous, useful life in the community. The five signs of a Sikh man are uncut hair, a special comb, a bangle, a dagger and a particular type of underwear. Orthodox Sikh men will wear turbans and grow a beard. Younger men are generally clean shaven. The Sikh temple or 'Gurdwara' serves three meals daily and most people will partake in one of these meals. Most Sikhs in Britain originate from the Punjab, but some come from East Africa. Their first language is Punjabi but many speak English.

Naming system All Sikh men have a first or personal name plus *Singh*. All women have a first or personal name plus *Kaur*. Additionally a Sikh family may adopt a hereditary family name.

Food restrictions For Sikhs this is a matter for each individual's conscience. As a group they are less strict than Hindus and Muslims, but for each Sikh their own self-imposed restrictions are binding. Some Sikhs, (especially women), are vegetarian, but many eat chicken, lamb and fish. They are unlikely to eat beef and even less likely to eat pork. Alcohol is forbidden, but its consumption is becoming increasingly common, particularly amongst men.

Festivals and fasting There are three main festivals in the Sikh calendar:

1 Baisakhi – the Sikh New Year's Day (April).
2 Diwali – the Festival of Light (October/November).
3 Birth of Guru Nanak – the founder of Sikhism (November).

Some devout Sikhs fast once or twice a week.

Dietary practices of Asian people

'Hot' and 'Cold' foods

This bears no relationship to the temperature or spiciness of a food or the temperature at which it is served. It is believed to be an inherent property of the food itself.

Hot foods are thought to increase body temperature, excite the emotions and increase activity. Conversely, *cold foods* reduce body temperature and impart strength and cheerfulness. Normally, a diet containing a mixture of hot and cold foods would be consumed. However, hot foods are generally restricted during 'hot' conditions (e.g. mangos are restricted during pregnancy). The intake of cold foods is controlled during 'cold' conditions (e.g. potatoes are consumed only in small amounts during lactation). This belief could be a potential problem if nutritious foods are restricted in vulnerable people. For example, dairy product consumption may be reduced in people who have asthma or arthritis. A consequently lower calcium intake may be significant in the elderly patient. Table 3.35 gives some examples of hot and cold foods, although all Asian groups do not necessarily agree on which foods come under which category.

Food preparation

1 Vegetables are cooked in fat or water.
2 Fat in the form of oil or *ghee* (clarified butter) is an integral part of Indian cooking. Spices and onions are often fried in fat before the main ingredients are added.
3 Spices are used individually (e.g. turmeric or *haldi*) or in specific combinations (e.g. *garam masala*). Curry powder, as used in Britain is not comparable. Freshly ground garlic, ginger and green chillies are commonly used.
4 Home-made pickles and chutneys often accompany main course dishes. These may contain *gur* (unprocessed rock sugar) and oil.
5 Yoghurt is served as an accompaniment with main meals either plain or spicy (*raita*). The yoghurt is often home made from whole milk.
6 Home made curd cheese (*paneer*) is quite unlike the cheese used in Britain. The nearest equivalent is cottage cheese.
7 Eggs are usually eaten hard boiled, curried or fried.
8 Considerable use is made of pulses, seeds and nuts.
9 Side salads, especially of raw onion and tomato, are frequently eaten at main meals. If dressed, a vinegar or lemon-based dressing would be used.
10 People from South India and Sri Lanka may use coconut (cream, milk or powder) in cooking.

Dietary constituents

Principal staple foods are wheat, rice and pulses. Dairy products are usually widely consumed. *Chapatis*, the main type of Indian bread, are generally made from 85% extraction wheat flour. They are unleavened and may contain oil and/or salt in the dough. Ghee is often spread on the surface of chapatis, particularly if they are prepared in advance of the meal. The thickness and size varies according to the region of origin. Gujarati chapatis are normally thin and small, whereas Punjabi chapatis tend to be thick and large.

Rice is often boiled, although fried varieties are eaten at weekends and special occasions. The consumption of brown rice is minimal, despite the fact that brown *basmati* rice is now widely available.

The wide variety of pulses comes in different colours, shapes and textures. They can be cooked to varying consistencies ranging from a watery soup to a thick puree or even a whole bean/lentil dish. Examples of commonly used pulses or *dahls* are *mung*, *urad*, *toor*, *masur*, *channa*, black eyed beans and kidney beans. People with diabetes may make a point of eating *karela*, a bitter vegetable which is known to have a hypoglycaemic effect (Baylis and Dattani 1986).

Table 3.35 Examples of 'hot' and 'cold' foods (Source: British Diabetic Association Asian Diet Information Pack)

Food group	Hot	Cold
Cereal		Wheat Rice
Green leafy vegetables		All
Root vegetables	Carrot Onion	Potato
Other vegetables	Capsicum Pepper Aubergine/brinjal	Most other vegetables including cucumbers beans, cauliflower marrow, gourds, ladies fingers or okra
Fruit	Dates Mango Pawpaw/papaya	All other fruits e.g. apple, orange, melon etc
Animal products	Meats — including chicken, mutton, fish	
Dairy products	Eggs	
Milk products		Milk and cream Curds or yoghurt Buttermilk
Pulses	Lentils	Bengalgram or chickpea Greengram peas, redgram
Nuts		All types including ground or peanuts cashew nuts
Spices and condiments	Chilli, green and powder Cinnamon Clove Garlic Ginger Hing Mustard Nutmeg Pepper	Coriander Cumin Cardomon Fennel or Variali Tamarind
Oils	Mustard	Butter, ghee or clarified butter coconut oil groundnut oil
Miscellaneous	Tea Coffee Honey Jaggery/brown sugar	

Indian sweetmeats are widely consumed during festivities, which are held frequently. Sweetmeats are prepared using a combination of sugar, ghee, full cream milk powder, nuts, flour and sweetened condensed milk. One small portion can provide 450 kcal (Govindji 1988).

Sugary drinks such as cola or Lucozade are consumed often (Peterson *et al* 1986) and sugar may be routinely added to Indian tea.

The meal pattern

Breakfast Yoghurt with rice or chapatis, *or* leftover curry and chapatis from the previous evening meal, *or* egg with bread *or* cereal with milk. Tea with hot milk and sugar. Poories and parathas (deep-fried Indian breads) may be consumed at weekends.

Main meals Rice or chapatis; meat or fish dish if acceptable; several vegetable or pulse dishes; pickles; side salad; yoghurt; fresh fruit such as mango, pawpaw or banana.

Variations occur within this pattern but in general the variety of dishes used is less than in a typical British menu cycle.

Snacks These are often deep fried and the oil is re-used. Examples are samosas, pakoras (e.g. onion bhajia) chevda (similar to Bombay mix).

Customs associated with meals

1 Hands are always washed before and after meals.

2 Many people like to rinse their mouths with water after a meal.

3 It is customary in Asia to use the right hand for picking up food at the table.
4 Strict vegetarians will not wish to use china or utensils which may have been in contact with meat or fish.

Many Asian cookery books give useful information on the food habits and customs of the country concerned.

Dietary management of diabetes and obesity

Dietary modification

Diabetes and obesity are common problems among Asians in the UK, where many Asians consume a high-fat, a low-fibre, high refined carbohydrate diet (Peterson *et al* 1986). Modification of the diet to make it in line with national dietary recommendations can be achieved by promoting traditional Asian eating habits. Table 3.36 provides some practical suggestions for dietary advice. Patients may not be keen to comply and are generally known to prefer medicines. Compliance can be enhanced if the foods promoted are widely available and acceptable to the group. For example, a strict Muslim is less able to reduce his intake of saturated fat if lean *Halal* meat is not available. It is important to find out which group predominates in the local area and tailor the advice accordingly.

Pulse dishes are high in soluble fibre, they have a low glycaemic index and a hypocholesterolaemic effect. There is a lack of accurate and comprehensive nutrition composition data on cooked Asian foods and assessment of dietary fibre is particularly difficult. However, the intake of fibre is likely to be higher than the UK national average of 20 g/day (Baylis and Dattani 1986).

Barriers to communication

Many clinics with substantial numbers of Asian patients did not provide facilities specifically for this group in the 1984 survey of British diabetic clinics (Goodwin *et al* 1987). Patient anxiety, lack of basic understanding of the condition and uncertainty about the need for dietary modification can act as strong deterrents to receiving instruction. Further, Asian patients may not feel respected, since they consider that they are given less time than white patients (Hawthorne 1990).

The health professional needs to win the trust and confidence of the patient. Any information given must make sense and the use of jargon or an inappropriate level of language is undesirable. Introducing names of some common Asian foods (Table 3.37) may improve rapport. Non-verbal communication is important, particularly if very little verbal understanding is apparent.

The use of an interpreter can be extremely valuable in cases where very little English is understood. When using interpreters, the following points should be borne in mind:
1 The interpreter may not understand what the dietitian is saying, therefore language needs to be appropriate to the interpreter as well as the patient.
2 The interpreter may not be able to translate accurately since some words may not have an equivalent in the Asian language.
3 It is not unlikely that the interpreter will give out some of his or her own advice, and may neglect to pass on some of the more important advice.
4 The patient may not feel comfortable relating to an interpreter if personal lifestyle and habits are being exposed.
5 Using a porter or a domestic worker in the hospital is undesirable. Time is usually limited and there is a lack of interest and commitment. The person may also be known to the patient and there may be class differences.
6 Using a member of the family may not always be appropriate. This is particularly the case when a young child is used as an interpreter, or when a man is used to

Table 3.36 Dietary advice for Asian diabetic or overweight patients (Govindji 1991)

Practical advice on reducing fat	Use less ghee or oil during cooking and in spreading. Measure the amount of fat added with tablespoons, and gradually reduce the total quantity used. Choose polyunsaturated oils (corn, sunflower or safflower oil), monounsaturated oils (olive oil, rapeseed or peanut oil) and polyunsaturated margarine or low-fat spreads wherever possible. Try making ghee with a mixture of butter and polyunsaturated margarine Save fried snacks for special occasions only Buy lean meat, trimming off any visible fat before cooking Eat boiled rice routinely, and fried rice only occasionally Choose low-fat dairy products
Practical advice on reducing sugar	Try to eat sweetmeats on special occasions only Do not add gur to curries and pickles Replace sugar and gur with artificial sweeteners e.g. aspartame Choose low-calorie and diet drinks in preference to sugared fizzy drinks
Practical advice on increasing fibre intake	Revert to traditional eating habits by including dahls, vegetarian dishes and wholemeal chapatis into meals as often as possible Choose wholemeal or granary bread, high-fibre breakfast cereals and brown rice in preference to the more refined low-fibre varieties Eat more vegetables, particularly with their skins (e.g. jacket potatoes) Choose fresh fruit instead of fruit juice

Table 3.37 Names of some common Asian foods (Peterson and Govindji 1988)

Indian breads	Chapati Paratha Naan Rotla
Sweetmeals (mithai)	Burfi Halwa Jalebi Gulab juman
Rice dishes	Biryani Pulau Kheer (dessert)
Fried snacks	Samosa Chevda Ganthia Sev Pakora Bhajia

interpret to a female patient. If using a member of the family, it is important to try to choose an equal. Even then, confidentiality and sensitivity is a problem.

A skilled interpreter is needed as part of the health care team. One-to-one teaching with the professional, the patient and the interpreter is ideal, although it may not be time or cost-effective. Teaching sessions may be valuable especially if the group uses a common language. In this case, one interpreter, and a video cassette in one language would be sufficient. If the group is varied, then Hindi would be the most appropriate language to choose since Indian films are produced in Hindi and these are generally widely understood. Non-attendance has been reported to be a problem and perhaps holding teaching sessions in local community centres would be more successful. If these are held in collaboration with a respected and well-known elder within the community, participation by local residents may be enhanced. It must not be forgotten, however, that some people within the group may not understand, or may not be confident enough, to share personal problems.

In a study by Hawthorne (1990) on Asian patients with diabetes, none of the men had been given dietary advice. Also, very few patients realized and understood the relationship between control of diabetes and complications.

There is some controversy over whether information in different Asian languages is useful. Some people believe that if patients can read their own language, they can generally also read English. This is not necessarily the case. If information in both languages is available, the patient is likely to prefer reading in his or her own language. Such material may not be requested, perhaps because it could be considered to be an insult to their intelligence.

There is a definite desire for more education, which suggests that the lack of knowledge by Asian patients is not due to indifference (Hawthorne 1990).

Dietary motivation

Many Asians who have lived in the UK for some time speak English fluently, and work as professionals integrating well within the host community. Factors which can affect motivation include lifestyle, budgets, hierarchy within the family and social pressures. A young daughter-in-law living within an orthodox extended family may not be able to modify her diet and cooking methods if her mother-in-law governs what is bought and how it is cooked. Similarly, a woman may not have a desire to lose weight if her husband finds rounded women more attractive. All dietary advice should be tailored to the individual. When counselling Asian patients, it is important to establish whether social pressures within the home govern that person's ability and desire to modify his or her diet.

Dietary advice should ideally involve discussion of the place food has within the household, who does the cooking and the shopping. It may be helpful for the dietitian to invite another member of the family to the dietary interview so that such information can be acquired. Diet sheets have limited use and a relaxed conversation with more interactive visual aids is likely to be more effective.

It is essential to stress that traditional Asian foods should be included regularly, and methods of cooking must be discussed in order to encourage low-fat meals. Follow-up as always is essential.

Appropriate teaching methods, effective educational material and a reliable, sensitive and confidential interpreter service are only a few of the areas which still need careful exploring.

3.9.2 Afro-Caribbean diets

The name Afro-Caribbean collectively refers to people of African descent who come from the many Caribbean islands. The majority of people from the Caribbean moved to the UK during the 1950s and 1960s, notably from Jamaica (HEA 1991).

When discussing the Caribbean diet, it is important to remember that the people of the Caribbean are not a homogeneous group. Dietary practices of each island have been influenced by different historical, political, social and geographical factors. For example, development of the sugar colonies brought many different cultures to the Caribbean (HEA 1991). Hence dietary practices will vary considerably and dishes with similar or the same name can contain different ingredients. Alternatively the same dish may have several names; Journey cakes are also called Jonny cakes (Douglas 1987).

Dietary constituents

Staples

These generally form the main part of the diet.

Cereals Cereals include rice, corn and cornmeal, oats and wheatbased foods such as pasta, cakes, bread (often West Indian bread).

Starchy fruits, roots and tubers A combination of two, three or perhaps four different starchy foods may be included as part of a meal.

Starchy fruit may include green banana, plantain, breadfruit.

Starchy roots and tubers may also be referred to as provisions, and include cassava, yam and sweet potato.

Peas, beans and nuts

Peas and beans A large variety of pulses are included in the diet, in stews, casseroles, one pot meals and as rice and peas.

Nuts and seeds A wide variety of nuts and seeds are eaten as part of a meal or as a snack. Examples include cashew nuts, almond, coconut, pumpkin, watermelon and sesame seeds.

Dark green leafy and yellow vegetables

These are used in soups, stews and one pot meals, often with meat and fish. Examples include callaloo (spinach), kale, peppers, karela, carrots. The name callaloo may be used as a collective term for all green vegetables.

Fruit

A large variety of fruit is eaten. Examples include pawpaw, guava, banana, pineapple. Some fruits are used as vegetables when unripe.

Animal foods and fish

Cows' milk and cheese Condensed and evaporated milk may be used in preference to fresh milk.

Eggs Eggs are generally used.

Fish A wide variety of fish is eaten.

Fats and oils

Butter, margarine and different types of oils are used. Coconut cream is used for flavour. Palm oil is also used to give flavour and colour to dishes.

The meal pattern varies with the individual or family. Traditional dishes may take a long time to prepare, and are more likely to be eaten at weekends and evenings. At weekends there is a tendency towards eating two meals, omitting lunch.

Methods of food preparation and cooking are generally passed down directly from the parents. The quantity of ingredients used varies with taste and the number of servings required. Snacks tend to be eaten as desired and include fruit, cream crackers, nuts, crisps and chocolate.

The above list outlines traditional Afro-Caribbean foods. A Birmingham study (Kenn *et al* 1986) on the nutritional intake of pregnant Afro-Caribbean women found that 31% ate traditional foods daily and 13% ate traditional foods 4–5 times a week. The main traditional foods consumed were cornmeal, coconut, green banana, plantain, okra and yam.

Many people also include a wide variety of European foods in their diet. The study in Birmingham showed that breakfast cereals, cakes, biscuits, crisps, burgers and chips were commonly consumed.

Religious beliefs

Religious beliefs also influence food choice, preparation and cooking methods. Although Afro-Caribbean people are generally Christian (Cruickshank and Beevers 1989), there are many faiths in the Caribbean. Two main religions which affect dietary practice are Seventh Day Adventism and Rastafarianism.

Seventh Day Adventists

Followers are often vegetarian. If meat and fish are eaten, pork is avoided as are fish without fins and scales. Alcohol and other stimulants (e.g. coffee and tea) are avoided.

Rastafarians

The degree of dietary restriction depends upon the individual. Many are vegetarian or vegan. The majority of followers will only eat 'ITAL' foods which are foods considered to be in a whole and natural state. Processed or preserved foods are excluded. Specific foods not consumed are pork, fish without fins and scales, fruit of the vine and stimulants (e.g. alcohol, coffee, tea).

Within the Afro-Caribbean community there are also widely and strongly held beliefs about diet and health which may influence dietary practices, e.g. use of herbal (bush) teas as a cure for disease (Springer and Thomas 1983).

Dietary problems

There has been very little research conducted into present dietary practices of the Afro-Caribbean community in Britain. It is thought that the Afro-Caribbean diet in the UK is high in fibre and lower in fat than the average UK diet. However, there are a number of areas of concern.

1 The prevalence of obesity is a striking feature of the

UK Afro-Caribbean population (Cruickshank and Beevers 1989).

2 A high fat intake may result from:
- The consumption of convenience, snack and fast foods;
- Some foods being fried before another method of cooking, such as steaming, is used;
- Large amounts of coconut cream which may be used in dishes such as rice and peas;
- The use of cheaper cuts of meat (e.g. trotters, tails) which have a high fat content.

3 Sugar intake may be high due to:
- Beverages such as carrot juice (homemade with condensed milk and sugar or honey);
- Glucose energy drinks, squashes, milk-based energy or malt drinks (e.g. Nutriment, Nourishment, Supermalt);
- Sweet snack foods being eaten, for example cakes (Caribbean and European), biscuits, sweets, and chocolate.

4 Salt intakes may be high if salt fish, salt pork, convenience and snack foods are consumed regularly.

5 Alcohol intake may be high, particularly in men (HEA 1991).

6 Rastafarians who exclude animal protein and do not replace this with other protein sources may be lacking in essential nutrients.

7 Infant feeding practices may cause malnutrition in Rastafarian children in the UK (Cruickshank and Beevers 1989; Springer and Thomas 1983).

However, in many respects the traditional dietary practices of Afro-Caribbean people follow guidelines for healthy eating and ensure good general nutrition.

3.9.3 West African diets

The majority of Africans in the UK originate from Nigeria and Ghana and have settled in major cities.

The foods consumed by West Africans are in general similar to those consumed by Afro-Caribbeans but the cooking methods differ. Cassava is used more frequently by West Africans in various dishes. Some commonly used dietary constituents are shown in Table 3.38.

The incidence of diabetes, hypertension and obesity is high in the West African community. General weight-reducing dietary advice is often necessary and areas which need to be highlighted are:

1 Reducing the amount of oil used in stews. Palm oil and palmnut oil are commonly used but are saturated fats; if possible a limited amount of sunflower, corn or groundnut oil should be used instead.

2 Reducing the amount of peanut butter used in soups.

3 Reducing the amount of fried foods such as fried fish or meat. Fish, for example snappers, may be stewed or baked instead of being fried.

4 The portion-size of green bananas, yam, ground rice and other starchy foods is often quite substantial and may need to be reduced.

5 Sugared drinks such as Lucozade should be avoided.

3.9.4 Chinese diets

Most of the Chinese in Britain originate from Hong Kong or South China; consequently many Chinese restaurants and takeaways serve food typical of that part of China although the cuisine of other regions can also be found.

Chinese food is becoming increasingly popular in the

Table 3.38 Dietary constituents commonly used in West African diets

		Examples	Cooking methods
Starchy vegetables	Ghana	Yam Green Bananas Plantain (called *fufu* when pounded)	Pounded and boiled or boiled whole
	Nigeria	Yam Green Bananas Cassava – pounded (*eba*)	As above Salt and hot water is added
Pulses	Nigeria	Blackeyed beans (*Akara*)	Cooked as a stew with palm or palmnut oil
Cereals	Nigeria/Ghana	Ground rice Whole rice Cornmeal	Boiled Boiled with sugar or salt
Typical meals may comprise:			
	Nigeria – Meat/fish + Eba (ground Cassava) + vegetable stew		
	Ghania – Meat/fish + Fufu (ground Cassava, yam or plantain) + soup		
	Desserts are not usually served		

UK and there is a growing number of people who venture beyond the better known 'Westernized' dishes to sample the diverse dishes of Chinese cuisine.

Dietary constituents

The people of the various regions in China have developed their own styles of cooking based on ingredients available locally. These schools of cooking are often named after the large cities such as Peking (Northern), Shanghai (Eastern), Szechuan (Western) and Canton (Southern) which regard themselves as the leading exponents of a particular approach to cookery.

In Northern China, wheat is the predominant cereal grown so noodles, dumplings, pancakes and Chinese-style breads (baked, steamed or fried and made from white flour) are staple foods. Sorghum and millet contribute to a lesser extent to the diet.

Peking cuisine developed around the royal court – hence emphasis is placed on the presentation of dishes and the exquisiteness of recipes. Liberal use is made of stronger flavoured ingredients such as peppers, garlic, ginger, leek and coriander. Oil is used lavishly in cooking and dishes are more energy-dense than those of other regions.

In Southern China, although wheat products are eaten, rice is the staple – either as the grain or made into different types of 'Pasta' such as rice sticks and noodles. Cantonese cuisine is known for its fresh and delicate flavours. Ideally, freshly bought ingredients are prepared the same day and cooked just before serving, using little oil or spicy seasonings.

It is becoming increasingly acceptable for pre-prepared foods to be bought. 'Dim Sum' is a special snack which originated in South China and which can be purchased ready-made and chilled. This dish consists of chopped meat, seafood and vegetables wrapped up in a wafer-thin coating of pastries or dough and then either steamed, braised, fried or boiled. Dim Sum differs from other kinds of Chinese eating since a variety of small savoury and sweet items are consumed throughout the meal.

In the West of China, Szechuan cooking is distinguished by the use of spices such as chilli, hot pepper oil and Szechuan peppercorn. Noodles and steamed bread are eaten in preference to rice. Food preservation by means of salting, drying, smoking and pickling is common.

Shanghai, a port in Eastern China does not have a cuisine of its own but successfully refines all the tastes of the surrounding provinces. Fresh fish and shellfish are important features of the diet, as are pork, cabbage and soya beans. Noodles are more common than rice and they are usually thick. Desserts are rich and oily. Dumplings and fritters are often served as accompaniments and a glutinous rice cake which can be stuffed with sesame, dates or black bean paste may be eaten.

Eating habits

The Chinese style of eating is a communal affair and one helps oneself to dishes placed in the centre of the table. The bite-sized pieces are easily picked by chopsticks. There is a sauce dish for each person. Dipping many foods into various complementary sauces enhances their flavour. For example, steamed chicken may be dipped into minced ginger, scallion and peanut oil. Roast chicken may be dipped into peppercorn-flavoured salt or Worcestershire sauce. Soy sauce and chilli sauce are also popular.

The Chinese like hot foods to be served very hot (in temperature). Salads are not commonly consumed. The midday or evening meal consists of the staple such as rice (usually boiled) or fried noodles with several main dishes – meat, poultry or fish. This will also often include a clear soup and at least one vegetable dish. Most vegetables are of the green leafy or gourd variety (e.g. Chinese broccoli, flowering cabbage and water melon). Traditionally, desserts were not usually eaten. However, with Western influence, fresh fruit – especially oranges – are now often eaten after a meal. Fruit is also eaten as a snack between meals, as are cakes, nuts and, in the summer, ice cream.

Soup provides a substantial meal as it can contain noodles, pieces of meat, fish, egg and vegetables. Fried rice is eaten usually only at the end of a special meal. Dim sum may be eaten as part of the midday meal.

Traditionally, breakfast consists of *congee*, steamed buns or noodles. The congee may contain soya bean sticks and nuts or chicken or fish. Nowadays many eat a Western-style breakfast such as egg and ham with toast, or breakfast cereals with milk, or any combination of Chinese and Western foods (such as cheese with Chinese bread). Some drink tea with milk.

Popular Western foods are beefburgers, pork chops, ham, bacon, peas, milk, butter, crisps and chips. They tend to be consumed mostly by children and young adults who either favour these foods or find them convenient. Lamb and frozen vegetables are not very popular.

Sweet liquid drinks, 'tong sui', are usually taken in the afternoon and may be included as part of the midday meal. Unrefined cane sugar forms the base to which a variety of ingredients may be added. These are usually made up of:

1 Sweet potato chunks and a little root ginger.
2 Red mung beans and dried citrus peel.
3 Soya bean shoots and nuts.
4 Beans, ground roasted peanuts and dried citrus peel.

The vegetarian style of eating is common in Chinese society. A major source of protein is the soya bean, processed into beancurd. Use is also made of a vast array of Chinese mushrooms and other types of fungi.

Festival food includes moon cakes, eaten to mark the 'August Moon Festival', which coincides with the end of the harvest year. These are sweetened, mashed lotus nuts which are encased in a thin, sweet pastry. Glutinous rice (sweet or savoury and sometimes stuffed with meat) is eaten at the time of the 'Dragon Boat Festival'. It is served wrapped in lotus leaves and then steamed.

Cooking methods

Most common cooking methods are quick and the freshness of the food makes a big difference to the taste of the meal. Cantonese cooking, in particular, relies on food being cooked as quickly as possible in as little oil as possible. Hence food is cut up into small, more or less equal portions to enable the heat from the cooking to penetrate the food quickly and evenly. Vegetable oil, especially peanut oil, is used in Chinese cookery.

Braising or stewing are slow cooking methods used to tenderise meat. Boiling is often used for soups and is also used for the rice where just sufficient water is added so that is it all absorbed. Foods are sometimes cooked in the steam generated by boiling rice, for example a savoury egg custard with minced pork. Steaming in a closed pan is used for whole birds or large pieces of meat. Usually, deep-fat frying is reserved for special dishes. Stir-frying is a quick cooking method carried out in a work with very little oil.

When roasting, grilling or boiling, the surplus fat is often skimmed off.

Root ginger, garlic and spicy onions are commonly used in food preparation. Dried unsalted vegetables and beans are also added to flavour meat and fish dishes.

Vegetables are rarely eaten uncooked (except as a garnish) and this includes salads. Most are lightly cooked via stir-frying, a method which helps conserve flavour and nutritional value.

Yin and yang

According to traditional Chinese medicine, good health depends on a balance of two opposite elements (in the body), yin and yang. In illness, the balance is disturbed and the body becomes too 'hot' (an excess of yang) or too 'cold' (an excess of yin). Each individual has a body base or equilibrium point. This is not a fixed point but varies according to the person's age and also during pregnancy and lactation. A person is seen as being healthy when his or her equilibrium is maintained.

A person's base can be shifted through diet, drugs, tonics, herbs and the weather. The healthy state is maintained (when the body is not invaded by an outside agent like a virus) by readjusting the base to equilibrium.

Diet is believed to play an important role in maintaining the individual's normal healthy balance and in correcting imbalances. Different foods have different properties – some are 'heating', some 'cooling' and some 'neutral'. Different cooking methods have different properties. A person whose body equilibrium was on the 'cold' side of the scale would avoid 'cold' foods. There are no hard and fast classifications as different Chinese people may define particular foods differently. It is important to discuss these when giving advice about nutrition and diet. A general classification is shown in Table 3.39.

The concept of yin and yang is particularly relevant in illness and pregnancy. Pregnancy is thought of as a 'hot' condition and a pregnant woman may cut down on red meat and fish. A traditional stew, *keung chow*, made from pigs' trotters and boiled eggs soaked in vinegar and ginger is given to a woman after childbirth to help recovery and in celebration of the birth of a child. For several weeks after childbirth, a women is encouraged to eat 'hot' foods to regain her strength.

Some health issues related to food habits and beliefs

1 Apart from yin and yang, there is a belief that certain foods and dishes have certain therapeutic qualities – for example, snakemeat combats rheumatism and female frogs are an antidote for asthma.

2 Monosodium glutamate is widely used in commercial Chinese cooking as a flavour enhancer and meat tenderizer. This can raise the sodium content of a meal.

3 Infant formula milk is seen as very 'hot', so a Chinese mother may want to give her bottle-fed baby 'cooling' drinks such as boiled water or barley water.

4 A lactating mother may want to eat 'cooling' foods because they may impart 'cool' properties to the breast milk.

5 Foods used during convalescence include steamed white fish, finely minced meat, congee and chicken essence.

6 Nasopharyngeal carcinoma (NPC) is a common form of cancer in south China and cases have been reported amongst the Cantonese in Britain. Studies show an associ-

Table 3.39 General guidelines on the Chinese classification of foods

	'Cold' Foods	'Neutral' Foods	'Hot' Foods
Food	Most fruit Vegetables Barley water Chinese herbal teas	White fish Rice, bread Papaya Orange	Oily fish, meat Alcoholic drinks Ginger, spices Some fruit e.g. mango, pineapple
Cooking method		Boiling Steaming Stir-frying	Deep frying Roasting

ation between Cantonese-style salted fish intake, especially during childhood, and NPC. Over 90% of cases in young Hong Kong Chinese were attributed to consumption of this food during childhood (Yu *et al* 1986). Case-control studies have also found that, besides salted fish, childhood exposure to other preserved foods is significantly related to NPC together with lower consumption of fresh fruit and vegetables during childhood (Yu *et al* 1989; Yan and Drettner 1989).

7 The traditional Chinese weaning diet has been shown to be suboptimal (Field and Baber 1973; Whyte 1972). This does not usually present a problem today as most infants at this stage are usually given adequate intakes of infant formula milk.

3.9.5 Vietnamese diets

Vietnamese civilization originates from the Chinese but adapted to become a distinctive Vietnamese tradition. France, as a colonial power, also exerted some influence on Vietnam.

Many of the Vietnamese community in Britain are ethnic Chinese and speak Cantonese. Some also speak Vietnamese or French and many now speak English.

Food habits

Given the strong Southern Chinese influence, many Cantonese dishes are familiar to the Vietnamese. Some, such as Vietnamese spring rolls, have been adapted. Chopsticks and bowls are used. The Chinese concept of yin and yang also plays a part in Vietnamese life. There are, however, major differences between the Chinese and Vietnamese cuisine and these lie in the seasonings used, the cooking methods employed and the differing emphasis on basic ingredients.

A commonly used Vietnamese seasoning is 'nuoc mam' – a fermented salted fish sauce. Nuoc mam is combined with garlic, chilli peppers, fresh lime and sugar to give a sauce which takes the place of salt at the table. In Britain, when this is not available, dark soy sauce is used instead. Other popular flavourings are vinegar, chilli sauce and monosodium glutamate.

Shallots are used in great abundance by the Vietnamese, as are fresh herbs such as lemon grass. Fresh, uncooked vegetables and salads are an integral part of many Vietnamese meals and lettuce, cucumber, coriander and mint (of which there are many varieties) are almost always included. Sliced green bananas may also be served.

Vietnam can be divided into three regions, each with its own cuisine. The food of the North, with a smaller variety of ingredients and spices, is somewhat lighter and less spicy. Black pepper is widely used as a condiment. Although seafood, particularly crab, is popular, fish constitutes a surprisingly minor part of the diet. Stir-fried dishes appear more frequently, perhaps due to greater Chinese influence.

The cuisine of the central area of Vietnam is famous for its highly decorative presentation of foods. Meals consist of small portions of many dishes. Foods are very spicy and there is frequent use of hot chilli peppers and shrimp sauce.

The Southern diet includes a great variety of vegetables, fruits, meat and game. A French influence is more apparent as shown in the fondues and there is more frequent use of vegetables such as white potatoes and asparagus. Sugar and sugar cane are used widely.

Although each region has its own style, the lines of distinction between them are blurred (Ngo and Zimmerman 1986). People from the North eat dishes typical of the South and vice versa.

Foods not popular amongst the Vietnamese are lamb, ox liver and tinned or cooked fruit.

Rice is the main staple and is served either boiled or fried at main meals. Rice grown in Vietnam is a useful source of iron and calcium. Vegetables, if cooked are done lightly and bear no comparison to British cooked vegetables. Vegetable oils or lard are used in stir-fry cooking. Butter and margarine are used sparingly and cheese, which is only eaten in small amounts, is processed. Hence the Vietnamese diet can be low in fat.

Barbecuing is an important cooking method in Vietnam and some dishes must be barbecued at the table. Simmering long, slow cooking in a covered pan, with liquid – over charcoal is also popular.

Other foodstuffs found in Vietnamese cuisines are cassava, coconuts, maize, peanut, soyabeans, sugar cane and sweet potatoes. Tea, coffee and fruit juice are the usual drinks, with alcohol kept for celebrations. Fresh milk is not available in Vietnam, but some use is made of evaporated and sweetened condensed milk. Lactase deficiency is fairly common amongst the Vietnamese, and may account for the limited use of milk and milk products in the traditional diet. Roast nuts, sweet potato, rice or noodle soup, rice with shreds of meat, spring rolls and fresh fruit are popular snacks between meals.

The Vietnamese calendar includes a number of festivals with associated traditional foods and meals. The main festival of New Year, in late January/early February, is celebrated over seven days. Rice cakes, soyabean soup, fruit and seeds are enjoyed, and the end of the celebrations is marked with a special feast.

Within the family, special ritual meals are associated with births, weddings, anniversaries and funerals.

Possible dietary problems

Lack of calcium

Calcium may be low in the diet of Vietnamese people in Britain because:

1 Rice grown in Vietnam contains much more calcium than the rice imported into Britain.

2 Fruit and vegetables in this country contain less calcium than some tropical varieties.
3 Milk and cheese are only consumed in small amounts, if at all.

Inadequate vitamin D

Low vitamin D intake has been identified in some Vietnamese children; in Vietnam their principal source of this nutrient in sunlight and oral supplements may be necessary for those living in Britain.

3.9.6 Jewish diets

Judaism is an ancient religion. Many people of the Jewish faith have been born in Britain of families which have been here for several generations; most have come from Europe and some from the Middle East. For the majority, English is their native language.

Naming system

This is the same as that used in Britain. In addition, Jewish people have a Hebrew name.

Jewish dietary laws

The Jewish people, like all other peoples, have food customs traditionally associated with their daily lives, their holidays and festivals. In addition to these, regulations are prescribed in a code of dietary laws (Kashrut), from the slaughter of animals used for food, to the kinds of dishes prepared for special holidays, festivals and the Sabbath. These food traditions have accumulated through the long, historic experience of the Jewish people. Maintenance of health and food hygiene underlie these laws.
1 The flesh of animals which may be used for food are quadrupeds that chew the cud and have cloven hoofs such as sheep, goats, deer and cattle. (Pork and all products of the pig are forbidden.)
2 Permitted birds are chicken, duck, goose and turkey. Birds of prey, which are more prone to disease than herbivorous birds, are forbidden.
3 Fish with scales and fins are allowed. Shellfish are not allowed as they are considered to be a source of disease. Fish does not have to be koshered in any way.
4 Meats must not be cooked with milk or milk derivatives, or be served at the same meal. Utensils, crockery, china pots and pans used for milk and meat must be stored, washed and dried separately.
5 Animals and birds must be slaughtered by the Jewish method; this procedure, which must be carried out by a trained and authorized person, entails a rapid cut with a sharp knife to sever the jugular vein and carotid artery. The meat is then salted and soaked in water to remove the blood and render it Kosher (permitted).

Festivals and fasting (the main holy days)

The seventh day of the week is the Sabbath, a day of devotions at synagogue and complete freedom from work. Sabbath begins at sundown on Friday and ends when the first star becomes visible on Saturday evening. On Friday night the Sabbath meal is served. No preparation of food is done on the Sabbath, but food prepared in advance is eaten.

The Jewish year is based on lunar calculations. The beginning of the Hebrew calendar is marked by the holiday called *Rosh Hashanah* (September). On the New Year it is customary to serve apple slices dipped in a bowl of honey, signifying the heart-felt yearning for a sweet and happy year.

Ten days after Rosh Hashanah is the Day of Atonement (*Yom Kippur*). This is the most Holy Day of the Jewish calendar. It is a fast day; no food or drink is permitted for 25 hours (from sundown to sunset).

Passover, which commemorates the exodus of Jews from Egypt, is celebrated for eight days in April. Unleavened bread (*Matzoa*) and cakes and biscuits made from Matzo-meal are eaten in place of leavened bread.

Sources of help

1 The British Diabetic Association Ethnic Working Party produces educational material for health professionals and Asian patients.
2 Local community leaders may help with general information, translation of leaflets and the establishment of contacts with relevant individuals or groups.
3 Dietetic departments in districts with specific cultural groups may develop diet sheets and nutrition education material. Many are willing to have their material used in other districts.
4 The Commonwealth Institute in Kensington High Street, London, has an excellent reference library and many publications on Commonwealth countries.
5 Individual embassies will often be helpful in supplying information on their own national diet and some offer translation facilities.
6 Black and Ethnic Minorities Food Working Party, c/o National Community Health Resource, 57 Charlton Street, London NW1 1HU.

Further reading

General

Brissenden R (1986) *South-east Asian food.* Penguin, London.
Chinese Food and Diet, National Extension College, Cambridge.
Henley A *Asian patients in hospital and at home.* King Edwards Hospital Fund, London.
Hill S (1990) *More than rice and peas.* The Food Commission, London.
Hom K (1984) *Ken Hom's Chinese cookery.* BBC Publications, London.
Lazarus HM *The ways of her household.* Jewish Memorial Council.

Leah WL *Jewish Cookery in Accordance with the Jewish Dietary Laws*.

Lo K *The Chinese cookbook*. Penguin, London.

McDermott MY *The Muslim guide*. The Islamic Foundation, Leicester.

Mares P *The Vietnamese in Britain*. National Extension College, Cambridge.

Ortis E *Caribbean cookery*. Penguin, London.

Singh D *Indian cookery*. Penguin, London.

Trainers' handbook for multiracial health care. National Extension College, Cambridge.

Food tables

Immigrant foods. Second supplement to McCance and Widdowson's *The composition of foods*. HMSO, London.

Wharton PA, Eaton PM and Day KC (1983) Sorrento Asian Food Tables. *Hum Nutr: Appl Nutr* **37a**, 378–402.

Gopalan C, Ramasastri BV and Balasubramanian SC (1982) *Nutritive value of Indian foods* 2e.

Training packs

British Diabetic Association. *Asian Information Pack*. Available from the Diet Information Service, British Diabetic Association, 10 Queen Anne Street, London W1M 0BD.

Henley A and Taylor C. *Asian names and records*. Available from the National Extension College, Brooklands Avenue, Cambridge CB2 1HN.

Henley A. *Asian foods and diets*. National Extension College, Cambridge.

References

Baylis J and Dattani J (1986) Dietary advice for Asian diabetics. *Practical Diabetes* **3**(4), 194–5.

Chandalia HB, Bhargav A and Kataria V (1987) Dietary pattern during Ramadan fasting and its effect on the metabolic control of diabetes. *Practical Diabetes* **4**(6), 287–90.

Cruickshank JK and Beevers DG (1989) *Ethnic factors in health and disease*. Butterworth, London.

Douglas J (1987) *Caribbean food and diet, food and diet in a multiracial society*. National Extension College, Cambridge.

Field EC and Baber FH (1973) *Growing up in Hong Kong*. Hong Kong University Press, Hong Kong.

Goodwin AM, Keen H and Mather HM (1987) Ethnic minorities in British diabetic clinics: a questionnaire survey. *Diabetic Medicine* **4**, 266–9.

Govindji A (1988) Spice of life. *Balance* **107**, 61–4.

Govindji A (1991) Dietary advice for the Asian diabetic. *Practical Diabetes* 8(5), 202–203.

Hawthorne K (1990) Asian diabetics attending a British hospital clinic: a pilot study to evaluate their care. *Br J Gen Pract* **40**, 243–7.

Health Education Authority (1991) Nutrition in minority ethnic groups: Asians and Afrocaribbeans in the UK. HEA, London.

Kenn J, Douglas J and Sylvester V (1986) Survey of infant feeding practices by Afro-Caribbean mothers in Birmingham. *Proc Nutr Soc* **45**(3), 87a.

Mather HM and Keen H (1985) The Southall diabetes survey: Prevalence of known diabetes in Asians and Europeans. *Br Med J* **291**, 1081–4.

McKeigue PM, Miller GJ and Marmot MG (1989) Coronary heart disease in South Asians overseas – a review. *J Clin Epidemiol* **42**, 597–609.

McKeigue PM, Shah B and Marmot MG (1991) Relation of central obesity and insulin resistance with high diabetes prevalence and cardiovascular risk in South Asians. *Lancet* **337**, 382–6.

Ngo B and Zimmerman G (1986) *The classic cuisine of Vietnam*. Penguin Books, Ontario.

Peterson DB, Dattani JT, Baylis JM and Jepson EM (1986) Dietary practices of Asian diabetics. *Br Med J* **292**, 170–71.

Peterson D and Govindji A (1988) Giving dietary advice to Asian diabetic patients. *Diabetic Med* **5**(7), 683–6.

Springer L and Thomas J (1983) Rastafarians in Britain. A Preliminary study of their food habits and beliefs. *Hum Nutr: Appl Nutr* **37a**, 120–27.

Thomas BJ (1988) Cultural minorities. In *Manual of dietetic practice*, Thomas BJ (Ed) pp. 307–312. Blackwell Scientific Publications, Oxford.

Yan L, Xi Z and Drettner B (1989) Epidemiological studies of nasopharyngeal cancer in the Guangzhou area, China. Preliminary report. *Acta Otolaryngologica* **107**(5–6), 424–7.

Yu MC, Ho JH, Lai SH and Henderson BE (1986) Cantonese-style salted fish as a cause of nasopharyngeal carcinoma: report of a case-control study in Hong Kong. *Cancer Research* **46**(2), 956–61.

Yu MC, Huang TB and Henderson BE (1989) Diet and nasopharyngeal carcinoma: a case-control study in Guagzhou area, China. *Int J Cancer* **43**(6), 1077–82.

Whyte RO (1972) *Rural nutrition in China*. Oxford University Press, Oxford.

3.10 Vegetarianism and veganism

Vegetarian diets are becoming increasingly popular. Health professionals may be concerned about the nutritional adequacy of some plant-based diets; however, with planning, most vegetarian diets are consistent with good nutrition and can provide health benefits and other advantages.

3.10.1 Types of vegetarian diets

In contrast to an *omnivorous* diet which includes all kinds of animal and plant foods, a *vegetarian* diet is one which excludes animal flesh (meat, poultry, fish, and shellfish) and other products of the animal carcass such as lard and gelatine. Most vegetarians also avoid animal-derived rennet (used to coagulate many hard and soft cheeses) and the insect-derived food colouring cochineal.

There are several types of vegetarian diets. The most common form is *lacto-ovo-vegetarian*, which excludes animal flesh but includes milk, milk products, and eggs as well as all plant foods; *lacto-vegetarians* also exclude eggs. The *partial or semi-vegetarian* diet is not strictly vegetarian but eliminates certain types of animal foods, often red meat, while including fish and perhaps poultry. A semi-vegetarian diet may be adopted for health reasons or may be part of a traditional religious or cultural pattern (see Section 3.9). In this chapter, the term 'vegetarian' will be taken to refer to lacto-ovo-vegetarians.

A *vegan* diet completely excludes all foods of animal origin, that is, milk and milk products, eggs, and honey, as well as animal flesh. Vegans also avoid the many food additives which are or may be of animal origin, such as whey, lecithin, and vitamin D_3. A vegan diet therefore is based on cereals and cereal products, pulses, vegetables, fruits, nuts, and seeds. Human breastmilk is acceptable for vegan babies.

Rastafarian diets in their strictest form can be almost vegan; however, milk and some types of fish may be acceptable. There are different types of *macrobiotic* diets, which are mainly vegan with a dependence on cereals, vegetables, and pulses but only limited intakes of fruit, nuts and seeds; a small amount of fish may be acceptable. Both Rastafarian and macrobiotic diets have additional restrictions on the types of food allowed, and have led to cases of nutritional deficiencies such as rickets and delayed growth and development in infants and children (Jacobs and Dwyer 1988).

A 1991 survey showed that over 6% of the British population consider themselves vegetarian: about 3.6 million people, with perhaps 20 000 vegans (Pink 1992). This represents a 120% increase in the number of vegetarians in the previous five years. In addition, half of the omnivores surveyed reported that they had reduced the amount of meat in their diet. Several surveys have shown that women are twice as likely as men to adopt a vegetarian diet, and there are higher rates among younger adults, teenagers, and children than among older adults. Vegetarians are evenly distributed throughout England, but fewer reside in Wales and Scotland. Vegetarians tend to be more highly educated than the general poulation, and from non-manual occupations, although increasing numbers of manual workers are becoming vegetarian.

People adopt vegetarian diets for a variety of reasons, including ethical and environmental concern for the use of world resources, animal welfare, religious and cultural reasons, and personal motivations of health, aesthetics, and economics. As a result, vegetarianism usually involves not just an eating pattern but a philosophy which affects the whole lifestyle. As an example, vegans may refuse immunizations which are produced using animals. Food attitudes which may accompany a vegetarian diet include an emphasis on whole, minimally processed, raw, or organically grown foods, avoidance of food additives, and elimination of alcohol and caffeine. Many vegetarians are well-informed about food and choose balanced diets with care; others may depend on a limited number of foods or on convenience products. Those people following a macrobiotic diet may be more concerned with the balancing of foods according to the defined properties of yin and yang than with their nutritional content.

Vegetarians are not a homogeneous group but come from a variety of social, cultural and educational backgrounds. Because of the wide variation in vegetarian practices, it is important that health professionals dealing with vegetarians investigate sympathetically the extent and variety of food exclusions and any associated food and health beliefs.

3.10.2 Health and nutritional status of people on vegetarian diets

Benefits and risks

Several research studies have shown that vegetarians have diets lower in fat, especially saturated fat, and higher in complex carbohydrates and dietary fibre than comparable omnivores (Abdulla *et al* 1981; Bull and Barber 1984; Lockie *et al* 1985). Vegan diets can be even lower in fat at 30–35% of energy, with saturated fat intakes of 5–7% of energy (Roshanai and Sanders 1984; Thorogood *et al* 1990; Sanders and Manning 1992). Thus vegetarians, and especially vegans, tend to approach more closely the diet recommendations of the NACNE and COMA Reports (NACNE 1983; DHSS 1984) than omnivores.

Epidemiological studies indicate that vegetarians tend to have lower weight (Sanders 1978a) and blood lipid levels (Thorogood *et al* 1990; Resnicow *et al* 1991) than omnivores, and lower rates of coronary heart disease, stroke, and certain cancers (Phillips and Snowdon 1986; Burr and Butland 1988). Evidence for the health benefits of vegetarianism has been reviewed by Dwyer (1988). It should be noted that these advantages are likely to be related to the lifestyle as well as to the diet of vegetarians, and that they could be achieved without eliminating meat from the diet (Dwyer 1991).

Vegetarian and vegan diets have been used for therapeutic purposes such as lowering blood cholesterol and treating angina, and also for treating hypertension, rheumatoid arthritis, obesity and asthma (Langley 1988). Vegetarians may also benefit by avoiding some of the risk of animal-related diseases and food poisonings.

The main area of concern regarding vegetarian diets is the small but important risk of a nutritional deficiency, particularly amongst population sub-groups with increased needs such as infants, children, and pregnant or lactating women. The inclusion of animal products alone does not ensure the adequacy of a diet; as with any eating pattern, the likelihood of a nutritional deficiency is higher in people who restrict the variety of foods that they eat. The nutrients of special concern to vegetarians are discussed in the next three sub-sections.

Macronutrients in vegetarian diets

Energy

Because most plant foods contain more water and fibre and less fat than foods of animal origin, vegetarian diets are usually less energy-dense than omnivorous diets. For adults, this may be a benefit and help in maintaining desirable weight. For those undergoing growth, or with a limited appetite, however, the bulkiness of vegetarian diets, particularly vegan diets, is a potential problem. For these people it is important to ensure sufficient energy intake to prevent the catabolism of dietary protein for energy. This can be accomplished by eating more of the energy-dense vegan foods such as nuts and nut spreads, pulses and dried fruits (and spreads made from them), soya milk, vegetable oils and margarines, and for lacto-ovo-vegetarians, milk and milk products.

There have been reports of protein-energy malnutrition, growth retardation, and delayed psychomotor development among infants and children fed on very restrictive macrobiotic and Rastafarian diets (Truesdell and Acosta 1985; Dagnelie *et al* 1989b). Inadequate energy in weaning foods and extended unsupplemented breastfeeding account for most of the cases (Jacobs and Dwyer 1988). Among vegan children on less restricted diets, two studies have shown normal growth and development, although the children tend to be lighter in weight and leaner than omnivores (O'Connell *et al* 1989; Sanders and Manning 1992). Lacto-ovo-vegetarian children appear not to differ from omnivores in growth (Sabate *et al* 1991).

Protein

Some people may be concerned about the protein adequacy of vegetarian diets, since plant foods are lower in protein than animal foods, and the protein is in a less utilizable form (see Section 2.2). However, the human requirement for protein is about 10% of energy intake or less, and many plant foods contain this level (pulses average over 25%, and cereals, nuts and seeds over 12%). An adequate amount of protein is not difficult to achieve on a moderately varied vegetarian diet, or a vegan diet, *as long as the energy intake is adequate*. Surveys of vegans consistently show protein intakes which meet recommended levels (Lockie *et al* 1985; Thorogood *et al* 1990). There is no health benefit in consuming a higher level of protein, as occurs with nearly all omnivorous diets, and there may be disadvantages in the form of increased burden on the kidney and increased excretion of calcium (DoH 1991). In addition, plant proteins are usually accompanied by fibre, whereas animal proteins tend to be accompanied by saturated fat.

The protein quality of vegetarian diets is sometimes questioned because the amino acid profile of plant proteins is less similar to the one required by humans than that of animal proteins. Theoretically a plant-based diet could be limited in the availability of some indispensable amino acids, restricting synthesis of body proteins for growth and development. Plant proteins, however, do contain all of the amino acids essential for humans, and different plant proteins together can supply any amino acid deficits in a particular food; this is referred to as protein complementation. Pulses with grains or pulses with nuts and seeds are traditional combinations; note that botanically, peanuts are pulses. For lacto-ovo-vegetarians, milk products or eggs complement any plant protein source.

In the past it was thought that vegetarians must carefully combine proteins from different plant sources *at each meal* for maximum use of indispensable amino acids. However, recent research has established that a diet which includes protein from two or more plant groups *every day*, along with the amino acid pool in the body, will be adequate in all the amino acids required by adults; precise protein complementation at every meal is unnecessary (American Dietetic Association 1988; Langley 1988). There has been less research on the effect of protein quality in diets of vegetarian children. Infants have a relatively high protein requirement and the consequences of deficiency at this age are serious. In view of this, it would be prudent to aim to include two complementary sources of plant protein at each meal for infants being weaned.

Fat

Vegetarian diets tend to be fairly low in fat, as long as there is not excessive intake of whole milk products, nuts, vegetable fats, and processed foods. Recently, there has been a concern expressed about the balance of fat types present in vegan diets (Sanders and Manning 1992). Vegan diets can be very high in linoleic acid, up to 60% of fat intake compared to less than 10% in omnivorous diets. This level may inhibit endogenous production of docosahexaenoic acid, which is absent from vegan diets. It is therefore recommended that vegans use soya, rapeseed, or olive oil and margarines rather than sunflower, safflower, or corn oil, in order to reduce the linoleic to alpha-linoleic ratio of the diet.

Carbohydrate

The diets of vegetarians are high in carbohydrate compared to those of omnivores (Bull and Barber 1984; Roshanai and Sanders 1984). Refined sugar usually accounts for a small proportion of dietary carbohydrate, although the intake of sugars from fruit may be quite high. One study found that vegan children were consuming 15% of their energy as sugar, mostly in the form of fruit juice (Sanders and Manning 1992).

Dietary fibre

Vegetarians generally have fibre intakes which meet or exceed the individual minimum DRV of 12 g/d non-starch polysaccharides and the NACNE recommendation of 30 g/d dietary fibre; most vegans have fibre intakes of 40 g/d or more (Roshanai and Sanders 1984; Thorogood *et al* 1990). While high intakes of fibre are recommended in general, an excessive level of fibre may be of concern in population sub-groups with high nutrient needs, since it adds to the bulk of the diet. In these cases, it may be necessary to recommend the replacement of some high fibre foods with more refined cereal products or an increased intake of energy-dense foods.

Another concern is that fibre and other components of plant foods, including phytic and oxalic acids, complex with the minerals in food and reduce their absorption in the intestine. Although this does occur experimentally, it has not been shown to compromise the mineral status of people with high fibre diets (DoH 1991). Phytates are found in appreciable amounts in wholegrain cereals, pulses, nuts, and seeds. While refining these foods removes some of the inhibitors of absorption, it also removes some of the minerals; one study showed that there was less net zinc absorption from white bread than from wholemeal bread (Turnlund 1982). The issue of whether vegetarians adapt to high levels of fibre and phytate in the diet over the long term is still contentious.

In the absence of research on very high fibre intakes, the Department of Health recommends an upper limit of 24 g/d of non-starch polysaccharide, or about twice the average British intake. Most vegetarians are below this level, but many vegans will exceed it; despite this, most vegetarians and vegans have adequate mineral status (see below). However, if mineral intakes are of borderline adequacy, it would be prudent to avoid excessive intake of foods which are fibrous, phytate-rich, or oxalate-rich (spinach, nuts, peanuts, chocolate, parsley, rhubarb). In particular, concentrated isolates of fibre and phytates such as wheat bran and bran-based breakfast cereals are not recommended. A proportion of phytate is inactivated by cooking and the leavening process (Robertson *et al* 1986), so cereals processed this way are preferable to raw forms. Inadequate mineral intake often accompanies a diet low in energy; modifying excessive intake of dietary fibre can help alleviate both problems.

Vitamins in vegetarian diets

Nutritional studies generally show that vegetarians have higher intakes of most vitamins than typical omnivores (Langley 1988). Lacto-ovo- and lacto-vegetarians do not systematically lack any particular vitamins in their diet; eating a varied diet remains the best advice for ensuring adequacy. For vegans, however, there are three vitamins of concern; sources of these vitamins are shown in Table 3.40.

Vitamin D

Dietary sources of vitamin D are limited to animal foods (egg yolk, fatty fish, liver) and fortified foods such as margarine and breakfast cereals. For most people in Britain, however, the main source is from the action of sunlight on the skin; blood levels in winter depend on exposure during the rest of the year. Vitamin D status in adults who spend sufficient time outdoors is usually adequate, but people with darker skin appear to have less ability to meet their requirements in this way (Clemens *et al* 1982). There have been several reports of rickets in children on Rastafarian and macrobiotic diets and some among Asians (Jacobs and Dwyer 1988; Dagnelie *et al* 1990). In some cases, therefore, supplemental vitamin D is recommended for both vegan and vegetarian children under two years old and pregnant and lactating women (DoH 1991). Cholecalciferol (vitamin D_3) is obtained from fish oil or lanolin; ergocalciferol (vitamin D_2) is the non-animal form acceptable to vegans, and is found in some fortified vegan margarines, soya milks and soya cheeses.

Table 3.40 Sources of vitamins which may be low in vegan diets (amount per 100 g)

Vitamin	Sources	Comments
Vitamin D	Exposure to sunlight	1–2 hours/week, more for elderly
	Fortified soya milk	Plamil (0.75 μg), Unisoy Gold (0.3 μg)
	Fortified cereal	Grape-nuts (4.4 μg)
	Fortified vegan margarines	(8 μg) Vitaquell, Tomor, Granose
	Fortified soya cheeses and soya yoghurts	(amount varies)
	Vitamin supplements	
Vitamin B_{12}	Fortified yeast extract	Tastex (50 μg), Barmene (50 μg), Natex (9 μg)
	Fortified soya milk	Plamil (1.6 μg), Unisoy Gold (0.6 μg)
	Fortified textured soya protein	Protoveg products (amount varies)
	Fortified cereals	Grape-nuts (5 μg)
	Vitamin supplements	
Riboflavin	Yeast extract	Tastex (2 mg), Barmene, Natex (7.5 mg)
	Wheat germ	(0.7 mg)
	Almonds	(0.8 mg)
	Grape-nuts	(fortified with 1.5 mg)
	Soya beans	(0.3 mg)
	Tempeh	(0.5 mg)
	Plamil soya milk	(fortified with 0.3 mg)
	Pumpkin, sunflower, sesame seeds, tahini	(all 0.2 mg)
	Mushrooms	(0.3 mg)
	Seaweeds:	
	kombu	(0.3 mg)
	nori	(1.3 mg)
	Avocado	(0.2 mg)
	Dried apricots, prunes	(both 0.2 mg)
	Carob flour	(0.5 mg)

Vitamin B_{12}

Cobalamins are synthesized only by bacteria, fungi, and some algae, and accumulate from microbial action in animals; plant foods contain no appreciable amounts unless they are contaminated by bacteria or insects. It has recently been shown that the microbial assay used for measuring the B_{12} content of foods is not specific for the form biologically active in humans. This means that several foods that were thought to have a high content of cobalamins actually contain mainly analogues which are not active, and may even compete with the active form for uptake (Herbert 1988). Fermented foods such as tempeh and miso, and algal products such as spirulina and nori cannot be relied on as sources of active B_{12} (Dagnelie *et al* 1991).

Long-term deficiency of vitamin B_{12} can deplete liver stores and lead to neurological damage; however, B_{12} deficiency in adult vegans is very rare (Sanders *et al* 1978b), and there may be protective mechanisms which act to conserve body stores. There have been isolated reports of low blood levels of B_{12} with associated neurological symptoms in exclusively breastfed infants of vegan mothers (Langley 1988) and also in people of all ages on macrobiotic or Rastafarian diets (Campbell *et al* 1982; Dagnelie *et al* 1989a). Others have reported low serum levels in vegan adults and low levels in the breastmilk of vegan mothers (Reddy and Sanders 1990; Specker *et al* 1990; Miller 1991). It is important that all vegans regularly include a reliable source of B_{12} in their diet, and particular care should be taken by children and pregnant and lactating women. The requirement for cobalamin is very small (the RNI is 1.5 μg/d for adults), and several vegan products are fortified; vitamin supplements which are free of animal products are also available. Sources of B_{12} which can be currently recommended are shown in Table 3.40; the Vegan Society (see The 'Useful Addresses' list at the end of this chapter) can advise on newer fortified products.

Riboflavin

Because the major sources of riboflavin are dairy products and meat, the intake of this vitamin is occasionally mentioned as a potential problem of vegan diets. Several studies in the last decade, however, have shown satisfactory intakes, even among vegan children and lactating women, who have increased requirements (Langley 1988; Helman and Darnton-Hill 1987). It remains prudent for pregnant and lactating women to ensure an adequate intake of riboflavin.

Minerals in vegetarian diets

There are several concerns regarding mineral adequacy of both vegetarian and vegan diets:

1 Many of the richest sources of the major minerals are animal foods.

2 The low energy intake of some vegetarians may result in mineral intakes of borderline adequacy.

3 The high fibre content of vegetarian diets may inhibit intestinal absorption of minerals some (Freeland-Graves 1988).

However, mineral adequacy can also be a problem in omnivorous diets which also contain constituents that may inhibit absorption, such as tannic acid in tea (DoH 1991). Sources of minerals possibly limited in vegan and vegetarian diets are shown in Table 3.41. Cereals and cereal products, although only moderately concentrated sources of minerals, are the major source overall in vegetarian and vegan diets due to the large amounts consumed.

Iron

Omnivorous diets derive about 60% of their iron from plant sources, while in vegetarian diets the proportion is over 90%. The iron found in plant foods, eggs and milk is in an inorganic (non-haem) form and has a much lower absorption rate from the intestine than the iron complexed with haem found in animal flesh. High levels of fibre, phytates, oxalates, and tannins in the diet also bind inorganic iron and reduce its bioavailability. The absorption of non-haem iron is increased up to four-fold when it is chelated with ascorbic acid, amino acids, or citric acid (Monsen 1988). A recent study, however, suggests that the effect of both enhancers and inhibitors of non-haem iron absorption in normal diets is less important than in laboratory test meals (Cook *et al* 1991).

In several surveys, iron intake of adult vegetarians and vegans has equalled or exceeded that of omnivores, iron status has been adequate, and iron-deficiency anaemia has not been more common than among omnivores (Sanders *et al* 1978b; Anderson *et al* 1981; Kelsay *et al* 1988), perhaps due to high intakes of vitamin C. However, two studies found low serum ferritin levels in a significant proportion of vegetarian women, showing poor iron storage status (Helman and Darnton-Hill 1987; Reddy and Sanders 1990). Another study of macrobiotic children showed low blood levels of haemoglobin and ferritin in 15% (Dagnelie *et al* 1989a). Meeting recommended iron intakes is a difficulty among many population groups; vegetarians with high needs should take the same precautions to ensure iron status as omnivores, that is, including rich sources of iron and vitamin C in the daily diet, and avoiding excessive intakes of inhibitors of iron absorption.

Zinc

Zinc is similar to iron in that its richest sources are animal foods, and high levels of fibre, phytates, and oxalates impair its bioavailability. In addition, a high intake of non-haem iron (Solomons and Jacob 1981), or calcium plus phytates (Harland *et al* 1988), characteristics which are not limited to vegetarian diets, may reduce the absorption of zinc. Several studies have shown that vegetarians and vegans, including children and pregnant women, generally have equal or higher dietary intakes of zinc than omnivores (Freeland-Graves 1988; Nieman *et al* 1989; Sanders and Manning 1992). Most studies of zinc status show that vegetarians and vegans have adequate blood levels, although lower than those of matched omnivores; inadequate plasma levels have been found in a minority (Anderson *et al* 1981; Sanders 1983). As with iron, it would be prudent for vegetarians as well as omnivores, especially lactating women, to include rich sources of zinc in the diet and avoid excessive intake of inhibitors.

Calcium

Because milk and milk products are a major source of calcium, the nutritional status of this mineral differs greatly between lacto-vegetarians and vegans. Lacto-vegetarians tend to have equal or higher calcium intakes (Bull and Barber 1984), and equal or greater bone densities than matched omnivores (Marsh *et al* 1988; Hunt *et al* 1989). Adult vegans appear to have intakes of calcium from plant sources which achieve or nearly achieve recommended levels, and satisfactory calcium status despite high levels of phytates in the diet (Langley 1988). High protein, sodium, and caffeine intakes lead to increased body loss of calcium, so vegans probably conserve more of their calcium intake than omnivores. The body also adapts to lower intakes of calcium by increasing the rate of intestinal absorption. Drinking water can be an important source of calcium which is not often accounted for; although the calcium content varies widely by locality, on average, drinking water provides 15% of the RNI in Britain (DoH 1991). Some studies of vegan children have shown intakes of calcium well below the RNI, although without deficiency symptoms (Sanders and Purves 1981). Calcium status is rarely a problem if vitamin D status is adequate. Particular care should be taken to include good food sources of calcium in the diets of vegan children and lactating women.

Table 3.41 Non-animal sources of minerals which may be low in vegan and vegetarian diets

Approximate amount providing					
100 mg Calcium		2 mg Iron		1 mg Zinc	
Tofu made with calcium chloride or sulphate, soya cheese	25 g	Soya flour	30 g	Peanuts, miso, soya flour	30 g
Tofu made with nigari, tempeh	70–85 g	Soya beans, tempeh, lentils	70 g	Soya cheese, tempeh	55 g
Fortified soya milk (Unisoy Gold, Plamil)	120 ml	Haricot, pinto, kidney beans, chickpeas, peanuts, peanut butter	80–100 g	Chickpeas, split peas, lentils	70–85 g
Soya, kidney, haricot beans	120–150 g	Peas, split peas	120–130 g	Haricot, pinto, soya beans, peas	100 g
Sesame seeds, brown (unhulled)	10 g	Sesame seeds, brown (unhulled)	15 g	Sesame, pumpkin, sunflower seeds, cashews	20 g
Almonds	40 g	Pumpkin seeds	20 g	Almonds	30 g
Hazelnuts	70 g	Sunflower seeds, pine nuts, cashews	35 g	Walnuts	40 g
Brown or white bread	100 g	Grape-Nuts	20 g	Wheat germ	5 g
Wholemeal bread	185 g	Wheat germ	25 g	Grape-Nuts	25 g
		Wholemeal bread	75 g	Wholemeal bread	55 g
		Brown bread	90 g	Brown rice	140 g
		White bread	125 g		
Dried figs	40 g	Parsley	25 g	Watercress	140 g
Parsley	50 g	Dried figs, dried apricots, raisins	50 g	Spinach	200 g
Spinach, watercress, kale	70 g	Prunes	70 g		
Spring greens	130 g	Watercress, kale	90–105 g		
		Spinach	125 g		
Kombu, wakame, nori seaweeds	15–25 g	Nori, wakame, kombu seaweeds	15 g	Kombu seaweed	15 g
Black treacle	20 g	Black treacle	20 g	Cocoa powder	15 g
Milk	75–90 ml	Breakfast cereals, fortified	30–50 g	Hard cheeses	30–50 g
Hard cheeses	20 g	Eggs	100 g	Breakfast cereals, fortified	50 g
Yoghurt	50–70 g			Eggs	75 g

3.10.3 Practical dietary advice for vegetarians

General considerations

Health professionals who counsel vegetarians should do so in a non-judgmental manner, considering their beliefs, attitudes and lifestyle, and be ready to provide reassurance that their diet can be consistent with good health and to suggest acceptable modifications if necessary. A helpful outline of a counselling process with vegetarians has been published (Johnston 1988). For adult vegetarians, the main advice is to include a variety of foods from the major food groups; and for vegans, also to ensure energy intake is adequate. Vegetarians should limit the intake of foods which are of low nutrient density. Different food guides can be devised for vegan and vegetarian adults which may be useful for evaluating diets or for educational purposes; one which has been shown to be adequate in energy, protein, calcium, iron, and riboflavin is presented in Table 3.42 (Mutch 1988).

Many vegetarian and vegan cookbooks are now available, including ones which are designed for people new to vegetarian diets or with limited cooking skills. Some are available from the relevant societies (see the end of this Section); others may be in local public libraries.

Table 3.42 Daily food guides for vegetarian children and adults

Food group	Serving size for children	Servings for children aged: 1–4 years	4–6 years	6 years–adolescent	Serving size for adults	Servings for adults (for pregnancy add one serving in each group)
Bread and rolls						
Preferably wholegrain	1 slice or roll	3	4	4–5	1 slice or roll; 30 g dry	5
Cereals						
Wheat flakes, wheat flour, bulgur wheat, wheat germ, rice, oatmeal, pasta, breakfast cereal	1–5 level tablespoons	1	2	2–3	cereal; 100 g cooked	
Vegetables and fruits						
Citrus: Oranges, orange juice, grapefruit, grapefruit juice, tangerines, satsumas	4–8 level tablespoons; 60–120 ml of juice	2 chopped	2	2	120 g; 120 ml juice	1
Dark green or deep orange: broccoli, spinach, kale, spring greens, watercress, carrots, dried apricots	4–6 level tablespoons	$\frac{1}{2}$ chopped	1	2–3	100 g cooked	1
Other vegetables and fruits: potato, tomato, apple, banana, raisins, sweetcorn, avocado	4–6 level tablespoons	3 chopped	4	5–7	100 g cooked or raw	5
Protein foods — a variety daily						
Pulses: lentils, soya, kidney and other beans, split peas, tofu, tempeh, peanuts, peanut butter	2–6 level tablespoons pulses;	3 chopped	3	3–4	100 g pulses; 30 g nuts and seeds	2
Nuts and seeds: sunflower, sesame, and pumpkin seeds; tahini; all nuts except coconut	1–3 level tablespoons nuts/seeds					
[Eggs, cheese for vegetarians]						
Milk						
Fortified soya milk Plamil, Unisoy Gold	250 ml	3	3	3–4	250 ml	2 (If omitted, add calcium and B_{12} sources and 2 more servings of protein)
[Cows' milk, yoghurt for vegetarians]						
Fats						
Vegetable oil and margarine, preferably rapeseed, soya, olive	1 level teaspoon	3	4	5	1 level teaspoon	3
[Butter, ghee for vegetarians]						
Other foods	1 level tablespoon each of: yeast extract (B_{12} fortified) and black treacle				Add extra servings of these and other foods to meet energy requirements	

Adapted from Truesdell and Acosta (1985) and Mutch (1988)

Vegetarians should be reminded to cook vegetables lightly in a minimum of water to retain nutrients; pressure cookers and microwave ovens save time as well as conserving nutrients. Cereals and dried pulses should be stored in airtight containers in a cool, dry, dark place; wholegrain flours go rancid more quickly than refined ones, so should be purchased in small amounts and stored in the refrigerator if possible. Although minimally processed foods should form the main part of the diet, vegetarian products and convenience foods are now widely available in supermarkets. Vegan convenience foods are less widely available but can be found in health food stores.

While, in general, a varied lacto-ovo-vegetarian diet is likely to be nutritionally adequate, health professionals should be alert to the needs of people who have newly adopted a vegetarian diet, or who are the only vegetarian in an omnivorous household. In addition vegetarians, and particularly vegans in the following groups, need to take some care in choosing their diet and may benefit from consultation with a dietitian.

Vegetarian population groups with special needs

Pregnant women

Well-planned vegetarian and vegan diets are adequate to maintain the health of both mother and child during pregnancy. General guidelines for planning diets in pregnancy are found in Section 3.1.2. The moderately increased requirements of protein, thiamin, and vitamin A, and more substantial increases in riboflavin, vitamin C and folate are not difficult to meet with varied vegetarian and vegan diets, provided that the recommended increase in energy intake is met. The bulkiness of a vegetarian diet may be a problem, particularly if energy intake is reduced due to appetite changes or morning sickness. A reduction in fibre intake and increase in energy-dense and nutrient-dense foods may be necessary; frequent smaller meals may also help. A food guide for pregnant vegetarians and vegans is shown in Table 3.42 which has been shown to meet the US RDAs for energy, protein, calcium, iron, and riboflavin (Mutch 1988).

Pregnant women with limited exposure to sunlight and those with dark skins are recommended to ensure a dietary intake of 10 μg/d of vitamin D, which may require a vitamin supplement (DoH 1991). Pregnant vegans should take particular care to ensure that their diet contains sufficient vitamin B_{12} from reliable sources; meeting the increased requirement for riboflavin also deserves consideration.

There is no recommendation for increased mineral intake in pregnancy; maternal stores and increased absorption are considered to balance higher needs. However, as mineral adequacy can be borderline in some vegetarian diets, this should also receive attention; if iron stores were low prior to pregnancy, supplementary iron is advisable.

Lactating women

Principles for diet planning during lactation are discussed in Section 3.3.1. The DRVs for energy, protein, and most B vitamins (including B_{12}) during lactation are increased 25% over those for non-pregnant women, with higher increases in riboflavin and vitamins A, C, and D. If this greater energy intake is achieved, varied vegetarian diets should also be able to meet the protein and vitamin requirements, given sufficient exposure to sunlight for vitamin D synthesis. As during pregnancy, those with dark skin or limited exposure to sunlight need to have an intake of 10 μg/d of vitamin D through diet or supplementation. Vegans should take extra care to ensure sufficient B_{12} intake from reliable sources to prevent deficiency in the breast fed infant, and perhaps pay extra attention to riboflavin intake.

The recommended intakes of calcium and zinc are about 80% higher than for non-pregnant women; there is no increase recommended in iron intake. These increased intakes were recommended in the absence of good data about the conservation of calcium and zinc in adaptation to lactation. It would be prudent for lactating vegetarians to include extra food sources of zinc and, for vegans, calcium also, and to avoid excessive intakes of fibre, phytates, oxalates, tannins and other inhibitors of mineral absorption.

Infants

The nutritional status of exclusively breast fed infants depends to a large extent on the nutrient stores and intake of the mother which, with some care, is adequate in both vegetarians and vegans. Iron supplementation is recommended for infants who are exclusively breast fed beyond 4–6 months. For those who choose to use infant formula, the only soya-based brand acceptable to vegans which is currently available in Britain is Farley's OsterSoy. Ordinary soya milk is not appropriate as the sole food of infants, since it is not fortified with iron and all appropriate vitamins. Vitamin D status in breast fed infants and those being weaned should be maintained by exposure of the face and hands to sunshine for two hours weekly (Specker *et al* 1985), or by supplementation (DHSS 1988). Vitamin D supplementation should be monitored by a health professional due to the risk of toxicity from an overdose.

Weaning on to solid foods should follow the same principles as for omnivorous babies (see Section 3.3.3). As weaning is a time of great nutritional vulnerability, very restrictive practices such as strict macrobiotic and Rastafarian diets carry a high risk of deficiencies, and are not recommended at this stage (Jacobs and Dwyer 1988). It is of the highest importance to ensure a sufficient energy intake in the weaning diet. The energy content of a vegetarian weaning diet can be improved by avoiding excessive intake of fibrous or watery foods such as very dilute porridges and many fruits and vegetables, and concentrating on cereal products, pulses, and vegetable fats; bananas and avocados are also relatively high in energy. Home-prepared foods are often more energy-dense than manufactured products; frequent feeding also aids energy intake.

Commonly-used first weaning foods such as cereals, fruit, and vegetables are suitable for vegans, although many packaged baby cereals are fortified with animal-derived vitamin D_3. Several manufactured baby foods are suitable for vegetarians, but fewer are completely free of animal products; these are listed in the Vegan Society's 'Animal-free shopper'. Later weaning foods appropriate for vegan babies are bread, mashed lentils, nut spreads such as peanut butter and tahini (not whole nuts), tofu, rice and pasta, soya formula, soya yoghurt and vegan margarine. Beans can also be used but, if they cause indigestion, they should be re-introduced after the age of 12 months. Vegetarians can include rennet-free cheese, yoghurt, and eggs (after nine months). Vegan infants may have low vitamin B_{12} stores at birth and may be receiving low levels in breastmilk, so it is crucial that the weaning diet contains foods fortified with B_{12}, such as fortified soya formula or Low Salt Natex yeast extract. It would also be prudent to aim to include two different sources of plant protein at each meal for vegan infants, to ensure maximum utilization of indispensable amino acids at this time of rapid growth.

Children

Children should be progressing toward a varied vegetarian or vegan diet by the age of 9–12 months; whole cows' milk or fortified soya milk can be introduced at this time. It is important to assure an adequate energy density and include a variety of protein foods daily for adequate growth, especially in vegan diets. Low fat, high fibre diets are not appropriate for children under two years; fibrous foods should not be eaten at the expense of more energy-rich foods (DoH 1991). Providing frequent, smaller meals and energy-dense snacks may be beneficial in increasing energy intake. The growth of young children, particularly vegans, should be monitored closely for early identification of any problems (Nutrition Standing Committee BPA 1988).

Adequate iron intake is a problem for children in general; good sources of iron should be included regularly and accompanied by vitamin C-rich foods. For children with limited sunlight exposure, 7 μg/d of vitamin D, from the diet or supplementation, is recommended until the age of two. Vegan children should have a reliable source of vitamin B_{12}. A food guide for vegan and vegetarian children is shown in Table 3.42 which has been shown to meet the US RDAs for energy, protein, riboflavin, vitamins D and B_{12}, and calcium, iron, and zinc (Truesdell and Acosta 1985). The Vegan Society maintains a 'Vegan families list' for mutual support of parents raising children on a vegan diet and lifestyle.

Adolescents

The nutritional needs of adolescents are described in Section 3.6.1. Vegetarians and vegans should take special care to meet the requirements of energy, protein, iron, calcium and B_{12} during the adolescent growth spurt; teenaged males have particularly high requirements for iron and calcium. Intake of foods providing energy but few other nutrients should be limited. There are health advantages in vegetarian and vegan diets in adolescence, such as low serum lipid levels and less risk of obesity (Jacobs and Dwyer 1988). Adolescence is a time when many adopt a vegetarian diet, often for ethical and environmental reasons, and perhaps within an omnivorous household. Such people may be particularly at risk of dietary deficiencies due to lack of knowledge, poor food choices, and lack of support. Basic nutrition books, cookbooks, and contacts with like-minded local people may provide help and are available through the Vegetarian Society and the Vegan Society, both of which have reduced price junior memberships.

Elderly people

There has not been much research on elderly vegetarians; the basic diet principles for this group are the same as for omnivores (Section 3.7). Two recent reports (Nieman *et al* 1989; Brants *et al* 1990) suggest that older vegetarians have more nutrient-dense diets than omnivores, but that they need to pay attention to intakes of vitamins D and B_{12}, iron, and zinc. Elderly people need a high exposure to sunlight, about one to two hours per day, in order to synthesize adequate vitamin D. As this may be difficult to achieve, an intake of 10 μg of Vitamin D daily, through diet or supplementation, is recommended. The incidence of absorption problems increases among elderly people, so that vitamin B_{12} uptake may become borderline even among non-vegans; regular use of reliable B_{12} sources is important. Older vegetarians benefit from being leaner than omnivores (Dwyer 1991), and from improved laxation due to a high fibre diet. The Department of Health, however, cautions against excessive intakes of non-starch polysaccharide and phytate in elderly people in general, whose diet may be marginal in mineral content. An excessive fibre intake may also prevent intake of adequate energy for those with limited appetites.

Useful addresses

These are good sources of nutrition and recipe books, magazines, and local contacts.

The Vegan Society, 7 Battle Road, St Leonards-on-Sea, East Sussex TN37 7AA.

The Vegetarian Society, Parkdale, Dunham Road, Altrincham, Cheshire WA14 4QG.

Further reading

The bean book. Rose Elliot (Fontana)
The new simply delicious. Rose Elliot (Fontana)
365 plus one vegetarian main meals. Janet Hunt (Thorsons)
Eva Batt's vegan cookery. Eva Batt (Thorsons)
The animal-free shopper. R Farhall, R Lucas, and A Rolfe (The Vegan Society)
A vegetarian in the family. Janet Hunt (Thorsons)
The teenage vegetarian survival guide. Anouchka Grose (The Vegetarian Society)
Rose Elliot's mother and baby book. Rose Elliot (Fontana)
A healthy pregnancy: a vegetarian approach. Sarah Brown (BBC Books)
Vegetarian catering. Richard Davies (available from the Vegetarian Society)
Choice: nutritional guidelines for vegetarian catering in schools and *4 week menu planner* (The Vegetarian Society)

References

Abdulla M, Andersson I, Asp N, Berthelsen K, Birkhed D, Dencker I, Johansson C, Jägerstad M, Kolar K, Nair BM, Nilsson-Ehle P, Nordén Å, Rassner S, Åkesson B and Öckerman P (1981) Nutrient intake and health status of vegans. Chemical analyses of diets using the duplicate portion sampling technique. *Am J Clin Nutr* **34**, 2464–77.

American Dietetic Association (1988) Position of the American Dietetic Association: Vegetarian diets – technical support paper. *J Am Diet Assoc* **88**, 352–8.

Anderson BM, Gibson RS and Sabry JH (1981) The iron and zinc status of long-term vegetarian women. *Am J Clin Nutr* **34**, 1042–8.

Brants HA, Lowik MR, Westenbrink S, Hulshof KF and Kistemaker C (1990) Adequacy of a vegetarian diet in old age. *J Am Coll Nutr* **9**,

292–302.

Bull NL and Barber SA (1984) Food and nutrient intakes of vegetarians in Britain. *Hum Nutr: Appl Nutr* **38A**, 288–93.

Burr ML and Butland BK (1988) Heart disease in British vegetarians. *Am J Clin Nutr* **48**, 830–32.

Campbell M, Lofters WS and Gibbs WN (1982) Rastafarianism and the vegans' syndrome. *Br Med J* **285**, 1617–18.

Clemens TL, Henderson SL, Adams JS and Hollick MF (1982) Increased skin pigment reduces capacity of skin to synthesize vitamin D_3. *Lancet* **i**, 74–6.

Cook JD, Dassenko SA and Lynch SR (1991) Assessment of the role of nonheme-iron availability in iron balance. *Am J Clin Nutr* **54**, 717–22.

Dagnelie PC, van Staveren WA, Vergote FJVRA, Dingjan PG, van den Berg H and Hautvast JGAJ (1989a) Increased risk of vitamin B-12 and iron deficiency in infants on macrobiotic diets. *Am J Clin Nutr* **50**, 818–24.

Dagnelie PC, van Staveren WA, Vergote FJVRA, Burema J, Van't Hof MA, van Klaveren JD and Hautvast JGAJ (1989b) Nutritional status of infants aged 4–18 months on macrobiotic diets and matched omnivorous control infants: a population-based mixed longitudinal study. II Growth and psychomotor development. *Eur J Clin Nutr* **43**, 325–38.

Dagnelie PC, van Staveren WA and van den Berg H (1991) Vitamin B-12 from algae appears not to be bioavailable. *Am J Clin Nutr* **53**, 695–7.

Dagnelie PC, Vergote FJVRA, van Staveren WA, van den Berg H, Dingjan PG and Hautvast JGAJ (1990) High prevalence of rickets in infants on macrobiotic diets. *Am J Clin Nutr* **51**, 202–8.

Department of Health (1991) *Dietary Reference Values for food energy and nutrients in the United Kingdom*. Rep Hlth Soc Subj 41. HMSO, London.

Department of Health and Social Security (1984) Committee on Medical Aspects of Food Policy. *Diet and cardiovascular disease* (The COMA Report). Rep Hlth Soc Subj 28. HMSO, London.

Department of Health and Social Security (1988) *Present Day Practice in Infant Feeding, Third Report*. Rep Hlth Soc Subj 32. HMSO, London.

Dwyer JT (1988) Health aspects of vegetarian diets. *Am J Clin Nutr* **48**, 712–38.

Dwyer JT (1991) Nutritional consequences of vegetarianism. *Ann Rev Nutr* **11**, 61–91.

Freeland-Graves J (1988) Mineral adequacy of vegetarian diets. *Am J Clin Nutr* **48**, 859–62.

Harland BF, Smith SA, Howard MP, Ellis R and Smith Jr JC (1988) Nutritional status and phytate : zinc and phytate × calcium : zinc dietary molar ratios of lacto-ovo vegetarian Trappist monks: 10 years later. *J Am Diet Assoc* **88**, 1562–6.

Helman AD and Darnton-Hill I (1987) Vitamin and iron status in 'new' vegetarians. *Am J Clin Nutr* **45**, 785–9.

Herbert V (1988) Vitamin B-12: plant sources, requirements and assay. *Am J Clin Nutr* **48**, 852–8.

Hunt IF, Murphy NJ, Henderson C, Clark VA, Jacobs RM, Johnston PK and Coulson AH (1989) Bone mineral content in postmenopausal women: comparison of omnivores and vegetarians. *Am J Clin Nutr* **50**, 517–23.

Jacobs C and Dwyer JT (1988) Vegetarian children: appropriate and inappropriate diets. *Am J Clin Nutr* **48**, 811–18.

Johnston PK (1988) Counselling the pregnant vegetarian. *Am J Clin Nutr* **48**, 901–5.

Kelsay JL, Frazier CW, Prather ES, Canary JJ, Clark WM and Powell AS (1988) Impact of variation in carbohydrate intake on mineral utilization by vegetarians. *Am J Clin Nutr* **48**, 875–9.

Langley G (1988) *Vegan nutrition: a survey of research*. The Vegan Society, Oxford.

Lockie AH, Carlson E, Kipps M and Thomson J (1985) Comparison of four types of diet using clinical, laboratory and psychological studies. *J Roy Coll Gen Pract* **35**, 333–6.

Marsh AG, Sanchez TV, Michelsen O, Chaffee FL and Fagal SM (1988) Vegetarian lifestyle and bone mineral density. *Am J Clin Nutr* **48**, 837–41.

Miller DR, Specker BL, Ho ML and Norman EJ (1991) Vitamin B_{12} status in a macrobiotic community. *Am J Clin Nutr* **53**, 524–9.

Monsen ER (1988) Iron nutrition and absorption: dietary factors which impact iron bioavailability. *J Am Diet Assoc* **88**, 786–90.

Mutch PB (1988) Food guides for the vegetarian. *Am J Clin Nutr* **48**, 913–9.

National Advisory Committee on Nutrition Education (1983). *Proposals for Nutritional Guidelines for Health Education in Britain*. (The NACNE Report) Health Education Council, London.

Nieman DC, Underwood BC, Sherman KM, Arabatzis K, Barbosa JC, Johnson M and Shultz TD (1989) Dietary status of Seventh-Day Adventist vegetarian and non-vegetarian elderly women. *J Am Diet Assoc* **89**, 1763–9.

Nutrition Standing Committee of the British Paediatric Association (1988) Vegetarian weaning. *Arch Dis Child* **63**, 1286–92.

O'Connell JM, Dibley MJ, Sierra J, Wallace B, Marks JS and Yip R (1989) Growth of vegetarian children: The Farm Study. *Pediatrics* **84**, 475–81.

Phillips RL and Snowdon DA (1986) Mortality among Seventh-Day Adventists in relation to dietary habits and lifestyle. *Plant Proteins: Applications, Biological Effects and Chemistry*. American Chemical Society. pp. 162–74.

Pink B (1992) Vegetarian Britain 2000. *The Vegetarian* March 1992, pp. 58–9.

Reddy S and Sanders TAB (1990) Haematological studies on pre-menopausal Indian and Caucasian vegetarians compared with Caucasian omnivores. *Br J Nutr* **64**, 331–8.

Resnicow K, Barone J, Engle A, Miller S, Haley NJ, Fleming D and Wynder E (1991) Diet and serum lipids in vegan vegetarians: a model of risk reduction. *J Am Diet Assoc* **91**, 447–53.

Robertson L, Flinders C and Ruppenthal B (1986) *The New Laurel's Kitchen*. Ten Speed Press, Berkeley, California.

Roshanai F and Sanders TAB (1984) Assessment of fatty acid intakes in vegans and omnivores. *Hum Nutr: Appl Nutr* **38A**, 345–54.

Sabate J, Lindsted KD, Harris RD and Sanchez A (1991) Attained height of lacto-ovo vegetarian children and adolescents. *Eur J Clin Nutr* **45**, 51–8.

Sanders TAB (1978a) The health and nutritional status of vegans. *Plant Fds Man* **2**, 181–93.

Sanders TAB (1983) Vegetarianism: Dietetic and medical aspects. *J Plant Foods* **5**, 3–14.

Sanders TAB, Ellis FR and Dickerson JWT (1978b) Haematological studies on vegans. *Br J Nutr* **40**, 9–15.

Sanders TAB and Manning J (1992) The growth and development of vegan children. *J Hum Nutr Diet* **5**, 11–21.

Sanders TAB and Purves R (1981) An anthropometric and dietary assessment of the nutritional status of vegan preschool children. *J Hum Nutr* **35**, 349–57.

Solomons NW and Jacob RA (1981) Studies on the bioavailability of zinc in humans: effects of heme and nonheme iron on the absorption of zinc. *Am J Clin Nutr* **34**, 475–82.

Specker BL, Black A, Allen L and Morrow F (1990) Vitamin B_{12}: low milk concentrations are related to low serum concentrations in vegetarian women and to methylmalonic aciduria in their infants. *Am J Clin Nutr* **52**, 1073–6.

Specker BL, Valanis B, Hertzberg V, Edwards N and Tsang RC (1985) Sunshine exposure and serum 25-hydroxyvitamin D concentrations in exclusively breast-fed infants. *J Pediatr* **107**, 372–6.

Thorogood M, Roe L, McPherson K and Mann J (1990) Dietary intake and plasma lipid levels: lessons from a study of the diet of health conscious groups. *Br Med J* **300**, 1297–301.

Truesdell DD and Acosta PB (1985) Feeding the vegan infant and child. *J Am Diet Assoc* **85**, 837–40.

Turnlund JR (1982) Bioavailability of selected minerals in cereal products. *Cereal Foods World* **27**, 152–7.

3.11 Chronic physical disablement

The United Nations (1975) has defined 'disabled person' to mean any person unable to ensure by himself or herself, wholly or partly, the necessities of a normal individual and/or social life, as a result of a deficiency, either congenital or not, in his or her physical or mental capabilities. This section considers the nutritional and dietetic problems of those with a chronic physical disability.

3.11.1 Aetiology and classification

Congenital disorders

Congenital disorders that can lead to feeding and nutritional problems include *cerebral palsy*, *muscular dystrophy* and *spina bifida*.

Cerebral palsy

Cerebral palsy is the term given to a group of non-progressive motor handicaps. It was first described in 1843 by Little (Bowley and Gardner 1980). It was initially assumed that the condition was associated with mental retardation. It was not until the 1930s that accurate assessment showed that 50% of children with cerebral palsy had a normal IQ.

The incidence of cerebral palsy varies between countries but it is usually around 2.0 per 1000 live births. The incidence of severely handicapped children with cerebral palsy has decreased due to improved antenatal and postnatal care.

Bowley and Gardner (1980) estimated that about one third of children with cerebral palsy are premature or of low birthweight. Abnormal labour and forceps delivery are more common in cerebral palsy than the normal population. About 15% of cases are due to damage acquired after birth, e.g. meningitis or head trauma. Very young or very old mothers appear to be more at risk from having a child with cerebral palsy.

Cerebral palsy can be classified according to clinical or neurological signs. These are spastic, athetoid, ataxic and mixed.

Spastic cerebral palsy accounts for about 75% of all cases. It is characterized by marked rigidity of movement and inability to relax muscles. One or all four limbs can be involved.

Athetoid cerebral palsy accounts for 10% of all cases and is also termed *dyskinesia*. It is characterized by frequent involuntary movements which may mask or interfere with normal movements of the body. Grimacing, dribbling and slurred speech commonly occur.

Ataxic cerebral palsy is characterized by poor body balance, difficulties in hand to eye co-ordination and control. It is a rare form of cerebral palsy.

About 10% of all cases are of a *mixed* type.

The extent of the handicap in people with cerebral palsy varies from mild handicap where the child learns to walk and talk and his or her movements are just clumsy, to severe handicap where individuals have little control of their arms, hands or legs. As cerebral palsy is a permanent and non-progressive condition the management of the child in the early years of life is of great importance, as is early diagnosis. Many children with cerebral palsy have difficulty with feeding as they often take a long time to learn feeding skills. These problems can persist into adulthood.

Muscular dystrophy

There are a number of disorders which can be called 'muscular dystrophy'. The common feature is a progressive degeneration of certain groups of muscles (Bannister 1985). All forms of muscular dystrophy are inherited and are distinguished by differences in the age of onset and variations in the distribution of the muscles affected.

The most common form is the pseudohypertrophic type which is usually inherited as a sex-linked recessive, although it can be the result of genetic mutation. The severe form of this muscular dystrophy is known as *Duchenne muscular dystrophy* and the milder form as *Becker muscular dystrophy*. Of the known cases of muscular dystrophy in the UK, 50% are boys with Duchenne muscular dystrophy. This form is carried on one of the X chromosomes of the mother. Any child born to a carrier mother will have a 25% chance of being an affected son or a carrier daughter. It is usually undetected at birth, unless there is a family history of the condition. Babies usually appear normal in early infancy, but may be late in starting to walk. As the disease progresses they become clumsy in walking and have difficulty in running, climbing stairs and getting up unaided after a fall. Boys are usually diagnosed at about the age of three (Ashworth and Saunders 1985). Muscles which exhibit pseudohypertrophy are mainly the calf muscles and occasionally the triceps and forearm muscles. The damaged muscle cells are replaced by fat and fibrous tissue and the muscle weakness gets progressively worse. Diagnosis is usually confirmed by abnormally high levels of serum creatine kinase. Most boys with Duchenne muscular dystrophy are unable to walk by the age of eleven. Eventually arm muscles become so weak that they are unable to push their own wheelchairs and have to rely on electric ones or their carers for mobility. As the weakness progresses the respiratory muscles are affected, considerably shortening the life expectancy.

Children with Duchenne muscular dystrophy have acquired feeding skills by the time the disease strikes, and arm muscle weakness does not usually prevent self-feeding. The main nutritional problem is weight gain due to immobility.

Clinical onset of the rarer forms of muscular dystrophy often occur later on in life, for example symptoms of dystrophia myotonica usually appear between the ages of 15 to 40 years. This type of muscular dystrophy is characterized by muscle weakness and myotonica. The myotonica leads to delayed muscular relaxation.

There are no treatments available to influence the course of the muscular dystrophies although physiotherapy may help to prolong the active life of boys with Duchenne muscular dystrophy. The pattern of inheritance of all the major forms of muscular dystrophy is now known, and this has meant that parents can now undergo genetic counselling. Tests have also been developed which can detect carriers of some of the muscular dystrophies.

Spina bifida

'Spina bifida' means an incomplete closure of the vertebral canal which is usually associated with incomplete closure of the spinal cord (Bannister 1985). There are two main types, *spina bifida cystica* and *spina bifida occulta.*

Spina bifida cystica This is the severe form and encompasses two lesions: *myelomeningocele* (where the main feature is a sac protruding through the vertebral opening which contains the flattened open spinal cord) and *meningocele* (where the defect is confined to a few vertebral segments and a protruding vertebral sac). The spinal cord is structurally normal and in a normal position. Both lesions occur mainly in the lumbosacral and thoracic regions, and are both characterized by weakness in the lower limbs, incontinence of urine and other abnormalities such as hydrocephalus and mental handicap (Ashworth and Saunders 1985).

In less severe cases of spina bifida, surgical repair of the spinal cord will be undertaken as well as reconstruction of the urinary tract. However, people with spina bifida may have permanent faecal and urinary incontinence.

Spina bifida occulta The milder form is characterized by a failure of fusion of one or more posterior vertebral arches, usually in the lumbosacral region. This is mainly seen as a depression which is covered by a dimple or tuft of hair. It is estimated that one in ten people have this condition, the vast majority of those will have no symptoms or problems (ASBAH 1990).

The defects found in spina bifida cystica occur in the early development of the embryo, the less severe spina bifida occulta can develop after 60 days. Spina bifida malformations occur in approximately 1 in 200 pregnancies (Bannister 1985) (see also Sections 2.6.2 and 3.1.1). The malformation can be detected by ultrasound scan and serum alpha-fetoprotein levels, usually taken around the 16–18th week of pregnancy. The incidence of spina bifida is decreasing; this can partly be explained by screening during pregnancy and the availability of termination and also by improved maternal nutrition.

Children with the severe forms of spina bifida usually have a poor prognosis. In the milder forms, weight gain due to immobility is the main nutritional problem.

Acquired conditions

Chronic physical disablement may also result from acquired conditions. The following are discussed in detail elsewhere:

- Head and spinal injuries (Section 5.3);
- Stroke (Section 4.21);
- Multiple sclerosis (Section 4.22);
- Arthritis (Section 4.29).

3.11.2 Feeding problems associated with chronic physical disablement

The process of eating has many social functions as well as being necessary to maintain our nutritional status. For people with acquired chronic physical disability (e.g. those with arthritis or upper limb paralysis caused by strokes and spinal injuries) it is important that feeding problems are overcome quickly in order to help the person regain self-confidence and self-respect.

General aspects

Positioning

The position of the child or adult with a physical disability for feeding is important. Patients with spinal injuries under traction may only be able to tolerate semi-solid food. Disabled people with poor head and trunk control should be well supported during feeding. The ideal feeding position depends on the type and degree of handicap and can be assessed by a physiotherapist. Many disabled people have individually designed chairs. Disabled people should not be fed in the lying position as it discourages swallowing and can cause choking. A good position for feeding cerebral palsied children helps to control chewing, swallowing and sucking (Davies 1986).

Self-feeding

The inability to feed oneself can be a source of great frustration and can be very demoralizing for the adult with acquired physical disabilities. Many feeding aids are available which will assist in regaining independent feeding. Occupational therapists will assess each individual and give advice on the most suitable aids. Equipment that is available include the following.

Non-slip mats These provide a non-slip base for plates and are particularly useful for people who have the use of one arm only (e.g. stroke victims or people with arthritis).

Dishes Dishes with wide bases which are less easily tipped up. 'Manoy' dishes have a higher wall on one side to enable food to be pushed against it.

Adapted cutlery Many disabled people have weak or stiff hand grips and are unable to hold conventional cutlery as it is often too thin and slippery. Ordinary cutlery can be adapted by enlarging the diameter of the handle with sponge or rubber tubing. Large spoons designed as cooking implements may be easier to hold. Plastic cutlery may be better for the cerebral palsied child with a bite reflex (see below) as such children can injure themselves if metal cutlery is used. Specially shaped cutlery is available for athritic patients who have little wrist movement.

Drinking aids Flexistraws are useful for disabled people who are unable to hold a cup, particularly tetraplegics. A plastic container with an airtight lid with a hole for the straw will prevent any spills if the container is knocked over. Special beakers with cutaway stems which can be lifted with the palm of the hand as well as the fingers are useful for those people with poor grip. Disabled children often find mugs with two handles easier to hold and encourage the maintenance of a stable and symmetrical position whilst drinking.

Occupational therapy departments will have details of all the feeding aids. Details can also be obtained from the Spastics Society, Disabled Living Foundation and Boots the Chemists (see the useful address list at end of this chapter).

Specific problems associated with cerebral palsy

Feeding problems are especially acute in children with cerebral palsy. Some parents spend as much as 4–6 hours each day feeding their cerebral palsied child. The experience of feeding may be unpleasant for both feeder and child, and can result in manipulative behaviour by the child (Jones 1989).

Correct feeding patterns are extremely important for the development of speech; usually children with feeding problems are referred to a speech therapist for assessment and treatment.

In severely disabled children, feeding problems can develop at birth if there is an insufficient sucking and/or swallowing reflex. Swallowing difficulties may be characterized by an abnormal pattern of tongue thrust. This occurs when the tongue protrudes from the mouth inhibiting food from being taken in. Some children also exhibit poor mouth closure due to lack of control of muscles in the mouth, which can cause excessive drooling. Alternative feeding (e.g. nasogastric feeding) can be used in very severe cases. A poor lip seal can be improved by placing food on alternate sides of the mouth, almost in the cheek pouch and not directly on the tongue.

Feeding problems may become more acute at the time of weaning. Usually weaning is delayed in severely disabled children; in some cases it can take up to five years before semi-solid foods are accepted (Webb 1980). Some children with cerebral palsy have extremely sensitive mouths and may develop spasm if the face is touched. This can become exaggerated if there is over stimulation during feeding, such as constant wiping of a dribbling child's wet mouth. Children can become tolerant to touch by gently stroking the face from the mouth outwards with a finger or soft object (Jones 1978).

Children with cerebral palsy commonly aspirate during feeding, which results in choking and coughing and causes lower respiratory tract infection (Jones 1989). Chronic aspiration can cause fibrotic changes in the lungs which can aggravate gastro-oesophageal reflux, which can also be present in severely disabled cerebral palsied children. Fear of the child choking can result in the carer delaying the introduction of semi-solid food (Davies 1986).

Some children have a tonic bite reflex. This is characterized by a strong clamping of the jaw on the spoon and delayed release of the bite, making spoon feeding difficult, as well as being very unpleasant for the child, especially if the spoon is metal.

The assessment of a person's abnormal feeding requires detailed observation of the following: the normal feeding position, consistency of the food offered, head and trunk control, abnormal mouth functions and a history of choking and aspiration. Recently developed techniques also allow for the detailed observation of abnormal swallowing reflexes (Jones 1989). Videofluoroscopy (see Chapter 4.21) developed by Logemann (Jones 1989) involves the person swallowing barium impregnated substances of varying consistencies, seated in different positions. X-ray images of the food bolus as it passes through the mouth and pharynx are recorded on videotape. Studies have shown that individual management of feeding disorders can be improved using this technique. Griggs *et al* (1989) studied 10 patients aged from nine months to 24 years and showed that the subjects tended to aspirate food in a paste rather than a liquid consistency. Recommendations based on the videofluoroscopic findings resulted in noticable improvements in mealtime behaviour and reduced coughing and choking.

3.11.3 Nutritional problems associated with chronic physical disablement

Nutritional problems of the chronic physically disabled include obesity or underweight, poor growth and constipation.

Obesity

Immobility results in decreased requirements for energy, particularly in such conditions as stroke, arthritis, muscular dystrophy, spina bifida and spastic cerebral palsy. Many disabled people eat more energy-dense foods as compensation; it is also common for parents to give their physically disabled children extra high energy snacks, also for compensation.

Dietetic intervention is based on the same principles as for the non-physically disabled (see Section 4.17.1), although weight loss may be slow due to immobility and extra encouragement and patience by the dietitian may be necessary. Patients can be weighed on chair scales if they are unable to stand (see Section 5.3). If it is impossible to use scales, skinfold thickness or mid-arm circumference measurements can be used as an indication of weight loss (see Sections 1.10.1 and 1.11.2).

Underweight

Some people who acquire physical disabilities are at risk from poor appetites which can cause weight loss. Depression, inability to shop, prepare and cook food can lead to an uninteresting and boring diet. Difficulties with feeding may be overcome by the use of the feeding aids discussed in Section 3.11.2, the subsection on 'self-feeding'. Physically disabled people in institutions can have low energy intakes due to lack of time to eat given by feeding helpers, inappropriate consistency of the food and poor positioning. Lack of choice and unattractive meals may also exacerbate the problem.

Studies on the growth of children with multiple physical handicaps, particularly those with cerebral palsy have shown low heights and weights. Aliakbari and Webb (1986) studied 16 children with cerebral palsy and found that 50% of the children were below the third centile for height-for-age and 80% were below weight-for-age. Nicholls (1990) found that there were highly significant differences in the heights and weights of 50 children with cerebral palsy under 11 years of age compared with their matched controls. The mean height and weight for the cerebral palsied children was on the 10th centile compared with the 50th centile for the matched controls. The energy intakes of the cerebral palsied was highly significantly lower than in the control group. Low energy intakes have been associated with feeding problems (Krick and Van Duyn 1984) and inability to communicate their need for food or to buy snacks or forage for food in the kitchen (*Lancet* 1990).

The energy intake of the physically disabled who are underweight can be increased by conventional methods, for example using supplements, fortifying food with skimmed milk powder, using energy-dense foods such as sugar, cream, spreading fats etc. If oral intake is insufficient to maintain an adequate energy intake, nasogastric or gastrostomy feeding can be instituted.

Inadequate nutrient intake

Physically disabled people can be at risk from poor intakes of certain nutrients. Chewing and swallowing difficulties can lead to low intakes of meat, fruit and vegetables which can result in low intakes of protein, iron and vitamin C. The physically disabled person with a low energy intake will be at risk from deficiencies of all nutrients unless the diet is of high nutrient density. Each individual person should be assessed by a dietitian and given advice on the nutrient content of the diet, appropriate to the consistency tolerated.

Constipation

Many physically disabled people have chronic constipation which is due to immobility and/or changes in gut motility (e.g. people with spinal injuries, cerebral palsy or multiple sclerosis). Many disabled people also develop a fear of defaecation because of pain or discomfort and for this reason may be reluctant to increase their fibre intake. Some physical disabilities such as spinal injuries and spina bifida cause faecal incontinence which may be treated by regular enemas. Once established it is difficult to stop this form of treatment.

Semi-solid or liquid diets used to feed the physically disabled with feeding problems tend to be low in fibre as well as other nutrients. The use of high fibre diets is only effective if there is sufficient liquid to absorb the fibre and soften the stools (Winstock and Evans 1987). However, many disabled people also have low fluid intakes, particularly if they are unable to communicate or indicate when they want to drink. The fibre content of a semi-solid or soft diet can be increased by the use of soft, high fibre breakfast cereals such as Weetabix soaked in milk, the addition of wholemeal breadcrumbs to food and the use of well cooked soft pulses and wholemeal spaghetti. Soft puréed fruit and vegetables can also be included.

3.11.4 Communication with people with a visual or aural handicap

Visual handicap

In the UK the common causes of visual handicap are cataracts, glaucoma, trauma and diabetic retinopathy. About one million people are registered as blind in the UK, and 600 000 people are registered as partially sighted. Persons registered as blind or partially sighted are mostly elderly and the majority of elderly visually handicapped people are female (DHSS 1988).

Verbal communication

1 Before you start talking to someone who is blind, gain the person's attention by using his or her name and by touching the person on the shoulder. Say who you are.
2 Before you leave, make sure the blind person knows you are going.
3 Do not shout.

Written communication

Reference material for people who are blind (See the 'Useful addresses' list at the end of this chapter)

1 The RNIB list 'A Feeling for Food: cookery books for the visually handicapped' gives details of books printed in Braille and on cassette. The RNIB will also provide a list of nutrition and diet related material in Braille or on cassette which are available for loan or for sale.

2 There are several reading services throughout the country (e.g. Ada Reading Services, see 'Useful addresses') who will tape written material. This is carried out on an individual basis and pre-recorded material is not usually available for sale.

3 The Braille Unit at HM Prison, Wakefield have a small library of nutrition, diet and cookery material available. The unit will transfer information in Braille on an individual basis but this service can be quite expensive.

4 The British Diabetic Association produces an information pack 'Vision and Diabetes' which includes details of the BDA literature available on tape and in Braille as well as practical advice.

Transcribing material for people with a visual handicap

Relative merits of Braille, Moon and tapes Only some visually handicapped people learn Braille. People who lose their sight in later years find it particularly hard to learn. Many elderly people learn 'Moon' which consists of simplified Roman letters.

Tapes are easy to carry and store and can also be understood by sighted helpers. They tend to be used mainly by the young because some of the elderly are discouraged by the technicalities of using them. Tapes can distract others whereas Moon and Braille can be read silently.

Transcription services are offered by the RNIB, HM Prison Wakefield and The Braille Unit, Aylesbury Youth Custody Centre.

Producing large print material The size of the print is not the only criterion on which the readability depends (Gardiner 1979). Other criteria include:
1 Contrast. Black on a white background with high density print is best. Photocopied material is often hard to read.
2 Spacing. Letters should be spaced so that the area between them is similar; the width of an 'o' should be left between words; and at least half the height of a letter should be left between lines.
3 Case. Words produced in lower case can be recognized by their shape more readily than those in upper case.
4 Style of print. There needs to be sufficient contrasting background within the letters.

Communicating with those who are deaf or hard of hearing

Listening through a hearing aid is rather like listening over a very bad telephone line. Sounds are distorted and there may be a lot of background noise. People with a hearing aid often lip-read as well. This requires a great deal of concentration.

When interviewing someone who is deaf or hard of hearing use the following techniques to help the person understand you:
1 Speak clearly and slowly and raise your voice slightly. Never shout. Do not over-exaggerate lip movements.
2 Try to ensure privacy and absence of distracting voices and sounds.
3 Face the deaf person directly. Make sure your face is well lit.
4 Do not hide your mouth with your hand or anything else.
5 Use gestures to make your meaning clear.
6 Do not expect a deaf person to listen to you and look at a diet sheet or other paper at the same time.

Sources of help

1 Speech and occupational therapists.
2 Technical officers for the blind employed by Social Services departments or voluntary organizations.

3 Boots the Chemists have a large selection of eating and cooking aids for the disabled.

4 Some branches of the Red Cross and St John Ambulance Brigade have eating and cooking aids available for hire.

Useful addresses

Action for Blind People (formerly London Association for the Blind), 14–16 Vernay Street, London SE16.

Ada Reading Services, 6 Dalewood Rise, Laverstock, Salisbury, Wiltshire SP1 1SF. Tel 0722 26987.

Association for Spina Bifida and Hydrocephalus (ASBAH), 42 Park Road, Peterborough PE1 2UQ. Tel 0733 555988.

British Diabetic Association, 10 Queen Anne St, London W1M 0BD. Tel 071–323 1531.

Disabled Living Foundation, 380–384 Harrow Road, London W9 2HU. Tel 071–289 6111.

Muscular Dystrophy Society, Natrass House, 35 Macauley Road, London SW4 0QP. Tel 071–720 8055.

Partially Sighted Society, Queens Road, Doncaster DN1 2NX. Tel 0302 323132 or 368998.

Royal London Society for the Blind, 105–109 Salisbury Road, London NW6 6RH. Tel 071–372 1551.

Royal National Institute for the Blind (RNIB), 224 Great Portland Street, London W1N 6AA.

RNIB Production and Distribution Centre, PO Box 173, Peterborough PE2 0WS. Tel 0733 370777.

Spastics Society, 12 Park Crescent, London W1N 4EQ. Tel 071–636 5020.

Talking Books (RNIB), 224 Mount Pleasant, Wembley, Middlesex.

Talking Newspaper Association for the UK, 90 High Street, Heathfield, East Sussex, TN21 8JD.

The Braille Unit, Aylesbury Youth Custody Centre, HM Prison, Brerton Road, Aylesbury, Bucks. Tel 0296 24435.

The Braille Unit, HM Prison Wakefield, 5 Live Lane, Wakefield WF2 9AG. Tel 0924 378282.

Further reading

Blockley J and Miller G (1971) Feeding techniques with cerebral palsied children. *Physiotherapy* **57**, 300–308.

Cordle M *Feeding can be fun*. Spastics Society, London.

Crump IM (1987) *Nutrition and feeding of the handicapped child*. Little Brown, Boston.

Finnie NR (1975) *Handling the young cerebral palsied child at home*. Heinemann, London.

Warner J (1981) *Helping the handicapped child with early feeding*. Winslow Press, Winslow, Bucks.

References

Aliakbari J and Webb Y (1986) Nutrient intakes of cerebral palsied children. *Proc Nut Soc Aust* **11**, 114.

ASBAH (1990) *Guide to services 1990/91*. Association for Spina Bifida and Hydrocephalus, Peterborough.

Ashworth B and Saunders M (1985) *Management of neurological disorders* 2e. Butterworths, London.

Bannister R (1985) *Brain's clinical neurology* 6e. Oxford University Press, Oxford and London.

Bowley AH and Gardner L (1980) *The handicapped child. Educational and psychological guidance for the organically handicapped* 4e. Churchill Livingstone, Edinburgh.

Davies E (1986) Appendix to chapter on children with cerebral palsy. In *Children with Neurological Disorders, Bk 1. Neurologically Handicapped Children, Treatment and Management*. Gordon N and McKinley I (Eds) pp. 61–75. Blackwell Scientific Publications, Oxford.

DHSS (1988) *Causes of blindness and partial sight among adults in 1976/77 and 1980/81 England*. HMSO, London.

Gardiner PA (1979) *ABC of Ophthalmology*. BMA Publications, London.

Griggs CA, Jones PM and Lee RE (1989) Videofluoroscopic investigation of feeding disorders of children with multiple handicap. *Develop Med Child Neurology* **31**, 303–308.

Jones AM (1978) Overcoming the feeding problems of the mentally and physically handicapped. *J Hum Nutr* **32**, 359–67.

Jones PM (1989) Feeding disorders in children with multiple handicaps. *Develop Med Child Neurology* **31**, 404–406.

Krick J and Van Duyn MAS (1984) The relationship between oral motor involvement and growth: a pilot study in a paediatric population with cerebral palsy. *J Amer Dietet Assoc* **84**, 555–9.

Lancet (1990) Growth and nutrition in children with cerebral palsy (Editorial). *Lancet* **335**, 1253–4.

Nicholls AM (1990) MPhil thesis, University of Wales.

United Nations (1975) *Declaration of the rights of disabled persons*. Annex IV. General Assembly Resolution 3447.

Webb Y (1980) Feeding and nutrition problems of physically and mentally handicapped children in Britain: a report. *J Hum Nutr* **34**, 281–5.

Winstock A and Evans S (1987) Food for the child with cerebral palsy. *Therapy Weekly* 8 January.

3.12 People with a learning disability

The term 'learning disability' is now used instead of 'mental handicap'. Dietitians new to this service are likely to find themselves surrounded by unfamiliar jargon created from different networks of staff, systems and practice. Provision of a dietetic service can only be effective by responding to local demands and using resources which are well understood.

Currently the emphasis of change is towards integration into mainstream services such as schools, ordinary housing or other community facilities. Generally, but not always, change in this particular field occurs at a slow pace. Accordingly dietitians may need to review their own expectations of time taken to effect nutritional change.

3.12.1 Background to the services for people with learning disabilities

Philosophy

Contemporary services are moving away from a medical emphasis to one based on social needs. This reflects the fact that people with a learning disability are not necessarily ill. Their needs, as service users, are for social integration and access to the everyday resources which the rest of the community take for granted.

Dietitians working in this service should become familiar with the principles of 'Normalization' (O'Brien and Tyne 1981) and 'Social Role Valorization' (Wolfensberger 1972) as they form the basis of service philosophy. Numerous social policy documents (see 'Further reading') have contributed to the present ideology of community care. This literature contains information which can enhance understanding of the services and the changes experienced by many people with learning disabilities.

Accommodation

Community care policy (DHSS 1989, see 'Further reading') has led the way for people to move from long-stay institutions into the community. Each authority has interpreted this in a different way and is at a different stage of implementation. For example, in some areas large institutions have closed completely, in others, these are in the process of closure while some authorities, owing to financial constraints, have postponed the process of rehousing for the time being. People are moving or have moved to a wide variety of housing funded by a number of agencies. Examples of housing available include larger units (10–25 people) such as NHS locally based hospital units (LBHU) and social service hostels, or smaller houses/flats owned by the NHS, social services, voluntary agencies such as Mencap, housing associations, private registered homes and consortiums. A large percentage of people live with their families and some people live independently in rented accommodation. Adult placement schemes exist for some people needing minimum support, and these may be normal tenant/landlord agreements with supervision from social services. The staff provision in each type of accommodation varies in response to the skills of individual people living there. As people acquire independence through new skills, staff support may alter.

The problems associated with the provision of suitable and desirable accommodation with appropriate staffing cannot be underestimated. The problem of locating and financing suitable accommodation in cities such as London is huge. People may have no choice but to continue living with their families or they may be rehoused inappropriately. This can cause immediate or future problems.

The concept of 'community care' relies upon good respite provision. Respite, or short term care, is a service offered to families allowing people to have planned breaks away from home. It is organized by health or social services or a family link scheme. However its availability varies nationally and financial constraints may result in inadequate provision.

Support services

Community mental handicap teams (CMHTs)

CMHTs were recommended by the National Development Team following the 1979 DHSS reports (see 'Further reading'). In line with the changes in terminology, some teams are known as 'specialist teams' or 'support teams'. CMHTs are currently funded either by the NHS or joint funded with social services and vary enormously in their composition and the type of service offered. Membership of a CMHT may include community nurses, psychologist, psychiatrist, occupational therapist, speech therapist, physiotherapist, social worker, manager, and administrative staff. Recently some teams have employed dietitians as integral members.

Some CMHTs work only with adults while others work with children as well. Similarly, CMHTs may only offer a service to people living in their own homes in the community. A team with a broader remit may encompass residential (agency funded hostels and houses) as well.

Generally the CMHT does not work with people living in institutions but liaison may occur with resettlement teams.

Resettlement team

This is a group of staff who facilitate a person's move from an institution to alternative accommodation. The team, usually based within the institution, consists of nurses and managers with likely input/liaison from psychologists, paramedical and social workers.

Staffing

The majority of staff working in all types of accommodation (institution or community) are care assistants with little or no formal training and the quantity and quality of inservice training varies between services. However the experience and skills of care assistants should not be underestimated. Care assistants are usually managed or led by Registered Nurses Mental Handicap (RNMH) (NHS), or social workers (social services) or managers from a variety of backgrounds in private or voluntary sectors.

Occupations

Valued employment for people with learning disabilities is difficult to find. Pathway Officers are employed by some Job Centres to actively seek employment to suit an individual's desires and skills. Some resettlement teams refuse to rehouse people from an institution without the provision of appropriate day care for each individual. Most people use the day services provided by social services. These centres may also be called Adult Training/Day Centres or Resource and Activity Centres. Again each local authority varies in the type of service it provides. The emphasis has moved away from the low paid light industrial work of 'training centres' to a social/education model which encourages people to develop the skills necessary for using local resources and enhance their functional and interpersonal skills.

3.12.2 Role of the dietitian in services for people with learning disabilities

This dietetic speciality is enjoying a period of growth. In 1992 65 dietitians were working in the field, although of these, 41% combine working in this field with other dietetic specialities including 26% who split posts with mental illness (BDA Mental Health Group figures). There are two distinct areas in which dietitians can work, long-stay institutions and the community. A dietitian taking up a new single-handed post cannot possibly be expected to do everything, and will need to decide which aspects have the greatest priority. If it is a new post, the dietitian's potential will be unknown to the majority of people working in and using the service and the first task will be to make others aware of the skills, and services which can be offered.

The role of the dietitian can encompass the following aspects:

Individual referrals

The nutritional requirements of people with a learning disability, like those of any other child or adult, need individual assessment. Individual nutritional care plans may be of particular help to those who are nutritionally at risk. These provide guidelines for when to contact the dietitian, for example when body weight falls below a certain level, thus enabling people to become responsible for their own or their client's care.

Many people with a learning disability are on a low income and the dietitian must be sensitive to the associated problems (see Section 3.8).

Frequently people with learning disabilities are unable to express their needs and feelings by direct verbal communication and this may initially be frustrating and bewildering to dietitians new to the service. Some clients overcome these difficulties by adopting and developing other ways of communication which listening and observation will soon identify. Some people may use food to communicate their feelings. This is important to remember during nutritional assessment when behaviour towards food may express an emotional need. There are those who can communicate verbally but need more time to do so effectively; always check that apparent inattention is not the result of hearing or sight impairment.

Speech therapists run courses on communication skills and sign languages such as Makaton for both individuals and professionals. Teaching aids may need adaptation and a good imagination will help overcome challenges presented when teaching those who use alternative forms of communication. The use of real food, meals, supermarkets and shops rather than food models or pictures are cognitively less confusing for those people who have difficulty with abstract concepts.

Teaching and educating clients, care staff and colleagues

Many clients are able to learn about and manage their own diets, however this can easily be overlooked by professionals (Cole 1990). Group work may be appropriate.

Educating care staff, both qualified and untrained, can be an extremely effective use of time. An induction course may be in operation for all new care staff, and this may be a good opportunity for a dietitian to raise awareness of the importance of food in everyone's life. On-going access to dietetic support and update training is also important.

Nutritional standards and monitoring

Setting nutritional standards such as menu planning, meal

choice, flexibility etc. are time consuming to establish but, once in operation, will raise awareness of the nutritional needs of individuals. Regular monitoring and evaluation of the standards can be performed by non-dietetic staff. This system is likely to be successful if it becomes part of an established in house monitoring system. Liaison with house staff and managers is crucial if the implementation and monitoring methods are to be realistic. A dietitian can then use this as a baseline for future in house training (Hay and Jeffereys 1992).

Nutrition education and healthy eating

People with learning disabilities have the same right to this information as the rest of the population. If a Food Policy is in existence, the dietitian can make people aware of its content thus enabling people to make informed choices.

Advocating for people to access medical services

People with communication difficulties or those living in institutions may not be able to ask for, or may not know of their rights to, existing medical services. The dietitian, in conjunction with other professionals, may be able to put forward a case for people to receive the medical services required. For example, blood tests may not be as readily available to those living in the community, and some people may not receive the level of care that our society now expects.

Liaison with other professions and agencies (e.g. social services)

In order to maximize the standard of care which each person receives, all 'professionals' must liaise. This avoids duplication of effort and unnecessary use of time. It also minimizes the number of visits to a person who may already have input from a variety of 'professionals'. Where many 'specialists' are involved in a client's care, case conferences or care reviews can bring them together to ensure a co-ordinated approach.

Liaison with other dietitians in the district

Good links with local dietitians working in different fields can be of enormous value to ensure continuity of dietetic care when clients are, for example, admitted to acute hospitals. It also helps to keep dietitians informed of events happening outside their own specialities.

3.12.3 Nutritional problems

The nutritional problems associated with long-stay institutions have been well documented (Fenton 1989; Macdonald *et al* 1989). In contrast, however, Cunningham *et al* (1990) report that the diets of 332 people living in five institutions were no different from the rest of the population. Although in theory problems such as dehydration, constipation and underweight should be reduced or eradicated as people move to the community, some may remain if clients and staff are not properly prepared and supported. A move from an institution to the community may also create new, or exacerbate existing, nutritional problems. For example the stress caused by moving from their home of perhaps 50 years may cause some people to stop eating. Alternatively, freely available food may cause a person to eat excessively and gain weight.

The nutritional problems which are most commonly encountered are detailed below.

Underweight

Apart from obvious medical causes such as cancer, there may be many reasons why someone is underweight. A few of the most common are as follows:

Anorexia

This may be caused by depression or environmental factors such as unappetizing food or people not being offered food which is to their liking.

Not eating enough

A person may simply not be eating enough either because they have not been offered enough food or because it may be dropped as a result of poor hand to mouth co-ordination, or wasted as a result of dribbling or drooling. In some instances, food may be being taken from them.

Ignorance

Professionals and carers may confuse a history of chronic low body weight with acceptable/ideal body weight. This belief is difficult to change. In addition they may prefer a lighter body weight which is obviously easier to lift and/or carry.

Lack of time

People may not be given sufficient time to finish the whole meal.

Increased requirements

These may be due to challenging behaviours, hyperactivity (Woods 1991) or some underlying medical problem.

Dysphagia and feeding problems

Chewing and/or swallowing problems and a fear of choking may make people frightened or unable to eat. Dysphagia (see Section 4.2.2) and feeding problems can occur for neurological or physical reasons, or as a side effect of certain drugs. The inappropriate sloppy, liquidized or puréed diets commonly given to people with these problems, result in unrecognizable, unpalatable diets of low nutrient density.

People with chewing and/or swallowing problems may not be underweight, but the fear of choking, the risk of aspiration and the consequent recurrent chest infections are very real problems. Speech therapists are often the best people to liaise with in these instances as their expertise lies in assessing oral-motor dysfunction in relation to feeding as well as speech.

The treatment of dysphagia in adults usually involves texture modification aimed at minimizing the risk of choking. In children, however, it may be possible to improve oral feeding skills (Evans Morris and Dunn Klein 1987). For some children and adults nasogastric or gastrostomy feeding may be the best option for reasons of safety, nutritional adequacy and improved quality of life. Positioning of the body is also a basic requirement of comfortable and safe eating and physiotherapists and occupational therapists can provide essential advice on this.

Constipation

Constipation is a common problem and is often, incorrectly, assumed to be a life long condition. Constipation may exacerbate other conditions: for example, many carers report that those people with severe epilepsy may have more frequent and/or more severe fits when constipated (personal communication).

Constipation is usually caused by one or more of the following:

Inadequate fluid

The occurrence of dehydration in institutions has been documented (Macdonald *et al* 1989). This may happen because drinks are not offered or consumed, for example poor lip closure affects liquid control in the mouth. Thickened fluids may help as these are easier to control and less likely to fall out of the mouth. A hot atmosphere will also increase fluid requirements.

Inadequate fibre

People may simply not be offered sufficient fibre-containing foods or not have been advised about appropriate choices. People with few or no teeth may have received a soft low-fibre diet for some time. Great care is needed when increasing dietary fibre in the diet of someone who has habitually eaten a very low-fibre diet, particularly if that person is unable to communicate discomfort.

Inadequate exercise

Those with physical disabilities may be unable to exercise; others may not be encouraged to take the opportunity.

As a side effects of drugs

Antipsychotic and antidepressant drugs may result in constipation. Chronic use of some laxatives without exploring alternative treatments may contribute to cathartic colon (Moriaty and Silk 1988).

Diarrhoea

Diarrhoea may be the result of poor bowel control, overflow, behavioural problems or food intolerance. The latter may be a genuine food intolerance; however some staff/carers may not recognize this, and regard it as part of the person. Some people with Down's syndrome have been reported to have a higher prevalence of coeliac disease than the rest of the population (Simila and Kokkonen 1990).

Overweight

There may be many reasons for people being overweight, for example lack of opportunity or ability to exercise, the side effects of anti-psychotic drugs, food regularly being used as a reward or palliative measure and some people may eat compulsively (see Section 4.24.3). Ideally people themselves must wish to lose weight or they will lack motivation. It goes without saying that factors such as exercise and lifestyle should also be taken into account. Medical reasons must also be considered, for example the link between Down's syndrome and thyroid dysfunction has been well documented (Kinnell *et al* 1987; Dinani and Carpenter 1990). More obscure disorders such as Prader-Willi syndrome are known to result in the person being overweight (Section 4.25).

Vomiting, regurgitation and rumination

Physical causes should be explored initially as these symptoms may be associated with conditions such as hiatus hernia. If the condition is behavioural in nature, other members of the multidisciplinary team, such as a psychologist, should become involved (Foxx *et al* 1979; Hewitt and Burden 1984; Rast *et al* 1985). In some instances, gross movements to a horizontal position, such as changing incontinence pads or giving physiotherapy, immediately after a meal may exacerbate these problems. Simply giving a person at least 30 minutes between the end of the meal and movement to a horizontal position may resolve the problem.

Drug-nutrient interactions

(See Section 2.10)

3.14.4 Developments in services for people with learning disabilities

With the move to community care and a 'needs-led service', there are many issues which a dietitian must consider if the service provided is to be successful.

Service systems

Each service will have developed its own unique set of systems and frameworks within which a dietitian will have to work. CMHTs/specialist teams usually hold regular referral meetings at which new clients are allocated a case worker and other clients are reviewed. Being part of these meetings enables a dietitian to obtain up-to-date information, identify people who may benefit from dietetic advice and receive support from other team members. Some teams have centralized case notes which all members use, thus providing a co-ordinated service for the client. The issue of writing up case notes needs careful consideration as Dyson (1986) has strongly criticized some professionals for their devaluing notations.

'Keyworker' or 'named person' systems exist in most residential settings. A particular member of staff is allocated special responsibility to ensure that a client's needs are met. Working with the identified keyworker and client can make all the difference to meeting a person's nutritional requirements. Systems such as 'Shared Action Planning', 'Life Planning', 'Personal Needs Profile' (PNP), 'Individual Personal Plan' (IPP), reviews and case conferences may also exist, particularly in residential settings. These systems all involve meetings to which relevant staff are invited to meet with the client, and possibly the client's family, to review and plan future or immediate needs. They help to identify clients' strengths and needs, emphasizing that they are developing as individuals, rather than being just one person in a particular residence. These forums provide an excellent opportunity for dietitians to negotiate and set realistic nutrition goals.

Control of caseloads

Developing caseloads is not common in dietetic practice; however, working alongside a CMHT/specialist team highlights the necessity to review this situation. Dietitians need to consider the number of clients that they can realistically and competently work for at any one time. Some teams are currently discussing this issue, preparing profiles of caseloads and establishing waiting lists.

People who challenge the service

'Challenging behaviour' is a contemporary term for people whose behaviour challenges the offered service. Some of these people may have mental health problems, others may be reacting to their environment, or to the side effects of medication. Authorities have responded in a variety of different ways by housing people in 'special units', employing special project teams or perhaps resettling in ordinary housing with a high staff ratio. The implications for dietitians are numerous but as yet unresearched. There could be a nutritional component to the behaviour; for example, is the person simply hungry, has a strict diet been imposed, does the person have untreated phenylketonuria (Harper and Reid 1987) or a food allergy?

Sensory stimulation

Longhorn (1988) and Sanderson and Gitsham (1991) have developed sensory curricula for people with profound learning disabilities and sensory loss. This approach enables people to use all their senses to understand and have some control over their environment. Used carefully, people can anticipate what will happen to them next. Dietitians have a lot to offer in guiding staff to apply this philosophy practically, for example, in enabling a person with a profound learning disability to identify their food preferences, to make food choices and participate in sensory baking (Mental Health Group, BDA, April 1992).

Conclusion

Dietitians working in this service have a great deal to offer to the service user. The position offers the opportunity to identify, plan, implement and evaluate individual nutritional plans and challenge current services to provide more opportunities concerning food and health. However dietitians should not be complacent and, in the future, when people realize their rights to good health through good food, must ask themselves whether people with learning disabilities still require segregated dietetic services.

Useful addresses

British Dietetic Association, Mental Health Group, 7th Floor, Elizabeth House, Suffolk Street, Queensway, Birmingham B1 1LS. Produces a comprehensive list of references, resources, literature and support organizations.

British Institute of Mental Handicap (BIMH), Wolverhampton Road, Kidderminster, Worcs DY10 3PP. Tel 0562 850251. Produces reference lists on current interest topics and a wide variety of training courses.

Down's Syndrome Association, 155 Mitcham Road, Tooting, London SW17 9PG. 081–682 4001.

MENCAP, 123 Golden Lane, London EC1Y 0RT. Tel 071–454 0454.

National Autistic Society, 276 Willesden Lane, London NW2 5RB. Tel 081–451 1114.

Open University, Department of Health and Social Welfare, Learning Materials Sales Office, PO Box 188, Milton Keynes MK7 6DH.

Spastics Society, 12 Park Crescent, London W1N 4EQ. Tel 071–636 5020.

Values in Action (VIA), (formerly Campaign for People with a Mental Handicap), Oxford House, Derbyshire Street, London E2 6HG. Contemporary literature on a range of service issues.

Further reading

Flynn M (1988) *Independent living for adults with mental handicap: A place of my own*. Cassells, London.

Kings Fund *An ordinary life: Comprehensive locally based services for mentally handicapped people*. Project Paper 24. Kings Fund, London.

Open University *Mental handicap: patterns for living*. p. 555. Open University, Milton Keynes. Available from the OU Learning Materials Sales Office.

Perske R, Clifton A, Mclean B and Ishler Stein J (1986) *Mealtimes for people with severe handicaps*. Paul Brooks, Baltimore and London.

Key social policy documents

DHSS (1971, reprinted 1979) *Better services for the mentally handicapped*. HMSO, London.

DHSS (1979) *Report of the Committee of Enquiry into Mental Handicap Nursing and Care* (The Jay Report). HMSO, London.

DHSS (1985) House of Commons, second report from the Social Services Committee. Session 1984–85, *Community care with special reference to adult mentally ill and mentally handicapped people 13–1*. HMSO, London.

DHSS (1989) *Caring for people: Community care in the next decade and beyond*. HMSO, London.

References

Cole A (1990) Teaching people how to manage their own 'special' diets: Some lessons from practice. *Mental Handicap* **18**, 156–9.

Cunningham K, Gibney M, Kelly A, Kevany J and Mulcahy M (1990) Nutrient intakes in long-stay mentally handicapped persons. *Br J Nutr* **64**, 3–11.

Dinani S and Carpenter S (1990) Downs syndrome and thyroid disorder. *J Mental Deficiency Res* **34**, 387–92.

Dyson S (1986) Professionals, mentally handicapped children and confidential files. *Disability, Handicap and Society* **1**(1), 73–87.

Evans Morris S and Dunn Klein M (1987) *Pre-feeding skills. Therapy skill builders*. Winslow Press, Winslow, Berks.

Fenton J (1989) Some food for thought. *The Health Service Journal*, June, 666–7.

Foxx RM *et al* (1979) A food satiation and oral hygiene punishment programme to suppress chronic rumination by retarded persons. *J Autism and Development Disorders* **9(4)**,

Harper M and Reid A (1987) Use of unrestricted protein diet in the treatment of behaviour disorder in a severely mentally retarded adult female phenylketonuric patient. *J Mental Deficiency Research* **31**, 209–212.

Hay F and Jeffereys K (1992) *A pilot study on the implementation strategies and monitoring of nutritional standards and services for people with learning disabilities*. Portsmouth and SE Hants HA, Portsmouth.

Hewitt K and Burden P (1984) Behavioural management of food regurgitation: parents as therapists. *Mental Handicap* **12**, 168–9.

Kinnell HG, Gibbs N, Teale JD and Smith J (1987) Thyroid dysfunction in institutionalised Downs syndrome adults. *Psychological Medicine* **17**, 387–92.

Longhorn F (1988) *A sensory curriculum for the very special child. A practical approach to curriculum planning*. Souvenir Press, London.

Macdonald NJ, McConnell KN, Stephen MR and Dunnigan MG (1989) Hypernatraemic dehydration in patients in a large hospital for the mentally handicapped. *Br Med J* **299**, 1426–9.

Mental Health Group, BDA (1992) Abstract from workshop on Sensory-stimulation, Gitsham & Jeffereys.

Moriaty KJ and Silk DA (1988) Laxative abuse. *Digestive Diseases* **6**, 15–29.

O'Brien J and Tyne A (1981) *The principle of normalisation: a foundation for effective services*. CMH/CMHERA, London.

Rast J *et al* (1985) Dietary management of rumination: four case studies. *Am J Clin Nutr* **42**, 95–101.

Simila S and Kokkonen J (1990) Coexistence of celiac disease and Down syndrome. *Am J on Mental Retardation* **95**(1), 120–22.

Sanderson H and Gitsham N (1991) *A holistic sensory approach – a guide to sensory stimulation for people who have profound learning disabilities*. Available from the Day Resource Centre, Slade Hospital, Headington, Oxford.

Wolfensberger W (1972) *The principle of normalisation in human services*. National Institute on Mental Retardation, Toronto.

Woods T (1991) Tackling low body mass index in people with severe learning difficulties. Abstract from BDA Mental Health Group Meeting, April 1991.

3.13 Sports nutrition

Coaches and athletes are becoming more and more aware of the role nutrition plays in improving both health and sports performance. Diet directly affects an athlete's ability to train and recover from training, to compete and keep on competing. 'An adequate diet, in terms of quantity and quality, before, during and after training and competition, will maximize performance. In the optimum diet for most sports, carbohydrate is likely to contribute about 60–70% of total energy intake and protein about 12%, with the remainder coming from fat' (Consensus Statement from the Conference on Foods, Nutrition and Sports Performance 1991).

Owing to the wide diversity of different sporting activities and the vastly differing demands placed upon the individual by their particular sport, level of performance and commitment, it is clearly beyond the scope of this chapter to provide detailed guidelines for every sport. However, there are two specific nutritional principles which are applicable to most sports irrespective of the standard of the participant:

1 The intake of sufficient dietary carbohydrate to maintain muscle glycogen levels during training and competition.
2 The intake of sufficient fluids to maintain normal thermoregulatory function during exercise.

3.13.1 Carbohydrate and exercise

In order to appreciate the relationship between diet and performance, it is helpful to summarize the effects of exercise on energy metabolism.

Energy metabolism during exercise

During exercise the working muscles convert stored energy into kinetic energy and heat – not unlike a combustion engine where the chemical energy (fuel) is transformed into mechanical energy. The energy needs of the muscles are covered by accelerating the rate of adenosine triphosphate (ATP) resynthesis to match the rate at which ATP is being utilized. ATP is produced when muscle cells metabolize carbohydrate and fatty acids in the presence of oxygen. This process is called aerobic metabolism. ATP can also be produced without the presence of oxygen but during this anaerobic metabolism, only carbohydrate can be utilized. Thus the two main fuels for muscle metabolism are carbohydrate and fat. The body's reserves of carbohydrate (as glycogen stores in muscle and liver) are limited but the bodily reserves of fat are for all practical purposes unlimited even in the leanest of athletes. Fatigue often coincides with depletion of the carbohydrate reserves.

It is important to appreciate the factors that influence fuel choices during exercise. These include exercise intensity and duration, training status and diet (Hargreaves 1991). As exercise intensity increases there is increased reliance on carbohydrate but as exercise duration increases there is a declining contribution from carbohydrates. This is partly due to the progressively depleted muscle glycogen and glucose as exercise continues but also to the increased availability of free fatty acids. Training enables the working muscles to take up more oxygen from the blood supply and produce more energy aerobically i.e. utilizing more free fatty acids and therefore sparing the limited glycogen stores.

What is important to appreciate is that whatever exercise is performed, some carbohydrate will always be used – the longer or harder the exercise, the greater the demands placed upon the carbohydrate stores of the body. One of the primary limitations to maintaining high rates of energy expenditure is the availability of glycogen to maintain the desired rate of ATP resynthesis. Without the contribution made by glycogen utilization, the rate at which ATP can be resynthesized is markedly reduced. The only way in which the imbalance in the rates of demand and supply can be redressed is by decreasing the demand for ATP (e.g. by slowing down the rate at which work is performed). Consequently, without adequate muscle glycogen reserves, the ability to perform high levels of work is markedly impaired. This has consequences not only in competition but more importantly in training. It is only through training that performance can improve and this can only be achieved if each training session is started with muscles well stocked with glycogen.

The role of carbohydrates in training

Every time an athlete trains, the amount of glycogen within the working muscles will fall. As these stores are limited, they must be restocked adequately before the next training session, or it will be started with lower than normal glycogen reserves. If the reserves are lower than normal, the point at which glycogen could become limiting may be attained more rapidly, impairing both the quality and quantity of training which can be accomplished within the training session. If the process of incomplete refuelling is repeated over successive days of training, a progressive depletion of glycogen stores within the working muscles will result and even the lightest exercise will become extremely difficult to complete. The feeling of continual lethargy and heavy tired muscles or incomplete recovery between training sessions and the over-training syndrome may all be related to trying to train with insufficient restocking of muscle glycogen.

The importance of muscle glycogen and blood glucose during exercise is demonstrated by the observations that muscle glycogen loading and glucose ingestion result in improved endurance exercise performance. In view of the importance of carbohydrates in exercise, replacing the glycogen reserves (particularly muscle glycogen following exercise) is a critical metabolic process in the recovery period. Exercise activates glycogen synthase in muscle but full restoration of muscle glycogen during recovery is dependent on an adequate intake of dietary carbohydrate (Hargreaves 1991).

Factors influencing the rate of glycogen repletion

The main factors influencing the rate of muscle glycogen synthesis are the type and amount of carbohydrate ingested and the timing of ingestion. Muscle glycogen becomes totally depleted after 2–3 hours of continuous exercise at intensities of 60–80% VO_2 max. (As an individual moves from rest to running the oxygen uptake increases in an almost linear fashion until the individual reaches a point where there is no further increase in O_2 consumption. This is the maximum O_2 uptake or VO_2 max for the individual. When the exercise intensity expressed as a % VO_2 max it is called the relative exercise intensity and it reflects the physiological and psychological demands on the individual.) Muscle glycogen can also be severely depleted after only 15–30 minutes of exercise at intensities of 90–130% VO_2 max when the exercise takes the form of intervals of 1–5 minutes exercise followed by rest, followed by exercise, rest etc (Coyle 1991). This type of short intermittent, high intensity exercise is a pattern found typically in many individual and team sports such as soccer, hockey and tennis. Many athletes who train daily need to increase their carbohydrate consumption if they are to avoid residual fatigue, poor performance and the over-training syndrome.

Glycogen is restored to the muscles at a rate of about 5% per hour and after exhaustive exercise up to 20 hours are needed to fully replenish muscle glycogen stores. During the first two hours after exercise, muscle glycogen resynthesis proceeds at the rate of 7% per hour. It is therefore essential that athletes consume sufficient carbohydrate during this time. It is generally recommended that athletes should aim to eat 50 g (for 70 kg body weight – adjustments should be made for actual body weight) carbohydrate during the first two hour period after exercise.

Dietary recommendations for training

Athletes whose diet is consistently high in carbohydrate with up to 70% of daily energy needs supplied by carbohydrate are better able to maintain their glycogen stores. In terms of quantitative amounts, an intake of 500–600 g is often quoted as the recommended amount for the replenishment of muscle glycogen stores on a daily basis. However this is more usefully expressed in terms of body weight as female athletes do not consume the same absolute amounts of carbohydrate as men. For athletes involved in heavy training schedules a daily intake of 8–10 g kg^{-1} b.wt may be necessary. Certainly daily training for one or more hours decreases muscle glycogen stores when carbohydrate intake is only 5 g kg^{-1} b.wt per day. This is essentially the same advice, but more so, that would be given to all members of the population and thus there is no conflict between eating for performance and eating for health. Moreover, an interest in sport may present the opportunity to introduce healthy eating to an otherwise non-compliant population, particularly the young adolescent.

Starchy and sugary carbohydrates appear to be equally effective in glycogen refuelling. Athletes with high energy requirements will be eating large amounts of carbohydrate and if they limit themselves to starchy foods, the diet will become excessively bulky. In guiding such athletes to include sugary sources of carbohydrate, care must be taken that fat intake is not greatly increased and that a healthy balance is achieved between the contribution of carbohydrate from these sources and the starchy sources. Athletes with lower energy needs will obtain carbohydrate primarily from starchy foods, fruit and fruit juices.

Many athletes find solid food immediately after exercise unacceptable and in order to achieve the required intake of carbohydrate during the first two hour period, drinks containing glucose, sucrose or maltodextrin in concentrations of 6 g/100 ml or higher may be more acceptable. There are many such commercial preparations available including Maxijul and Maxim. After the initial two hour period, 50 g (or the body weight equivalent) of carbohydrate should continue to be consumed every two hours. However as such frequent meals are not usually practical, subsequent meals should take this into account. Meals should thus contain sufficient carbohydrate to cover the time interval before the next meal (i.e. 150 g for a 6 hour interval, 250 g for a 10 hour interval etc.) The reader is strongly recommended to read Coyle (1991) for a more detailed account of this important topic.

The practical constraints placed on athletes by their lifestyle can make it difficult for them to achieve a balanced, healthy diet high in carbohydrates. These constraints are specific to each individual athlete and should be taken into account when giving advice. A single standardized set of dietary guidelines will result in poor compliance!

For example, one of the greatest difficulties facing the athlete is simply fitting in the purchase, preparation and consumption of relatively large amounts of food with training travel, competition and employment/education. Many athletes rely heavily on the use of confectionery and convenience foods to satisfy their appetite. If athletes remove such foods from their usual diet in order to improve the overall quality of the diet, alternative sources of carbohydrate of comparable density must be included or total carbohydrate intake will fall considerably. Ease and speed of preparation of meals are important considerations.

General recommendations during preparation for competition

The most important nutritional consideration is ensuring that the athlete arrives at the competition fully recovered from training with at least normal glycogen stores. Training will result in substantially lowered glycogen stores – thus, the first consideration is to taper the training load over the week preceding competition to allow repletion. Consumption of a diet containing 350–450 g carbohydrate per day combined with rest should result in normal muscle glycogen stores within 3–4 days; whilst consumption of a high carbohydrate diet will result in significantly greater than normal increases in muscle glycogen (Sherman 1983). Such increases are comparable to those increases in glycogen achieved using the traditional carbohydrate loading technique of prolonged exhaustive exercise and three days on a very low carbohydrate, high protein high fat diet followed by three days on a very high carbohydrate diet. The latter technique can result in inadequate glycogen repletion through poor dietary management (Wootton *et al* 1981). Therefore, the best approach would be for athletes to consume a high carbohydrate diet at all times and then simply taper their training in preparation for competition.

Such increases in glycogen stores not only benefit the endurance athlete such as the marathon runner, triathlete, distance cyclist etc., but may be of help in tournament situations where competition lasts for several days. Starting the competition with high glycogen stores may help to offset the progressive depletion of muscle glycogen stores with each bout of competition. One possible disadvantage of increasing glycogen stores is the commensurate increase in body weight through the associated storage of water with glycogen. This may be an important consideration where an athlete competes in a weight category sport such as judo, boxing etc. Supercompensating muscle glycogen stores may also improve performance during maximal exercise of short duration (Maughan 1990).

The pre-competition meal should be carbohydrate-based, low in fat, protein and fibre and readily digested so that it does not cause any gastrointestinal discomfort. It is generally recommended that approximately 200–300 g of carbohydrate should be ingested during the four hours before competition. Where performance may be limited by carbohydrate availability, the use of carbohydrate feeding immediately prior to and during exercise can be considered. The effect of carbohydrate taken as a special feed during the last hour before exercise begins has been reported in a number of studies. The concern that sugar feedings can cause insulin induced hypoglycaemia seem less well-founded (for review see Coyle 1991) and there is now little support for the idea that such feedings prior to exercise impair performance.

Consuming carbohydrate during endurance events and high intensity intermittent exercise such as soccer and hockey ensures that sufficient carbohydrate is available in the later stages of competition where otherwise lack of carbohydrate could lead to fatigue and poor performance. It is better to ingest carbohydrate at regular intervals throughout exercise (where the sport permits) than to wait until signs of fatigue. Glucose, sucrose and maltodextrin seem equally effective in prolonging the onset of fatigue. In most situations, fluids are easier to ingest than solid foods. Appropriate volumes and concentrations should be used depending on the circumstances, preferences and need for fluid replacement. High concentrations of carbohydrate impair fluid absorption. It is therefore important to assess the likely cause of fatigue – lack of fuel or dehydration – and provide the appropriate solution to delay the onset of fatigue. For a more detailed account the reader is recommended to read Coyle (1991).

3.13.2 Fluid balance

Thermoregulation during exercise

Humans are very inefficient when it comes to converting the energy stored in food into mechanical work. Only about 20–25% of the available energy stored in carbohydrate or fat is actually converted into a form which the muscles can actually use to contract and generate force. The remaining 70–80% is lost as heat. During exercise, when the rate of energy utilization increases, the rate of heat production will also increase. In order to prevent an excessive rise in body temperature (hyperthermia) the body must lose this additional heat. It can do this by several mechanisms, the most important of which is through the evaporation of sweat on the surface of the skin.

Although sweating is a very effective way of losing heat, care must be taken to ensure that this process is not impaired through dehydration. Sweat is simply a dilute version of blood. Thus when sweating is prolonged or pronounced, the body loses both water and electrolytes. The loss of electrolytes is much less than the loss of water and does not represent an immediate problem. It does not appear to be necessary to replace these electrolytes during exercise – if anything the concentration of the major electrolytes in plasma tend to increase during exercise. Food eaten after exercise will replace any electrolyte losses – the use of salt tablets should be strongly discouraged. Water loss will cause serious problems if no attempts are made to replace the lost fluid.

The body needs to balance the losses and intake of fluids in order to maintain the capacity to regulate body temperature. Where sweat losses greatly exceed replacement, the circulatory system is unable to cope and skin blood flow falls. With this comes a reduction in sweating and a reduction in the ability to lose heat, thus body temperature will rise with potentially fatal consequences. Considerable care should be taken to ensure adequate hydration before, during and after exercise so as to avoid thermal distress. These principles apply equally to both training and competition as progressive depletion of the body water can occur over several days of insufficient fluid intake in the same way as the progressive depletion of glycogen. It should also be remembered that these points apply equally to all sportsmen and women – not just marathon runners – and especially to those exercising indoors. The rate of sweating depends on a number of factors – work rate, environmental temperature, humidity, body surface area, hydration status, training status, acclimatization and clothing (Brouns 1991) and these should be taken into account when considering volume and concentration of fluids to be ingested. The addition of some carbohydrate and sodium speeds up the absorption of water and thus the process of rehydration. The carbohydrate also provides an additional source of fuel for the working muscles. There are now several commercial preparations available that athletes can use for rehydration (e.g. Gatorade, Isostar, Lucozade Sport). Athletes can also make their own by making up a 50:50 solution of fruit juice and water with a pinch of salt or by dissolving 4–8 g glucose or glucose polymer in 100 ml hot water and adding a small pinch of salt (any flavouring should be 'sugar free'). Where rehydration is a priority the carbohydrate content is low; where provision of additional fuel is paramount a higher concentration of glucose can be used. For a review of this subject see Maughan (1991).

Dietetic advice concerning fluid balance

Before exercise

The athlete should be fully hydrated prior to taking any exercise – training or competition; sporting activities should never be started in a dehydrated state. Large amounts of alcohol the night before should be avoided. In any situation but especially where opportunities for intake during events are likely to be restricted, there is a need to be fully hydrated before competition begins. This can be achieved by having a high intake of fluid in the days running up to competition. (A useful check is to ensure that urine is pale in colour.) In the last 10–30 minutes before competition 400–600 ml of fluid should be drunk. Drinking earlier than this can cause problems because of the need to urinate once the event has started.

During exercise

There is no advantage in taking fluids during exercise lasting less than 30 minutes but fluid intake should be encouraged in all other situations. Drinking should be encourage at an early stage and *before* thirst has developed; in some sports a cyclist's water bottle may be a useful piece of equipment. Frequent ingestion of small amounts of fluids keeps up the rate of gastric emptying which can be a limiting factor in water absorption. Athletes are often encouraged to consume up to 150 ml fluid every 15 minutes but in reality the amount of fluid ingested will depend on losses through sweating and will be affected by palatability and tolerance to fluid in the stomach (Brouns 1991). Athletes should use training sessions to get used to drinking during exercise. Cold drinks were believed to be better than warm because they left the stomach faster but recent reports have cast doubt on the importance of temperature (Maughan 1991). The athlete's own preference is the best guide – a larger volume is more likely to be consumed if the athlete finds the drink palatable.

Heat build-up can be minimized by splashing water on the skin during exercise which will cause heat loss via evaporation. Sporting activities in warm climates require careful preparation and sufficient time for acclimatization before competition.

Following exercise

Rehydration should start immediately and not some hours after the event, particularly when repeated bouts of exercise have to be performed. Drinking plain water after exercise results in a rapid fall in the plasma sodium concentration and in plasma osmolality. This has the effect of reducing the sensation of thirst and of stimulating urine output which in turn delays rehydration. More effective rehydration may well be achieved with the use of fluids which contain sodium. Athletes should carry their own supply of fluid in their kit bag and not rely on fluids always being available at events.

3.13.3 Other considerations

The energy expenditure due to physical activity can account for 25–35% of the daily energy turnover up to 75% during intense training of long duration. Energy intakes can therefore vary from 1500 kcal per day for young female gymmnasts to 6000–7000 kcal per day for Tour de France cyclists. In sports where a specific body image is required (e.g. female gymnastics, bodybuilding, dancing) or where a sport requires the athlete to compete in a weight category (e.g. judo, wrestling, boxing, lightweight rowing), athletes will often restrict energy intake to lose weight or maintain a particular body composition.

Athletes who repeatedly restrict energy intake for competition, then regain weight afterwards (weight cycling) may find it increasingly harder to lose weight though regaining weight becomes easier. Female athletes who follow intensive training progammes while restricting energy intake may experience other related problems such as menstrual dysfunction (including amenorrhea), decreased bone density and iron deficiency anaemia (Westerterp and Saris 1991). Lower energy intakes may also be associated with low intakes of vitamins. There is also the potential risk that élite female athletes competing in weight category sports or sports where weight or body composition is relevant for performance may present with eating disorders.

Rapid weight loss in days before competition to 'make weight' is also achieved in some sports by increasing rather than tapering training, fasting or vomiting, restricting fluids and by the use of saunas, sweat suits, laxatives and diuretics. Such practices will lead to diminished body reserves which more than offset any advantages of competing in a lower weight category. Long term planned weight reduction programmes are essential if athletes are to maintain training and not impair their performance.

Where high energy intakes are required, it is still important to provide a high proportion of carbohydrate for maximal power output and not to rely on increasing the intake of more energy dense fatty foods. The lifestyle of athletes often limits the amount of time available to eat and for those athletes requiring a high energy intake it is not practical to recommend that the carbohydrate is provided solely by starchy, unrefined foods such as wholegrain cereals, potatoes and pulses. In such cases the diet will need to be supplemented with sources of simple carbohydrate in solid or liquid form, including such products as Maxijul and Maxim.

Protein

Many atheletes believe they must eat large amounts of protein to build muscles and increase strength, yet most expert committees on nutrition throughout the world have not provided additional allowances of protein for active individuals when recommending dietary protein intakes. Experimental evidence collected over the last 15 years seems to indicate that regular exercise does increase protein needs. Several factors including the composition of the diet, total energy intake, the type, intensity and duration of exercise, ambient temperature, gender and maybe even age can influence protein requirements.

Definitive dietary recommendations for different types of sport are not yet available but current evidence suggests that strength or speed athletes require 1.2–1.7 g protein/kg body weight per day and endurance athletes 1.2–1.4 g protein/kg body weight per day (Lemon 1991). Unless total energy intake is insufficient to meet requirements such quantities of protein can be meet by a diet providing 12–15% energy from protein. The high energy intakes typical of most athletes makes these recommendations easy to attain without any dietary manipulation. Athletes at the lower end of the energy intakes range may require dietary manipulation to achieve their protein requirements. Vegetarian athletes may also need some guidance to ensure adequate protein intake, particularly those also consuming low energy diets.

Fat

Unlike glycogen which can only be stored in limited amounts, fat is not a limiting factor for exercise. Even the leanest of competitors (male and female endurance athletes have only about 7–10% of their body weights as fat) has a large reserve of fat for energy. There is no need to supplement the normal diet with additional fat, indeed intakes of more than 30% energy from fat are likely to indicate an inadequate intake of carbohydrate.

Vitamins

Vitamin supplements do not enhance the performance of athletes who are already consuming an adequate diet. However there may be situations where intakes should be increased by altering the diet or recommending the use of supplementation e.g. poor eating habits giving rise to limited intakes, restriction of food intake to maintain low body weight. Athletes who need to consume high energy intakes may be including foods of low nutrient density in order to achieve their energy intake without too much bulk. In both extremes of energy intake it may be necessary to recommend the use of a vitamin supplement but without megadosing (van der Beek 1991).

Minerals

Particular attention should be paid to iron and calcium intakes. Some athletes are predisposed to poor iron status due to low intakes of iron because of restricted food intakes or because dietary iron is predominantly in the form of non-haem iron. Such at risk groups of athletes should be detected as early as possible and monitored for iron depletion. Treatment may include iron supplementation as well as dietary modification to maximize iron absorption.

Female athletes with amenorrhoea or dysmenorrhoea have an increased risk of developing osteoporosis because of the reduced levels of bone-protecting oestrogen. Improved calcium intakes are particularly important in athletes with low bone density, menstrual irregularities and low calcium intakes since stress fractures are particularly common in this group of athletes (Clarkson 1991).

Ergogenic aids

Ergogenic aids are substances that supposedly raise athletic performance above what would normally be expected, i.e. that will give the athlete that competitive edge. Substances that are claimed to be ergogenic aids include bee pollen, ginseng, royal jelly, guarana, coenzyme Q_{10} and many many more. By their very nature the list is forever changing.

There is a definite lack of any scientific evidence to support the performance enhancing claims for these substances. Taking such substances is unlikely to have any effect on performance except as a result of a placebo effect. Ergogenic aids can be expensive but, more importantly, little is known about the possible side effects or toxic levels of these substances. Commercially produced preparations can contain impurities which may be harmful or illegal (banned substances). Athletes should be encouraged to accept training programmes, technique, good diet, good equipment, adequate rest and sleep and the right mental approach as the effective ways to aid performance.

Weight control

The aim of a weight loss diet for an athlete is to decrease the body's fat store without affecting the glycogen, water or lean body mass content. It is essential that the diet contains sufficient carbohydrate to restock the glycogen stores between each training session. The diet must therefore be very low in fat and provide all the essential nutrients in a total energy intake that will achieve the desired weight loss. Rapid weight loss by dietary or non-dietary methods should be discouraged if loss of performance due to dehydration and glycogen depletion is to be avoided (for review see Smith 1984).

In gaining weight, an athlete will want to increase lean body mass rather than body fat content. Muscle mass is determined by the training effect and the best dietary advice for an athlete desiring to gain weight is to ensure an adequate diet with a high proportion of carbohydrate to support training. A conscious effort should be made to keep up food intake, meals should not be missed and high carbohydrate snacks should be included between meals whenever possible.

Useful addresses

Sports Nutrition Foundation, National Sports Medicine Institute of the UK, c/o Medical College of St Bartholomew's Hospital, Charterhouse Square, London EC1M 6BQ. Tel 071–250 0493.

Sports Nutrition Service, Department of Physical Education and Sports Science, Loughborough University, Loughborough, Leics LE11 3TU. Tel 0509 263171 ext 4251.

The National Coaching Foundation, 4 College Close, Becket Park, Leeds LS6 3QH. Tel 0532 744802.

Further reading

Bean A and Smeaton I (1990) *Nutrition and sports performance*. Community Nutrition Group Information Sheet No 18, September 1990.

Wootton S (1988) *Nutrition for sport: eating to improve performance*. Simon and Schuster

Katch FI and McArdle WD (1988) *Nutrition, weight control and exercise*. Lea and Febiger, Philadelphia.

Clark N (1990) *Nancy Clark's sports nutrition guidebook*. Leisure Press, (Human Kinetics Publishers Inc.)

References

Brouns F (1991) Dehydration – rehydration: a praxis oriented approach. *J of Sp Sci* **9**, 143–52.

Clarkson PM (1991) Minerals: exercise performance and supplementation in athletes. *J of Sp Sci* **9**, 91–116.

Coyle EF (1991) Timing and method of increased carbohydrate intake to cope with heavy training, competition and recovery. *J of Sp Sci* **9**, 29–52.

Final Consensus Statement (1991) *J of Sp Sci* **9**, iii.

Hargreaves M (1991) Carbohydrates and exercise. *J of Sp Sci* **9**, 17–28.

Lemon PWR (1991) Effect of exercise on protein requirements. *J of Sp Sci* **9**, 53–70.

Maughan R (1990) Effects of diet composition on the performance of high density exercises. In *Nutrition et Sport*. Monod H (Ed) pp. 200–211. Masson, Paris.

Maughan R (1991) Fluid and electrolyte loss and replacement in exercise. *J of Sp Sci* **9**, 117–42.

Sherman WM (1983) Carbohydrate metabolism. In *Ergogenic aids in sport*. Williams MH (Ed) pp. 3–26. Human Kinetics Publishers, Champaign.

Smith NA (1984) Weight control in the athlete. In *Nutritional aspects of exercise. Clinics in sports medicine*. Hecker AL (Ed) pp. 693–704. WB Saunders, Philadelphia.

van der Beek EJ (1991) Vitamin supplementation and physical exercise performance. *J of Sp Sci* **9**, 77–89.

Westerterp KR and Saris WHM (1991) Limits of energy turnover in relation to physical performance, achievement of energy balance on a daily basis. *J of Sp Sci* **9**, 1–15.

Wootton SA, Shorten MR and Williams C (1981) Nutritional manipulation of metabolism for the purpose of sport. In *Applied Nutrition I*. Bateman EC (Ed) pp. 60–64. John Libbey, London.

Section 4 **Therapeutic dietetics for disease states**

4.1 Disorders of the Mouth

Healthy teeth and gums are important for good digestion. Dental caries, periodontal disease and poorly fitting dentures are often implicated in malnutrition and indigestion. When giving dietary advice it is important to ensure that the patient can masticate his or her food adequately.

4.1.1 Dental caries

Dental caries results from demineralization of the enamel surface of the tooth by acids produced from dietary sugars by microbial action. Initially mineral disappears from the sub-surface of the tooth and if this process is not checked or reversed, a cavity will develop in which more bacterial growth can occur causing further dissolution of enamel and progression of the lesion into the dentine and towards the pulp. Eventually the tooth may be lost.

Causation

The factors which determine the extent of dental caries are:

The bacterial flora of the mouth

Dental caries does not occur in the absence of the appropriate bacteria. *Streptococcus mutans* is probably the most significant organism for initiating lesions. It converts sucrose into glucan, a viscous and sticky polymer which adheres to the surface of the tooth. This enables other acid-forming bacteria such as lactobacilli to colonize the tooth and once the critical pH of 5.5 is reached, the enamel will begin to dissolve.

Substrates for acid production

The presence in the mouth of fermentable sugars, such as sucrose and glucose, is essential for the development of dental caries. Within minutes of their consumption, such sugars cause the pH in dental plaque to fall below the critical pH (5.5) for enamel dissolution. This fall in pH will occur irrespective of the amount of sucrose consumed or its source, and the normal oral pH of 7.0 will only be restored about 30 min after the sugar has been finally swallowed. The quantity of sugar eaten is therefore less important than the time taken to consume it and the interval before more is taken. Normal pH will return sooner if an item is consumed quickly rather than sipped or sucked slowly. For example, a sugar-rich drink consumed rapidly will cause less damage than one containing less sugar but sipped over a period of time. A packet of sweets eaten at frequent intervals during the day will result in acid conditions in the mouth for most of that period; if the same sweets are eaten all at once, the normal pH can be restored within half an hour. The type of sugar-containing food eaten is also relevant to caries formation; items which are sticky and can leave residues in the teeth (e.g. toffees, dates or raisins) can also result in cariogenic conditions persisting in the mouth for extended periods of time.

The acidity of foods eaten

Acid foods (such as citrus fruits or juices) inevitably lower the mouth pH and hence produce cariogenic conditions. Cola drinks are particularly acidic and thus even sugar-free cola is still potentially damaging to teeth (but to a lesser extent than the sugar-containing type). Finishing a meal with an alkaline food (such as cheese, milk or peanuts) can help to raise the pH of the mouth.

The resistance of the teeth

There is considerable variability in the resistance of tooth enamel to decay. Those with crowded teeth or poorly developed enamel are most vulnerable. Fluoride can markedly increase enamel resistance since it results in the formation of fluorhydroxyapatite crystals in the tooth matrix which are more resistant to acid erosion than unfluoridated hydroxyapatite. The maximum benefit from fluoride is obtained if it is available during the period of tooth formation, i.e. before the tooth erupts through the gum. Once the tooth has emerged, further protection can be obtained from topical or dietary fluoride.

Oral hygiene

Proper cleansing of the teeth and gums by means of brushing and flossing is essential to remove plaque and accumulation of debris at the base of the teeth which can lead to gum inflammation (gingivitis). Patients undergoing radiotherapy to the head and neck or chemotherapy may be more susceptible to dental caries and good oral hygiene is essential throughout their treatment.

Treatment and prevention of dental caries

Fillings

Fillings do not prevent caries but merely repair the damage caused. Caries can still occur around or alongside fillings if preventative measures are not observed.

Oral hygiene

Correct and regular brushing and flossing of the teeth and gums is essential to help prevent both caries and gum disease.

Diet and fluoride supplementation

Complete exclusion of fermentable sugars from the diet is neither practical nor desirable since they are present in many nutritious foods (e.g. fruits) as well as in manufactured confectionery. However, children should be discouraged as far as possible from consuming sugar-rich drinks and sweets and ideally these should only be eaten at meal times and the teeth cleaned afterwards. In practice, most children do eat sweets at other times and if this cannot be prevented then they should at least be taught to avoid the sticky or slowly sucked items, and that their intake of all sweets should be 'few and far between'.

The availability of adequate fluoride, either systemically or topically, is important. This can be obtained in several ways.

Drinking water Some parts of the country have a naturally high level of fluoride in the drinking water; other areas add fluoride artificially to the water supply. A water fluoride content of 1.0–1.5 ppm has been shown to reduce significantly the incidence of dental caries.

Fluoride supplements These are available in either tablet or liquid form, the latter being especially useful for babies and young children who will benefit most from fluoride supplementation. However, before these supplements are given it is essential to check the local fluoride water content since too high a fluoride intake can cause mottling of the teeth. Local dentists are usually the best people to advise as to whether supplements would be beneficial. If the fluoride content of the local water supply is less than 0.3 ppm, the fluoride supplements listed in Table 4.1 should be given.

If the fluoride content of the local of water supply is between 0.3–0.7 ppm, no supplements should be given below the age of 2 years. Thereafter, only half of the recommended levels of supplementation described in Table 4.1 should be given.

If the fluoride content of water exceeds 0.7 ppm, additional fluoride supplements are probably unwise.

Table 4.1 Recommended levels of fluoride supplements for 'at risk' children

Age	Fluoride supplement (mg/day)
2 weeks–2 years	0.25
2 years–4 years	0.5
4 years–6 years	1.0

Fluoride toothpastes Tooth enamel will accrue fluoride from toothpaste to some extent and thus be strengthened further, but the benefit will be less if fluoride was not already available systemically during the stage of tooth formation.

Topical fluoride Fluoride can be 'painted' on to teeth in the form of a varnish or, more commonly, a gel and this can be a useful way of remineralizing enamel in the precavitation stage of decalcification. Routine applications can be beneficial to children, particularly those on long term medication which is syrup-based.

Fluoride mouth rinses These also arrest decalfication, encourage remineralization and will increase the benefit from a fluoride toothpaste. Mouth rinses are more suitable for adults than children (who tend to swallow them).

Fissure sealing

In children, the vulnerable biting surfaces of the teeth can be coated with a thin layer of plastic sealant. This is a very effective way of preventing decay especially on molars where the deep grooves readily accumulate plaque and are not easily accessible to the toothbrush. This procedure can only be carried out by a dentist and ideally should be performed as soon as the crown of each permanent tooth emerges (i.e. around the age of six years). If left later than this, the coating will also seal in any decay process which has already commenced and this may cause more damage than if the tooth is left alone.

4.1.2 Periodontal disease

Healthy gums can withstand hard usage. The massaging effect of chewing unrefined foods helps to keep both the teeth and gums healthy. A soft diet, rich in refined carbohydrate, tends to stick round the teeth and forms an ideal medium for bacterial growth causing the gum margin to become red and inflamed (gingivitis). Histological changes in the gingival crevice can be seen within 2–4 days after stopping normal oral hygiene. It is therefore particularly important that the teeth and gums of those who are acutely ill or unable to care for themselves are cleansed regularly.

Deficiencies of certain vitamins, particularly vitamin C, may produce similar inflammation and the teeth may become loose from the lack of cement which normally holds them to the jaw. However, lack of vitamin C is not usually a common factor in the cause of periodontal disease. The disease is treated by improved oral hygiene and antibiotic therapy if necessary. The amount of refined carbohydrate eaten should be reduced and unrefined carbohydrate increased as the condition of the gums improves.

Periodontal disease and dental caries are frequently seen together, though this is not always the case. Both can be prevented if children are taught how to care for their teeth as part of the foundation of good eating habits. It is most important that dentists, doctors, dietitians, health educators and school teachers work together to provide sound advice in antenatal clinics, children's clinics and schools.

4.1.3 Mouth lesions related to nutritional deficiencies

Deficiencies of practically all the vitamins of the B group have an effect on the soft tissues of the mouth. A sore mouth and pain on eating may lead to anorexia and result in multiple nutritional deficiencies.

Angular stomatitis

Angular stomatitis is an infection of the skin at the corners of the mouth and responds rapidly to large doses of riboflavin and sometimes pyridoxine. It also occurs in iron deficiency anaemia. A common cause of angular stomatitis is ill-fitting dentures. Radiotherapy to the head and neck can also cause angular stomatitis and lesions of the oral mucosa (see Section 4.34.2).

Cheilosis

Cheilosis is a zone of red denuded epithelium at the line of closure of the lips. It is seen in people with pellagra and often associated with angular stomatitis. It is not likely that a lack of one specific vitamin or nutrient is the sole cause and a good mixed diet with multivitamin therapy should help to improve the condition.

Scurvy

A lack of vitamin C causes weakening of periodontal fibres and the teeth may become loose and fall out. The gums become tender and bleed easily. Treament is by vitamin therapy and sources of vitamin C should be included in the diet regularly.

Vitamin A deficiency

Deficiency of vitamin A may cause hypoplasia in the enamel and dentine of the teeth of children.

Vitamin D deficiency

Deficiency of vitamin D causes defective calcification of the dentine of the teeth and may increase susceptibility to dental caries. Eruption of the teeth may be delayed in children with rickets. Vitamin D therapy should be given and good sources of vitamin D taken in the diet, together with exposure to sunlight where possible.

Patients with lesions of the mouth resulting from vitamin deficiencies should find a soft or even liquid diet more acceptable to take. Very hot, cold, salty or spicy foods should be avoided until the lesions have healed (Table 4.2).

Anaemia

Iron deficiency and pernicious anaemia both result in changes in the tongue causing it to become very red, sore and smooth. The deficiencies should be corrected by iron and vitamin B_{12} as appropriate and a soft diet taken until the condition improves.

4.1.4 Oro-facial granulomatosis

Oro-facial granulomatosis (OFG) is a term which describes a number of related conditions of the mouth. These include Melkersson-Rosenthal syndrome, cheilitis granulomatosa, sarcoidosis and the oral manifestations of Crohn's disease (Wiesenfeld *et al* 1985). The presenting features of OFG include enlargement of the lips, diffuse facial swellings, gingival hyperplasia, oral ulceration and mucosal tags. A review of possible aetiologies of OFG by Ferguson and MacFadyen (1986) included dental infection and hypersensitivity to streptococcal infection or another environmental factor. Treatments have included intralesional and systemic use of steroids, radiotherapy, anti-

Table 4.2 Advice for patients with a sore mouth or throat

1	Meals should be small and frequent
2	A soft, semi-solid diet or nourishing fluids may be better tolerated than solid foods
3	Very hot, salty and spicy foods such as peppers, curries or bottled sauces should be avoided
4	Food should be eaten lukewarm or cold rather than hot
5	Well chilled foods and drinks may be soothing
6	Acid fruits and fruit juices (such as orange, grapefruit, lemon or tomato juice) should be avoided as they may sting the mouth and throat
7	Dry meals should be avoided; plenty of sauce or gravy should be added to meals
8	Strong alcoholic drinks (such as spirits and sherries) should be avoided
9	Protein and energy supplements should be used as directed
10	Ill-fitting dentures should be removed when eating
11	Care should be taken with oral hygiene; teeth should be brushed with a soft brush and the mouth rinsed with a mouthwash after each meal
12	Smoking and smoky atmospheres should be avoided
13	All medications should be taken as directed

inflammatory drugs and surgical reduction. All appear to be ineffective as long term therapy, although temporary relief is possible.

More recently the use of an elimination diet and food reintroduction programme has been described by Haworth *et al* (1988), based on the technique developed for patients with Crohn's disease. Use of energy or more complete supplements should be considered in all cases, but particularly in children.

4.1.5 Disorders of the salivary glands

Inflammation of the parotid glands due to either the mumps virus or bacterial infection may make chewing and swallowing painful and difficult. A high protein, high energy fluid diet using either commercially available sip feeds, liquidized foods or a combination of both should be given until the inflammation subsides (see Section 1.13.3).

Salivary calculi cause pain and difficulty on eating. A soft or high protein, high energy fluid diet should be consumed (see Section 1.13.3). Removal of the stones is usually by surgical excision and the diet gradually regraded to normal as the mouth heals.

4.1.6 Fractured jaws and oral surgery

Patients with fractured jaws are likely to require wiring of the jaws. Jaw wiring may also be required in some cases of oral surgery. In both cases nutritionally complete commercially available liquid feeds are the most suitable means of providing nutrition (Section 1.13.3). If patients can sip these through a straw and consume adequate fluid, energy and protein, they should be encouraged to do so. In most cases the jaws remain wired for approximately 6–8 weeks. Many patients can be managed successfully at home taking a high protein, high energy fluid diet. Variety is important and a range of savoury and sweet nourishing fluids should be recommended together with liquidized meals if the patient wishes and is able to take them. However if they are unable to suck or unwilling to take adequate amounts, a nasogastric tube may need to be passed to provide nutritional support until oral fluids can be taken (see Section 1.13.4).

As the wires are relaxed and ultimately removed, the diet should be regraded from nourishing fluids to a liquidized, soft or semi-solid diet, with protein and energy supplements if indicated, until a normal diet can be taken.

Careful attention should be given to oral hygiene as protein and energy-containing fluids are an ideal medium for bacterial growth.

Patients whose jaws are wired for the treatment of frank obesity obviously do not require a high energy intake. This use of jaw wiring in obesity is discussed in Section 4.17.1.

4.1.7 Cancer of the mouth and pharynx

Cancer of the mouth and pharynx cause difficulties in chewing and swallowing food and many patients experience anorexia and weight loss. These tumours are treated by surgical excision and/or radiotherapy. Chemotherapy may also be used.

Prior to treatment a soft, semi-solid or fluid diet should be given. If the mouth is sore, very hot, cold, salty and spicy foods should be avoided (Table 4.2). Protein and energy supplements may be required to help prevent further weight loss and maintain nutritional status. If an inadequate oral diet is consumed, nasogastric feeding may be required (see Section 1.13.4).

The benefit of pre-operative feeding is debatable and early surgery may be preferred with nutritional support provided post-operatively. Where surgery is required it may necessitate extensive reconstruction of the face and mouth (e.g. Commandos procedure) resulting in severe disfiguration. At the time of surgery a nasogastric tube should be inserted and feeding using a commercially prepared enteral feed commenced post-operatively once gastric emptying is established (see Section 1.13.4). A soft, high protein, high energy light diet should be introduced when oral diet is tolerated and enteral feeding via the nasogastric tube phased out. These patients require regular and practical dietetic advice in order to encourage their interest in, and adequate consumption of, food.

Radiation of the mouth will cause tender, swollen tissues and management should be by either nasogastric feeding or sip feeding using nutritionally complete enteral feeds. There are many side effects and problems associated with radiotherapy (see Section 4.34.2). Radiotherapy to the mouth may damage the taste buds and alter taste sensitivity. It may also result in a dry mouth due to lack of saliva. The resistance of the teeth to dental caries is also reduced and particular attention should be given to oral hygiene and the protection of the teeth. The treatment can also have profound psychological, physiological and nutritional side effects. 'Post-irradiation mouth blindness' (MacCarthy-Leventhal 1959) may persist for some time after the completion of treatment.

4.1.8 Cancer of the larynx

As well as causing difficulty in speaking and hoarseness of the voice, carcinoma of the larynx may also result in difficulty in eating and swallowing solid foods.

At the time of laryngectomy, a nasogastric tube should be inserted and nutritional support provided using a nutritionally complete enteral feed (see Section 1.13.4). Nasogastric feeding is usually continued for a minimum of ten days. Once healing has taken place a soft, light diet plus protein and energy supplements should be introduced as nasogastric feeding is phased out. Patients requiring radiotherapy may need to continue with this diet, but most

Table 4.3 Dietary management of disorders of the oral cavity

Oral condition	Eating difficulty	Treatment	Dietary management
Dental caries	Pain on eating, loss of teeth	Dental treatment ? Fluoride protection Oral hygiene	Reduction of sugar in diet, especially sugary snacks between meals. General nutrition education
Periodontal disease	Pain on chewing and eating	Oral hygiene ? Antibiotics	Gradual increase in unrefined foods and reduction in soft, sugary foods. General nutrition education
Vitamin deficiencies Associated dental/oral problems	Sore, painful mouth, poorly developed or loose teeth	Vitamin replacement therapy	Regular intake of vitamins in diet to achieve RNI. Soft, semi-solid diet if mouth is sore
Anaemias – iron – vitamin B_{12}	Red, inflamed tongue, pain on eating	Iron and vitamin B_{12} therapy	Increase iron and B_{12} content of the diet to achieve RNI. Pharmaceutical supplements may still be required
Inflammation of the salivary glands	Pain on eating	Antibiotic therapy if required	Soft, semi-solid or liquidized diet; protein, and energy supplements as indicated
Salivary stones	Pain on eating	Surgical excision	Protein and energy supplements as indicated
Fractured jaws and oral surgery	Unable to eat	Jaw wiring	High protein, high energy fluids, plus liquidized meals if desired, sipped through a straw. May require nasogastric feeding
Cancer of the mouth, pharynx and larynx	Difficulty and pain on eating. Dysphagia, anorexia	Surgery, radiotherapy and chemotherapy	Pre-treatment – sip feeding or nasogastric feeding Post-operation – nasogastric feeding and then gradual introduction to soft diet plus protein and energy supplements
Crohn's disease of the mouth	Sore, painful mouth	Steroid therapy	Soft, semi-solid or liquidized diet. Protein and energy supplements as required. Sip feeding or nasogastric feeding if indicated

should be encouraged to resume a normal diet. Some patients may still experience difficulty in swallowing and require dilatation to improve the situation. A frequent check should be kept on nutritional intake as some patients may exist on a very limited range of soft foods and drinks. Patients in whom the parathyroid gland is also removed will need appropriate calcium and vitamin D therapy.

4.1.9 Oral Crohn's disease

Crohn's disease is primarily an inflammatory disorder of the small bowel (see Section 4.8), though lesions can occur anywhere along the gastrointestinal tract from the mouth of the anus. Crohn's disease of the mouth may result in multiple lesions in the oral mucosa and on the lips either as part of a generalized condition or without other gut involvement (Tyldesley 1979). The mouth is sore, making eating painful and difficult. During an acute attack, a soft or fluid diet should be advised and hot, salty and spicy foods should be avoided (Table 4.2). Nutritional support provided by supplementary sip feeding or nasogastric tube feeding may be needed if the oral diet is inadequate (see Section 1.13).

General dietary advice for patients with oral disorders is summarized in Table 4.3.

Further reading

Davidson S, Passmore R, Brock JF and Truswell AS (1979) *Human nutrition and dietetics*, pp. 304, 389–96. Churchill Livingstone, Edinburgh.

Department of Health (1989) Sugars and dental caries. In *Dietary sugars and human disease*. Rep Hlth Soc Subj 37, pp. 16–20. HMSO, London.

Dickerson JWT and Lee HA (1988) *Nutrition in the clinical management of*

disease, pp. 212–3. Edward Arnold, London.
Mason DK and Chisholm DM (1975) *Salivary glands in health and disease.* WB Saunders, London.
Levine RS (1985) *The scientific basis of dental health education. A policy document.* Health Education Council, London.
Stones HH (1962) *Oral and dental disease*, pp. 47–71. Livingstone, Edinburgh.

References

Ferguson MM and MacFadyen EE (1986) Oro-facial granulomatosis – a 10 year review. *Ann Acad Med Singapore* **15**(3), 370–79.
Haworth RJP, MacFadyen EE and Ferguson MM (1988) Dietary modifications in oro-facial granulomatosis. In *Dietetics in the 90s. Role of the dietitian/nutritionist.* Moyal MF(Ed) pp. 221–4. John Libbey Eurotext, Paris.
MacCarthy-Leventhal EM (1959) Post-radiation mouth blindness. *Lancet* **ii**, 1138–9.
Tyldesley WR (1979) Oral Crohn's disease and related conditions. *Br J Oral Surg* **17**, 1–9.
Wiesenfeld D, Ferguson MM, Mitchell DN, MacDonald DG, Scully C, Cochran K and Russell RI (1985) Oro-facial granulomatosis – a clinical and pathological analysis. *Q J Med New Series* **54**(213), 101–113.

4.2 Disorders of the oesophagus

The oesophagus is a muscular tube about 25 cm in length. The function of the oesophagus is relatively simple, i.e. the transport of food from the mouth to the stomach. The upper oesophageal sphincter lies below the pharynx, and the lower oesophageal sphincter at the gastro-oesophageal junction. Various mechanical factors help to prevent the reflux and regurgitation of food from the stomach (Fig. 4.1) though reflux of acid gastric contents occurs in most people from time to time without causing undue discomfort.

4.2.1 Acid reflux, oesophagitis, heartburn and hiatus hernia

Acid reflux, oesophagitis and heartburn

The refluxed contents of the stomach may contain partly digested foods, acid, pepsin and possibly bile and pancreatic enzymes (Fig. 4.2). It is probably this combination which causes mucosal damage and oesophagitis. Symptoms develop if reflux becomes frequent and the mucosa of the oesophagus becomes sensitive to the acidic reflux.

Symptomatic reflux may occur after operations in the gastro-oesophageal region (e.g. truncal vagotomy and proximal partial gastrectomy). The main symptom of reflux is heartburn which is felt sub-sternally and may be accompanied by regurgitation of acid fluid into the mouth. Heartburn occurs after meals and may be aggravated by bending, lying flat, lifting or straining. A gain in body weight will also aggravate heartburn. Meals which are high in protein increase sphincter pressure and reduce the likelihood of reflux and heartburn. Fatty meals, chocolate, coffee, alcohol, spicy foods and citrus juices lower the sphincter pressure and may induce reflux.

The aims of the drug treatment of reflux are as follows:

1 To reduce acid by use of antacids.
2 To reduce reflux by increasing sphincter tone.
3 To increase mucosal resistance.

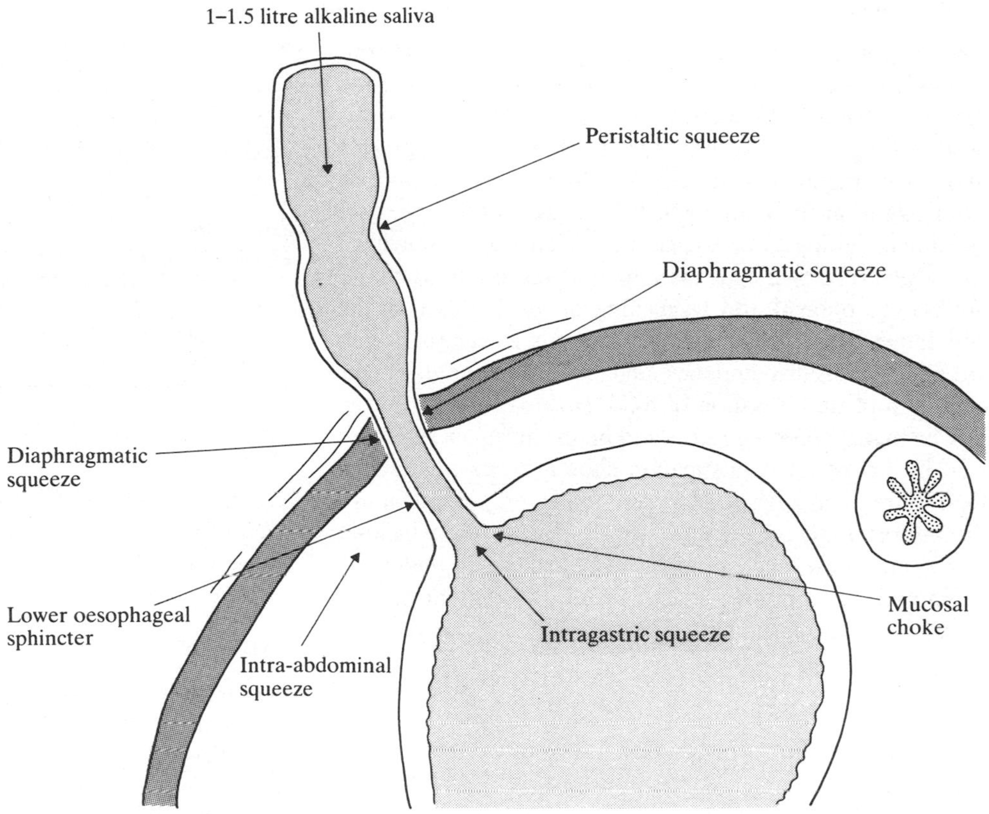

Fig. 4.1 Factors preventing the reflux and regurgitation of food from the stomach

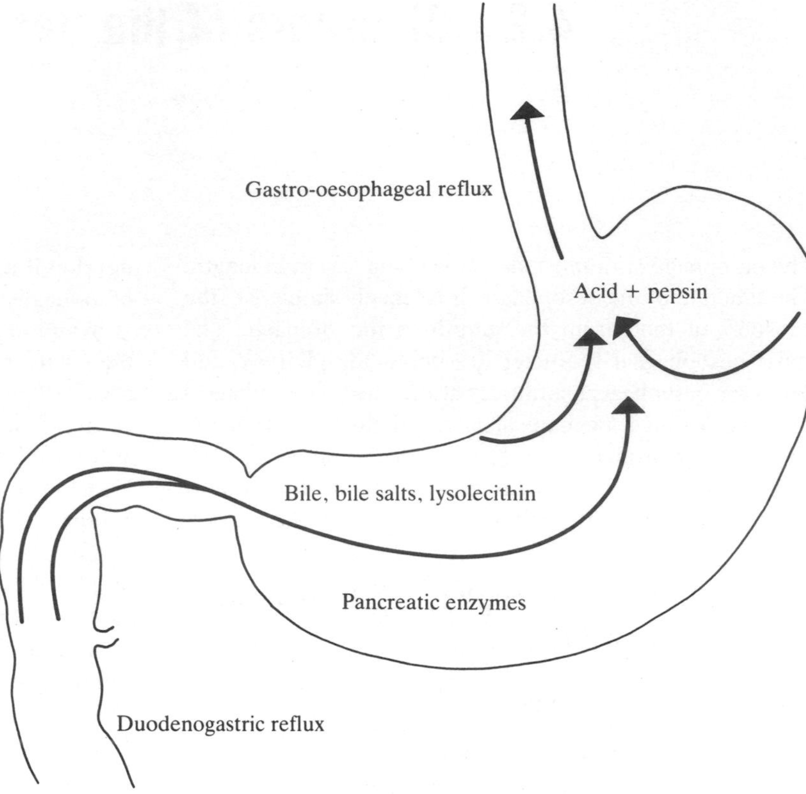

Fig. 4.2 Constituents of gastro-oesophageal reflux

Hiatus hernia

The diaphragm has several openings through which the abdominal viscera can enter the thorax. The opening for the oesophagus, the hiatus, is loosely attached to the oesophagus. In middle age this attachment weakens and in overweight patients additional abdominal weight puts an extra strain on the hiatus which herniates. Pregnancy and chronic coughing can also act in a similar way. A low fibre diet which results in constipation causes straining when the bowels are opened and weakening of the hiatus (Burkitt and James 1973). The major symptoms of hiatus hernia are those of reflux and oesophagitis and patients might complain of the sensation of food 'sticking'.

The management of reflux and hiatus hernia is summarized in Table 4.4. Constipation should be avoided and a high fibre diet advised. Certain foods may cause more discomfort than others and 'stick'. These often include salad items, new bread and rich, heavy cakes and puddings. If pain and discomfort persists, surgical treatment may be required to correct a hiatus hernia.

Table 4.4 The management of hiatus hernia and acid reflux

Measures which may help	Things to avoid
1 Losing weight, if overweight	1 Smoking
2 Eating small, frequent meals	2 Eating large meals
3 Eating foods which are known to be well tolerated	3 Eating late at night
4 Standing upright and bending correctly	4 Eating very hot, very cold or very spicy foods, fatty foods, chocolate, onions, cucumber
5 Propping up the bed by approximately 4 inches, e.g. a household brick under each leg at the head end	5 Strong coffee and alcohol
6 Taking all medicines regularly as prescribed by the doctor	6 Stooping, bending from the waist or lying completely flat
	7 Tight fitting underwear, skirts or trousers

4.2.2 Dysphagia

Dysphagia is a difficulty or a discomfort in swallowing and may be due to oropharyngeal or oesophageal problems. A number of benign conditions as well as malignant lesions make the swallowing of food difficult or painful.

Details of the normal swallowing process and techniques used to assess dysphagia (e.g. videofluoscopy) are given in Section 4.21.1.

Benign stricture

Chronic persistent gastro-oesophageal reflux may result in a benign peptic stricture. Strictures may at first be due to muscular spasm following mucosal injury. Intubation with wide bore nasogastric tubes may predispose a patient to benign stricture.

The first symptom is usually difficulty in swallowing

solid foods. The foods which usually cause problems include white bread, beef and roast potatoes. Dysphagia with solid foods may soon progress to dysphagia with semi-solids and liquids (Table 4.5). Appetite is usually reduced and severe weight loss may be reported. Sadly, many patients seem to suffer these difficulties for some time before seeking or obtaining help and may be dehydrated and malnourished on presentation. Some patients who are very depleted may need intravenous fluid replacement and nutritional support prior to treatment which is usually by oesophageal dilatation. Following dilatation, swallowing should be improved though most patients still need to choose their foods carefully. Some patients may require repeated dilatations and should be observed closely for possible oesophageal perforation. Younger patients fit for surgery may undergo thoracic surgery to reduce reflux and dilate the stricture.

As with many gastrointestinal disorders, dysphagia is often affected by anxiety. Anxious patients should be helped to relax and encouraged to discuss their problems with the appropriate counsellors.

It is important to treat gastro-oesophageal reflux adequately to prevent recurrence of the stricture.

Sideropenic dysphagia

(Patterson-Kelly or Plummer-Vinson Syndrome) Sideropenic dysphagia results from iron deficiency. The condition is relatively rare, occurs more commonly in women and may be associated with hiatus hernia, oesophagitis or partial gastrectomy. Relief is gained by medicinal iron and advice on an iron-rich diet to maintain body iron stores.

Table 4.5 The dietary management of dysphagia

Stages of dysphagia	Dietary management
Dysphagia to solids	Small, frequent meals. Soft to semi-solid foods. Day-old wholemeal bread and crispbreads or biscuits may be tolerated. Protein and energy supplements if necessary (see Section 1.13.3)
Dysphagia to semi-solids	Liquidized meals or liquid meal replacement preparations. Protein and energy supplements. If severely depleted or intake nutritionally inadequate, may require fine bore nasogastric tube and enteral nutrition (see Section 1.13.4)
Dysphagia to liquids	May need rehydration with intravenous solutions. Enteral nutrition via a fine bore nasogastric tube if intubation possible. If severely depleted and completely dysphagic, TPN prior to treatment may be needed (see Section 1.15)

Malignant stricture of the oesophagus

Carcinoma of the oesophagus is more common in the elderly and is seen more frequently in men than in women. The lower third of the oesophagus is the most common site and the upper third is the least common site.

Patients may present with loss of body weight, dysphagia and chest pain on eating. The extent of weight loss is related to the degree and duration of the dysphagia.

The diagnosis of cancer of the oesophagus is by barium swallow, endoscopy, biopsy and brush cytology. When patients present with symptoms, the disease is often advanced. Once symptoms have developed deterioration may occur rapidly, changing from dysphagia with solids to dysphagia with liquids. Patients may appear poorly nourished and cachectic. The dietary management of the dysphagia is the same as for benign peptic stricture of the oesophagus.

A brief diet history will reveal the recent changes in dysphagia and highlight which particular foods are most difficult for the patient to chew and swallow. There is seldom need for an accurate nutritional analysis of food intake to be calculated. Patients who are severely depleted and dehydrated will need rehydration with intravenous fluids. If a soft diet can be taken, protein and energy supplements should be used (see Section 1.13.3). If fluids only can be taken, nutritional support should be provided by sip feeding or nasogastric feeding using a fine bore tube (see Section 1.13.4). In patients who are dysphagic to fluids, it may not be possible to pass a fine bore tube and total parenteral nutrition (TPN) may be required to provide pre-operative nutrition (see Section 1.15).

In the majority of patients with cancer of the oesophagus, palliative therapy is all that can be offered. The controversy about the relative value of surgery and radiotherapy continues (Earlam and Lunha-Melo 1980a; 1980b) and treatment is by radiotherapy, chemotherapy, laser therapy, surgery or the insertion of a prosthetic tube (Celestin or Atkinson tube, see Fig. 4.3) through the tumour.

Disagreement also exists about the relative value of pre- and post-operative nutrition. Whilst pre-operative nutrition may reduce the risk of post-operative complications (Moghissi *et al* 1977), some surgeons may operate shortly after diagnosis has been confirmed and provide nutritional support either enterally or parenterally in the early post-operative period (Russell 1984). Whichever method of treatment is to be offered to the patient, the dietitian should be available to give advice as early as possible.

Surgical treatment

Surgical treatment of carcinoma of the oesophagus may be by limited or total oesophagectomy or oesophago-gastrectomy, depending on the site and extent of the lesion. In some cases, a length of colon may be substituted for the excised oesophagus.

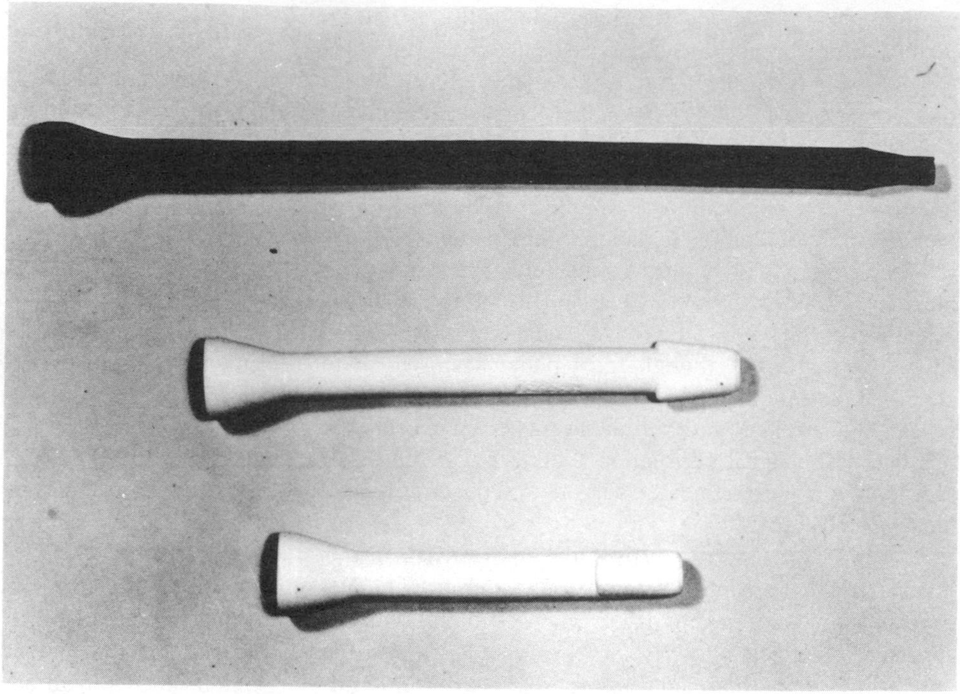

1 Celestin tube

2 Medium length Atkinson tube

3 Short length Atkinson tube

Fig. 4.3 Prosthetic tubes

Post-operative nutrition is required to promote wound healing and maintain nutritional status. This has been achieved successfully by either jejunostomy feeding or TPN. Assessment of nutritional requirements should be made and most patients will require approximately 2500 kcal and 12–14 g of nitrogen, together with adequate vitamins, minerals and trace elements (see Section 1.12).

The integrity of the anastamosis should be confirmed before an oral diet is introduced. Oral fluids followed by a light diet should be phased in as enteral nutrition or parenteral nutrition is phased out. Regular dietetic advice and supervision should be offered, both during hospitalization and following discharge.

Post-operative nutritional problems can include:

1 Poor appetite.
2 Early satiety.
3 Fear of eating, particularly foods which were difficult to eat pre-operatively.
4 Difficulty in maintaining body weight.
5 Nausea.
6 Reflux.

Dietary treatment of these problems is summarized in Table 4.6.

As with all carcinomas it is very difficult to regain body weight. Patients should not be expected to achieve their pre-illness weight. The dietary aims should be to prevent further weight loss and maintain the quality of life. A gain in weight should be regarded as a bonus.

Table 4.6 Dietary advice for post-oesophagectomy patients

1	Meals should be small and frequent
2	Fluids should be consumed separately from meal times, e.g. 1 hour before or 1 hour after eating
3	Protein intake can be increased with supplements such as Build-up, Complan or Fortimel taken between meals (see also Section 1.13.3). Skimmed milk powder can be incorporated into foods such as sauces, milks and custards
4	Energy intake can be increased by supplements of glucose polymers, sugar, Hycal and Fortical
5	Patients should be encouraged to relax before and after eating
6	Food should be chewed well
7	Reflux can be minimized by avoiding eating late in the evening and by sleeping with two to three pillows or with the head of the bed raised on household bricks

Treatment by radiotherapy

Radiation of oesophageal carcinoma may be used as the sole treatment, in combination with chemotherapy or following surgery. During a course of radiotherapy, the tissues will become oedematous, inflamed and swollen, making dysphagia worse and the patient possibly unable to swallow liquids. This stage is usually temporary but as these patients are already often malnourished and may have lost a lot of body weight it is best to pre-empt the situation. The passing of a fine bore nasogastric tube at the start of the treatment when there is sufficient space to do so enables nutritional support to be given if dysphagia worsens and nutritional intake is inadequate. The tube need not be used if the patient can achieve an adequate intake orally.

Reintroduction of a normal diet should be gradual and protein and energy supplements should be used. Most patients continue on a soft diet as they will often still experience some difficulties with swallowing and may be afraid to try foods with which they associate problems.

Insertion of prosthetic tubes

When radical surgery is contraindicated because of metastatic spread or because the patient is elderly and too frail, a palliative procedure should be considered. The establishment of satisfactory swallowing will enable the patient to be managed at home. A prosthetic tube may be inserted at laparotomy or by an endoscopic technique using light sedation. The tubes most commonly used are the Celestin tube or the Atkinson tube (short, medium or long length) (Fig. 4.3).

These tubes provide an opening through the tumour but the diameter of the tubes is relatively small (approximately that of the index finger). The insertion of these tubes carries with it a risk of perforation of the oesophagus and death. If perforation is suspected, introduction of an oral diet should be delayed and TPN may need to be instigated until the site has healed and an oral diet can be introduced. The internal lining of the tubes is specially coated to facilitate the passage of food through them but care should be taken when eating. Dietary guidelines for patients will a prosthetic tube are summarized in Table 4.7.

More and more patients are seeking the help of alternative methods of treating their cancer (see Section 4.34.3). These methods usually involve a vegetarian diet consisting largely of raw fruits, vegetables and cereals. Any patients who have prosthetic tubes inserted must be advised of the hazards of eating such a diet which will undoubtedly block their tube.

Radiotherapy following the insertion of a prosthetic tube

This combination of treatment is occasionally used. During radiotherapy, dysphagia may recur and a fine bore tube can be passed through the oesophageal prosthetic tube to provide nasogastric feeding throughout the period of treatment, until an oral diet may be resumed.

Occasionally the prosthetic tube may need to be replaced if the tumour has grown and obstructed the entrance or the exit of the tube. This procedure carries a high risk of mortality.

Table 4.7 Dietary guidelines for patients with a prosthetic tube

1	Meals should be small and frequent and, if necessary, soft, semi-solid or liquidized
2	Meat should be very tender, minced or liquidized
3	Food should be chewed well. If the patient has dentures, ensure that they fit properly
4	Meals should be accompanied by plenty of sauces, gravy or custard
5	New bread should be avoided. Day-old wholemeal bread and crispbreads crumble more easily and are usually better tolerated
6	Nourishing fluids (such as milk, Horlicks, Ovaltine and Bournvita) should be taken between meals
7	Protein and energy supplements (such as Complan, Fortimel, Build-up, Maxijul, Fortical or Hycal) should be used
8	A good source of vitamin C (such as Ribena) should be included in the diet
9	After eating a meal, a fizzy drink (such as soda water or lemonade) should be consumed to help clear the tube of any food particles
10	Should the tube block, the patient should be advised NOT to panic but to take sips of fizzy drinks, walk around, jump up and down and take more fizzy drinks. If the blockage persists, the hospital gastric clinic or casualty department will be able to clear it. Patients should be reassured that if their tube does block, they will come to no harm

4.2.3 Other disorders of the oesophagus

Perforation and caustic burns

If the oesophagus perforates spontaneously or is perforated as a result of dilatation, intubation or oesophagoscopy, any foods consumed would enter the thoracic cavity which would need to be drained by suction. The perforation may be allowed to heal naturally or may need surgical repair. Patients should be 'nil by mouth' and an alternative means of feeding instituted, such as TPN, nasogastric feeding or jejunostomy feeding (see Sections 1.13 and 1.15). If a nasogastric tube is to be used it should be inserted at the time of surgical repair.

Household cleaning agents such as caustic soda or industrial acids or alkalis taken accidentally or deliberately destroy the oesophageal mucosa and may also damage the muscle coats of the oesophagus. The area must be totally rested and intravenous fluids provided. If an oral diet has to be withheld for more than six or seven days, enteral feeding from a site below the level of damage (if necessary via a gastrostomy or jejunostomy) or TPN should be commenced.

Pharyngeal pouch

The mucosa of the pharynx may protrude through the triangular space formed by the cricopharyngeus and the inferior pharyngeal constrictor muscles. A pharyngeal pouch may occur and cause symptoms of dysphagia with regurgitation, particularly of fluids. This may occur some hours after a meal and especially when lying flat which increases the risk of pulmonary aspiration. Surgical correction and post-operative nasogastric feeding is the usual treatment.

Achalasia

Achalasia is characterized by the inability of the lower oesophageal sphincter to relax after a swallow, and weak peristalsis of the oesophagus. It is relatively uncommon. Food collects in the oesophagus, causing discomfort and eventually may pass through the sphincter by the action of gravity and the weight of food consumed. Regurgitation of food is common but lacks the bitter taste of acid or bile which is typical of reflux. Aspiration of food from the oesophagus may lead to pneumonia. As food collects it can irritate the mucosa and cause oesophagitis and pain. Loss of weight is uncommon unless the patient becomes afraid to eat. Relief may be obtained by following a typical gastric regimen (see Table 4.9 in Section 4.3). A semi-fluid diet can also be beneficial and the patient may find that standing up several times during a meal, drinking a glass of water and exhaling hard may help to force food into the stomach. If these measures are ineffective, surgical myotomy or mechanical dilatation may give permanent relief.

Further reading

Atkinson M (1983) The oesophagus. In *Recent advances in gastroenterology* 5. Bouchier IAD (Ed) pp. 1–20. Churchill Livingstone, Edinburgh.

Davidson S, Passmore R, Brock JF and Truswell AS (1979) *Human nutrition and dietetics* 7e. pp. 396–7. Churchill Livingstone. Edinburgh.

Dickerson JWT and Lee HA (1988) *Nutrition in the clinical management of disease*, pp. 213–15. Edward Arnold, London.

Hunt RH (1981) *Disorders of the oesophagus*. Update Post-Graduate Centre Series. Update Publications, London.

References

Burkitt DP and James PA (1973) Low residue diets and hiatus hernia. *Lancet* **ii**, 128–30.

Earlam R and Lunha-Melo JR (1980a) Oesophageal squamous carcinoma i: A critical review of surgery. *Br J Surg* **67**, 381–90.

Earlam R and Lunha-Melo JR (1980b) Oesophageal squamous carcinoma ii: A critical review of radiotherapy. *Br J Surg* **67**, 457–61.

Moghissi KN, Hornshaw J, Teasdale PK and Dawes EA (1977) Parenteral nutrition in carcinoma of the oesophagus treated by surgery: nitrogen balance and clinical studies. *Br J Surg* **64**, 125–8.

Russell CA (1984) Fine needle catheter jejunostomy in patients with upper gastrointestinal carcinoma. *Appl Nutr* **11**, 1–7.

4.3 Disorders of the stomach and duodenum

Diseases of the gastrointestinal tract account for almost one-third of the medical referrals to hospital and disorders of the stomach and duodenum constitute a large proportion of these.

The stomach functions as a reservoir for food received from the oesophagus and plays a role in the digestion and absorption of nutrients. It is sensitive to pain and thermal sensations. Gastric disease, and particularly the surgical treatment of gastric disease, are likely to have considerable effects on gastric function and nutritional intake.

4.3.1 Gastric and duodenal ulcer

It has been common practice to describe gastric and duodenal ulcers as peptic ulcers and include them under this one heading. However, there is much to suggest that they are separate diseases and have a different aetiology.

Gastric ulcers are less common than duodenal ulcers. Normally, there is a balance between factors which attack the gastric mucosa and those which protect it (Table 4.8). Ulcers may be single or multiple, acute or chronic, large or small. They are usually associated with normal or reduced gastric acid and pepsin output. Confirmation of diagnosis is made by upper gastrointestinal endoscopy.

A duodenal ulcer, like a gastric ulcer, is a defect in the mucosa. It may be single or multiple, superficial or deep. The majority of duodenal ulcers occur in the duodenal cap and duodenitis is invariably present. Ulceration may also occur in the pyloric antrum which may, in time, cause pyloric stenosis.

The cause of duodenal ulcers is not fully understood. Hypersecretion of acid, nocturnal acid secretion and the rapid delivery into the duodenum of acid contents which are inadequately buffered by pancreatic secretion of bicarbonate, are all precipitating factors. It has been suggested that certain occupations may predispose to peptic ulcers and factors such as stress, irregular meals, eating quickly and inadequate mastication may contribute to ulcer development.

Table 4.8 Factors affecting the gastric mucosa

Destructive factors	Defensive factors
Hydrochloric acid	Epithelial cell barrier
Pepsin	Mucus
Psychogenic factors	Gastric blood flow
Gastric irritants, e.g. alcohol	Cell regeneration
Duodenal and biliary reflux	Regulation of acid secretion
Nicotine and tobacco tars	
Analgesics and anti-inflammatory drugs	

Treatment of gastric and duodenal ulcers

Relief of symptoms

Many different dietary regimens have been used. In the past, very strict diets consisting of frequent milk drinks interspersed with antacids sometimes resulted in patients becoming severely malnourished. Other patients have spent years on boiled fish and milk with very little benefit. Ingelfinger (1966) recommended a more normal diet to 'let the ulcer patient enjoy his food'. A bland or gastric diet comprised of small, frequent meals interspersed with snacks may relieve the symptoms of dyspepsia (Table 4.9). However, such a regimen may not necessarily accelerate the healing of an ulcer.

Table 4.9 The general principles of a gastric diet

1 Meals should be small, frequent and regular
2 Fried foods should be avoided
3 Strong tea, coffee and alcohol should be avoided
4 Mucosal irritants such as spices, pickles, black pepper, vinegar or mustard should be avoided
5 Any food known to cause dyspepsia should be avoided
6 Very hot or very cold foods should be avoided: air is swallowed which may aggravate dyspepsia
7 Smoking must be stopped
8 Aspirin should not be taken. Paracetamol will provide analgesia without acting as a gastric irritant

Healing of the ulcer and prevention of recurrence

The drug treatment of gastric ulcer and duodenal ulcer may include antacids, anticholinergic drugs or H_2 receptor antagonists (e.g. cimetidine, ranitidine). H_2 receptor antagonists have now become the routine treatment for benign gastric and duodenal ulcers. Their widespread use has enabled ulcers to heal whilst allowing patients to eat a more normal diet. However certain guidelines should be followed:

1 Regular meals should be eaten, preferably little and often.

2 Strong tea and coffee should be taken in moderation only.

3 Any food known to cause dyspepsia should be avoided.

4 Alcohol and aspirin should be avoided.
5 Smoking must be stopped.

Complications of gastric and duodenal ulcers

The most common complications are:
1 Haemorrhage.
2 Perforation.
3 Penetration into adjacent tissues or organs.
4 Obstruction, e.g. pyloric stenosis and gastric outlet obstruction.

These complications will require surgery, either as an emergency or, in some cases, electively. Surgery, for patients who have failed to respond to medical treatment, prevents recurrence in most cases. A number of gastric reconstructions may be undertaken dependent on the site and extent of the ulcer. Partial gastrectomy (Billroth I, Billroth II or Polya operations) (see Fig. 4.5) may result in two-thirds to three-quarters of the stomach being removed and may have a higher incidence of post-operative mechanical or nutritional problems (see Section 4.3.3 below). These operations are however rarely performed nowadays for peptic ulcer. Truncal vagotomy (Fig. 4.4a) may be combined with gastroenterostomy, gastro-jejunostomy or pyloroplasty. Patients may suffer problems of gastric stasis and delayed stomach emptying, dumping syndrome or diarrhoea. Highly selective vagotomy (HSV) or proximal gastric vagotomy (PGV) is a refinement of selective vagotomy (Fig. 4.4b,c). In this operation the parietal cell mass alone is denervated and the mobility and drainage of the stomach is preserved. There are a number of advantages of this procedure; the stomach itself is not opened or reconstructed and diarrhoea, dumping, nausea and vomiting are relatively rare. The nutritional status of the patient is better and oral intake may be resumed in the early post-operative period.

Pyloric stenosis

Pyloric stenosis stems from scar tissue resulting from duodenal ulcers around the pyloric channel. Gastric emptying is delayed and food debris collects in the stomach, obstructing the pylorus. Retained food in the stomach tends to ferment and cause the characteristic bad breath associated with pyloric stenosis.

Patients complain of discomfort, nausea, vomiting and anorexia. Food debris must be removed from the stomach by gastric lavage. Once the stomach has been emptied, a

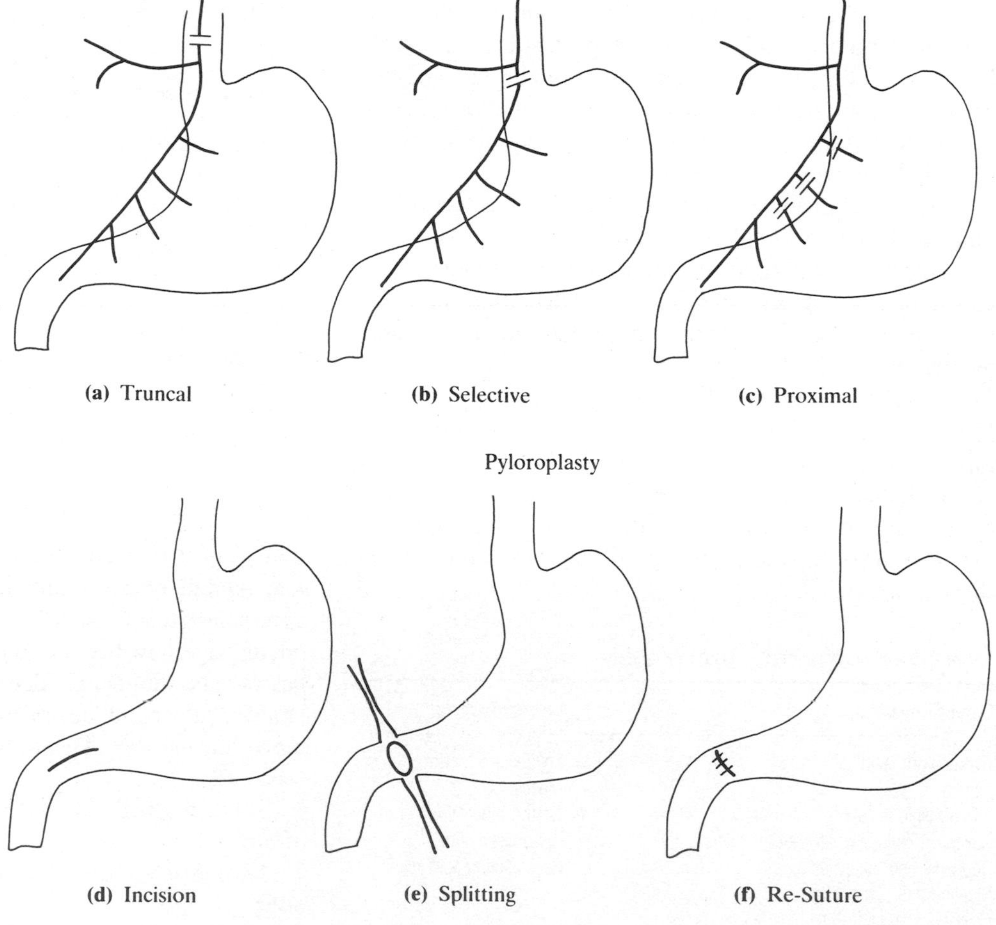

Fig. 4.4 The different vagotomies

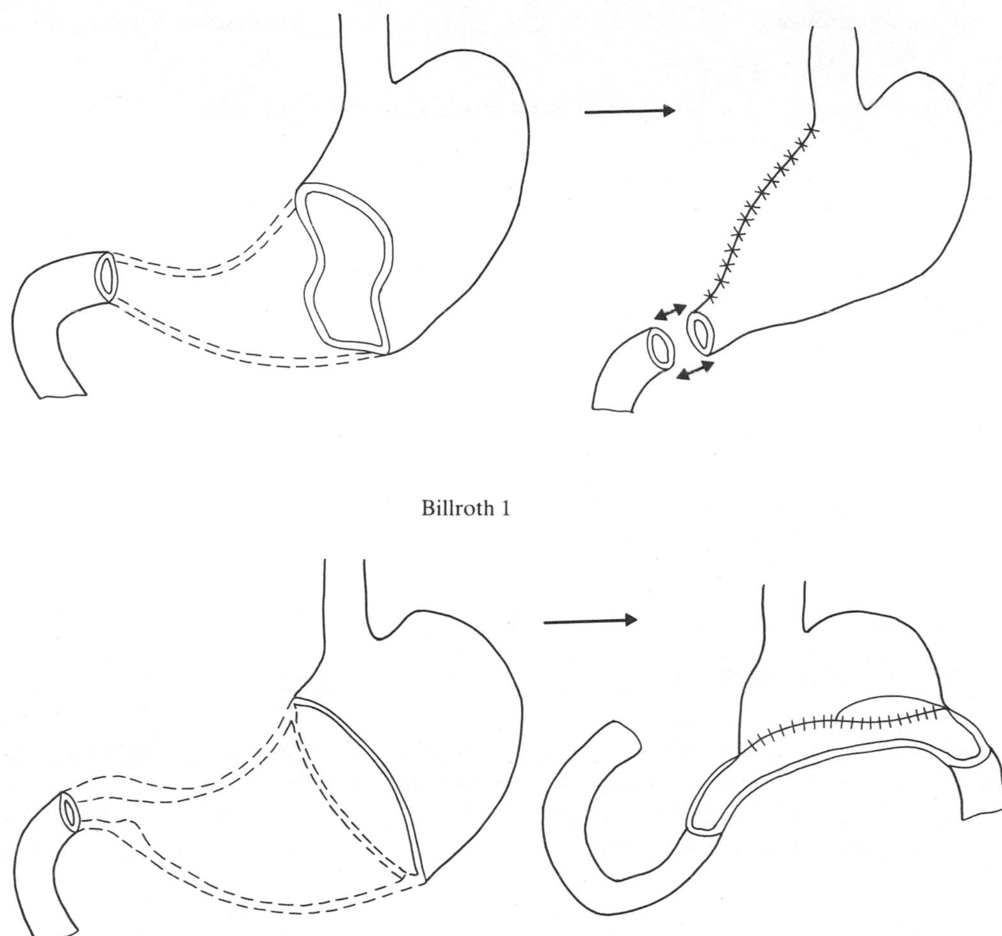

Fig. 4.5 Partial gastrectomy

high protein, high energy fluid diet, taken either orally or administered via a nasogastric tube, may be well tolerated prior to surgery. Occasionally, if the stenosis is severe and the patient nutritionally depleted. TPN may be instigated pre-operatively (see Section 1.15). This should be replaced post-operatively by enteral nutrition in the form of jejunostomy feeding – the jejunal catheter being placed at the time of surgery.

Post-operatively, gastric retention may still occur for some days. If the introduction of oral fluids and diet has to be withheld for more than about seven days post-operatively, nutritional support should be provided by nasojejunal, jejunostomy or parenteral feeding (see Sections 1.13, 1.15).

4.3.2 Carcinoma of the stomach

Carcinoma of the stomach affects mainly middle-aged or elderly people and is seen more often in men than in women. Unfortunately, most treatments are palliative as a permanent cure can only be achieved by radical surgery before metastasis has occurred. Early diagnosis is difficult and on presentation most patients complain of pain on eating, nausea, vomiting, anorexia and severe weight loss.

If the carcinoma is resectable, a total or partial gastrectomy may be performed (Figs. 4.5 and 4.6). Lesions in the cardia of the stomach will be treated surgically by an oesophago-gastrectomy. A jejunostomy catheter should be positioned to provide post-operative nutritional support. When gastrectomy is contraindicated, a gastroenterostomy may relieve symptoms and allow the patient to be managed at home eating such foods as can be tolerated with the addition of protein and energy supplements.

Pre-operative feeding may be undertaken in severely malnourished patients. Enteral feeding via fine bore nasogastric tube may be tolerated; if not, parenteral nutrition should be considered (see Sections 1.13, 1.15).

4.3.3 Nutritional problems following gastric surgery

Disturbances in gastric function (Table 4.10) often occur following gastric reconstruction and have an effect on nutritional intake and nutritional status. Some of these

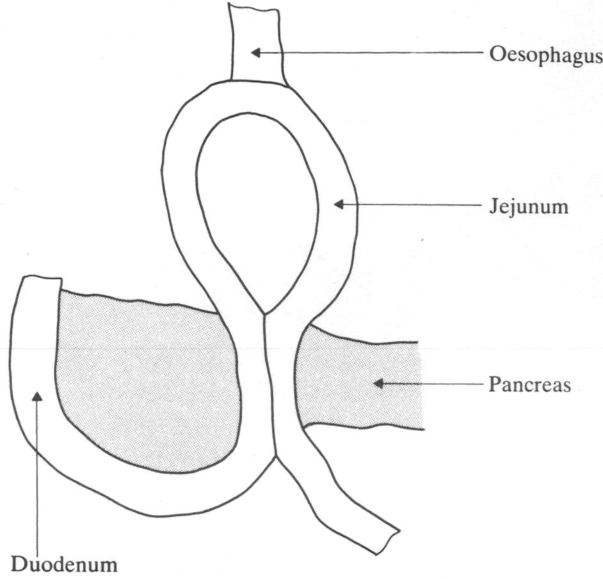

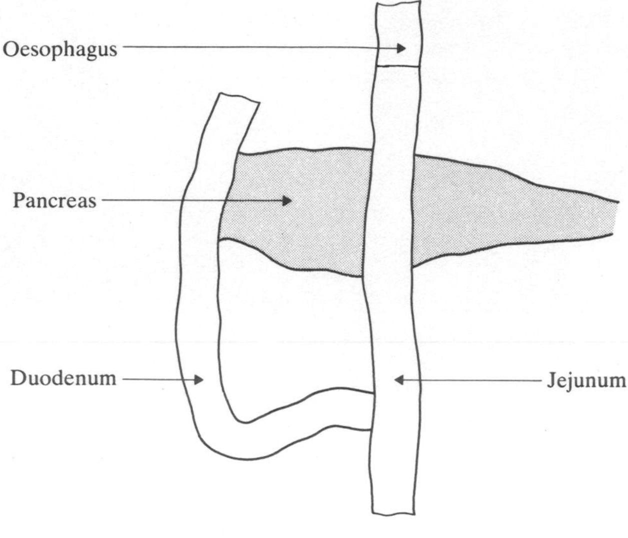

Fig. 4.6 Anatomy after a total gastrectomy

problems occur soon after eating and may be described as early or post-cibal syndromes; others develop later due to long term effects of disturbed gastric function. These may be described as late symptoms (Table 4.11).

Early symptoms

Small stomach syndrome

The majority of patients experience early satiety and may feel distended and uncomfortable during or after eating.

Table 4.10 Changes in gastric function following gastric resection and reconstruction (Celestin 1981)

Rapid emptying of the stomach remnant
Rapid secretion of hydrochloric acid and pepsin
Reduced secretion of intrinsic factor
Reduced secretion of pancreatic enzymes
Inadequate mixing of food with enzymes and bile
Reduced absorption of certain food substances, especially protein and fat
Rapid absorption of glucose
Abolition of the normal pH gradient in the alimentary canal
Increased intestinal mobility
Altered bacteriological state of the intestine (occasionally)
Effects related to the creation of the afferent loop

Table 4.11 Post-gastrectomy syndromes

Early symptoms	Late symptoms
Small stomach	Weight loss and malnutrition
'Dumping syndrome'	Calcium malabsorption
Diarrhoea	Anaemia
Bile vomiting	

This occurs particularly after total and partial gastrectomy. It may also occur after vagotomy and pyloroplasty. Small, frequent meals should be eaten and fluids should be consumed separately from solid food.

'Dumping syndrome'

Early dumping This occurs soon after eating and the symptoms include hypotension, tachycardia, diminished pulse volume and giddiness. The cause is thought to be due to the rapid and early delivery of a hyperosmolar meal into the jejunum. The symptoms usually settle 2–3 months after surgery, but in the meantime may be relieved by avoiding liquids at meal times and taking limited amounts of refined sugars. A glucose polymer is often better tolerated as an energy supplement than sucrose or glucose. Small meals containing protein and fat also help to reduce the incidence of dumping.

Late dumping Some patients may experience symptoms about two hours after a meal either in addition to early dumping or alone. The symptoms are similar to those of hypoglycaemia, i.e. feeling weak, faint, cold and sweaty and are usually corrected by eating carbohydrate. The cause of late dumping is probably due to an over-production of insulin by the pancreas in response to elevated blood glucose levels following rapid absorption from the upper small intestine. Again, symptoms can be relieved by eating less sugar and refined carbohydrates at meal times and consuming fluids separately from solid foods.

Diarrhoea

Diarrhoea frequently occurs following vagotomy or total gastrectomy. The problem may be alleviated by codeine phosphate or loperamide, and should disappear 1–2 months after surgery.

Bile vomiting

Pancreatic and biliary secretions may accumulate in the afferent loop and, after a meal has left the stomach, can enter the gastric remnant causing nausea and vomiting. Treatment is surgical and involves reducing the size of the afferent loop.

Late symptoms

Following gastric reconstruction, long term follow-up of patients is important to identify early signs of nutritional disturbances and to ensure that an adequate diet is being taken.

Weight loss and malnutrition

Weight loss is a well known consequence of gastric surgery and is a result of reduced food intake. Patients are often afraid to increase their food intake and frequently experience early satiety. Such patients should be reassured and encouraged to take small, frequent meals with protein and energy supplements (see Section 1.13.3). Malnutrition and malabsorption resulting in steatorrhoea may be due to poor mixing of food with pancreatic enzymes and bile, or possibly pancreatic insufficiency or bacterial overgrowth in the afferent loop. Reduction in dietary fat content may be beneficial.

Calcium malabsorption

Significant malabsorption of calcium occurs after gastrectomy and can cause osteomalacial bone changes (Eddy 1971). Inadequate intake of calcium will aggravate the situation and calcium and vitamin D supplements should be given.

Anaemia

Iron deficiency anaemia occurs in almost half the patients following partial gastrectomy. It may be due to a poor iron intake, inadequate conversion of ferrous iron to ferric iron or the bypassing of the duodenum and upper jejunum in patients with gastroenterostomies.

Megaloblastic anaemia due to vitamin B_{12} deficiency may occur in partial or total gastrectomy due to reduction or loss of intrinsic factor. This may only be severe in patients who survive five years after total gastrectomy but can be prevented by vitamin B_{12} therapy.

Table 4.12 Dietary advice following gastric reconstruction

1. Small, frequent, regular meals should be eaten
2. Fluids should be taken between meals
3. Excess quantities of sugar, glucose and sweet sugary foods should be avoided
4. Excess fat should be avoided
5. Small amounts of vegetables and fruit should be eaten — these are bulky and may result in early satiety. A vitamin C supplement should be taken
6. Eating late at night should be discouraged
7. Protein and energy supplements should be advised as indicated
8. Good sources of calcium and vitamin D should be advised
9. Iron, folic acid and vitamin B_{12} supplements should be prescribed as appropriate

Impaired absorption of folate occurs in some gastrectomy patients (Elsborg 1974) though folate deficiency is a much less important cause of anaemia. However, routine folic acid supplements are given occasionally.

General dietary advice following gastric reconstruction is summarized in Table 4.12.

4.3.4 Gastritis

Gastritis is an inflammatory lesion of the gastric mucosa and may be an acute, erosive gastritis or a chronic, atrophic gastritis. Alcohol, drugs such as aspirin, other chemical irritants and occasionally foods infected with pathogens may be associated with acute gastritis. Chronic gastritis may follow repeated attacks of acute gastritis and is more common in patients who smoke and drink alcohol heavily.

Iron deficiency anaemia may result from repeated bleeding, and pernicious anaemia may result from reduced production of intrinsic factor and consequent reduced absorption of vitamin B_{12}.

The symptoms of acute gastritis are nausea, pain and vomiting. The treatment should concentrate on resting the stomach, preventing dehydration and restoring electrolyte balance. Water, with or without glucose, or diluted fruit juices may be taken hourly if tolerated. Regeneration of healthy mucosa should occur in 2–5 days.

Chronic gastritis is relieved by resting the inflamed gastric mucosa and removing or correcting the cause of gastritis, such as faulty eating habits, smoking, drinking and drugs. Iron and vitamin B_{12} deficiencies should be corrected and once symptoms have disappeared, patients may return gradually to a normal diet. They should be urged to correct inappropriate eating habits and to stop smoking and drinking.

Further reading

Davidson S, Passmore R, Brock JF and Truswell AS (1979) *Human nutrition and dietetics* 7e, pp. 398–402. Churchill Livingstone, Edinburgh.

Dickerson JWT and Lee HA (1988) *Nutrition in the clinical management of disease*, pp. 216–21. Edward Arnold, London.

Hunt R (1981) *Disorders of the stomach and duodenum*. Update Post-Graduate Centre Series. Update Publications, London.

References

Celestin LR (1981) Postgastrectomy and postvagotomy problems. In *Basic gastroenterology* 3e. Read AE, Harvey RF and Naish JM (Eds) pp. 104–14. Wright, Bristol.

Eddy RL (1971) Metabolic bone disease after gastrectomy. *Am J Med* **50**, 442–9.

Elsborg L (1974) Malabsorption of folic acid following partial gastrectomy. *Scand J Gastroenterol* **9**, 271–4.

Ingelfinger FJ (1966) Let the ulcer patient enjoy his food. In *Controversy in internal medicine*. WB Saunders, Philadelphia.

4.4 Disorders of the pancreas

Nutritional abnormalities are a common finding in patients with pancreatic disease. Many patients have a degree of malabsorption, caused by pancreatic exocrine insufficiency. Undernutrition may be caused by a number of factors; poor dietary intake, reduced appetite and the presence of malabsorption have all been implicated. Moreover, nutritional treatment may be further complicated by the onset of diabetes mellitus, although this endocrine abnormality is usually transient in an acute exacerbation of the disease.

4.4.1 Acute pancreatitis

The pancreas is protected against its own enzymes by their synthesis as pro-enzymes. Acute pancreatitis develops when activated pancreatic enzymes are liberated within the pancreatic system. The clinical features of pancreatitis result from the autodigestion of tissue and the toxic effects of digestion products. Elevated serum and urinary amylase concentration remain one of the main diagnostic criteria in acute pancreatitis. Recent advances in imaging techniques – computerized tomography (CT) and endoscopic retrograde cholangiopancreatography (ERCP) – have assisted in both the diagnosis and treatment of pancreatic disease.

The aetiology of acute pancreatitis is associated with biliary tract disease, alcohol abuse, trauma and, rarely, hyperlipidaemia. The main symptom of this disorder is pain, and treatment with simple analgesia is often ineffective. Nausea and vomiting frequently occur and may be precipitated by a large meal and/or alcohol consumption. The majority of patients who have mild or moderate attacks of pancreatitis recover without the need for intensive or invasive therapy. However, the mortality rate in approximately 20% of patients is still considered to be unacceptably high (McMahon 1990).

Conservative management of the patient with acute pancreatitis includes resting the pancreas and maintaining fluid balance. Traditionally, nutrition was withheld in an attempt to reduce pancreatic secretions, although this may further exacerbate the presence of any pre-existing malnutrition. The role of nutritional support in these patients remains an area of controversy, but the use of appropriate nutritional support (total parenteral nutrition, jejunostomy) may be a useful adjunct in patient management. In severe forms of the disease, patients may develop complications such as pancreatic pseudocysts or abscesses and the presence of continuing retro-peritoneal inflammation may restrict nutritional support to the intravenous route (see Section 1.15). If surgical intervention is indicated the surgeon may at the time of operation elect to insert a feeding jejunostomy. Post-operatively this facilitates use of the gut without stimulating the production of pancreatic secretions. Early enteral nutrition may be important in maintaining gut integrity and minimising bacterial translocation (Alverdy *et al* 1988; 1990). It has been suggested that the enteral feed of choice for this patient group is a peptide regimen and reports imply that such feeds are better tolerated when compared with their whole protein counterparts (Ziegler *et al* 1990). The evidence to date is inconclusive and there is no physiological reason why these patients are unable to tolerate a whole protein regimen. There is general agreement that oral feeding should be witheld until pain, tenderness and fever have reduced (Ranson 1984). Once the patient is able to tolerate an oral diet the enteral/parenteral regimen should be reduced in a stepwise manner. Low fat diets are frequently prescribed in acute pancreatitis and may be well tolerated during the first few days of oral feeding. However, this reduction of fat intake may significantly reduce overall energy intake, an important consideration in this nutritionally depleted patient group. The incorporation of medium chain triglycerides (MCT) may be useful in increasing the energy content of the diet. Once the episode of acute pancreatitis has resolved the patient should be able to tolerate a normal diet.

An integral component of patient care in this group is regular nutritional assessment (see Section 1.11). Care must be taken when interpreting changes in serum albumin concentrations in this group as a low serum albumin concentration may be a reflection of the severity of disease rather than of nutritional depletion.

In summary, these patients often require aggressive nutritional therapy and, as a consequence, the dietitian is a key member of the care team.

4.4.2 Chronic pancreatitis

This may follow repeated attacks of acute pancreatitis or may be associated with chronic inflammation of the biliary tract. There is a strong relationship between alcohol consumption and the risk of developing chronic pancreatitis. Nutritional problems, diagnostic techniques and treatment are similar to those previously described. The more disabling features of the disease are pain, malabsorption, weight loss and steatorrhoea. Malnutrition may be severe, in part due to the chronic nature of the disease combined with years of alcohol abuse.

Pancreatic enzyme supplementation is the cornerstone of treatment in long term patient management and its function is twofold; firstly to assist in pain control and secondly to reduce malabsorption. Steatorrhoea does not occur until the enzyme output of the exocrine pancreas is reduced by more than 90% (Di Mango *et al* 1973). The use of enzyme supplementation may also aid the stabilization of insulin requirements among diabetic patients. These pancreatic enzyme supplements contain amylase, trypsin and lipase although the lipase content determines their effectiveness (average dose 10 000–12 000 units lipase/meal). Furthermore, the efficacy of these enzymes supplements is improved by simultaneous administration of H_2 receptor antagonists, since these enzyme preparations are known to become inactivated at a pH of less than 4.

One of the main practical problems in the management of these patients is poor compliance, in terms of taking medication and in abstinence from alcohol.

General dietary guidelines for patients with chronic pancreatitis are summarized in Table 4.13. Regular clinical, nutritional and biochemical assessments are all important in assessing the severity of disease and in establishing an appropriate treatment plan.

Table 4.13 Guidelines for the dietary management of chronic pancreatitis

1	Alcohol should be avoided
2	Meals with a high fat content should be avoided as they may increase the frequency and intensity of pain. In severe cases of steatorrhoea, medium chain triglycerides (MCT) may be used to maintain energy intake.
3	Nitrogen and energy intake should be adequate
4	Blood glucose should be regularly monitored
5	Vitamin and mineral supplementation may be required. In particular, supplements of the fat soluble vitamins, folic acid and calcium are often given
6	Pancreatic enzymes should be taken with all foods and the amount taken at each meal adjusted according to the quantity of food eaten and the fat content of meal

4.4.3 Cancer of the pancreas

Epidemiological evidence suggests that the incidence of pancreatic carcinoma is increasing in the Western World. Genetic, occupational and dietary factors have all been implicated (Shearman and Finlayson 1989). Several studies have related coffee consumption to pancreatic cancer although a recent control study (Carter 1990) from Milan showed that there was no significant association.

Diagnosis of pancreatic carcinoma is usually made using imaging techniques and if the tumour is situated at the head of the pancreas then radical surgical resection (Whipple's) may be undertaken; but if the tumour is sited in the tail of the pancreas, there may be little indication for surgical intervention and palliative measures to relieve jaundice may be appropriate.

Aggressive diet therapy is indicated only in the pre- and post-operative management of those patients undergoing major surgery. Intravenous and/or a jejunostomy regimen may be prescribed and one should not forget that in the post-operative period these patients may require enzyme supplementation and insulin.

For those patients with irresectable disease, nutritional care is as described in Sections 4.34 and 4.36. In the majority of patients who receive palliative treatment, the main aim is to relieve jaundice, by endoscopically siting a stent in the biliary tree.

The outlook for those patients diagnosed with pancreatic carcinoma is dismal, with less than 10% of patients surviving to five years. This includes those patients who undergo surgery.

References

Alverdy JA, Aoys E and Moss MD (1988) Total parenteral nutrition promotes bacterial translocation from the gut. *Surgery* **104**, 185–90.

Alverdy JA, Aoys E and Moss MD (1990) Effect of commercially available chemically defined liquid diets on the intestinal microflora and bacterial translocation from the gut. *JPEN* **14**, 1–6.

Carter DC (1990) Cancer of the pancreas. *Current opinion in Gastroenterology* **6**, 775–9.

Di Mango EP, Go VLW and Summerskill WHJ (1973) Relations between pancreatic enzyme outputs and malabsorption in severe pancreatic insufficiency. *N Eng J Med* **288**, 813–15.

McMahon MJ (1990) Acute pancreatitis. *Current Opinion in Gastroenterology* **6**, 757–62.

Ranson JHC (1984) Acute pancreatitis: pathogenesis, outcome and treatment. *Clinics in Gastroenterology* **13**, 843.

Shearman DJC and Finlayson ND (1989) Carcinoma and other tumours of the pancreas. In *Diseases of the Gastrointestinal Tract* 2e pp. 1101–1116. Churchill Livingstone, Edinburgh.

Ziegler F, Ollivier JM, Cynober L, Masini JP, Caudray Lucas C, Levy E and Gibourdeau J (1990) Efficiency of enteral nitrogen support in surgical patients: small peptide versus non-degraded proteins. *Gut* **31**, 1277–83.

4.5 Cystic fibrosis

Cystic fibrosis (CF) is a generalized hereditary condition in which there is widespread dysfunction of exocrine glands. It is characterized by chronic pulmonary disease, pancreatic enzyme deficiency and abnormally high concentration of electrolytes in the sweat.

The incidence of CF in Caucasians is approximately 1 in 2500 live births (BPA 1988), but its incidence in non-Caucasians is much rarer, and estimated to be around 1 in 20 000 in black populations and 1 in 100 000 in Oriental populations (Corey *et al* 1988). Exciting advances have been made in the knowledge of the genetics of CF over the last three years. The condition has been shown to be caused by an abnormality of a single gene in the middle of chromosome 7. It appears that several different mutations may affect the same gene and these may account for varying clinical features, although 70% of the CF population share the same specific defect, i.e. delta 508 mutation (RCP 1990).

Symptoms usually begin in infancy and in Britain there is currently a 50% survival up to the age of 20 years; mortality is substantially greater for females than for males under 20 years of age (BPA 1988). The overall survival rate in Britain is not as good as in some of the other countries and many CF centres in the USA, Canada and Australia report an 80% survival to 19 or 20 years (Goodchild 1987).

Progressive malnutrition and poor growth are common features of CF and they represent a serious problem. A wide range of nutritional deficiencies has been described; the most common including energy malnutrition and fat-soluble vitamin malabsorption, particularly vitamins A and E.

4.5.1 Dietary problems associated with cystic fibrosis

Nutritional problems result from:

1 Pancreatic insufficiency.
2 Low energy intake.
3 Increased energy expenditure associated with:
   - Pulmonary infections;
   - Increased work of breathing;
   - The basic gene defect?

Pancreatic insufficiency

It is estimated that this is present in 85–95% of patients with CF (Kelleher 1987).

The severity of steatorrhoea is variable. In some patients, even when they appear to be taking sufficient quantities of pancreatic enzymes, there can still be a significant malabsorption of fat, nitrogen and fat-soluble vitamins contributing to a deterioration in nutritional status. Murphy *et al* (1991) estimate that up to 10.6% of dietary energy may be lost in the stools. Patients who are pancreatic sufficient appear to have better growth and lung function.

Low energy intake

For the last 10 years, CF patients have been recommended to eat a high energy diet, but recent studies monitoring energy intake demonstrate that patients rarely eat in excess of the DHSS (1979) or WHO (1985) Recommended Daily Amounts (Buchdahl *et al* 1989; MacDonald *et al* 1989; Thompson *et al* 1990). The reasons to explain the poor energy intake are many, but by far the commonest cause is anorexia which so frequently accompanies a chest infection. Children with CF may be accused of being pernickity and unco-operative when a low grade chest infection may turn out to be the cause of their poor appetite. In direct contrast, however, emphasis about weight gain and food may heighten parental anxiety with regard to feeding and may result in undue pressure being exerted at meal and snack time, making the feeding process less pleasant and this may result in behavioural feeding problems and food refusal on the part of the child. In addition, poor use of dietary supplements, lack of financial resources, adherence to a normal 'healthy' diet (i.e. a high fibre, low fat, low sugar diet), dislike of fatty foods and, fortunately now to a lesser degree, the outdated recommendation in some residual pockets of the country to follow a low fat diet, all contribute to an inadequate energy intake.

Increased energy expenditure

Patients with severe pulmonary disease tend to have higher energy expenditures. However, increased levels of energy expenditure are also seen in CF patients with normal pulmonary function. This increased resting energy expenditure in CF has been particularly associated with the increased work of breathing associated with pulmonary disease, infection and, possibly, it may be due to the molecular defect of the disease itself (Buchdahl *et al* 1988). Laboratory studies have suggested that the primary CF defect might be associated with an energy-requiring mechanism at the intracellular level, possibly within the mitochondria (Durie and Pencharz 1989).

4.5.2 Dietary management of cystic fibrosis

It is important to provide the CF patient with the optimum diet to enable the potential for growth to be fulfilled and resistance to infection maximized. Specific diet therapy should be determined individually, taking into account age, activity, weight, clinical condition, food preferences and tolerances.

Energy

It is accepted that energy requirements are generally increased due to steatorrhoea and pulmonary infection. As a general guideline, it has been arbitrarily recommended that energy intake be increased by up to 50% above the 1979 RDA in patients with CF, although Pencharz *et al* (1989) now consider a more realistic recommendation to be 120% of the (1979) RDA for the majority of CF patients. However, because of the heterogeneity of these patients, it is difficult to give precise recommendations and patients need to be assessed individually. Occasionally, a patient can grow in a normal fashion by consuming no more than the RDA for energy for normal healthy people. On the other hand, patients with advanced pulmonary disease may need 50–60% more than the normal intake of energy.

In order to achieve a high energy intake, the first step is to maximize energy intake from ordinary foods. A good variety of energy-rich foods should be encouraged such as full cream milk, cheese, meat, full cream yoghurt, milk puddings, bread generously covered with butter or margarine, cakes and biscuits. High fibre foods are bulky and not energy-dense and therefore not particularly suitable. Regular meals and frequent snacks are important. This type of dietary advice directly opposes normal healthy eating recommendations and, not surprisingly, it is common to find resistance to it by parents, older patients, school teachers and even some health professionals, particularly dentists (MacDonald *et al* 1991). An essential part of the dietitian's role is not only to apply this dietary advice to the specific needs of an individual patient, but also to ensure that all professional personnel connected with CF understand fully the rationale for this dietary treatment and that they are all giving consistent messages with regard to diet.

Protein

Although the exact protein requirements are unclear, it is generally accepted that the protein intake should be increased to compensate for excessive loss of nitrogen in the faeces and sputum and to support the accretion of amino acids in growing tissue (Beddoes *et al* 1981). It has been suggested that at least 15–20% of the energy intake should come from protein sources (Farrell and Hubbard 1983). In practice, protein intakes are usually high and do not need special supplementation.

Fat

Fat is the most concentrated source of energy in the diet and it is now widely accepted that it should be encouraged liberally and should provide approximately 35–40% of the total energy intake.

Traditionally, fat restriction has been widely advocated for CF in order to reduce steatorrhoea, increase protein absorption and improve the character of the stools. However, there is no objective data supporting this practice and fat restriction reduces the intake of energy and essential fatty acids. There is now evidence that patients who consume normal fat intakes exhibit better growth and the percentage fat malabsorption is not increased by a higher intake (MacDonald *et al* 1984).

In the past, medium chain triglycerides (MCT) have been used as a replacement oil in CF diets because shorter chain fatty acids (fewer than 12 carbon atoms) can be absorbed in the absence of pancreatic lipase and bile salts (Dodge and Yassa 1980). Although MCT oil has been shown to improve the character of the stools, it is unpalatable, inconvenient to use and it still needs the concurrent administration of pancreatic enzymes to aid absorption (Durie *et al* 1980); its use is generally no longer recommended in CF.

Dietary supplements

If growth is still suboptimal or to compensate for poor nutrition during an acute infection, effective use should be made of the wide range of commercial dietary supplements that are now available (Table 4.14). Unfortunately their use is inconsistent in CF, both by health professionals and by patients, and it is not uncommon to find their use discontinued soon after initiation by the patients themselves. The quantity and timing of dietary supplements is important in childhood so as not to impair appetite and decrease nutrient intake from normal foods. It is not uncommon to find young children taking large quantities of glucose polymer in drinks and then refusing most solid

Table 4.14 Useful energy supplements in the treatment of cystic fibrosis

Product category	Product (manufacturer)
Glucose polymers	Caloreen (Clintec), Maxijul (SHS) Liquid Maxijul (SHS), Polycal (Cow & Gate Nutricia), Polycose (Abbott)
Glucose drinks	Hycal (Beechams), Fortical (Cow & Gate Nutricia)
Fortified Milk Shake Drinks	Liquisorb (Merck), Fortisip (Cow & Gate Nutricia) Ensure Plus (Ross), Paediasure (Ross), Build-Up (Nestlé), Fresubin (Fresenius)

foods. The quantity recommended in CF is age dependent (Littlewood and MacDonald 1987) and a useful guide is given in Table 4.15.

Enteral feeding

Overnight enteral feeding is being used more frequently as a method of providing nutritional support in CF when nutritional status cannot be maintained with an oral high energy diet. Short term enteral feeding in CF appears to have no benefit on long term nutritional status, but long term feeding over months and years has been shown to improve both nutritional status and growth, even though there may be a time period of up to six months before there is an increase in linear growth velocity. Even pulmonary function may decline at a slower rate.

A wide variety of formulae, delivery techniques and methods of pancreatic enzyme administration are being used. Enteral feeds used include elemental, whole protein with an energy density of both 1 kcal/ml and 1.5 kcal/ml, and high fat feeds such as Pulmocare (Ross). It has been hypothesized that low fat elemental formulae are better absorbed in CF, but these feeds are expensive, have a high osmolality and generally have a lower energy density than whole protein feeds. It has been shown that steatorrhea is no greater on whole protein feeds than on elemental formula (Kane and Black 1989) and, in one recent study, a higher net protein deposition was associated with a higher protein non-elemental formula than an elemental formula (Pelkanos *et al* 1990).

In practice, most CF patients over 20 kg will tolerate an energy-dense (1.5 kcal/ml) whole protein feed providing approximately 1000 kcal overnight. Children weighing less than 20 kg should be provided with a 1.0 kcal/ml whole protein paediatric feed such as Nutrison Paediatric (Cow & Gate Nutricia) or Paediasure (Ross), supplying about a third of their energy requirements.

Feeds that supply 1.5 kcal/ml are higher in protein than the 1.0 kcal/ml feeds and are unsuitable for the younger age groups (MacDonald *et al* 1991).

The method of enzyme administration varies from centre to centre and no single method seems to be better than another. The majority of centres in Britain give enteric coated microspheres such as Creon (Duphar) or Pancrease (Cilag) orally. Enzymes are sometimes given at the beginning of the feed and again before the patient goes to sleep, or at the beginning, midway and at the end of feeding, or all at the beginning. The dosage of pancreatic enzymes is arbitrary and can be calculated by comparing the amount of enzyme normally given with a meal of a certain fat content, and the fat content of the feed.

For long term feeding, gastrostomy is now usually the preferred route of choice in CF. A number of complications have been associated with nasogastric feeding, particularly the dislodgement of the nasogastric tube following coughing and physiotherapy, and difficulty in inserting the nasogastric tubes. However, gastrostomy feeding is not without complications and leakage around the site, particularly with the button gastrostomy, and local infections are proving a common problem.

Table 4.15 Energy content of dietary supplements for children with cystic fibrosis

Age	Energy content of dietary supplement
1–2 yrs	200 kcal
3–5 yrs	400 kcal
6–10 yrs	600 kcal
11 yrs	800 kcal

Fat-soluble vitamins

Deficiencies of vitamins A, D, E and K are well documented. Biochemical deficiency is not always accompanied by clinical effects, but it is reasonable to correct it when demonstrated (Dodge and Yassa 1980).

Vitamin A

Vitamin A deficiency in CF has been well documented in the literature. Night blindness (O'Donnell and Talbot 1987), xerophthalmia, bulging fontanelles and increase intracranial pressure have all been associated with vitamin A deficiency (Eid *et al* 1990).

Daily supplementation of 8000 iu (2400 μg) is currently advised (Congdon *et al* 1981). Monitoring of blood levels ensures that adequate supplementation has been prescribed. However, if this is not possible, 8000 iu/day usually restores the plasma levels to normal.

Vitamin D

Although rickets is rarely seen in CF, subclinical deficiency has been noted (Littlewood *et al* 1980) and a daily supplement of 20 μg (800 iu) is advisable for patients with pancreatic insufficiency.

Vitamin E

Vitamin E deficiency in CF has been associated with severe neurological malfunction (Kelleher 1987). Plasma levels are generally low, but can be corrected by giving a daily supplement varying from 50 mg for infants to 200 mg for adults.

Vitamin K

Deficiency of this vitamin has been noted in patients with liver disease and in young infants with CF, causing bleeding due to hypoprothrombinaemia (Farrell and Hubbard 1983). A supplement is only necessary if deficiency has been demonstrated.

Water-soluble vitamins

With the exception of vitamin B_6 (Kelleher 1987) there is little evidence of water-soluble vitamin deficiency and routine supplementation is not recommended.

Trace minerals

Serum iron levels are frequently low in CF patients but iron supplementation is not routinely recommended. There is some suggestion that mucoid strains of *pseudomonas aeruginosa* may be more stable under iron-limited conditions (Kelleher 1987), although there is no known correlation between presence of pseudomonas and serum ferritin levels. Low plasma zinc levels have also been reported (Dodge 1983).

Salt

To avoid salt depletion in patients with CF, it is clear that salt supplements are required in hot environments when exposure to the sun and/or physical exertion causes increased sweating (di Sant'Agnese and Hubbard 1984). However, the problem of salt loss is only of major concern during heat waves and in hot climates, and there is no good rationale for the traditional practice of recommending routine consumption of salty foods and aggressive use of the salt pot (Farrell and Hubbard 1983).

4.5.3 Feeding infants with cystic fibrosis

Infants with pancreatic insufficiency who have been diagnosed by a CF screening procedure usually thrive on a normal energy intake, i.e. 100–120 kcal/kg in conjunction with pancreatic enzymes. Breast milk or normal infant formula milks are suitable feeds. If weight gain is inadequate, or if a meconium ileus has resulted in surgery and short bowel syndrome, the energy requirements may be as high as 150–200 kcal/kg (MacDonald *et al* 1991). To achieve this energy intake in infants who are failing to thrive, the addition of a glucose polymer such as Maxijul (SHS) or Polycal (Cow & Gate Nutricia) and a 50% long chain fat emulsion such as Calogen (SHS) to a normal infant formula milk is necessary. If the infant has a temporary disaccharide intolerance following surgery for a meconium ileus, a lactose free, protein hydrolysate feed such as Pregestimil (Mead Johnson) or PeptiJunior (Cow & Gate Nutricia) may be necessary with or without the use of additional energy supplements.

It is necessary to give pancreatic enzymes with all infant formula milks including breast milk. Unfortunately neither the pancreatin powders or the newer enteric coated microsphere enzyme preparations are ideal to administer to a baby. Both the enteric coated granules and pancreatin powder can be mixed with a little breast or formula milk, but it should not be added to the full bottle. Apart from the pancreatin powder being largely ineffective (Beverley *et al* 1987), if the baby dribbles the milk with this enzyme in it around its mouth it will cause a skin irritation. However the enteric coated granules when given in a little milk from a spoon may cause choking. So far, the best method of administering the enteric coated granules to a milk-fed infant is to mix them with a small amount of fruit puree which will hold these enzymes in a gel and they can then be given at the beginning of the feed.

4.5.4 Pancreatic enzymes

Exogenous pancreatic enzymes are available in powder, tablet or capsule form (Table 4.16), but by far the most common preparations in use are the enteric coated microsphere granules of pancrealipase available in capsule form.

Table 4.16 Pancreatic enzyme preparations available in the UK

Product (Manufacturer)	Composition (per g of powder/granules or per capsule/tablet) BP units		
	Lipase	Protease	Amylase
Powder			
Pancrex V (Paines & Byrne)	25 000	1400	30 000
Capsules			
Pancrex V '340 mg' (Paines & Byrne)	8 000	430	9 000
Pancrex V '125 mg' (Paines & Byrne)	2 950	160	3 000
Tablets			
Enteric-coated tablets			
Pancrex V (Paines & Byrne)	1 900	110	1 700
Pancrex V Forte (Paines & Byrne)	5 600	330	5 000
Enteric-coated granules			
Pancrease (Cilag)	5 000	350	3 000
Creon (Duphar)	8 000	210	9 000
Nutrizym GR (Merck)	10 000	650	10 000

Table 4.17 General guidelines for the use of pancreatic enzyme preparations

1 Give with every meal; during rather than all before or after

2 Give extra enzymes (e.g. 1–2 capsules or tablets) with fatty or large snacks and milky drinks

3 Do not give enzymes with squash, lemonade, fruit or boiled and jelly sweets

4 Mix powdered enzyme either with a little soft food or jam or honey. Do not sprinkle over a complete meal

5 The enteric-coated microsphere capsules e.g. Pancrease (Cilag) and Creon (Duphar) can be swallowed whole. Where swallowing is difficult the capsules may be opened and the contained microsphere taken with liquids or mixed with foods such as jam, honey, yogurt or mashed potato. They should not be crushed or chewed

6 Increase the enzyme dose (e.g. by 1–2 capsules or tablets) if the stools are loose, fatty or occur more than twice daily

There are three which are currently marketed in the UK. These include Pancrease (Cilag), Creon (Duphar) and Nutrizym GR (Merck). These enzymes have been shown to be more effective than the powdered or enteric-coated tablet enzymes (Beverley *et al* 1987; Williams *et al* 1990). The granules can be mixed with a little food, but should not be chewed, or the capsules can be swallowed whole. The granules do not taste or smell; neither do they alter the consistency of the food.

The optimal dose varies for each patient and does not necessarily bear a relationship to the intake of dietary fat. Although faecal fat estimations can help to determine the enzyme dose, in practice this is usually decided by bowel habits and abdominal discomfort. Enzymes should be administered with all meals and fatty snacks. Guidelines for using pancreatic enzymes are summarized in Table 4.17.

Useful address

The Cystic Fibrosis Research Trust, 5 Blyth Road, Bromley, Kent BR1 3RS.

Further reading

Goodchild MC and Dodge JA (1985) *Cystic fibrosis manual of diagnosis and management*. Baillière Tindall, London.

References

Beddoes V, Laing S, Goodchild MC and Dodge JA (1981) Dietary management of cystic fibrosis. *Practitioner* **225**, 557–60.

Beverley DW, Kelleher J, MacDonald A, Littlewood JM, Robinson T and Walters MP (1987) Comparison of four pancreatic extracts in cystic fibrosis. *Arch Dis Childh* **62**, 564–8.

British Paediatric Association (BPA) Working Party on Cystic Fibrosis (1988) Cystic fibrosis in the United Kingdom 1977–1985: an improving picture. *Br Med J* **297**, 1599–602.

Buchdahl RM, Cox M, Fulleylove C, Marchant JL, Tomkins AM, Brueton MJ and Warner JO (1988) Increased resting energy expenditure in cystic fibrosis. *J Appl Physiol* **64**(5), 1810–16.

Buchdahl RM, Fulleylove C, Marchant JL, Warner JO and Brueron MJ (1989). Energy and nutrient intakes of cystic fibrosis. *Arch Dis Childh* **64**, 373–8.

Congdon P, Bruce G, Rothburn MM, Clarke P, Littlewood JM, Kelleher J and Losowsky M (1981) Vitamin status in treated patients with cystic fibrosis. *Arch Dis Childh* **56**, 708–14.

Corey M, McLaughlin FJ, Williams M and Levison H (1988) A comparison of survival, growth and pulmonary function in patients with cystic fibrosis in Boston and Toronto. *J Clin Epidemiol* **41**, 583–91.

Department of Health and Social Security (1979) *Recommended daily amounts of food energy and nutrients for groups of people in the United Kingdom*. Rep Htlh Soc Subj 15. HMSO, London.

di Sant'Agnese PA and Hubbard VS (1984) The pancreas. In *Cystic fibrosis*, Taussig LM (Ed) pp. 230–95. Thieme-Stratton, New York.

Dodge JA (1983) Nutrition. In *Cystic fibrosis*, Hodson ME, Norman AP and Batten JC (Eds) pp. 132–43. Baillière Tindall, London.

Dodge JA and Yassa JG (1980) Food intake and supplementary feeding programmes. In *Perspectives in Cystic Fibrosis*, Sturgess JM (Ed) pp. 125–136. Imperial Press, Mississauga.

Durie PR, Newth CJ, Forstner GG and Gall DG (1980) Malabsorption of medium chain triglycerides in infants with cystic fibrosis; correction with pancreatic enzyme supplements. *J Paediatr* **96**, 862–4.

Durie PR and Pencharz PB (1989) A rational approach to the nutritional care of patients with cystic fibrosis. *J Royal Soc Med* Suppl 16(82), 11–20.

Eid NS, Shoemaker LR and Samiec TD (1990) Vitamin A in cystic fibrosis. Case report and reviews of the literature. *J Paed Gastroenterol Nutrition* **10**, 265–269.

Farrell PM and Hubbard VS (1983) Nutrition in cystic fibrosis: vitamins, fatty acids and minerals. In *Textbook of Cystic Fibrosis*. Lloyd-Still JD (ED) pp. 263–92. John Wright, Bristol.

Goodchild MC (1987) Nutritional management of cystic fibrosis. *Digestion* **37**(Suppl 1), 61–7.

Kane RE and Black P (1989) Glucose intolerance with low-medium-high carbohydrate formulas during night-time enteral feeding in cystic fibrosis patients. *J Ped Gast Nutrition* **8**, 321–6.

Kelleher J (1987) Laboratory measurements of nutrition in cystic fibrosis. *J Royal Soc Med* Suppl 15(80), 25–9.

Littlewood JM, Congdon PJ, Bruce G, Kelleher J, Rothburn M, Losowsky MS and Clarke PCN (1980) Vitamin status in treated cystic fibrosis. In *Perspective in Cystic Fibrosis*. Sturgess JM (Ed) pp. 166–71. Imperial Press, Mississauga.

Littlewood JM and MacDonald A (1987) Rationale of modern dietary recommendations in cystic fibrosis. *J Royal Soc Med* Suppl 15(80), 16–24.

MacDonald A, Holden C and Harris G (1991) Nutritional strategies in cystic fibrosis: current issues. *J Roy Soc Med* **84**(Suppl 18), 28–35.

MacDonald A, Kelleher J, Miller MG and Littlewood JM (1984) Low, moderate or high fat diets for cystic fibrosis. In *Cystic fibrosis: Horizons*. Lawson D (Ed) pp. 395. John Wiley, Chichester.

MacDonald A, Williams J and Weller P (1989) Is a normal diet adequate for CF patients? Abstracts of the 16th Annual Meeting of the European Working Group for Cystic Fibrosis, Prague, p. 74.

Murphy JL, Wootton SA, Bond SA and Jackson AA (1991) Energy content of stools in normal healthy controls and patients with cystic fibrosis. *Arch Dis Childh* **66**, 495–500.

O'Donnell M and Talbot JF (1987) Vitamin A deficiency in cystic fibrosis: case report. *Br J Ophthalmology* **71**, 787–90.

Pelkanos JT, Holt TL, Ward LC, Cleghorn GJ and Shepherd RW (1990) Protein turnover in malnourished patients with cystic fibrosis: effects of elemental and non-elemental nutritional supplements. *J Pediatric Gast Nutrition* **10**, 339–43.

Pencharz PB, Benall G, Corey M, Durie P and Vaisman N (1989) Energy intake in cystic fibrosis. *Nutrition Reviews* **47**(1), 31–2.

Royal College of Physicians (1990) *Cystic fibrosis in adults. Recommendations for care of patients in the UK*. RCP, London.

Thompson JM, O'Rowe A, Dodge JA and McCraken KJ (1990) Energy balance and macronutrient digestibility in 30 patients with cystic fibrosis (abstract). *Paed Pulmonology* Supp 5, 264.

Williams J, MacDonald A, Weller PH, Fields J and Pandov H (1990) Two enteric coated microspheres in cystic fibrosis. *Arch Dis Childh* **65**, 594–7.

World Health Organization (1985) *Protein and energy requirements*. Tech Rep Ser 724. WHO, Geneva.

4.6 The malabsorption syndrome

There are a number of reasons why a defect in absorption of one or more nutrients may occur and these are summarized in Table 4.18. Although dietary therapy or nutritional supplementation may be indicated it is important that the primary disorder is recognized and treated.

4.6.1 Diagnostic features of malabsorption

Principal clinical features of the malabsorption syndrome include diarrhoea, abdominal distension, flatulence and nutritional deficiencies, although not all of these need be present. In steatorrhoea the stool is pale, malodorous, greasy and unformed whereas in carbohydrate malabsorption the diarrhoea tends to be watery and frothy due to the presence of fermented sugars. The nutritional features may include those of fluid and electrolyte loss, weight loss and other specific nutritional deficiencies.

The diagnosis of fat malabsorption is confirmed using the standard 3-day faecal collection. The upper limit of daily fat excretion is normally taken as 7 g or 20 mmol/24 hours. A very high faecal fat excretion (50 g or more) is suggestive of pancreatic insufficiency and symptoms can be relieved with pancreatic enzymes. Unless the steatorrhoea is severe, the loss of faecal fat is of little nutritional importance compared with the concomitant loss of other nutrients, particularly the fat-soluble vitamins A, D, E and K as well as calcium and magnesium. Specific nutritional deficiences may also occur as a result of disease or resection of a specific part of the gastrointestinal tract as will be appreciated from Fig. 4.7 which shows absorption sites.

4.6.2 Dietary treatment of malabsorption

Whatever the cause of malabsorption the principles of dietary therapy remain the same:

1 Dietary treatment of the primary disorder, e.g. coeliac disease.

2 The daily replacement of large losses of fluid and electrolytes.

3 The restoration of optimal nutritional state, by supplementation if necessary.

Fat malabsorption

Restriction of dietary fat should not be pursued too enthusiastically in patients with steatorrhoea as energy deficiency is a common consequence of severe malabsorption disorders. Fat restriction is indicated when:

1 The patient finds the symptoms socially and personally unacceptable despite optimum drug therapy for steatorrhoea.

2 The steatorrhoea is severe enough to lead to electrolyte disorders or mineral deficiencies.

3 There is a defect in fat transport and clearance from the lymphatic system as in abetalipoproteinaemia, intestinal lymphangectasia, chylouria or chylothorax.

Figure 4.8 shows the major steps involved in fat absorption and metabolism. If a low fat diet is prescribed to control symptoms, the usual fat intake of the patient needs to be determined. If this exceeds 100 g/day, the fat intake should be reduced by about 50%. If the fat intake is less than 100 g, 40–50 g of longchain triglycerides (LCT) may be prescribed to see if symptoms improve. Restrictions below 40 g are not practical and if prescribed should not be continued if symptoms do not improve. Where fat restriction is indicated but adequate energy provision is also desirable, medium chain triglycerides (MCT) and glucose polymers may be used (see Section 1.13). LCT should continue to provide 10–20% of energy requirements in a form which will ensure an adequate provision of linoleic acid. In the absence of pancreatic lipase and bile salt activity, absorption of MCT is about one third of normal. A proportion of MCT is able to enter the mucosal cell directly as a triglyceride, where it can be hydrolysed by a mucosal lipolytic system. The medium chain fatty acids then pass into the portal vein.

In some individuals, rapid intraluminal hydrolysis of MCT may result in osmotic diarrhoea; if this is the case then the MCT should be administered at a slower rate. MCT can be delivered as an oil in a dose up to 15 ml orally four times per day. This provides about 460 kcal/day. The oil can be given on its own or mixed with fruit juice to help obscure the taste. When MCTs are used for cooking they should not be heated above 150–160°C or their palatability is altered. Complete enteral feeds containing MCT can be used as a supplement, for example, Peptisorb (Merck), Liquisorbon MCT (Merck), MCT Pepdite 2+(SHS). Although as an energy substrate MCT may have some metabolic advantages over LCT, there appears to be no clinical advantage to be gained, in terms of absorption, from the use of MCT in the LCT-tolerant patient. When a LCT fat restriction is employed, particularly for the malnourished individual, it must be ensured that the resultant diet is adequate in protein, minerals, vitamins and trace elements. Suitable low fat supplements may be needed.

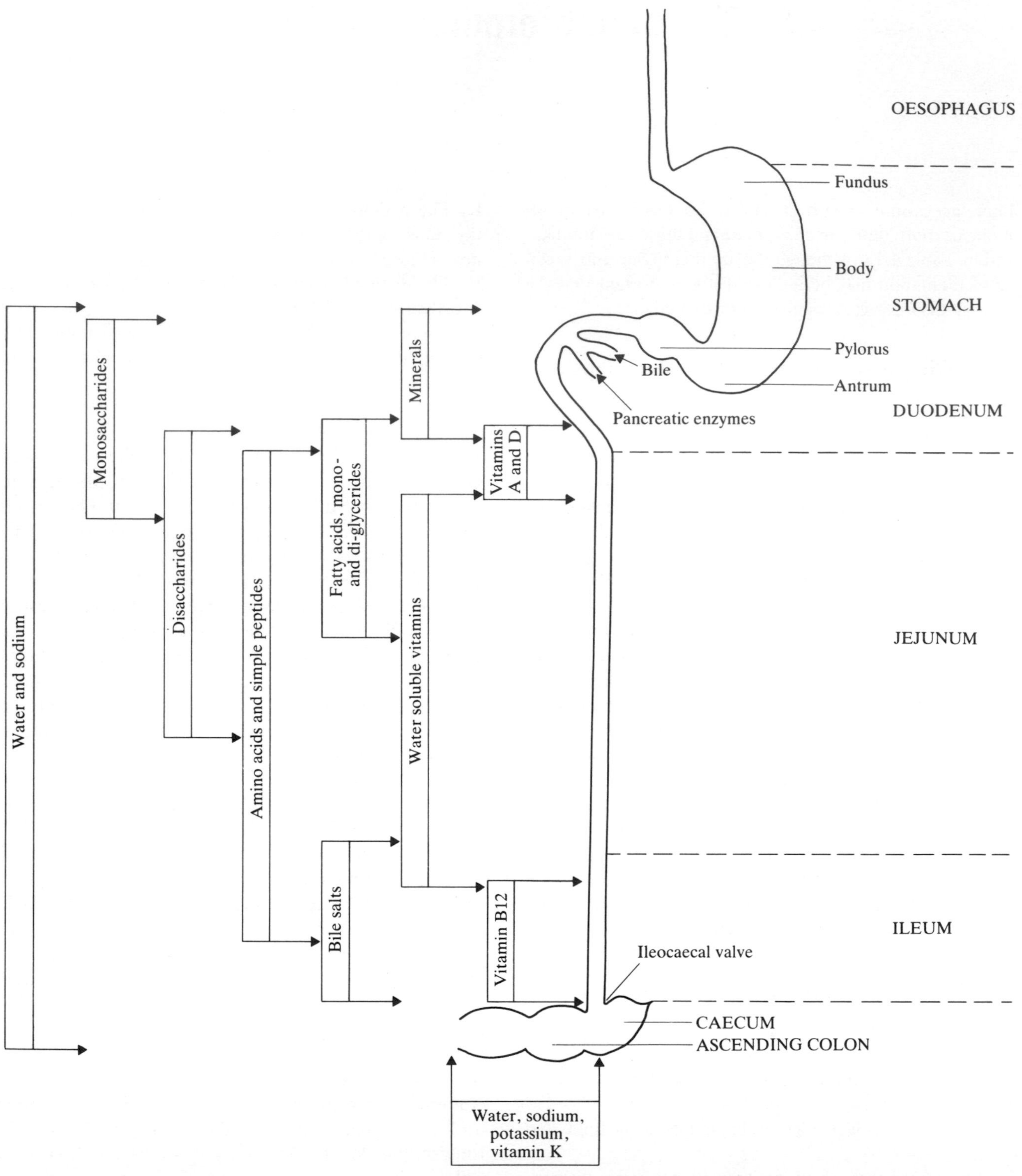

Fig. 4.7 Principal absorption sites for nutrients.

Carbohydrate malabsorption

Diagnosis can be confirmed with the relevant disaccharide tolerance test. This estimates the enzyme activity by measuring a rise in the level of blood glucose after administering a standard oral loading dose of the disaccharide.

The breath hydrogen test measures hydrogen which is one of the products metabolized by colonic bacteria from undigested sugars. Its concentration in the exposed air is determined by gas chromatography and is measured at intervals after the patient has ingested the test disaccharide.

In secondary disaccharide deficiency, treatment consists

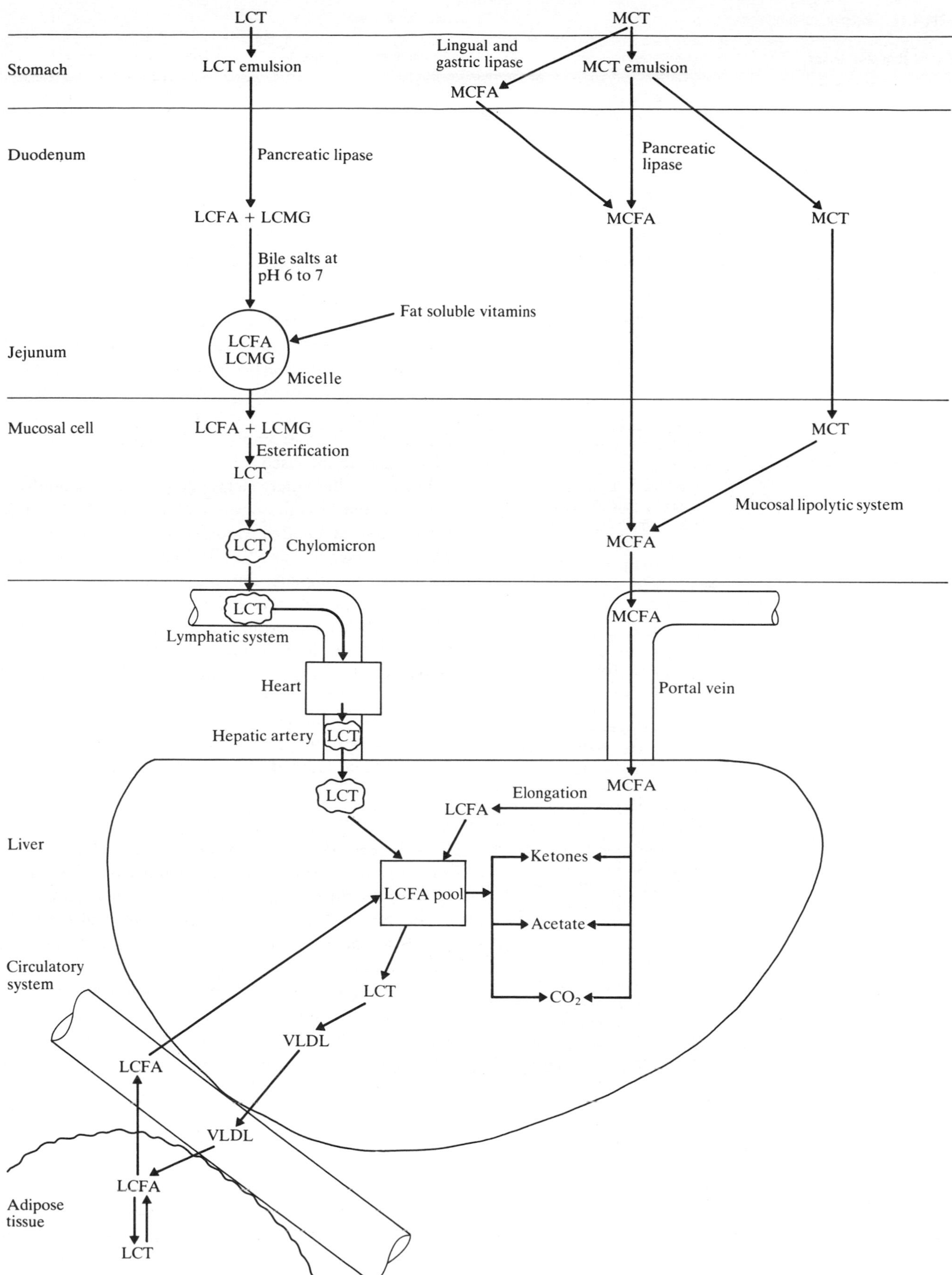

Fig. 4.8 Absorption and metabolism of long chain and medium chain triglycerides. LCT = long chain triglyceride; MCT = medium chain triglyceride, LCFA = long chain fatty acids; LCMG = long chain monoglyceride; VLDL = very low density lipoprotein.

Table 4.18 Causes of malabsorption

Reduced absorptive surface	Intestinal or gastric resection Villous atrophy, e.g. coeliac disease, tropical sprue Gastro-colic and jejuno-colic fistulae Inflammatory bowel disease Infiltration – amyloid, scleroderma, lymphoma Protein-energy malnutrition Vascular insufficiency Mucosal damage by drugs or irradiation
Intra-luminal causes	Pancreatic insufficiency – chronic pancreatitis, cystic fibrosis, (a deficiency of pancreatic lipase and pancreatic bicarbonate are implicated) High pH in duodenum – achlorhydria Low pH in duodenum – Zollinger-Ellison syndrome Bile salt deficiency – obstructive jaundice
Infection	Blind loop syndrome – bacterial deconjugation of bile salts resulting in steatorrhoea. There may also be some competition by bacteria in the small intestine for available nutrients. Bacterial growth may also lead to secondary disaccharide and monosaccharide intolerance Parasitic infestations Acute enteritis
Enzyme deficiencies	Disaccharidase deficiency Primary alactasia and primary sucrose-isomaltose deficiency. A permanent lactose or sucrose-free diet is required. Secondary lactase deficiency and occasionally sucrose-isomaltose deficiency. A temporary lactose-free diet is required. The primary disorder must also be treated. Typical causes include gastrointestinal infection, reduced absorptive surface, gastrointestinal tract trauma, protein intolerance and protein-energy malnutrition Racial or late-onset lactase deficiency is common in certain ethnic groups, e.g. Africans, American negroes, Indians, Chinese and others. The incidence in UK Caucasians in small at around 6%. There is a variable degree of tolerance to lactose and a symptomatic approach to treatment should be taken Specific deficiency of one or more pancreatic enzymes including isolated lipase deficiency, combined lipase and proteolytic enzyme deficiency and trypsinogen deficiency Enterokinase deficiency
Impairment of fat transport and clearance	Congenital lymphangectasia, retroperitoneal fibrosis, congestive heart failure, lymphoma Abetalipoproteinanaemia
Impairment of monosaccharide transport	Primary – a rare congenital malabsorption of monosaccharides has been reported involving a disturbance in the active transport of glucose and galactose. Strict adherence to a diet free of all carbohydrates other than fructose is necessary throughout infancy Secondary – Malabsorption of all monosaccharides may occur in infants following surgery, protein-energy malnutrition or gastroenteritis

principally of reducing the dietary intake of the malabsorbed sugars combined with specific therapy for the primary disorder e.g. acute enteritis, chronic alcoholism, non-tropical sprue. In practice control of dietary lactose is usually sufficient; only when maltase and sucrase deficiency is severe is it necessary to restrict maltose and sucrose. As the primary disorder improves, the restriction of dietary lactose should be eased.

In cases of hereditary lactase deficiency most adults can tolerate about 12 g/day or more of lactose. The use of low lactose milk and coffee whiteners may be substituted for whole milk (see Section 2.14.4). In children a lactose-free, nutritionally complete formula is required. A detailed dietary history will reveal the major sources of lactose which can be eliminated and substituted with foods containing no lactose. Tolerance can be increased when small amounts of lactose are taken with other foods and distributed among daily meals.

Sucrase-isomaltase deficiency may be hereditary or a secondary disorder. Foods with a sucrose content above 2% should be avoided. Restriction of starch is not usually necessary.

Congenital malabsorption of monosaccharides This is rare. It involves a disturbance in the active transport of the monosaccharides glucose and galactose. The diet must be free of all starch, disaccharides, glucose and galactose. For infants a fructose-based formula such as Galactomin 19 (Cow and Gate Nutricia) may be used. All oral medicines must be carbohydrate-free. The diet should be nutritionally adequate in all other respects and vitamin and mineral supplementation may be necessary. Strict adherence to the diet is required during infancy though in later years limited quantities of milk and sucrose may be added.

Secondary malabsorption of all monosaccharides This may occur in infants following surgery, protein-energy malnutrition or gastroenteritis. An initial period of intravenous fluids is often necessary to correct water and electrolyte imbalances. This will be followed by a carbohydrate-free formula during which there should be careful monitoring for signs of hypoglycaemia. The problem is thought to be one of monosaccharide malabsorption, since disaccharidase activity is normal. The ability to tolerate carbohydrates slowly recovers and a monosaccharide such as glucose or fructose may be added to the diet in increasing increments of 1% of normal carbohydrate intake. These children are often underweight and gravely ill and parenteral nutrition may be life saving if resumption of adequate oral nutrition is delayed. The detailed dietary management of carbohydrate malabsorption in infants and children is discussed by Francis (1986).

Protein malabsorption

Malabsorption states in which there is a deficiency of enzymes involved in protein digestion, e.g. pancreatic proteolytic enzyme, trypsinogen, or enterokinase deficiency are not indications for the dietary restriction of protein. When increased protein losses occur due to an enteropathy or malabsorption, a high protein intake (0.5–1.5 g/kg/day) should be prescribed to allow for the decreased efficiency of absorption. If fat malabsorption is present, high protein foods must be selected which are also low in fat. Protein supplements can be used along with non-protein calories in the form of carbohydrate (see Section 1.13.3).

Further reading

Dickerson JWT and Jones MH (1982) Malabsorption. *Nursing* **2**, 113–7.

Losowsky MS, Walker BE and Kelleher J (1974) *Malabsorption in clinical practice*. Churchill Livingstone, Edinburgh.

Reference

Francis DEM (1986) *Diets for sick children* 4e. Blackwell Scientific Publications, Oxford.

4.7 Coeliac disease

Coeliac disease is a condition in which the lining of the small intestine is damaged by gluten, a protein found in wheat and rye. Coeliacs are also affected by similar proteins present in barley and possibly oats. The damage which occurs considerably impairs the absorption of nutrients from the small intestine causing wasting and ultimately severe illness resembling malnutrition.

4.7.1 Causation

Despite a great deal of research, exactly why or how gluten harms the intestine is unknown. It is known that the fraction of gluten responsible for the damage is gliadin, but gliadin is itself a mixture of proteins. Work is in progress to identify the toxic elements and it is now known that the alpha, beta, gamma and omega fractions are all harmful to coeliacs.

There are several theories about the pathogenesis of gluten intolerance in coeliac disease. Recent workers have concentrated on the hypothesis that an abnormal immunological response is the most likely cause, while an earlier view was that gluten, or a component of it, was intrinsically toxic and that coeliacs lacked essential detoxifying enzyme systems. Neither these, nor other hypotheses, adequately explain the wide variety of ways in which the condition presents, or the complete age range over which diagnosis is now made following appearance of clinical symptoms. Whether these variations in age and symptoms reflect differences in individual sensitivity to gluten, or differences in exposure to causal events and environmental factors is unknown, but they do suggest a multifactorial process combining with a genetic predisposition to the condition.

A number of studies have shown that, in spite of running in families (coeliacs have an estimated 1 in 10 chance of a member of their family having or developing the condition), the disease is not inherited as a dominant characteristic. Although the mode of inheritance is not clear, susceptibility is associated with HLA B8 and DR3.

It has been estimated (McCrae 1969) that the coeliac condition affects approximately one person in 1850 in the UK, but it is likely that many cases remain undiagnosed and that the true incidence is higher (Swinson and Levi 1980). There are known variations in the incidence of coeliac disease in different populations. A very high incidence of one in 300 has been reported in the West of Ireland (Mylotte *et al* 1973), whereas the condition is virtually unknown in Negro and Oriental populations.

4.7.2 History of the condition

The word 'coeliac' is derived from the Greek word koiliakos which means 'suffering in the bowels'. The coeliac condition was first described nearly 1800 years ago in the writings of the Roman physician, Aretaeus of Cappadocia. He mentioned fatty diarrhoea, loss of weight, pallor and food passing undigested through the body. He also said 'that bread is rarely suitable for giving (coeliac children) strength'. It was not until 1888 that Samuel Gee of St Bartholomew's Hospital in London gave the second classic description and a clear clinical account of the condition.

Early this century a few physicians drew attention to the harmful effect of carbohydrate in coeliac disease and the 'banana diet' – a diet low in carbohydrate except for ripe bananas – was recommended. However, no real progress in recognizing and treating the disease was made until after the Second World War. In 1950, Professor Dicke, a Dutch paediatrician, described how coeliac children had benefited dramatically during the war when wheat, rye and oat flours, which were unavailable, were replaced by maize or rice; while at the end of the war, the children relapsed when wheat flour was air-lifted into Holland. This work was confirmed and extended by Professor Charlotte Anderson in Birmingham, who extracted the starch from wheat flour and found that the remaining gluten was the harmful part.

Since the 1950s, therefore, a gluten-free diet has been the treatment for coeliacs. In 1954 Paulley, a physician in Ipswich, described an abnormality of the lining of the small intestine found during an operation on an adult coeliac patient. This abnormality was the existence of an inflammatory condition, resulting in the loss of the villi from the mucosa of the small intestine and hence considerably reducing the surface area available for nutrient absorption. Treatment with a gluten-free diet usually results in the 'flat' lining of the coeliac intestine returning to the normal state as the villi grow again. On the whole, the younger the patient the more dramatic the improvement, provided that the diet is followed rigidly.

The development of biopsy tubes (in particular by Dr Margot Shiner in 1956 and Colonel Crosby, an American army officer, who designed the 'Crosby capsule' (Crosby and Kugler 1957) which removes a small section of intestinal mucosa for microscopic examination of the villi) resulted in jejunal biopsy becoming the standard technique for diagnosis of coeliac disease.

4.7.3 Diagnosis

The coeliac disorder can manifest itself at any age. In children, symptoms usually become apparent between three and five months after eating gluten, although in a few cases this interval may be shorter. After being weaned on to solids containing gluten, a normal baby who has thrived well initially on milk begins to refuse feeds and stops gaining weight. The next stage is actual weight loss and the child gradually becomes irritable, listless and develops a large abdomen or pot-belly. The stools become abnormal and are either large, pale and smell offensive or they may be loose, later developing into diarrhoea. Vomiting may also occur. If this state of affairs continues, the baby will quickly become wasted, especially around the buttocks, and may eventually develop acute diarrhoea and dehydration and become seriously ill.

In a few cases children do not show symptoms until they are older, when they present with a poor appetite and failure to grow. These children are obviously much more difficult to diagnose, as there are many other possible reasons for these symptoms. Various investigations can be undertaken for malabsorption (see Section 4.6), but a definite diagnosis can only be established by an intestinal biopsy. In the hands of experienced operators this is not a traumatic procedure, and can usually be completed within a couple of hours.

Thirty years ago, coeliac disease was almost exclusively a paediatric condition. Now it is much more prevalent in adults than in children.

Annual statistics issued by the Coeliac Society of the United Kingdom show that the percentage of newly-diagnosed children joining the Society has decreased in the last decade from 25% of the total new membership in 1981 to 15% in 1991. In fact, more adults over 60 are now being diagnosed in a year than children under 16. In 1991, 2716 newly-diagnosed coeliacs joined the society: 404 (15%) were children and 2312 (85%) were adults, of whom 541 were over 60 including 35 octogenarians.

Data from a number of sources worldwide, with the exception of Sweden (Ascher *et al* 1991), confirm that the incidence in infants is declining, possibly due to delayed introduction of solids combined with a reduction of gluten in weaning foods and prolonged breast-feeding (Greco *et al* 1985). It is not clear whether the declining incidence in childhood will be followed by an increase in diagnosis in later years. The number of adults being diagnosed is continually on the increase as more doctors become aware of the many different ways in which the condition can present itself in later life.

The majority of adult coeliacs consult their doctors not because of gastrointestinal symptoms but because of problems such as breathlessness, fatigue or just because they feel more tired at the end of the day than they used to. The difficulty for the general practitioner is that almost any chronic illness can start in this way. In the case of coeliacs, the fatigue and breathlessness is usually due to the anaemia which results from poor absorption of iron and folic acid. Deficiency of other essential nutrients such as calcium may also occur. The diagnosis is first suspected from the clinical evidence of symptoms or on the results of routine blood tests; it is then confirmed by jejunal biopsy. A smaller proportion of adult coeliacs see their doctors complaining of symptoms which arise directly from the effects of gluten on the small intestine, such as diarrhoea, abdominal fullness, discomfort, pain or vomiting. The diarrhoea is usually caused by inadequate absorption of dietary fat and the stools are pale, bulky, offensive and may be difficult to flush down the lavatory. It is this last feature which is sometimes more troublesome to patients than the increase in the number of bowel actions.

4.7.4 Treatment

The gluten-free diet always excludes wheat, rye and barley, but the use of oats is controversial. Some coeliacs are undoubtedly intolerant to oats and must avoid them, but others can tolerate them well and suffer neither obvious ill-effects nor microscopic changes on biopsy. Without conclusive evidence as to whether or not oats are harmful, medical opinion is divided but many leading authorities tend to err on the side of caution and exclude oats from the gluten-free diet.

The gluten-free diet must be followed strictly and it is now strongly recommended that it is continued for life. Careful studies, particularly in Bristol and Birmingham, have shown that patients with coeliac disease are at greater risk than the general population of developing malignant neoplasms, particularly lymphomas, although more rarely some cancers of the bowel may occur.

Although it has been suspected for many years that taking a strict gluten-free diet might reduce the cancer risk, it is only recently that evidence to support this has been forthcoming. Holmes (1989) followed up a group of coeliac patients over a period of 15 years and found clear evidence that the risk of tumour development in coeliacs who adhere to a strict gluten-free diet for at least five years is no greater than for anyone else in the general population.

Many doctors who run large coeliac clinics are convinced that the number of coeliacs developing cancer is decreasing, and probably as a result of the wider use of strict gluten-free diets in recent years.

Clearly prevention is better than cure and dietitians should therefore be very positive about the protection against malignancy conferred by following a life-long gluten-free diet. In addition, it is hoped that chronic nutritional deficiencies, relapses and infertility will also be avoided.

Avoidance of gluten

There are two sources of gluten in the diet – the obvious

and the less obvious. Firstly, it occurs in foods obviously made from wheat flour such as ordinary bread, cakes; biscuits, pastries and pies (Section 2.14.1). Secondly, it occurs in manufactured or processed foods including a whole range of convenience foods in which wheat flour is used either as an ingredient or as a filler. It is through eating foods in the second category that most dietary indiscretions occur.

To help fill the gap in the diet left by the omission of common gluten-containing foods, excellent gluten-free products are specially manufactured for patients with coeliac disease and dermatitis herpetiformis. Details of these can be found in Section 2.14.1. Many of these products are available to patients on prescription. A current list of prescribable products is given in Table 2.74 (in Section 2.14.1) and up-to-date lists can be obtained from the Coeliac Society or found in Monthly Index of Medical Specialities (MIMS) (Borderline Substances Appendix). Coeliac patients are not normally exempt from prescription charges unless they are in the general categories for exemption (such as children, pregnant or lactating mothers or old age pensioners). Since many items are likely to be needed, non-exempt patients may find that a prescription 'season ticket' (prepayment of charges) may be worthwhile. Details of this can be found on form FP95 available from Post Offices.

General dietary considerations

At diagnosis many coeliacs are anaemic and may also exhibit varying degrees of malnutrition. Immediately after treatment has started, there will be a phase of tissue growth and regeneration, and requirements for iron, folic acid and other vitamins will increase. Supplementation will be required and may need to be continued for several months. When full recovery has occurred and the patient is well established on a full and varied gluten-free diet, no further supplementation is usually necessary.

Apart from restriction of gluten the diet must be adequate in all other respects for normal growth and development. In general there need be no restriction of milk or dairy products, eggs, meat, fish, vegetables, fruit, rice or maize (corn).

Role of the dietitian

Following a gluten-free regimen is a life-long measure for the coeliac and it is vital that good dietary foundations are laid at the onset of treatment. Poor teaching or inadequate explanations will leave the patient confused and unable to follow the diet correctly. Months of ill-health can result.

In addition to teaching the essentials of a gluten-free diet to the patient and family, dietitians are also likely to be asked by patients for further information about coeliac disease or to clarify various points raised during their consultation with the doctor. It is important to reassure the patient or, in the case of a child, the parents, that a gluten-free diet will restore normal health.

Patients should be encouraged to adopt a positive attitude to their diet and think about all the foods they *can* eat instead of dwelling on those which are no longer suitable. Showing patients the 100-page long gluten-free foods list published by the Coeliac Society is a useful way of illustrating this point.

Dietitians should remind their patients to keep up-to-date with information about their diet and in particular to use *only* current gluten-free manufactured food lists since the ingredients of products do change.

It is also important to stress to patients the need for regular follow-up and for them to see a dietitian when they attend an out-patient or coeliac clinic. Patients who have done well initially often become complacent about their diet and do not take so much trouble over it; gradually they become under par, often without realizing it, and an astute dietitian will pick this up.

4.7.5 Complications

Secondary intolerances

In a few isolated cases, secondary disaccharide intolerance may occur and it is necessary to restrict lactose and sucrose as well as gluten (see Section 2.14.1 and Table 2.25). This is, however, a temporary condition and usually only affects children who are severely wasted. Special dietetic advice is required and milk substitutes will be required for a period of 2–3 months. In certain areas it has become common place to restrict milk as well as gluten in newly diagnosed coeliac children. There is no scientific support for making this a routine procedure and merely makes the dietary regimen more restrictive and more difficult to follow.

Constipation

Some coeliacs regularly complain to their dietitian that they are constipated and care needs to be taken in assessing whether this is really the case. Many coeliacs do become obsessed with their bowels and may think they are constipated when they are not; others feel that because their diet cannot contain wheat bran, their fibre intake is bound to be lower than it should be.

Fibre intake can be increased by either soya bran or rice bran or by an increase in fruit, vegetable and nut intake, together with the consumption of commercial high fibre gluten-free foods (see Section 2.14.1).

Weight problems

It may seem ironic, when one of the main concerns of the coeliac before diagnosis is weight loss and wasting, that after diagnosis and subsequent treatment, excessive weight gain can become an even greater long term problem. After diagnosis coeliacs usually feels so much better on their gluten-free diet that appetite and interest in food returns. Excessive weight gain is therefore not surprising. A weight reducing diet, in line with an ordinary weight reducing diet, should be advised.

Diabetes mellitus

An increase in the incidence of coeliac disease in diabetics and a more frequent occurrence of diabetes in coeliac patients have been reported (Koivisto *et al* 1977). Gluten-free diabetic diets are therefore not uncommon. Gluten-free products have a similar carbohydrate content to ordinary foods and can therefore be substituted easily into a conventional dietary regimen for diabetes.

4.7.6 Special needs of particular groups

The gluten-free diet causes different problems with different age-groups.

Infants

Apart from choosing baby foods which are gluten-free, there is no need for a mother to feed or treat her baby differently from any other baby. Parental attitudes are extremely important, and if the parents accept their child's coeliac condition and gluten-free diet as a way of life, so will the child.

Pre-school children

In this age-group it is generally easier if the whole family eat gluten-free foods; difficulties at meal times are guaranteed if different members of the family have different things on their plate. Other children's parties need not be a problem if the situation is explained to the appropriate mother beforehand and the coeliac child sent to the party with suitable gluten-free food. Food for their own birthday parties should all be gluten-free. Playgroups present few problems since the children are usually only allowed to eat food under supervision so it is not difficult to ensure that the coeliac child is only allowed to eat gluten-free snacks.

Parents should be aware that Play-doh is 40% ordinary flour and that similar home-made substances used by most playgroups contain ordinary flour as the main ingredient. Although flavourings are usually added to give an unpleasant taste, small children do have a tendency to put things in their mouths.

Children

Parents should be reassured that they will be able to cope easily with social occasions such as eating out, parties, holidays, school dinners, and all school activities. Invitations to eat at other children's houses should be accepted. The coeliac child will soon get used to the idea that he takes his own gluten-free bread, for example, with him, and that this, for him, is a normal procedure. When entertaining at home, gluten-free food can be provided for everyone, which helps the child to feel secure.

A child soon learns to eat only those foods which are familiar which means in effect that they are gluten-free. 'If in doubt, leave it out' should be the child's motto. Occasional dietary accidents and indiscretions may occur (as may also happen with adults!) and cause minor symptoms, but these will usually clear up within a few days. Such episodes can act as a useful warning against further dietary deviations.

Teenagers

During adolescence many children may rebel against their parents and coeliacs are no different; it is important to the coeliac teenager to be one of the crowd and to do the same sort of things as his or her friends. Many stray off their diet, eating foods such as fish and chips, pies, hamburgers or pizzas. Those who become ill after doing so are usually wary of future indiscretions, but there is a problem with those teenagers who seem to have a high degree of gluten tolerance and can get away with dietary indiscretions without any obvious symptoms, although damage to the intestinal mucosa will still occur (Kumar *et al* 1979). Parents should be advised to keep their wayward children on the straight and narrow as much as possible, but should be warned not to become obsessional about the diet as this is likely to lead to further behaviour problems. Most teenagers have good appetites and may extremely hungry because of inadequate school lunches; providing extra food from home may help prevent the tendency for their children to fill up with unsuitable foods from nearby shops.

Adults

The motto for adults is to 'be prepared'. They should carry supplies of gluten-free foods in their cars, briefcases and shopping bags.

Some canteens will provide gluten-free meals and most will certainly save or put aside a naturally gluten-free meal for a coeliac *if* they are aware of the person *and* the nature of the diet. In many large companies, food for evening and night shift workers is often left in a cooler to be microwaved by the worker when he takes his meal break. It may be possible for a gluten-free labelled meal to be left for the coeliac; alternatively, the worker concerned may have to provide his own food.

Elderly people

Many elderly patients find it difficult to change the eating habits of a lifetime overnight but others do so very successfully, because they find that retirement gives them more time to experiment with cooking.

Some meals-on-wheels services provide gluten-free diets but others do not, patients will need to make enquiries.

As the coeliac population gets older, more emphasis will need to be given to the provision of gluten-free diets in retirement, nursing and old people's homes. It is a constant worry to many elderly coeliacs that they may have difficulty in obtaining a balanced, acceptable gluten-free diet if or when they become institutionalized.

4.7.7 General problems which may arise

Eating away from home

Although many coeliacs opt for self-catering holidays, there is no reason why holidays in hotels or guest houses should not be successful if a coeliac is prepared to explain the essence of his diet and to be careful in the choice of his food. The Coeliac Society produces lists of holiday hotels and guest houses in Britain where a gluten-free diet can be guaranteed and also publishes information leaflets for most foreign countries. When away on holiday or just travelling, coeliacs should be encouraged to take supplies of bread, biscuits, wafers or crackers so that they always have gluten-free foods available.

Most airlines departing from the UK will agree to supply a gluten-free diet if it is ordered beforehand when the ticket is booked. Stopovers and refuelling stops on long-haul flights can be a problem as different caterers, who may not be familiar with gluten-free diets, will be responsible for re-provisioning the aircraft. Coeliacs should be warned that, theoretically, gluten-free meals may be available but that these are often supplemented with gluten-containing rolls and ordinary crackers by over-enthusiastic cabin staff who consider that a tray looks incomplete without them.

Eating in other people's homes can be hazardous and coeliacs should always tell their hosts of their gluten-free diet requirements when the invitation is offered and not when they arrive on the doorstep. Most buffet food is unlikely to be gluten-free and coeliacs should be warned of this and encouraged to eat something beforehand or take food with them; the effects of drinking alcohol on an empty stomach can be disastrous!

Other people's attitudes

One of the greatest problems experienced by coeliacs is the attitude of friends or relatives who cannot, or will not, understand the need for a strict gluten-free diet. Coeliacs should be encouraged to explain their diet simply and briefly to other people. Friends and relatives are often eager to help the patient comply with the diet when the diagnosis is initially made, especially if the person concerned has been obviously ill; problems tend to arise later when a patient becomes fit and well and many relatives then feel that the diet need not be so strictly complied with. Grandparents can often be the most difficult in this respect – 'surely one biscuit won't hurt' said in front of a grandchild, can make life extremely difficult for parents.

Many coeliacs have found that showing the Coeliac Society's video about the condition to their relatives has been helpful.

Ignorance of medical and nursing personnel

Dietitians should explain to coeliacs that, statistically, they are likely to be the only coeliac patient in the care of their GP, and it is therefore a little unfair to expect their doctor to have complete knowledge of all the gluten-free foods or even all those available on prescription. The same argument applies to hospitals and hospital staff (unless the patient attends a children's hospital or one with a coeliac clinic); the nursing and catering staff may only have a very limited knowledge of the condition and its treatment. If a coeliac knows that he has to go into hospital, it is sensible and helpful if he contacts the hospital dietitian and ward sister in advance and then also takes with him into hospital gluten-free bread and biscuits. Coeliacs should be warned that in specialist units such as orthopaedic or obstetric, they may have to fend for themselves and explain the condition and their diet to all personnel, even the doctors.

Minor ailments

Patients should be warned not to blame all their medical problems on their coeliac condition, as coeliacs are not immune to all other disorders. Mothers tend to attribute all incidences of diarrhoea in their coeliac child to dietary indiscretions whereas it is often just a minor tummy upset which is going around.

Pharmaceutical preparations

A few pharmaceutical preparations including some on prescription do contain gluten. This is not a great problem since wheat or wheat flour is rarely used as an excipient by the pharmaceutical industry. Any pharmaceutical preparation which causes an exacerbation of coeliac symptoms should be checked for possible gluten content. Unfortunately there is confusion in the terminology used, as pharmaceutical manufacturers generally refer to the protein in maize starch (the most commonly used excipient) as maize 'gluten'. This is of course suitable for coeliacs.

It may be difficult to differentiate between symptoms such as diarrhoea related to coeliac disease and diarrhoea as a known side-effect of the medication is question.

Useful addresses

The Coeliac Society

In the UK, the Coeliac Society exists to help those who

have coeliac disease or dermatitis herpetiformis. The Society produces a booklet listing brands of gluten-free manufactured foods which is invaluable for all coeliacs. This comprehensive list is published annually and is up-dated every six months via the Society's magazine. Information is also available on BBC Ceefax (contact the Coeliac Society for more details).

It is in a coeliac's own interest to keep the Food List up-to-date and, to facilitate this, the Society now has a Food List Hot Line. This is a telephone line dedicated to the Food List and used solely for updating it by playing a recorded message of deletions and amendments. The service is available 24 hours a day, every day for the cost of a normal call on 0494 473510.

Deletions, amendments and additions to the Food List are always available from the Coeliac Society Office on receipt of a stamped addressed envelope.

The Coeliac Society also produces a handbook giving information about the condition and its treatment, recipe books, a magazine *The Crossed Grain*, holiday information, a video about coeliac disease and many other services. There are about 50 local groups of the Coeliac Society. The Society's address is: The Coeliac Society, PO Box 220, High Wycombe, Bucks HP11 2HY. Tel 0494 437278.

Further reading

The coeliac handbook The Coeliac Society, High Wycombe.

Rawcliffe P and Rolph R (1985) *The gluten-free diet book.* Martin Dunitz, London.

References

Ascher H, Krantz I and Kristiansson B (1991) Increasing incidence of coeliac disease in Sweden. *Arch Dis Childh* **66**, 608–11.

Crosby WH and Kugler HW (1957) Intraluminal biopsy of the small intestine: intestinal biopsy capsule. *Am J Dig Dis* **2**, 236–41.

Dicke WK (1950) Coeliacki. MD Thesis, University of Utrecht, The Netherlands.

Gee S (1888) On the coeliac affliction. *St Bartholomew's Hospital Reports* **24**, 17.

Greco L, Mayer M, Grimaldi M *et al* (1985) The effect of early feeding on the onset of symptoms in coeliac disease. *J Paed Gastroenterol Nutr* **4**, 52–5.

Holmes GKT (1989) Malignancy in coeliac disease – effects of a gluten-free diet. *Gut* **30**, 333–8.

Koivisto VA, Kuitunen P, Tiilikainen A and Akerblom HK (1977) HLA antigens in patients with juvenile diabetes mellitus, coeliac disease and both of the diseases. *Diabet Metab* **3**, 49.

Kumar P, O'Donoghue D, Stenson K and Dawson A (1979) Re-introduction of gluten in adults and children with treated coeliac disease. *Gut* **20**, 743.

McCrae WM (1969) Inheritance of coeliac disease. *J Med Genet* **6**, 129–31.

Mylotte M, Egan-Mitchell B, McCarthy CF and McNicholl B (1973) Incidence of coeliac disease in the west of Ireland. *Br Med J* **1**, 703–5.

Paulley JW (1954) Observations on the aetiology of idiopathic steatorrhoea. *Br Med J* **2**, 1318–21.

Shiner M (1956) Jejunal biopsy tube. *Lancet* **1**, 85.

Swinson CM and Levi AJ (1980) Is coeliac disease underdiagnosed? *Br Med J* **281**, 1258–60.

4.8 Inflammatory bowel disease (Crohn's Disease and ulcerative colitis)

4.8.1 Inflammatory bowel disease

Inflammatory bowel disease (IBD) includes a wide range of disorders of the intestine. The two main diseases in this category are Crohn's disease (CD) and ulcerative colitis (UC) for which no specific aetiological agent can be identified. These two diseases share many clinical and laboratory features but it remains unclear as to whether they are related or two independent conditions.

Clinical features

Patients with both UC and CD suffer from chronic inflammation of the bowel wall. CD is often associated with granulomas and deep fissuring ulceration and can affect any part of the gastrointestinal tract from the mouth to the anus. Only CD affects the small bowel, usually the terminal ileum, but both CD and UC occur in the colon. The inflammation in CD is often discontinuous with the inflamed areas being separated by normal bowel whereas UC is a disease of the large bowel which predominantly affects the rectum and left colon with continuous inflamed mucosa.

Both diseases are characterized by periods of remission and relapse and can affect any age group although they most frequently occur in young adults. Inflammatory bowel disease occurs more often in North America and Europe than other parts of the world. The incidence of IBD in high incidence countries is about 5–20 per 100 000 population. UC has remained approximately stable in many geographical areas while the incidence of CD continues to rise. The cause of both diseases remains unknown though various possible mechanisms have been suggested including genetic factors, immune mechanisms and bacterial or viral agents.

Sugar and fibre are two dietary components which have been implicated as risk factors in CD. Thornton *et al* (1979) compared the diet of newly diagnosed Crohn's patients with a control group and found they ate nearly twice as much sugar, and less fibre in the form of fruit and vegetables. Two similar studies of patients with UC found no difference in sugar intake between cases and control subjects (Thornton *et al* 1980; Martini *et al* 1980) but this has been disputed by Bianchi *et al* (1985). It is difficult to draw any firm conclusions from this evidence particularly as all studies have used retrospective dietary questionnaires.

Symptoms and diagnosis

Patients usually suffer from abdominal pain and a disturbed bowel habit, particularly diarrhoea. Weight loss and anaemia may be additional features. In patients with CD the presence of blood and mucus in the stools can indicate colonic disease whereas steatorrhoea would suggest small bowel involvement. Additional complications may be present in active disease. These include inflammation in joints, skin lesions such as erythema nodosum, aphthous ulcers in the mouth and iritis. The diseases may be complicated by the development of abscesses, fistulae and strictures.

Although blood tests are not diagnostic they can help to indicate the presence and severity of inflammation. The erythrocyte sedimentation rate (ESR), C-reactive protein, α1-antichymotrypsin and orosomucoid indicate the level of disease activity. A low serum albumin is common. Diagnosis is confirmed by barium studies, endoscopy, radio-labelled leucocyte scintiscans and histology.

Inflammatory bowel disease and pregnancy

IBD usually has no deleterious effect on pregnancy though active disease may reduce fertility. The natural course of the disease is not affected, indeed many patients find pregnancy to have a beneficial effect on their disease. If a relapse does occur this can be treated safely with corticosteroids and sulphasalazine.

Nutritional status of patients with IBD

Nutritional deficiencies are more common in severe Crohn's disease than in ulcerative colitis. During a severe attack patients may suffer from anorexia, fear of eating, and nausea. These factors contribute to the nutritional deficiencies summarized in Table 4.19.

Once inflammation is suppressed by medical therapy, appetite returns, catabolism is diminished and loss of nutrients reduced.

4.8.2 Ulcerative colitis

Management of an acute relapse

The aim of treatment is to induce remission as quickly as possible. Patients with a severe relapse admitted to hospital may be given intravenous fluids with potassium sup-

Table 4.19 Common nutritional deficiencies in patients with IBD

Nutritional deficiencies	Cause	Suggested treatment
Protein-losing enteropathy	Increased nitrogen losses. Catabolic effects of chronic inflammation	Corticosteroid therapy and elemental diet
Inadequate energy intake	Decreased appetite	Whole protein liquid supplements. Glucose polymers
Reduced fat absorption	Resection of 30 cm of distal ileum causing bile salt malabsorption. Small bowel bacterial overgrowth	Cholestyramine Reduced fat diet
Vitamins D and K	Bile salt deficiency	Vitamin supplements
Acquired disaccharidase deficiency	Small bowel disease	Low lactose diet
Iron	Chronic blood loss	Oral iron
Folic acid	Impaired absorption from diseased bowel. Sulphasalazine	Folate supplements
Vitamin B_{12}	Resection of 60 cm ileum. Small bowel bacterial overgrowth	B_{12} injections
K, Na, Zn	Persistent diarrhoea and vomiting	Fluid and electrolytes. Antidiarrhoeal agents
Ca, Mg	Short bowel syndrome. Malabsorption and chronic diarrhoea	Ca, Mg supplements

plements in cases of hypokalaemia. A blood transfusion may be necessary for anaemia. Intravenous hydrocortisone or oral prednisolone may be used as the medical treatment. If symptoms fail to improve surgery may be needed.

Diet in acute relapse

Total parenteral nutrition (TPN) may be used for the patient with UC who is severely malnourished, especially pre-operatively. Enteral feeding may be required if patients have suffered weight loss following an acute attack. Neither TPN nor enteral nutrition in acute UC has been shown to affect the course of the underlying disease (Gassull *et al* 1986). Patients suffering from a mild or moderate attack, or after recovery from a more severe attack have often lost weight and should be given practical dietary advice on increasing the energy and protein content of their diet. Commercial whole protein supplements may be useful during this stage.

Management of patients in remission

Drug therapy

Sulphasalazine (containing 5-amino salicylate) is used for long term maintenance treatment to reduce the frequency of relapses. Side effects, which include skin rashes, anaemia, headaches, nausea, vomiting and loss of appetite, can occur in 10–15% of patients.

Folate deficiency may occur as sulphasalazine inhibits folate absorption. Several new forms of 5-amino salicylate are under review including mesalazine and olsalazine which have fewer side effects.

Corticosteroids which have been used in the acute stage of the disease can usually be tailed off when the disease reaches remission; a maintenance dose of sulphasalazine is continued.

Diet during remission

Patients who are symptom-free should be encouraged to eat a normal diet with adequate amounts of protein, energy, vitamins and minerals. A diet high in fibre can be prescribed without causing relapse and can be beneficial in patients with distal colitis who may relapse if they become constipated. In cases of steroid-induced diabetes mellitus, sources of extrinsic sugars should be restricted but care should be taken not to jeopardize the energy content of the diet.

Milk-free diet

A milk-free diet has only been found to be beneficial in one small clinical trial (Wright and Truelove 1965). This interesting controlled trial found that twice as many patients on a milk-free diet remained well for one year, as those on a normal diet. This work has not been repeated but some patients with UC do have alactasia and a milk-free diet may be prescribed during an acute attack in which case a nutritionally complete milk substitute must be prescribed

(Section 2.14.4). In the long term, patients should be advised to include milk in their diets for nutritional benefit and should only exclude it if alactasia is present.

Elemental diets and food intolerance

Neither elemental diets nor TPN have been found to be effective in UC (Dickinson *et al* 1980; McIntyre *et al* 1986; Munkholm-Larson *et al* 1989). As these treatments exclude normal food completely from the diet, it can be assumed that food intolerance is not a factor in UC. Patients should therefore be discouraged from following a restricted diet which could result in an inadequate nutritional intake.

Essential fatty acids

Essential fatty acids are precursors of prostaglandins which have a major role in inflammatory processes. Eicosopentaenoic acid (EPA) is derived from the n-3 series of fatty acids found naturally in fish oil and inhibits the production of mediators of inflammation derived from arachidonic acid metabolism. A small controlled pilot study (McCall *et al* 1989) found a significant improvement, both histologically and symptomatically, in UC patients given fish oil containing 3–4 g EPA daily for 12 weeks. In a randomized controlled double-blind crossover trial (Lorenz *et al* 1989), disease activity fell in UC patients given fish oil supplements for three months but the results did not reach statistical significance.

Further controlled studies need to be undertaken with n-3 fatty acids before any recommendations can be made.

Surgical treatment

About 5–10% of patients with UC have persistent symptoms which cannot be controlled effectively with drugs, and have a colectomy resulting in an ileostomy. A recently developed alternative to the ileostomy is an ileal-anal anastomosis, or Parks pouch, where a reservoir is made out of the lower small bowel and is then joined to the anus allowing closure of any ileostomy and normal defaecation.

Dietary management following surgery

During the first 2–3 weeks after surgery, the ileostomy excreta may be very watery and of a large volume, between 1200–2000 ml/day (normal effluent volume is about 750 ml/day). Sufficient fluid and salt must be taken to compensate for large losses. It is advisable for the patients to avoid too much fibre until the ileum has adapted or in the case of the ileal-anal anastomosis, two weeks after the ileostomy has been closed (Raymond and Becker 1986). Fibre can then be gradually increased to a level to suit the patient. Once the ileum has adapted, patients should be advised to eat a diet as varied as possible, and to avoid only those foods which consistently upset them.

4.8.3 Crohn's disease

Management of active disease

Drug therapy

Corticosteroids (e.g. oral prednisolone) are widely used for treating active disease. Patients are slowly weaned off high doses over 2–3 months though it is often impossible to withdraw steroids completely. Surgical intervention may be needed if patients do not respond to corticosteroids. Sulphasalazine can be used in cases of colonic Crohn's disease.

In difficult cases, some physicians may choose to use immunosuppressive drugs such as azathiaprine or cyclosporin. These toxic drugs are often ineffective and have many side effects some of which can be serious. The search for alternative effective medical treatment is continuing and dietary treatment remains a primary therapy.

Dietary therapy for active Crohn's disease

Total parenteral nutrition (TPN) This is known to be an effective method of inducing remission in acute Crohn's disease (Reilly *et al* 1976; Driscoll and Rosenberg 1978; Dickinson *et al* 1980). The mechanism is uncertain but could be due to improved nutritional state, removal of dietary antigens, a change in gut flora or simply due to bowel rest. In a prospective randomized controlled trial, Greenberg *et al* (1988) reported that patients taking oral food as well as TPN achieved remission as quickly as those on TPN alone, but the numbers studied in this trial were small. Although TPN is effective in treating active Crohn's disease it is invasive, expensive and requires supervision by a specialized nutrition team to prevent complications such as infection. Patients who have responded to TPN often relapse after returning to normal eating (Ostro *et al* 1984).

Enteral nutrition Remission can be achieved more economically with few complications by elemental diets (ED) (Hunter 1985). These nutritionally complete diets contain protein in the form of amino acids. Comparable remission rates in patients have been achieved with ED as with corticosteroids (O'Morain *et al* 1980, 1984; Saverymutto *et al* 1985).

Growth arrest may occur in children with Crohn's disease and can be reversed with a parenterally or enterally supplemented diet. Elemental diets are effective in promoting growth and allow the withdrawal of corticosteroids which can impair growth (Sanderson *et al* 1987).

Practical details and some of the problems associated with elemental diets are discussed in Section 4.31.6. These diets are unpalatable and all staff involved with the patient should give a great deal of support and encouragement, especially during the first few days when nausea and headaches may occur. Once symptoms start to improve, patients usually find the diet more acceptable. If ED is not tolerated orally it can be fed nasogastrically by continuous feeding over 24 hours.

Elemental diet should be continued until remission is achieved. The time to induce remission varies; the average in one group of patients was nine days (Hunter 1985) but may be as long as four weeks (Teahon *et al* 1990).

Whole protein nasogastric feeds have also been used to treat active disease. Using an oligopeptide feed, 52% of patients achieved remission, however this treatment was not as successful as corticosteroids (Locks *et al* 1988). A randomized controlled trial comparing a polymeric diet to an elemental diet found that ED produced remission in 72% compared to 36% of those taking the polymeric feed (Giaffer *et al* 1990). Other workers have found up to 90% of patients receiving ED succeeded in achieving remission (Kelly *et al* 1989; Teahon *et al* 1990). These results indicate that elemental diets are more successful than whole protein feeds in inducing remission in active Crohn's disease. One preliminary study suggests that feeds containing short chain peptides (Pepdite 2+) may also be effective (Middleton *et al* 1991).

Identification of food intolerances in Crohn's disease

The majority of patients who achieve remission following TPN or ED are often maintained on steroids or may relapse after a relatively short period of time. Some patients with Crohn's disease may have food intolerances. Neither TPN or ED contain any potential food antigens and this could be the reason for their effectiveness. It has been claimed that identification of food intolerances may prolong remission (Alun Jones *et al* 1985).

Food intolerance can only be identified in patients with active disease who respond to an elemental diet. During feeding with elemental diet, all medication for Crohn's disease is tailed off to ensure that remission is related to food withdrawal and to prevent masking any subsequent reaction once food testing begins. Elemental diet should be mixed with distilled or mineral water to eliminate the possibility of tap water intolerance. No other food or drink is allowed during this time. When patients are symptom-free and remission has been confirmed biochemically, foods are reintroduced daily one at a time. Patients need to continue taking some elemental diet during the first few weeks of testing as a nutritional supplement. Foods which are most likely to cause problems are not tested until later and are interspaced with those that are unlikely to precipitate symptoms. The reintroduction order used in Cambridge is shown in Table 4.20 (Hunter 1985). Foods need to be tested in large portions 2–3 times a day to ensure reactions are not missed. After each six foods, patients are advised to continue with these for three further days before testing the next batch. This is to ensure that the tested foods are safe as reactions may develop slowly.

Table 4.20 Order of food reintroduction for patients with Crohn's disease

1	Chicken
2	Pears
3	Rice
4	Carrots
5	White fish
6	Runner beans
7	Beef
8	Peas
9	Turkey
10	Tap water
11	Banana
12	Milk
13	Tomatoes
14	Tea
15	Cauliflower
16	Apple
17	Lamb
18	Lettuce
19	Pork
20	Yeast tablets
21	Potatoes
22	Butter
23	Eggs
24	Coffee beans
25	Leeks
26	Cane sugar
27	White wine
28	Oranges
29	Brussels sprouts
30	Beet sugar
31	Wheat
32	Onion
33	Parsnips
34	Cheddar cheese
35	Mushrooms
36	Corn
37	Spinach
38	Grapefruit
39	Plain chocolate
40	Grapes
41	White bread
42	Courgettes or marrow
43	Soya beans
44	Cabbage
45	Oats
46	Rhubarb
47	Instant coffee
48	Honey
49	Melon
50	Celery
51	Lemon
52	Olive oil
53	Turnip or swede
54	Yoghurt
55	Broccoli
56	Rye bread
57	Monosodium glutamate
58	Prawns or shrimps
59	Saccharin tablets

Patients must keep a detailed diary of all foods eaten and the time at which any symptoms, such as abdominal pain and diarrhoea, occur. Care should be taken when testing cereals, particularly wheat, which may take a week or more to react. If a reaction is provoked, only the foods known to be safe are eaten until symptoms clear. It may be wise to avoid the three previous foods which were reintroduced. If a reaction is severe the patient should be advised to return to ED until better. Foods which cause symptoms must be avoided until tested again at a later date.

The food reintroduction process can be very slow; patients need to be motivated and to have a lot of support from a dietitian for the diet to be successful. The resulting food intolerances vary greatly but those foods most frequently found to provoke symptoms are wheat, dairy products, corn, brassicas, yeast, tomatoes, eggs and citrus fruit (Hunter 1985).

When food intolerances have been identified a dietitian must assess the final diet, recommend relevant supplements and give ideas for substitute foods. If the diet is so restricted as to be unacceptable, it may be necessary for the medical team to prescribe a small dose of corticosteroids so that the diet can be expanded.

Nutritional management of Crohn's disease during remission

Those patients maintained in remission with drug therapy need to follow a diet that is well planned and nutritionally adequate. No benefit can be obtained from avoiding specific foods unless the food intolerance regimen has been strictly followed.

A variety of diets have been claimed to prolong remission. Heaton *et al* (1979) found patients on a high fibre diet had fewer admissions to hospital than a group of matched control patients. A large multi-centre double-blind controlled study, however, did not find any significant difference in remission rates between patients taking a high fibre diet and those on a low fibre diet (Ritchie *et al* 1987). No recommendations can be made therefore about the level of fibre intake required by Crohn's patients, and patients should be advised to find the amount that is suitable for them.

Patients who have small bowel resections may experience fat malabsorption. If a low fat diet is prescribed, care should be taken in replacing the energy in the diet with a more readily absorbable source (e.g. carbohydrate and possibly medium chain triglycerides). Fat-soluble vitamins may need to be given.

Useful address

National Association for Colitis and Crohn's Disease (NACC), 98A London Road, St Albans, Herts AL1 1NX.

References

Alun Jones V, Dickinson RJ, Workman E, Wilson AJ, Freeman AH and Hunter JO (1985) Crohn's disease: maintenance of remission by diet. *Lancet* **2**, 177–80.

Bianchi Porro G and Panza E (1985) Smoking, sugar and inflammatory bowel disease. *Br Med J* **291**, 971.

Dickinson RJ, Ashton MG, Axon AT, Smith RC, Yeung CK and Hill GL (1980) Controlled trial of intravenous hyperalimentation and total bowel rest as an adjunct to the routine therapy of acute colitis. *Gastroenterology* **79**, 1199–204.

Driscoll RH Jr and Rosenberg IH (1978) Total parenteral nutrition in inflammatory bowel disease. *Med Clin North Am* **62**, 185–201.

Gassull MA, Abad A, Cabre E, Gonzalez-Huiz F, Gine JJ and Dolz C (1986) Enteral nutrition in inflammatory bowel disease. *Gut* **27**(Suppl 1), 76–80.

Giaffer MH, North G and Holdsworth CD (1990) Controlled trial of polymeric versus elemental diet in treatment of acute Crohn's disease. *Lancet* **335**, 816–19.

Greenberg GR, Fleming CR, Jeejeebhoy KN, Rosenberg IH, Sales D and Tremaine WJ (1988) Controlled trial of bowel rest and nutritional support in the management of Crohn's disease. *Gut* **29**, 1309–1315.

Heaton KW, Thornton JR and Emmett PM (1979) Treatment of Crohn's disease with an unrefined-carbohydrate, fibre-rich diet. *Brit Med J* **2**, 764–6.

Hunter JO (1985) The dietary management of Crohn's disease. In *Food and the gut*, Hunter JO, Alun Jones V (Eds) Baillière Tindall, Eastbourne.

Kelly SM, Thuluvath P, Fotherby K, Crampton J and Hunter JO (1989) Elemental diet is an effective treatment of acute Crohn's disease. *Scand J Gastroenterol* **24** (S158), 148.

Locks H, Steinhardt HJ, Klaus-Wenz B, Baver P and Malchow H (1988) Enteral nutrition verses drug treatment for the acute phase of Crohn's disease. *Gastroenterology* **94**, A267.

Lorenz R, Weber PC, Szimnau P, Heldwein W, Stasser T and Loeschke K (1989) Supplementation with n-3 fatty acids from fish oils in chronic inflammatory bowel disease – a randomized placebo-controlled, double-blind, cross-over trial. *J International Med* **225**(Suppl 1), 225–32.

McCall TB, O'Leary D, Bloomfield J and O'Morain CA (1989) Therapeutic potential of fish oil in the treatment of ulcerative colitis. *Alimentary Pharmacology Therapeutics* **3**, 415–24.

McIntyre PB, Powell-Tuck J, Wood SR, Lennard-Jones JE, Lerebours E, Hecketsaveiler P, Galmiche JP and Colin R (1986) Controlled trial of bowel rest in the treatment of acute colitis. *Gut* **27**, 481–4.

Martini GA, Stenner A and Brandes WJ (1980) Diet and ulcerative colitis. *Brit Med J* **280**, 1321.

Middleton SJ, Riordan AM and Hunter JO (1991) Peptide based diet as an alternative to elemental diet in the treatment of acute Crohn's disease. Proceedings from BSG, 10–12 April 1991. *Gut* April, T144.

Munkholm Larsen P, Rasmussen D, Ronn B, Munck O, Elmgreen J and Binder V (1989) Elemental diet: A therapeutic approach in chronic inflammatory bowel disease. *J International Med* **225**, 325–31.

O'Morain C, Segal AW and Levi AJ (1980) Elemental diets in the treatment of acute Crohn's disease. *Brit Med J* **281**, 1173–5.

O'Morain C, Segal AW and Levi AJ (1984) Elemental diet as primary therapy of acute Crohn's disease: a controlled trial. *Brit Med J* **288**, 1859–62.

Ostro MJ, Greenberg GR and Jeejeebhoy KN (1984) TPN and complete bowel rest in the management of Crohn's disease. *Gastroenterology* **86**, 1203.

Raymond J and Becker J (1986) Ileoanal pull-through: A new surgical alternative to ileostomy and a new challenge in diet therapy. *J Amer Dietet Assoc* **86**, 663–5.

Reilly J, Ryan JA, Strole W and Fischer JE (1976) Hyperalimentation in inflammatory bowel disease. *Am J Surg* **131**, 192–200.

Ritchie JK, Wadsworth J, Lennard-Jones KE and Rodgers E (1987) Controlled multicentre therapeutic trial of an unrefined carbohydrate, fibre rich diet in Crohn's disease. *Brit Med J* **295**, 517–20.

Sanderson IR, Udeen S, Davies PSW, Savage MO and Walker-Smith JA (1987) Remission induced by an elemental diet in small bowel Crohn's disease. *Arch Dis Childh* **62**, 123–7.

Saverymutto S, Hodgson HJF and Chadwick VS (1985) Controlled trial comparing prednisolone with an elemental diet plus non absorbable antibiotics in active Crohn's disease. *Gut* **26**, 994–8.

Teahon K, Bjarnason I, Pearson M and Levi AJ (1990) Ten years' experience with an elemental diet in the management of Crohn's disease. *Gut* **31**, 1133–7.

Thornton JR, Emmett PM and Heaton KW (1979) Diet and Crohn's disease: characteristics of the pre-illness diet. *Brit Med J* **2**, 762.

Thornton JR, Emmett PM and Heaton KW (1980) Diet and ulcerative colitis. *Brit Med J* **280**, 293.

Workman E, Hunter JO and Alun Jones V (1988) *The Allergy Diet*. Optima, London.

Wright R and Truelove SC (1965) A controlled therapeutic trial of various diets in ulcerative colitis. *Brit Med J* **2**, 138.

4.9 Disorders of the colon

4.9.1 Irritable bowel syndrome

Irritable bowel syndrome (IBS) is a common gastrointestinal condition accounting for between 33–70% of referrals to gastrointestinal clinics in Britain (Drossman *et al* 1977; Harvey *et al* 1983). IBS is characterized by a change in bowel habit which may be either diarrhoea, constipation or an alternation of both these conditions. Abdominal pain or distension may be present and spasm of the bowel may be detected at sigmoidoscopy. The diagnosis of IBS is made by excluding any organic disease after radiological investigations, biochemical tests and mucosal biopsies are shown to be normal.

IBS is not a single entity but has many possible causes including stress, hyperventilation and air swallowing, food intolerance, musculoskeletal problems and hormonal imbalances during the menstrual cycle. This variety of causes has resulted in no single treatment being totally effective. The treatments which have been found to be helpful for IBS patients include antispasmodic drugs, bulking agents, tranquillizers, psychotherapy (Svedlund *et al* 1983), hypnotherapy (Harvey *et al* 1989), evening primrose oil (gamma linolenic acid) in menstrually related IBS (Cotterell *et al* 1990), physiotherapy, diets high and low in fibre and exclusion diets.

Dietary treatment

High fibre diets

Wheat bran has been used to treat IBS for many years. Manning *et al* (1977) showed that the addition of 7 g of wheat bran to the diet of IBS patients for six weeks resulted in a significant improvement of symptoms. This result however has not been confirmed in placebo controlled trials; Lucey *et al* (1987) found equal benefit from both bran and placebo biscuits. In a another study Cann *et al* (1984) found constipation to be the only symptom to show a significant response to bran when compared with placebo. Wheat bran and other non-starch polysaccharides may therefore be of benefit to those patients with constipation but other patients may find bran can exacerbate symptoms of distension, flatulence, diarrhoea and abdominal pain.

Ispaghula, a bulking agent made from viscous polysaccharide, has been shown to be effective in increasing stool weight (Prior and Whorwell 1987), and improve symptoms of constipation. Kumar *et al* (1987) found 20 g of ispaghula/day to be the optimal quantity for improving symptoms.

Some patients with abdominal distension and flatus may benefit from avoiding brassicas, legumes, apples, grapes and raisins (Friedman 1989). If a low fibre diet is effective the gradual addition of both soluble and insoluble fibre should be advised to help the patient find a tolerable level of fibre.

Food intolerance in IBS

There is now considerable evidence that food intolerance is one of the common causes of IBS (Lessof *et al* 1980; Alun Jones *et al* 1982; Hunter *et al* 1985; Nanda *et al* 1989; Riordan *et al* 1990). The use of an exclusion diet has been shown to be effective in treating between 48–67% of IBS patients (Hunter *et al* 1985; Nanda *et al* 1989; Riordan *et al* 1990). The differences in success rates is probably due to patient selection.

In order to detect food intolerances, an exclusion diet is prescribed for two weeks (Table 4.21) (Workman *et al* 1984; see also Section 4.31). The patient is assessed symptomatically at the end of two weeks. If there has been no improvement, patients should be advised to return to a normal diet. If symptoms have cleared, the foods which have been excluded are reintroduced one at a time at two-day intervals in the order shown in Table 4.22. When a food precipitates a recurrence of symptoms, patients are advised to return to the previous safe foods and to resume testing only when they are again symptom free. Patients need to keep a daily symptom diary recording the new food tested and the presence or absence of symptoms. They must be closely supervised by a dietitian during this stage to ensure the diet is followed correctly.

Many foods have been found to cause symptoms of IBS and foods causing symptoms in 20% or more of a study of 122 patients are shown in Table 4.23 (Hunter 1985). The number of foods which affected each patient in this study varied from very few to more than 20. The resulting diets must be assessed nutritionally by a dietitian and relevant supplements advised.

Detection of food intolerances

Immunological abnormalities have not been found in patients with food intolerances (Lessof *et al* 1980; Alun Jones *et al* 1982).

Skin testing or the detection of 1gE serum antibodies

Table 4.21 The Cambridge exclusion diet

	Not allowed	Allowed
Meat	Preserved meats, bacon, sausages	All other meats
Fish	Smoked fish, shellfish	White fish
Vegetables	Potatoes, onions, sweetcorn	All other vegetables
Fruit	Citrus fruit	All other fruit
Cereals	Wheat, barley, oats, corn, rye	Rice, tapioca, millet, buckwheat
Oils	Corn oil, vegetable oil	Sunflower oil, soya oil safflower oil, olive oil
Dairy	Cows' and goat's milk Butter, most margarines, yoghurt, cheese, eggs	Soya milk Milk free margarine
Beverages	Tea, coffee Fruit squashes, orange juice, grapefruit juice Alcohol Tapwater	Herbal teas Apple, pineapple, tomato juice Mineral water
Miscellaneous	Chocolate Yeast, vinegar Preservatives	Carob Salt, herbs, spices Sugar, honey

Table 4.22 Reintroduction order for IBS patients as suggested by Workman *et al* (1984)

1	Tapwater
2	Potatoes
3	Cow milk
4	Yeast
5	Tea
6	Rye
7	Butter
8	Onions
9	Eggs
10	Oats
11	Coffee
12	Chocolate
13	Barley
14	Citrus fruit
15	Corn
16	Cheese
17	White wine
18	Shellfish
19	Yogurt
20	Vinegar
21	Wheat
22	Nuts
23	Preservatives

Table 4.23 Percentage of IBS patients intolerant to particular foods (Hunter 1985)

Food	%
Wheat	60
Corn	44
Milk	44
Cheese	39
Oats	34
Coffee	33
Rye	30
Eggs	26
Butter	25
Tea	25
Citrus	24
Barley	24
Yogurt	24
Chocolate	22
Nuts	22
Onions	22
Potatoes	20
Preservatives	20

cannot therefore be used to identify food intolerances. Various other tests such as vega machine, hair analysis and cytotoxic tests have no scientific justification. Food intolerance has been suggested to be related to a change in faecal flora (Bayliss *et al* 1984) resulting from antibiotics and surgery. Changes in faecal flora have been seen in IBS patients when challenged with symptom-provoking foods (Wyatt *et al* 1988). It remains to be seen whether changes in the faecal flora can indicate the presence of food intolerance.

The only reliable method of detecting food intolerance at present is by use of an exclusion diet under medical and dietetic supervision.

4.9.2 Constipation

Constipation is the delayed transit of faeces which results in them becoming hardened and difficult to pass. The consequent straining can precipitate and exacerbate conditions such as haemorrhoids and anal fissure.

In the past, the excessive and inappropriate use of laxatives to regularize bowel function has frequently been counter-productive and has resulted in an atonic, poorly functioning colon. It is now recognized that dietary measures should be the primary form of treatment and laxatives should be used only as an adjunct to dietary therapy where there are complicating factors.

Dietary treatment

Simple constipation can usually be remedied by
1 Increasing the intake of dietary fibre, of both cereal and vegetable origin (see Section 2.5).
2 Increasing fluid intake, both with and between meals.

Dietary fibre acts by absorbing fluid and thus producing a soft bulky stool; it also encourages beneficial bacterial action in the bowel.

Although it is relatively simple to increase the fibre intake of a motivated adult, it can be difficult in those with conservative eating habits, in particular the very young and the very old. Elderly people, especially those with dentures, may reject fibre-rich foods on the grounds that they are too difficult to chew and leave irritating residues in the mouth. Children who live mainly on white bread, tinned spaghetti and refined rice-based breakfast cereals are unlikely to greet the sudden advent of fresh fruit and vegetables, wholemeal bread and fibre-rich breakfast cereals with much enthusiasm. This is one reason why healthy eating habits should be encouraged from childhood and, in addition, that the whole family should consume such a diet so that the child sees this as the norm.

In both of these groups, changes should be introduced gradually. If wholemeal bread is disliked, a high-fibre white bread may be more acceptable. Cooked and pureed fruit may be preferred to raw fruit. Vegetables can be 'hidden' in casseroles or pies. Wholemeal flours and cereals can be incorporated into home-baked products.

Bulk-forming preparations and laxatives

Bulk-forming preparations

Patients who cannot, or will not, consume sufficient dietary fibre for adequate bowel function may require an additional bulk-forming preparation. Unprocessed wheat bran, taken either in tablet form or added to foods or liquids, is one of the most effective. Ispaghula, sterculia or methylcellulose are suitable alternatives for those who cannot tolerate bran. However, it is vital that sufficient fluid intake accompanies the use of these bulking agents to avoid the risk of faecal impaction or intestinal obstruction. It is also important to remember that bran impairs the absorption of iron, calcium, zinc and other trace elements and prolonged supplementation should be avoided, especially in the elderly.

Laxatives

Faecal softeners (e.g. dioctyl sodium sulphosuccinate) or lubricants (e.g. liquid paraffin) are sometimes useful for the management of haemorrhoids or anal fissure. However, patients should be strongly discouraged from the regular use of liquid paraffin without medical direction as it can cause a number of severe side effects in addition to impairing the absorption of fat soluble vitamins.

Osmotic laxatives These act by maintaining a volume of fluid in the bowel by osmosis, have occasional medical uses but must never be used on a regular basis. Preparations such as magnesium carbonate, magnesium hydroxide and magnesium sulphate (Epsom salts) all have a very rapid purgative action (the latter within 2–4 hours).

A less drastic and more acceptable laxative effect can be achieved with lactulose, a disaccharide which is unabsorbed and hence exerts an osmotic effect. Lactulose results in softer, bulkier motions within 1–2 days and is particularly useful for re-establishing bowel habits in constipated children or in patients following treatment for an impacted bowel. Lactulose is also a useful preparation for the elderly when constipation does not respond to fibre supplementation alone owing to deterioration in bowel muscle function. Lactulose should be administered in gradually decreasing doses over a period of a few days, ideally with a concomitant increase in dietary fibre and fluid intake.

Stimulant laxatives (such as senna, fig, castor oil, bisacodyl or danthron) which act by increasing intestinal motility should not be used routinely, and preferably not at all, without medical direction. Some preparations (e.g. sodium picosulphate) are a useful way of achieving bowel evacuation prior to investigative or surgical procedures (see Section 6.3).

4.9.3 Diverticular disease

Diverticular disease is a common disorder of the large bowel. Early stages of the disease can be identified in 15% of people over the age of 50 years. There is usually a history of constipation which results in increased colonic pressure, straining to pass hard faeces and rupture of the bowel wall to form small pockets – diverticuli. Inflammation and bacterial overgrowth in diverticuli may result in diarrhoea.

Dietary treatment

Patients should benefit from a high fibre diet together with increased fluid intake. The addition of bran or bran products may be particularly beneficial in those patients with constipation.

4.9.4 Colorectal carcinoma

Colorectal carcinoma is a major cause of death in the UK. This common cancer is up to eight times more prevalent in the Western World than in developing countries (Boyle *et al* 1985). The aetiology of this debilitating disease has been linked to a number of dietary factors. For example, it has been suggested that a high intake of non-starch polysaccharides (NSP) may play a protective role against colonic cancer (Drasar and Jenkins 1976). The original hypothesis was that a diet high in NSP added bulk to stools, diluting potential carcinogens and reducing transit time through the colon. However, other workers have suggested that the relationship is much more complex and, whilst NSP may be protective, the apparently simple relationship between NSP intake and colonic carcinoma may result from foods high in NSP containing other substances which are protective against cancer development (Mastromarino *et al* 1976). For example, it has been suggested from animal work by Wattenberg and Loub (1978) that the protective effect of certain vegetables may be attributed to their indole content.

Colonic tumours may be categorized using Duke's classification. Each category has a different prognosis and this in turn will influence the type of nutritional therapy used. Duke's classification of Colonic Carcinoma is as follows:

1 Duke's A: Isolated tumour, no lymph node involvement.
2 Duke's B: Spread of the tumour into the pericolic tissue, no lymph node involvement.
3 Duke's C: Lymph node involvement.
4 Duke's D: Presence of distant metastases.

Treatment of this disease is by surgical removal of the tumour.

Dietary treatment

Due to the presence of the tumour combined with a reduced dietary intake, many patients present with some degree of protein energy undernutrition. If possible, patients should receive appropriate nutritional support during the pre-operative period and this may be parenteral and/or enteral nutrition (see Sections 1.13 and 1.15). However, the time available for nutritional repletion is influenced by the need to excise the tumour as well as the patient's general condition. Nutritional support should be prescribed according to requirements and regular biochemical and anthropometric assessments undertaken.

Useful address

IBS Network, GUT Reaction Newsletter, Susan Backhouse, c/o Voluntary Action Sheffield, General Office, 69 Division Street, Sheffield S1 4GE.

References

Alun Jones V, McLaughlan P, Shorthouse M, Workman E and Hunter JO (1982) Food intolerance: a major factor in the pathogenesis of irritable bowel syndrome. *Lancet* **2**, 1115–17.

Bayliss CE, Houston AP, Alun Jones V, Hishon S and Hunter JO (1984) Microbiological studies on food intolerance. *Proc Nutr Soc* **43**, 16a.

Boyle P, Zaridze DG and Smas M (1985) Descriptive epidemiology of colorectal cancer. *Int J Cancer* **36**, 9–26.

Cann PA, Read NW and Holdsworth CD (1984) What is the benefit of coarse wheat bran in patients with irritable bowel syndrome? *Gut* **24**, 168–173.

Cotterell JC, Lee AJ and Hunter JO (1990) Double-blind cross-over trial of evening primrose oil in women with menstrually-related irritable bowel syndrome. *Omega-6-Essential Fatt Acids: Pathophysiology and Roles in Clinical Medicine* pp. 421–6. AR Liss Inc, New York.

Drasar BS and Jenkins DJA (1986) Bacteria, diet and large bowel cancer. *AJCN* **29**, 1410–16.

Drossman DA, Powell DW and Sessions JT (1977) The irritable bowel syndrome. *Gastroenterology* **73**, 811–22.

Friedman G (1989) Nutritional therapy of irritable bowel syndrome. *Gastr Clinics N America* **18**, 513–24.

Harvey RF, Hinton RA, Gunary RM, Barry RE (1989) Individual and group therapy in the treatment of refactory irritable bowel syndrome. *Lancet* **1**, 424–5.

Harvey RF, Salih SY and Read EA (1983) Organic and functional disorders in 2000 gastroenterology outpatients. *Lancet* **1**, 632–4.

Hunter JO, Workman E and Alun Jones V (1985) The role of diet in the management of irritable bowel syndrome. *Topics of Gastroenterology* **12** Gibson PR and Jewell DP (Eds) Blackwell Scientific Publications, Oxford.

Hunter JO (1985) The dietary management of Crohn's disease. In *Food and the gut*. Hunter JO, Alun Jones V (Eds) Baillière Tindall, Eastbourne.

Kumar A, Kumar N, Vij JC, Sarin SK and Anand BS (1987) Optimum dosage of ispaghula husk in patients with irritable bowel syndrome — correlation of symptom relief with whole gut transit time and stool weight. *Gut* **28**, 150–55.

Lessof MH, Wraight DG, Merrett TG, Merrett J and Buisseret PD (1980) Food allergy and intolerance in 100 patients. *Quart J Med* **195**, 259–71.

Lucey MR, Clark ML, Lowndes JO and Dawson AM (1987) Is bran efficacious in irritable bowel syndrome. A double-blind, cross-over study. *Gut* **28**, 221–5.

Manning AP, Heaton KW, Uglow P and Harvey RF (1977) Wheat fibre and the irritable bowel syndrome: A controlled trial. *Lancet* **2**, 417–18.

Mastromarino A, Reddy BS and Wynder EL (1976) Metabolic epidemiology of colon cancer: enzyme activity of fecal flora. *AJCN* **29**, 1455–60.

Nanda R, James R, Smith H, Dudley CRK and Jewell DP (1989) Food intolerance and the irritable bowel syndrome. *Gut* **30**, 1099–104.

Prior A and Whorwell PJ (1987) Double-blind study of ispaghula in the irritable bowel syndrome. *Gut* **28**, 1510–13.

Riordan AM, Cotterell JC, Pickersgill CS, Workman E and Hunter JO (1990) Evaluating an exclusion diet in the treatment of patients with irritable bowel syndrome. *J Hum Nutr Dietet* **13**, 362–3.

Svedlund J, Sjodin I, Ottosson JO and Dotevall G (1983) Controlled study of psychotherapy in irritable bowel syndrome. *Lancet* **2**, 589–91.

Wattenberg LW and Loub WD (1978) Inhibition of polycytic aromatic hydrocarbon-induced neoplasia by naturally occurring indoles. *Cancer Res* **38**, 1410–13.

Workman E, Alun Jones V, Wilson AJ and Hunter JO (1984) Diet in the management of Crohn's disease. *Hum Nutr: Appl Nutr* **38A**, 469.

Workman E, Hunter JO and Alun Jones V (1988) *The allergy diet*. Optima, London.

Wyatt GM, Bayliss CE, Lakey AF, Bradley HK, Hunter JO and Alun Jones V (1988) The faecal flora of two patients with food related irritable bowel syndrome drawing challenge with symptom provoking foods. *J Med Microbiol* **26**, 295–9.

4.10 Intestinal surgery and resection

Elective or emergency surgical procedures are frequently embarked upon in patients with inflammatory or neoplastic bowel disorders. The bowel is an important metabolic organ and it is therefore not surprising that patients present with some degree of protein energy malnutrition. Consequently, the dietitian plays a key role in their nutritional care.

4.10.1 Intestinal resection

During intestinal resection, the diseased segment of bowel is resected and an anastomosis formed using the two unaffected ends of bowel. Following resection of the small bowel, intestinal adaptation and hypertrophy of the intestinal brush border occurs. In patients with more than 100 cm of small bowel remaining, a normal diet should be well tolerated. However, in cases where less than 100 cm of small bowel remain the absorptive function of the bowel is significantly reduced and patients develop short bowel syndrome.

Short bowel syndrome

In the early post-operative period, patients will require TPN (see Section 1.15). However, enteral nutrition should be introduced as soon as possible, either orally or naso-gastrically using an elemental or whole protein feed (see Section 1.13). During this stage attention should be paid to the patient's fluid and electrolyte requirements. Most elemental feeds contain low concentrations of sodium, and intestinal absorption of fluid and electrolytes has been shown to improve if at least 70 mmol of sodium/1 are administered (Spiller *et al* 1982). Enteral feeding should be gradually replaced by a light, low residue diet. Once a significant oral diet has been introduced, energy and protein intake may be increased by the use of dietary supplements (see Section 1.13.3 and Appendix 6). The enzyme lactase may be depressed with short bowel syndrome and lactose loads should therefore be avoided.

Fat malabsorption may aggravate diarrhoea and increase malabsorption of fat soluble vitamins and minerals such as calcium. If a low fat diet is advised, the energy deficit should be corrected by the use of supplementary carbohydrates and possibly MCT (see Chapter 1.13 and Appendix 6).

Persistent diarrhoea can result in fluid and electrolyte deficiencies and an adequate intake should be ensured to restore fluid and electrolyte balance. Patients with a permanent ileostomy in whom the absorptive capacity of the colon is bypassed will also have increased requirements for fluid and electrolytes.

Iron, folate supplements and vitamin B_{12} injections may be required to prevent anaemia, and bile salt malabsorption should be controlled by the use of cholestyramine.

Close dietetic supervision of these patients is important, particularly during the early stages until intestinal adaptation has taken place and the patient is able to take a nutritionally adequate diet.

4.10.2 Colostomy and ileostomy

Following intestinal resection, a colostomy or ileostomy may be performed. The gut is brought out to the surface of the abdomen and a prominent stoma fashioned.

A variety of stoma bags are manufactured and a stoma therapist should be available to advise the best type of appliance for each patient. The bag is fitted over the stoma and the intestinal effluent collected in it and discarded regularly. If the rectum is left *in situ*, a mucus fistula will be formed on the surface of the abdomen to allow drainage.

Dietary treatment

Patients should follow as normal a diet as possible but individuals may find certain foods cause the stool consistency and odour to be unacceptable and these foods should be avoided. Foods which pass through unaltered need not be avoided unless they cause embarrassment to the patient by suddenly filling the bag and causing it to leak. Patients may also prefer to avoid foods which tend to cause flatulence (e.g. onions, lentils, beans and sprouts), but a moderately high fibre intake should be encouraged in order to ensure efficient functioning of the stoma.

Patients with ileostomies may initially lose both electrolytes and fluid and require an increased intake of these for at least 6–8 weeks after which time the ileum appears to adapt and losses decrease. Diarrhoea may exacerbate the electrolyte imbalance and extra potassium (via fruit juices) and sodium (via extra salt on food or salty beverages such as soup or Bovril) should be consumed. Alternatively, supplementary electrolytes can be given.

Useful address

Ileostomy Association of Great Britain and Ireland, Amblehurst House, Chobham, Woking, Surrey GU24 8PZ.

Reference

Spiller RC, Jones BJM and Silk DBA (1982) Influence of sodium content of enteric diets on water absorption from the human jejunum. *JPEN* **6**, 342.

4.11 Liver and biliary disease

Dietary therapy plays a major role in the clinical management of patients with liver and biliary disease. The dietitian is an integral member of the medical team providing nutritional expertise.

Objectives of nutritional support are to administer nutrients in the correct quantity and form, to treat the clinical symptoms, correct specific deficiencies, promote hepatocyte regeneration and restore and maintain nutritional status.

Although there have been many recent advances in the medical aspects of liver disease, little attention has been given to nutritional management. It is clear that nutritional support is beneficial for patients with acute liver disease but whether good nutrition significantly alters the course of chronic liver disease and subsequent mortality is still unclear (Mendenhall *et al* 1985). Nutritional deficiencies commonly arise in patients with chronic hepatobiliary disease which may adversely affect hepatic function, perpetuate liver injury and ultimately affect prognosis. Factors limiting nutritional support are given in Table 4.24.

Nutritional management is based entirely on the patient's clinical condition irrespective of the underlying liver disease. Specific dietary modifications are necessary to treat the complications of liver disease (e.g. ascites, steatorrhoea and encephalopathy) and to alleviate symptoms creating a better sense of well-being. The physical signs of liver disease are illustrated in Fig. 4.9.

Although opinions on the optimal type of diet and the most effective method of delivery may vary between liver units, there is a general consensus on management. In all instances diets must be tailored to suit each patient and often in practice a compromise has to be made between enforcing formal dietary restrictions and maintaining an adequate nutrient intake. Each patient must be individually assessed and nutritional therapy regularly monitored and evaluated.

4.11.1 Anatomy and function of the liver

The liver is the largest organ in the body and comprises one fiftieth of the total body weight. The liver has a double blood supply – the portal vein brings venous blood from the intestines and the spleen, and the hepatic artery supplies the liver with arterial blood.

The liver cells (hepatocytes) comprise about 60% of the total liver weight. Bile canaliculi form a network between the hepatocytes which eventually form the common hepatic duct. This connects to the gall bladder via the cystic duct. The gall bladder stores and concentrates hepatic bile (Fig. 4.10 and 4.11).

Table 4.24 Factors limiting nutritional support in patients with liver disease

Ascites, oedema
Steatorrhoea, diarrhoea
Vomiting, nausea
Active bleeding
Unpalatable diets and treatment
Encephalopathy
Alcohol withdrawal
Repeated investigation
Altered taste sensation

The liver plays a central role in metabolism and nutrition (Table 4.25). Irrespective of its aetiology, liver dysfunction will give rise to a variety of nutrient imbalances which may result in several clinical manifestations. The degree of disturbance is related to the severity of the liver disease, its activity and aetiology.

4.11.2 Classification of liver disease

Liver disease may be divided simply into either acute or chronic. An acute episode may also be superimposed on to pre-existing chronic disease.

Acute liver disease

This may be caused by viruses or toxins (including alcohol and drugs (Table 4.26). Development of severe hepatic dysfunction occurs within six months of the first symptoms and in the absence of any pre-existing liver disease. When these features develop very quickly (within eight weeks of the first symptoms), the condition known as fulminant hepatic failure (FHF) occurs. This condition is rare but carries a high mortality rate; a patient who survives FHF will usually go on to make a full recovery (Katelaris and Jones 1989). These patients often require intensive nutritional support.

Chronic liver disease

This may be caused by a variety of agents (Table 4.27) in particular drugs such as alcohol, infections such as acute hepatitis, and autoimmune diseases such as primary biliary cirrhosis and chronic active hepatitis.

Chronic liver disease will give rise to cirrhosis which

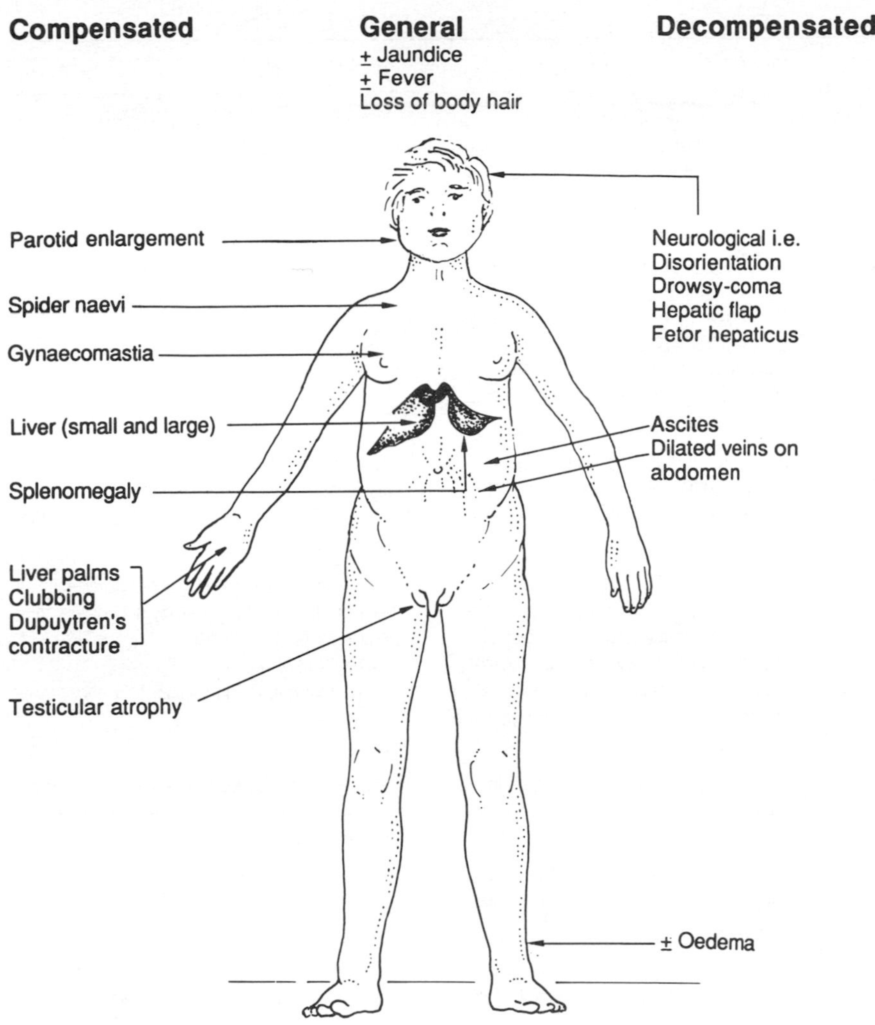

Fig. 4.9 The physical signs of liver disease

reflects the pathological state of the liver, characterized by fibrosis, nodular regeneration and disturbance of normal hepatic architecture. The severity of the cirrhosis can be described by the use of Child's classification (Child and Turcott 1964).

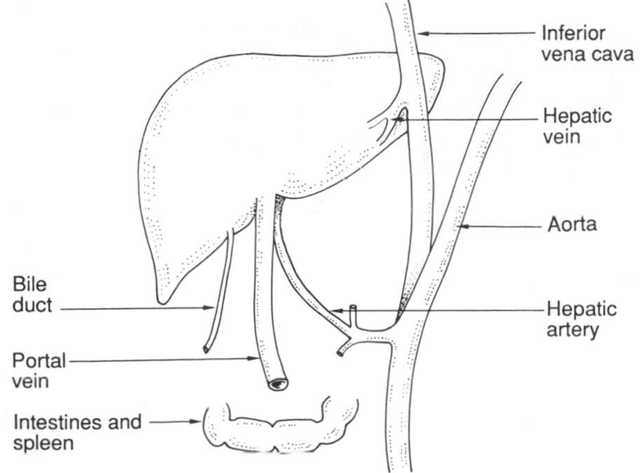

Fig. 4.10 The liver anatomy

Cirrhosis does not always cause symptoms, in which case it is said to be 'well compensated' i.e. although the liver is damaged, it is still able to function normally.

When cirrhosis forces the liver to become 'decompensated', blood flow to and from the liver is impaired and portal hypertension develops. This may give rise to a variety of clinical entities (Table 4.28) including ascites,

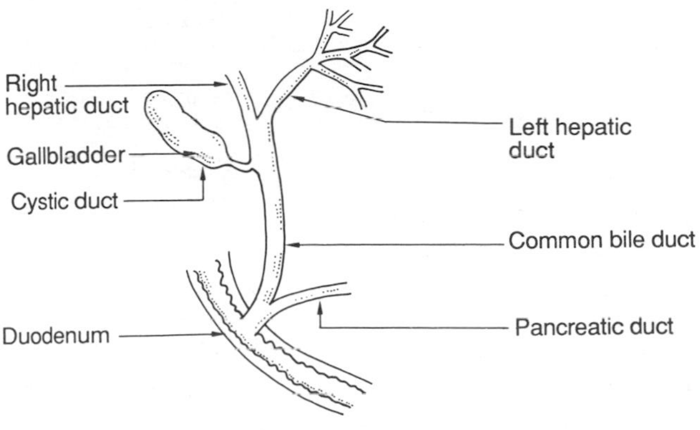

Fig. 4.11 The biliary tree

Table 4.25 Major functions of the liver

Function	Role of the liver	Effect of damage
1 Carbohydrate	Maintaining glucose homeostasis. Stores glycogen and mobilizes glucose in response to hypoglycaemia	In fulminant hepatic failure hypoglycaemia is common. In chronic liver disease fasting hyperglycaemia and glucose intolerance occur
2 Protein	(a) Utilizes amino acids for protein synthesis and glyco-neogenesis. (b) Deaminates amino acids into urea for excretion (c) Regulates supply of amino acids to peripheral tissues for e.g. muscles Major site of synthesis of plasma albumin, prothrombin, fibrinogen and clotting factors V, VII, IX, X, XII	Reduced synthesis of plasma proteins (e.g. albumin and prothrombin) causes hypoalbuminaemia and prolonged clotting time (INR)
3 Lipid fat	Production of triglycerides and lipoprotein formation. Phospholipid and cholesterol synthesized. NEFA synthesis and degradation. Ketogenesis	Reduced flow of bile salts leads to fat malabsorption (steatorrhoea)
4 Vitamins	Stores A, B, K, B_{12}, folate Vitamin K required by hepatic cells for the production of prothrombin and Factor VII The liver contains enzymes which convert tryptophan to nicotinic acid. The methylation of methonic acid and the 25-hydroxylation of Vitamin D occurs in the liver	Absorption of vitamins A&D are impaired but, owing to liver stores, deficiency only occurs in long standing cholelithiasis Clotting time is prolonged Possible vitamin D and calcium deficiency
5 Detoxification of drugs	Responsible for deactivation of drugs in cytochrome p450 system	Drug effects are potentiated — liver patient will require minimal drug therapy and close drug level monitoring
6 Inactivation of hormones	Oestrogens, corticosteroids, and other steroid hormones are conjugated in the liver and excreted in the urine	Care with steroid dosage
7 Biliary excretion	Production of bile (a mixture of inorganic salts, bilirubin, bile acids, cholesterol and alkaline phosphatase)	Elevated bilirubin levels result in jaundice and fat malabsorption will cause steatorrhoea

Table 4.26 Some causes of acute liver disease

Viral infections	Virus A, B, C – (the latter previously known as non A-non B) Epstein Barr virus Cytomegalovirus Yellow fever virus
Non-viral infections	Toxoplasmosis *Leptospira* *Coxiella burnetti*
Drugs	Paracetamol Halothane
Alcohol	
Poisons	e.g. Amanita phalloides Aflatoxin Carbon tetrachloride
Other	Complications of pregnancy e.g. 'acute fatty liver of pregnancy'

jaundice and encephalopathy and these provide the focal point for dietary therapy.

4.11.3 Investigation of liver disease

Investigative tests can be divided into:

1 Tests to assess liver function.
2 Imaging techniques to examine hepatobiliary anatomy.
3 Liver biopsy for histological examination.

Liver function tests

These are markers of liver disease and are not actual tests of function *per se*. These tests are usually abnormal in hepatobiliary disease and, while recognized patterns of test abnormalities occur in some diseases, considerable overlap occurs. They are useful to the dietitian in monitoring clinical progress but have no direct relevance *per se* to any dietary prescription. Reference ranges are given in Table 4.29.

Table 4.27 Aetiology of chronic liver disease

Drugs and toxins	Alcohol Methotrexate Methyldopa Isoniazid Prednisolone
Infections	Hepatitis B, C, D *Schistosoma japonicum*
Autoimmune diseases	Chronic active hepatitis Primary biliary cirrhosis
Metabolic disorders	Wilson's disease Haemochromatosis Alpha-1-antitrypsin deficiency Carbohydrates (galactosaemia; Type IV glycogen storage disease) Amino acids (tyrosinosis) Urea cycle (ornithine transcarbamylase deficiency) Lipids (abetalipoproteinaemia) Porphyria
Biliary obstruction	Atresia Mucoviscidosis Gallstones Strictures Sclerosing cholangitis
Vascular disorders	Chronic right heart failure Budd-Chiari syndrome Veno-occlusive disease Hereditary telangiectasia
Miscellaneous	Neonatal hepatitis syndrome Indian childhood cirrhosis Intestinal bypass Sarcoidosis Cystic fibrosis Carolis syndrome
Cryptogenic	Unknown aetiology

Imaging techniques

The main aim of these is to delineate the anatomy and to look for any abnormality in the liver and biliary tree. They include plain X-ray ultrasonography, computerized tomography (CT) cholecystogram endoscopy and endoscopic retrograde cholangiopancreatography (ERCP).

Liver biopsy

This is the only means by which a diagnosis can be confirmed. A biopsy needle is inserted into the liver and a small sample of liver tissue can be removed and examined microscopically.

4.11.4 Nutritional assessment of patients with liver disease

It is advisable to assess nutritional status before initiating nutritional support so that there is a rational basis for dietary advice. Continuing evaluation is also necessary to monitor the effects of dietary intervention and ensure that deficiencies do not arise as a result of inadequate or ill-conceived dietary advice (Blackburn *et al* 1977).

Nutritional status may best be assessed by combining the results of clinical examination, anthropometric measurements and some biochemical tests. However, nutritional status is extremely difficult to determine in these patients as liver disease may severely affect the validity and interpretation of the standard tests. A combination of clinical, nutritional, anthropometric and biochemical assessments will be required therefore.

Clinical observation will determine the degree of muscle wasting and loss of subcutaneous fat, and the presence of ascites, oedema and jaundice.

A dietary history should be obtained although in alcoholic liver disease this may be difficult to obtain, especially the amount of alcohol ingested. Relatives may be able to provide some clarification (Watson *et al* 1984). Nevertheless even a rough guide will facilitate and confirm identification of possible nutrient deficiencies and serve as useful guide for meal planning. It should be borne in mind that patients with liver disease are likely to have increased nutritional requirements.

Anthropometric measurements may be useful in assessing long term changes in individual patients, but comparison with standard values should be avoided. Mid-arm muscle

Table 4.28 Effects of cirrhosis

Portal hypertension and gastrointestinal haemorrhage (oesophageal/gastric varices)
Ascites oedema
Portosystemic encephalopathy
Renal failure
Hepatoma (primary liver cell carcinoma)
Jaundice

Table 4.29 Reference ranges for the main liver function tests (NB these ranges vary between hospitals)

Test	Normal range
Bilirubin	5–17 μmol/l
Alkaline phosphatase	100 iu/l
Aspartate aminotransferase	40 iu/l
Alanine aminotransferase	40 iu/l
Prothrombin time	12–16 seconds
International Normalized ratio (INR)	1.0–1.2
Albumin	30–52 g/l
Total protein	60–80 g/l
Gamma glutamyl transpeptidase (Gamma GT)	10–48 iu/l

Table 4.30 Guide for assessing fluid weight

Guide for assessing weight of ascites		Guide for assessing weight of peripheral oedema	
Minimal	−2.2 kg	Mild	−1.0 kg
Moderate	−6.0 kg	Moderate	−5.0 kg
Severe	−14.0 kg	Severe	−10.0 kg

Source: James (1989)

circumference and mid-arm muscle mass are difficult to interpret as fluid shifts and changes in hydration status often occur. Body weight must be interpreted with care as oedema and ascites may mask true body weight. A guide for assessing fluid weight is given in Table 4.30. Loss of intravascular fluid with a concurrent decrease in lean body mass may cause further problems.

Biochemical values need to be interpreted with caution. Malnutrition, and also the presence of hepato-renal syndrome (renal failure with severe oliguria due to hypovolaemia, hyponatraemia and changes in acid base balance), will affect creatinine excretion. Furthermore an accurate 24-hour urine collection may be difficult to obtain.

The hepatic transport proteins (albumin, transferrin, thyroxine binding prealbumin, and retinol binding protein) are manufactured in the liver. In liver disease their validity as nutrition parameters is questionable. Only 25% of hepatocytes need to be functioning to maintain normal albumin production; serum albumin levels appear therefore to correlate better with the degree of liver damage than with nutritional status (Merli *et al* 1987).

The presence of hepato-renal failure and a compromised urinary output may affect the validity of nitrogen balance.

Biochemical assessment of trace element and vitamin status is difficult and often may not be routinely available.

The use of any one of these nutritional parameters in isolation to determine nutritional status is useless and as many as possible should be used.

4.11.5 Dietary management of specific aspects of liver disease

Malnutrition

The majority of patients with chronic liver disease requiring hospitalization are severely to moderately malnourished, especially those with an alcohol-related aetiology. Not only is protein-energy malnutrition present but deficiencies of minerals, electrolytes and trace elements are also seen. The severity of malnutrition may be related to the degree, length and clinical manifestations of the liver disease.

Factors contributing to deficiency are summarized in Table 4.24 at the beginning of this section and include an inadequate dietary intake, malabsorption and maldigestion superimposed on a hypercatabolic state. Hospitalization may initially perpetuate nutrient deficiency because of repeated investigations, active bleeding or sedation for alcoholic withdrawal. Imposition of severely restrictive and unpalatable diets may reduce nutrient intake.

Dietary management

Basal energy requirements should be calculated with appropriate adjustment for fluid retention. A stress factor of 1.5 together with the appropriate activity factor are required to promote weight gain, spare protein and meet increased metabolism. Dietary fat should be given as tolerated with the inclusion of medium chain triglycerides (MCTs) wherever needed. Sufficient protein should be provided for hepatic regeneration while at the same time, avoiding the development of encephalopathy (see the subsection below on Portalsystemic encephalopathy).

Ascites

Ascites is the presence of a protein-rich fluid in the peritoneal cavity and is a common feature of liver disease. The actual mechanism of production of ascites is unclear but it probably results from a combination of the effects of liver failure and portal hypertension. Plasma aldosterone is increased and this initiates sodium and water retention. This results in an expanded extracellular fluid which overflows into the peritoneal cavity due to increased portal pressure, reduced plasma oncotic pressure (low albumin) and impaired lymph drainage. Oedema usually occurs and, in about 6% patients, a pleural effusion as well.

Ascites may develop slowly over the course of several months or suddenly due to decompensation of liver function, for example as a result of a variceal bleed, infection, alcohol binge or diuretic imbalance. Unless ascites is slight, hospital admission is usually necessary for diagnosis and treatment.

Malnutrition is common in ascitic patients as they are often anorexic due to the physical discomfort of a distended abdomen. Conventional treatment consists of diet therapy, bed rest and diuretics.

Sodium restriction

Restriction of dietary sodium is essential in the treatment of ascites. While this may not be effective alone, sodium restriction will enhance and hasten the effects of diuretics. The degree to which sodium should be restricted is variable and ranges from 22 mmol sodium/day to a No Added Salt regimen (60−80 mmol sodium/day). Examples of sodium restricting diets are given in Table 4.31 (see also Section 2.7.1). Very low sodium diets (22 mmol) are often unpalatable, and difficult to follow unless under hospital supervision. However one advantage may be that, as the patient has become accustomed to a very low intake in

Table 4.31 Salt restricted diets

1 No added salt	This restricts sodium intake to between 60–80 mmol per day. A pinch of salt may be used in cooking, but none must be added to food at the table. The following foods should be avoided: Bacon, ham, sausages, pâté Tinned fish and meat Smoked fish and meat Fish and meat pastes Tinned and packet soups Sauce mixes Tinned vegetables Bottled sauces and chutneys Meat and vegetable extracts, stock cubes Salted nuts and crisps Soya sauce Monosodium glutamate Some breakfast cereals, biscuits and cakes Cheese – up to 4oz per week Bread – up to 4 slices per day
2 40 mmol sodium diet	In addition to the foods listed above under No Added Salt, the following restrictions apply: No salt to be used in cooking or at table Salt-free butter or margarine must be used Milk should be restricted to 300 ml daily Only 4 slices of bread permitted per day – extra must be salt-free Breakfast cereals must be free from added salt
3 22 mmol sodium diet	As above but replace ordinary bread with salt-free bread

hospital, he or she may more readily follow a No Added Salt diet at home. A lower sodium intake will also resolve the ascites more quickly which in turn will help to improve appetite more rapidly (Gauthier *et al* 1986). In practice, a 40 mmol sodium diet is more acceptable and more easily managed, together with a fluid restriction of 1–1.5 litres daily. Choice and quantity of food and drink still needs to be carefully controlled and usually necessitates provision of meals from a special diet kitchen.

The rationale of this diet therapy needs to be clearly explained to the patient, nursing staff and relatives to ensure compliance. Regular patient contact and monitoring of food intake via food record charts are useful ways of assessing the adequacy of energy and protein intakes. Appropriate supplementation with proprietary products such as Fortical or Polycal (Cow and Gate Nutricia) and Caloreen (Clintec) may be necessary. Once the ascites has been reasonably controlled (often not to complete dryness) sodium intake can be increased to the level of a No Added Salt regimen (60–80 mmol/day). This should be reviewed before discharge, taking account of the patient's social situation and cooking facilities. Care should also be taken that no medications containing sodium (e.g. antacids) are used.

Salt substitutes consisting of potassium compounds, for example Ruthmol (Cantassium), can add flavour and improve palatability of a salt-restricted diet. Careful monitoring of potassium levels is required and their use is contraindicated in hyperkalaemic patients with electrolyte imbalance following diuretic therapy and also in hepatorenal syndrome. All patients should be advised to avoid 'Lo Salt' and preparations still containing an appreciable amount of sodium, as well as those containing ammonium salts.

Diuretics

The aim of diuretic therapy is to block sodium conserving mechanisms within the kidney. Distal diuretics such as spironolactone or amiloride are used initially but some patients with resistant ascites require a powerful loop diuretic such as frusemide. It is vital to monitor weight carefully during the diuretic phase so that weight loss does not exceed more than one kilogram per day. Rapid ascitic loss may precipitate complications such as hepatorenal syndrome, encephalopathy and electrolyte disturbance. Dietetic expertise is required to distinguish between fluid and flesh weight loss.

Hyponatraemia can occur in patients on very low sodium intakes. Intravenous salt-poor albumin (several units daily) may be effective temporarily in relieving hyponatraemia by increasing the intravascular volume. Dietary sodium should not be increased or saline infused as this will result in fluid retention and pulmonary oedema.

Fluid restriction

Fluid intake may be restricted to 1–1.5 litres per day depending on the degree of ascites and response to treatment. This may severely limit nutritional support and patients need to be given high energy, low sodium fluids. Mineral waters and low-calorie drinks may not only contain large amounts of sodium but are also devoid of calories. Accurate recording of fluid balance is vital to avoid patients abusing restrictions.

Intravenous infusions, e.g. to administer antibiotics, may also make a significant contribution to the daily fluid intake and further constrain the amount which can be taken orally. Regular review is necessary to ensure that nutritional intake is maximized.

With resolution of ascites, fluid restrictions may be relaxed on discharge.

Bed-rest

Unless ascites is only mild, bed-rest is required to increase renal perfusion and potentiate a diuresis.

Paracentesis

Therapeutic paracentesis and drainage is being used increasingly in the treatment of tense or gross ascites. Combined with a moderate sodium restriction (50–

60 mmol/day) and appropriate albumin replacement (because paracentesis fluid is rich in protein), this is quicker and more effective in reducing ascites than conventional therapy (Gines *et al* 1987). A sodium restriction at this level and diuretic therapy are usually necessary to prevent sodium accumulation. The risk of electrolyte imbalance, renal impairment and encephalopathy are common to both paracentesis and diuretic therapies, though the latter is still preferred for patients most at risk of complications (Franco *et al* 1983).

Ultrafiltration and re-infusion

In this procedure, ascitic fluid is removed via a peritoneal dialysis catheter, filtered and returned intravenously to the patient.

A Leveen shunt where a long tube is used to connect the peritoneal cavity with the jugular vein may sometimes be given to patients with refractory ascites. Inspiration sucks the ascitic fluid from the peritoneum and into the superior vena cava. There are many complications with this technique, notably disseminated intravascular coagulation and infection. Sodium and fluid restrictions are also still required.

Portalsystemic encephalopathy (PSE)

There is no agreed consensus about either the pathogenesis or the treatment of hepatic encephalopathy.

The term PSE refers to a chronic neuropsychiatric syndrome secondary to liver cirrhosis. A similar acute encephalopathy can also occur in acute fulminant hepatic failure. Encephalopathy is potentially reversible although a small number of patients remain chronically encephalopathic. The factors which precipitate PSE are shown in Table 4.32.

The mechanism is unknown but several factors are known to play a part. In cirrhosis, blood bypasses the liver via the collaterals, and the toxic metabolites pass into the systemic circulation and then reach the brain to precipitate encephalopathy. Many toxic substances have been suggested as the causative factor including fatty acids, mercaptans, false neurotransmitters and especially ammonia. Increased blood levels of aromatic amino acids (tyrosine and phenylalanine) with a corresponding reduction in levels of branched chain amino acids (valine, leucine and isoleucine) also contribute.

Plasma ammonia levels are frequently raised in encephalopathic patients due to ammonia production by bacteria in the gut and the liver failing to convert sufficient ammonia into urea. Ammonia may alter the blood-brain barrier and allow toxins to interfere with cerebral metabolism.

Table 4.32 Factors precipitating portalsystemic encephalopathy (PSE)

High dietary protein/protein overload
Gastrointestinal/variceal haemorrhage
Constipation
Infection
Diuretic therapy
Drugs e.g. sedatives
Paracentesis (large amounts)
Hypokalaemia
Portocaval shunt operations
Surgery
Diarrhoea/vomiting

Dietary treatment

Restriction of dietary protein (see Section 2.2.7) is a fairly accepted method of treatment for encephalopathic patients but the level of restriction varies between liver units. Generally a low protein diet should only be prescribed when management of encephalopathy is severe enough to ignore the ensuing deleterious effect on the nutritional state.

It is essential to determine the cause and degree of encephalopathy before deciding on the level of protein restriction. Clinical assessment includes pychometric tests e.g. (connecting numbers or drawing stars) and electroencephalogram. Very sick patients in coma (grade 4/5) often receive no nutritional support. Some energy should be given in order to minimise catabolism even if all protein is withheld. This may be administered either nasogastrically or intravenously within fluid constraints using either 20% dextrose peripherally or 50% dextrose if there is a central line. Salt-poor albumin may also be given.

This regimen is intended only for the short term (24–48 hours) and nutrition therapy should be reviewed on a daily basis. A protein-free regimen should not be continued for more than 48 hours as the ensuing gluconeogenesis will exacerbate encephalopathy. As a guide, 20–40 g of protein should then be given. If this is administered enterally, a continuous feed should be given rather than a single bolus dose of protein. It is difficult to give specific levels of protein, and each patient should be reviewed individually and on a regular basis taking into account the patient's clinical state and requirements. Close consultation with the medical and nursing team is vital. The dilemma of how much protein to give is frequently resolved by either an improvement in the patient's encephalopathic state or by the intervention of death.

As the patient recovers, protein intakes may be increased to 40 g per day; this is the minimal amount required to maintain essential body functions and promote tissue repair. Increments of 5–10 g/day should then be added with careful clinical observation to determine protein tolerance. The aim is to give 1 g per kg body weight initially, after deducting surplus fluid weight (O'Keefe *et al* 1981).

Quantity, quality and timing are important. Soft, small, easy to eat meals are necessary. Patients often limit their own intake due to anorexia.

Supplements such as Polycal, Fortical (Cow and Gate

Nutricia) or Caloreen (Clintec) are often necessary to ensure adequate energy intakes. If ascites is present, sodium and fluid restrictions are necessary.

The quality of protein may be important and protein from milk or vegetable sources may be better tolerated than animal protein because it contains smaller amounts of methionine and aromatic amino acids (Greenburger 1977; Fenton *et al* 1966). In practice many patients with liver disease appear to dislike meat (no established reason) and a high vegetable diet may be poorly tolerated due to bulk flatulence and diarrhoea.

The timing of protein meals may also be important. Traditionally, patients were advised to distribute their protein intake as small meals throughout the day in order to minimize encephalogenesis, but recently it has been shown that a late evening meal improves the efficiency of nitrogen metabolism in cirrhotic patients (Swart *et al* 1989).

As the patient improves, protein intake can gradually be increased as tolerated – usually to 65–75 g per day which will achieve positive nitrogen balance. Very high protein intakes are unnecessary.

Accurate monitoring of food intake, with a regular review of clinical state is vital to make appropriate dietary adjustments. In the chronically encephalopathic patient, sufficient protein is required to prevent catabolism whilst at the same time avoiding encephalopathy. These patients present a challenge as they are often malnourished, anorexic and may not appreciate the importance of dietary restrictions.

Branched chain amino acids

The branched chain amino acids (BCAA) i.e. valine, leucine and isoleucine may have a role in the management of encephalopathy. However, the use of BCAA given either intravenously or nasogastrically in acute coma, or orally in chronic coma, is controversial and has been the subject of numerous publications (Wahren *et al* 1983; Falccadori *et al* 1984; Cerra *et al* 1985). The rationale for their use is to decrease aromatic amino acids in plasma by promoting muscle protein synthesis thus allowing a greater nitrogen intake in otherwise protein intolerant patients. There is no evidence to suggest that giving BCAA supplements to patients who do not have encephalopathy is beneficial (Horst *et al* 1984).

Products currently available are all nutritionally incomplete and all are relatively low in sodium. Taken orally they are poorly tolerated because of their unpalatability even if flavoured. They are also expensive and because of this they are not widely used except in encephalopathic patients requiring additional nitrogen.

Jaundice and steatorrhoea

Jaundice is detectable when the serum bilirubin is greater than 30–60 μmol/l.

Table 4.33 Causes of cholestatic jaundice

Extrahepatic	Common duct stones
	Carcinoma:
	head of pancreas
	ampulla
	bile duct
	Biliary stricture
	Pancreatitis ± pseudocyst
	Sclerosing cholangitis
Intrahepatic	Viral hepatitis
	Drugs
	Alcoholic hepatitis
	Cirrhosis – any type
	Pregnancy
	Recurrent idiopathic cholestasis
	Some congenital disorders

Both chronic and acute liver disease can give rise to jaundice. Table 4.33 lists some of the major causes.

Traditionally jaundiced patients have been advised to follow a low fat diet perpetuating the incorrect myth that fat is bad for the liver. Fat restriction is only indicated in patients with marked steatorrhoea and in those who experience discomfort on eating fatty foods. Some patients, especially those with hepatitis, do discover that fatty foods are poorly tolerated and will self-limit their intake.

Fat is a significant energy source and appropriate compensation adjustment must be made with the use of predominantly carbohydrate-based supplements. MCT may be useful as it is partially water-soluble, so does not require bile for emulsification. It will provide energy and permit flexibility in cooking. Details of the practical advice for MCT use may be found in Section 4.6.2.

In prolonged cholestasis, fat-soluble vitamins and calcium may be necessary.

Oesophageal varices

These are grossly enlarged veins in the oesophagus and fundus of the stomach due to increased portal venous pressure. Haemorrhage from them carries a high risk of mortality. Acute bleeds may be managed by using either a Sengstaken-Blakemore tube to compress the veins, vasopressin to produce vasoconstriction, surgery or sclerotherapy. One litre of blood contains 70–80 g of protein causing temporary decompensation with encephalopathy, and protein intake may need to be monitored.

No other specific dietary therapy is indicated but a soft diet is advisable 24 hours post sclerotherapy. Repeated sclerotherapy may cause scarring and some difficulty in swallowing.

4.11.6 General nutritional considerations in the management of liver disease

Nutrient delivery

Oral feeding

It is preferable to provide nutritional support through the oral route wherever possible. Often a compromise has to be made between enforcing a strict diet and achieving an adequate nutrient intake. Proprietary products used either as a sole provider of nutrition or more commonly as supplements play a crucial role in providing nutritional support (see Section 1.13.3). Accurate monitoring of food intake is important to assess adequacy of the oral route.

Nasogastric/parenteral nutrition

Patients who are unable to consume an adequate oral intake to meet their nutritional needs but who have a functioning gut, should be tube-fed (see Section 1.13.4).

The presence of varices is no longer a contraindication as fine bore tubes are well tolerated. The most important issue concerns the selection of the most appropriate formulae.

In uncomplicated liver disease, any standard polymeric feed such as Osmolite (Ross) or Nutrison (Cow & Gate Nutricia) may be used. If fluid volume is restricted and energy needs increased then a high energy feed is preferable, such as Ensure Plus (Ross).

If ascites is present, fluid and sodium restrictions are advisable (e.g. 40 mmol sodium, 1500 ml). Commercially available low sodium feeds such as Nutrison Low Sodium (Cow & Gate Nutricia), may contain insufficient energy and need to be supplemented with a carbohydrate source such as Fortical, Polycal (Cow & Gate Nutricia). Alternatively a homemade feed may be prepared from specific nutrient modules. It is essential to check the adequacy of vitamin and mineral content.

Initiation and advancement of tube feeding should proceed very slowly, the concentration and volume gradually being increased to the desired level based on the patient's tolerance. The suggested regimen should be tailored to the requirements of the individual patient and composition of the feed reviewed regularly and modified in light of clinical changes. The protein intake of encephalopathic patients may need to be restricted.

If a patient with fat malabsorption requires tube feeding, an MCT based feed – such as Pepti 2000 (Cow & Gate Nutricia), Trisorbon (Merck) – should be given. However in the presence of ascites, severe encephalopathy and bleeding varices with the possible insertion of a Sengstaken-Blakemore tube, parenteral feeding (TPN) may be indicated. This method has been reported to be more effective in the earlier stages of liver disease but may also run the risk of inducing complications such as septicaemia which, in these already immunocompromised patients, may prove fatal. It is also known that TPN may induce liver dysfunction even in normal patients causing fatty infiltration and cholestasis. The exact cause of this is unclear but may be related to excessive glucose administration (Baker and Rosenberg 1987; Fisher 1989).

In patients with liver disease and no history of encephalopathy, parenteral infusions of standard L-amino acids formulations are indicated. In the presence of encephalopathy, a consensus is emerging that a more modified amino acid mix containing less phenylalanine, tyrosine and methionine but increased amounts of arginine and the BCAA, is advisable (Silk 1988).

TPN should be carefully monitored with daily measurements of urea and electrolytes. Specific considerations in liver patients are fluid volume, electrolyte balance, nitrogen source and amount (depending on fluid volume) with adequate vitamins and minerals. Recent research suggests that a 10% infusion of Intralipid (Kabi) may be safely tolerated (Forbes and Wicks 1990).

Vitamins and minerals

Irrespective of the aetiology of the liver disease it should be assumed that deficiencies of most vitamins occur (Table 4.34).

Factors leading to deficiency are:

1 Inadequate dietary intake.
2 Abnormal metabolism.
3 Increased requirements.
4 Increased losses.

Parenteral vitamin supplements should be given initially with folic acid and intramuscular vitamin K if clotting is prolonged. This should be followed by maintenance therapy of a balanced oral multivitamin preparation with folic acid.

In the presence of prolonged cholestasis, fat-soluble vitamins are necessary with careful regulation in order to avoid toxicity. Administration of single agents should be avoided, even to correct a specific abnormality, as this may create a metabolic imbalance. When normal eating patterns have been re-established then oral supplements may be discontinued.

There has been little work done on the status of trace elements in liver disease. Oral supplements of trace elements given in amounts to meet the RNI may be advisable although not essential.

4.11.7 Transplantation

Liver transplantation is now an accepted treatment for patients with end stage liver disease in whom conventional therapy has failed (McMaster and Buist 1989). The main indications for transplantation are given in Table 4.35. As survival rate is improving the indications are widening to include patients with either alcoholic hepatitis or those with chronic disease who have no serious disease of other

Table 4.34 Vitamin and Mineral replacement therapy

Vitamin	Comments	Recommended dosage
A	Large hepatic stores–deficiency occurs in chronic alcoholic and long standing cholestasis e.g. Primary Biliary Cirrhosis (PBC)	100.00 i.u of monthly intramuscular injection for jaundiced PBC patients with 25 000 i.u daily orally as disease progresses
D	Deficiency in long standing cholestasis – impaired skin photolysis by bilirubin and poor absorption	100 000 i.u vitamin D as monthly intramuscular injections
E	Little known	3–15 mg tocopherol per day, orally
K	Poor absorption in chronic or acute liver disease – exacerbated by cholestyramine. Deficiency causes prolonged clotting time	If clotting time is >1.5, recommend 10 mg vitamin K intramuscularly daily until coagulation improves
B_1,B_2,C	Deficiency more common in patients with alcoholic liver disease but also occurs in other types	IV Multibionta (Merck) initially, followed by oral supplement
Folic acid	Most common vitamin deficiency in all patients with liver disease	10 mg intramuscular folic acid initially, followed by 10 mg orally/day

Mineral	Comments	Recommended dosage
Iron	Deficiency is more common in alcoholic and crytogenic liver disease – main cause is gastrointestinal bleeding and poor intake	200 mg ferrous sulphate tds orally
Calcium	Deficiency most common in patients with steatorrhoea and long standing cholestasis	Recommend 1.5 g calcium per day orally
Zinc and magnesium	Little known – magnesium excretion is increased with diuretic therapy	15 mg zinc orally with 350 mg magnesium per day

organs but despite abstinence from alcohol, still suffer from chronic encephalopathy or intractable ascites (Neuberger 1989; Kumar *et al* 1990).

A detailed nutritional assessment before transplantation is crucial because patients with end-stage liver failure are frequently malnourished. Poor nutrition is a major risk factor associated with a poor prognosis of liver transplantation (Shronts *et al* 1987; Diecco *et al* 1989). Timely and appropriate nutritional intervention can then be planned and implemented.

Table 4.35 Indications for liver transplantation

1 Chronic liver disease (commonest)	e.g.	Chronic active hepatitis Progressive primary biliary cirrhosis Primary sclerosing cholangitis Budd Chiari syndrome Haemochromatosis
2 Acute liver failure	Resulting from:	Viral hepatitis Idiosyncratic drug reactions Wilson's disease
3 Metabolic disorders	e.g.	Alpha-1-antitrypsin deficiency
4 Malignant disease		Primary hepatic and bile duct malignancy

Aggressive nutritional support appears to be an important component in perioperative care and dietary advice should be given according to the presenting symptoms (Hehir *et al* 1985).

Post-operative management is similar to that of any critically ill patient undergoing major surgery. Ventilatory support is required initially, as is immunosuppressive therapy. Liver rejection may become evident, usually within 5–7 days of transplantation. Nutritional support varies between liver units. In some, TPN is commenced immediately and is continued until an adequate oral intake can be achieved (usually seven days). In other centres, TPN is instigated only if patients are unable to tolerate a reasonable intake after 4–5 days post surgery, either orally or nasogastrically.

TPN is not continued any longer than is necessary because of the risk of infection in an already immunocompromised patient. The patient can then commence a high protein, high energy diet. Appetite may be slow to return and, if inadequate, tube feeding may be indicated. Patients should be encouraged to consume a free diet and reassured that it is safe for them to do so. Occasionally ascites persists and a sodium restriction may be necessary. Post-operatively, nutritional intake may be inhibited by a fear of eating due to previous dietary restrictions, by infection and by altered taste sensation due to drug therapy.

Hyperglycaemia is common during the first four to five days post-operatively and is controlled by insulin; no dietary restriction is usually necessary. In some patients, steroid-induced diabetes may in time develop and additional dietary measures may then be needed. Increased appetite due to steroid therapy and liberation of food intake may often result in excessive weight gain and appropriate advice should be given. Unless alcohol is implicated in diagnosis of the liver disease, alcohol may be allowed as per recommended safe limits.

4.11.8 Other types of liver disease

Neoplastic disease of the liver

Benign tumours are rare. Primary malignant tumours, such as hepatocellular carcinoma, commonly arise as a complication of longstanding cirrhosis.

The liver is the most common site of metastatic deposits. Dietary advice given should be according to symptoms present.

Storage diseases

Wilson's disease

Wilson's disease is an inherited disorder characterized by abnormal copper transport and storage mechanisms resulting in excessive copper depositions in body tissues, including the liver, causing cirrhosis. Low copper diets are rarely used in adults.

Haemochromatosis

This usually affects males over the age of 45 years and its aetiology remains unclear. Excessive iron absorption occurs over many years, which is deposited it tissues particularly in the liver. Treatment is by regular venesection; dietary iron restriction is unnecessary.

4.11.9 Disorders of the biliary tree

Gallstones

Gallstones may present in various ways. The most common and characteristic are either acute cholecystitis or obstruction of the common bile duct (cholangitis). Patients may complain of flatulence and an intolerance to fatty foods, jaundice and pain. No evidence exists that any particular diet influences gall bladder or gallstone disease. A low fat diet is often prescribed but has not been evaluated satisfactorily. It seems reasonable to adjust fat intake according to individual tolerance level. High fibre diets do not appear to prevent the recurrence of gallstones (Bouchier 1990).

Cholangiocarcinoma

Cholangiocarcinomas can be extrahepatic or intrahepatic giving rise to jaundice. Palliative therapy for the former consists of passing a stent (a thin plastic tube) during endoscopic retrograde cholangiopancreatography.

A free diet should be encouraged, and a fat restriction imposed only if patients are symptomatic on consuming fat. These patients are usually malnourished and require a high protein, high energy diet.

Primary sclerosing cholangitis

This results from the inflammation and fibrosis of the bile ducts leading to multiple areas of narrowing throughout the biliary system. The cause is unknown and 50% of patients have inflammatory bowel disease.

Active nutritional support is required as these patients are frequently malnourished. Restriction of fat may be appropriate if steatorrhoea occurs.

Useful address

Recently a liver patients support group has been established in London and it is envisaged that a network of local groups may also be formed throughout the UK. The aim is to provide advice, contacts and to fundraise on behalf of liver patients and their families.

More information may be obtained from:

The Liver Support Group, Academic Dept of Medicine, 10th Floor, Royal Free Hospital, London NW3 2QG.

Further reading

British Dietetic Association, Liver Interest Group (1990) *A practical guide to nutrition in liver disease.* BDA, Birmingham.

Keohane PP, Attrill H, Grimble G, Spiller R, Frost P and Silk DBA (1983) Enteral nutrition in malnourished patients with hepatic cirrhosis. *JPEN* 7, 346–50.

Johnson PJ (1989) *The laboratory investigation of liver disease.* Baillière Tindall, Eastbourne.

Morgan MY (1990) Branched chain aminoacids in the management of chronic liver disease – facts and fantasies. *J Hepatology* **11**, 133–41.

Sherlock S (1989) *Diseases of the liver and biliary system* 6e. Blackwell Scientific Publications, Oxford.

Wright R (1989) *Liver and biliary disease.* Baillière Tindall, Eastbourne.

References

Baker AL and Rosenberg IH (1987) Hepatic complications of total parenteral nutrition. *Am J Med* **82**, 489–97.

Blackburn GL, Bistrian B, Maini B, Schlamm H and Smith M (1977) Nutritional metabolic assessments of the hospitalised patient. *J Parent Ent Nutr* **1**, 11–22.

Bouchier IAD (1990) Gallstones. *Br Med J* **300**, 592–7.

Cerra FB, Cheung NK, Fischer JE, Kaplowitz N, Schiff ER, Dienstag JL, Bower RH, Mabry CD, Leevy CM and Kiernan T (1985) Disease-specific amino acid infusion in hepatic encephalopathy. *JPEN* **9**, 288–95.

Child CG and Turcott JB (1964) Surgery and portal hypertension. In *The liver and portal hypertension*, Child CG (Ed) p. 500. WB Saunders, Philadelphia.

Diecco SR, Wiener EJ, Weisner RH, Southorm PA, Plevak DJ and Krom RAF (1989) Assessment of nutritional status of patients with end stage liver disease undergoing liver transplantation. *Mayo Clinic Proceedings* **64**, 95–102.

Falccadori F *et al* (1984) BCAA enriched solution in hepatic encephalopathy. In *Hepatic encephalopathy in chronic liver failure*, pp. 311–21. Plenum Press, New York.

Fenton JCB, Knight EJ and Humpherson PL (1966) Milk and cheese diet in portal-systemic encephalopathy. *Lancet* **i**, 164–5.

Fisher RL (1989) Hepatobiliary abnormalities associated with total parenteral nutrition. *Gastroenter Clin N Amer* **18**, No. 3.

Forbes A and Wicks C (1990) Fulminant hepatic failure nutrition and fat clearance. *Recent Advances in Nutriology* **1**, 67A.

Franco D, Charra M, Jeambrun P, Belghiti J, Bismuth H, Cortesse A and Sossler C (1983) Nutrition and immunity after peritoneovenous drainage of intractable ascites in cirrhotic patients. *Am J Surg* **146**, 652–7.

Gauthier A, Levy VG, Quinton A, Michel H, Rueff B, Desios L, Durbec JP, Fermanian J and Lancrenon S (1986) Salt or no salt in the treatment of cirrhotic ascites – a random mixed study. *Gut* **27**, 704–709.

Gines P, Arroyo V, Quintero E, Planas R, Bory F, Cabrera J, Rimola G, Viver J, Camps J and Jimenez W (1987) Comparison of paracentesis and diuretics in the treatment of cirrhosis with tense ascites. *Gastroenterology* **93**, 234–41.

Greenburger NJ (1977) Effect of vegetable and animal protein diets in chronic hepatic encephalopathy. *Dig Dis* **22**, 845–55.

Hehir DJ, Jenkins RL, Bistrian B and Blackburn G (1985) Nutrition in patients undergoing orthotopic liver transplantation. *J Parent Ent Nutr* **9**(6), 695.

Horst D, Grace ND, Conn HO, Schiff E, Schenker S, Viteri A, Law D and Atterbury CE (1984) Comparisons of dietary protein with an oral BCAA supplement in chronic portal systemic encephalopathy. *Hepatology* **4**, 279–87.

James R (1989) Nutritional support in alcoholic liver disease: a review. *J Hum Nutr Dietet* **2**, 315–23.

Katelaris PH and Jones DB (1989) Fulminant hepatic failure. *Med Clin N Amer* **73**(4), 955–70.

Kumar S, Stauber RE, Gavaler JS, Basista MH, Dinozans VJ, Schade RR, Rabinovitz M, Tarter RE, Gordon R and Starzi TE (1990) Orthotopic liver transplantation for alcoholic liver disease. *Hepatology* **II**(2), 159–64.

McMaster P and Buist LJ (1989) Liver transplantation. *Hospital Update* **89**, 1528.

Mendenhall CL *et al* (1985) A co-operative study of alcoholic hepatitis 111. *J Parent Ent Nutr* **9**, 590–96.

Merli M, Romiti A, Riggio O, Capocaccia L (1987) Optimal nutritional indexes in chronic liver disease. *J Parent Ent Nutr* **2**, 130–34.

Neuberger JM (1989) Transplantation for alcoholic liver disease. *Br Med J* **299**, 693–94.

O'Keefe SJD, Abraham R, El-Zayadi A, Marshall W, Davis M and Williams R (1981) Increased plasma tyrosine concentrations in patients with fulminant hepatic failure associated with increased plasma tyrosine flux and reduced hepatic oxidation capacity. *Gastroenterology* **81**, 1017–24.

Silk DBA (1988) Parenteral Nutrition in patients with liver disease. *J Hepat* **7**, 269–77.

Shronts EP, Teasley KM, Theole SL and Cerra FB (1987) Nutritional support of the adult liver transplant candidate. *J Am Dietet Assoc* **87**, 441–51.

Swart GR, Zillikens MC, Van Vuure JK and Van Den Berg JWO (1989) Effect of a late evening meal on nitrogen balance in patients with cirrhosis of the liver. *Br Med J* **299**, 1202–203.

Wahren J, Denis J, Dersurmont P, Eriksson LS, Escoffier JM, Gauthier AP, Hagenfeldt L, Michel H, Opolon P, Paris JC and Veyrac M (1983) Is intravenous administration of BCAA effective in the treatment of hepatic encephalopathy? *Hepatol* **3**, 475–80.

Watson CG, Tilleslejor B, Hoodecheck-Schaw B, Pikel J and Jacobs L (1984) Do alcoholics give valid self reports? *J Studies Alcohol* **45**, 344–8.

4.12 Paediatric liver and biliary disorders

4.12.1 Common paediatric liver and biliary disorders

Extrahepatic biliary atresia

Extra hepatic biliary atresia (EHBA) is the commonest life-threatening liver disorder to present in infancy; 33% of those investigated for jaundice are diagnosed as having extra hepatic biliary atresia.

EHBA is a progressive disease which is defined as the complete inability to excrete bile due to obstruction, destruction, or absence of the extra hepatic bile ducts. This leads to bile stasis in the liver with progressive inflammation and subsequent fibrosis.

The aetiology is unknown but it is not a congenital condition. It affects at least 1 in 20 000 liveborn infants (Mowat 1987). These infants are normal at birth and have satisfactory postnatal weight gain. An infant with biliary atresia usually presents with mild prolonged jaundice beyond 14 days, and the colour of the stools may fluctuate from a normal colour to very pale.

Bile drainage can be restored by the 'Kasai' operation which bypasses the blocked ducts (portoenterostomy). Success can be as high as 90% as judged by those whose serum bilirubin returns to normal after the operation (Ohi *et al* 1985). Such surgery must be done before eight weeks of age otherwise the prognosis is very poor (Mieli-Vergani *et al* 1989), the majority of children dying before the age of two years unless liver transplantation is considered.

The most common application of extrahepatic biliary atresia is ascending cholangitis which can cause fever, jaundice and deteriorating liver function functions. Cholangitis can lead to increased nutritional requirements due to malabsorption and fever complicated by associated anorexia (see below).

Malabsorption is secondary to reduced or absent bile flow and abnormal bile constituents. It often improves within the first year after the Kasai. However, it can have a profound effect on fat digestion, as bile acids are necessary for micelle formation. Ascites and hypoalbuminaemia are common in these children (see below).

Oesophageal varices are an indication of portal hypertension and cirrhosis. They can present in children with extrahepatic biliary atresia as early as 12 months or younger.

Alpha-1-antitrypsin deficiency

The genetic deficiency of the glycoprotein alpha-1-antitrypsin can cause varying degrees of liver disease in infancy and can present with cholestasis. The most severe form of alpha-1-antitrypsin deficiency is an infant presenting in the first four months of life with conjugated hyperbilirubinaemia. Approximately 17% of those investigated for jaundice are diagnosed as having alpha-1-antitrypsin deficiency.

Infants may have a low birth weight, but appear well apart from jaundice and slow weight gain. Others show irritability, marked failure to thrive, vomiting, biochemical and haematological changes such as low platelet count and prolonged prothrombin time. Up to 10% present with serious bleeding due to vitamin K malabsorption.

The exact physiological role of alpha-1-antitrypsin is unknown. The liver disease is thought to be secondary to the uninhibited action of proteases which are critical in the inflammatory response.

Diagnosis is made by protease inhibitor (Pi) phenotyping. Phenotype Pi ZZ indicates alpha-1-antitrypsin deficiency.

The liver disease can be so severe that cirrhosis develops rapidly and 25% of these children would die in infancy or early childhood without liver transplantation.

Management is dependent on the severity of the condition. Cirrhosis and portal hypertension are common complications and the resultant ascites is the main factor to determine treatment (see below).

Neonatal hepatitis

Approximately 30% of infants presenting with conjugated hyperbilirubinaemia have a neonatal hepatitis with no cause found. Neonatal hepatitis is associated with infections caused by bacterial toxins or viruses including cytomegalovirus (CMV). Toxins such as drugs in pregnancy or labour, immunological incompatibility between infant and mother, prematurity associated with one or more blood transfusions (Kubota *et al* 1988) and vascular abnormalities are all possible causes of neonatal hepatitis.

Infants with neonatal hepatitis are treated medically. It is important to monitor these infants even though the jaundice can clear and liver function tests return to near normal by the age of six months. Some infants have gone on to develop cirrhosis in later life.

If an infant exhibits failure to thrive and/or malabsorption, dietary intervention is needed with respect to the infant formula given. Energy supplementation is sometimes required, while fluid restriction is rare.

Intrahepatic biliary hypoplasia

Biliary hypoplasia is an absence or reduction in the number of bile ductules seen in portal tracts within the liver. A genetic aetiology is suggested. Fibrosis occurs rapidly progressing to biliary cirrhosis.

Infants present with cholestasis followed by severe pruritis. Medical treatment of complications improves prognosis. Dietary treatment involves that mainly for failure to thrive (see below). Before transplantation became available, children often died from liver failure by the age of three years.

Alagille's syndrome

In this disorder, biliary hypoplasia is associated with cardiovascular, skeletal, facial and ocular abnormalities. A genetic aetiology is suggested but the inheritance is complicated.

The estimated incidence is one in 100 000 live births: 10% have cyanotic heart disease as the main problem; 50% show 'butterfly like' vertebrae on X-ray, although this does not seem to affect spinal growth; 20% are prematurely born or small-for-gestational-age. Chronic cholestasis dominates clinically (Alagille 1985). Conjugated hyperbilirubinaemia presents followed by pruritus and finally, (in severe cases) xanthelasma which usually appears by two years of age.

Chronic malabsorption of fat is common and sometimes contributed to by exocrine pancreatic insufficiency. Severe growth retardation may be partly due to malabsorption. Dietary treatment is essential as soon as diagnosis is made. Many children need intensive treatment including nasogastric feeding. However, improving nutritional status can result in severe pruritis, and full medical supervision is essential.

For many children medical management controls the symptoms. If cirrhosis develops then liver transplantation is the only treatment.

Autoimmune liver disease

Autoimmune liver disease is a chronic aggressive hepatitis with or without cirrhosis. It is usually controlled by immunosuppressive therapy.

Age at diagnosis varies widely. It is rare before six years and is most common between 10 and 30 years. Over 70% of cases are females. Frequently the presentation is of lethargy, anorexia and fever as well as the more common features of liver disease.

As methods of diagnosis and treatment improve, the prognosis is encouraging; 80% can go on to develop cirrhosis but, with continued steroid treatment, this is rarely fatal.

Dietitians are frequently involved with these children who suffer from weight loss and anorexia when first investigated. While on steroids, excessive weight gain is occasionally a problem; steroid-induced diabetes is less common.

Fulminant hepatic failure

Fulminant hepatic failure is the rapid onset of acute and severe liver dysfunction with encephalopathy. The aetiology is unknown. It is described more fully within Section 4.11 on adult liver and biliary disease (see especially Section 4.11.2.) The child can be jaundiced and ascites is common. Dietary treatment of symptoms is an essential part of treatment, and can help to stabilize the condition (see below).

Congenital cholestatic liver disease

Liver disease with cholestatic features has been described in a number of distinct familial syndromes.

Malabsorption and jaundice can be the first symptoms starting within the first year of life. Pruritis is severe. Portal hypertension leading to bleeding varices can develop. Failure to thrive due to steatorrhea and diarrhoea are prominent features and require dietary intervention (see below).

The longest recorded life span of children with this condition is 18 years. Liver transplantation is the only effective long term treatment.

Wilson's disease

Wilson's disease is an autosomal recessive condition. It may present with liver involvement in childhood or neurological involvement in the adult (Walshe 1990). It is fatal without treatment. Early treatment is relatively safe and effective.

In children with Wilson's disease there are defects in copper handling, so little copper is excreted in the bile and caeruloplasmin is not produced at the normal rate. Copper collects in the liver, poisoning the hepatocytes, and is also deposited in other organs.

Most symptoms appear before puberty. These can begin with nausea and malaise going on to jaundice and ascites. Occasionally the hepatic illness is very acute.

Treatment is by penicillamine given orally and taken for life. Zinc sulphate is also given to prevent copper reaccumulation. Some liver units still advocate a low copper diet avoiding chocolate, nuts, cocoa, shellfish and mushrooms. Yet with the use of penicillamine, the need for such restriction is questionable.

If there is no improvement after two to three months of adequate treatment, liver transplantation must be considered. Some units use a scoring system of liver function tests with prothrombin time as an assessment of prognosis without transplantation (Mowat 1987).

Other family members should be screened and treated appropriately.

4.12.2 Nutritional assessment

Nutritional assessment of a child with liver disease is important in order to set dietary goals. There is no single ideal method of nutritional assessment and therefore a combination of methods is required. Weight for height measurements overestimate nutritional status due to organomegaly and ascites. However serial measurements of weight and girth will distinguish fat and muscle accumulation from fluid overload. Anthropometry including triceps skinfold thickness (TSF) and mid-arm circumference (MAC) should be carried out regularly to obtain serial measurements. This will give a trend in the degree of muscle wasting and fat loss over a period of time (Sokol and Stall 1990).

Circuit indirect calorimetry with gas analysis by mass spectrometry is being used in some centres to determine resting energy expenditure (REE). Infants and children can be assessed over a period of 10 to 15 minutes whilst asleep or resting (Pierro *et al* 1989).

4.12.3 Treatment of the complications of liver disease in children

Jaundice

Jaundice is a feature of a number of liver disorders. As a sole symptom it does not warrant dietary manipulation; however, it is usually present in conjunction with a number of complications which may require dietary intervention.

Fat malabsorption

Fat absorption may be as low as 40% of the total fat ingested (Kaufman *et al* 1987) and this will result in poor absorption of energy, fat-soluble vitamins and essential fatty acids. Dietary fat, however, should not be restricted. Children with liver disease have greatly increased requirements for energy and, since they may also be anorexic and nauseous, an energy-dense diet is required. This is difficult to achieve without inclusion of fat, and dietary fat should be encouraged to tolerance.

Dietary treatment of fat malabsorption in infants

A cholestatic infant should be changed from an ordinary infant formula to a specialized formula containing a higher proportion of medium chain triglyceride (MCT). MCTs are liberated by intraluminal triglyceride hydrolysis and are less dependent on bile acids for absorption. They can also be oxidized peripherally.

Long chain triglyceride (LCT) should contribute at least 3% of total energy intake to provide essential fatty acids (EFA) (Kaufman *et al* 1987). Pregestimil (Mead Johnson) containing 42% fat as MCT, Pepti Junior (Cow & Gate Nutricia) containing 50% fat as MCT, or MCT Pepdite 0–2 (Scientific Hospital Supplies) containing 83% fat as MCT are all suitable. MCT Pepdite is supplemented with essential fatty acids. Other hydrolysed protein formula such as Prejomin (Milupa) are not suitable as they contain little MCT. Portagen (Mead Johnson) has 85% fat as MCT, but is not supplemented with EFA (Kaufman *et al* 1987). Transition to a higher MCT formula should be done gradually so that the infants gets accustomed to the taste of the feed.

Breast fed babies who are failing to thrive should be provided with supplementary Pregestimil/Pepti Junior feeds. Breast feeding should be stopped in the infant who continues to fail to thrive. 150–200 ml of formula feed per kg of expected weight should be given. This provides 100–130 kcal/kg and may be sufficient to maintain growth. Many infants will require more, and regular nutritional assessment is essential.

Dietary treatment of fat malabsorption in children

Children over 12 months of age will frequently tolerate more LCT, and manipulation of dietary fat is not necessary unless the child has severe steatorrhea or feels nauseous on a high fat diet. However, fat should only be restricted to the level of tolerance as unnecessary fat restriction will make dietary goals difficult to achieve.

An energy-dense diet aiming for 140–160% of the Estimated Average Requirement (EAR) for energy should be given to take account of malabsorption.

Failure to thrive

Children with liver disease require around 160–200% of the normal requirements for energy and protein (Charlton *et al* 1992). It is estimated that 55–80% of children with liver disease have growth failure (weight for height < 90% of expected) (Cohen and Gartner 1971; Weber and Roy 1972). This is due to increased requirements, malabsorption and anorexia.

Anorexia is particularly prominent in children with ascites and hepatosplenomegaly. Nausea may be common due to the large amount of medication required, and behavioural food refusal is as much a feature of children with liver disease as it is of other children with chronic disorders.

Dietary treatment of failure to thrive in infants

In an infant with severe failure to thrive, in whom catch-up growth is needed, it may be necessary to achieve extremely high energy and protein intakes. This may be done in several ways.

Increasing the volume of feed This may be appropriate if the infant is not on a fluid restriction. A fine bore nasogastric tube may be used if the feeds cannot be completed orally. Feeds can be administered by bolus gravity feeding, or by continuous 'top up' feeding overnight using an enteral feeding pump. Where possible, the feeds should be given in part at least by bottle, to maintain oral stimulation. In an infant with end stage liver disease, this may not be possible and continuous nasogastric feeding using an enteral feeding pump (Kangaroo, Abbott) may be necessary (Charlton *et al* 1992).

Supplementing the energy content of feeds This will need to be done in the majority of infants if a large volume of feed is not tolerated (e.g. due to vomiting, fluid restriction or if nasogastric completion of the feed is not thought to be desirable). *Carbohydrate* may be added in the form of glucose polymer such as Maxijul (Scientific Hospital Supplies), Caloreen (Clintec), Polycal (Cow & Gate Nutricia) to 1 g/100 ml feed initially, and increased by 1 g/100 ml daily to 6 g/100 ml as tolerated. *MCT* may be added as a 50% emulsion (Liquigen, Scientific Hospital Supplies) 0.5 g being added initially (1 ml Liquigen/100 ml feed) and this increased to 2.5 g (5 ml emulsion/100 ml feed) as tolerated. Alternatively, Duocal (Scientific Hospital Supplies) may be used as a combined fat/ carbohydrate supplement (see above).

Sucrose may also be used as part of the carbohydrate supplement. This may improve the taste of the feed and enable a larger volume of feed to be completed orally.

Supplementing the protein content of the feed This may be necessary in order to achieve dietary goals.

The value of branched chain amino acids (BCAA) as a protein supplement is a subject of much discussion and controversy. Recent evidence suggests that BCAA supplemented feeds may help to improve nutritional status in children, possibly because BCAA are preferentially utilized by skeletal muscle (Achord 1988). Generaid (Scientific Hospital Supplies) may be added to the feed to achieve a protein intake of 3–4 g/kg; if BCAA are not felt to be necessary, Maxipro HBV (Scientific Hospital Supplies) may be used at similar concentrations.

Using suitable weaning solids These will provide valuable additional energy and protein. Weaning foods should be started at 3–4 months of age. Solids may be energy supplemented with a carbohydrate polymer or Duocal (Scientific Hospital Supplies).

Full fat cows' milk may be included in the diet from six months of age in the form of yoghurt/milk puddings. Cows' milk should not be given as a drink in preference to the specialized formula feeds. Attention should be paid to the volume of specialized feeds consumed during weaning to ensure that sufficient quantities are taken.

Dietary treatment of failure to thrive in children

A high energy and protein intake may be possible with ordinary diet and mid-meal snacks if the child has a good appetite. Refined carbohydrates as sugar, jam, sweets, drinks, cakes and biscuits, and fat as full fat cows' milk, fried foods, butter, cream, full fat yoghurts and cheese should be encouraged.

It is frequently not possible to achieve the desired intake by diet alone, and dietary supplements may be necessary. Maxijul (SHS), Caloreen (Clintec), Polycal (Cow and Gate Nutricia), Duocal (SHS), Hycal (Smith Kline Beecham) and Fortical (Cow & Gate Nutricia) may be used as energy supplements at a dilution which provides 20–25 g carbohydrate/100 ml. Useful combined energy and protein supplements include Fresubin (Fresenius), Liquisorb, Liquisorbon MCT (Merck), Fortisip (Cow & Gate Nutricia) and Ensure (Ross). These provide 3–5 g protein and 100–150 kcal/100 ml.

If a child has severe anorexia, it may be necessary to feed enterally to achieve dietary adequacy. This may be given either continuously using an enteral feeding pump or as an overnight supplement. A whole protein, LCT fat feed may be tolerated. Suitable choices are Nutrison Paediatric (Cow & Gate Nutricia), Paediasure (Ross), or an adult enteral feed, modified as appropriate for age. Occasionally a feed with a higher MCT:LCT ratio may be needed. Pepdite 2+ (Scientific Hospital Supplies) or Liquisorbon MCT (Merck) are appropriate choices.

A child who has been taking Pregestimil (Mead Johnson) or Pepti-Junior (Cow & Gate Nutricia) in infancy may continue to take it into childhood, either as a drink or an enteral feed. This should be supplemented with protein/ fat and carbohydrate as appropriate for age.

Ascites

The development of ascites is a feature of a number of liver disorders and should be managed aggressively. Treatment consists of a combination of sodium and fluid restriction plus diuretics.

Dietary treatment of ascites in infants

If fluid restriction is required (80–100 ml/kg) this will restrict the intake of all nutrients and concentration of the feeds will be necessary.

When an infant is well established on Pregestimil (Mead Johnson) or Pepti-Junior (Cow & Gate Nutricia), the feed should be supplemented to give 3–4 g protein/kg and 140–160 kcal/kg within the volume allowed. Sodium intakes are reduced to 1.2–1.5 mmol/kg by this feed regimen.

Some centres advocate a modular approach to feeding to meet the sodium restriction. This should be based on five ingredients.

A low sodium protein source e.g. Maxipro HBV (SHS)/Generaid (SHS) given at a level which provides 3–4 g protein/kg.

Carbohydrate in the form of a glucose polymer is used at an initial level of 12 g/100 ml, although it is often necessary to achieve higher concentrations.

Fat as a combination of LCT emulsion (Calogen, Scientific Hospital Supplies) and MCT emulsion (Liquigen, Scientific Hospital Supplies) is used at a level of 5 g fat/100 ml.

Full vitamins and minerals should be added. A combined low sodium, low potassium, vitamin and mineral supplement is useful. Paediatric Seravit (Scientific Hospital Supplies) will provide complete vitamin and mineral intake, 8 g being required for infants up to six months of age, and 12 g for those over six months.

Electrolytes should be added. Potassium chloride solution must be added to 2–3 mmol/kg. Sodium chloride solution is added to the restricted level. This feed must be introduced in a diluted form and built up to full strength over 4–5 days.

It may be possible to increase energy density further by the addition of more glucose polymer and fat emulsion to tolerance. Extremely high carbohydrate levels (20 g/100 ml) may be tolerated, but extreme caution should be used in concentrating feeds to this level.

Energy supplemented solids will provide additional energy without fluid, and should be encouraged.

Dietary treatment of ascites in children

Fluid restriction (50 ml/kg) with or without sodium restriction may be necessary to control ascites. Restriction to 'no added salt' level is usually sufficient.

Restriction of fluid and sodium will often have a deleterious effect on appetite and favourite foods within the restriction should be offered.

Restriction of fluids will limit the quantity of fluid supplements or enteral feed which can be given, and these should be as energy dense as tolerated. Fluids should be spread over the day and may be offered as Hycal/Fortical ice lollies.

Any fluids offered should be supplemented with a glucose polymer at 20–25 g/100 ml.

Oesophageal varices

Portal hypertension will lead to the development of oesophageal varices which may need endoscopic injections if they bleed.

Immediately afterwards, the child is started on clear fluids, then milk, and soft diet is continued for 10 days or until the child is reinjected, whichever occurs first. This may then be discontinued if there are no complications.

Enteral feeding using a fine bore polyurethane tube may still be undertaken in the presence of varices.

Pruritus

Pruritus is a symptom of bile salt accumulation and may be distracting and uncomfortable for the child. It may be controlled by drugs (phenobarbitone, rifampicin or cholestyramine) or by the application of evening primrose oil.

If cholestyramine is used, it may interfere with fat-soluble vitamin absorption, and supplements of these should be administered separately from the cholestyramine.

Encephalopathy

Encephalopathy is diagnosed more on clinical status, as an increased ammonia level can be difficult to interpret. As yet there is little evidence to suggest that BCAA will reverse an encephalopathic state, although it may be possible to achieve a higher protein intake and improve nutritional status without deterioration of mental state with the use of a BCAA supplemented diet (Keohane *et al* 1983; McCullough *et al* 1989).

Dietary treatment of encephalopathy in infants and children

At the start of chronic encephalopathic symptoms protein should be decreased to 1.5–2.0 g/kg for 48 hours and then increased back up to 3–4 g/kg if an improvement is seen.

In acute onset encephalopathy, restriction to 0.5 g protein/kg may be needed. Regular evaluation is necessary and protein should not be restricted in an asymptomatic child.

Children in encephalopathic coma (grade 4/5) should have dietary protein removed for 24–48 hours. Protein should then be introduced gradually at 0.5 g protein/kg/day, possibly as a combination of BCAA and aromatic amino acids. This will need to be administered by a nasogastric tube. Throughout the coma state, a high energy intake should be ensured with a carbohydrate/fat mixture given either nasogastrically or intravenously. This will minimize muscle breakdown which will worsen the coma state.

4.12.4 General nutritional aspect of management

Behavioural food refusal

Behavioural food refusal is a symptom of many chronic

disorders in children and makes achieving dietary goals difficult. It may be minimized by maintaining an oral intake wherever possible. Even in a child requiring total enteral feeding, oral food and drinks should be offered at mealtimes to maintain the normal mealtime routine. Wherever possible the child should eat and drink with other children to promote the social aspects of mealtimes. Behavioural food refusal is difficult to manage and may require input from clinical psychologist, speech therapist and occupational therapist.

Vitamin, mineral and essential fatty acid deficiencies

All infants and children with liver disease require a complete vitamin supplement daily; 5 ml Ketovite liquid and 3 Ketovite tablets (Paines & Byrne) should be given. Water-soluble vitamin deficiencies are rare in infants and children with liver disease. The daily supplements are usually sufficient.

Fat-soluble vitamin deficiencies are a feature of long standing or severe liver disease. Vitamin A, D, E and K should be given orally in large doses as a water miscible preparation (Silverberg and Davidson 1970). With modern preparations intramuscular vitamins are only needed in severe cholestatic disease. Suggested dose levels of fat-soluble vitamins are given in Table 4.36. However, these do vary between centres.

Rickets may be present combined with vitamin D deficiency and an adequate intake of calcium and phosphorus should be ensured. Supplements may be necessary, at a level of 1 mmol/kg/day of both calcium and phosphate. These may need to be increased further according to clinical response.

Iron deficiency may be due to poor dietary intakes and possible losses of iron through bleeding. Supplementation may be needed. Zinc is required for the hepatic synthesis of retinol binding protein and zinc deficiency should be excluded if vitamin A deficiency occurs (Morrison *et al* 1978; Suita *et al* 1987).

Essential fatty acid deficiencies may be seen in children with severe fat malabsorption or who have been on a very low fat diet for long periods. Supplements in the form of sunflower or safflower oil may be used.

Table 4.36 Suggested dose levels of fat soluble vitamins for use in severe liver disease

Vitamin A	5000–15 000 i.u. daily given in suspension (Children with Alagille's syndrome: 50 000 i.u. intramuscularly monthly)
Vitamin D	50 ng/kg up to a maximum of 1 μg/day given as 1-alpha-25hydroxy cholecalciferol (alpha calcidol)
Vitamin E	100–500 mg b.d. as alpha tocopheral acetate suspension (Ephynal ®, Roche)
Vitamin K	5–10 mg/day given as menadiol sodium phosphate (Synkavit ®, Roche)

On commencement of fat soluble vitamin supplements, serum levels should where possible be monitored regularly to ensure correct dosage

4.12.5 Nutritional support in paediatric orthotopic liver transplantation

Since the development of the surgical procedure in 1963, human orthotopic liver transplantation has progressed to become a primary therapeutic option in the management of end-stage liver disease in children (Goulet *et al* 1987).

Nutritional care of the patient pre- and post the waiting period is vital for increasing the chances of patient survival, both during the wait for a donor organ and in the transplant recovery phase (Stuart *et al* 1989). The goal of any intermediate therapy, therefore, is to support or improve nutritional status and to slow down the inevitable deterioration of this group of children (Goulet *et al* 1987; Kaufman *et al* 1989).

Immediate post-transplant considerations

Post-transplantation, with the restoration of normal liver function, the eventual nutritional goal is to convert all children to a normal diet for their age and away from the special formulations that were necessary prior to transplantation (Byer and Shaw 1988a).

Infants and children have markedly reduced body reserves of energy compared to adults (Grant and Todd 1987). The demands made on these energy reserves immediately post-transplant are great, emphasizing the need for rapid introduction of nutritional support.

Total parental nutrition (TPN)

The use of TPN post-transplantation varies between centres. TPN is administered either to all transplant recipients for a short period post-surgery, or only to children who have:

1 Complications post transplant.
2 TPN prior to surgery.
3 Severe pre-transplant malnutrition.

The feeding regimen is initiated within 24–48 hours of the procedure, and attempts to provide the calculated nitrogen and energy needs of the child; however, with fluid restrictions and high volume drug infusions so often necessary immediately post-transplant, the volume available for TPN is severely limited. Use is made therefore of the more concentrated parenteral solutions, in particular Aminoplex 24 (Geistlich). This is infused alongside dextrose (40–50% dextrose is generally well tolerated). Insulin is administered as indicated by regular blood glucose monitoring. Lipid can be a useful concentrated energy source and is administered as 20% Intralipid (Kabivitrum) at an initial rate of 0.5 g fat/kg body weight.

The ratio of nitrogen to non-protein energy should be maintained at around 1 g : 200 kcal if possible, thus ensuring the correct utilization of amino acids for tissue growth and repair.

Vitamin supplements are given parenterally as 10 ml of Multibionta (Merck) every other day, and 10 mg vitamin K and 5 mg folic acid daily. Trace elements are also given on alternate days (Addenbrooke's Hospital 1990). Sodium and potassium are administered according to daily electrolyte levels. Calcium and phosphate requirements can often be high particularly after the catabolic phase is overcome (Addenbrooke's Hospital 1990).

Enteral nutrition

Oral feeds are started as soon as bowel movements show that ileus has resolved.

As with any child who has undergone major abdominal surgery, oral feeds start with water or dextrose at 5 ml/hour and progress as rapidly as tolerance allows to a formula suitable to the child's age. If TPN has been employed, the volume is reduced in proportion to the amount of energy provided by the oral route. The method of choice is for full strength formula in small volumes rather than larger volumes of graded concentrations.

All children post-transplant require fluid restriction. The provision of the required volume of standard formula that would provide the child's calculated requirements is often not possible. The use of energy supplements (as described above) is indicated.

In the early stages of recovery the child is given bolus feeds hourly, slowly increasing to 3 or 4 hourly. In the younger infant attempts are made to mimic the child's normal feeding pattern or to establish one if a pattern had not previously existed. All children are encouraged to take their bolus feeds orally if possible. Occasionally the child's condition prevents oral administration of the formula and continuous nasogastric infusion is necessary. As the child's condition improves, nasogastric infusion is restricted to during the nighttime hours, thus allowing the child to be bolus-fed during the day or, more importantly, to encourage food intake at mealtimes.

At this stage some transplant patients may exhibit a transient malabsorptive phase. The cause is often unclear, although malabsorption due to pre-transplant malnutrition or manipulation of the bowel during surgery and the administration of immunosuppressive drugs may play a part (Byer and Shaw 1988b). The volume of feed administered should be decreased or the formula changed to one more suited to malabsorption. If this is unsuccessful, TPN will need to be reintroduced and, at a later stage, tolerance to food tested by oral challenge.

Infants The choice of an oral feed is dependent upon the age of the child and on the type of feed utilized pre-transplant.

The oral feed of choice for infants is a highly modified formula such as Premium (Cow & Gate Nutricia) or SMA Gold Cap (Wyeth). Medium chain triglyceride rich formulas such as Pregestimil (Mead Johnson), Pepti Junior (Cow & Gate Nutricia), or the specific paediatric hepatic feed Generaid Plus (Scientific Hospital Supplies) are utilized only if the child is intolerant to a highly modified formula, displays a transient lactose intolerance or if malabsorption was a major problem prior to transplant. The MCT formulae are continued until liver function tests normalize and diarrhoea settles, at which time the child can be switched to a highly modified formula. In practice, few children prove to be intolerant to standard formulae and their use produces a much needed boost to a child's parents as they see their child take 'normal' foods, probably for the first time.

Young children Young children are encouraged to take ordinary cows' milk and diet. Should lactose intolerance or pre-transplant malabsorption prove a problem, the procedure described in the previous paragraph is followed. Frequently, poor oral intake is supplemented with overnight infusions of specialized paediatric enteral formulas such as Paediasure (Ross) or Nutrison Paediatric (Cow & Gate Nutricia), or with standard adult formulae modified to provide the appropriate ratio of protein and energy. The older child is particularly well tolerant of formulae providing 1.5 kcal/ml.

Progression to normal diet

The ultimate nutritional aim in paediatric liver transplantation is to return the child to a diet that is normal for his or her age. This transition often proves to be an extremely long and stressful process, particularly for the child's parents.

Accepting the fact that pre-occupation with weight gain, nasogastric feeding and strict sodium restrictions are no longer necessary post-transplant, is a difficult process for parents. However, once this is understood the opposite problem is encountered. Parents, on realizing that their child can eat normally, expect the process to happen immediately after the transplant and often get distressed at the length of time the child takes to adapt a normal eating pattern.

Many children have never exhibited hunger, and indeed many have delayed feeding development, having been dependent upon nasogastric feeding for so long. When this is the case, particularly in biliary atresia patients, the skills of a speech therapist can be of great benefit.

The child is encouraged to take a regular meal pattern with frequent high energy snacks. Crisps, chocolate and sweets do have a short term part to play at this stage and are not actively discouraged.

Meals and fluids should be routinely supplemented with energy supplements and parents should be given appropriate guidance. On discharge the majority of children return home on normal diets with no additional formulations. Some younger children still require energy supplements, but these are invariably removed after one to two months.

Those children with delayed feeding development often improve rapidly at home.

Useful address

Children's Liver Disease Foundation (CHILD), 138 Digbeth, Birmingham B5 6DR.

Further reading

Christie ML, Sack DM, Pomposelli J and Horst D (1985) Enriched branched chain amino acid formula versus a casein based supplement in the treatment of cirrhosis. *J Parenter Enter Nutr* **9**, 671–8.

Fitzgerald JF (1988) Cholestatic disorders of infancy. *Pediatr Clin North Am* **35**(2), 357–73.

Hehir DJ, Jenkins RL, Bistrian BR and Blackburn GL (1985) Nutrition in patients undergoing orthotopic liver transplantation. *J Parent Ent Nutr* **9**, 695–700.

Novak DA, Balistreri WF (1985) Management of the child with chronic cholestasis. *Paediatric Annals* **14**(7), 488–92.

Singer JC (1990) Alagille's Syndrome – information for patients and their families. Children's Liver Disease Foundation 40–42 Stoke Road, Guildford. GU1 4HS

Smith J, Horowitz J, Henderson JM and Heymsfield S (1982) Enteral hyperalimentation in under nourished patients with cirrhosis and ascites. *Am J Clin Nutr* **35**, 56–72.

References

Achord JL (1988) Nutrition in liver disease. *Current Opinion in Gastroenterology* **4**, 499–505.

Addenbrooke's Hospital Children's Liver Transplantation Protocol (March 1990).

Alagille D (1985) Management of paucity of interlobular bile ducts. *J Hepatol* **1**, 561.

Byer SW and Shaw BW Jr (1988a) Liver transplantation therapy for children, Part I. *J Paed Gast Nutr* **7**, 157–66.

Byer SW and Shaw BW Jr (1988b) Liver transplantation therapy for children, Part II. *J Paed Gast Nutr* **7**, 797–815.

Charlton CPJ, Buchanan E, Holden C *et al* (1992) Intensive enteral feeding in advanced cirrhosis: reversal of malnutrition without precipitation of hepatic encephalopathy. *Arch Dis Childh* **67**(5), 603–7.

Cohen MI and Gartner LM (1971) The use of medium chain triglycerides in the management of biliary atresia. *J Paedit* **79**, 379–84.

Goulet OJ *et al* (1987) Preoperative nutritional evaluation and support for liver transplantation in children. *Transplant Proceedings* **19**, 3249–55.

Grant A and Todd E (1987) *Enteral and parenteral nutrition*. Blackwell Scientific Publications, Oxford.

Kauffman SS, Murray ND, Wood RP, Shaw BW Jr and Vanderhoof JA (1987) Nutritional support for the infant with extrahepatic biliary atresia. *J Paediat* **110**, 679–86.

Keohane PP, Attrill H, Grimble G, Spuler R, Frost P and Suk DBA (1983) Enteral nutrition in malnourished patients with hepatic cirrhosis and acute encephalopathy. *J Parent Ent Nutr* **7**, 346–50.

Kubota A, Okada A, Nezu R, Kamata S, Imura K and Takagi Y (1988) Hyperbilirubinaemia in neonates associated with total parenteral nutrition. *J Parent Ent Nutr* **12**(6), 602–6.

McCullough AJ, Mullen KD, Smanik EJ, Mousah Tabbaa and Szauter K (1989) Nutritional therapy and liver disease. *Gast Clin N America* **3.18**(3), 619–43.

Mieli-Vergani G, Howard ER, Portman B and Mowat AP (1989) Late referral for biliary atresia – missed opportunities for effective surgery. *Lancet* **1**, 421–23.

Morrison SA, Russel RM, Carney EA and Oause V (1978) Zinc deficiency: a cause of abnormal dark adaption in cirrhotics. *Am J Clin Nutr* **31**, 276.

Mowat AP (1987) *Liver disorders in childhood*. 2e. Butterworths, London.

Ohi R, Hanamatsu M, Mochizuki I, Chiba T and Kasai M (1985) Progress in the treatment of biliary atresia. *World J Surg* **9**, 285–93.

Pierro A, Koletzko B, Carnielli V, Superina RA, Roberts EA, Filler RM, Smith J and Heim T (1989) Resting energy expenditure is increased in infants and children with extrahepatic biliary atresia. *J Pediatr Surg* **24**(6), 534–38.

Silverberg M and Davidson M (1970) Nutritional requirements of infants and children with liver disease. *Am J Clin Nutr* **23**, 604–613.

Sokol RJ and Stall C (1990) Anthropometric evaluation of children with chronic liver disease. *Am J Clin Nutr* **52**, 203–8.

Stuart S, Kaufman SS, Scivner DJ and Guest JE (1989) Preoperative evaluation, preparation, and timing of orthotopic liver transplantation in the child. *Seminars in Liver Disease* **9**(3), 176–83.

Suita S, Ikeda K *et al* (1987) Zinc status and its relations to growth retardation in children with biliary atresia. *J Pediatr Surg* **XXII**(5), 401–405.

Walshe JM (1990) Wilson's disease (hepatocellular degeneration). *Research Trust for Metabolic Diseases in Children Newsletter* **3**(4), 9–11.

Weber A and Roy CC (1972) The malabsorption associated with chronic liver disease in children. *Pediatrics* **50**(1), 73–83.

4.13 Renal Disease

The aims of management of the patient with renal failure are to maintain residual renal function, to keep blood chemistry within normal limits and, in the case of children, to promote growth, all with the least possible disruption to family life.

With all patients in renal failure, six aspects of the diet need to be considered:

1 Protein.
2 Sodium.
3 Fluid.
4 Potassium.
5 Phosphorus.
6 Energy.

In addition, the carbohydrate intake may need to be adjusted and the diet must be nutritionally adequate in respect of all other minerals and vitamins. In patients with urinary calculi the intake of calcium, oxalate and vitamins C and D must also be considered. It is therefore clear that each patient must be treated individually according to their prevailing nutritional and clinical requirements, and their biochemical and clinical status carefully monitored.

4.13.1 The nephrotic syndrome (NS)

The nephrotic syndrome has four essential features:

1 Oedema.
2 Proteinuria greater than 5 g/l in adults.
3 Hypoalbuminaemia.
4 Hypercholesterolaemia and hypertriglyceridaemia.

The hypercholesterolaemia is secondary to hypoalbuminaemia (Lewis 1976).

The nephrotic syndrome is not a diagnosis of a particular renal disease and can occur in the following conditions.

Glomerulonephritis (GN) Patients with GN can present with the nephrotic syndrome, an acute nephritic syndrome (facial swelling, haematuria, hypertension and granular casts in the urine), asymptomatic proteinuria or as acute or chronic renal failure (CRF). Fifty per cent of patients on renal replacement therapy have some form of GN as their underlying aetiology. GN can be subdivided into several different types and since the years of Richard Bright (c. 1830) the classification of GN has been the subject of changing concepts. Pathological findings do not always correlate with clinical symptoms (Table 4.37).

Table 4.37 Classification of glomerulonephritis (GN)

Pathological features	Clinical symptoms
Minimal change GN	Most common type of GN in children. Occasionally occurs in adults Selective proteinuria. Good prognosis, rarely progresses to CRF. Usually responds to steroids and/or cyclophosphamide
Membranous GN	May be associated with malaria, malignancy and drugs such as gold and penicillamine. Often progresses to end stage renal failure (ESRF)
Focal sclerosis	Usually progresses to ESRF
Focal and segmental GN	Occasionally presents as nephrotic syndrome. May progress to ESRF
Mesangio-capillary GN	Presents as nephrotic syndrome or acute nephritic symptoms
Mesangio-proliferative GN	This may present with a variety of clinical presentations
Rapidly progressive GN	Rapidly progresses to ESRF. Epithelial crescents in glomeruli seen on biopsy. May be associated following streptococcal infection, polyarteritis nodosa or Wegener's granulomatosis

Renal vein thrombosis This can be a cause or a complication of the nephrotic syndrome.

Systemic lupus erythematosis (SLE) This is a multi-system disease which may present with fever, arthritis, rashes, leucopenia, positive anti-nuclear factor (ANF), positive DNA binding and low complement 3 and complement 4 (C3 and C4). Some patients will develop renal manifestations which usually present initially as the nephrotic syndrome, later progressing to end stage renal failure (ESRF).

Amyloidosis Occasionally patients with amyloidosis will present with the nephrotic syndrome, those who do usually develop ESRF.

Congenital nephrotic syndrome There are several different aetiologies (Barratt 1985).

Clinical presentation of the nephrotic syndrome

The first symptom is usually a rapid increase in body weight (up to 30 kg) due to oedema. In children, facial and abdominal oedema are usual but in adults, leg oedema predominates. White transverse bands develop on the nails if the syndrome becomes chronic.

Patients' urine often froths excessively on micturition owing to the presence of albumin. The proteinuria is caused by an increased permeability of the glomerular basement membrane (GBM) to protein. This may lead to hypoalbuminaemia (the degree of proteinuria and serum albumin levels are only loosely related) and a decreased plasma osmotic pressure causing fluid to be lost from the intravascular spaces thus lowering plasma and blood volumes, cardiac output and blood pressure. This in turn is thought to activate homeostatic responses involving plasma renin and aldosterone which lead to salt and water retention as a secondary response. Many patients with NS do not show the expected drop in plasma volume nor raised plasma aldosterone or renin levels. Dorhout Mees *et al* (1984) suggest there may be some other renal abnormality at glomerular level in addition to a protein leak, such as increased reabsorption of sodium and a possible stimulation of renin which is inappropriate for the requirements of the circulation.

Medical treatment of the nephrotic syndrome

One of the main objectives in treating the nephrotic syndrome is to reduce the oedema using diuretics such as frusemide and bumetanide. These can cause potassium to be excreted in large quantities and patients may need potassium supplementation. Spironolactone, a potassium sparing diuretic, can be used but care must be taken to monitor potassium levels. If the oedema is resistant to diuretics, salt-poor albumin is sometimes administered, but this is very expensive. It acts by temporarily increasing plasma osmotic pressure and producing a diuresis. If haemodialysis facilities are available, ultrafiltration may be used to remove fluid. Too rapid fluid removal may induce acute renal failure. If on biopsy there appears to be vascular damage in the glomeruli, the patient may be anticoagulated and given dipyridamole. Patients with minimal change GN invariably respond to steroids. Patients with other forms of GN, depending on biopsy findings, may be given azathioprine, prednisolone, cyclophosphamide and/or plasmapheresis to try to arrest the destructive process.

Dietary treatment of the nephrotic syndrome

Protein

Traditionally, high protein (>100 g/day), low sodium diets were used, but there is now a general consensus that these diets are not appropriate. High protein diets were used in an attempt to maintain serum albumin concentration (Epstein 1917). However a number of studies have shown that increasing the protein intake merely increases the losses in the urine (Farr 1938) and that maintaining a good energy intake is more important for maintaining a positive nitrogen balance (Blainey 1954; Manos *et al* 1983; Kaysen *et al* 1986; Mansy *et al* 1989).

Manos *et al* (1983) were able to achieve a positive nitrogen balance on diets containing 1 g protein/kg ideal body weight (IBW) and 200 kcal (840 kJ) per gram of dietary nitrogen. Kaysen *et al* (1986) compared two isocaloric diets providing 0.8 g protein/kg/IBW/day and 1.6 g protein/kg/IBW/day in nine patients. Albumin synthesis was greater on the higher protein intake but so was the proteinuria. Average plasma albumin increased on the lower protein diet due to a decrease in protein losses into the urine. Mansy *et al* (1989) found similar results in 12 patients following low, normal and high protein diets. They advocated abandoning high protein diets and suggested that, pending the results of long term trials of protein restricted diets, a normal diet containing 1 g protein/kg ideal body weight should be recommended.

A low protein diet (0.6 g protein/kg ideal body weight/day) may be indicated in those patients in whom progressive renal failure has developed, as indicated by a serum creatinine of 400–500 μmol/l. Regular follow up of these patients is essential to ensure both protein and energy intakes are as prescribed.

Sodium

Sodium restriction used to play a central role in the management of the oedema associated with nephrotic syndrome, however, the use of more powerful diuretics now makes this unnecessary in the majority of patients. A 'No Added Salt Diet' is now generally advised, particularly in those patients who are also advised to limit their fluid intake.

Energy

Malnourished patients should be encouraged to consume a minimum of 35 kcal (146 kJ)/kg ideal body weight/day. Those in an acute phase of their illness have poor appetites and may need sip feeds or high energy drinks in order to achieve this. Patients on long term steroid therapy may need to limit their energy intake once they go into remission to prevent unwanted flesh weight gain.

Lipids

Hyperlipidaemia is present in most nephrotic patients and total serum cholesterol and triglyceride levels may be considerably elevated. The magnitude of the hyperlipidaemia is related to the albumin concentration (Appel 1985) but its pathogenesis is incompletely understood.

The degree of atherosclerotic risk as a consequence of the hyperlipidaemia is uncertain but it seems sensible to advise patients to modify their fat intake by using polyunsaturated fats and reducing their intake of saturated fats.

The effectiveness of such a diet in reducing hyperlipidaemia in nephrotic patients, however, has not been investigated.

4.13.2 Acute renal failure (ARF)

ARF is a syndrome in which the kidneys are unable to excrete the products of metabolism. This leads to a rapid increase in serum urea and creatinine concentrations in patients with previously normal renal function. Urine output in the majority (98%) of cases drops to less than 400 ml/day and the patient is classed as oliguric. If urine production ceases altogether, the patient is termed anuric. Occasionally patients who present with ARF maintain or even increase urine output (Polyuric ARF). Some patients with ARF may have acute tubular necrosis (ATN). Patients may occasionally be in ARF for as long as six weeks.

Causes of ARF

Many patients will have more than one possible cause:
1 Shock, dehydration leading to hypotension, e.g. accidents, surgery or gastrointestinal bleeding.
2 Impaired vascular supply, e.g. renal artery thrombosis or aortic aneurysms.
3 Drugs and poisons, e.g. antibiotics, aminoglycosides, carbon tetrachloride, ethylene glycol, paraquat and paracetamol.
4 Intravascular coagulation, e.g. septicaemia or post-partum ARF.
5 Haemolysis (transfusion reactions or drugs).
6 Myoglobinuria (traumatic and non-traumatic).
7 Intrinsic renal disease.
8 Obstruction, e.g. bilateral renal calculi, bilateral papillary necrosis or malignancy (such as cancer of the cervix or bladder).

Treatment of ARF – General principles

This will depend on the facilities available, the aetiology of ARF and the clinical condition of the patient. In the past, the high morbidity and mortality rates were related to infections and inadequate nutrition and negative nitrogen balance often resulted from unnecessarily restricted protein intakes.

Immediate treatment of ARF

1 If the ARF is due to dehydration, rehydration of the patient using intravenous fluids is essential. In dehydration the urinary sodium concentration will be <20 mmol/l. Patients who, after volume repletion, have a low cardiac output may benefit from a dopamine infusion. If there is no response to all these measures it is likely that ARF has become established.
2 Hyperkalaemia. This is managed initially by administering glucose and insulin intravenously which temporarily pushes potassium back into the cells. Dialysis is needed to remove it. Exchange resins (such as resonium A and calcium resonium) given rectally or orally can reduce further absorption of potassium from the gastrointestinal tract but act slowly and thus the enteral or parenteral administration of potassium may need to be restricted.
3 Obstruction. This must be relieved by either surgical means or pericutaneous nephrostomies.

Long term management of ARF

Patients with ARF can be divided into three groups according to the degree of catabolism of their underlying disease (Lee 1980) (Table 4.38). Normocatabolic patients (Group A), e.g. patients with obstructive uropathy or drug reaction, may be managed conservatively with a protein and fluid restricted diet, while catabolic patients (Group B), e.g. post-surgery and hypercatabolic patients, (Group C) e.g. multiple trauma, or road traffic accident victims, will need a high protein diet and some form of renal replacement therapy. The type of replacement therapy used will depend on the needs of the patients and the facilities available.

Replacement therapy in ARF

Acute peritoneal dialysis

This can be performed on a general medical or surgical ward as it requires little specialist equipment. A rigid catheter is placed into the peritoneal cavity through a stab incision; 1–2 litres of dialysate is run in and left to dwell for 10–15 minutes and then drained out. Cycles are carried out continuously for several days. Fluid is removed by osmosis and waste metabolites (e.g. urea, creatinine, potassium) by diffusion. Protein and amino acids also lost into the dialysis effluent to the extent of 25 g protein and 15 g of amino acids per 40 litres of dialyses exchange (i.e. per day) (Lee 1980) and a high protein diet is therefore required. Some of the glucose from the dialysate will be absorbed and this must be considered when estimating

Table 4.38 Classification of patients with acute renal failure

Group	Daily blood urea rise (mmol/l*)	Protein breakdown (g N/day)
A Normocatabolic (ARF usually due to 'medical' causes)	4–8	10–14
B Moderately raised catabolism ('surgical')	8–12	14–24
C Hypercatabolic (severe multiple trauma/septicaemia)	>12	>24

* Gastrointestinal bleeds may make these figures invalid

energy requirements. Peritoneal dialysis is less efficient than haemodialysis and is therefore used for less catabolic patients.

Continuous haemofiltration

The use of continuous haemofiltration as a method of renal replacement therapy is increasingly being carried out in intensive care units in District General Hospitals. Vascular access is required, using either a shunt or subclavian catheter so that blood can be passed through a filter, placed beside the patient's bed. Fluid is removed by ultrafiltration and the waste products dissolved in the plasma are dragged across the membrane of the filter with the fluid flow i.e. by convection. Large volumes of fluid (3–20 litres) are removed daily which gives ample space to feed patients adequately with either enteral or parenteral feeds. Unfortunately haemofiltration is unable to clear the toxic waste production of hypercatabolic patients who may need occasional haemodialysis as well. Alternatively, continuous haemodialysis may be used which combines the simultaneous use of filtration and dialysis.

There is a small loss of amino acids in all forms of filtration. Large losses of electrolytes can occur which may need replacing in enteral/parenteral feeds.

Haemodialysis

Haemodialysis (see Section 4.13.3, Subsection on 'Replacement therapy in CRF') provides the most rapid clearance of waste products from the body and is used for the most hypercatabolic patients. Daily or alternate day dialysis is required to remove waste products and allow adequate fluid space for enteral or parenteral feeding.

Intermittent haemofiltration

See the paragraphs on this subject in the subsection on 'Replacement therapy in CRF' (Section 4.13.3).

Dietary treatment of ARF

Normocatabolic patients (Group A)

These patients can usually be managed conservatively (i.e. no replacement therapy). Some patients with urological obstruction recover renal function rapidly once the obstruction is relieved and may require no dietary intervention.

Protein Patients in this group are non-catabolic so they can be managed on a diet providing 0.6–0.7 g protein (70% high biological value)/kg ideal body weight/day. This should prevent an excessive rise in blood urea level. A lower protein intake is not recommended as it will inevitably lead to negative nitrogen balance.

Sodium The intake will depend on the patient's state of hydration. Patients who are oedematous, anuric or oliguric will require a fluid restriction and foods with a high sodium content should be avoided as they will exacerbate thirst. Sodium intake should also be reduced if the patient is hypertensive. Sodium should not be restricted if the patient is polyuric.

Fluid Once the fluid balance has been corrected, the daily fluid allowance is normally 500 ml plus the equivalent of the previous day's urine output and gastrointestinal losses. It is important that the patient is weighed daily to check fluid balance.

Potassium The intake should normally be reduced to 0.6–0.7 mmol/kg ideal body weight/day unless serum levels are below 4.5 mmol/l. Some polyuric patients may not need a restriction.

Phosphate Intake will normally need to be limited to 700 mg/day. This will automatically be achieved with the protein restriction advocated.

Energy A minimum of 35 kcal (146 kJ)/kg ideal body weight/day should be consumed. Glucose polymers or Duocal (SHS) may be added to drinks and puddings to help achieve this and glucose drinks such as Hycal, Lucozade (Smith Kline Beecham) encouraged within the fluid allowance. Patients should be encouraged to suck boiled sweets and eat low protein biscuits between meals. Anorexic patients may require sip feeding using feeds with a relatively low protein but high energy content such as Fortisip (Cow & Gate Nutricia) or Fresubin (Fresenius). Occasionally nasogastric feeding may be necessary (see the subsection below on 'Enteral Feeding in ARF').

Dietary restrictions are usually relaxed once renal function begins to recover. If however serum urea and creatinine levels continue to rise on this therapy, or if the patient becomes fluid overloaded, some form of replacement therapy will be needed. Protein requirements will increase with all types of replacement therapy and intakes must be adjusted accordingly. In this case treat as Type B patients.

Catabolic and hypercatabolic patients (Groups B and C)

These patients will need replacement therapy and the type used will govern the amount of nutritional support given. Only a few patients in groups B and C will be able to meet their nutritional requirements from normal foods; the majority will require either enteral or parenteral feeding. Ileus of the gastrointestinal tract is frequent and results in the need for parenteral nutrition. Many patients have concurrent respiratory failure and will require artificial ventilation.

The first priority when a patient in either category is admitted is to decide on a method of replacement therapy and insert either a peritoneal dialysis catheter or establish vascular access for renal replacement therapy and administering drugs, blood and albumin. A line for feeding may also be needed. The patient's fluid balance will need to be corrected before nutritional support can be given.

Protein/nitrogen Low protein diets do not play a role in the management of these patients. A high protein intake is required because of the catabolism resulting from the underlying disease coupled with the protein losses due to peritoneal dialysis or the catabolic effect of haemodialysis (Feinstein and Massry 1988). Nitrogen requirements can be calculated using standard formulae but care must be taken that excessive nitrogen is not given leading to unnecessary urea generation and its consequent osmotic and uraemic effects (Raman 1990). The majority of patients in Group B will need 0.2 g N (1.2 g protein)/kg ideal body weight/day, while those in Group C will need 0.3 g N (1.8 g protein)/kg ideal body weight/day. However, an upper limit of 20 g N/day has been suggested as the liver is unable to metabolize more than this (Allison 1984).

Sodium The amount needed will depend on the clinical state of the patient and mode of replacement therapy. Patients on haemodialysis generally require 50–100 mmol/day while patients on haemofiltration may require 150–240 mmol/day.

Fluid This needs to be sufficient for adequate nutrition. There is usually no problem if the patient is on continuous haemofiltration but patients on haemodialysis may need more frequent dialysis in order to permit adequate enteral (minimum 1–1.5 l) or parenteral (minimum 2 l) feeds.

Potassium Serum levels will indicate requirements. Some conditions result in pronounced hyperkalaemia, e.g. rhabdomyolysis where muscle breakdown releases potassium into the serum, while other conditions, e.g. gastrointestinal fistula, may cause potassium loss and hypokalaemia. The type of replacement therapy will also affect requirements. With haemodialysis, requirements range from 20–80 mmol/day while with haemofiltration 80–180 mmol/day may be needed. The higher intakes are generally used as patients recover and become anabolic.

Phosphate Hyperphosphataemia is a problem initially but low levels can occur once haemodialysis or more particularly haemofiltration is established and the patient becomes anabolic. Requirements vary from 0–50 mmol/day.

Energy An adequate energy intake is vital to prevent further catabolism. Energy balance has been correlated with the outcome of ARF (Feinstein *et al* 1981; Mault 1983). The average metabolic rate in AFR is stated to be 20–60 per cent above normal (Mault 1983; Raman 1990). A minimum of 35 kcal (146 kJ/kg)/kg ideal body weight is recommended (see Parenteral Feeding in ARF, below).

Vitamins Water-soluble vitamins are lost during dialysis and should therefore be prescribed but caution should be used with vitamin C as large doses may cause oxalosis in ARF (Friedman *et al* 1983). Fat-soluble vitamins (except vitamin K) are not required (Feinstein and Massry 1988).

Parenteral feeding in ARF (Groups B and C)

Nutrients

Nitrogen source An amino acid solution containing a well balanced profile of both essential and non-essential amino acids (e.g. Vamin, Kabi Pharmacia) should be used. Some studies have claimed that specific solutions of essential amino acids are necessary in ARF (Solossol *et al* 1978; Cerra *et al* 1982), but these claims have not been substantiated. It is thought that some non-essential amino acids may become essential in the hypercatabolic patient as the liver may not be capable of adequate amino acid synthesis (Raman 1990). If fluid space is a problem, using a solution which has 9 or 12 g nitrogen/500 ml may be advantageous. Note must be made of the electrolyte content of the solutions used and if necessary an electrolyte free solution chosen.

Energy Ideally this should come from a mixture of lipid and glucose. A maximum of 2000 kcal (8400 kJ)/day should be provided by glucose as quantities above this can result in excessive carbon dioxide production and cause problems in ventilated patients. Glucose absorbed from dialysate fluid, and glucose present in haemofiltration replacement fluid should be included in the calculations.

Lipid clearance is impaired in ARF (Drumal *et al* 1983) and blood clearance of lipids should be checked. Quantities above 500 ml 20% Intralipid (Kabi Pharmacia)/day should be used with caution. Propolol (Diprovan) is a sedative increasingly being used in intensive care units. It is administered as a 10% lipid IV infusion at 10–50 ml/hour. Patients on this drug must have the energy and lipid provided by it included their daily calculated intake.

Minerals Most patients will require one vial of Addamel (Kabi Pharmacia) daily. If the patient becomes hypercalcaemic then Addamel can be changed to Additrace (Kabi Pharmacia) which contains no calcium or magnesium. Electrolytes should be supplied according to serum levels and mode of replacement therapy.

Vitamins Water-soluble vitamins (e.g. one vial Solivito N, Kabi Pharmacia) should be given daily. Fat-soluble vitamins (except vitamin K, 10 mg of which is usually given weekly IM) are not normally required until recovery phase (Feinstein and Massry 1988).

Administration

Ideally TPN should be given as a 'Big Bag' as this allows all the nutrients to be given at an equal rate and reduces the need for insulin. Administering the lipid slowly over 24 hours is less likely to cause problems such as obstructed haemofilters and will reduce the incidence of impaired lipid clearance.

Enteral feeding in ARF (Groups A, B and C)

The composition of the feed will depend on the frequency and type of replacement therapy. Patients treated conservatively may have a fluid restriction of one litre per day and therefore require a concentrated feed. This should be given through a feeding pump over at least 18 hours with the concentration increasing to 2 kcal (9 kJ)/ml over several days. 1.5 kcal/ml commercial feeds can be modified by adding a fat emulsion such as Calogen (SHS) or a neutral liquid glucose polymer or Duocal (SHS). There are amino acid mixtures marketed specifically for patients with renal failure, but these have a high osmotic load. It is doubtful whether they have any advantage over conventional feeds (Lee 1980). Patients on replacement therapy can usually be managed successfully on a normal commercial feed choosing the one with the most appropriate electrolyte content. However a new feed, Nepro (Ross) has recently been introduced for feeding dialysis patients. It contains 2 kcal/ml and has a moderately high protein, low potassium content.

Oral food/sip feeding

Great care must be taken to make sure the patient's nutritional intake is adequate. Many patients will not have eaten anything for several weeks, are frequently anorexic and/or nauseated and taste thresholds may be affected. Supplements will be essential and the most useful are those providing 1.5 kcal/ml with a relatively low phosphate content (e.g. Fortisip, Cow & Gate Nutricia). Individual care plans incorporating any food the patient will actually consume are necessary and daily food records should be kept to assess progress.

Diuretic (recovery) phase of ARF

As renal function improves dietary restrictions may be lifted and replacement therapy phased out. Nutritional support is still vital as most patients will have lost muscle mass due to catabolism. Extra electrolytes will probably be required as well as an increased fluid intake.

Monitoring

Serum biochemistry This should be monitored daily to enable appropriate adjustments to be made to parenteral/ enteral nutrition.

Anthropometric measurements These are of limited use in acutely ill patients as they are difficult or impossible to do accurately.

Complications

Protein malnutrition will occur if catabolic patients are put on low protein diets.

Muscle loss is almost inevitable in hypercatabolic patients as it is impossible to meet their requirements.

4.13.3 Chronic renal failure (CRF)

CRF is the irreversible destruction of kidney tissue by disease, eventually resulting in the death of the patient if not treated by dialysis, haemofiltration or transplantation. CRF has a variety of aetiologies, the most common of which are listed in Table 4.39.

The treatment of CRF can be divided into several types: conservative management (i.e. prior to needing renal replacement therapy), dialysis, haemofiltration and transplantation. Dietary treatment is discussed in detail in each section but is summarized in Table 4.40.

Conservative management of CRF

This is usually a combination of medical and dietary treatment depending on the clinical state of the patient at time of referral and the preferences of the consultant in charge. Policies vary widely. Some patients are referred at a relatively early stage in the course of CRF whilst others may not present until requiring urgent dialysis treatment, either in end stage renal failure or during an 'acute on chronic' episode.

Table 4.39 Aetiology of chronic renal failure

Glomerulonephritis (GN) — see Table 4.37 for subdivisions
Pyelonephritis (CPN) (reflux nephropathy)
Polycystic disease of the kidney (PCK)
Hypertension
Diabetic nephropathy
Myeloma
Obstruction (stones, prostatic enlargement)
Analgesic nephropathy
Systemic lupus erthymatosis (SLE)
Unknown aetiology

Table 4.40 Dietary management of adults with chronic renal failure

	Protein/day[1]	Sodium/day[2]	Potassium/day[2]	Phosphorus/day[3]	Energy/day[4]	Fluid/day[5]
Conservative management	0.6 g/kg ideal body weight; 70% HBV	Normal unless severe hypertension or fluid overload then no added salt (NAS) (80–100 mmol). Salt losers require an increased intake	Unrestricted unless serum level above normal then reduce to 30–40 mmol. Do not encourage excessive intake.	Restricted to <700 mg (23 mmol)	35 kcal (146 kJ)/kg ideal body weight	Unrestricted unless oedematous or in ESRF and oliguric. Then reduce to 500 ml plus equivalent to previous day's urine output (PDUO)
Haemodialysis	1–1.2 g/kg ideal body weight	Usually NAS (80–100 mmol)	<1 mmol/kg ideal body weight	Restricted to <1000 mg (33 mmol)	35 kcal (146 kJ)/kg ideal body weight. Reduce if obese	500 ml plus equivalent to PDUO
Chronic haemofiltration	1–1.2 g/kg ideal body weight	Usually NAS	<0.8 mmol/kg ideal body weight	Restricted to <1000 mg (33 mmol)	35 kcal (146 kJ)/kg ideal body weight	500 ml plus equivalent to PDUO
Continuous ambulatory peritoneal dialysis (CAPD)	1.2–1.5 g/kg ideal body weight	Usually NAS	Do not encourage excessive intake. May need restricting	Restricted to <1200 mg (40 mmol)	70% absorption of dialysate dextrose therefore reduce to 25–30 kcal/kg ideal body weight. Reduce if obese	700 ml plus equivalent to PDUO
Continuous cyclic peritoneal dialysis (CCPD)	1.2–1.5 g/kg ideal body weight	Usually NAS	Restrict intake on day off CCPD	Restricted to <1200 mg (40 mmol)	As for CAPD	700 ml plus equivalent to PDUO
Long term intermittent peritoneal dialysis (IPD)	1.2–1.5 g/kg ideal body weight on dialysis	Unrestricted on dialysis unless hypertensive	Normal on dialysis	Restricted on dialysis to <1200 mg (40 mmol)	As for CAPD on dialysis	Unrestricted on dialysis unless fluid overloaded
	0.7–0.8 g/kg ideal body weight on inter-dialysis days	Usually NAS on inter-dialysis days	40 mmol/day on inter-dialysis days	Restricted on inter-dialysis days to <700 mg (23 mmol)	35 kcal (146 kJ/kg) ideal body weight on inter-dialysis days	500 ml plus equivalent to PDUO on inter-dialysis days

[1] Section 2.2; [2] Section 2.7.1; [3] Section 2.7.1; [4] Section 2.1; [5] Section 2.9

Medical treatment (conservative management)

Aims of conservative medical management

The aims of conservative medical management are as follows.

1 *To retrieve some or all of the lost renal function by identifying and treating its cause(s)*

- Hypertension. This is both a cause and a complication of CRF. The early treatment of it can slow the progression of renal deterioration or lead to an improvement in renal function.
- Urinary tract infections. These should be treated concurrently.
- Urinary tract abnormalities. These should be corrected wherever possible.
- Iatrogenic causes. The use of certain drugs to treat renal impairment (e.g. tetracyclines, NSAIDs) may lead to a rapid decline in renal function. Some of this loss may be recoverable.
- Dehydration. This may lead to a deterioration in renal function which may be reversible when the patient is rehydrated appropriately.

2 *Correction of acidosis* Acidosis results from the diminished ability of the kidney to excrete hydrogen ions produced from the metabolism of dietary protein. It can contribute to hyperkalaemia and recent evidence suggests that it causes an increase in protein breakdown. Correction may lead to a lowering of serum urea and nitrogen excretion and reduced protein breakdown (Jenkins *et al* 1989a). It is normally corrected in the predialysis patient by giving sodium bicarbonate (Papadoyannakis *et al* 1984). Reducing protein intake will help reduce the acid load.

3 *Prevention of uraemic bone disease* Hyperphosphataemia has been implicated as a possible factor causing progression of renal failure (Maschio *et al* 1982) and some physicians may request a low phosphorus diet. However, the more generally accepted problem is the role of hyperphosphataemia in renal osteodystrophy. When GFR is less than 15 ml/min (normal adult value 60–120 ml/min) hyperphosphataemia is usual and results in hypocalcaemia and

secondary hyperparathyroidism. In order to correct the hyperphosphataemia, a reduction of dietary phosphorus to 600–700 mg (20–23 mmol/day) will be needed (see Section 2.7.2). Patients on a low protein diet will automatically achieve an intake at this level but phosphate binding drugs may also be required to maintain serum phosphate in the desired range (<2 mmol/l and >0.9 mmol/l). Until recently the most common drug used was aluminium hydroxide. However, there is now great concern regarding aluminium intoxication. As well as being a cause of dementia in renal patients, there is evidence implicating aluminium in bone disease (Andres 1990) and it may also lead to a diminished response to recombinant human erythropoietin therapy. A study by Jenkins *et al* (1989b) showed that low dose aluminium hydroxide (<6 Alucaps/day) was not associated with aluminium bone disease. However, the use of aluminium hydroxide has now been stopped by many nephrologists. The most frequently used alternative in the United Kingdom is calcium carbonate (Calcichew, Shire; Titralac, 3M Health Care). The usual dosage is either one Calcichew or three Titralac taken with each protein containing meal. Other phosphate binders, e.g. calcium acetate (Schmitt 1991), calcium citrate (Molitoris *et al* 1989) are being tested but are not yet in routine use. If hypercalcaemia is a problem, patients may benefit from the combined use of calcium carbonate and aluminium hydroxide.

Serum calcium (adjusted to albumin) levels should be maintained within the normal range (2.1–2.6 mmol/l). If serum calcium levels are low, when serum phosphate levels are <2.0 mmol/l, vitamin D should be prescribed. Either 1.25 dihydroxy vitamin D_3 (Calcitriol) or its analogue one-alpha calcidol should be prescribed (0.25 μg bd initially). Serum calcium levels must be monitored as vitamin D overdosage leads to hypercalcaemia.

4 *Correction of anaemia* Normal kidneys produce erythropoietin which stimulates the bone marrow to produce erythrocytes. With loss of renal parenchyma, insufficient erythropoietin is produced and anaemia develops. Haemoglobin levels may fall to 5–7 g/dl. Until recently the only therapy was blood transfusions but the latter given frequently may lead to iron overload. In the past few years recombinant human erythropoietin (r-HuEPO) has become available for use with dialysis patients. This has led to a marked improvement in quality of life with haemoglobin levels maintained around 10 g/dl without iron overload. It is currently on trial in pre-dialysis patients. r-HuEPO therapy's main drawback is cost (between £1000–£4000/patient/year in 1992). Reported side effects include hypertensive encephalopathy and thrombosis of vascular access. Ferritin levels need checking before administration and iron and folate intake may need supplementation (Bennett *et al* 1991). Hyperkalaemia has also been reported.

Monitoring renal function

This can be done in a variety of ways. Both creatinine clearance and glomerular filtration rate (GFR) can be measured but in a clinical setting serum creatinine is the most commonly used indicator. Serum creatinine will remain within the normal range until more than 50% of

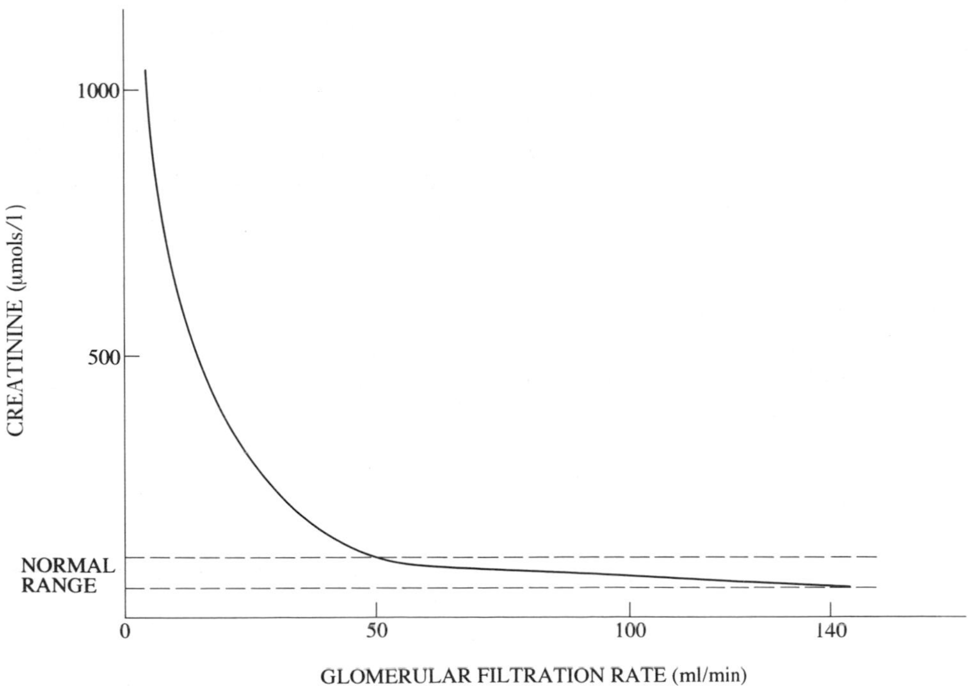

Fig. 4.12 Graph to show rising serum creatinine with decreasing GFR

renal function is lost (see Fig. 4.12). As renal function deteriorates, serum creatinine will start to rise, the rate accelerating as end stage renal failure is reached (creatinine >1000 μmol/l). Serum urea is not a good marker of renal failure as it is affected by diet, drugs (e.g. steroids and tetracyclines), gastrointestinal bleeds, catabolism, blood transfusions and dehydration.

Dietary treatment of patients with CRF (Conservative management)

Aims of conservative nutritional management

The aims of nutritional therapy in the patient managed conservatively are:

1 To maintain or improve nutritional status.
2 To reduce uraemic toxicity.
3 To retard the rate of progression of renal deterioration.

Protein In the 1960s Giovannetti and Maggiore (1964) and Giordano (1963) showed that diets containing 0.24 g protein/kg body weight/day were successful in diminishing symptoms of uraemia and preventing death by reducing protein metabolism to a minimum. The Italian diets were modified by Berlyne *et al* (1966) for use in the UK. These diets were often started in end stage renal failure and many patients went into negative nitrogen balance partly due to their inability to consume the whole diet and meet their high energy requirements.

By the mid 1970s, these diets had fallen from favour partly because of the increased availability of dialysis. An editorial in the *British Medical Journal* (1975) stated that 'the imposition of an unpalatable diet solely in an imperious attempt to improve biochemical profile was neither reasonable nor kind'. Thus patients were started on dialysis earlier and dietary management generally only offered to those not selected for replacement therapy. The aim of the diet was palliative, to reduce uraemic symptoms such as vomiting, nausea, pruritus, fatigue, weakness and anorexia and was generally 40 g protein/day.

There has been renewed interest in low protein diets since the early 1980s following Brenner's hyperfiltration theory (Brenner *et al* 1982). Many human studies have suggested that protein restricted diets not only alleviate uraemic symptoms but also markedly reduce the rate of progression of renal disease (Barsoti *et al* 1981; Maschio *et al* 1982; Alvestrand *et al* 1983; Bennett *et al* 1983; El Nahas *et al* 1984; Rosman 1984). However there has been some controversy over how progression of renal failure is measured and whether other factors e.g. frequent clinic visits, improved blood pressure control have also influenced progression. A study by Ihle *et al* (1989) showed that low protein diets (0.4 g/kg body weight/day) were successful in slowing down the progression of renal disease as measured by GFR. A multi-million dollar long term controlled study 'Modification of Diet in Renal Disease' is currently being carried out in the USA sponsored by the National Institute of Health. It was due for completion in 1992 and analysis the following year.

The role of diet in slowing down the progress of CRF remains controversial (El Nahas and Coles 1986) and some nephrologists disagree with it while others advocate it. Where used, it is commonly instigated when serum creatinine levels reach 400–500 μmol/l. The most common level of protein restriction used is 0.6 g protein/kg ideal body weight/day. Kopple and Coburn (1973) showed that patients with CRF maintained on diets containing 0.6 g protein (60–70% HBV)/kg ideal body weight and 37 kcal/kg ideal body weight remained in positive nitrogen balance. This level of protein restriction is well accepted by most patients and has been shown to have no nutritional adverse effects as well as reducing the rate of progression of functional deterioration (Oldrizzo *et al* 1989). These diets have been shown to be almost as effective as very low protein diets (15–20 g of protein/day) supplemented with keto analogues and/or essential amino acids (Hirschberg and Kopple 1988). In this latter dietary strategy, there is no need for the protein to be HBV so the patient is permitted a wider choice of foods containing low quality protein. This approach is therefore considered by some people to be less restrictive but it probably depends on individual patients' preference. The EAA/keto analogues are expensive and many patients find them unpalatable. However the amino acid supplement, Dialamine (SHS), which is orange flavoured, is generally well accepted.

Many patients can be maintained successfully on conservative management for periods of up to ten years, but the rate of progression of renal failure depends on individual factors and the underlying aetiology of the disease.

Sodium and fluid Patients with CRF cannot respond normally to changes in sodium intake. The quantity of sodium excreted each day by patients with CRF is fixed between 60–100 mmol and this amount will continue to be excreted even if dietary sodium is restricted. It is important therefore to prevent negative sodium balance which ultimately leads to dehydration. Some patients are 'salt losers' and require additional sodium which can be given as sodium bicarbonate or sodium chloride. Sodium restriction is necessary only if the patient is oedematous or severely hypertensive. A restriction if required should normally be 60–100 mmol/day. Patients on protein restricted diets will automatically have reduced their sodium intake to some extent.

Most patients with CRF will have nocturia and sometimes polyuria. With the loss of renal parenchyma, the remaining nephrons function under a constant osmotic load and the kidney loses its ability to produce a concentrated urine. It is important that the patient does not become dehydrated. However, in end stage renal failure the urine volume may drop and oedema develop. Fluid intake should then be restricted to 500 ml/day plus the equivalent of the previous day's urine output.

Potassium Potassium levels do not normally rise until end stage renal failure, usually just after the patient starts dialysis. However, a small percentage of patients will develop raised serum potassium levels earlier (>5.5 mmol/l). In most cases this is due to iatrogenic causes such as drugs, especially potassium-sparing diuretics or drugs containing potassium, for example ACE (angiotensin-converting enzyme) inhibitors (e.g. Captopril/Enalapril), some effervescent tablets and most isphagula bulking agents. Blood transfusions and general anaesthesia can also elevate serum potassium and haemolysed blood samples will give falsely elevated results. Excessive dietary intakes of fruit, vegetables and other high potassium foods can also be the cause. Hyperkalaemia (serum K > 6.0 mmol/l) is the most dangerous of all electrolyte disturbances in patients with CRF as untreated it may lead to cardiac arrest.

When a potassium restriction is necessary a dietary history will reveal if there is an obvious cause such as an excessive intake of potatoes, fruit juice, bananas. If not, fruit and vegetables should be restricted to a maximum of two, 4 mmol exchanges of each spaced out during the day. In addition one serving of potatoes can be allowed. The potassium content of potatoes and root vegetables can be reduced by cutting them into $\frac{1}{2}$inch slices and boiling twice (Bower 1989). The cooking water should be thrown away each time. Steaming, roasting, pressure cooking, (stir) frying or microwaving of vegetables should be avoided unless they are par-boiled first, as these methods do not reduce the potassium content significantly. Other high potassium foods should be restricted to give a total intake of 0.6–0.7 mmol/kg ideal body weight/day.

If the patient is not already on a protein restriction then milk, yoghurt and milk-based products e.g. Complan will also need restricting as they are particularly high in potassium. Table 2.35 in Section 2.7.1 lists high potassium foods.

Potassium exchange resins, Calcium Resonium or Resonium A are sometimes given on a short term basis but most patients find them unpalatable and they are expensive.

Phosphorus The protein restriction will automatically reduce phosphorus intake. High phosphorus foods (listed in Table 2.40 Section 2.7.2) should only be taken occasionally. Eggs should be limited to one per day.

Energy In diets providing 30–45 g protein/day, an energy intake of 35–40 kcal (146–158 kJ)/kg ideal body weight is needed to achieve positive nitrogen balance. This can only be achieved by using glucose polymers and prescribable low protein foods (Hadfield 1992). Without these a low protein diet will usually only provide 1200–1500 kcal/day.

Low protein flour can be made into extra 'free' bread, biscuits, cakes and crumbles. The choice of commercially available, low protein biscuits has improved in recent years, the wafer type and low protein crackers being very popular. Low protein pastas are also useful as fillers. Proprietary low protein products are discussed in Section 2.2.7.

Increased variety can be achieved by making custard, blancmange, and milk type puddings with coffee creamers (Coffeemate or Coffee Compliment; $\frac{1}{2}$oz. to 10 fl.oz water or 15 g to 250 ml water). White sauces can be made in a similar way using cornflour or low protein flour instead of ordinary flour. (Recipes can be found in *Enjoying food on a renal diet* edited by M Vennegor.)

Most patients will not eat sufficient low protein foods to meet their energy requirements and therefore an additional 400 kcal should be prescribed as a glucose polymer or glucose drink. Ordinary boiled sweets, barley sugars and glacier mints are also good sources of energy, as are fizzy drinks (most of which are low in potassium).

A large percentage of patients with CRF will have hyperlipidaemia and therefore it is unwise to encourage an excessive intake of animal fat. Cholesterol intake will automatically be lowered by the protein restriction. Many patients will use corn oil for frying and polyunsaturated fat for cooking (White Flora shortens low protein pastry) and most will use a margarine high in polyunsaturated fat instead of butter, but some double cream does help the palatability of the diet.

Obese patients should be given a diet containing approximately 1500 kcal (1250 kJ)/day. Strict reducing diets will lead to catabolism and a rise in serum urea levels and they should not be used until the patient is on dialysis.

Fibre Wholemeal bread is normally encouraged within the protein allowance. Bran should be used with caution as the absorption of potassium and phosphorus from it varies between patients. If patients are constipated small amounts of bran enriched foods should be allowed but serum levels of potassium and phosphate must be monitored. Fluid should be encouraged, unless on a fluid restriction.

Vitamins and minerals There are no clear guidelines for supplementation but a recent report suggests that intakes of iron, calcium, zinc, thiamin riboflavin and folate are borderline on a low protein diet and should be supplemented (Hadfield 1992).

Monitoring dietary treatment

It is important that patients who are advised to follow low protein diets are seen regularly so that biochemistry can be assessed, and any necessary changes in the diet (such as potassium intake) made. The importance of adhering to the diet should be reinforced regularly and patients given help and encouragement to follow what can be a monotonous regimen.

Serum biochemistry can be used to check compliance. The ratio of urea : creatinine is individual for each patient but should fall on commencing a low protein diet. An increase in the ratio may indicate poor compliance but steroids or catabolic states may also lead to an increase. Since the main sources of phosphate in the diet are protein foods, an elevated serum phosphate may be an indicator of poor compliance and warrant further investigation.

Protein catabolic rate (PCR) can be calculated if an accurate 24 hour urine specimen can be collected for urea estimation at the same time as a serum urea measurement is made (Wendland 1987).

Complications of dietary management

Protein malnutrition Serum albumin, protein and transferrin levels should be checked regularly. If any are low or falling, assess whether the patient is consuming an adequate energy intake and that he or she is not reducing protein intake below 0.6 g protein/kg ideal body weight/day.

Weight loss Many patients have difficulty in maintaining an adequate energy intake. Serial mid-arm circumference measurements are useful in assessing whether a change in weight is due to fluid or flesh loss or gain (Bennett *et al* 1986) since patients with CRF can easily become dehydrated or oedematous.

Hyperkalaemia This can result from patients eating large quantities of fruit and vegetables, or drugs (see the paragraph on Potassium above).

Dehydration If a sodium restriction is imposed unnecessarily, dehydration can occur.

Replacement therapy in CRF

Haemodialysis and haemofiltration

Haemodialysis (HD) Major advances have taken place with dialysis equipment with increased use of microprocessor technology. Most artificial kidneys are now disposable although they are often reused for economy. Many of the membranes used are 'high flux' allowing dialysis hours to be reduced to three 2–5 hour sessions instead of the normal 4–5 hours three times a week. A few units still use two 6-hour dialysis sessions a week.

The process of haemodialysis requires the transport of blood and dialysate on either side of a semi-permeable membrane. Products of metabolism, e.g. urea, creatinine, potassium, phosphorus, are removed by diffusion and fluid by convection (ultrafiltration) through the semi-permeable membrane. Normal serum levels of calcium, sodium, magnesium and chloride are maintained by regulating the level of ions in the dialysis fluid.

Blood access is normally achieved by creating an arterio-venous fistula in the arm, by joining an artery and vein together. This must be done several weeks before dialysis is needed. When dialysis is necessary two needles are inserted in the fistula and blood is pumped from the body through the dialyser and then returned to the patient. Subclavian catheters or arterio-venous shunts provide temporary access and can be used immediately.

Machine intermittent haemofiltration (HFM) In haemofiltration, blood is pumped from the body in a similar manner to HD but instead of passing through an artificial kidney it passes through a haemofilter. Fluid is removed by ultrafiltration and metabolic breakdown products are dragged through the membrane at the same time by convection. Replacement fluid is required to maintain blood volume. There is a large fluid exchange of 20–30 litres. A machine with a microprocessor controls the accurate balancing and monitoring systems which are needed. HFM is more expensive than HD and is normally reserved for those patients who do not tolerate HD, e.g. those with severe cardiovascular problems.

Dietary management of haemodialysis patients

Patients on regular haemodialysis therapy need to adhere to some dietary and fluid restrictions to prevent the build up of protein metabolites, phosphate, potassium and fluid between each dialysis.

Protein Most patients are allowed 1–1.2 g protein/kg ideal body weight/day of which 70% should be from HBV sources. This increase in the recommended protein intake compared to the predialysis patient is to make up for the small loss of amino acids during dialysis and the catabolism resulting from the dialysis (Alvestrand 1988).

The diet for a 65 kg man would be made up of 7×7 g or 8×6 g protein exchanges plus cereal based protein. The latter is not normally restricted as long as it is low in potassium and phosphate. The other dietary restrictions needed (e.g. potassium and phosphate) will also limit the type of HBV protein exchanges taken. No more than two should come from dairy produce. The protein should be spaced out over the day.

Sodium This is normally restricted to control thirst and hypertension. A 'no added salt' diet (80–100 mmol/day) is generally used even in those with severe hypertension in whom drugs rather than very low sodium diets are generally advocated. A list of foods high in sodium is given in Section 2.7.1, Table 2.31.

A few patients may not need a sodium restriction if they continue to pass good urine volumes. Foods with a high sodium but low potassium content e.g. bacon, low potassium snack foods, Oxo, are normally allowed during dialysis as they can help prevent cramps and hypotension.

Fluid In order to prevent pulmonary oedema and hypertension, it is important that the inter-dialytic weight gain is kept below 2 kg and preferably nearer to 1 kg. In small patients this may need to be even less. In adults a daily fluid allowance of 500 ml plus that equivalent to the amount of urine passed the previous day will prevent fluid overload.

Patients should be reminded of the hidden sources of fluid in foods such as jelly, custard, soups and gravies. The patient can be given useful hints to limit fluid intake, e.g. using a smaller cup or sucking an ice cube instead of having a drink. During hot weather, pyrexia, or diarrhoea and vomiting, an increased fluid allowance will be needed.

Potassium The risk of hyperkalaemia is high. Potassium intake should be restricted to 1 mmol/kg ideal body weight/day. This can be achieved by avoiding very high potassium foods, restricting fruit and vegetables to 2 × 4 mmol exchanges of each/day and keeping to the prescribed protein intake for HD. (See under Potassium restriction (p. 425) in the section on Conservative management above for further information.)

Patients should be discouraged from eating high potassium foods during dialysis since, due to its short duration, immediate post dialysis potassium levels may be acceptable, only to rise later when the potassium is absorbed (a large proportion from the large bowel).

Phosphorus Dietary phosphorus restriction is becoming increasingly important due to problems of toxicity being encountered with phosphate binders (see under 'Aims of conservative medical management in Section 4.13.3, CRF). Intake should be <1000 mg (33 mmol)/day in order to prevent hyperphosphataemia. The main source of dietary phosphorus are the protein foods (especially milk, cheese, egg yolks, offal and tinned fish) and most raising agents. These foods should be restricted or avoided.

Energy An intake of 35 kcal (146 kJ)/kg ideal body weight is recommended for the majority of patients. Approximately 70% of dialysis patients have lipid abnormalities (Golper 1984) and cardiovascular disease remains a major cause of death in the dialysis population. Patients should therefore be encouraged to use polyunsaturated margarine rather than butter and to use a polyunsaturated oil when cooking. Animal sources of saturated fat will be already limited by the phosphorus restriction.

Overweight patients should be encouraged to lose flesh weight but most will encounter difficulties as there are few foods they can fill up on and fluid must be restricted. Patients who are underweight or who are acutely ill may need energy supplements such as glucose polymers (for further advice see under Acute Renal Failure). If appetite is poor, sip feeds may be needed, e.g. Fortisip which provides 1.5 kcal/ml. Care must be taken with the potassium and phosphorus content of sip feeds. Although a 'free' diet may, in theory, encourage an increased nutritional intake in the malnourished patient, in practice it leads to the consumption of 'forbidden' foods low in energy but high in potassium, salt and water. Time spent giving patients individualized advice is likely to be more beneficial than free choice.

Fibre Some wholemeal bread should be included in the diet and most patients will tolerate 4 slices without it having an adverse effect on serum potassium and phosphate levels. However bran and bran-enriched foods should be avoided.

Vitamins and minerals It is normal practice to supplement patients with water soluble vitamins i.e. B complex, folic acid and C. 'Leaching' of vegetables to reduce potassium and small dialysis losses lead to a diet deficient in folic acid and containing only borderline amounts of vitamins B_1, B_2, B_6 and C (Bennett *et al* 1985). However large doses of vitamin C should not be given as this can lead to high serum levels of oxalate (Pru *et al* 1985). Iron supplements should be prescribed according to the patients' serum ferritin and iron levels.

Monitoring of haemodialysis patients

Serum biochemistry should be monitored regularly and appropriate action taken as necessary. Urea kinetic modelling can be used to assess protein intake by calculating protein catabolic rate (Wendland 1987; Forrest 1990). Serial anthropometric measurements can be used to identify changes in flesh weight (Bennett *et al* 1986).

Continuous ambulatory peritoneal dialysis (CAPD) and continuous cyclic peritoneal dialysis (CCPD)

Since its conception by Popovich *et al* (1976), the use of CAPD has grown rapidly as a form of renal replacement therapy. It mimics the normal kidney by providing continuous dialysis with steady state biochemistry.

In CAPD a silastic catheter is surgically inserted into the peritoneal cavity. Dialysate is allowed to flow into the peritoneum, allowed to dwell for 4–6 hours and then drained out. Three to five 1.5–3 litre exchanges are carried out each day, the patient being able to follow a normal life between dialysate exchanges. The dialysate contains glucose and small quantities of electrolytes. Excess fluid is removed by osmosis. Several strengths of dialysate are routinely used, 1.36%, 2.27% and 3.86% glucose. The higher glucose concentrations will remove more fluid. Metabolic toxins are removed by diffusion. As the removal is continuous, these patients may have a more liberal intake of certain foods than patients on HD.

In *continuous cyclic peritoneal dialysis (CCPD)* a machine cycles 4–8 exchanges of 1–2 litres of dialysate at night, instead of manual daytime exchanges.

Dietary requirements for CAPD patients

Protein Amino acids, 1.7–3 g/day and protein 5–15 g/day (Blumenkrantz *et al* 1981; Rubin *et al* 1981; Heide *et al* 1983; Sandoz *et al* 1986) are lost into the dialysate effluent. Protein losses increase during peritonitis. If these losses are not compensated, hypoalbuminaemia will result (Bennett *et al* 1990). Studies have shown that a daily protein intake of 1.2–1.5 g/kg ideal body weight is necessary to maintain positive nitrogen balance for patients on CAPD (Kopple and Blumenkranz 1983). Elderly patients, vegetarians and those with a poor appetite often need a protein supplement in order to achieve this. Supplements should be low in phosphorus and relatively concentrated e.g. Maxisorb (SHS), Maxipro (SHS) and Protein Forte (Fresenius). Vipro (SHS) and amino acid supplements such as Dialamine (SHS) may be useful in vegans. During episodes of peritonitis when appetite is reduced, supplements are essential.

Sodium Foods which taste salty should normally be avoided by oliguric patients as they create thirst.

Fluid As it is important to prevent dehydration or fluid overload, weight should be measured daily. Sudden changes in weight reflect changes in fluid balance. A fluid restriction is usually necessary in anuric and oliguric patients. Some patients continue to pass good volumes of urine while others become virtually anuric after 1–2 months on CAPD.

Potassium The risk of hyperkalaemia is lower in CAPD than HD due to continuous dialysis. However some patients will need to restrict their intake, especially if they are on erythropoietin. All patients should be advised to avoid an excessive intake of fruit and vegetables. Patients who have serum potassium levels > 5.5 mmol/l should restrict their intake to 1.2 mmol/kg ideal body weight/day (see Section 2.7.1.)

Phosphorus Uraemic bone disease is a problem in CAPD patients as in other patients undergoing replacement therapy and conservative management for CRF (see above). A dietary phosphorus restriction of <1200 mg (40 mmol)/day will be needed (Kopple and Blumenkrantz 1983). This necessitates limiting milk to 300 ml/day; eggs to one per day and only occasionally eating cheese, offal and shellfish.

Energy Many patients lose weight prior to starting dialysis and may need to regain flesh weight initially. However, continued weight gain should be prevented. The oral energy intake should be reduced to 25 kcal (110 kJ)/kg ideal body weight since the patient will absorb approximately 300 kcal (1250 kJ) daily from isotonic dialysate. Reducing the intake of sugar and sugar-containing foods as well as reducing energy intake will also prevent accelerated hypertriglyceridaemia (Turgan *et al* 1981) but overweight patients may need to reduce energy intake further.

Fibre It is important that constipation is prevented as this can lead to poor dialysate drainage. Patients should be actively encouraged to take wholemeal bread and wholegrain or bran-enriched cereals as part of their diet.

Vitamins and minerals If appetite is normal there is probably no need to supplement water soluble vitamins. However if appetite is poor, or energy intake restricted, a multivitamin supplement should be prescribed. Low vitamin B_{12} levels have been reported (Bennett *et al* 1985) particularly in vegetarians or those on Ranitidine (H_2 antagonist).

Monitoring of CAPD patients

See the section on 'Haemodialysis', above.

Complications of CAPD patients

Hypoalbuminaemia This is likely to occur in severe episodes of peritonitis and other acute illnesses where appetite is reduced. Aggressive nutritional support should be instigated early using high protein supplements, e.g. Protein Forte (Fresenius), Maxisorb (Scientific Hospital Supplies), Fortipudding (Cow and Gate). If sip feeding and oral foods are not tolerated nasogastric feeding using high protein feeds, e.g. Clinifeed Protein Rich (Roussel) should be started. Occasionally, in patients with severe vomiting or ileus, parenteral nutrition becomes essential. Regular nutritional monitoring, with protein supplementation to high risk patients can reduce the incidence of hypoalbuminaemia (Bennett *et al* 1990).

Intermittent peritoneal dialysis (IPD)

IPD has become less common since the introduction of CAPD. Patients on IPD are usually dialysed using hourly exchanges for a period of 48–72 hours once a week. A relatively liberal diet should be encouraged during dialysis ensuring that at least 1.2 g/kg ideal body weight is consumed to compensate for losses into the dialysate. On non-dialysis days, a diet providing 0.7–0.8 g protein and 0.7 mmol potassium/kg ideal body weight/day is normally allowed. Fluid will also need to be restricted off dialysis to

500 ml plus the equivalent of the previous day's urine output. Sodium is restricted to avoid thirst and control blood pressure (approximately 80 mmol/day). Phosphorus intake should be reduced to <800 mg/day.

Transplantation

Patients look forward to a successful kidney transplant with its relative freedom from dietary and fluid restrictions. However, the immunosuppressive therapy given can have multiple metabolic side effects. Prednisolone therapy is associated with obesity, glucose intolerance and hyperlipidaemia whilst hyperkalaemia and hyperlipidaemia may be a problem with cyclosporin A (Hunsicker 1988).

Following transplantation the patient should be encouraged to eat a high protein diet 1.3–1.5 g/kg ideal body weight with 30–35 kcal/kg/day (Hunsicker 1988). This will help negate the protein catabolism of steroid therapy and improve wound healing. A moderate potassium restriction (1 mmol/kg/day) may be necessary.

Once good renal function is established and steroid levels are reduced general healthy eating advice should be given to prevent excessive weight gain and hyperlipidaemia; 60% of transplant patients have hyperlipidaemia (Cramp 1982) which has been shown to respond to dietary therapy (Shen *et al* 1983).

Patients who go on to develop chronic rejection may extend the life of the transplanted kidney by protein restriction (Feehally *et al* 1986).

Further reading

Vennegor M (1982) *Enjoying food on a renal diet.* Oxford University Press, Oxford.

References

Allison SP (1984) Nutritional problems in intensive care. *Hospital Update* Dec, 1001–1002.

Alvestrand A, Ahlberg M, Furst P and Bergstrome J (1983) Clinical results of long term treatment with low protein diet and a new amino acid preparation in patients with chronic uraemia. *Clin Neph* 19(2), 67–73.

Alvestrand A (1988) Nutritional requirements of haemodialysis patients. In *Nutrition and the Kidney*, Mitch W E and Klahr S (Eds) pp. 180–97, Little Brown, Boston/Toronto.

Andress DC (1990) Aluminium bone disease in chronic renal failure. *Seminars in Dialysis* 3(1), 27–9.

Appel GB (1985) The hyperlipidaemia of the nephrotic syndrome: relation to plasma, albumin concentration, oncotic pressure and viscosity. *N Engl J Med* **312**, 1544–8.

Barratt TM (1985) In *Postgraduate Nephrology*, Marsh F (Ed) pp. 467–8. Heinemann Medical, London.

Barsoti G, Guiducci A, Ciardella F and Giovannetti S (1981) Effects on renal function of a low nitrogen diet supplemented with essential amino acids and ketoanalogues and of haemodialysis and free protein supply in patients with chronic renal failure. *Nephron* **27**, 113–117.

Bennett SE, Edmunds M, Feehally J and Walls J (1991) Nutritional status of haemodialysis patients on recombinant human erythropoietin therapy. *J Renal Nutr* **1**(3), 125–9.

Bennett SE, Robinson C and Walls J (1990) Is peritonitis a major factor in protein status in CAPD? *EDTNA ERCA Journal* **8**, 15–17.

Bennett SE, Russell GI and Walls J (1983) Low protein diets in uraemia *Br Med J* **287**, 1344–1345.

Bennett SE, Russell GI and Walls J (1986) Serial anthropometry as an adjunct to the assessment of 'dry' weight in patients receiving dialysis therapy. *Dialysis and Transpl* **15**(3), 148–51.

Bennett SE, Smith BA, Feehally J and Walls J (1985) Vitamin and mineral supplementation in chronic haemodialysis patients. *Proc European Dialysis Transplant Nurses Assoc/European Renal Care Assoc* **14**, 157–61.

Berlyne GM, Janabi KM and Shaw AB (1966) Dietary treatment of chronic renal failure. *Proc Roy Soc Med* **665**, 7.

Blainey JD (1954) High protein diets in the treatment of the nephrotic syndrome. *Clin Sci* **13**, 567.

Blumenkrantz MJ, Gahl GM, Kopple JD, Fauder AV, Jones MR, Kessel M and Coburn JW (1981) Protein losses during peritoneal dialysis. *Kidney Int* **19**, 593–602.

Bower J (1989) Cooking for restricted potassium diets in dietary treatment of renal patients. *J Hum Nutr Diet* **2**(1), 1, 31–38.

Brenner BM, Meyer TW and Hostetter TH (1982) Dietary protein intake and the progressive nature of kidney disease: the role of haemodynamically mediated glomerular injury in the pathogenesis of progressive glomerular sclerosis in ageing, renal ablation and intrinsic renal disease. *N Engl J Med* **307**, 652–9.

British Medical Journal (1975) Editorial: Low protein diets in chronic renal failure. *Br Med J* **iv**, 486.

Cerra FB, Upson D, Angelico R, Wiles C, Lyons J, Faulkenbach L and Paysinger J (1982) Branched chain amino acids support post-operative protein synthesis. *Surgery* **92**, 192–8.

Cramp DG (1982) Plasma lipid alterations in patients with chronic renal disease. *CRC Crit Rev Clin Lab Sci* **17**, 77.

Dorhout Mees EJ, Geers AB and Koomans HA (1984) Blood volume and sodium retention in the nephrotic syndrome. A controversial path of physiological concept. *Nephron* **36**, 201–211.

Drumal W, Laggner A, Widhalm K, Kleinberger G and Levz K (1983) Lipid metabolism in acute renal failure. *Kidney Int* **24**(Suppl 16), S139–S142.

El Nahas AM, Masters-Thomas A, Brady SA, Farrington K, Williamson V, Hilson AJW, Varghese Z and Moorhead J (1984) Selective effect of low protein diets in chronic renal failure. *Br Med J* **289**, 1337–41.

El Nahas AM and Coles GA (1986) Dietary treatment of renal failure; ten unanswered questions. *Lancet* **1**, 597–600.

Epstein AA (1917) Concerning the causation of oedema in chronic parenchymatous nephritis: method for its alleviation. *Am J Med Sci* **54**, 638–47.

Farr LE (1938) The assimilation of protein by young children with the nephrotic syndrome. *Am J Med Sci* **195**, 70–83.

Feehally J, Harris KPG, Bennett SE and Walls J (1986) Is chronic renal transplant rejection a non-immunological phenomenon? *Lancet* **II**, 486–8.

Feinstein EI, Blumenkrantz MJ, Healy M, Koffler A, Siberman H, Massry SG and Kopple J (1981) Clinical and metabolic responses to parenteral nutrition in acute renal failure – a controlled double blind study. *Medicine* **60**, 124–37.

Feinstein EI and Massry SG (1988) Nutritional therapy in acute renal failure. In *Nutrition and the kidney* Mitch WE and Klahr S (Eds) pp. 80–103. Little Brown, Boston/Toronto.

Forrest C (1990) The use of urea kinetic modelling in the renal dietitians' quality assurance programme. *Artery* Dec, 3–7.

Friedman AL, Chesnelof RW and Gilbert EF (1983) Secondary oxalosis as a complication of parenteral alimentation in acute renal failure. *Am J Clin Neph* **3**, 248.

Giordano C (1963) Use of exogenous and endogenous urea for protein synthesis in normal and uraemic subjects. *J Lab Clin Med* **62**, 231–40.

Giovannetti S and Maggiore Q (1964) A low nitrogen diet with proteins of high biological value for severe chronic uraemia. *Lancet* **1**, 1000–1003.

Golper TA (1984) Therapy for uraemic hyperlipidaemia. *Nephron* **38**, 217–25.

Hadfield C (1992) Nutritional adequacy of a low protein diet. *J Renal Nut* **2**(3) Suppl 1 (July), 37–41.

Heide B, Pierratos A, Khanna R, Pettit J, Ogilvie R, Harrison J, McNeil K and Oreopoulos DF (1983) Nutritional status of patients undergoing CAPD. *Peritoneal Dialysis Bull* **3**(3), 138–42.

Hirschberg R and Kopple JD (1988) Requirements for protein, calories and fat in the predialysis patient. In *Nutrition and the kidney*, Mitch WE and Klahr S (Eds) pp. 131–154. Little, Brown & Co, Boston/Toronto.

Hunsicker LG (1988) Nutritional requirements of renal transplant patients. In *Nutrition and the kidney*, Mitch WE and Klahr S (Eds) pp. 224–38. Little Brown & Co, Boston/Toronto.

Ihle BU, Becker GJ, Whitworth JA, Charlwood RA and Kincard-Smith PS (1989) The effect of protein restriction on the progression of renal insufficiency. *N Engl J Med* **321**, 1773–7.

Jenkins D, Burton PR, Bennett SE and Walls J (1989a) Metabolic consequences of correcting acidosis in uraemia. *Nephrol Dial Transplant* **4**, 92–5.

Jenkins DAS, Gouldersbrough D, Smith GD and Crowie JF (1989b) Can low dosage aluminium hydroxide control the plasma phosphate without bone toxicity? *Nephrol Dial Transplant* **4**, 51–56.

Kaysen GA, Gambertoglio J and Jiminez I (1986) The effect of dietary protein intake on albumin homeostasis in nephrotic patients. *Kidney Int* **29**, 572–7.

Kopple JD and Blumenkrantz MJ (1983) Nutritional requirements for patients undergoing continuous ambulatory peritoneal dialysis. *Kidney Int* **S16**, S295–S302.

Kopple JD and Coburn JW (1973) Metabolic studies of low protein diets in uraemia I. Nitrogen and potassium. *Medicine* **52**, 583.

Lee HA (1980) Nutritional support in renal and hepatic failure. In *Practical nutritional support* pp. 275–82. Pitman Medical, London.

Lewis B (1976) *The hyperlipidaemias: clinical and laboratory practice*, p. 21; p. 31. Blackwell Scientific Publications, Oxford.

Manos J, Harrison A, Jones M, Adams PH and Mallick NP (1983) Protein/calorie balance in the nephrotic syndrome. *Kidney Int Suppl* **24**, S347.

Mansy H, Goodship THJ, Tapson JS, Hartley GH, Keavey P and Wilkinson R (1989) Effect of high protein diet in patients with the nephrotic syndrome. *Clin Sci* **77**, 445–51.

Maschio G, Oldrizzi R, Tessitore N, D'Angelo A, Valvo E, Lupo A, Loschiavo C, Fabris A, Gammaro L, Rugia C and Panzetta G (1982) Effects of dietary protein and phosphate restriction on the progression of early renal failure. *Kidney Int* **22**, 371–6.

Mault JR (1983) Starvation a major contributor to mortality in acute renal failure. *Trans Am Soc Artif Intern Organs* **28**, 510.

Molitoris BA, Proment DH, Mackenzie TA, Huffler WH and Alfrey AC (1989) Citrate: A major factor in the toxicity of orally administered aluminium compounds. *Kidney Int* **36**, 949–53.

Oldrizzo L, Rugiu C and Maschio G (1989) The optimal protein intake in patients with early chronic renal failure. In *The progressive nature of renal disease: myths and facts*, Oldrizzo L, Maschio G, Rugiu C *et al* (Eds) 75, pp. 203–208. Kager, Basel.

Papadoyannakis NJ, Stefanidis CJ and McGowan M (1984) The effect of correction of metabolic acidosis on nitrogen and potassium balance of patients with chronic renal failure. *Am J Clin Nutr* **40**, 623–7.

Popovich RP, Moncrief JW, Decherd JF, Bomar JB and Pyle WK (1976) The definition of a novel portable/wearable equilibrium dialysis technique. *Abstr Trans Am Soc Artif Intern Organs* **5**, 64.

Pru C, Eaton J and Kjellstrand C (1985) Vitamin C intoxication and hyperoxalaemia in chronic dialysis patients. *Nephron* **39**, 112–16.

Raman VG (1990) General principles of parenteral nutrition. In *A handbook of parenteral nutrition*, Lee HA, Venkat-Raman G (Eds) pp. 27–52. Chapman and Hall, London.

Rosman J, Terwee P, Meijer S, Piers-Becht T, Sluiter W and Donker A (1984) Prospective randomised trial of early dietary protein restriction in chronic renal failure. *Lancet* **2**, 1291–6.

Rubin J, Nolph K, Arfania D, Prowant B, Fruto L, Brown P and Moore H (1981) Protein losses in continuous peritoneal dialysis. *Nephron* **28**, 218–21.

Sandoz P, Vallance D, Winder AF and Walls J (1986) Protein and amino acid losses from the peritoneum during CAPD and CCPD. In *Frontiers in peritoneal dialysis*. Maher JF and Winchester J (Eds) p. 446. Field and Rich, New York.

Schmitt J (1991) Selecting an appropriate phosphate binder. *J Renal Nut* **1**(1), 38–40.

Shen SY, Lukens CW, Alongi SV, Sfeir RE, Dagher FJ and Sadler JH (1983) Patient profile and the effect of diet therapy on post-transplant hyperlipidaemia. *Kidney Int* (Suppl) **16**, S147–52.

Solossol CI, Joyeux H, Solassol CL, Pujol H and Romieu C (1978) Chirurgie regionale des concers du pariorees. *Chirurgie* **104**, 131–40.

Turgan C, Feehally J, Bennett SE, Davies TJ and Walls J (1981) Accelerated hypertriglyceridaemia in patients on continuous ambulatory peritoneal dialysis – a preventable abnormality. *Int J Art Org* **4**(4), 158–160.

Wendland BE (1987) Urea kinetic modelling: the role of the dietitian. In *Aspects of renal care 2*, Monkhouse PM (Ed) pp. 158–64. Baillière Tindall, London.

4.14 Gout and renal stones

4.14.1 Gout

The role of purines in human disease has been of importance since the discovery that uric acid (to which they are metabolized) was a component of some renal stones and that serum uric acid levels were elevated in patients with gout. Hyperuricaemia may be primary or secondary, but whatever its aetiology it reflects either overproduction of purines, reduced renal clearance of uric acid or a combination of both.

The most common manifestation of hyperuricaemia is gout which appears to be a familial disease. Allopurinol inhibits the enzyme xanthine oxidase which is responsible for the conversion of xanthine and hypoxanthine to uric acid. This causes the serum uric acid to fall and the excretion of its precursors to be increased since they are more soluble and have a higher renal clearance rate than uric acid. Allopurinol is now used regularly in the treatment of gout, reducing the need for a strict low purine diet. Dietary purines are responsible for only a small part of the excess uric acid which accumulates in gout. However, it does no harm to reduce the intake of purines especially as the foods which are rich sources (such as fish roes, sardines, crab, anchovies, sprats and offal) are not difficult to avoid (see Table 2.61, in Section 2.11.4). Patients with chronic gout should be advised to attain ideal weight by gradual dieting. Fasting or strict dieting will increase serum uric acid levels. The diet should be reduced in fat, refined sugar and animal protein with emphasis on vegetable protein, fibre and unrefined carbohydrate. Over-indulgence in food or alcohol must be avoided. Fluid intake should be at least 1–2 l/day to facilitate the passage of any small stones in the renal tract.

4.14.2 Renal stones

Waste products of metabolism and excess ions in a soluble form are disposed of by the kidney but certain combinations of ions, because they are only sparingly soluble in urine, may precipitate and become lodged in a narrow section of the urinary tract forming a nucleus around which a stone may grow.

Diagnosis is rarely difficult because the symptoms are so painful, ranging from dull loin pain if the stone is in the renal pelvis to agonising colic if it is lodged in the ureter.

In the UK the prevalence of urinary tract stone disease is relatively low about 1.5% (Currie and Turner 1979). The annual incidence of stone formation is around 7 per 10 000 of the population with a male/female ratio of about 2:1. The incidence of upper urinary tract stones containing calcium appears to be related to affluence (Robertson *et al* 1980; 1981a) and one dietary component implicated is animal protein. This is substantiated by the findings that the prevalence of stone disease in vegetarians is only about 50% of that in the general population (Robertson *et al* 1981b). A high intake of animal protein increases the urinary excretion of calcium and oxalate and the accompanying increase in purine intake increases uric acid excretion. These three products are all known risk factors for the formation of calcium-containing renal stones.

Stone formation is more common in hot climates. Low urine volume is the most likely cause but an increased exposure to ultra violet light which is known to increase the intestinal absorption of calcium from the diet may be a contributing factor and also account for the seasonal variation seen in this country (Robertson *et al* 1975).

Some workers have found that the concentration of inhibitors of crystallization of calcium salts in urine is lower in stone formers than the rest of the population (Robertson *et al* 1976). The inhibitors identified include citrate, glycoproteins, glycosaminoglycans and Tamm Horsfall glycoprotein. There may also be an inhibitor (not yet identified but certainly a macromolecule) which can reduce the rate of crystallization of urates and uric acid in urine (Sperling *et al* 1965; Porter 1966).

Environmental factors may be just as important as the concentration of inhibitors in determining stone formation but before aetiology and treatment can be specified the types of renal stones must be classified.

Classification of renal stones

Stones can be classified according to their chemical constituents. There are four main types: calcium, uric acid, magnesium ammonium phosphate together with calcium phosphate ('infection' stones), and cystine. In addition there are some rare forms but these account for less than 0.1% of all stone occurrence.

Calcium stones

In the UK, 70% of all stones contain calcium, about 50% contain pure calcium oxalate and the remainder are a mixture of calcium oxalate and calcium phosphate. In about 80% of cases there is no underlying cause and the stone can be described as idiopathic. In the remaining

20%, the stone is secondary to some other factor. The causes of secondary calcium stone disease are discussed later in this section.

Idiopathic calcium stone disease

Risk factors are listed below.

1 Sex. Men are particularly susceptible and account for 85% of cases.

2 Age. It occurs most commonly between the ages of 20 and 50 years but the incidence rises in the fourth decade.

3 Occupation. Cooks, below-deck sailors and heavy metal workers all have a greater than average incidence of calcium oxalate stones which may be linked with environmental factors. Hot working conditions may cause dehydration and heavy metal workers, for example, are often advised to consume a lot of milk and therefore have a high calcium intake.

4 Social class. The incidence is greater in social classes I and II and as previously suggested the higher protein intake in these groups may contribute to stone formation.

5 Diet. Dietary factors which may be involved in idiopathic hypercalciuria include calcium, vitamin D, fluids, fibre, protein, sodium and refined carbohydrate.

The role of excessive vitamin D intake is obvious, as is that of a low fluid intake. However the independent influence of other dietary components is unclear. For many years it has been assumed that a high calcium intake increases the risk of stone formation. It now appears that this may not be the case. A high calcium intake tends to reduce urinary oxalate excretion, an effect which is likely to lessen the risk of stone formation (see point 8 below). A major prospective study on a cohort of 45 619 men (Curhan *et al* 1993) has recently reported that a high dietary calcium intake actually decreased the risk of symptomatic kidney stones.

The role of protein is also uncertain. A high animal protein intake will lower urinary pH and, although urinary pH *per se* is not a major risk factor, calcium oxalate is less soluble in acid conditions. Dietary protein may have a more specific role; Tschope *et al* (1983) have reported that feeding certain amino acids increased urinary calcium and oxalate levels in normal subjects. Fellstrom *et al* (1983) have reported that a high protein intake fed to stone formers increased urinary saturation and decreased urinary citrate levels (an inhibitor to stone formation) and pH.

6 Increased intestinal absorption of calcium. This can occur in people consuming a diet containing normal amounts of calcium and although it could be due to increased plasma levels of 1,25 dihydroxycholecalciferol or parathormone, both are usually normal in idiopathic hypercalciuria. Increased calcium absorption could also be a result of a decreased intake of dietary phosphate, fat, phytate or fibre.

7 Reduced tubular reabsorption of calcium. Some workers have reported a relatively high incidence of this (25% – Pak *et al* 1974; 65% – Coe *et al* 1975) but hypercalciuria alone does not cause calcium stone disease.

8 Increased urinary oxalate. Oxalate is absorbed by a passive process, with sodium oxalate being more readily absorbed than the insoluble calcium oxalate.

Finch *et al* (1981) found the amount of oxalate absorbed from different foods varied between 1.3% from strawberries to 22% from tea. The amount of fat and calcium in the diet will alter the percentage of oxalate which is absorbed. Fat will bind with calcium in preference to oxalate thus a high fat diet will result in more oxalate being available for absorption. In contrast, a high calcium intake will result in less free oxalate and hence less being absorbed.

The same authors have also shown that it is possible to increase the urinary oxalate excretion in normal subjects, from a mean of 0.17 mmol/24 hours by between 0.05 and 0.38 mmol/24 hours by adding various high oxalate foods (in normally consumed quantities) to a previously low oxalate diet. This indicates that dietary oxalate can be responsible for up to two-thirds of urinary oxalate. Oxalate crystals were found in the urine of the subjects when they ate the high oxalate foods and there is evidence that a raised urinary oxalate level is an important risk factor in the recurrence of calcium oxalate stones. Robertson and Peacock (1980) found that the rate of recurrence of idiopathic calcium oxalate stones was highly related to the urinary oxalate level, but only weakly related to the urinary calcium level.

9 Urinary uric acid. Total urinary uric acid output is usually normal in stone formers but the concentration is increased. This is thought to reduce the activity of the macromolecular inhibitors.

Diagnosis of idiopathic hypercalciuria

A range of tests and questions is needed to establish the cause and type of stone.

24-hour urine collection An accurate 24-hour urine collection is needed to diagnose any type of stone. It is especially important in idiopathic hypercalciuria that this is done with the patient at home consuming their normal diet and carrying out their usual activities. In hospital a patient's diet and fluid intake can vary greatly from that at home. For example, a normal ward diet may contain 500–800 mg calcium, and if the patient usually consumes well over 1 g per day, any dietary hypercalciuria may disappear in hospital. Similarly, a patient at home may consume a large amount of one particular high oxalate food which is not present on the hospital menu, so dietary hyperoxaluria will disappear.

Dietary history It is very important to determine the past and present intake of all relevant nutrients to establish if hypercalciuria is of dietary origin or due to hyperabsorption.

Hypercalciuria on a low or normal calcium diet indicates hyperabsorption. Vitamin D is present in many proprietary multivitamin preparations and fish liver oil capsules available over the counter in health food and chemists shops, so patients should be specifically asked about self-medication as they may not even realize they are taking vitamin D supplements.

Social history Patients should be asked about past and present occupations to establish whether environment is likely to have caused long periods of dehydration. At risk jobs have been described previously and Caucasians who have worked abroad in a hot climate are at similar risk as a stone may have been formed during a period of dehydration many years previously, and has since been growing slowly. Alternatively, a period of bed rest sometime in the past may be responsible since this can lead to mobilization of calcium from the bones and thus to hypercalciuria.

Early morning urine calcium/creatinine ratio This is a useful diagnostic procedure because if after overnight starvation, the urine calcium/creatinine ratio is above 0.5 it probably indicates failure of tubular reabsorption of calcium.

Treatment of idiopathic hypercalciuria

Dietary treatment There are different schools of thought as to which dietary restrictions are necessary to treat idiopathic hypercalciuria and, more importantly, to prevent the recurrence of stones.

1 Calcium. Although dietary calcium restriction has been the mainstay of treatment for the prevention of renal stones, compliance with calcium restriction may be poor in the long-term (Baker and Mallinson 1979) and, in addition, its effectiveness as a treatment is questionable (Goldfarb 1988) and may be detrimental to bone mass (Fuss *et al* 1990a; 1990b). Reduced bone mineral content (BMC) has been reported in idiopathic renal stone formers who had been following a low calcium diet (352 ± 20 mg) for about 10 years (±0.7 years) (Fuss *et al* 1990a). The reduction in BMC was as pronounced as that observed in hyperparathyroid stone formers. Although comparison with normal subjects showed that idiopathic renal stone formers had lower than average BMC values whether or not they restricted calcium intake, those on a low calcium diet were found to have a lower BMC in the distal radius than those on a free diet (Fuss *et al* 1990b). Several situations may lead to this, one or more of which may be present in idiopathic renal stone formers (Fuss *et al* 1990a):

- Idiopathic hypercalciuria, if not compensated by an adequate calcium supply, will lead to negative calcium balance;
- Hypophosphataemia in idiopathic renal stone formation is associated with increased resorption and decreased formation of bone;
- Elevated circulating levels of 1,25 dihydroxyvitamin D can induce bone resorption and result in negative calcium balance, especially if associated with a low calcium diet. Goldfarb (1988) has suggested that a reduction in dietary protein, sodium and oxalate is a preferable dietary strategy to calcium restriction.

2 Oxalate. Although most urinary oxalate is derived from metabolic pathways, reducing dietary oxalate does lower renal oxalate excretion especially where dietary oxalate intake was previously high (Goldfarb 1988). Advice to avoid rich sources of oxalate (see Table 2.60 in Section 2.11.3) should therefore be given.

3 Fluid. A high fluid intake helps to maintain a dilute urine and should be encouraged in all patients with stones. Extra care to drink plenty of fluids must be taken in hot weather and especially when going on holiday to a hot climate. There is no necessity for a patient to purchase a water-softener.

4 Protein/sodium. High dietary protein and sodium intakes lead to increased urinary calcium excretion (see Section 4.28, Osteoporosis), and patients regularly consuming large amounts of either should be given appropriate guidance for reducing their intake.

5 Sugar and refined carbohydrates. There is some evidence that a reduction in the intake of sugar and refined carbohydrate is beneficial (Rao *et al* 1982) but, rather than eliminate them from the diet, it is more conducive to compliance to recommend a reduction in intake in line with that advocated for the rest of the population.

Non-dietary treatment Thiazide diuretics such as bendrofluazide or chlorthalidone would appear to be a preferable treatment to a low calcium diet (Fuss *et al* 1990b). These diuretics act on the renal tubules causing greater reabsorption of calcium, putting the patient into positive calcium balance and reducing urinary calcium without increasing urinary oxalate. They are a cheap, easy and effective treatment but occasionally have the unfortunate side effect of causing diabetes.

Cellulose phosphate used to be given to reduce hypercalciuria. It complexes with calcium in the gut, reducing its absorption and therefore its urinary excretion. However, it was more expensive than diuretics, had to be taken with all meals, cause an increase in urinary oxalate levels and may therefore have even increased the risk of stones. In addition, it had some side effects, notably gastric discomfort and diarrhoea, and is therefore no longer prescribed.

Secondary calcium stone disease

Causation and treatment Secondary calcium stone disease usually results from one of the following:

1 Primary hyperparathyroidism. The treatment of primary hyperparathyroidism is a parathyroidectomy. How-

ever, if the parathyroidectomy is delayed or unsuccessful a low calcium diet can be prescribed to lower plasma and urine calcium levels. In some cases surgical removal of the stone may be required.

2 Medullary sponge kidney. Because of the abnormal anatomy of the kidney, these patients make stones when the urinary calcium concentration is normal and should therefore reduce their calcium output below the level used for the treatment of idiopathic hypercalciuria (see above).

3 Renal tubular acidosis (RTA). This is a rare condition, caused by primary or secondary damage to the renal tubules. The patient cannot produce an acid urine, because of a failure of bicarbonate reabsorption and calcium phosphate stones are formed. Renal tubular acidosis can be treated by the use of alkalis and/or diet:

- Alkalis are given to return the serum bicarbonate and pH to within the normal range.
- Diet. A diet rich in animal protein will cause a more acid urine, so patients should be advised to reduce their animal protein intake. Some patients may choose to make radical changes to their diet and become vegan since such a diet can have a dramatic effect in reducing symptoms. They should be given help to make sure their diet is nutritionally balanced.

4 Primary hyperoxaluria. This is caused by an inborn error of glyoxylic acid metabolism. Glyoxylic acid is normally transaminated to glycine or glycolic acid but if the necessary enzymes are absent, oxalic acid will be produced. The absence of two enzymes has been identified – alanine: glyoxalate aminotransferase resulting in Type I, and D-glycerate dehydrogenase resulting in Type II hyperoxaluria. The majority of cases are Type I.

The full biochemistry of oxalic acid and glyoxylic acid metabolism is not known but in patients with primary hyperoxaluria the production and excretion of oxalic acid is vastly increased. Calcium oxalate is insoluble, so renal stones readily occur, and in addition, oxalosis (oxalate deposition in soft tissues) is common. When this happens the prognosis is very poor. Treatment of primary hyperoxaluria is outlined below

- Pyridoxine. This is the only known effective treatment for primary hyperoxaluria. In doses of up to 1 g per day, pyridoxine has been shown to reduce urinary oxalate excretion from 1.4 mmol/24 hours to nearly normal (upper limit 0.5 mmol/24 hours; Rose 1979). Not all patients respond to pyridoxine and work is in progress to see if other substances are effective in non-responders.
- Fluid. The same regimen should be advised as for patients with uric acid stones and patients encouraged to drink enough to produce at least 3 litres urine/24 hours.
- Diet. Patients should be advised to follow a low oxalate diet. A list of foods high in oxalate which should be avoided is given in Table 2.60, Section 2.11.3.
- Increase solubility of calcium oxalate. Both magnesium hydroxide and disodium hydrogen phosphate can be given for this purpose.
- Liver transplant. As the enzymes responsible for primary hyperoxaluria are only located in the liver, a liver transplant will correct the abnormality. This has been carried out in a few patients and results are encouraging.

5 Secondary hyperoxaluria. There are several causes of secondary hyperoxaluria:

- Treatment of hypercalciuria. (See idiopathic hypercalciuria.)
- Intestinal bypass and bowel disease. In both these circumstances steatorrhoea may be present in which case the calcium in the gut will bind with fatty acids and be unavailable for binding with oxalate. Thus more oxalate is available for passive absorption. Gregory *et al* (1975) found that of 435 patients given an ileal bypass for obesity, 60% developed hyperoxaluria and 6% suffered from calcium oxalate stones. Treatment revolves around reducing the steatorrhoea by prescribing a low fat diet. MCT oil has no effect on oxalate absorption and therefore can be used in patients with bowel disease to improve the palatability of the diet and increase the energy intake. A diet low in oxalate will also help to reduce the hyperoxaluria.
- Excess vitamin C intake. This can lead to hyperoxaluria as ascorbic acid can be converted in the body to oxalic acid. However, it only happens when megadoses of vitamin C are taken, for instance as a 'cold cure', or as sometimes prescribed in cases of malabsorption, a procedure which must be avoided if hyperoxaluria occurs. A patient being investigated for hyperoxaluria should always be asked about any self-medication with vitamins or tonics.

6 Vitamin D overdose. This will cause increased intestinal absorption of calcium.

7 Immobilization. If prolonged, immobilization leads to bone resorption and consequent hypercalcaemia and hypercalciuria.

Uric acid stones

There is a high incidence of uric acid stones in industrialized societies which may indicate an environmental factor in their aetiology. However, only a small percentage of uric acid stone formers have a raised urinary uric acid attributable to a higher intake of purines from a diet rich in animal protein. More often, uric acid stone formers have a low urinary pH, and below pH 5.3, spontaneous precipitation of uric acid can occur.

Treatment of uric acid stones

Diet If a patient with uric acid stones has hyperuricosuria, they should be advised to avoid purine-rich foods (see Table 2.61, Section 2.11.14). However, the necessity for such a diet has been mainly superseded by the use of allopurinol.

Fluid intake As with all types of stones, a high fluid intake is beneficial. A daily urine output of at least 2 litres should be the target since precipitation will not occur when urine concentration is below the supersaturation level for uric acid.

Alkalis Above pH 6, urine is unlikely to be supersaturated with uric acid, so treatment with alkalis to raise urine pH is useful. A combination of substances such as sodium or potassium bicarbonate or citrate can be used. The amount of alkali needed varies with the patient's diet, as a higher protein intake results in a more acid urine. A reduction in animal protein may therefore be a useful measure in some cases.

Allopurinol This substance blocks the action of the enzyme xanthine oxidase in the pathway oxidizing hypoxanthine to urate and has few side effects. It is very successful in preventing uric acid stone formation.

'Infection' stones (stones containing magnesium ammonium phosphate and calcium phosphate)

Chronic infection of the urinary tract with a urea-splitting organism is a very common cause of urinary stones. The organisms break down urea producing ammonia which causes an alkaline urine. Magnesium ammonium phosphate and calcium phosphate are extremely insoluble in alkali conditions and will crystallize spontaneously.

Treatment of infection stones

1 Surgery. Initially the stone must be surgically removed and any anatomical cause of the infection corrected.
2 Eradication of infection. Antibiotics must be used but results are often poor unless the stone is removed, as the source of infection is often within the stone itself.
3 Acidification of the urine. Ammonium chloride, ascorbic acid and methionine have all been used.
4 Urease inhibitor. It has been shown that it is possible to inhibit the action of the urea-splitting enzyme, urease, in the bacteria in the kidney, thus preventing ammonia release. The substance used is acetohydroxamic acid (1 g/day), but it is not as yet in general use in the UK.

Diet has little role in the treatment of these stones, but patients should be advised against an excessive calcium intake. On *very rare* occasions an acid ash diet may be indicated if it is not possible to acidify the urine by other methods. Generally this means a high intake of animal protein foods and minimal intake of fruit and vegetables, avoiding potatoes totally.

Cystine stones

This is a very rare type of kidney stone. It is caused by an autosomal recessive genetic disorder of renal tubular reabsorption of cystine, lysine, arginine and ornithine resulting in an increased concentration of cystine in the urine (see Table 4.41). The limit of solubility of cystine at pH range 5–7 at 37°C is 1250 μmol/l, so homozygous cystinurics readily precipitate cystine.

Treatment of cystine stones

Dilution of urine The patient should be instructed to drink enough fluid to pass at least 3 litres of urine each 24 hours, including getting up at night to pass urine. Approximately 600 ml of fluid should be drunk at bedtime and another 600 ml during the night. This treatment is simple, and, if complied with, will prevent the recurrence of stones.

Alkalinization of urine Sodium bicarbonate can be given to increase the urinary pH to 7–7.4. The extra sodium may also help by making the patient thirsty thus encouraging them to drink. However, since calcium may precipitate round the cystine stones in an alkaline urine making it impossible to dissolve the stones with D-penicillamine, alkalinization of the urine is no longer pursued so vigorously.

D-penicillamine This forms a more soluble complex with cystine and is a very effective treatment for cystinuria. It is, however, toxic, causing rashes, fever, iron depletion and proteinuria in a few patients. Sometimes nephrotic syndrome can develop. Another substance which forms an insoluble complex with cystine is Thiola (alpha-mercaptopropionylglycine). This has been shown to be effective and may have fewer side effects than D-penicillamine but is not widely available in the UK.

Diet Cystine is a non-essential amino acid and is synthesized in the body from methionine. A diet low in

Table 4.41 Urinary concentration of cystine

Patient	Cystine concentration (μmol/l)
Normal	10–100
Heterozygous cystinurics	200–600
Homozygous cystinurics	1400–4200

methionine will reduce urinary cystine. However, the diet is restrictive and difficult to follow. Animal protein is limited to 30 g/day from meat, fish, cheese and eggs, in addition to the protein contained in 300 ml milk. The remaining protein requirements are met by vegetable protein. The diet should only be used as a last resort when other treatments have failed.

Rare forms of stone disease

There are a number of uncommon forms of urinary stone disease which account for a very small percentage of all cases. These include xanthine, silica and 2,8 dihydroxyadenine stones but they are not amenable to dietary manipulation.

References

Baker LRI and Mallinson JW (1979) Dietary treatment of idiopathic hypercalciuria. *Br J Urology* **51**, 181–3.

Coe FL, Lawton RL, Goldstein RB and Tembe V (1975) Sodium urate accelerates precipitation of calcium *in vitro*. *Proc Soc Exp Biol and Med* **149**, 926–9.

Curhan GC, Willett WC, Rimm EB and Stamfer MJ (1993) A prospective study of dietary calcium and other nutrients and the risk of symptomatic kidney stones. *New Engl J Med* **328**, 833–8.

Currie WJC and Turner P (1979) The frequency of renal stones within Great Britain in a gouty and non-gouty population. *Br J Urol* **51**, 337–41.

Fellstrom BG, Danielson B, Karlstrom H, Lithell BJ, Ljunghall B and Vessby B (1983) The influence of a high dietary intake of purine-rich animal protein on urinary urate excretion and supersaturation in renal stone disease. *Clin Sci* **64**(4), 399–405.

Finch AM, Kasieles GP and Rose GA (1981) Urine composition in normal subjects after oral ingestion of oxalate-rich foods. *Clin Sci* **60**, 411–8.

Fuss M, Pepersack T, Bergman P, Hurard T, Simon J and Corvilain J (1990a) Low calcium diet in idiopathic urolithiasis: a risk factor for osteopenia as great as in primary hyperparathyroidism. *Br J Urology* **65**, 560–3.

Fuss M, Pepersack T, Van Geel J, Corvilain J, Vandewalle J, Bergmann P, and Simon J (1990b) Involvement of low-calcium diet in the reduced bone mineral content of idiopathic renal stone formers. *Calcif Tissue Int* **46** 9–13.

Goldfarb S (1988) Dietary factors in the pathogenesis and prophylaxis of calcium nephrolithiasis. *Kidney Int* **34**, 544–55.

Gregory JG, Starkloff EB, Miyai K and Schoenberg HW (1975) Urological complications of ileal bypass operation for morbid obesity. *J Urol* **113**, 521–4.

Pak CYC, Ohata M, Lawrence EC and Snyder W (1974) The hypercalciurias. *J Clin Invest* **54**, 387–400.

Porter P (1966) Colloidal properties of urates in relation to calculus formation. *Res Vet Sci* **7**, 128–37.

Rao PN, Prendiville V, Buxton A, Moss DG and Blacklock NJ (1982) Dietary management of urinary risk factors in renal stone formers. *Br J Urol* **54**, 578–83.

Robertson WG and Peacock M (1980) The cause of idiopathic calcium stone disease: hypercalciuria or hyperoxaluria? *Nephron* **26**, 105–10.

Robertson WG, Peacock M, Marshall RW, Speed R and Nordin BEL (1975) Seasonal variations in the composition of urine in relation to calcium stone formation. *Clin Sci Mol Med* **49**, 597–602.

Robertson WG, Peacock M, Marshall RW, Marshall DH and Nordin BEL (1976) Saturation-inhibitor index as a measure of the risk of calcium oxalate stone formation in the urinary tract. *New Engl J Med* **294**, 249–52.

Robertson WG, Peacock M, Heyburn PJ and Hanes FA (1980) Epidemiological risk factors in calcium stone disease. *Scand J Urol Nephrol* (Suppl)**53**, 15–28.

Robertson WG, Peacock M, Heyburn PJ, Hanes FA and Swaminathan R (1981a) The risk of calcium stone formation in relation to affluence and dietary animal protein. In *Urinary calculus*, Brockis JG and Finlayson B (Eds) pp. 3–12. PSG Publishing, Littleton, Mass.

Robertson WG, Peacock M, Marshall DM and Speed R (1981b) The prevalence of urinary stone disease in practising vegetarians. *Fortschritte der Urologie und Nephrologie* **17**, 6–14.

Rose GA (1979) *Urinary calculus disease*, Wickham JEA (Ed) p. 119. Churchill Livingstone, Edinburgh.

Sperling O, De Vries A and Keelem O (1965) Studies on the aetiology of uric acid lithiasis. Urinary non-dialysable substances in idiopathic uric acid lithiasis. *J Urol* **94**, 286–92.

Tschope E, Ritz E, Schmidt-Gayk H and Knebel L (1983) Different effects of oral glycine and methionine on urinary lithogenic substances. *Proc Eur Dial Transplant Assoc* **20**, 407–410. London.

4.15 Diabetes and renal disease

Diabetic nephropathy affects between 25 and 40% of insulin dependent diabetic (IDD) patients (Andersen *et al* 1983, Krowleski *et al* 1985). A similar proportion of non-insulin dependent diabetic (NIDD) patients develop proteinuria (Hasslacher *et al* 1989) – although 30% of these may have non-diabetic proteinuria (Parving *et al* 1990) where the decline of renal function is less predictable. Afro-Caribbeans and Asian Indians in the UK appear to have a greater risk of developing proteinuria (Grenfell *et al* 1988). Approximately 600 cases of end stage renal failure occur in diabetic patients every year in the UK and it is rapidly becoming the most common cause of end-stage renal failure (ESRF) (Joint Working Party 1988).

The development of persistent proteinuria in both IDD and NIDD patients is associated with early mortality from cardiovascular disease (Jarrett *et al* 1984; Mogensen and Christensen 1984; Borch-Johnsen and Kreiner 1987). It has been estimated that the risk of developing coronary artery disease is 15 times higher in IDD patients with proteinuria compared to those without proteinuria (Krowleski 1987).

There is considerable scope for a dietary role in ameliorating the progressive hypertension, hyperlipidaemia, albuminuria and renal insufficiency of diabetic nephropathy, but at present lack of firm evidence prevents the construction of precise guidelines.

4.15.1 Incipient nephropathy

The presence of microalbuminuria (urinary albumin excretion of 20–200 μg/min or 30–300 mg/day) predicts the development of persistent proteinuria and the progressive decline in renal function (Mogensen and Christiansen 1984). The development of microalbuminuria appears to be related to the degree of glycaemic control; patients who develop this complication have been shown to have a higher level of glycosylated haemoglobin than those who remain normoalbuminuric. Microalbuminuria may also be associated with increased blood pressure and adversely elevated serum lipids (Wiseman *et al* 1984; Jensen *et al* 1988; Mattock *et al* 1988; Jones *et al* 1989; Watts *et al* 1989); although these may be a consequence of increased insulin resistance rather than a causative factor *per se*.

The development of persistent proteinuria has also been shown to be related to the level of hyperglycaemia during the first 15 years of diabetes (Krowleski *et al* 1985). However genetic susceptibility also appears to play a role since not all those with poor glycaemic control will develop renal disease.

Strict blood glucose control has been shown to reduce the albumin excretion rate in both IDD and NIDD patients with microalbuminuria (Vasquez 1984; Bending *et al* 1985) and to prevent the progressive increase in albumin excretion in IDD patients (Feldt-Rasmussen 1986).

Diet and the development of diabetic nephropathy

Dietary protein is known to influence renal function and protein restriction is an important component in the management of renal failure. Recently it has been suggested that a high protein intake may be linked with the development of nephropathy and concern has been expressed over the relatively high protein intake of some diabetics in Western countries.

However, there are no large scale or prospective studies examining the potential dietary contribution to the development of nephropathy in diabetes. Cross-sectional studies have been published in small groups of IDD subjects. Watts *et al* (1988) reported that 15 microalbuminuric IDDs consumed significantly more fat, expressed as grams and percentage of total energy, and a smaller percentage of energy from carbohydrate than a well matched group of normoalbuminuric patients. Nyberg *et al* (1987) showed no differences in protein intake between patients with and without nephropathy although the range of intake was wide in both categories.

Pending more research in this area, it seems prudent for microalbuminuric patients to concentrate on achieving good glycaemic control by means of a diet which is relatively low in saturated fat and with a protein content which does not exceed average consumption levels (British Diabetic Association 1991). If hyperlipidaemia becomes evident, additional fat modification and, if appropriate, more intensive weight reducing measures may be necessary. In addition, a reduction in salt intake may be helpful in the treatment of hypertension (Dodson *et al* 1984).

4.15.2 Established renal disease

Dietary intervention

Protein

There are now many studies showing that a reduction in protein intake can reduce the generally linear decline in renal function which is seen in most renal diseases. Patients with primary glomerular disease and those whose proteinuria is reduced by diet may benefit most from protein restriction (El Nahas *et al* 1984; Rosman and ter Wee 1989).

Recently there have been a limited number of studies in (mainly insulin-dependent) diabetic patients (Walker *et al* 1989; Zeller *et al* 1991) demonstrating that a restricted protein diet (0.6–0.7 g/kg ideal body weight) significantly reduces the rate of decline of glomerular filtration rate (GFR) and, in most cases, the albumin excretion rate (Ciavarella *et al* 1987; Yue *et al* 1988).

What is not known is at what stage protein restriction should be introduced, at what level, or whether restriction of animal and vegetable protein have the same effect. Traditionally, low protein diets have contained 70–75% HBV protein in order to maintain nitrogen balance. There is some preliminary evidence that vegetable protein may not have the same deleterious effect on renal function as animal protein (Williams *et al* 1987; Bilo *et al* 1989; Kontessis *et al* 1990). In the USA, it is currently recommended that protein intake is held at 0.8 g/kg for all diabetics. A similar reduction in protein intake to these levels may be advisable for all patients in this country with proteinuria and a reduced GFR or raised creatinine level.

In most people, this can be achieved by reducing portion sizes of animal protein foods thereby maintaining a high carbohydrate, high fibre diet but decreasing the intake of phosphate and saturated fat. If necessary, fruit consumption can be increased to provide additional calories but minimal protein. Patients with high energy requirements may need supplements of low protein products such as bread, pasta or biscuits.

If a stricter low protein diet is required at lower levels of GFR, a system of protein exchanges can be incorporated into the diabetic diet (Dodds and Keen 1990). It is recommended that at least 50% of protein comes from HBV sources i.e. for a 42 g protein diet: 3 × 7 g protein exchanges and 9 × 10 g carbohydrate exchanges (with an emphasis on high fibre foods) each providing about 2 g LBV protein. The remaining carbohydrate should come from fruit (until a potassium restriction intervenes) and low protein products. This regimen has the additional benefit of increasing the P/S ratio and decreasing plasma cholesterol levels without apparent deterioration of nutritional status (Walker *et al* 1989; Zeller *et al* 1991).

Fibre

Dietary fibre can reduce plasma urea levels by inhibiting colonic bacterial ammonia generation and increasing faecal nitrogen (Rampton *et al* 1984). In a small group of diabetic patients, a moderate protein intake (12%) consumed as part of a high carbohydrate (50%), high fibre (65 g) diet resulted in similar plasma urea and creatinine levels as a lower protein diet (9%) containing 40% carbohydrate and 22 g fibre. Glycaemic control and serum cholesterol level also improved on the high fibre diet over the 10 day period, although a less desirable increase in serum phosphorus also occurred which is a common consequence of a high fibre diet (Parillo *et al* 1988). However, despite this and the fact that this level of fibre intake is difficult to sustain in this country, the potential benefits from an increased fibre intake (in particular, soluble fibre) on serum lipids, blood glucose control and cardiovascular risk should not be ignored in this group of patients.

Potassium

Hyperkalaemia due to retention of dietary potassium is not normally a problem until GFR is markedly reduced (<10–15 ml/min). However, insulin deficiency or angiotensin-converting enzyme (ACE) inhibitors may precipitate hyperkalaemia earlier in diabetic patients and a potassium restriction may become necessary. Plasma potassium levels should be closely monitored to determine the degree of restriction required for the individual patient as this is one of the most difficult blood parameters to maintain.

Other diet-related aspects of established renal disease

Insulin requirements

Insulin requirements normally decline as renal failure progresses. The half-life of insulin is prolonged as the functional renal mass decreases and there is an increased risk of hypoglycaemia. As patients become progressively uraemic, it is likely that reduced appetite also plays a role in reducing insulin requirement.

Uraemia increases insulin resistance and insulin requirements may fall on introduction of a low protein diet despite an adequate energy intake (Aparicio *et al* 1989; Gin *et al* 1989).

Glycosylated haemoglobin

Once uraemia has developed, glycosylated haemoglobin is no longer a reliable measure of the preceding long term blood glucose control. HbA1 will be elevated due to the presence of carbamylated haemoglobin which is detected by ion-exchange chromatography (Fluckiger *et al* 1981).

In patients on haemodialysis there is increased red cell turnover, anaemia is common and transfusions may be necessary. All of these reduce HbA1, giving a false impression of better blood glucose control.

Diabetic complications

Patients with diabetic nephropathy often suffer from other long term complications. The majority of patients will have co-existent retinopathy and neuropathy which, if severe, may affect the ability for self-care. All patients have an increased risk of cardiovascular mortality.

Blindness Retinopathy is always present in advanced diabetic nephropathy and as many as one third of patients may be blind at the start of renal replacement therapy, although this proportion should lessen as treatment for retinopathy becomes more effective. This handicap obviously affects rehabilitation but there is no evidence that the outcome of renal failure treatment is adversely affected by blindness. A number of aids for monitoring blood glucose or changing dialysis solution bags are available for visually handicapped people.

Dietary treatment may undergo frequent changes as the diabetic patient progresses through possibly a reduced protein diet, potassium and/or phosphate restriction to the higher protein diet on continuous ambulatory peritoneal dialysis (CAPD) and back to 'healthy eating' if transplanted. For blind diabetic patients living alone, dietary advice can be recorded on cassette to enable them to listen at home. Food models may also be useful to demonstrate portion sizes.

Gastropathy Gastric neuropathy, with diarrhoea, nausea, vomiting and anorexia, although rare, can play a prominent role in the development of malnutrition in the dialysed diabetic patient. There may be decreased gastric secretion and delayed gastric emptying which results in a feeling of fullness and inability to consume the necessary food.

Diabetic diarrhoea and vomiting are difficult to assess in uraemic patients and frequently improve after treatment. If urea levels are stable the initial management of gastropathy should include small frequent feeding with a reduction in the fat content which tends to delay gastric emptying.

If vomiting continues to be a problem, metoclopramide, which accelerates gastric motility and acts as an anti-emetic, is effective in some patients (Feldman and Schiller 1983).

Delayed transit time, decreased dietary fibre, inactivity and the administration of phosphate binders, all contribute to the development of constipation in these patients which is also a frequent complication of neuropathy in diabetes. If an increase in dietary fibre is not feasible due to the phosphate and potassium content, laxatives may be prescribed.

Dialysis

The diabetic is likely to develop fluid retention, nausea, vomiting, anorexia and anaemia earlier than a non-diabetic (Watkins 1985), and dialysis or transplantation may need to be initiated sooner.

General dietary aspects

In the patient with a combination of end stage renal failure and diabetes, diet plays a crucial role in management. The nutritional needs and constraints imposed by the dialysis have to be met and, in addition, diet and insulin therapy must remain balanced in order to obtain the best possible blood glucose control. The increased risk of catabolism and hyperkalaemia if the blood glucose level is not well controlled, as well as the high prevalence of complications, place an additional burden on the patient and the renal diabetic diet is one of the most difficult to follow.

It is important to make the diet as liberal as feasible in order to maintain reasonable compliance. However, nutritional balance and fluid control must also be maintained and some previously 'free' foods such as clear soups, sugar-free drinks and low calorie vegetables may have to be limited.

The principles of dietary treatment are generally the same as those in non-diabetics (see Section 4.13) and only those areas which are specific to the diabetic will be covered here.

Dietary inadequacies

Diabetic patients are more prone to develop malnutrition due to the increased incidence of gastric neuropathy and consequent poor tolerance of many energy-dense foods.

It is important to monitor oral intake and nutritional status on a continual basis when the patient is catabolic, for example with peritonitis. It may be necessary to start enteral, or even parenteral, feeds in conjunction with voluntary food intake in order to prevent tissue wasting and consequent delay in recovery. Careful monitoring of glycaemia and adjustment of insulin therapy is important to preserve the nutritional status.

Adequate energy must be consumed in order to maintain body weight and ensure that protein is available for anabolic purposes. Dialysis patients tend to be less active than the average individual, and diabetic dialysis patients, who often have limited vision, severe peripheral neuropathy and/or vascular disease, can be even more sedentary. The prescribed energy intake should reflect the patient's current weight and level of activity. If underweight, 30–40 kcal/kg will be necessary to achieve an optimal weight but some patients are obese and 25 kcal/kg is more appropriate in order to reduce weight gradually while sparing protein.

Continuous ambulatory peritoneal dialysis (CAPD)

This is now the most common form of treatment for diabetic patients needing renal replacement therapy in this country.

Glycaemic control

One advantage of CAPD for diabetic patients is the infusion of insulin into the peritoneal cavity with the dialysis fluid. It is absorbed mainly into the portal circulation, simulating physiological insulin secretion more closely than systemic injections. Blood glucose control with this method is generally good although doses are around double the predialysis level due to adsorption onto the bag and incomplete absorption (less than 50%) across the peritoneum. With intraperitoneal insulin, each exchange is generally carried out before meals so that peak insulin levels coincide with nutrient absorption and postprandial hyperglycaemia is minimized (Khanna *et al* 1988). If carefully trained, diabetic patients can soon adjust their insulin dose as necessary with lower doses at night and more insulin in a hypertonic bag. The incidence of peritonitis is no higher than in non-diabetics (Khanna *et al* 1988).

Nutrient intake

Protein It may be difficult for some patients to consume sufficient protein and a protein supplement may be necessary to maintain serum albumin.

Carbohydrate Since glucose is used as an osmotic agent in the dialysate, complications such as obesity, hypertriglyceridaemia and premature atherosclerosis tend to be exacerbated in diabetics. The dialysate provides a potential load of 75–210 g glucose, although there is a wide individual variation in the percentage which will be absorbed. At an average absorption of 70% from dialysate:

21 3.86% glucose provide approximately 55 g carbohydrate (205 kcal).
21 1.36% glucose provide approximately 20 g carbohydrate (80 kcal).

This reduces the need for additional carbohydrate in the diet which should be derived from high fibre carbohydrate foods in order to minimize glycaemia and avoid constipation. However, plasma phosphate levels should be closely monitored.

Fluid Fluid overload can be avoided if blood glucose control is adequate and sodium intake is limited to <2 g (60 mmol) per day, in order to minimize thirst.

The use of hypertonic bags should be limited as this increases protein losses in the dialysate and the risk of hypertriglyceridaemia. Some patients continue to pass good volumes of urine while others become virtually anuric. A fluid restriction of 700 ml plus the volume of urinary output usually prevents fluid accumulation.

Peritonitis

During episodes of peritonitis there are increased protein losses which are exacerbated if hypertonic bags are used. If the patient is not maintaining an adequate intake, additional high protein supplements will be required or, if this is not tolerated, parenteral nutrition may be necessary (Khanna *et al* 1988).

Haemodialysis

In the diabetic, there can be considerable problems in maintaining vascular access for haemodialysis owing to the likelihood of arterial disease. Other disadvantages of this procedure for diabetic patients are the tighter fluid restriction and generally poorer glycaemic control.

Dietary management during the first few weeks of haemodialysis may be difficult. The insulin requirement varies with changes in appetite, food intake and physical activity, although it is generally increased compared to the pre-dialysis level. Small, frequent meals and sliding-scale soluble insulin may be helpful at first (Schmidt *et al* 1985).

In spite of this, it is often hard to achieve good blood glucose control and the resultant thirst may exacerbate the difficulty of maintaining a fluid restriction of 500 ml/day plus the urinary output. Strategies which may help make this more acceptable to the patient include the use of a small cup, drinking only at set times and the provision of refreshing drinks such as iced lemon tea and ice cubes to suck. Rinsing with cold water or a spray of artificial saliva may be useful for a dry mouth.

Insulin dependent patients should be advised to use concentrated carbohydrates such as honey, glucose tablets or sugar cubes to counteract hypoglycaemia rather than liquid sources such as Lucozade or fruit juices.

Transplantation

Following transplantation the diet should not be changed until the transplanted kidney is shown to be functioning well and dialysis can be stopped.

After transplantation, myocardial infarction remains a major cause of morbidity and mortality, emphasizing the continued importance of surveillance of the serum lipids. Polyunsaturated and monounsaturated fats should be encouraged as part of a 'prudent' diet resembling that recommended to all diabetic patients. Sodium restriction may be helpful in the control of blood pressure and some degree of energy restriction may be recommended if dry weight gain is rapid (Schmidt *et al* 1985).

Hyperkalaemia may continue to be a problem in a minority of patients treated with cyclosporin A, particularly in diabetics with low renin-aldosterone secretion.

Further reading

American Journal of Kidney Disease (1989) **1**, 1–44. Several articles on preventing the kidney disease of diabetes mellitus.

Diabete & Metabolisme (1990) **16**, 453–69. Three articles on protein restriction in diabetic nephropathy.

Mogensen CE (Ed) (1988) *The kidney and hypertension in diabetes mellitus*. Martinus Nijhoff, Boston.

Reddi AS and Camerini-Davalos RA (1990) Diabetic nephropathy; an update. *Ann Intern Med* **150**, 31–43.

References

Andersen AR, Christiansen JS, Åndersen JK, Kreiner S and Deckert T (1983) Diabetic nephropathy in Type 1 (insulin-dependent) diabetes: an epidemiological study. *Diabetologia* **25**, 496–501.

Aparicio M, Gin H, Potaux L, Bouchet J-L, Morel D and Aubertin J (1989) Effect of a ketoacid diet on glucose tolerance and tissue insulin sensitivity. *Kidney Int* **36**(Suppl 27), S231–235.

Bending JJ, Viberti GC, Bilous RW and Keen H (1985) Eight-month correction of hyperglycaemia in IDDM is associated with a significant and sustained reduction of urinary albumin excretion rates in patients with microalbuminuria. *Diabetes* **34**(Suppl 3), 69–73.

Bilo HJG, Schaap GH, Blaak E, Gans ROB, Oe PL and Donker AJM (1989) Effects of chronic and acute protein administration on renal function in patients with chronic renal insufficiency. *Nephron* **53**, 181–7.

Borch-Johnsen K and Kreiner S (1987) Proteinuria: value as a predictor of cardiovascular mortality in insulin-dependent diabetes. *Br Med J* **294**, 1651–4.

British Diabetic Association, Nutrition Sub-Committee (1991) Dietary recommendations for people with diabetes; an update for the 1990s. *J Hum Nutr Dietet* **4**, 393–412.

Ciavarella A, Di Mizio G, Stefoni S, Borgnino L and Vannini P (1987) Reduced albuminuria after dietary protein restriction in insulin-dependent diabetic patients with clinical nephropathy. *Diabetes Care* **10**, 407–413.

Dodds RA and Keen H (1990) Low protein diet and conservation of renal function in diabetic nephropathy. *Diabete & Metabolisme* **16**, 464–9.

Dodson PM, Pacy PJ, Bal P, Kubicki AJ, Fletcher RF and Taylor KG (1984) A controlled trial of a high fibre, low fat and low sodium diet for mild hypertension in Type 2 (non-insulin-dependent) diabetic patients. *Diabetologia* **27**, 522–6.

El Nahas AM, Masters-Thomas A, Brady SA, Farrington K, Wilkinson V, Hilson AJM, Verghese Z and Moorhead JF (1984) Selective effect of low protein diets in chronic renal diseases. *Br Med J* **289**, 1337–41.

Feldman M and Schiller LR (1983) Disorders of gastric motility associated with diabetes mellitus. *Ann Intern Med* **98**, 378.

Feldt-Rassmussen B, Mathiesen ER and Deckert T (1986) Effect of two years of strict metabolic control on progression of incipient nephropathy in insulin-dependent diabetes. *Lancet* **2**, 1300–4.

Fluckiger R, Harmon W, Meier W, Loo S and Gabbay KH (1981) Haemoglobin carbamylation in uraemia. *N Eng J Med* **304**, 823–7.

Gin H, Aparicio M, Potaux L, Bouchet JL and Aubertin J (1989) Reduced albuminuria and improved insulin sensitivity after dietary protein restriction in IDDM patients. *Diabetes Care* **12**, 369–70.

Grenfell A, Bewick M, Parsons V, Snowden S, Taube D and Watkins PJ (1988) Non-insulin-dependent diabetes and renal replacement therapy. *Diabetic Med* **5**, 172–6.

Hasslacher C, Ritz E, Wahl P, Michael C (1989) Similar risks of nephropathy in patients with Type I or Type II diabetes mellitus. *Nephrol Dial Transplant* **4**, 859–63.

Jarrett RJ, Viberti GC, Argyropoulos A, Hill RD, Mahmud U and Murrells TJ (1984) Microalbuminuria predicts mortality in non-insulin-dependent diabetes. *Diabetic Med* **1**, 17–19.

Jensen T, Stender S and Deckert T (1988) Abnormalities in plasma concentrations of lipoproteins and fibrinogen in Type 1 (insulin-dependent) diabetic patients with increased urinary albumin excretion. *Diabetologia* **31**, 142–5.

Joint Working Party on Diabetic Renal Failure (1988) Renal failure in diabetics in the UK: deficient provision of care in 1985. *Diabetic Med* **5**, 79–84.

Jones SL, Close CF, Mattock MB, Jarrett RJ, Keen H and Viberti GC (1989) Plasma lipid and coagulation factor concentrations in insulin-dependent diabetics with microalbuminuria. *Br Med J* **298**, 487–90.

Khanna R, Mactier R and Oreopoulos D (1988) Continuous Ambulatory Peritoneal Dialysis in uremic diabetics. In *The kidney and hypertension in diabetes mellitus*. Mogensen CE (Ed) pp. 331–9. Martinus Nijhoff, Boston.

Kontessis P, Jones S, Dodds R, Trevisan R, Nosadini R, Fioretto P, Borsato M, Sacerdoti D and Viberti GC (1990) Renal, metabolic and hormonal responses to ingestion of animal and vegetable proteins. *Kidney Int* **38**, 136–44.

Krowleski AS, Warram JH, Christlieb AR, Busik EJ and Kahn CR (1985) The changing natural history of nephropathy in Type 1 diabetes. *Am J Med* **78**, 785–94.

Krowleski AS (1987) Magnitude and determinants of coronary artery disease in juvenile-onset, insulin-dependent diabetes mellitus. *Am J Cardiol* **59**, 750–5.

Mattock M, Keen H, Viberti GC, El-Gohari MR, Murrells TJ, Scott GS, Wing JR and Jackson PG (1988) Coronary heart disease and urinary albumin excretion rate in Type 2 (non-insulin-dependent) diabetic patients. *Diabetologia* **31**, 82–7.

Mogensen CE and Christiansen CK (1984) Predicting diabetic nephropathy in insulin-dependent patients. *N Eng J Med* **311**, 89–93.

Nyberg G, Norden G, Attman PO, Aurell M, Uddebom G, Arvidsson LR, Lenner R and Isaksson B (1987) Diabetic nephropathy; is dietary protein intake harmful? *J Diabetic Compl* **1**, 37–40.

Parillo M, Riccardi G, Pacioni D, Iovine C, Contaldo F, Isernia C, De Marco F, Perrotti N and Rivellese A (1988) Metabolic consequences of feeding a high-carbohydrate, high fibre diet to diabetic patients with chronic kidney failure. *Am J Clin Nutr* **48**, 255–9.

Parving HH, Gall MA, Skott P, Jorgensen HE, Jorgensen F and Larsen S (1990) Prevalence and causes of albuminuria in non-insulin-dependent diabetic (NIDDM) patients. *Kidney Int* **37**, 243.

Rampton DS, Cohen SL, Crammond V de B, Gribbons J, Lilburn MF, Rabet JY, Vince AJ, Wager JD and Wrong OM (1984) The treatment of chronic renal failure with dietary fibre. *Clin Nephrol* **21**, 159–63.

Rosman JB and ter Wee PM (1989) Relationship between proteinuria and response to low protein diets early in chronic renal failure. *Blood Purif* **7**, 52–7.

Schmidt L, Davies M and Barbosa J (1985) Nutritional aspects of diabetic kidney disease. In *Nutrition and diabetes*. Jovanic L and Peterson CM (Eds) pp. 89–92. Alan Liss, New York.

Vasquez B (1984) Sustained reduction of proteinuria in Type 2 (non-insulin dependent) diabetes following diet-induced reduction of hyperglycaemia. *Diabetologia* **26**, 127–33.

Walker JD, Bending JJ, Dodds RA, Mattock MB, Murrells TJ, Keen H and Viberti GC (1989) Restriction of dietary protein and progression of renal failure in diabetic nephropathy. *Lancet* **ii**, 1411–15.

Watkins PJ (1985) Diabetic nephropathy; prevalence, complications and treatment. *Diabetic Med* **2**, 7–12.

Watts GF, Gregory L, Naoumova R, Kubal C and Shaw KM (1988) Nutrient intake in insulin-dependent diabetic patients with incipient nephropathy. *Eur J Clin Nutr* **42**, 697–702.

Watts GF, Naumova R, Slavin BM, Morris RW, Houlston R, Kubal C and Shaw KM (1989) Serum lipids and lipoproteins in insulin-dependent diabetic patients with persistent microalbuminuria. *Diabetic Med* **6**, 25–30.

Williams AJ, Baker F and Walls J (1987) Effect of varying quantity and quality of dietary protein intake in experimental renal disease in rats. *Nephron* **46**, 37–42.

Wiseman MJ, Viberti GC, Mackintosh D, Jarrett RJ and Keen H (1984) Glycaemia, arterial pressure and microalbuminuria in Type 1 (insulin-dependent) diabetes mellitus. *Diabetologia* **26**, 401–405.

Yue DK, O'Dea J, Stewart P, Conigrave AD, Hosking M, Tsang J, Hall B, Dale N and Turtle J (1988) Proteinuria and renal function in diabetic patients fed a diet moderately restricted in protein. *Am J Clin Nutr* **48**, 230–4.

Zeller K, Whittaker E, Sullivan L, Raskin P and Jacobson HR (1991) Effect of restricting dietary protein on the progression of renal failure in patients with insulin-dependent diabetes mellitus. *N Eng J Med* **324**, 78–84.

4.16 Diabetes mellitus

4.16.1 Aims of dietary treatment

The main aims of dietary therapy in the treatment of diabetes are:

1 To abolish primary symptoms by achieving blood glucose levels as close to the normal range as possible, whilst maintaining optimal nutrition.

2 To minimize the risk of hypoglycaemia in diabetics treated with insulin and certain oral hypoglycaemic agents.

3 To achieve weight loss in the obese.

4 To minimize the risk of long term microvascular and macrovascular complications.

4.16.2 Dietary principles

Normalization of blood glucose and lipids may help delay or prevent the onset of long term complications (Pirart 1978; Seviour *et al* 1988). The risks of microvascular and macrovascular complications are more apparent in type I and type 2 diabetes respectively. The maintenance of near-normal glycaemia is important for the prevention of microvascular complications. Normalization of other metabolic parameters (e.g. lipids) may be just as important for prevention of macrovascular complications.

The belief that good diabetes control can only be achieved by means of carbohydrate restriction is no longer held. Traditional low carbohydrate diets led to a corresponding high fat intake since foods such as meat, cheese and nuts were allowed freely (Thomas 1982). This may have contributed to the increased incidence of macrovascular complications. In 1982, the British Diabetic Association reviewed the epidemiological evidence to date and published its first dietary policy document. This paper placed more emphasis on controlling total energy content, increasing complex carbohydrate intake and reducing dietary fat (Nutrition Sub-Committee of the British Diabetic Association 1982). Essentially identical policies by diabetes associations in many other countries and by the Nutrition Study Group of the European Association for the Study of Diabetes (1988) followed. The British Diabetic Association (1991) has more recently published an update to these recommendations entitled 'Dietary recommendations for people with diabetes: an update for the 1990s'. The broad recommendations of this document are given in Table 4.42. This paper suggested some changes in emphasis as a result of the new scientific evidence that had come to light regarding, for example, sucrose, monounsaturated fats and glycaemic index.

Table 4.42 Summary of nutritional recommendations for people with diabetes for the 1990s (Nutrition Sub-Committee, British Diabetic Association 1991)

	Recommendations for diabetes
Energy	At a level which attains/ maintains a BMI in the region of 22
Carbohydrate	
(% energy)	50–55%
Added sucrose or fructose (g/day)	<25 g
Dietary fibre (g/day)	>30 g
Total fat (% energy)	30–35%
Saturated fatty acids	<10%
Monounsaturated fatty acids	10–15%
Polyunsaturated fatty acids	<10%
Protein (% energy)	10–15%
Salt (g/day)	
Normotensive	<6 g
Hypertensive	<3 g
'Diabetic' foods	None (avoid)

Energy

In dietary terms, the energy content of the diet in relation to energy requirement probably has the greatest influence on long term diabetes control. Around 75% of people with non-insulin dependent (Type 2) diabetes are overweight (Salans 1987; Lean *et al* 1990). Reducing energy intake in the obese type 2 patient has been shown to be effective in helping blood glucose return close to the normal range (Weinsier *et al* 1974). Weight reduction also promotes a decrease in insulin resistance.

A diet history, crude and inaccurate as it may be, is still considered an appropriate starting point for the dietary consultation. It helps to create rapport and also gives an indication of general food consumption patterns. However, some more appropriate estimation of energy intake and requirements should ideally be performed. Various methods have been suggested (Lean and James 1986) and estimation of basal metabolic rate and daily expenditure may be more appropriate (see Table 4.43).

There is a possibility of prescribing too low an energy intake which may cause the patient to make up the deficit with inappropriate foods. For most overweight Type 2

Table 4.43 Estimation of Daily Energy Expenditure by use of equations

Method:	BMR can be calculated from the modified Schofield equations (DoH 1991) given in Section 2.1.1 A ready reference table based on these equations giving the BMR according to a person's age, sex and weight can be found in Appendix 4. The BMR should then be multiplied by the factor for the appropriate Physical Activity Level (PAL) (see Section 2.1.1)
Example:	75 kg housewife aged 50 years. BMR = (8.3 × 75) + 846 = 1468 kcal/day Daily energy expenditure = BMR × PAL = 1468 × 1.5 = 2203 kcal/day

patients, actual energy requirements may be higher than expected (Lean and James 1986).

Realistic targets should be set by both patient and dietitian, and regular follow up and counselling should form a routine part of the dietary management. Weight loss of between 1–2 lbs (½–1 kg) per week is good progress. It is not necessary for patients to have their diet quantified and general advice based on sensible meal planning is less complicated.

People who are of normal weight should be maintained at their current energy intake with emphasis on the amounts of various nutrients that they should aim to include. The terminology used when prescribing a diet for diabetes is percentage of total energy, the totals of carbohydrate, protein and fat making up 100%.

Carbohydrate

A high complex or unrefined carbohydrate diet has been recommended for people with diabetes since 1982. The BDA suggests that carbohydrate should provide between 50–55% of dietary energy and that most of this carbohydrate should be taken in the form of fibre-rich polysaccharides. Table 4.44 gives an example of how this level of carbohydrate can be achieved.

Dietary fibre

Previous recommendations on fibre implied that all types of dietary fibre, i.e. both insoluble (cereal) fibre and soluble (viscous) fibre, promoted similar beneficial effects on blood glucose control. Although both types have small hypoglycaemic effects, recent studies have consistently shown that the soluble fibre and other similar leguminous fibres are more effective in improving blood glucose, glycosylated haemoglobin and serum lipid concentrations (Fuessl *et al* 1987; Vinik and Jenkins 1988). Examples of sources of soluble and insoluble fibre are given in Table 4.45.

Table 4.44 Example of how to provide approximately 50% of energy as carbohydrate assuming a daily energy intake of 1600 kcalories

Food	Serving size
Branflakes	30 g
Semi-skimmed milk	½ pint
Wholemeal bread	4 medium slices
Fruit	3 average sized pieces
Biscuits	2
Potatoes	3 medium (180 g)
Sweetcorn	3 tablespoons (90 g)

Foods high in both types of fibre have the additional advantage of being bulky and therefore promoting satiety. This, coupled with the fact that fibre is often associated with low energy foods, can assist weight loss. The fibre component of the diet appears to be essential to the effectiveness of the high carbohydrate diet and the British Diabetic Association recommends that a total of 30 g dietary fibre (or 18–20 g non-starch polysaccharide) be consumed daily.

The amount of fibre present in a food, the food form (i.e. whether it is intact as in whole fruit, or disrupted, as in puréed fruit), the temperature of the food and the water content are only some of the factors which influence the glycaemic effect of a food. A mixture of carbohydrate and fibre generates a smaller rise in glycaemia than the same type and amount of carbohydrate consumed alone. Thus, an apple has less effect on blood glucose than apple juice (Haber *et al* 1977); a high fibre cereal has a less glycaemic effect than cornflakes even when it contains four times the quantity of sugars (Jenkins *et al* 1983). Such studies, and in particular the work of Jenkins and colleagues have led to the concept of the 'glycaemic index' – i.e. the glycaemic response to individual foods in relation to that of glucose.

Glycaemic index = 3 hour glucose area (food)/3 hour glucose area (glucose or bread) × 100
(Where 'glucose area' = the area under the three-hour post-prandial blood glucose curve.)

Table 4.46 lists the glycaemic index of some common foods. It has been hoped that a system based on these glycaemic indices could replace the conventional carbohydrate exchange scheme based solely on analytical content.

Table 4.45 Examples of foods which primarily contain either soluble or insoluble fibre

Soluble fibre	Insoluble fibre
Beans e.g. baked beans kidney beans	Wholemeal bread
Lentils e.g. orange lentils, green gram	Wholemeal breakfast cereals e.g. 'Weetabix'
Peas	Brown rice
Oats	Wholemeal biscuits and crispbreads
Oranges, apples	Wheat bran

Table 4.46 The glycaemic index of some common foods using glucose as the reference (Fuller 1990). Reproduced with permission

Food	Glycaemic index
Maltose	100+
Glucose	100
Carrots, parsnips, baked potato	90–100
Cornflakes, instant potato, honey	80–90
Wholemeal bread, white bread, white rice, 'Weetabix', broad beans, apple (puree), swede	70–80
White bread standard	70
Brown rice, muesli, 'Shredded wheat', rye biscuits, bananas, raisins, new potato, digestive biscuit, sweetcorn, sucrose	60–70
Pastry, white spaghetti, oats, peas, bran cereal	50–60
Wholemeal spaghetti, sweet potato, baked beans, oranges, orange juice, grapes, porridge	40–50
Butter beans, haricot beans, kidney beans, soya beans, lentils, apple (whole), ice cream, milk products, peach	Below 40

However in practice this has been difficult to achieve. Glycaemic index studies have not always given consistent results, possibly because the glycaemic effect of a food can vary according to the way it is cooked or processed (e.g. as a result of the formation of resistant starch). Furthermore, to date most studies have been carried out on single foods and there is evidence that these effects may differ when these foods are consumed as part of a mixed meal.

However, it seems sensible to give advice on the inclusion of as many low glycaemic index foods as possible within the context of an appropriate mixed diet.

Sugars

It is still wise that people with diabetes avoid concentrated sources of sugar (such as sugar-rich foods or drinks). It was traditionally assumed that simple sugars (e.g. sucrose or glucose) were absorbed more rapidly than starch, but it is now known that starch and glucose have a similar rate of absorption and glycaemic effect. The glycaemic index of sucrose is only 86% that of white bread, and 60% that of glucose owing to the fructose content of sucrose (Jenkins *et al* 1984). The glycaemic index of some foods which contain sucrose is lower than that of some foods which contain only complex carbohydrate.

The British Diabetic Association has produced a policy statement on the role of sucrose and fructose in the diabetic diet (Nutrition Sub-Committee BDA 1990). This paper suggests that it is no longer necessary or appropriate to limit sucrose in the diet of well controlled, non-obese, normo-lipidaemic patients to a greater extent than that recommended for the general population. Fruit juices, biscuits, reduced-sugar jam have all been allowed as part of the diabetic diet and yet the inclusion of sucrose in home baking has traditionally not been recommended. The BDA policy is now to permit a maximum of 25 g of sucrose for use in baking daily provided it is consumed as part of an overall diet low in fat and high in dietary fibre and that its consumption is distributed throughout the day. The 25 g limit has been proposed for two reasons:

1 To reduce the risk of over-consumption leading to excess energy intake and obesity.

2 Since this is the same quantity previously recommended for fructose as a bulk sweetener to be used in baking.

Patients who prefer to use fructose may continue to do so, but it is considered preferable on economic, social and culinary grounds to use sucrose instead.

Artificial sweeteners (such as aspartame, saccharin, acesulfame K) should remain the sweeteners of choice for drinks, cereals, milk products and other desserts where the bulking and creaming qualities of sucrose are not required.

Consumption of refined sugars in general should be limited since they are often associated with high energy foods, and also since they may predispose to dental caries. A restriction of refined sugar should be particularly recommended to individuals with hypertriglyceridaemia.

Fat

The Committee on Medical Aspects of Food Policy (COMA) has recommended that total fat intake should average 30% of dietary energy, with 10% arising from saturated fatty acids, 12% from monounsaturated fatty acids and around 6% from polyunsaturated fatty acids (DoH 1991). Trans-fatty acids should not exceed 2%. This dietary regimen aims to reduce the risk of developing cardiovascular disease.

People with diabetes, particularly non-insulin dependent diabetes, have an increased risk of developing cardiovascular disease. It is therefore especially important for people with diabetes to keep to a low fat (particularly a low saturated fat) diet. The British Diabetic Association now recommends that total fat should be restricted to 30–35% of total energy with, ideally, no more than 10% energy from saturates, 10% from polyunsaturates and 10–15% from monounsaturates. The main emphasis is to reduce saturated fat intake by controlling the amount of full fat dairy products, fatty meat and saturated cooking/spreading fats in the diet. A reduction in saturated fatty acid intake is associated with a reduction in LDL and total cholesterol (Keys *et al* 1965). Saturated fat intake and not dietary cholesterol exerts the principal influence on serum cholesterol. However, restriction of saturated fat to around 10% of total energy is usually associated with a cholesterol intake of around 300 mg. Table 4.47 suggests ways of reducing saturated fat intake.

Higher intakes of total fat in Mediterranean countries have been linked with lower rates of heart disease (James *et al* 1988). Although cultural and environmental factors may largely account for this, the high monounsaturated fat intake (mainly from olive oil) may also be relevant. People

Table 4.47 Advice for reducing saturated fat intake

1	Buy lean meat and trim off visible fat. Choose fish and poultry (without the skin) more often or replace meat with pulses such as beans and lentils
2	Try using a low or reduced-fat spread rather than butter or margarine. Monounsaturated or polyunsaturated versions are preferable
3	Use as little oil in cooking as possible. Choose an unsaturated oil such as olive oil, rapeseed oil, corn oil or sunflower oil
4	Use low fat dairy products e.g. semi-skimmed or skimmed milk, low fat yoghurt, half-fat hard cheese or cottage cheese
5	Cut down on crisps, cakes, pastries and biscuits
6	Grill, steam, poach, boil or microwave food rather than frying it. Alternatively, fry in a non-stick pan without adding any fat
7	Eat fewer manufactured meat products such as beefburgers, sausages and pies

with diabetes are now advised to include monounsaturated oils (such as olive, rapeseed, peanut oil) and spreads in preference to polyunsaturated versions (Govindji 1991a). Very high intakes of polyunsaturated fats are not advised since this may be potentially damaging due to an increased production of lipid peroxides (Stringer *et al* 1989). This may be important in diets which are low in fruit and vegetable content since the antioxidant vitamin intake will be correspondingly low. Although there is no direct evidence on the role of antioxidants, low intakes of fruit and vegetables have been linked to increased rates of heart disease in the general UK population (Kushi *et al* 1985; James *et al* 1988; Gramenzi *et al* 1990). The World Health Organization (WHO 1990) recommends that around 400 g of fruit and vegetables (excluding potatoes) should be consumed daily. This recommendation is applicable to diabetics also and can be achieved by having two medium portions of vegetables and two pieces of fruit per day.

The overweight Type 2 patient often has raised blood triglyceride levels. The use of long chain polyunsaturated omega-3 fatty acids from fish oils in individuals with diabetes is still experimental, but these fatty acids do appear to have a beneficial effect on triglyceride levels. Populations with a high fish consumption have been shown to have a reduced incidence of heart disease (Gramenzi *et al* 1990). Although fish oil supplements are not recommended for people with diabetes (Govindji 1991b), it is appropriate to advise patients to eat more fish, particularly oily fish, at least once or twice a week.

Protein

Restriction of dietary protein can reduce albuminuria and glomerular filtration rate in patients with early nephropathy (Viberti 1988). Although current evidence is weak, it is sensible to recommend that people with diabetes avoid higher than average protein intakes, and a maximum intake of around 12% of dietary energy would seem appropriate for patients with early nephropathy (see Section 4.15.1). Any limitation of protein intake is likely to be more important in Type 1 diabetes where nephropathy is more common.

Salt

Hypertension is a recognized risk factor for ischaemic heart disease and stroke. Dietary modification can contribute to an improvement in hypertension and also nephropathy. Individuals with diabetes should ensure that they do not consume more salt than the non diabetic population. A high intake of manufactured foods (such as breakfast cereals, cheese, salty snack foods, even bread) can lead to a high sodium intake. Total salt consumption should be limited to 6 g per day (Nutrition Sub-Committee, BDA 1991).

Alcohol

The general recommendations for alcohol are as follows:

1 Never drink and drive.

2 Men should drink no more than three units of alcohol daily and women no more than two. Two to three days a week should be alcohol-free.

3 Alcohol inhibits gluconeogenesis and can increase the risk of hypoglycaemia in people taking insulin or sulphonylureas. People with diabetes should therefore not drink alcohol on an empty stomach and should also ensure that some food is taken either with the drink or afterwards, since the hypoglycaemic effect of alcohol can last for several hours.

4 For people on carbohydrate allowances, the carbohydrate content of alcoholic drinks should not be counted.

5 Alcohol-free or low alcohol drinks are now widely available. They are useful for people who wish to drive and they do not have the disadvantages listed in point 3 above. However, many are high in readily absorbed carbohydrate and should therefore be treated like a sugary drink and taken in moderation. Some low alcohol drinks are low in carbohydrate also, and these are better choices.

6 Low calorie mixers are recommended for spirits. The combination of alcohol and a sugar-containing mixer can trigger reactive hypoglycaemia.

7 If alcohol is consumed regularly, the energy intake should be taken into account. Patients on weight-reducing diets should ideally drink no more than one unit of alcohol daily and no more than five times per week.

8 Patients should be warned that hypoglycaemia can mimic drunkenness; if the breath smells of alcohol, this may prevent people offering help. People with diabetes should therefore always carry some form of diabetic identification.

Diabetic foods

In the era of the traditional carbohydrate restricted diet,

these foods provided a welcome treat to people who had a taste for sweet foods. However, a recent discussion paper on diabetic foods (Thomas and Nutrition Sub-Committee BDA 1992) concluded that 'these products have no place in the current management of diabetes'.

Some of the products surveyed in this report were found to be higher in fat than their non-diabetic equivalents and although some were lower in energy, would not offer a significant calorie saving. With the introduction of a more liberal policy on sucrose, it is recommended that small amounts of ordinary foods should be used in preference. The availability of low sugar and low calorie manufactured products in supermarkets at competitive prices make the avoidance of diabetic foods even more justifiable.

4.16.3 Diet prescription

Regular meals

Eating regularly can help prevent hypoglycaemia in people treated with insulin and some oral hypoglycaemic agents. The introduction of more flexible pen-injecter regimens has allowed people to inject smaller doses of insulin more frequently in response to small frequent meals and snacks.

Snacks in-between meals can be used to complement an otherwise low carbohydrate intake. In this case healthy snacks, such as fruit or reduced fat milk, are advisable.

Carbohydrate exchanges

All meals and snacks should contain some kind of carbohydrate. Carbohydrate exchange lists can help some people regulate their carbohydrate intake. However, since the glycaemic response is governed by many other factors, precise carbohydrate exchanges suggest a degree of precision which is unlikely to be realized in practice. Furthermore, imposing a 'daily carbohydrate allowance' implies a degree of restriction and yet carbohydrate intake is to be encouraged. Carbohydrate exchanges also give no indication of the fat, protein or energy content of a food and hence tend to draw attention away from these other dietary components. For these reasons, as well as the fact that it can be a complicated system, there has been a reduction in the use of formal exchange lists. Some people with Type 1 diabetes still like to use an exchange list; it gives them confidence that they are in control of their diabetes and able to prevent hypoglycaemia. However, simpler systems based on household measures and general meal planning advice may result in a more appropriate dietary intake and, ultimately, better diabetic control. Such general meal planning advice should encompass the following guidelines:

1 Control energy intake.
2 Eat regular meals and snacks.
3 Eat a variety of foods.
4 Use appropriate cooking methods.
5 Include as many low glycaemic index foods as possible.
6 Encourage low fat, high complex carbohydrate foods.
7 Eat more fruit and vegetables, particularly those containing soluble fibre.

4.16.4 Special considerations for Type 1 diabetics

The diet should be formulated in accordance with the general guidelines outlined in the previous section, i.e. once energy requirements have been established the relative percentages of nutrients can be calculated. The eating habits should be assessed first and the insulin regimen chosen subsequently to fit in with the patient's lifestyle and preferred social and food habits. Food consumption as well as insulin type, dose and frequency should be reviewed during regular follow-up sessions. Dietary measures which may slow down the progression of microvascular diseases should be directed more strongly at people with Type 1 diabetes (Nutrition Sub-Committee, BDA 1991).

Balancing food with insulin

Regular meals and snacks are required to balance the peak extrinsic insulin activity and hence to prevent hypoglycaemia. Insulin dosage needs to be matched with the daily carbohydrate intake and thus complex carbohydrate foods should be distributed throughout the day. A carbohydrate exchange system can be adopted to help the patients gauge their carbohydrate intake. Alternatively, simple advice using household measures and meal planning advice can also ensure an even distribution of carbohydrate. The practice of weighing foods accurately is unnecessary. The main aim of the diet is to eat roughly the same amount of carbohydrate at around the same time every day and also to teach people how to adapt this diet in different circumstances.

Insulins

Up until about the last 10 years, bovine (beef) and porcine (pork) insulins have been used to treat Type 1 diabetes. Human insulin is now becoming increasingly more popular and more widely available. This is a synthetic product which has been manufactured using genetic engineering. The main advantage of this type of insulin is that it is less immunogenic than the animal insulins. Many patients have been transferred from pork or beef insulin to the human version. However, there have been complaints about the loss of hypoglycaemic warning signs when using human insulin. In 1989 the British Diabetic Association set up a Human Insulin Working Party of experts in diabetes including a representative from the Committee on Safety of Medicines. The working party has commissioned research on how people react to human and pig insulins.

Conventional insulin regimens

Most patients are managed on at least two injections per day. This will usually consist of a combination of short-acting (clear) and intermediate-acting (cloudy) insulins administered half an hour before both breakfast and the evening meal. The short-acting insulin controls the rise in blood glucose levels after breakfast and the evening meal, and the intermediate-acting insulin controls the rise in blood glucose after lunch. The latter also helps to maintain a normal basal blood glucose level during the night. Table 4.48 shows a selection of insulins which were marketed in the UK in 1990; current information on insulin availability can be found in *MIMS*.

Multiple injection regimens

The introduction of pen-injection devices has led to an increasing popularity in the use of multiple injection techniques, commonly four injections daily. One dose of a long-acting insulin is injected usually at bedtime – this gives a continuous background supply of insulin. Quick-acting insulin is then taken before each meal. This system allows for greater flexibility with timing of meals and is particularly suitable for people who work shifts or need to travel a lot.

Insulin pumps

These first became available in the late 1970s. The pump is worn outside the body and it constantly provides a slow trickle of short acting insulin throughout the day and night. The pump can be set to deliver additional doses of insulin before meals and snacks. The patient must be highly motivated since day-to-day decisions on insulin dosage need to be made and frequent daily monitoring of blood glucose is necessary. Therefore, a great deal of effort is required when using the pump and, since the introduction of pen-injection devices, these pumps have become less popular.

Whichever regimen is chosen, patients should ideally be sufficiently confident to conduct regular self-monitoring

Table 4.48 A selection of insulins available in the UK (Gale and Tattersall 1990). Reproduced with permission

Trade name	Source	Type	Manufacturer
Fast-acting			
Velosulin	P	S	Nordisk/Wellcome
Human Actrapid	H(emp)	S	Novo
Human Velosulin	H(emp)	S	Nordisk/Wellcome
Humulin S	H(crb)	S	Lilly
Intermediate-acting			
Semitard MC	P	SL	Novo
Human Insulatard	H(emp)	I	Nordisk/Wellcome
Human Protaphane	H(emp)	I	Novo
Humulin I	H(crb)	I	Lilly
Human Monotard	H(emp)	L	Novo
Long-acting			
Human Ultratard	H(emp)	UL	Novo
Humulin Zn	H(crb)	L	Lilly
Mixtures			
Initard (50% Fast 50% NPH)	P	S/I	Nordisk/Wellcome
Mixtard (30% Fast 70% NPH)	P	S/I	Nordisk/Wellcome
Human Initard	H(emp)	S/I	Nordisk/Wellcome
Human Mixtard	H(emp)	S/I	Nordisk/Wellcome
Actraphane (30% Sol 70% NPH)	H(emp)	S/I	Novo
Humulin MI (10% SOL 90% NPH)	H(crb)	S/I	Lilly
Humulin M2 (20% Sol 80% NPH)	H(crb)	S/I	Lilly
Humulin M3 (30% Sol 70% NPH)	H(crb)	S/I	Lilly
Humulin M4 (40% Sol 60% NPH)	H(crb)	S/I	Lilly

P = Pork; S = Soluble; L = Lente; I = Isophane; H = Human; SL = Semilente; emp = chemically modified from pork insulin; crb = manufactured by recombinant DNA technology; UL = Ultralente of blood glucose and self-adjustment of insulin doses. The diabetes care team is a valuable source of help and encouragement in this respect.

Hypoglycaemia

Hypoglycaemia occurs when the blood glucose falls below 3 mmol/litre and is most likely to occur in insulin dependent diabetics. The causes of hypoglycaemia are delayed or missed meals or snacks, strenuous activity, alcohol and too much insulin (or sometimes sulphonylureas). Signs and symptoms vary but tend to include shakiness, palpitations, double or blurred vision, confusion, weakness, dizziness, aggression, and irritability. If untreated, loss of consciousness and convulsions can occur. Table 4.49 gives examples of quick-acting carbohydrate sources which can be used to treat hypoglycaemia. This must be followed by a slower-acting carbohydrate food such as a sandwich, biscuits or fruit to prevent blood sugar dropping again. People with Type 1 diabetes should always carry diabetic identification as well as some form of sugar in case of emergency.

Exercise

As well as the general benefits of lowering blood pressure and blood lipids, regular exercise may reduce insulin requirements and improve overall blood glucose control. In Type 1 diabetes, exercise can affect blood glucose levels in two main ways. If blood glucose control is poor and there is insufficient insulin, the adrenaline released as a result of the exercise can make blood glucose levels rise. On the other hand, if blood glucose is reasonably well controlled, there is usually an adequate supply of insulin. Here the main danger of exercise is hypoglycaemia.

It is important that the insulin is not injected into the limb involved in the exercise (e.g. the thigh before running) since its absorption may then be enhanced. The abdomen is the preferred site before exercise because it absorbs insulin more consistently.

In order to avoid low blood sugar, extra carbohydrate is required before the activity. Alternatively, dosage of the preceding insulin injection can be reduced but care needs to be taken not to reduce this too much. Sometimes both adjustments are made. The extra carbohydrate can be eaten as part of the last meal before exercise (e.g. an extra 20 g of complex carbohydrate) or as a quick snack immediately prior to more intense activity. This would take the form of a quick-acting carbohydrate food such as a bar of chocolate. Top-ups of carbohydrate may be needed for endurance exercise and it is imperative that extra carbohydrate is consumed after exercise since its hypoglycaemic effect can last for several hours (MacDonald 1987). Alcohol will obviously exacerbate any hypoglycaemia.

Table 4.49 Examples of quick-acting carbohydrate sources which can be used to treat hypoglycaemia

Foods to provide 10 g quick acting carbohydrate	
Sugar or glucose	2 level teaspoonfuls
Honey, jam or syrup	2 level teaspoonfuls
Glucose tablets	3 tablets
Lucozade	50 ml/2 fl oz
Fizzy drink (sugar-containing)	100 ml/4 fl oz
Orange juice	100 ml/4 fl oz

Illness

The body's natural response to illness is to produce more glucose and hence blood glucose levels tend to rise. There is an increased risk of ketoacidosis and it is vital that the usual amount of insulin is taken regardless of whether or not the patient is eating. An even distribution of carbohydrate in some form should be encouraged, although it is unlikely that the usual carbohydrate intake will be attained. Table 4.50 gives examples of some suitable sources of carbohydrate. Intake of fluids should be increased to prevent dehydration. Blood glucose should be measured at least four times a day.

Table 4.50 Examples of suitable sources of carbohydrate which can be used during illness (British Diabetic Association 1988)

Fluids to provide 10 g carbohydrate	Standard Lucozade, or similar glucose drink	50 ml/2 fl oz
	Grape juice (natural, bottled)	50 ml/4 fl oz
	Fruit juices (natural, unsweetened), 1 wine glass	100 ml/4 fl oz
	Coke or Pepsi, 1 wine glass	100 ml/4 fl oz
	Lemonade, or similar carbonated drink	150 ml/6 fl oz
	Milk, 1 cup	200 ml/8 fl oz
	Soup (thickened creamed e.g. chicken) 1 cup	200 ml/8 fl oz
	Soup (tomato tinned), $\frac{1}{2}$ cup	100 ml/4 fl oz
Foods to provide 10 g carbohydrate	Ice cream (plain), 1 scoop or small brickette	50 g/2 oz
	Natural yoghurt, 1 pot	150 g/5 oz
	Complan	3 level tblsp
	Drinking chocolate, Ovaltine, Horlicks or similar malted drink	2 heaped tsps
	Sugar or glucose	2 level tsps
	Honey, jam or syrup	2 level tsps
	Oster rusks (Glaxo Farley)	2 rusks
	Glucose tablets	3 tablets
Other useful carbohydrate-containing foods		Carbohydrate content
	Build-up (Carnation), 1 envelope	25 g
	Slender (Carnation), 1 envelope	20 g
	Sweetened fruit yoghurts, 1 pot) 150 g/5 fl oz)	25–30 g

4.16.5 Special considerations for Type 2 diabetes

Body weight

About 75% of Type 2 diabetic patients are overweight (Salans 1987; Lean *et al* 1990). One of the major aims of dietary therapy in this group should therefore be for the individual to achieve and maintain a desirable weight. The benefits of this include a reduction in hyperglycaemia, hyperlipidaemia and hypertension. Furthermore, weight loss is the only factor which has been shown to improve life expectancy in Type 2 diabetics (Lean *et al* 1990).

The general dietary guidelines need to be incorporated into a controlled energy intake and continuous encouragement and counselling are required. Realistic targets for weight loss should be set and intermediate goals with 'rewards' may increase motivation. Standardized printed weight-reducing diet sheets are of little value; time and effort is needed to find a suitable slimming strategy for each person.

Cardiovascular disease is a major cause of mortality in this group and restriction of saturated fat should be given greater emphasis in Type II patients where lipid abnormalities are more common (Nutrition Sub-Committee, BDA 1991).

Oral hypoglycaemia agents (OHAs)

There are two major types of OHAs:

1 Sulphonylurea tablets. These:
   - Stimulate the pancreas to produce insulin;
   - Increase the body's sensitivity to insulin.

2 Biguanide tablets. These:
   - decrease absorption of glucose from the intestine;
   - increase the uptake of glucose by the body tissues.

Although it is beneficial for everyone to eat regularly, in patients treated with sulphonylureas the timing of meals is especially important in order to prevent hypoglycaemia. In addition, complex carbohydrate should be distributed evenly throughout the day.

Patients treated by diet alone can be more flexible regarding the timing of carbohydrate intake, but the importance of regular meals comprised of the right types of foods (and if overweight, limited in energy content) should still be stressed.

4.16.6 Dietary management of children with diabetes

In the UK diabetes occurs in about 0.2% of children by the age of 16 years and in about 0.06% of pre-school children (Nutrition Sub-Committee, BDA 1989). Diagnosis of diabetes in a child is a traumatic experience for the whole family and parents are often very worried about the diet. Education must be a gradual process and, ideally, should extend to the whole family. It is helpful and important to take into account the social, ethnic and symbolic significance of food within the family while attempting to modify eating habits.

The basic nutritional requirements for children with diabetes are the same as those of the same age who do not have diabetes. Enough energy needs to be given to allow for growth and yet to prevent obesity. Vitamin supplements are required for children under 5 years of age.

Meal planning

General considerations

Children have variable energy demands which makes timing and distribution of meals more difficult to regulate. General guidelines on the amounts of food needed to match various activities can be given, but getting the balance right is largely a process of trial and error. With experience and a growing knowledge of food values and insulin action, families become more confident about changing the meal or snack size or altering the insulin dose to suit the circumstances.

Food fads and food refusal are common habits of any toddler and when these occur in a diabetic child cause great anxiety to parents. Small frequent meals throughout the day should help to prevent hypoglycaemia but, if necessary, a glucose-containing drink can be offered. Above all, the parents need to learn not to focus too much attention on the issue during such periods and not to try to force their child to eat as this will make the problem worse. Regular blood glucose testing can provide valuable reassurance.

Older children will both need and want to learn more about their dietary needs. Issues such as school meals and the need for carbohydrate top-ups etc. will also need to be addressed.

During adolescence, growth patterns and nutrient requirements change rapidly. Alterations in dietary habits such as more snacking, fast foods, vegetarianism etc. may also be apparent.

Adolescents are often keen to take full control of their diabetes. Explanations of glycaemic control and self-adjustment of insulin and food need to be given at this stage. Guidance on alcohol can also be incorporated into the dietary advice. The doctor and dietitian need to be seen as people who are on their side, willing to give help and support when needed.

Carbohydrate

The average UK intake of carbohydrate is around 45% of dietary energy – this should be maintained for the diabetic child, and unrefined sources encouraged. However inclusion of too many bulky foods which are low in energy may jeopardize nutritional intake in some children. High fibre breakfast cereals can gradually replace sugar-coated low fibre ones. Bread intake is to be encouraged and parents can be advised to experiment with the many different kinds of whole grain and soft grain breads which are available. Pasta, potatoes, rice and baked beans are suitable and are usually liked by children.

Sweets and chocolates need not be banned altogether. It is important for the child with diabetes to feel 'one of the group' and it should not be necessary to isolate the diabetic child. Ideally, fruit, low fat yoghurts, cereal bars and plain biscuits can be recommended in preference, but a small chocolate biscuit bar at breaktimes is unlikely to jeopardize diabetes control, particularly since children are often active during such times. Isolated sources of readily absorbed carbohydrate such as sugar-rich drinks should be avoided (except when used to treat hypoglycaemia, illness or before exercise). The incorporation of non-nutritive sweeteners in low calorie drinks, diet yoghurts and desserts has resulted in a choice of products which are suitable for the diabetic and non-diabetic alike. Diet drinks and yoghurts are indeed becoming increasingly more popular among the non-diabetic population, and hence feelings of isolation need not prevail.

It is sensible to limit sugar consumption (especially between meals) due to its link with dental caries. 'Tooth-friendly' sweets and chocolates are now available. The nutritive sweetener *Isomalt* used in these products has been shown to be non-cariogenic (See Section 2.13). The BDA is of the opinion that although sweets and chocolates should not be encouraged, it is probably preferable for a child to choose a 'tooth-friendly' version rather than a standard version. It is hoped that the laxative effect of Isomalt will limit consumption.

Artificial (non-nutritive) sweeteners can be used to sweeten drinks and breakfast cereals, milk puddings and certain desserts. Since these sweeteners do not have the same technical bulking qualities as sucrose, their use in home baking is limited. They are not permitted for use in food or drink especially prepared for babies.

As with other Type 1 diabetics, quantity and timing of carbohydrate is important. Regular meals and snacks are advisable and a carbohydrate exchange system may or may not be used. Distributing food throughout the day solely on the basis of its carbohydrate content has limitations. Too rigid an application of a food exchange system can detract from the more important advice on sensible meal planning, so a careful balance needs to be sought. An understanding of the carbohydrate exchange system can be valuable to the paediatric dietitian even if it is used simply as a basis for giving out more simple dietary instruction. A flexible approach is required, dependent on the dietary principles used in a particular health authority and on the needs of the patient. Simpler terminology such as 'swaps' or 'choices' may be useful.

Fat

The general principles of fat reduction can be applied in the diets of young children. Alternative cooking methods to frying, choosing lean meat and removing the skin from poultry are sensible ways of reducing saturated fat intake. Changing to lower fat dairy products is not advisable before the age of two years. Even at this age, semi-skimmed milk can be introduced only if the rest of the diet is nutritionally adequate. Skimmed milk should not be used until five years since it provides insufficient fat-soluble vitamins and energy.

Dietary education in children

Education needs to be a gradual process to allow the child and parents to adapt at their own pace. Regular follow-up is of paramount importance since dietary requirements will vary according to growth and activity.

Basic first-line advice may incorporate the following (Magrath *et al* 1993):

1 Eat regular meals and if necessary, between meal snacks.

2 Make a special effort to eat some breakfast.

3 Choose foods you are familiar with, and eat them according to appetite.

4 Don't eat sweets and sugar or drink ordinary pop, squash or large quantities of fruit juice. *Drink* low calorie pop, squash or water.

5 If you are hungry, ask for more food from the swop lists (see Table 4.51).

6 Do carry glucose sweets when away from home e.g. at school or when travelling.

Table 4.51 provides an example of how a child with diabetes can be started on a suitable meal plan. General portion size advice can be given instead of quantitative information on carbohydrate content.

Many schools have never had the experience of being responsible for a child with diabetes and they will need detailed guidance. Understanding of diabetes will therefore often be limited and a contact person at the diabetic clinic can be a vital helpline for the school teacher. The British Diabetic Association produces youth and school information packs which can be a great source of help to the carers. The Association also organizes holidays for diabetic children as well as parent/child weekends. Such activities can provide a valuable learning experience for all participants (including the dietitian).

Families and children are more receptive in their own environment, and so a home visit by the dietitian can be invaluable. This also enables the dietitian to assess the family's understanding of the diet and to see how they have adjusted. As children approach adolescence they should be encouraged to take full responsibility for their diet so that when the time comes to leave home they have a reasonable understanding of the diet.

Table 4.51 Meal planning for children with diabetes

SWOP LIST I	At each mealtime choose 2 foods (at least) from this list:	Bread: Wholemeal White Rice Pasta Breakfast cereal Milk Yoghurt Fruit
SWOP LIST II	Choose in-between meal snacks from this list:	Cereal bars Biscuits Fruit Savoury snacks Bread Milk

4.16.7 Dietary management of diabetes in pregnancy

Diabetes in pregnancy can be classified into two groups:
1 Gestational diabetes which occurs for the first time in pregnancy.
2 Women with existing diabetes who subsequently become pregnant.

In both groups, maintenance of blood glucose levels to as near normal as possible is essential to ensure normal growth and development of the fetus.

Gestational diabetes

Gestational diabetes develops after about 20 weeks of pregnancy as a result of insufficient circulating insulin and hence a raised blood glucose level. Tests for glycosuria are generally conducted at each antenatal visit, but a routine glucose tolerance test (GTT) is indicated in women who have previously had gestational diabetes or if there is diabetes in the family. The GTT is usually conducted early in the third trimester.

Dietary management

Many patients with gestational diabetes are obese and energy intake needs to be reduced sensibly (for example, to around 1500–1800 kcal per day). General meal planning advice, which ensures adequate intake of calcium, iron and vitamin C is necessary.

Insulin may not be prescribed initially, but in patients with severe hyperglycaemia, a combination of short and intermediate-acting insulin may be given. Self-blood glucose monitoring is desirable.

In over 90% of cases, the diabetes disappears after the baby is born. However, there is a greater risk of developing diabetes in later life and it is therefore important that these patients are encouraged to lose weight (and maintain the lost weight) post-pregnancy.

Pregnancy in women with pre-existing diabetes

Maintenance of near-normal blood glucose levels *before* and during pregnancy can help reduce the incidence of congenital abnormalities. Diet, insulin and exercise need to be carefully monitored, ideally prior to conception. Maternal hyperglycaemia will tend to enhance insulin secretion in the fetus resulting in a larger baby. This may cause problems at delivery and in the neonatal period. Patients therefore need to be taught how to conduct regular home blood glucose testing and self-adjustment of insulin and diet. Regular dietary follow-up is essential, paying particular attention to energy and nutrient intake.

Dietary management

Smaller frequent meals are usually more acceptable during pregnancy particularly if there is any morning sickness or heartburn. To match this, more frequent insulin administration will be required and multiple insulin regimens with home blood glucose monitoring can improve the level of glycaemic control.

Energy requirements will need to be assessed in order to ensure a steady total weight gain of around 10–12 kg. Although it is important to guard against excessive weight gain, strict energy reduction is not recommended. A relatively high intake of complex carbohydrate foods (which will also help relieve constipation) and fewer fatty foods within a generally healthy diet is recommended. Supplements of iron and folate (and vitamins A and D in Asian vegetarian women) should be prescribed as necessary.

Nausea and sickness are often accompanied by a loss of

appetite. Biscuits, fruit and glucose-containing drinks may be helpful in the short term. Food cravings and increased appetite as the pregnancy advances can lead to sudden changes in food intake and blood glucose levels. Hence, dietetic support needs to be available throughout the pregnancy.

Following the delivery, insulin and dietary requirements return to the pre-pregnancy state. Women not wishing to breast feed can be guided on a steady weight loss pattern.

Breast feeding and diabetes

Diabetic women who decide to breast feed need to take extra carbohydrate in order to prevent hypoglycaemia. A total of around 50 g carbohydrate (as lactose) can be secreted from breast milk daily and a certain amount of extra unrefined carbohydrate will therefore be required. The carbohydrate content of the bedtime snack will need to cover the needs of night time feeds. Hypoglycaemia is more likely to occur prior to a feed or if the baby is a slow feeder. A snack is required before each feed and many nursing mothers will keep a glass of milk at their side whilst feeding, since breast feeding is often accompanied by thirst. Regular blood glucose monitoring is essential.

4.16.8 Education

Teaching aids

As with any dietary modification, the diet sheet needs to be tailored to the individual in order to cause minimal disruption to daily life. In addition to the standard blank diet sheet, there are various other teaching aids which can be used:

1 Accompanying the diet sheet with basic recipes and suggestions on home recipe modification can be helpful.

2 A system of cards which can be given out at intervals to consolidate new advice may be more effective than giving out all the information in one booklet.

3 Plastic food models can provide a useful adjunct to written information and can be particularly appropriate for patients who do not speak English well and also for children. Afro-Caribbean and Asian replica foods are available.

4 Teaching packs for professionals, slides and photographs can provide a more visual approach.

5 Videos and audio cassettes either viewed at home by patients or in group teaching sessions are extremely useful.

6 Advances in food labelling have done much to increase consumer awareness of food composition and information on take-away foods is now also available. Many supermarkets produce nutrition education booklets.

7 The British Diabetic Association (BDA) has over 400 branches throughout the UK. These support groups help patients to exchange views and problems and also to keep up to date with developments in diabetes. The BDA also produces a wide range of educational material.

Dietary compliance

Ideally, dietary modifications should be made prior to the prescription of an appropriate insulin regimen. The patient needs to be educated in order to have a full understanding of diabetes, and how food, activity and possibly medication influence blood glucose. This awareness can help the patient to look after his or her own diabetes.

Dietary compliance is difficult to measure. Comparing actual versus prescribed carbohydrate intake fails to take account of justifiable variation in intake according to activity level. Testing dietary knowledge can also be of limited value; what people know and what they do in practice are not necessarily the same. Ultimately compliance can only be evaluated in terms of the effect of the diet on parameters of diabetic control.

Giving out information on all aspects of the diet at one consultation may be too much for patients to take in, especially if they have not yet come to terms with the diagnosis of diabetes. The first visit may therefore be more effective if it is used simply as an opportunity to create rapport between patient and dietitian and instil confidence. Basic first line advice can be given at this stage and this can be followed up with a little more detail at subsequent visits.

Continuous motivation is vital. Since people are striving for a negative objective – freedom from complications – it is difficult to sustain belief in the importance of diet. It is nevertheless a message which must be emphasized.

Further research is required to develop more interactive and effective approaches to dietary education.

The era of the traditional restricted diabetic diet may have led to an image of the dietitian as someone who makes the patient feel guilty at each visit. The dietitian today needs to be seen as an approachable and supportive person who is not going to be judgemental. Fears need to be allayed and guidance and encouragement should be ongoing.

Many diabetes centres have now been established throughout the UK and medical and paramedical members of the diabetes care team can provide more comprehensive education and clinical advice.

The dietitian's role is not only one of giving dietary advice: experience of counselling and a sound understanding of the psychology of eating behaviour can be a great asset.

Useful address

British Diabetic Association, 10 Queen Anne Street, London W1M 0BD. Tel 071–323 1531.

Further reading/resources

Useful books for patients

British Diabetic Association (1990) *Countdown* 7e. British Diabetic Association, London.

Day JL, Brenchley S and Redmond S (1992) *Living with non insulin dependent diabetes* 2e. Medikos, Crowborough.

Govindji A and Myers J (1992) *The essential diabetic cookbook*. Thorsons, London.

Sonksen P, Fox C and Judd S (1991) *Diabetes at your fingertips*. Class Publishing, London.

Video cassettes

Sharing and caring, for parents. (1992) Running time 17 minutes. British Diabetic Association.

It's only natural, healthy eating with diabetes. (1992) Running time 20 minutes. British Diabetic Association.

A new start, for people treating their diabetes with diet or tablets. (1992) Running time 19 minutes. British Diabetic Association.

It's my life, for teenagers. (1992) Running time 22 minutes. British Diabetic Association.

Breaking away for 17–25 yrs. (1992) Running time 20 minutes. British Diabetic Association.

A way of life, for people who are taking insulin. (1992) Running time 22 minutes. British Diabetic Association.

So you have diabetes? How to eat for health. A 12 minute video with dialogue in Hindi and accompanying notes in English/Gujarati, English/Urdu, English/Punjabi. Produced by Brent Nutrition and Research Group in association with Brent Health Education Team.

What can we eat? A 5 minute education programme for patients in a GP waiting room. Produced by Farmitalia Ltd in association with the British Diabetic Association.

Considering diet and diabetes. A 10 minute education programme for GPs. Produced by Farmitalia in association with the British Diabetic Association.

References

British Diabetic Association (1988) Coping when you are ill and on tablets or diet alone. Leaflet.

Department of Health (1991) *Dietary Reference Values for food energy and nutrients for the United Kingdom*. Rep Hlth Soc Subj 41. HMSO, London.

Fuessl HS, Williams G, Adrian TE and Bloom SR (1987) Guar sprinkled on food: effect on glycaemic control, plasma lipids and gut hormones in non-insulin dependent diabetic patients. *Diabetic Med* **4**, 463–8.

Fuller N (1990) The Glycaemic Index – how dietary carbohydrates raise the blood glucose. *Diabetic Nursing* **1**(5), 3–5.

Gale E and Tattersall R (1990) Choosing an insulin regimen. *Diabetes: clinical management*. Longman (PTE) Ltd, Singapore.

Govindji A (1991a) A matter of fat. *Balance* **125**, 54–6.

Govindji A (1991b) Sounds fishy? *Balance* **124**, 56–8.

Gramenzi A, Gentile A, Fasoli M, Parazzini F and Vecchia CL (1990) Association between certain foods and risk of acute myocardial infarction in women. *Br Med J* **300**, 771–3.

Haber GB, Heaton KW, Murphy D and Burroughs LF (1977) Depletion and disruption of dietary fibre. *Lancet* **ii**, 679–82.

James WPT, Ferro-Luzzi A, Izaksson B and Szostak WB (1988) *Healthy nutrition*. WHO Regional Pub 24. World Health Organization, Copenhagen.

Jenkins DJA, Wolever TMS, Jenkins AL, Thorne MJ, Lee R, Kalmusky J, Reichert R and Wong GS (1983) The glycaemic index of foods tested in diabetic patients: a new basis for carbohydrate exchange favouring the use of legumes. *Diabetologia* **24**, 257–64.

Jenkins DJA, Wolever TMS, Jenkins AL, Josse RG and Wong GS (1984) The glycaemic response to carbohydrate foods. *Lancet* **2**, 388–91.

Keys A, Anderson JT and Grande F (1965) Serum cholesterol response to changes in the diet, in particular saturated fatty acids in the diet. *Metabolism* **14**, 775.

Kushi LH, Lew RA, Stare FJ, Ellison CR, el Lozy M, Bourke G, Daly L, Graham I, Hickey N, Mulcahy R and Kevaney J (1985) Diet and 20-year mortality from coronary heart disease. The Ireland-Boston Study. *N Engl J Med* **312**, 811–18.

Lean MEJ, Powrie JK, Anderson AS and Garthwaite PH (1990) Obesity, weight loss and prognosis in Type 2 diabetes. *Diabetic Med* **7**, 228–33.

Lean MEJ and James WPT (1986) Prescription of diabetic diets in the 1980s. *Lancet* **i**, 723–5.

MacDonald MJ (1987) Post-exercise late-onset hypoglycaemia in insulin-dependent diabetic patients. *Diabetes Care*, **10**, 584–8.

Magrath G, Hartland B and Nutrition Sub-Committee, British Diabetic Association (1993) *Dietary recommendations for children and adolescents with diabetes – an implementation paper*. In press.

Nutrition Study Group, European Association for the Study of Diabetes (EASD) (1988) Nutritional recommendations for individuals with diabetes mellitus. *Diab Nutr Metab* **1**, 145–9.

Nutrition Sub-Committee, British Diabetic Association (1989) Dietary recommendations for children and adolescents with diabetes. *Diabetic Med* **6**, 537–47.

Nutrition Sub-Committee, British Diabetic Association (1982) Dietary recommendations for diabetics for the 1980s. *Hum Nutr: Appl Nutr* **36A**, 378–94.

Nutrition Sub-Committee, British Diabetic Association (1991) Dietary recommendations for people with diabetes: an update for the 1990s. *J Hum Nutr Dietetic* **4**, 393–412.

Nutrition Sub-Committee, British Diabetic Association (1990) Sucrose and fructose in the diabetic diet. *Diabetic Med* **7**, 764–9.

Pirart J (1978) Diabetes Mellitus and degenerative complications, a prospective study of 4400 patients observed between 1947 and 1973. *Diabetes Care* **1**, 168–88.

Salans LB (1987) Obesity and non-insulin dependent diabetes mellitus. In *Recent advances in obesity research V*, Berry EM, Blondheim SH, Eliahou HE and Shafrir E (Eds) pp. 26–32. John Libby, London.

Seviour PW, Teal TK, Richmond W and Elkeles RS (1988) Serum lipids, lipoproteins and macrovascular disease in non-insulin dependent diabetics: a possible new approach to prevention. *Diabetic Med* **5**, 166–71.

Stringer MD, Gorog PG, Freeman A and Kakkar VV (1989) Lipid peroxides and atherosclerosis. *Br Med J* **298**, 281–98.

Thomas BJ (1982) Patterns of Nutritional intake in diabetics and non-diabetics: Relationship with vascular disease and its pathogenesis. PhD thesis, London University.

Thomas BJ and the Nutrition Subcommittee, British Diabetic Association (1992) British Diabetic Association's discussion paper on the role of 'Diabetic' foods. *Diabetic Med* **9**, 300–306.

Viberti GC (1988) Low protein diet and progression of diabetic kidney disease. *Nephrol Dial Transplant* **3**, 334–9.

Vinik AI and Jenkins DJA (1988) Dietary fibre in the management of diabetes. *Diabetes Care* **11**, 160–73.

Weinsier RL, Seeman A, Herrera HG, Assal J-P, Soeldner JS and Gleason RE (1974) High and low carbohydrate diets in diabetes mellitus study of effects on diabetic control, insulin secretion and blood lipids. *Ann Intern Med* **80**, 332–41.

World Health Organization (1990) *Diet, nutrition and prevention of chronic diseases*. Tech Rep Ser 797. WHO, Geneva.

4.17 Obesity

Aspects of energy intake, requirements and expenditure are discussed in Section 2.1.

4.17.1 Obesity in adults

Identifying the problems

Classification of obesity

The Quetelet index or body mass index (BMI) is a useful way of classifying obesity:

$$\text{BMI} = \frac{\text{weight (kg)}}{\text{height}^2\ \text{(m)}}$$

(measured in indoor clothing and without shoes).

Garrow and Webster (1985) propose that grades of obesity be defined as follows:

		BMI
1	Grade O	20–24.9
2	Grade I	25–29.9
3	Grade II	30–39.9
4	Grade III	>40

Grade O indicates a 'desirable' weight range and Grade III indicates severe obesity.

The equivalent of the 1983 Metropolitan Height and Weight tables in terms of BMI over the range from the minimum for 'small frame' to the maximum for 'large frame' is 21.0–26.0 for men and 19.7–26.0 for women.

The aim of any treatment regimen is initial weight loss and future weight maintenance. Active treatment should be geared towards those people in obesity Grades II and III as they are likely to have the most serious medical and psychological problems. It is recommended that Grade I obesity be treated if any of the following factors are present:

1 Adult below 50 years of age.
2 Hypertension.
3 Hyperlipidaemia.
4 Diabetes.
5 Distribution of fat is central.

When calculating an obese patient's 'target weight', although Grade O represents 'desirable' or 'acceptable healthy' weight, it is worth considering the age of onset of obesity. Those patients whose obesity stems from childhood may have grown through the 'desirable' weight range during late childhood and early adolescence and only ever been at an obese weight since that time. Attempts at dieting may have resulted in weight loss only to have been followed by rapid weight gain. This presents a problem in that these patients have no concept of themselves at normal body weight and therefore have unrealistic expectations of such. Patients who becomes obese in adult years and have maintained a normal weight previously do, at least, have a mental picture of themselves and therefore more realistic expectations. Frequently these patients will carry photographs of themselves at their own 'target' weight. So, by taking a weight history, a realistic 'target' weight (or weight range) can be established which, although perhaps not in Grade O, can be seen to be achievable by the patient.

However, the BMI only indicates the degree of severity of the obesity, it does not reveal what the underlying problems are. There are many reasons why energy intake may have exceeded requirement (poor eating habits, behavioural and psychiatric problems, low energy requirements) and disentangling the relevant factors in each individual case are fundamental for ultimate success in achieving and maintaining weight reduction.

Obtaining background information

It is useful to try to include some of the following questions at the first appointment:

1 Why does the patient want to lose weight? Is it for him/herself or because of pressure from other family members? Are there health reasons?
2 What is the patient's own target weight? Has it ever been achieved? Is the presenting weight the highest weight the patient has been? Is there a weight which the patient has maintained for any period of time?
3 What are the previous attempts at dieting? Why have previous diets failed? What is the maximum length of time the patient has been 'on a diet'? What is the maximum weight loss which has been achieved? Has any weight loss ever been maintained?
4 What rate of weight loss is the patient expecting or hoping for?
5 What are the patient's expectations of the anticipated weight loss?
6 Is the patient working? Is it full time/part time/shift work? Does the job involve travelling/living away from home?
7 What is the family structure? Are other members of the family overweight? Do the family eat regular meals together

or is there a casual attitude towards food or meal times creating a more erratic pattern? Who does the shopping/cooking? Are the other family members interested in the patient losing weight?

Obtaining dietary information

Careful investigation into a person's usual eating habits will provide many valuable clues to the cause of the energy imbalance and hence give indications of how this may best be tackled. It is thus well worth the investment in time.

Methods of obtaining dietary information, and the problems associated with them, have been discussed in detail in Section 1.7. Points which are particularly relevant to the assessment of the intake of obese people are summarized below.

Dietary history/24-hour recall Though a dietary history cannot be totally relied upon, careful and skilful questioning can provide a reasonable estimate of energy intake and a picture of eating habits in obese patients.

The simplest method of finding out what people have been eating is to ask them what food and beverages they have consumed over the past 24 hours. This relies upon the assumptions that:

1 People will remember what they have eaten.
2 A 24 hour period is representative of their general energy intake.
3 They are willing to disclose what they eat.

It is the latter point which must, in particular, be watched when assessing the intake of obese people; most of them will be very sensitive about the amount and type of food they eat (even if there is no reason to feel guilt). In order to help distinguish between a genuinely low intake and a fabricated one, the 24 hour recall must be substantiated with information which acts as a cross-check (e.g. weekly food shopping, family meal patterns and meals eaten away from home). Questions relating to eating habits must be phrased in an open rather than a suggestive manner, for example 'Do you eat breakfast?' rather than 'What do you eat for breakfast?'.

Assessment of portion size must also be done with care. Some obese people may have a different concept of an 'average' portion compared with non-obese people. Food models are useful as they present the patient with a visual picture.

The dietitian must also enquire whether the patient's weight is static or changing (either decreasing or increasing) at the time of the interview since this is obviously relevant to the assessment of energy requirement.

Food diary This involves patients in recording their own food and beverage consumption for a number of days. It has the advantage of not being dependent on memory and covering a longer time span than the 24 hour recall, but carries the risk of a reduced or unrepresentative food intake as a result of having to record everything consumed (Black *et al* 1985; Prentice *et al* 1986).

Obese patients should be given (rather than supplying their own) record sheets, ideally divided into columns for recording the quantity and type of item consumed since this gives a clearer idea of the sort of information required. Additional guidelines on how to measure food intake (by means of scales, household measures, packet or can size) should also be given. It must be emphasized that the record should be made *at the time* of consumption and not at the end of the day (or even several days!). At the end of the recording period, the patient's weight should be checked; sudden weight loss is strongly suggestive of dietary alteration.

It must be remembered that neither the dietary recall nor the food diary will provide a totally accurate measure of dietary intake. Both methods are subject to distortion and atypicality and probably underestimate 'true' intake (Acheson *et al* 1980), especially in obese people (Prentice *et al* 1986; Southgate 1986). Nevertheless, providing that the limitations are borne in mind, they are useful indicators of energy intake. Whichever method is used it is essential that obese patients are urged to give as accurate a picture as possible of their usual food intake — however 'bad' they might think this is — since it is only by being truthful that the dietitian will be able to help them.

Behavioural aspects of food intake

Most people do not eat to satisfy hunger, but in response to other feelings. This may be particularly so in people who are overweight. A group of 20 women at a slimming club (BMI 26–34) were asked why they ate and gave the following reasons: hunger, boredom, comfort, stress, tiredness, habit, availability, anger and to be sociable. On further discussion the majority of them decided that hunger came at the bottom of the list (Bowyer, personal communication).

Food diaries can be used to explore why and where people eat as well as what they are eating. A record sheet suitable for recording this information is shown in Table 4.52. Patients can be asked to describe how they feel before and after eating and with accurately kept records patients can begin to learn about their own eating behaviour. The dietitian must take time to discuss with the patient methods of dealing with some of the reasons given, e.g. boredom, socializing or habit. Any change of behaviour of this type could help towards long term weight maintenance.

This type of record keeping may or may not identify the patient who is bingeing (i.e. consuming large quantities of food at one time) or a 'restrained' eater. The restrained eater is one who is constantly dieting in order to control his or her body weight. If the diet is 'broken' by consumption of a high calorie food or drink which the dieter considers

Table 4.52 Suggested format for recording eating patterns

Day Date Time	Where	Who with	Food and drink consumed	Comments and feelings e.g. hunger, anxiety, enjoyment, anger

'taboo' it usually leads to abandonment of the diet and eating in excess (Ruderman and Wilson 1979). Thus while bingeing may be the consequence of emotional upsets, it may also be the response to a very restrictive diet (Marcus *et al* 1985). Establishing regular meal patterns is important as is discussion of the foods considered taboo together with education that the occasional extra does not mean the end or waste of several days' or weeks' effort.

A morbidly obese person may suffer many prejudices, discrimination at work and low self-esteem. It may be that the individual does have some deep-rooted emotional, psychological problems or may be clinically depressed. If this is suspected, dietitians should refer back to the referring agent with the recommendation for psychological or psychiatric assessment. Psychological counselling may be needed prior to dietetic intervention, or liaison between the dietitian and psychotherapist may be another approach.

Tackling the problem

A standardized diet sheet handed out to all obese patients irrespective of their problems is of no therapeutic value whatsoever. Instead, the dietitian must work from a basic dietary outline and employ different strategies in order to create an individualized treatment programme tailored to the needs of the patient. Dietitians must also be prepared to educate their obese patients, not only in nutrition, but in relevant basic physiology, i.e. how their bodies work. Some patients have strong preconceived ideas about their obesity and may believe that no diet will work for them because their body 'defies the laws of physics' or 'has a slow metabolism' or because of their 'glands'. These are beliefs patients carry with them as they are referred from professional to professional and create a barrier to effective action by them.

The basis on which any obesity treatment should be planned is one of change; the concept of being 'on a diet' should be discouraged as it is the time of being 'off the diet' which causes the damage. The long term goal is to change habits, attitudes and behaviour by encouraging the patient to maintain the short term goals which have been achieved.

Responsibility

So often a patient's 'weight problem' is presented in such a way as if it is the responsibility of the professional and not the patient to solve the problem. In part, this is due to the manner in which obesity is managed and patients wanting someone else to cure it. Typically, a patient goes to the GP who provides a low energy diet sheet and on a return visit, if the patient has lost no weight, the GP refers the patient to a dietitian on the patient's insistence that the diet didn't work. If the dietitian's advice 'doesn't work' then the patient goes back to the GP for the next referral on to an obesity clinic and so the situation continues. The end result of these referrals is reaffirmation for the patient that his/her 'weight problem' cannot be solved by any dietary intervention given by any professional. Many chronic dieters have a long list of diets they have tried which 'didn't work'. However, in many of these patients, little attempt will have been made to help them discover the fundamental reasons for their weight problem.

The emphasis with any obesity treatment programme should be on permanent change – change of eating habits, attitudes, behaviour and perhaps even lifestyle – if patients are to have any chance of losing weight effectively and then maintaining the weight achieved. Health professionals should take time and effort to uncover the real nature of the problem and advise on how this can be remedied; the responsibility for acting on this advice then lies with the patient alone.

The reducing or low energy diet

There is an extensive amount of literature continually trying to provide the avid obese reader with the 'reducing diet that works' published as books (many reaching the best seller list), in women's magazines and in national newspapers. Many rely on gimmicks, and most food constituents in the nation's diet have been the focus of restraint at some time. However, ultimately the only reducing diet which works is one which achieves a sustained reduction in energy intake and such a reducing diet will only be beneficial if it provides a balanced nutrient intake.

General considerations When prescribing a reducing diet, the following factors must be borne in mind:

1 The diet must provide the body with all the essential nutrients, vitamins and minerals necessary to maintain health, without meeting the patient's total energy requirements.

2 The diet must be sufficiently flexible to take into

account a patient's taste, financial status and religious restrictions and must be adapted to their lifestyle.

3 The diet must be acceptable to the patient, but the patient must also understand that if the present energy intake is maintaining the obesity there must be substantial change initially, in order to lose weight, and permanently to maintain a lower weight.

4 The diet must be presented to the patient as a basis for long term change of eating habits and *not* a short term crash diet.

5 An energy deficit of 1000 kcal (4.2 MJ)/day below requirement will achieve an approximate weight loss of 1 kg/week. For many patients this will be the maximum, practical deficit achievable and for most it will be less than this.

6 The physiological responses of the body to weight loss such as sensitivity to cold and increased tiredness are frequently reported by patients and they need to be reassured that these will resolve.

Energy content and dietary composition

1 Many obese patients claim to be unable to lose weight on a daily intake of either 1000 kcal (4.2 MJ) or 800 kcal (3.4 MJ). James (1983) reports not to have yet found a single value for total energy expenditure over 24 hours below 1200 kcal (5 MJ) using whole body calorimetric studies on adults whether of normal weight, obese of underweight. The lowest oxygen uptake recorded by Pilkington (personal communication) is 161 ml/min which equates to an RMR of approximately 1100 kcal (4.7 MJ)/ 24 hours. The usual energy intake of each individual will provide the best guide to what the energy content of the weight reducing diet should be.

2 The importance of a regular meal pattern should be emphasized and most people should consume a minimum of three meals per day. This is partly because the metabolic rate is increased after each eating episode (thermogenic effect of food) but also because an unstructured meal pattern lends itself to erratic eating and the likelihood of consuming excess food. Many obese patients feel they are doing themselves good by missing a meal whereas in practice the energy saving is usually more than compensated for by nibbling throughout the day. Many patients accommodate between-meal snacks by cutting down at their next meal which in turn does not satisfy them sufficiently leading to further between-meal eating or bingeing. At the onset of treatment the meal pattern, as well as the content of the meals themselves, should be arranged to suit the patient's lifestyle and once agree should not be altered.

3 Bread, cereals and potatoes are still thought to be 'fattening' by many people and this misconception must be clarified. Fibre-rich sources of carbohydrate such as wholemeal bread, cereals and potatoes have a low energy density, are inexpensive, easily available, good sources of protein, vitamins and minerals and help provide satiety. They should be included with every meal. The use of carbohydrate exchange lists is sometimes useful – not so much for the purpose of restricting intake but to ensure that adequate amounts of these foods are consumed. This cannot be overemphasized as many obese people have been 'brainwashed' into restricting these foods.

4 Protein content must be adequate to meet daily requirements. Although weight loss may be faster if protein intake is restricted, this will be achieved at the expense of loss of lean body mass, rather than adipose tissue (Garrow *et al* 1981). All energy restricted diets should contain approximately 15% of energy in the form of protein. Guidelines are needed for recommended portion sizes of the protein-rich foods, e.g. meat, fish, cheese, eggs, milk, yoghurt and pulses to be included in the low energy diet.

5 With an energy value of 9 kcal (38 kJ)/g, fat is a very concentrated source of energy in any person's diet. Reduction in fat intake is vital if a significant energy saving is to be made. The percentage of energy from fat in a reducing diet should be as low as is achievable for palatability. All fat-rich foods should be avoided. Low fat spread can be used instead of butter or margarine and should be included in a measured quantity. Patients often find it more useful to know what quantity of fat will last a period of time, e.g. 1 week, rather than a daily amount. Adding fat to food (e.g. butter on vegetables), cooking in fat (e.g. frying or roasting) or consuming fat-containing sauces, gravies or batter should be avoided. However, ideas for alternative foods or cooking methods should also be given.

6 Fruit and vegetables should be included daily as they are valuable sources of fibre, vitamins and minerals.

7 Although energy-rich foods such as sweets, chocolates, cakes, etc. cannot be recommended for inclusion on a low energy diet, the use of the words 'fattening' 'bad' or 'forbidden' as a means of describing them should be avoided. Obese patients frequently regard these foods in this way and the guilt feelings produced by one lapse in this direction can lead patients to assume that they have 'failed' and that their dietary efforts have been in vain.

It should be stressed to patients that, for example, one bar of chocolate or one cake will not cause uncontrollable weight gain; it will only add the equivalent energy intake to that day's total intake. Weeks or even months of effort must not be abandoned simply because of lapses on one day. Identification of the 'taboo' foods of a restrained eater should be made so that some may be included in the diet plan. Dietary restrictions of any kind create craving for those foods 'not allowed'. Only the most superhuman will be able to resist totally the constant temptations.

8 It should be impressed clearly upon patients that short term (daily) fluctuations in weight are due to changes in *water* balance and that the changes in fat weight are small and slow. For this reason, patients should be discouraged from weighing themselves more than once a week. They should also not allow a sudden increase in weight after a

dietary indiscretion to discourage them from continuing with the attempt to lose *fat*.

9 Lists of both 'foods which can be eaten freely' and 'foods to avoid' based on low and high energy dense food respectively are helpful to patients. However, these lists should be practical and reasonably balanced in length; a long list of pleasant-tasting 'foods to avoid' accompanied by an 'unrestricted' list comprised only of items such as salt, pepper, mustard and low calorie squash will not help the patient's morale.

Education of the patient in choosing the foods that comprise a 'healthy' diet is important so that if he or she is hungry the most suitable option may be selected, for instance, a bowl of cereal with semi-skimmed milk rather than a cheese sandwich during the evening. Whilst this may appear to be stating the obvious, it is better to let the patient know that they may eat if hungry rather than risk non-compliance through being on a diet that removes all choices.

Motivation

Adequate motivation is a vital component of a successful weight loss programme. The reasons people give for wishing to lose weight are numerous and range from purely aesthetic reasons to very defined medical reasons. The associated complications and risks of obesity include diabetes mellitus, coronary heart disease, hypertension and premature death. Conditions exacerbated by obesity include osteoarthritis and respiratory disease. All of these complications can be improved by weight loss (RCP 1983).

Motivation may initially be very high, but within a very short period of time the resolve fades because these ultimate goals concerning health or appearance seem to be so far into the future and so out of reach. It becomes difficult to balance the long term benefits with the immediate satisfaction of eating.

Support from a partner, spouse or other family members can increase motivation substantially. Re-educating the eating habits of the whole family often secures a better chance of change rather than focusing solely on the individual who is 'on a diet'. Dietitians should involve other family members more often as ideas about supportive behaviour vary enormously. Many obese female patients feel their husbands/partners continually 'nag' them about their weight and about any food eaten which is considered 'fattening'. This can drive them to begin eating secretly. Hence a further problem arises of the husband/partner only then seeing the patient eat correctly and frugally yet losing no weight! So, the patient should be encouraged to define what behaviour from other family members will be supportive to the patient's own motivation, e.g. compliments, non-food treats, change of family eating behaviour. Every overweight patient must want to lose weight for him/herself and this must be the prime motivation. The situation where a patient claims to be losing weight for the dietitian should be avoided. Time and effort should be put into helping obese patients to find and secure their own motivational goals.

Rate of weight loss

Excess energy is stored in the body predominantly as adipose tissue. Any weight losing programme should result in the utilization of these adipose tissue stores with minimum loss of other important body tissue such as the lean body mass.

Many obese patients who seek tratment view a successful outcome as one which produces the 'greatest weight loss in the shortest period of time'. The following facts provide evidence as to why this may be impossible or undesirable:

1 Adipose tissue has an energy value of approximately 7000 kcal (29 MJ)/kg therefore a deficit of 1000 kcal (4.2 MJ)/day below requirement will achieve a weight loss of approximately 1 kg per week.

2 Garrow (1980) has shown that a more rapid weight loss than this, for example, over 3 kg/week, is effected by increased loss of lean body mass.

3 The RMR, (which contribute the greatest percentage to total energy expenditure) falls during weight loss as an adaptive response to a reduced energy intake. Therefore the rate of weight loss decreases with time for the same reduction in energy intake.

4 The initial rapid weight loss which patients experience when first reducing their energy intake, particularly from restricting carbohydrate, is due to the utilization of the body's glycogen stores and consequent loss of water. This can create motivation and resolve at the beginning of a reducing diet, but as the body begins to utilize its adipose tissue stores a decrease in the rate of weight loss is inevitable. Patients can become disillusioned very easily by this and the expected pattern of weight loss, and if possible the reason for it, should be clearly explained by the dietitian at the onset of dietary treatment.

Exercise

It is generally acknowledged that some exercise is beneficial to general health and well-being and people are being encouraged to include regular exercise in their lives. To many obese people 'exercise' means either stripping down to a minimum of clothing in a gymnasium or swimming pool or jogging around the park and, not surprisingly, most are unwilling to contemplate any of these. However, most are unaware that significant amounts of 'exercise' can be performed by means of ordinary daily tasks, e.g. walking up the stairs rather than using a lift; walking to the shops instead of taking the bus or car and finding some household task to do instead of watching television.

The severely obese have particular problems because they have difficulty with breathing, joints and balance. Increasing the level of activity should be taken slowly and the type of activity geared to each patient's capabilities. Once the patient starts to lose weight and adapts to the level of activity, the amount and degree of difficulty of the tasks performed can be increased, e.g. walking briskly, walking further and using the stairs more.

Although exercise will not in itself contribute a great deal to weight loss directly, it undoubtedly increases a sense of well-being and helps divert attention from food and hence is a valuable part of any weight reducing regimen. Some patients enjoy, as well as benefit from, a formalized exercise programme and this can be planned with the help and advice of a physiotherapist.

Realistic goals and expectations of treatment

Successful weight loss often brings its own problems. It should be stressed that it will not be easy going, that there may be setbacks and periods of weight plateaux. The most successful dieters do not allow setbacks to alter their ultimate goal. Some people can gain motivation and support from a slimming club (see Section 4.17.3 below).

Maintenance of weight loss

The patients who achieve their target weight may need some education as to how their energy intake may be increased in order to maintain their weight. They should be aware that their new weight brings a lower RMR than their obese weight (Garrow and Webster 1989) and that they will not be able to return to their previous eating habits. It may be some time before the patient feels confident about controlling his or her weight and support should be offered during this period.

Radical treatment approaches to obesity

Several radical approaches have been used in the treatment of severe obesity. All present problems to the medical and surgical teams involved and require skilled dietetic help.

Jejuno-ileal bypass

This long established surgical procedure involves the anastomosis of a short length of the proximal jejunum to a short length of the terminal ileum, hence bypassing a large segment of the small intestine. The most recent operations include a cholecystojejunostomy, in which the end of the excluded segment is anastomosed to the gall bladder. It has been found that the length of small intestine remaining in continuity and therefore available for the digestion and absorption of food should be less than 50 cm.

The operation carries many medical and surgical complications which include 'bypass enteritis', electrolyte disturbances, renal stones, liver damage, inflammatory skin and joint disease and mineral and vitamin deficiencies (e.g. iron, folic acid, vitamin B_{12} and vitamin D). Many of the complications are severe enough to warrant reversal of the operation and are not always confined to the early post-operative period. There is a mortality rate of 3–4% (Bray *et al* 1977; McFarland *et al* 1985).

The weight loss after bypass approximates 35% of pre-operative weight, the majority of which occurs during the first year (Pilkington 1980). After this time body weight is maintained but there may be some weight regained. It is frequently assumed this weight loss occurs due to severe malabsorption and many obese patients request the operation thinking they can eat as much as they like and still lose weight. However, it has been shown that the weight loss is due largely to a self-imposed reduction in food intake in order to avoid the unpleasant side effect of diarrhoea which tends to occur after an over-liberal fat and fluid intake (Pilkington *et al* 1976; Bray *et al* 1976). Patients who are unable to alter their food intake may have such severe complications that reversal becomes essential in order to prevent death.

The procedure also carries a risk of renal stone formation arising from the increased formation of calcium soaps with unabsorbed fatty acids in the gastrointestinal tract. The consequent reduction in intraluminal calcium ions results in less oxalate being bound and passive oxalate absorption being increased, particularly in the colon (Stauffer 1977). A high calcium, low oxalate, low fat (<40 g/day) intake can prevent excessive oxalate excretion via the kidneys.

Jejuno-ileal bypass is now virtually obsolete as a method of treating severe obesity due to the serious side effects and consequent life-long follow-up.

Gastric surgery

Because of the side effects associated with the jejuno-ileal bypass, surgeons have searched for another operation to offer to the severely obese. Mason introduced the gastric bypass in America in 1966 which was based on the Billroth II gastrectomy. Modifications of this bypass have been performed over the years and recent techniques in gastroplasty (leaving a passage along the greater or lesser curvature of the stomach without bypassing it) now involve stapling the stomach to create a very small upper pouch with a reinforced stoma through the staple line. Foods and fluids then pass from the upper pouch through to the remainder of the stomach. As there is no interruption of the gastrointestinal tract food is digested in the normal way. The aim of the procedure is to limit the quantity of food and fluids taken at any one time by producing early satiety. The size of the uper pouch is important if maximum weight loss is to be achieved and Mason (1980) suggested 50 ml as the optimum capacity. Complications associated with large upper pouches include vomiting, stomal ulcer and inadequate weight loss. The other criterion for successful outcome of gastric bypass and gastroplasty is a reinforced small stoma to prevent its dilatation. Mason (1980) reported an average weight loss of 30% of initial weight if the specifications of upper pouch size and reinforced stoma are met.

Post-operatively, once patients are able to tolerate sips of fluid, they should commence on a soft puréed diet. Small portions of food (one or two tablespoons) are essential to prevent disruption of the staple line and allow time for healing. Too large a portion may cause pain, discomfort or vomiting, leaving the patient unwilling to try eating, so food and drink should be alternated for this reason. It is important to commence this regimen while the patient is still in hospital.

As the total energy is low the patient should be encouraged to eat 'nutritionally dense' foods such as puréed porridge, puréed meat or fish, runny soft-boiled egg, strained yoghurt, mashed potato, puréed vegetables, fruit juice or puréed fruit, strained soup. One pint of milk should be consumed daily and vitamin and mineral supplements are usually necessary.

Once discharged from hospital, the patient should be encouraged to increase the variety of food, gradually introducing solids. With time the patient is able to tolerate larger portions and it may be appropriate to decrease snacks or advise on lower calorie choices. The range of food should expand though some patients may be unable to tolerate certain foods (Abraham and Owen 1988). Some find, for instance, that bread appears to 'stick' although they are able to manage crackers or toast. Many find that chocolates or crisps are readily tolerated whilst fruit is more difficult! Patients should be encouraged to find their food tolerances by trial and error.

Rapid weight loss during the post-operative period, whilst encouraging to the patient, may give cause for concern. There is sometimes a conflict of interests between the patient and the dietitian especially when the patient perceives the fast weight loss as the 'norm' and becomes despondent when the rate slows down.

The dietitian has an important role in the management of these patients ensuring that there is an adequate nutritional intake and education of eating habits. Counselling is important so that the patients are aware of the limitations imposed on their eating habits and do not see the stapling as an easy option.

Very low calorie diets

Very low calorie diets (VLCDs) are defined by the COMA report (DHSS 1987), as 'commercially produced nutrient preparations providing less than about 600 kcal (2.5 MJ) per day, marketed for use as a total food substitute'.

VLCDs are attractive to the dieter with promises of large weight losses as a result of the energy deficit. However the role of VLCDs in the treatment of obesity remains controversial.

Effects on lean body mass Reports were made in the 1970s of deaths of individuals on VLCDs (Isner *et al* 1979) as a result of cardiac arrythmias. This led to changes in the formulation of these products. Claims are made that the current composition of VLCD allows rapid weight loss whilst preserving lean body mass. This remains one of the areas of controversy. Nitrogen balance studies are difficult to undertake as a number of factors influence the outcome and there is a wide variation in individual response (Wadden *et al* 1983; Apfelbaum *et al* 1987). Garrow *et al* (1989) compared the rates of weight loss and nitrogen loss between a very low calorie diet and a milk diet on a metabolic ward, and demonstrated that there was a greater nitrogen loss on the VLCD. This indicated that the extra weight loss seen with VLCD was at the expense of lean body mass. It has been suggested that the lower the BMI, the shorter the duration of time that an individual can diet safely on a VLCD; in other words, the more obese the person, the greater the conservation of lean body mass (van Itallie and Yang 1984).

Recommendations for safe use of VLCDs It is recommended that VLCDs should only be used for those individuals who are massively or morbidly obese and should not be followed for a period of greater than four weeks (Apfelbaum *et al* 1987; DHSS 1987). Prolonged use is inadvisable and there should be an interval of two months before a VLCD is repeated (Apfelbaum *et al* 1987).

Patients following VLCDs should:

1 Have had a recent medical and electrocardiogram.
2 Be examined weekly by a physician.
3 Have their electrolyte levels monitored at least fortnightly.
4 Have their energy intakes increased during periods of rapid weight loss.

(Wadden *et al* 1990)

The decision to recommend VLCDs should not be taken lightly; they should not be used by pregnant or breast feeding women, children, or the elderly. Their use is also contraindicated in individuals with:

1 Cardiac disorders.
2 Cerebrovascular disease.
3 Hepatic or renal disease.
4 Hyperuricaemia.
5 Psychiatric disturbance.
6 Porphyria.

(DHSS 1987; Wadden *et al* 1990)

Compliance and effectiveness of VLCDs Whilst there is no doubt that an individual on a very low calorie intake will lose weight, the difficulty in compliance remains. Outpatients on VLCDs do not always, as might be expected, lose more weight than those given a conventional 800 kcal diet. However, patients on either regimen who have had their jaws wired tend to lose more weight than those who have not, suggesting that compliance is a factor, and that without jaw-wiring it is easy to cheat!

Concern regarding VLCDs Most of the concern is over the fact that VLCDs are available to the general public and, although recommendations governing their use may be made, there is no guarantee that these will be followed. These products are attractive to the mildly obese although are probably only suitable for the morbidly obese; in addition most of the studies investigating their effects and safety have been conducted in those with severe obesity.

VLCDs are sold by agents of the manufacturers (Garrow 1989) and frequently, these individual are not medically supervised. In addition, there may be some people who are so pleased with a fast weight loss that they choose to ignore the health warnings. All patients on VLCDs should be followed up and warned of the dangers of prolonged use (Apfelbaum *et al* 1987). The patients must then be advised on the foods that they should eat, either to maintain their weight loss or to continue losing weight.

Gastric balloon

The gastric balloon or bubble is another medical device used in the treatment of obesity. It is placed in a deflated state into the stomach via an endoscope and then inflated using air, water or a combination of both. The aim is to reduce the gastric volume and consequently the intake of food. It remains in place for a temporary period and is then deflated and removed.

Early satiety has been reported in obese patients with the inflated balloon, however there was no significant difference in weight loss over a three month period between those patients with a balloon and others who had a sham procedure (Hogan *et al* 1989). Each group took part in a weight loss programme which included a weight reducing diet, behaviour modification and exercise.

In another trial, where obese patients had an inflated balloon for six months, only 20% could maintain their weight loss (Worner *et al* 1989).

Side effects are reported and these include nausea, abdominal pain and vomiting. These usually disappear in most (but not all) patients in the first two weeks.

Hogan *et al* (1989) suggest that that balloon 'offers no additional benefits over standard weight loss therapy in the short term treatment of obesity in motivated patients'.

4.17.2 Obesity in children

Aetiology

As with adults, there are many factors contributing to obesity in children:

1 Hormonal causes (these are rare).

2 Hereditary tendency. Obesity tends to run in families, possibly due to lifestyle and eating habits, but also as a consequence of genetic factors. Eating habits should be watched closely in these families so that any potential problem can be diagnosed and corrected at an early stage.

3 Feeding habits in infancy. Breast fed babies are thought to be less likely to become overweight children that those who are bottle fed (although with the introduction of more modified feeding formulae in recent years, this difference may be less likely to occur). However, the incorrect use of artificial formulae, early weaning and inappropriate weaning foods may contribute to the development of obesity.

4 Emotional factors. Food for many children is a source of comfort; unhappy children may therefore eat more than happier children. Food is often used as a bribe or reward or as a replacement for love and attention and the least nutritious foods are usually chosen. Grandparents and separated parents tend to use sweets or chocolates to gain a child's confidence, favour and love.

5 The general lifestyle. This may exacerbate a tendency to acquire excess weight, e.g. lack of exercise resulting from travelling everywhere by car, watching television for prolonged periods and not participating in any active leisure pursuits. Children who are already obese often try to avoid games and sports at school because they are embarrassed by their physique.

Treatment

This will only be successful if the child wants to lose weight. Co-operation of the parents and other close family members is essential to ensure success.

Explaining *why* a child should achieve a more normal weight is important, i.e. the health risks attached, attitude of peers.

Dramatic weight loss is not desirable for children and, in general, it is better if they 'hold' or 'grow into' their weight. This must also be carefully explained to the parents and child who can otherwise become very discouraged by the absence of any weight loss and apparent lack of progress.

Children still require a healthy varied diet whilst reducing weight. A high fibre diet may help achieve satiety in addition to its other benefits. During growth spurts, and with the onset of menstruation in girls, adequate intakes of calcium, protein and iron are essential. Very low energy diets are not suitable for any child.

It is very important that overweight children are not made to feel any more different than is necessary either at home or at school.

At home

Children and parents should be encouraged to look at the family lifestyle and eating habits generally and make modifications for the whole family. As well as benefiting the family's health, such measures may also help prevent other members of the family becoming overweight. All members of the family should be encouraged to:

1 Not add sugar to drinks and cereals.

2 Use a low calorie sweetener if necessary.

3 Choose a high fibre breakfast cereal and avoid sugar-coated varieties.
4 Choose wholemeal bread.
5 Eat more fruit and vegetables.
6 Only eat chips once a week at most – jacket potatoes with or without fillings are often just as popular with children.
7 Only eat crisps once or twice a week at most.
8 Eat fewer cakes, biscuits, puddings and sweets.
9 Choose low calorie squash and soft drinks.
10 Choose tinned fruits in natural juice and natural fruit juices instead of sweetened varieties.

At school

Snacks taken to school should ideally be fruit, but this is not always popular or practical; the occasional bag of crisps or small chocolate wafer biscuit is acceptable.

School meals present problems as many items are fried, but discussion with school cook or head teacher may result in a better choice of foods being offered generally; the health visitor or community dietitian may be able to exert some influence if the school is unresponsive to a request from the parents. Packed meals brought from home may be a better alternative in some cases.

Tuckshops in school could be encouraged to offer healthier alternatives for children to purchase, e.g. fresh fruit, muesli bars, plain biscuits and low calorie drinks.

Overweight children are often reluctant to participate in sports due to teasing, but should be encouraged to take some form of regular exercise. This can be in the form of walking, cycling or swimming as well as the traditional sporting activities.

Guidance on spending pocket money may be necessary and children should be advised not to spend it on sweets or crisps but to save it up to buy a book, toy or game instead. Relatives and friends should be encouraged to give gifts other than sweets.

Birthday parties

Parties can be regarded as a permissible treat but it is still possible to include plenty of suitable foods, for example:
1 Wholemeal bread used in the sandwiches.
2 Low calorie squash or soft drinks.
3 Natural fruit juice.
4 Various interesting salads using fruit, nuts, raw vegetables, pulses, brown rice and pasta in attractive presentations.
5 Dried fruit, nuts and raisins.
6 Fresh fruit salad.
7 Yoghurt-based desserts.
8 Birthday cake – this could contain a fruit filling or be a fruit flan or fruit cake.
9 Savoury flans with wholewheat pastry.
10 Filled jacket potatoes.

Group therapy

This may be helpful with some children but this option is not available in every locality. Topics for discussion can include all aspects of healthy living and eating and not just slimming, i.e. exercise, dental health, hygiene and general healthy eating habits. They should also provide plenty of activities which involve the child and hold his interest, e.g. food diaries, scrap books, paintings and posters, practical cookery, games or quizzes.

Overweight children are often fussy eaters who require a great deal of encouragement. Attractive presentation of food and the choice of a wide variety of foods are essential. It is important for the child to realize that healthy eating is interesting and enjoyable.

With children especially, family co-operation is important and they must be given praise for the changes in their diet and lifestyle that they achieve rather than punished for what they do not. It is important that the child does understand the need for weight loss and has the family's support. In some cases, where weight loss is unachievable through non-compliance, it may be appropriate to accept this rather than turn the child into a 'failed dieter' and hope that, in the late teens or early twenties, the child will wish to lose weight for his or her own reasons.

4.17.3 Setting up a slimming club

The following information is directed towards setting up a slimming club within the structure of the NHS. The guidelines could also be adapted to apply to a private or commercial slimming club.

Advantages and disadvantages of slimming clubs

Advantages

They are an efficient use of dietitians' time because more patients are advised more regularly. This is especially true if the club is run by a non-dietitian with occasional input from the dietitian. Another advantage is that members of the group gain more support from sharing a common aim.

Disadvantages

The patient has less individual dietetic attention. There is a risk that some members will attend for solely social reasons rather than in a serious attempt to slim.

Aims and target group

It is important to be clear about the aims of the club. As well as the general aims of weight loss and improved health, there may be others, such as off-loading outpatient commitments or all GP referrals. Any planning will also depend on the target group. It may be all those with a weight problem or a more specific group, e.g. children or men. These points should be clarified so that they can be referred to while planning and used for evaluation later.

Type of club

Most commercial slimming clubs operate an open club; this runs indefinitely and members can join at any time. It has the advantage that a constant supply of new members will replace defaulters. Closed courses are more suitable for a structured educational programme (Seddon *et al* 1981), possibly including behavioural modification techniques (Long *et al* 1983). These have a set number of sessions (usually between ten and sixteen) and every member joins at the same time. This helps bond the group together and enables the leader to have a specific short term commitment. The disadvantages of set courses is that some members may default, decreasing the size of the group, and some may wish to rejoin every subsequent course preventing the input of new applicants. The answer may be to provide another course which follows on with less frequent, shorter sessions. As there is usually a higher drop-out rate, a central club taking members from several courses is one way of keeping numbers fairly steady.

Management backing

Consultation at an early stage with the appropriate General Manager or equivalent, is essential to discuss finance, personnel, premises, publicity and policy decisions. Further meetings will be needed to approve more definite plans.

Finance

For a club run as part of the NHS dietetic service, financial allocations must be approved and monitored by the General Manager or equivalent. Charging a fee may be necessary either to cover sundry expenses such as refreshments, leaflets and film hire, or for substantial funding of the project including hire of premises, payment of leader, speakers' fees and possibly insurance. If the club is aimed at health education, it is usually permissable to charge even if it is held on health service premises. A self-financing, but non-profit-making club can still charge considerably less than commercial organizations. Paying a fee in advance will also encourage attendance.

Club membership

A club membership of approximately 20 is a manageable size, but alows for some defaulting. The method of publicizing to potential members will depend on the target group. Some clubs only enrol members with a medical referral. It would not be regarded as a breach of professional conduct for a State Registered Dietitian to give general nutritional and dietetic advice to a group without individual referral (CPSM Dietitians Board Statement 1990). In the event of a dietitian actually being the club leader, it would obviously be their professional responsibility to ensure that each patient's GP is aware of their membership of the slimming club (Bond 1983). For example, the GP could be notified by a standard letter.

The club can be publicized by notifying relevant personnel, and by notices in GP surgeries, health clinics, out-patient departments and non-NHS premises such as libraries. The local newspaper might also mention it in a slimming feature.

Club leaders

Dietitians from the local dietetic department may be interested in being club leaders. The advantage of the closed course system is that there can be more than one leader, each running a different course. Some health visitors or clinic nurses welcome the opportunity to run a club but may benefit from an instruction course beforehand. Alternatively, the leadership could be shared, with a dietitian only taking certain sessions. Another possibility is to charge a fee and use it to pay dietitians who are looking for part time or evening work. Long *et al* (1983) also describe a group led by a dietitian/clinical psychologist team.

Organization

The organization of a slimming club can be time-consuming. Telephone enquiries, enrolling members, publicity, planning programmes, booking films and speakers, ordering leaflets can add to the load of a busy dietetic department. It may be worthwhile to pay an organizer to do this (e.g. one of the leaders), possibly using a home telephone as a base for enquiries.

It may also be helpful to form a small planning group including dietetic, medical, nursing, health education and administrative input. Once the club is established this group can be convened periodically to review progress.

Premises and timing

Most people prefer an evening club due to work and family commitments, though some mothers and senior citizens may favour the daytime.

Evening clubs need well-lit premises with adequate public transport. Health centres, clinics, the hospital or rented halls may be suitable.

It is essential to have accurate scales, preferably the bar type, which are serviced regularly. Health clinics are usually equipped with these and may have other useful equipment such as audio visual aid facilities and floor exercise mats.

It is usually best to plan weekly sessions of around $1\frac{1}{2}$–2 hours duration on a convenient day, allowing six to eight weeks before the commencement date for publicity, enrolment and programme planning.

Programme planning

Whether a structured course or an open club is decided upon, planning the sessions is important to ensure variety and a balance of topics.

The first half of the session should concentrate on recording members' weights and discussing their problems. It should be remembered that weighing a group of people takes time, 20 people take at least half an hour and much longer on the first session when height is measured and the target weight is determined as well. The second half of the session should be devoted to a different topic each week – videos, quizzes and talks including some by outside speakers such as a doctor, physiotherapist, psychologist or beautician. As well as visual aids such as videos, posters and slides, use real food where possible, e.g. a demonstration of the pros and cons of various slimming products borrowed from a local chemist or a tasting session of favourite low calorie recipes.

Giving members their own copy of the programme will encourage attendance. In addition to the diet sheet and a weight record card, the teaching should be endorsed with leaflets on recipes, exercise, calorie counting, a week's menu and helpful hints. Home made handouts are improved by using a cartoon picture or logogram on coloured paper; alternatively, there is a choice of printed material available (refer to BDA list of leaflets and posters). Instead of a comprehensive diet sheet at the first session, step-by-step advice cards could be given out for the first few weeks. Although financial limitations will influence the use of visual aids and leaflets, their cost per head is usually relatively small compared to other expenses.

Some useful suggestions for improving the programme content may come from members, especially if a questionnaire is circulated. The Trim-in pack produced by Portsmouth Health Authority is a helpful resource.

Evaluation

It is important to evaluate whether the original aim is being achieved and to review weight loss and attendance rates. It can be useful to refer to published studies of slimming clubs in the UK showing average weight loss and average attendance:

9.7 kg in 25.7 weeks (Ashwell and Garrow 1975)
4.4 kg in 7.1 weeks (Seddon *et al* 1981)
5.4 kg in 8.4 weeks (multi-course attenders)
3.82 kg in 6.8 weeks (single course attenders) (Bush *et al* 1988)
4.6 kg in 13 weeks
6.9 kg in 13 weeks with behaviour therapy (Long *et al* 1983)

Levy *et al* (1986) give a helpful table comparing statistics from slimming clubs in different countries. The leaders should keep clear records of weight and height (in metric units), age and possibly occupation for evaluation or for use in research studies.

References

Abraham R and Owen ERTC (1988) Dietetic management of patients after vertical banded gastroplasty. *J Hum Nutr Dietet* **1**, 9–13.

Acheson KJ, Campbell IT, Edholm OG, Miller DS and Stock MJ (1980) The measurement of food and energy intake in man – an evaluation of some techniques. *Am J Clin Nutr* **33**, 1147–54.

Apfelbaum M, Fricker J and Igoin-Apfelbaum L (1987) Low and very-low-calorie diets. *Am J Clin Nutr* **45**, 1126–34.

Ashwell M and Garrow JS (1975) A survey of three slimming and weight control organisations in the UK. *Nutrition (London)* **29**, 347–56.

Black AE, Prentice AM and Coward WA (1985) Validation of the 7-day weighed diet record by comparison against total energy expenditure. In *Proceedings of the British Dietetic Association Study Conference*, Keele University, April 1985, p. 25.

Bond S (1983) *The professional approach*. British Dietetic Association, Birmingham.

Bray GA, Barry RE, Benfield JR, Castelnuovo-Tedesco P and Rodin J (1976) Intestinal bypass surgery for obesity decreases food intake and taste preferences. *Am J Clin Nutr* **29**, 779–83.

Bray GA, Greenway FL, Barry RE, Benfield JR, Fiser RL, Dahms WT, Atkinson RL and Schwartz AA (1977) Surgical treatment of obesity. A review of our experience and an analysis of published reports. *Int J Obesity* **1**, 331–67.

Bush A, Webster J, Chalmers G, Pearson M, Penfold P, Brereton P and Garrow JS (1988) The Harrow Slimming Club: report on 1090 enrollments in 50 courses, 1977–1986. *J Hum Nutr Dietet* **1**, 429–36.

Council for Professions Supplementary to Medicine, Dietitians Board Statement of Conduct (1990)

DHSS (1987) Committee on Medical Aspects of Food Policy. *The use of very low calorie diets in obesity*. HMSO, London.

Garrow JS (1980) Combined medical-surgical approaches to the treatment of obesity. *Am J Clin Nutr* **33**, 425–30.

Garrow JS (1989) Very low calorie diets should not be used. *Int J Obesity* **13**(2), 145–7.

Garrow JS, Durrant ML, Blaza S, Wilkins D, Royston P and Sunkin S (1981) The effect of meal frequency and protein concentration on the composition of the weight lost by obese subjects. *Br J Nutr* **45**, 5–15.

Garrow JS and Webster J (1985) Quetelet's index (W/H) as a measure of fatness. *Int J Obesity* **9**, 147–53.

Garrow JS and Webster JD (1989) Effects on weight and metabolic rate of obese women at a 3.4 MJ (800 kcal) diet. *Lancet* **i**, 1429–31.

Garrow JS, Webster JD, Pearson M, Pacy PJ and Harpin G (1989) Inpatient–outpatient randomized comparison of Cambridge Diet versus Milk Diet in 17 obese women over 24 weeks. *Int J Obesity* **13**, 521–9.

Hogan RB, Johnston JH, Long BW, Sones JQ, Hinton LA, Bunge J and Corrigan SA (1989) A double blind, randomized, sham controlled trial of the gastric bubble for obesity. *Gastrointestinal Endoscopy* **35**(5), 381–5.

Isner JM, Sours HE, Paris AL, Ferrans VJ and Roberts WC (1979) Sudden, unexpected death in avid dieters using the liquid protein modified fast diet. Observations in 17 patients and the role of the prolonged QT interval. *Circulation* **60**, 1401–12.

James WPT (1983) Energy requirements and obesity. *Lancet* **2**, 386–9.

Levy S, Pierce JP, Dembecki N and Cripps A (1986) Self-help group behavioural treatment for obesity. An evaluation of Weight Control workshops. *Med J Aust* **145**, 436–8.

Long CG, Simpson CM and Allot EA (1983) Psychological and dietetic counselling combined in the treatment of obesity: a comparative study in a hospital out-patient clinic. *Hum Nutr: Appl Nutr* **37A**, 94–102.

Marcus MD, Wing RR and Lamparski DM (1985) Binge eating and dietary restraint in obese patients. *Addictive Behaviors* **10**, 163–8.

Mason EE (1980) In *Surgical management of obesity*, pp. 29–39. Academic Press, London.

McFarland RJ, Gazet JC and Pilkington TRE (1985) A 13 year review of jejuno-ileal bypass. *Br J Surg* **72**, 81–7.

Pilkington TRE, Gazet JC, Ang L, Kalucy RS, Crisp AH and Day S (1976) Explanations for weight loss after jejuno-ileal bypass in gross obesity. *Br Med J* **1**, 1504–5.

Pilkington TRE (1980) In *Surgical management of obesity*, pp. 171–8. Academic Press, London.

Prentice AM, Black AE, Coward WA, Davies HL, Goldberg GR, Murgatroyd PR, Ashford J, Sawyer M and Whitehead RG (1986) High levels of energy expenditure in obese women. *Br Med J* **292**, 983–7.

Royal College of Physicians of London (1983) Obesity. *J R Coll Physicians Lond* **17**(1), 3–58.

Ruderman AJ and Wilson GT (1979) Weight, restraint, cognitions and counterregulation. *Behav Res Therapy* **17**, 581–90.

Seddon R, Penfound J and Garrow JS (1981) The Harrow Slimming Club: analysis of results obtained in 249 members of a self-financing, non-profit making group. *J Hum Nutr* **35**, 128–33.

Southgate DAT (1986) Obese deceivers? *Br Med J* **292**, 1692–3.

Stauffer JQ (1977) Hyperoxaluria and calcium oxalate nephrolithiasis after jejuno-ileal bypass. *Am J Clin Nutr* **30**, 64–71.

van Itallie TB and Yang M-U (1984) Cardiac dysfunction in obese dieters: a potentially lethal complication of rapid, massive weight loss. *Am J Clin Nutr* **39**, 695–702.

Wadden TA, Stunkard AJ and Brownell KD (1983) Very low calorie diets: their efficacy, safety and future. *Ann Intern Med* **99**, 675–84.

Wadden TA, van Itallie TB and Blackburn GL (1990) Responsible and irresponsible use of very-low-calorie-diets in the treatment of obesity. *J Am Med Assoc* **263**(1), 83–5.

Worner H, Weschler JG, Wenzel H, Swobodnik W, Kurrle P, Janowitz P, Splitt S and Ditschuneit H (1989) Long term results after treatment of obesity with the intragastric balloon. *Int J Obesity* **13**(1), 210 (Abstract).

4.18 Hypertension

In young healthy adults the average systolic blood pressure is approximately 120 mm mercury (Hg) and average diastolic blood pressure 80 mm Hg. In Western societies blood pressure rises gradually with age so that the average blood pressure of a 65 year old is 160/90. This makes the definition of hypertension difficult, but it is usually accepted that essential hypertension (high blood pressure which is not secondary to a pre-existing medical condition) is present and classified as 'mild' when the diastolic pressure is between 90 and 105, 'moderate' between 105 and 120 and 'severe' when it exceeds 120 mm Hg (BNF 1981).

The advisability of treating mild or borderling hypertension and the feasibility of preventing its occurrence are controversial matters which are strongly debated (Brown *et al* 1984a, 1984b; de Wardener 1984, Rosenberg and Coleman 1984) and not clearly established.

However, the benefits of treating moderately severe hypertension are generally agreed and threshold values for the initiation of treatment have fallen steadily in most Western countries over the past two decades (*Lancet* 1984). As the number of people being treated increases so the use of non-pharmacological therapy becomes more attractive due to the cost and possible side effects of drug treatment.

Weight reduction and sodium restriction are the cornerstone of non-pharmacological therapy but more recently the dietary intakes of calcium and potassium have been implicated and may also have to be considered.

Weight reduction in hypertension

Weight loss by dietary restriction provides a cheap ethical means of treating hypertension and the association between obesity and hypertension is undisputed. It has been shown that hypertension is twice as prevalent in young overweight individuals and 50% more prevalent in older obese subjects than in control subjects within the normal weight range (Stamler *et al* 1978).

Patients who adhere to a diet are also more likely to follow a drug regimen and therefore have blood pressure which is easier to control (Hovell 1982) but nonetheless studies investigating the effect of weight loss on hypertension strongly suggest it is effective and all hypertensive patients who are overweight should be encouraged to lose weight. Methods of weight reduction are described in Section 4.17.

Sodium and potassium

One of the best known treatments in relation to sodium reduction for hypertension is the Kempner rice-fruit diet (Kempner 1948) which, although initially successful in over 50% of cases, is so rigid that few could adhere to it as outpatients and it is rarely used.

The effects of both drastic and moderate sodium restriction in patients who are clearly hypertensive are well established (Parijs *et al* 1973; Haddy 1980) but the effect in borderline hypertensives has until recently been less clear. However, detailed analysis of published data from 24 different communities (involving 47 000 people) has shown that there is an association between blood pressure and sodium intake which increases with age and is independent of factors such as body weight, level of physical activity, intake of alcohol, calcium and potassium, and mental stress (Law *et al* 1991a). Further analysis of 14 of these studies, making allowance for the variation in daily sodium intake, confirmed the strength of the association between sodium intake and blood pressure (Frost *et al* 1991). The same group (Law *et al* 1991b) also looked at the effects of intervention trials of salt reduction. Analysis of the results from 68 cross-over trials and 10 randomized trials showed that in all age groups, and in people with either normal or high blood pressure, trials of salt reduction lasting for five weeks or longer lowered blood pressure as predicted. The greatest fall in blood pressure occurred in older age groups and in those with the highest systolic blood pressure. It would therefore seem prudent to advise a moderate salt restriction to all hypertensive patients.

Some workers have claimed that blood pressure reduction caused by energy restriction is independent of sodium intake (Sowers *et al* 1982) but have failed to realize that the energy-reduced diet was also lower in sodium. Others have shown that either moderate weight reduction or a modest sodium restriction (70 mmol/day) produce substantial lowering of blood pressure in obese subjects with borderline hypertension (Gillum *et al* 1983) and the effect is greater if the two are combined. However, Fagerberg *et al* (1984) found that weight loss lowered blood pressure only when patients restricted both their energy and sodium intake.

There is considerable evidence from animal experiments that there is a genetic variation which determines individual sensitivity to sodium. This has been elegantly substantiated in human studies by Skrabai *et al* (1981) who showed that in 20 normotensive subjects (ten with a family history of hypertension) a reduction in salt intake from 200 to

50 mmol/day significantly reduced the rise in blood pressure induced by various doses of noradrenaline. Twelve subjects (eight with a family history of hypertension) responded to salt restriction with a fall of either diastolic or systolic blood pressure of at least 5 mmHg. A high potassium intake (200 mmol/day) reduced diastolic blood pressure by at least 5 mmHg in ten of the subjects, seven of whom had a family history of high blood pressure.

Studies in young adults with and without a family history of hypertension have shown that whereas a high sodium intake causes an increased blood pressure in both groups, a high potassium intake only reduces blood pressure in those with a family history of hypertension (Parfrey *et al* 1981).

Calcium

There has been recent interest in the effect of calcium on blood pressure and Belizai *et al* (1983) showed that a daily supplement of 1 g calcium significantly reduced diastolic blood pressure in healthy individuals within a few weeks. Castenmiller *et al* (1985) have also found that in normotensive subjects, mean systolic and diastolic blood pressures were lower in subjects on a high calcium intake (4.1 mmol/MJ; 686 mg/1000 kcal) than those on a lower calcium intake (3.2 mmol/MJ; 535 mg/1000 kcal).

Dietary recommendations

Although not all factors are fully established the following recommendations can be made for the non-pharmacological treatment of hypertension:

1 All overweight hypertensive individuals should adhere to a suitable weight reducing regimen.

2 The sodium intake of both the obese and non-obese hypertensive should be reduced. This should not be extreme and should require only that no salt be used either in cooking or at the table and that highly salted foods, as described in Section 2.7.1, should be avoided.

3 A reduced sodium intake can be made more palatable by the liberal use of fresh fruit and vegetables. This will also increase the potassium intake and may be of additional benefit.

4 There is, as yet, insuffient evidence to make recommendations on the calcium content of the diet. However, care should be taken to ensure that all patients, especially post-menopausal women, are consuming at least the recommended daily intake of calcium.

References

Belizai JM, Vilar J and Peneda O (1983) Reduction of blood pressure with calcium supplementation in young adults. *J Am Med Assoc* **249**, 1161–5.

British Nutrition Foundation (1981) *Salt in the diet*. Briefing paper No 2.

Brown JJ, Lever AF, Robertson JIS, Semple PF, Bing RF, Heagerty AM, Swales JD, Thurston H, Leadingham JGG, Laragh JH, Hansson L, Nicholls MG and Espiner AE (1984a) Salt and hypertension. *Lancet* ii, 456.

Brown JJ, Lever AF, Robertson JIS, Semple PF, Bing RF, Heagerty AM, Swales JD, Thurston H, Ledingham JGG, Laragh JH, Hansson L, Nicholls MG and Espiner EA (1984b) Salt and hypertension. *Lancet* ii, 1333–4.

Castenmiller JJM, Mensink RP, van der Heyden L, Kouwenhoven T, Hautvast JGAJ, de Leeuw PW and Schaafsma G (1985) The effect of dietary sodium on urinary calcium and potassium excretion in normotensive men with different calcium intake. *Am J Clin Nutr* **41**, 52–60.

de Wardener HE (1984) Salt and hypertension. *Lancet* **ii**, 688.

Fagerberg B, Andersson OK, Isaksson B and Bjomtorp P (1984) Blood pressure control during weight reduction in obese hypertensive men: separate effects of sodium and energy restriction. *Br Med J* **288**(i), 11–6.

Frost CD, Law MR and Wald NJ (1991) By how much does dietary salt reduction lower blood pressure. II – Analysis of observational data within populations. *Br Med J* **302**, 815–8.

Gillum RF, Elmer PJ and Prineas RJ (1981) Changing sodium intake in children. *Hypertension* **3**, 698–703.

Haddy FJ (1980) Mechanism, prevention and therapy of sodium dependent hypertension. *Am J Med* **69**, 746–58.

Hovell MF (1982) The experimental evidence for weight loss treatment of essential hypertension: a critical review. *Am J Public Health* **72**, 359–68.

Kempner W (1948) Treatment of hypertensive vascular disease with rice diet. *Am J Med* **4**, 545–77.

Lancet (1984) Editorial: Diet and hypertension. *Lancet* **ii**, 671–3.

Law MR, Frost CD and Wald NJ (1991a) By how much does dietary salt reduction lower blood pressure. I – Analysis of observational data among populations. *Br Med J* **302**, 811–15.

Law MR, Frost CD and Wald NJ (1991b) By how much does dietary salt reduction lower blood pressure. III – Analysis of data from trials of salt reduction. *Br Med J* **302**, 819–24.

Parfrey PS, Candon K, Wright P, Vandenburgh MJ, Holly JMP, Goodwin FJ, Evans SJW and Ledinghain JM (1981) Blood pressure and hormonal changes following alteration in dietary sodium and potassium in young men with and without familial predisposition to hypertension. *Lancet* **i**, 113–7.

Parijs J, Joosens JV and Van de Linden (1973) Moderate sodium restriction and diuretics in the treatment of hypertension. *Am Heart J* **85**, 22–34.

Rosenberg E and Coleman BR (1984) Diet and hypertension. *Lancet* **ii**, 1334.

Skrabai F, Aubeck J and Hortnagi H (1981) Low sodium/high potassium diet for prevention of hypertension: probable mechanism of action. *Lancet* **ii**, 895–900.

Sowers JR, Nyby M and Stern N (1982) Blood pressure and hormone changes associated with weight reduction in the obese. *Hypertension* **4**, 686–91.

Stamler R, Stemler J, Reidlinger WF, Algera G and Roberts RH (1978) Weight and blood pressure. *J Am Med Assoc* **240**, 1607–10.

4.19 Hyperlipidaemia

Hyperlipidaemia, (or hyperlipoproteinaemia) means the presence in the blood of abnormally high concentrations of lipids (cholesterol and triglycerides), or lipoproteins. Reference values are given in Table 4.53.

Dietitians can be involved with patients with hyperlipidaemias to varying degrees, from specialized lipid clinics to occasional referrals from general practitioners.

Dietary advice is central to the treatment of all hyperlipidaemic patients and can reduce blood cholesterol by up to 25% in polygenic hyperlipidaemia (these results, however, will not usually be achieved in familial hyperlipidaemias). Total cholesterol level is associated with the development of coronary heart disease (CHD); trials of cholestyramine in middle aged men have shown that a 1% reduction in plasma cholesterol may result in a 1–2% reduction in CHD incidence (Haines 1989).

Raised serum triglyceride, especially fasting levels of Very Low Density Lipoprotein (VLDL) triglyceride, have been shown to predict CHD incidence but this is thought to reflect the inverse association between VLDL and High Density Lipoprotein (HDL), in particular with HDL cholesterol which may be an independent risk factor for CHD. However abnormally raised triglyceride levels do result in an increased risk of acute pancreatitis.

Periodically the effectiveness of intervention in patients with hyperlipidaemia is questioned. It has been suggested that the reduced cardiovascular mortality following cholesterol-lowering intervention may be accompanied by an increase in non-cardiovascular death rates (Muldoon *et al* 1990). Lipid lowering dietary advice has also recently been described as being insufficiently rigorous, and subsequently having little impact on serum cholesterol concentrations (Ramsey *et al* 1991). Nevertheless, the weight of evidence is in support of appropriate intervention; major studies like the Oslo Study offer reassuring results for dietetians involved in this important area of dietetics (Hjerman *et al* 1981).

Table 4.53 Reference and suggested 'healthy' ranges for plasma lipids in adults under 60 years

	Reference* range mmol/l	Suggested range mmol/l
Total Cholesterol	3.5–7.8	<5.2
LDL cholesterol	2.3–6.1	<4.0
HDL cholesterol	0.8–1.7	>1.15
Triglycerides	0.7–1.8	0.7–1.7

* The reference interval is calculated from the mean of an apparently healthy population plus and minus two standard deviations.
However sex and age differences need to be considered:
1 *Sex difference* Triglycerides are higher in men than women. HDL levels are higher in women than men.
2 *Age difference* Lipids e.g. cholesterol may increase with age, consequently a value in the reference range of 7.0 mmol/l would be much more noteworthy in a person of 25 years than one of 55 years.

4.19.1 Normal lipid metabolism

An appreciation of normal lipid metabolism is essential for an understanding of hyperlipidaemias.

Lipids such as cholesterol and triglyceride are insoluble in water and are therefore transported around the body bound to proteins (apoproteins or apolipoproteins). These water soluble complexes are called lipoproteins and are classified according to density. As density increases, the amount of protein and phospholipid associated with the lipoprotein also increases; thus HDL contains as much phospholipid as cholesterol.

1 *Chylomicrons* transport dietary triglyceride from the intestine into the blood.

2 *Very Low Density Lipoproteins* (VLDL) are synthesized by the liver; these carry triglyceride produced by the liver to other tissues.

3 *Intermediate Density Lipoproteins* (IDL) are derived from partially degraded VLDL. They are short-lived intermediates.

4 *Low Density Lipoproteins* (LDL) are formed from VLDL and transport cholesterol from the liver to peripheral tissues. Sixty per cent of total cholesterol is found in LDL. It is LDL cholesterol which is most closely associated with heart disease.

5 *High Density Lipoproteins* (HDL) transport excess cholesterol from cells to the liver for excretion in bile. High levels are, therefore, beneficial and are inversely related to CHD.

Dietary triglyceride undergoes intestinal hydrolysis to monoglycerides and is formed into micelles with bile salts and cholesterol. These are absorbed into small intestinal mucosal cells and resynthesized to triglycerides. These are then combined with apoproteins and pass into the lymphatic system entering blood via the thoracic duct.

VLDL is produced by the liver. VLDL and chylomicrons have parallels in their metabolism. Both are triglyceride rich, and this triglyceride is gradually hydrolysed by lipoprotein lipase; the resulting fatty acids are used for energy production (in muscle) or re-esterified and stored as triglyceride in fat cells. Glycerol is metabolized by the liver. As triglyceride is removed from the chylomicron, some of the more soluble components are used for HDL synthesis and the chylomicron remnant is taken up by the liver. In VLDL the removal of triglyceride transforms it into IDL and then into LDL which enters the cells after binding with LDL receptors. As with the chylomicrons, some of the more soluble components released during this conversion of VLDL to LDL are used for HDL synthesis.

Hyperlipidaemia results from either an overproduction, or an inadequate removal, of particular lipoproteins. For example, in hypertriglyceridaemia, it is the lipoprotein VLDL (containing triglyceride) which is being overproduced.

4.19.2 Diagnosis

Procedures and interpretation

A diagnosis of hyperlipidaemia should not be based on a single elevated value; there is considerable day-to-day variation in cholesterol and triglycerides.

It is customary clinical practice to measure non-fasting cholesterol levels since there is relatively little change in serum cholesterol from the fasting to fed state, and it is clearly more convenient for the patient. However some people show a marked increase in serum cholesterol following a fat-rich meal. If a non-fasting total cholesterol level exceeds 6.5 mmol/l, a repeated measurement on a fasting sample should be made a week or so later. Fasting triglyceride and HDL cholesterol should be assessed at the same time. LDL cholesterol can be estimated using the Friedwald formula:

$$\text{LDL cholesterol} = \text{Total cholesterol} - \text{HDL cholesterol} - \left(\frac{\text{Triglyceride}}{2.2}\right)$$

It is essential to know the patient's HDL level so that the ratio of total to HDL cholesterol, can be calculated and the risk of CHD assessed (Table 4.54). Patients with a raised total cholesterol resulting from high HDL cholesterol, are at little or no excess risk of CHD, and do not, therefore, need strict dietary control (Neil *et al* 1990).

If hyperlipidaemia is found, the possibility of this being secondary to other conditions such as hypothyroidism, renal impairment and diabetes, should then be considered. Only when these causes have been eliminated can a diagnosis of primary hyperlipidaemia be made and appropriate treatment be planned. Fredrickson's classification of hyperlipidaemia is illustrated in Table 4.55; however, other classifications exist, for example that introduced by Goldstein and Fredrickson (Ball and Mann 1988).

Table 4.54 Ratio of total cholesterol to HDL cholesterol illustrating CHD risk

Ratio	CHD Risk
<3.5	Low
3.5–4.5	Medium
>4.5	High

Appropriate dietary, and if necessary drug, treatment can then begin together with any other measures which may reduce the CHD risk from factors such as hypertension, smoking, obesity, lack of exercise, stress and excessive alcohol intake.

Reliability of results

Individual variation in blood tests is to be expected. However, variation within biochemistry departments also exists, and needs to be considered when interpreting results. Typically the coefficient of variation (for biological and analytical reasons) is about 4%. When relying on desk-top cholesterol measuring devices, variability can be greater, and participation in an external quality control assurance scheme is essential.

When assessing a change in cholesterol, for example before and after three months of dietary therapy, the precision of the method will give some guidance as to whether a fall in level is significant. The appropriate department of Clinical Chemistry or Chemical Pathology which generates the results can give guidance on this.

Population (or mass) screening versus selective (or opportunistic) screening

Population screening has major financial implications and since such a programme would be expected to reveal a quarter of the population having total cholesterol concentrations exceeding 6.5 mmol/l (Mann *et al* 1988) there are probably insufficient manpower resources for the necessary support (including dietetic support) for such a programme. There are additional drawbacks to mass screening. Screening should not take place within three months of a myocardial infarction or acute illness, since such events distort results (Mann and Ball 1985). There is also the danger that, in mass cholesterol screening, results would be considered in isolation rather than with other modifiable and non-modifiable risk factors. For all these reasons it is felt by many that any finance available would be more wisely channelled into a complementary strategy combining, firstly, the targeting of high risk groups and, secondly, a National Intervention Programme promoting the principles of healthy living, including healthy eating, which would help to reduce cholesterol levels.

However with selective testing, cases of heterozygous familial hypercholesterolaemia can be missed (King's Fund 1989; Tunstall-Pedoe 1989).

4.19.3 Lipid policies and guidelines

The formulation of district lipid guidelines is of great value

Table 4.55 Classification and features of hyperlipoproteinaemias

Type	Lipoprotein(s) elevated	Serum cholesterol	Serum triglyceride	Primary (genetic) causes	Secondary causes	Notes
I	Chylomicrons	Normal or slightly raised	Very high	**1** Lipoprotein lipase deficiency **2** Apoprotein C II deficiency (Apoprotein CII activates lipoprotein lipase)	Alcoholism	Rare As a result of 1 and 2, chylomicrons can not be broken down, so levels are grossly elevated
IIA	LDL	Raised	Normal	Familial hypercholesterolaemia **1** Homozygous form is severe **2** Heterozygous form mild to moderately severe Apoprotein β receptor deficiency	**1** Hypothyroidism **2** Nephrotic syndrome	**1** Heterozygous form relatively common **2** Enhanced risk of CHD in both types but especially in homozygous form which has a poor prognosis As a result of Apoprotein β receptor deficiency, the removal of LDL by cells is impaired causing raised circulating LDL and thus raised total cholesterol
IIB	LDL and VLDL	Raised	Raised	Familial combined hyperlipoproteinaemia	**1** Hypothyroidism **2** Nephrotic syndrome **3** Affluent living	**1** Most common form of hyperlipoproteinaemia **2** Carries enhanced risk of CHD
III	IDL ('broad beta')	Raised	Raised	Familial dysbetalipoproteinaemia Apoprotein E3 deficiency (Accumulation of remnant particles, partially degraded VLDL or IDL)		Uncommon
IV	VLDL	Normal or slightly raised	Raised	**1** Mild familial hypertriglyceridaemia **2** Tangier disease	**1** Diabetes or glucose intolerance **2** Obesity **3** Excessive alcohol **4** Renal failure **5** Advanced liver disease	**1** Common **2** May predispose to atherosclerosis
V	Chylomicrons and VLDL	Moderately raised	Very high	Severe familial hypertriglyceridaemia	**1** Diabetes (poorly controlled) **2** Uraemia	Rare

to primary health care teams offering advice on screening, elimination of secondary causes of hyperlipidaemia, diagnosis of primary hyperlipidaemia, treatment and available resources. Dietetic departments should formulate a strategy for patients with hyperlipidaemia (see Table 4.56) which should be used in conjunction with the district's lipid policy, to ensure consistent and accurate dietary advice (BDA 1990).

Some effort must also be directed into the training of primary health care teams to ensure continuation of consistent and accurate information in the community (Francis *et al* 1989).

4.19.4 Dietary treatment of hyperlipidaemia

Dietary guidance for hyperlipidaemia based on Fredrickson-type classification

The dietary treatment of each type of hyperlipoproteinaemia is outlined below. However, these should not be interpreted as strict rules but as guidelines to be considered in conjunction with the relevant factors (e.g. lipid abnormalities, body weight and any associated disease state) in each case.

Type I

The aim of treatment is to reduce chylomicron formation.

1 *Severely restrict fat intake*, usually to about 25–35 g/day. As a consequence of this, the following dietary aspects must also be considered:

- Energy. The reduction in fat intake inevitably results in a diet low in energy. If the patient is overweight (*not* usually a feature if the disorder is familial) then this does not matter. But in children and normal-weight adults, the energy deficiency may need to be rectified with medium-chain triglycerides (MCT); these do not form chylomicrons.
- Essential fatty acids (efa). The daily fat allowance should include sufficient quantities of a polyunsaturated fat or oil to prevent efa deficiency.

Table 4.56 An example of a hyperlipidaemia strategy

OXFORDSHIRE HEALTH AUTHORITY NUTRITION AND DIETETIC DEPARTMENT
DIET CARE – ACTION PLAN

CONDITION	CATEGORY	LEAFLET	ACTION	REFERRAL TO DIETITIAN
Elevated Lipids In all cases exclude: Diabetes, Hypothyroidism Excess Alcohol, Pharmaceutical side effects	*(a) Obesity* irrespective of lipid levels	Follow positive action for Obesity ▷		If response to diet fails to: (a) achieve weight loss (b) reduce lipid levels
	(b) 5.2–6.5 mmol/litre	**Healthy Eating Booklet (HEA) or Natural Eating + Practical Approach Healthy Eating with Meal Plan**	No further action unless risk factor profile alters	
TARGET LEVEL Cholesterol 5.2 mmol	*(c) 6.6–7.5 mmol/litre*	**Lipid Lowering Dietary Advice Booklet**	+ Low saturated fat diet/use of polyunsaturated fat/fibre/reduction of alcohol and sugar if appropriate. Monitor diet at 6 and 12 weeks	Refer if help required or if diet fails to reduce lipid levels after 12 weeks
	(d) >7.6 mmol/litre	**Lipid Lowering Dietary Advice Booklet**	+ Advice on saturated fat/use of polyunsaturated fat/fibre/ reduction of alcohol and sugar if appropriate	**AND** The FIRST available appointment to see dietitian together with a lipid profile

Reproduced with the permission of Oxfordshire Health Authority Nutrition and Dietetic Department

- Fat-soluble vitamins. Supplementation may be necessary in order to prevent deficiencies.
- Palatability/acceptability. These are particular problems with a diet of such low fat content. The use of MCT supplements may be helpful.

Type IIa

The aim of treatment is to reduce LDL and total serum cholesterol.

1 *Reduce total fat intake and in particular the consumption of saturated fat.* This measure has the most impact on LDL and total cholesterol levels.

2 *Increase the ratio of polyunsaturated and monounsaturated fats to saturated fats.* Monounsaturated fats, formerly believed to have a neutral effect on cholesterol levels, are now thought to lower total cholesterol but without the accompanying fall in HDL which can occur on diets rich in polyunsaturates (Ernst *et al* 1980; Mensink 1987). However, this dietary strategy is less important than total fat restriction. Its main value is that the substitution of polyunsaturated/monounsaturated fats and oils for more saturated alternatives may assist dietary acceptability.

3 *Reduce dietary cholesterol in some cases.* Cholesterol is synthesized endogenously hence the influence of dietary cholesterol on serum cholesterol is relatively small. The dietary cholesterol level must be reduced to below 300 mg/day to have any significant effect and this is almost impossible to achieve with other than a vegetarian diet. Restriction of dietary cholesterol is therefore not important in patients with mild or moderate Type IIA hyperlipoproteinaemia. However unusually high intakes of dietary cholesterol should be corrected (e.g. more than 3–4 eggs/week are normally consumed). In patients with severe homozygous Type IIA, characterized by grossly elevated serum cholesterol levels, complete avoidance of cholesterol-rich foods (see Section 2.3) may be necessary.

There is, however, evidence that 20–25% of the population may be non-compensators with regard to dietary cholesterol and may therefore benefit from a dietary cholesterol intake below 200 mg/day (McNamara 1990).

4 *Soluble fibre* (for example contained in pulses) has a mildly hypolipaemic effect and its consumption should be encouraged (Tredger *et al* 1991).

Type IIB

The aims of treatment are to reduce LDL and total serum cholesterol and to reduce VLDL and total serum triglycerides.

1 *Attain/maintain normal weight.* If overweight, attainment of normal weight is the first priority. Dietary measures 2 and 3 below will automatically produce a diet of reduced energy content.

2 *Reduce fat intake.* For those of normal weight, some polyunsaturated and monounsaturated fats and oils can be substituted for saturated fats.

3 *Increase soluble fibre intake.*

4 *Reduce refined carbohydrate intake.* Depending on the level of dietary energy required, the resulting energy deficit should be replaced by complex carbohydrate.
5 *Reduce alcohol intake* if this is excessive.

Type III

The aims of treatment are to reduce total serum cholesterol and total serum triglycerides. Dietary treatment is the same as for Type IIB.

Type IV

The aim of treatment is to reduce the production of endogenous triglycerides.
1 *Achieve/maintain normal body weight.* The majority of these patients are overweight and require energy restriction. This should be achieved primarily by measures 2 and 3 below.
2 *Restrict carbohydrate*, particularly from refined sources. A maximum of 45% of dietary energy should be comprised of carbohydrate, principally from complex sources.
3 *Alcohol* should be restricted.

Type V

The aims of treatment are to reduce serum chylomicron and VLDL triglyceride.
1 *Achieve/maintain normal body weight.*
2 *Restrict fat intake* to a maximum of 30% of dietary energy.
3 *Increase the proportion of polyunsaturated/monounsaturated fats.*
4 *Reduce the intake of refined carbohydrate.*
5 *Exclude alcohol.*

Dietary guidance for elevated levels of cholesterol and/or triglyceride

For the dietitian involved with hyperlipidaemic patients on an irregular basis, it may be simpler to use the following guide which relates directly to the patients lipid profile.

Raised cholesterol levels alone (normal triglyceride)

If the patient has a body mass index (BMI) above the acceptable range, correcting this should be the first line of treatment.

With patients of an acceptable body weight dietary advice should aim to:
1 Reduce total fat intake (to a maximum of 30% of total energy from fat).
2 Increase the proportion of polyunsaturated and mono-unsaturated fats, to saturated fats.
3 Moderate intake of dietary cholesterol.
4 Increase dietary fibre intake particularly soluble fibre.
5 Increase complex carbohydrate intake to ensure any energy deficit resulting from the reduced fat intake is met.

Raised triglyceride levels alone (normal cholesterol)

A BMI above the normal range should be corrected. In patients of an acceptable bodyweight, dietary advice should aim to:
1 Reduce/avoid alcohol.
2 Reduce/avoid refined carbohydrate.

If Type 1 hyperlipidaemia is suspected then a severe reduction in long-chain dietary fats will be necessary. The use of medium chain triglyceride (MCT) oils may need to be considered since these do not form chylomicrons.

Raised cholesterol and raised triglyceride levels

If the patient has a BMI above the normal range, correcting this should be the first line of treatment. With patients of an acceptable bodyweight, dietary advice should aim to:
1 Reduce total fat intake.
2 Increase the proportion of polyunsaturated and mono-unsaturated fats, to saturated fats.
3 Moderate intake of dietary cholesterol.
4 Increase dietary fibre intake, particularly soluble fibre.
5 Reduce/avoid alcohol.
6 Reduce/avoid refined carbohydrate.
7 Increase complex carbohydrate intake to ensure any energy deficit is met.

Secondary dietary considerations

Antioxidant vitamins

Adequate dietary sources of the protective antioxidant vitamins (A, C and E) are advised. Experimentally, these inhibit the oxidation of LDL and their subsequent break-down and formation of fatty streaks or atheroma in the arteries.

'Grazing'

The consumption of a low fat, high fibre diet in a 'grazing' pattern (i.e. little and often) has been reported to lower total cholesterol levels (Southgate 1990).

Garlic

Garlic has been reported to be helpful in reducing total cholesterol and triglyceride levels, and increase HDL. Additionally it is claimed to possess an antithrombotic effect (Fulder 1989; Mansell and Reckless 1991). However more evidence is needed before garlic supplements can be recommended to patients.

Oily fish

Consumption of oily fish 2–3 times weekly is advisable since this will increase intake of omega-3 fatty acids which have been reported to reduce total cholesterol, reduce triglyceride concentrations, increase HDL levels, decrease platelet adhesiveness and improve arterial wall characteristics (Wolmarans *et al* 1988; Burr 1989; Wahlquist *et al* 1989).

It is important for dietitians to remember that dietary advice must be *positive*, *palatable*, *practical* and *possible*. It must include alternative food choices, recipes and cooking techniques, within the limitations of the patient's financial and social circumstances, if continued motivation and adherence to a new lifestyle concept is to be maintained. Follow-up is essential to maintain support and encouragement and to offer further advice tailored to subsequent blood results.

Other modifications of lifestyle, for example, smoking, should also be addressed. Regular gentle exercise should be encouraged since this will aid any weight loss required, and may also improve the lipid profile by an increase in HDL and a reduction in triglycerides (Wood *et al* 1976; Ruys *et al* 1989).

4.19.5 Drug treatment

Widespread use of lipid lowering drugs is not recommended, and drug treatment should never be embarked upon before dietary modification as a sole treatment has been shown to give an inadequate response.

Diet should always be continued alongside drug treatment. The lipid lowering drugs of which one or more (but not fibric acid derivatives and HMG CoA reductase inhibitors) may be used to treat diet resistant patients (O'Connor *et al* 1990; Medicines Resource Centre 1991) are described below. However for those dietitians dealing on an infrequent basis with hyperlipidaemias, the most commonly encountered drugs are summarized in Table 4.57.

Bile acid sequestrants (anion exchange resins)

(e.g. Questran ®, Colestid ®)

These are first line drugs for hypercholesterolaemia in the form of either a powder or granules which are added to water or fruit juice. They are not systemically absorbed and have a good safety record. Their effectiveness is, however, constrained by their unpalatability, and gastrointestinal side effects may be experienced. They may reduce fat-soluble vitamin and iron status, and interfere with the absorption of other drugs.

Bile acid sequestrants act by binding bile acids in the intestine, thereby reducing their reabsorption and this leads to increased bile acid synthesis, utilising cholesterol. The consequent intracellular depletion of cholesterol results in an increase in LDL receptors on the hepatocytes and increased uptake of LDL cholesterol from the circulation, ultimately resulting in a reduced total cholesterol and LDL level.

The effect on the lipid profile is:

1 A reduction in total and LDL cholesterol (not in homozygous familial hypercholesterolaemia).
2 A neutral effect on HDL.
3 A possible increase in triglycerides.

Table 4.57 Summary of drugs used to treat hyperlipidaemias

Drug	Usage
1 Bile acid sequestrant/anion exchange resin	First line drug for hypercholesterolaemia
2 Fibric acid derivative/fibrate	First line drug for mixed hyperlipidaemia
3 HMG CoA reductase inhibitor/ statins	Second line drug for hypercholesterolaemia

Fibric acid derivatives (fibrates)

(e.g. Bezafibrate and Gemfibrozil)

These are first line drugs for mixed hyperlipidaemias. They function systemically and side effects include gastrointestinal symptoms, and gallstones. Their mode of action is uncertain, however their effect is thought to be mediated through one or more of the following: increased excretion of cholesterol into bile, increased lipoprotein lipase activity, decreased endogenous cholesterol synthesis, and increased LDL receptor activity.

The effect on the lipid profile is:

1 A reduction in triglyceride, by lowering VLDL.
2 Some reduction in total and LDL cholesterol.
3 An increase in HDL.

Hydroxymethylglutaryl coenzyme A (HMG CoA) reductase inhibitors) (statins)

(e.g. Simvastatin, Provastatin)

These are second line drugs for patients with a total cholesterol level above 7.8 mmol/l. They function systemically, but their long term safety has not yet been fully established. Regular liver function tests are recommended. Patients may complain of muscular aches, and there is an increased incidence of cataracts.

These drugs reduce cholesterol biosynthesis in the liver by inhibiting the enzyme hydroxymethylglutaryl Coenzyme A reductase; the reduced intracellular cholesterol consequently leads to an increased expression of LDL receptors, increasing LDL uptake, and reducing total cholesterol.

The effects on the lipid profile are:

1 A reduction in total and LDL cholesterol (not in homozygous familial hypercholesterolaemia).
2 A moderate reduction in triglyceride.
3 An increase in HDL.

Nicotinic acid derivatives

(e.g. Acipimox)

Although used widely in the USA, this is not commonly used in the UK. Side effects include gastrointestinal symptoms and flushing.

The mode of action is uncertain but it is believed to decrease VLDL synthesis by increasing lipoprotein lipase activity and by reducing the availability of free fatty acids for the production of VLDL.

The effects on the lipid profile are:

1 A marked reduction in triglyceride through a reduction in VLDL.
2 A reduction in total and LDL cholesterol.
3 An increase in HDL cholesterol.

Omega-3 fatty acid derivatives

(e.g Maxepa ®)

Long term efficiency and safety of these marine oils has not been established. Their mode of action is via decreased hepatic VLDL synthesis and increased lipoprotein lipase activity.

The effects on the lipid profile are:

1 A reduction in triglycerides.
2 Occasionally, a smaller reduction in total cholesterol.

These marine oils also inhibit platelet aggregation.

Useful address

Family Heart Association, Wesley House, 7 High Street, Kidlington, Oxford, OX5 2DH.
Tel 08675 70292.

Further reading

Ball M and Mann J (1988) *Lipids and heart disease. A practical approach.* Oxford University Press, New York.

Longstaff R and Mann J (1986) *The healthy heart diet book.* Marin Dunitz, London.

Thompson GR (1989) *A handbook of hyperlipidaemia.* Current Science Ltd, London.

References

Ball M and Mann J (1988) *Lipids and heart disease. A practical approach.* Oxford University Press, New York.

British Dietetic Association (1990) *Guidelines to dietitians on the management of adults found to have a high blood cholesterol level.* BDA, Birmingham.

Burr ML (1989) Effects of changes in fat, fish and fibre intakes on death and myocardial reinfarction: Diet and reinfarction trial (DART). *Lancet* **2**, 757–61.

Ernst N, Bowen P, Fisher M, Schaefer EJ and Levy RI (1980) Changes in plasma lipids and lipoproteins after a modified fat diet. *Lancet* **ii**, 111–113.

Francis J, Roche M, Mant D, Jones L and Fullard E (1989) Would primary health care workers give appropriate advice after cholesterol testing? *Br Med J* **298**, 1620–22.

Fulder S (1989) Garlic and the prevention of cardiovascular disease. *Cardiology in Practice* **7**(3), 30–35.

Haines AP (1989) Dietary advice for lowering plasma cholesterol – general practitioners need to know more. *Br Med J* **298**, 1594–5.

Hjerman I, Holme I, Velve Byre K and Leren P (1981) Effect of diet and smoking intervention on the incidence of coronary heart disease. *Lancet* **2**, 1303–310.

King's Fund Centre (1989) Blood cholesterol measurement in the prevention of coronary heart disease. The Sixth King's Fund forum consensus statement. King's Fund, London.

Mann J and Ball M (1985) Hyperlipidaemia. *Medicine International* **2**(14), 580–84.

Mann J, Lewis B, Shepherd J, Winder AF, Fenster S, Rose L and Morgan B (1988) Blood lipid concentrations and other cardiovascular risk factors: distribution, prevalence and detection in Britain. *Br Med J* **296**, 1702–706.

Mansell P and Reckless J (1991) Garlic. *Br Med J* **303**, 379.

McNamara DJ (1990) Dietary cholesterol: effects on lipid metabolism. *Current Opinion in Lipidology* **1**, 18–22.

Medicines Resource Centre (1991) Hyperlipidaemia Part 1 and Part 2. *Med Rec Bull* **2**(9) October, and (11) December. pp. 33–5; pp. 41–3.

Mensink R (1987) Effect of monounsaturated fatty acids versus complex carbohydrates on high-density lipoproteins in healthy men and women. *Lancet* **1**, 122–4.

Muldoon M, Manuck S and Matthews K (1990) Lowering cholesterol concentrations and mortality a quantitative review of primary prevention trials. *Br Med J* **301**, 309–313.

Neil HAW, Mant D, Jones L, Morgan B and Mann JI (1990) Lipid screening: is it enough to measure total cholesterol concentration? *Br Med J* **301**, 584–6.

O'Connor P, Feely J and Shepherd J (1990) Lipid lowering drugs. *Br Med J* **300**, 667–72.

Ramsay LE, Yeo WW and Jackson PR (1991) Dietary reduction of serum cholesterol concentration: time to think again. *Br Med J* **303**, 953.

Ruys T, Shaikh M, Nordestgaard BG, Sturgess I, Watts GF and Lewis B (1989) Effects of exercise and fat ingestion on high density lipoprotein production by peripheral tissues. *Lancet* **2**, 1119–21.

Southgate DAT (1990) Nibblers, gorgers, snackers and grazers. *Br Med J* **300**, 136–7.

Tredger JA, Morgan LM, Travis J and Marks V (1991) The effects of guar gum, sugar beet fibre and wheat bran supplementation on serum lipoprotein levels in normocholesterolaemic volunteers. *J Hum Nutr Dietet* **4**, 375–84.

Tunstall-Pedoe H (1989) Who is for cholesterol testing? *Br Med J* **298**, 1593–4.

Wahlquist M, Lo CS and Myers KA (1989) Fish intake and arterial wall characteristics in healthy people and diabetic patients. *Lancet* **2**, 944–6.

Wolmarans P, Benadé AJS, Rossouw JE and Kotze TJvW (1988) The effect of fatty fish and red meat on plasma lipids in healthy human volunteers. In *Dietetics in the 90s. Role of the dietitian/nutritionist*, Moyal MF (Ed) pp. 155–8. John Libbey, London.

Wood PD, Haskell W, Klein H, Lewis S, Stern MP and Farquhar JW (1976) The distribution of plasma lipoproteins in middle-aged male runners. *Metabolism* **25**, 1249–57.

4.20 Coronary heart disease

4.20.1 Prevalence of coronary heart disease

Coronary heart disease (CHD) is the major cause of mortality and morbidity in the UK. Northern Ireland and Scotland hold the unenviable position of being top of the world league table for CHD (Fig. 4.13).

In 1988, CHD accounted for one in every three deaths in men and one in every four in women (i.e. 27% of all deaths in the UK). These figures represent an average of 480 deaths per day or 175 793 per year from heart disease. The majority of these deaths are in individuals of 65 years of age or over, however one third of premature deaths in men and one in seven of those in women are caused by CHD.

Although CHD death rates in the UK are very high and cause concern, the morbidity rate is equally important. In Britain in 1985 there were 186 980 hospital admissions for CHD, and in 1986–87 CHD caused the loss of 40.5 million working days, 37.4 million of which were lost to men. These figures do not take into consideration the impact on the quality of life and human and social costs of the disease (Wells 1987).

CHD is perceived as a disease of affluence; however it is more prevalent in lower socioeconomic groups in affluent countries (Marmot *et al* 1978; Tunstall-Pedoe *et al* 1989a; Marmot *et al* 1991). The social inequalities in health were highlighted by the Black Report in 1980 and the Health Divide Report in 1987 (Black 1988; Whitehead 1988).

The term 'coronary heart disease' represents a group of clinical disorders including angina pectoris, acute myocardial infarction and sudden ischaemic death. The pathological basis of CHD is atherosclerosis, a proliferative process which ultimately results in narrowing of the blood vessels, subsequent impairment of blood flow and thrombosis. It is the concurrence of atherosclerosis and thrombosis which results in infarction.

4.20.2 Pathogenesis of coronary heart disease

Atherosclerosis

The blood vessels most likely to suffer from atherosclerosis are the aorta, the coronary arteries and the femoral and cerebral arteries. Atherosclerosis in the latter two arteries is associated with intermittent claudication and stroke; the latter is discussed in more detail in Section 4.21.

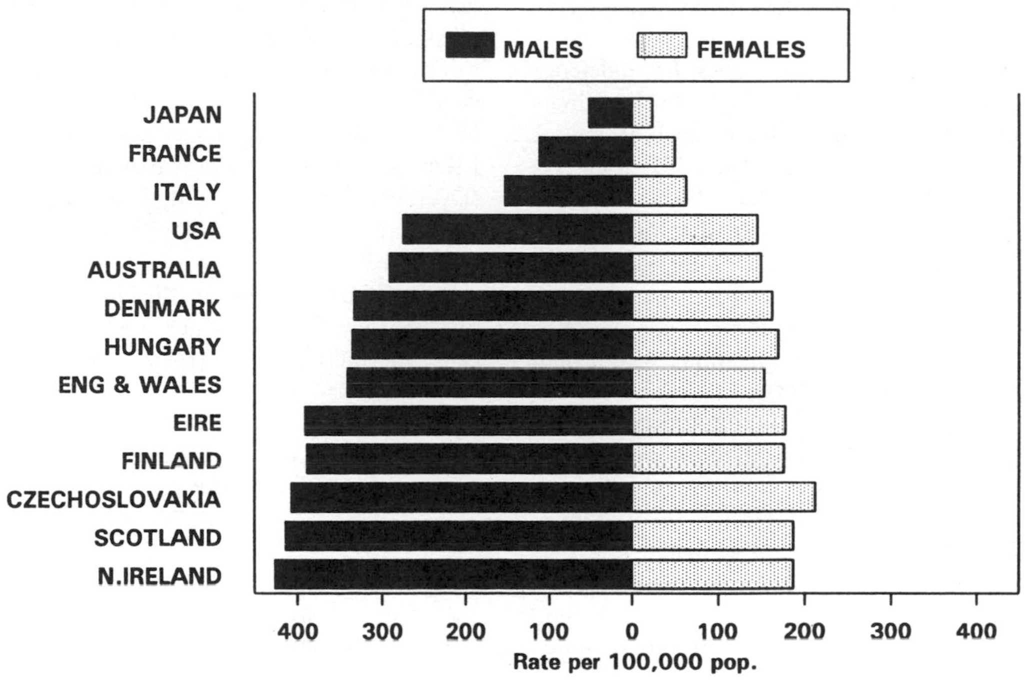

Fig. 4.13 Coronary heart disease death rates for selected countries, all ages, 1986 (Data has been standardized to a European population). Source: World Health Organization 1988.

Fatty streaks, which are made up of lipid filled monocytes and macrophages, running longitudinally along the internal surface of the arteries may be seen in children of primary school age. The relationship of these fatty streaks to the second stage of atherosclerosis (i.e. fibrous plaques) is not clear, but it seems to be dependent on a number of risk factors such as serum cholesterol, cigarette smoking, blood pressure. These are discussed in more detail below.

The plaques are white lesions, they are often raised and may protrude into the lumen of the artery. Endothelial cells, platelets, tissue macrophages and smooth muscle cells all play a role in the formation of the lipid-rich plaques. It is believed that the endothelial cell lining of the artery may be altered structurally or functionally by hyperlipidaemia. Subsequent to this alteration a chain of further changes occur, i.e. lipid filled monocytes enter the endothelium and smooth muscle cells proliferate. Damage to the endothelium results in platelet activation. The activated platelets release thromboxane which causes platelet aggregation and the contraction of smooth muscle cells within the arterial wall. As the plaques develop the outer fibrous layer may become hardened and a number of large plaques may coalesce to occlude the vessel and obliterate the normal structure and function of the artery.

There are numerous theories as to how plaques are formed, however the most interesting and recent theory is the 'free radical theory'. Free radicals are reactive chemical compounds, which can cause lipid peroxidation. Peroxidized lipids may damage the arterial endothelium and cause the proliferation of smooth muscle cells. Low density lipoproteins (LDL – see Section 4.19) are particularly susceptible to peroxidation; macrophages in the endothelial lining absorb peroxidized LDL and thus may cause fatty streaks.

Evidence suggests that the body does have defence mechanisms against lipid peroxidation in the form of circulating antioxidants vitamin E (alpha tocopherol), vitamin A (beta carotene) and vitamin C (Gey *et al* 1987; Riemersa *et al* 1990; Gurr 1991, Riemersa *et al* 1991). (See also Section 2.6.2.) However, it is possible that other components of the foods which contain these vitamins (such as fibre and minerals) may also play a part.

It is for this reason that there is now an increased interest in the vitamin intake of populations with a high incidence of CHD (Smith *et al* 1989).

Thrombogenesis

Thrombosis is a recognized pathological element of myocardial infarction and sudden death (Meade 1985). A thrombus is formed at the site of a large atheromatous plaque and may totally occlude the blood vessel. The platelet cells have a key role in thrombus formation; if they are exposed to damaged tissue they become 'activated'. The activated platelets produce thromboxane which promotes platelet aggregation and vasoconstriction. Simultaneously the blood vessel wall produces prostacyclin which inhibits platelet aggregation and is a vasodilator.

During the 1970s, studies on Greenland Inuit and Japanese fishermen revealed that both groups had a very low incidence of CHD (Dyerberg and Bang 1979; Dyerberg 1981; Dyerberg and Bang 1982; Kagawa *et al* 1982). These two population groups ate large quantities of fish and the low incidence of CHD was attributed to the anti-thrombotic effect of the n-3 polyunsaturated fatty acids (PUFA) in fish oil. Several studies have suggested an inverse relationship between fish oil consumption or eicosapentaenoic acid levels and CHD (Hirai *et al* 1980; Kromhout *et al* 1985; Wood *et al* 1987).

Arachidonic acid is the common substrate for the formation of aggregatory thromboxane A_2. In people who eat large quantities of fish, eicosapentaenoic acid replaces arachidonic acid in the platelets; this greatly reduces the production of thromboxane A_2 and the small amount of thromboxane A_3 produced is inactive. Fish oils also reduce VLDL production and thus reduce serum triglyceride levels. Raised triglycerides are believed to increase platelet stickiness, which may contribute to thrombosis.

The effect of fish oils on serum cholesterol is variable and depends on the type of supplementation and the individual's characteristics (Herold and Kinsela 1986). It is also postulated that fish oils may have a beneficial effect in reducing the adherence of monocytes which is necessary for atheroma formation (Glomset 1985; Lee *et al* 1985).

The active fatty acids in fish oils are eicosapentaenoic (EPA) 20:5 n-3 and docosahexaenoic (DHA) 22:6 n-3. The levels of these fatty acids in fish varies considerably between types of fish, seasons of the year and whether the fish is wild or farmed. Equally the fatty acid content of fish oil supplements varies considerably (Table 4.58).

There is much debate as to the quantity of fish which would have to be consumed to be protective. An intake of 1–2 g of EPA daily has been suggested. Greenland Eskimos consume approximately 6 g EPA per day (Dyerberg 1981). Exler and Weihrauch (1969) estimated that a daily consumption of 250 g of oily fish would supply 1.5 g of EPA.

A study on post myocardial infarction patients found that two oily fish meals per week reduced two-year all-cause mortality by 29% (Burr *et al* 1989). Therefore the

Table 4.58 The comparative amounts of fish or fish oil which will provide approximately 1 g of eicosapentaenoic acid

Cod	=	500 g
Mackerel	=	100 g
Salmon	=	100 g
Trout	=	200 g
Herring	=	100 g
Shrimp	=	400 g
Maxepa	=	3 g
Cod liver oil	=	55 g

evidence to date would suggest that post-cardiac individuals should be encouraged to eat fish and particularly oily fish. Fish is a good substitute for fatty meats or high fat cheeses at mealtimes.

The use of fish oil and fish oil capsules to supplement EPA intake should be treated more cautiously; there is a possibility of vitamin A and D overdosage and there has also been some concern expressed as to the efficacy of the refined oils. There are no studies of the long term benefit of fish oil and it should not be recommended for general consumption.

Aspirin has also been found to have an anti-thrombotic effect; it inhibits the metabolism of arachidonic acid and the subsequent production of thromboxane A_2.

4.20.3 Risk factors associated with the development of CHD

In 1981 Hopkins and Williams classified 246 factors which were associated with the occurrence of CHD. However only a small number of these are believed to be causative, but they act in a multiplicative rather than additive manner which greatly increases the risk of CHD. The main risk factors may be classified as modifiable and non-modifiable (Table 4.59).

Cigarette smoking

Cigarette smoking is one of the major risk factors for coronary heart disease. It has been estimated that cigarette smoking may be responsible for more that 20% of CHD deaths in the UK and 30% in the USA (HEA 1990). Cigarette smokers have a twofold greater incidence of CHD than non-smokers; heavy smokers have a fourfold greater incidence. There is a consistent dose response relationship between the risk of developing CHD and the number of cigarettes smoked per day.

The incidence of smoking in the UK has been declining over the last 20 years. In 1972, 52% of men smoked in Great Britain; this level had reduced to 33% in 1988. For women, the incidence decreased from 41% to 30% in the same period of time.

There is a large socioeconomic relationship in smoking incidence. In 1986, in Northern Ireland 34.1% of 16–64 year old males and 29.6% of females were current cigarette smokers (at least one cigarette per day). In non-manual male workers this level was 26.6%, in manual workers 38.1% and 55.2% of unemployed males smoked cigarettes daily. In females the rates were 24.7%, 38.2% and 44.1% respectively. The number of cigarettes smoked per day also increased with decreasing socioeconomic group (Evans *et al* 1990).

Table 4.59 Risk factors for CHD

Modifiable	Non-modifiable
Cigarette smoking	Sex
Raised cholesterol	Age
High blood pressure	Genetics
Overweight	
Lack of exercise	
Stress	

The definite mechanism by which cigarette smoking increases the risk of CHD is not clear. It is known that *nicotine* increases the heart rate, blood pressure and myocardial oxygen demands. Simultaneously *carbon monoxide* produced by smoking, results in an increase in the carboxyhaemoglobin level, which reduces the blood's capacity to carry oxygen. Smoking is also a source of *oxygen free radicals* which exert their cytotoxic effect by causing peroxidation of membrane phospholipids. Smoking also increases platelet stickiness and the tendency for thrombosis to occur.

Individuals who smoke have higher levels of total cholesterol and lower levels of protective high density lipoprotein (HDL) cholesterol than non-smokers. Smokers tend to exercise less, drink more alcohol, eat more chips and processed meats and use more salt and sugar. The majority also consume less eicosapentaenoic acid, linoleic acid and vitamin C, all of which are believed to be protective for CHD (Fehily *et al* 1984; Wood *et al* 1987; Fulton *et al* 1988; Oliver 1989; Whichelow *et al* 1991).

The increased risk of CHD from smoking is substantially reduced 10 years after cessation in those who had smoked less than 20 cigarettes per day. In heavier smokers, the residual risk of developing CHD is proportional to the length of time the smoker had smoked cigarettes and the quantity smoked (Strong and Oalmann 1990).

Serum cholesterol

The level of an individual's serum cholesterol is largely dependent on his or her nutritional intake and the metabolic response of that individual to his or her diet and lifestyle. In general the body absorbs approximately 40% of dietary cholesterol. The dietary intake of fat and particularly saturated fat has a major effect on serum cholesterol levels. Dietary cholesterol does not have the profound effect on serum cholesterol that was formerly believed. Raised serum cholesterol and particularly LDL cholesterol is one of the major risk factors for CHD. In 1982 the WHO Expert Committe on the Prevention of Coronary Heart Disease stated that they 'knew of no population in whom CHD was common that did not also have a relatively high average serum cholesterol level'. The 'Seven Countries Study' carried out on 12 000 men in 18 population groups showed a strong correlation between the mean serum cholesterol of a population and the mortality rate from CHD. The higher the cholesterol level in the blood the greater the risk of CHD (Rose and Shipley 1986). The Helsinki Heart Study showed that (using Gemfibrozil, a lipid lowering drug) there is a 1:3 relationship between cholesterol lowering and fall in CHD incidence i.e. for every 1% fall in cholesterol there is a 3% decrease in CHD incidence (Frick *et al* 1987); the Lipid Research Clinic Trial showed a 1:2 relationship (Lipid Research Clinics Program 1984).

The optimal level of serum cholesterol is difficult to set because of the gradient of risk, however it is believed that the risk of heart attacks is lowest at levels below 5.2 mmol/l in people over 30 years of age, and below 4.7 mmol/l in those under 30 years of age (National Forum for CHD Prevention 1988). An upper desirable limit of cholesterol of 5.2 mmol/l has also been agreed by the US Consensus Conference (1985), the European Atherosclerosis Society (1987) and the British Cardiac Society (1987).

In Britain, the range of cholesterol levels is large, the average total cholesterol level of 25–59 year old males and females were 5.9 mmol/l and 5.8 mmol/l respectively in one large study (Mann *et al* 1988). In Northern Ireland 58% of all males (12–64 years old) and 55% of females have a cholesterol level greater than 5.2 mmol/l. In the older age group (i.e. 55–64 years of age), these figures are 82% and 93% respectively (Evans *et al* 1990).

Many factors influence cholesterol levels; overweight or obesity are associated with a higher total cholesterol level, higher LDL cholesterol and lower HDL cholesterol. Overweight is also associated with raised triglyceride levels, which have an inverse relationship with protective HDL.

Cholesterol levels tend to be higher in professional men although CHD rates are lower (Marmot *et al* 1978; Pocock *et al* 1987; Tunstall-Pedoe *et al* 1989b).

Blood cholesterol levels increase with age in Western societies (but not all countries in the world). Hormone levels also have an influence; prior to the menopause, women tend to have lower average cholesterol levels than males, however after the age of 50 years the reverse situation occurs. HDL cholesterol levels are significantly lower in lower socioeconomic groups and the unemployed. There is still some debate as to the effect of a moderate alcohol intake (i.e. 1–2 units per day) in increasing HDL cholesterol and reducing coronary risk status. Exercise does appear to elevate HDL cholesterol (see the section on Exercise below). Brewed, unfiltered coffee has been reported to increase LDL levels (Thelle *et al* 1983; Bonaa *et al* 1988; Thelle 1991).

Other factors influence the cholesterol level, including the time of year, time of day, menstrual cycle, medication and it is for this reason that treatment for hyperlipidaemia should not be instituted on the basis of one measurement.

In recent years, it has been suggested that a low serum cholesterol may increase the risk of cancer. However, it is also possible that a low cholesterol level may be a consequence, rather than a cause of cancer. The Committee on Medical Aspects of Food Policy (COMA) panel on Dietary References Values reviewed the available data and stated that 'the balance of the evidence is against a specific predisposing effect of low blood cholesterol to cancer' (DoH 1991).

Blood pressure

High blood pressure or hypertension (defined as systolic or diastolic blood pressure greater than 160 mm Hg and 95 mm Hg respectively) is a consistent contributing factor in atherosclerosis. It is believed that the hypertension creates conditions which encourage the development of atheroma.

A large British study found that approximately 10% of women and 15% of men aged 25–59 years had hypertension (Mann *et al* 1988). Approximately 50% of hypertensive individuals have abnormal lipid profiles (Castelli and Anderson 1988; Feher and Lant 1991).

Blood pressure is influenced by a number of factors such as genetics; obesity, alcohol, salt and possibly fat intake (see Section 4.18 Hypertension).

Overweight

There has been much debate as to whether obesity is an independent risk factor for CHD or whether its major impact is due to its association with elevated blood pressure and cholesterol (Ashley and Kannel 1974), increased production of LDL cholesterol (Kesaniemi and Grundy 1983) or decreased glucose tolerance and insulin resistence (Jarrett 1986).

Overweight individuals have a twofold increase in the risk of developing CHD (RCP 1983; HEA 1990).

Increasing BMI has a positive relationship with serum LDL cholesterol, blood pressure and triglycerides and a negative effect on HDL cholesterol. A central distribution of excess adipose tissue is believed to be more of a risk for CHD than peripherally distributed fat (Larsson *et al* 1984; Baumgartner *et al* 1987; Donohue *et al* 1987). Individuals with a central fat distribution are sometimes referred to as having an 'apple shape figure' as opposed to a 'pear shaped' figure, the waist to hip ratio will be greater than 1.0 in males or more than 0.8 in females.

Most studies show an increasing proportion of the population carry excess weight with increasing age.

Exercise

It is generally agreed that exercise has a significant protective effect against CHD (Morris 1983; Slattery *et al* 1989). Exercise not only helps to maintain a desirable body weight but the endorphins released during exercise also inhibit appetite. Regular vigorous exercise helps to raise HDL cholesterol (La Porte *et al* 1983), possibly as a result of a decrease in the catabolism of HDL cholesterol rather than an increase in synthesis (Herbert *et al* 1984).

The conditioning effect of regular exercise increases the work efficiency of the heart muscle and reduces blood pressure.

Exercise is strongly linked to socioeconomic group.

Those in the higher socioeconomic groups take more exercise and participate in sport more regularly.

Stress

The influence of stress and behaviour types in the causation of CHD has been debated for several years; 50% of the differences in CHD rates between different employment grades of staff in the Whitehall Study of Civil Servants could not be accounted for by standard risk factors (Marmot *et al* 1978).

It is known that the physiological response to stress is to release 'catecholamines' which in turn promote fat breakdown and energy release and an increase in cholesterol synthesis. However some of the major difficulties with stress are its imprecise definition, difficulty of measurement and individualistic nature. There is a need for more research into the potential contribution of stressful life events, stress at work, poor social support and unfavourable socioeconomic circumstances to the incidence of CHD.

Some people use cigarettes, food or excess alcohol as a crutch in coping with stress, and this may influence their risk status.

Sex and age

The incidence of the symptoms of CHD increase rapidly with age. It is probable that this is a result of the cumulative effects of cigarette smoking, raised blood cholesterol, hypertension and other factors over time (Shaper 1988).

The majority of deaths in females from CHD occur in the 75 plus years age group, this is largely due to the protective effect of the female hormones during the productive years and lower smoking rates in adult women. Men under 65 years of age have three and a half times the risk of developing CHD as women in the same age group.

Genetics

CHD does tend to cluster in families and there has been great interest in the relative effects of nature and nurture. The genetic background of individuals can influence their likelihood to develop hypertension, abnormal lipids, diabetes or obesity. Familial hyperlipidaemia and other genetically determined dyslipidaemias are discussed in Section 4.19. The importance of environmental influences regardless of genetic background have been shown in studies of Japanese who emigrated to the USA. It has been suggested that the very low risk of CHD in Japan is not transferable with individuals who emigrate and adopt Western cultures and lifestyle patterns (Marmot *et al* 1975).

Indians, Pakistanis, Bangladeshis and Sri Lankans living in the UK have particularly high rates of CHD – 25% higher than the whole UK population. The high mortality rates cannot be explained simply by differences in diet, blood pressure or cigarette smoking. It is known that Southern Asians do have an increased tendency to develop diabetes mellitus and this factor, obesity and the stress of changing cultures may have some influence.

4.20.4 Diet and the prevention of coronary heart disease

It is vitally important that all interventions are properly planned, monitored and evaluated. Although the health gains of many programmes will only manifest themselves in the long term, short term achievable goals should also be set and monitored. Dietitians whether in clinical or preventive work should evaluate their work and share their findings with colleagues.

There are three categories of prevention, primary, secondary and tertiary. The time at which the intervention takes place dictates whether it is primary, secondary or tertiary in nature.

Primary prevention

Primary prevention is aimed at healthy people in an effort to promote health and prevent disease occurring. Programmes aimed at changing lifestyle practices in order to prevent CHD are primary prevention. Many of these programmes now exist e.g. Change of Heart, Look After Your Heart and the Kilkenny Health Project. An important element in all of these programmes is that they aim to bring about a change in behaviour not merely a change in knowledge. Health promotion should facilitate positive health choices, by making healthy choices easy choices. The social and economic environment must be conducive to health and projects such as Heartbeat Wales, the WHO Healthy Cities Project, and the WHO Health For All 2000 programme, endeavour to achieve this through lay participation, multisectoral collaboration and the elimination of inequalities in health.

Dietitians, and particularly those working in the community, play a very important role in primary health promotion. They have the knowledge and skills to convert scientific nutritional messages into practical healthy eating advice. Dietitians also have an important advocacy role; they can and should influence the creation and implementation of nutrition strategies and policies.

Secondary prevention

This is concerned with the early detection of illness and the prevention of a further deterioration in health or restoration to a former state of good health. The existence of CHD screening clinics has grown substantially in recent years and the introduction of the new General Medical Practitioner Contract in the UK in 1990, allowing payment for these clinics, has encouraged their growth. Dietitians may be employed to give nutritional counselling to people identified to be 'at risk' for CHD or they may be requested to provide nutrition training and updating to other members of the Primary Care or hospital team, who provide general first line nutrition advice to individuals.

Secondary nutrition education must be very positive and practical in nature. It is vitally important that all of the nutrition advice given to the patient is consistent and it is for this reason that dietitians should communicate freely and regularly with other members of the health care team. Several studies have shown that the level of practical nutritional knowledge on CHD prevention held by health care workers is inadequate (Francis *et al* 1989).

Most patients who have been diagnosed as having angina, or who have been found to be 'at risk' of CHD, will need more than one consultation with a dietitian to achieve a reduced serum cholesterol, reduced weight or blood pressure. At each consultation achievable dietary goals should be mutually agreed and progress monitored.

Tertiary prevention

This is targeted at individuals who have a distinct disease, and aims to help rehabilitate individuals and help them to maximize their quality of life. Since the relatives of those affected or threatened by CHD are a highly motivated group, secondary and especially tertiary prevention schemes are a good opportunity to influence the lifestyle of the whole family.

Many individuals who have had a heart attack will need counselling and support to enable them to return to an active and productive lifestyle. Some people will be very anxious about what they should or should not do and the provision of an interdisciplinary team approach can do much to improve a coronary patient's self-confidence and quality of life (Cornett and Watson 1984). The dietitian should be a member of the rehabilitation team and should provide practically-oriented nutritional advice and support.

In 1989 fewer than 30% of District Health Authorities in the UK were providing a coronary rehabilitation programme. In an effort to facilitate those wishing to set up such a programme the Coronary Prevention Group (1989) published a booklet on this subject.

Evidence to support the prevention of CHD

CHD is a multi-risk factor disease. Therefore the perfect trial to show the impact of altering the diet alone, and consequently reducing CHD can never be undertaken.

Drug trials have shown that it is possible to reduce serum cholesterol and consequent deaths from CHD. However, one of the worrying factors in these drug trials was that deaths from non-cardiovascular causes, largely accidents and violence, increased thus preventing all-cause mortality being significantly reduced (Lipid Research Clinics Program 1984; Frick *et al* 1987, Muldoon *et al* 1990; Oliver 1991). Secondary prevention drug trials, have shown that it is possible to reduce cholesterol levels and impede atherosclerotic progress (Levy *et al* 1984) or even cause plaque regression (Blankenhorn *et al* 1987).

Dietary studies have shown that serum cholesterol may be reduced by dietary change. The National Diet Heart Feasibility Study in 1960 showed a reduction in cholesterol of 12%, 13% and 3% respectively for diets containing 30%, 34% and 35% of energy from fat and a P:S ratio of 1:4, 1:8 and 0:4 respectively (The National Diet Heart Study Report 1968). The Finnish Mental Hospital Trial also showed that it was possible to alter cholesterol levels and reduce CHD incidence significantly by dietary intervention, using a six year crossover trial (Miettinen *et al* 1972).

Secondary prevention dietary trials have not provided conclusive evidence about the impact of nutrition education in post infarction patients. The DART study only achieved a 3–4% fall in cholesterol levels and no reduction in CHD mortality over a two year period, despite intensive dietary education (Burr *et al* 1989).

The majority of intervention trials to date have been multifactorial in nature or have targeted high risk individuals. It is very difficult with lifestyle intervention programmes to prevent 'contamination' of control or intervention groups by factors extraneous to the study, therefore the method of research must be kept in mind when considering the results.

Although the Oslo Study (Hjermann *et al* 1981) and European Collaborative Trial (WHO 1983, 1986) both showed it was possible to reduce mortality consequent to a screening and multifactorial intervention programme, the Multiple Risk Factor Intervention Trial (MRFIT Research Group 1982) did not show a significant difference in mortality between the control and intervention groups.

The North Karelia Project was an example of a community intervention programme. A detailed Health Promotion Programme was undertaken utilizing community groups and their networks, the media, workplaces, schools and many other venues. It showed that a public health education campaign could lead to substantial changes in behaviour patterns. The project did not provide absolute proof of the specific effect of dietary changes, however, it did provide a model for community intervention programmes (Puska *et al* 1985).

Based on the preceding information and many other research findings, the American Heart Association, World Health Organization, National Advisory Committee on Nutrition Education (NACNE) and Committee on Medical Aspects of Food Policy (COMA) have put forward dietary recommendations for the prevention of CHD.

Dietary recommendations for the prevention of CHD

There has been much debate as to whether it is better to utilize a population strategy or a high risk strategy in the prevention of CHD (i.e. to give everyone preventative advice or only advise those screened and found to be 'at risk'). However, most people would agree that the two are not mutually exclusive and indeed complement each other.

The general nutrition promotion message for CHD prevention is identical to that outlined in Chapter 1.1. The one dietary area not already discussed which has received a lot of attention recently is the influence of non-starch polysaccharide (dietary fibre) in reducing the risk of CHD.

Several studies have shown an inverse relationship between dietary fibre intake and CHD incidence (Kromhout *et al* 1982; Kushi *et al* 1985; Khaw and Barrett-Connor 1987). There is growing evidence of the hypocholesterolaemic effect of dietary fibre (Miettinen 1987). It is the soluble fibre found in beans, peas, lentils, oatmeal and fruit that has a lipid lowering effect. Insoluble fibre found in cereals does not effect lipid levels (Stasse-Wolthuis *et al* 1980). Van Horn and Anderson both found that adding oat bran or oatmeal to a lipid lowering diet increased the percentage decrease in cholesterol achieved (Anderson *et al* 1984; Van Horn *et al* 1986).

A review of studies utilizing soluble dietary fibre supplements showed that the average reduction in plasma total cholesterol would be 6–19% in hypercholesterolaemic individuals (Kris-Etherton *et al* 1988). Soluble dietary fibre decreases total and LDL cholesterol but has very little effect on HDL cholesterol. It is not clearly understood how fibre brings about its influence, although an increase in faecal bile acid excretion and decreased lipid absorption have been put forward as two possible mechanisms (Miettinen and Tarpila 1977).

The general recommendation that the population should eat more fibre is therefore important too for CHD prevention. Hypercholesterolaemic individuals should be particularly encouraged to increase their intake of soluble fibre.

All smokers will be advised to stop smoking to reduce their risk of CHD. The dietitian must be sympathetic to the problems encountered by many people trying to stop smoking. One of the common sequelae to smoking cessation is weight gain, in a small proportion of individuals the weight gained can be substantial (Williamson *et al* 1991). Although the benefits of smoking cessation outweigh the risks of weight gain, the aesthetic problems posed by weight gain may weaken the individual's resolve to stop smoking. Appropriate advice and counselling should be given to individuals trying to stop smoking to prevent or limit weight gain (see Section 4.17.1).

4.20.5 Coronary care

Patients admitted to coronary care units (CCUs) may be in contact with hospital services for the first time in their lives or be repeating earlier visits. Therefore, the needs of patients in CCUs are very varied. Ideally, the normal hospital menu should provide a light choice for those who are 'poorly' on admission, offering small, regular appetizing meals.

For those who are able to eat normally, there should be a 'healthy heart' menu choice, low in total fat, using polyunsaturated fat for cooking and spreading, high in dietary fibre from breakfast cereals, bread, fruit, vegetables, and encouraging the consumption of lean meats, oily fish and white fish.

If the patient is overweight, encouragement should be given to start a reduced energy diet to enable weight loss, during admission or once home. Special diets, if necessary, should be requested by medical staff soon after admittance.

Some patients have raised blood glucose levels immediately post-heart attack. This should not be taken as indicative of diabetes until a fasting blood glucose, taken several days post-heart attack, has been considered.

If the patient requires advice or re-education relating to diet (or other aspects of lifestyle), this should start as soon as possible as incentive tends to be high in someone who has recently had a heart attack. However, patients may be in a stressed state in the first few days of recovery and so may not remember advice given. Any dietary education should include written information and there should be a process for following the patient's progress, if required.

Many coronary care units offer multidisciplinary education sessions for groups of patients post-heart attack, often called 'after care groups'. Dietitians can use these group settings to continue to discuss healthy eating and answer questions. Relatives often attend these sessions. The room in which sessions are held, often the ward day room, can be used to display diet and lifestyle information.

Discussion points which dietitians may wish to include in group sessions are:

1 Energy balance – and the importance of achieving/maintaining ideal body weight. Patients may become less active after a heart attack, their lifestyle may change if they are not working, or they may give up smoking, all of which could lead to an increase in weight, so even patients who are not overweight may benefit from advice on weight control after a heart attack.

2 Fat intake (reduce saturated, increase polyunsaturated) – and the importance of reducing the total amount of fat in the diet to approximately 35% of the energy intake. Patients may have many questions about cholesterol and types of fat to use. Oily fish, fruit, vegetables, and food sources of antioxidants should be encouraged.

3 Fibre in the diet – a higher intake of fibre should be encouraged by promoting the use of wholemeal bread, wholegrain cereals, pasta and pulses, and fruit and vegetables.

4 Sugar intake – particularly in relation to weight control; identifying ways in which the individual can reduce sugar intake.

5 Alcohol consumption – advice given should be consistent with that given by medical staff.

6 Smoking and its effect on weight control.

7 General nutritional aspects – such as meal frequency (small regular meals are better than infrequent large ones)

or how to choose wisely when eating out or for special occasions.

Patients remain in hospital for a relatively short time post-heart attack. Fasting plasma lipids are carried out routinely in most CCUs but the results may not be available until just before, or after, discharge from the hospital. Many nutrition and dietetic departments have arranged that general healthy eating information is given to the patients by ward nursing staff and those with raised lipids are referred by the medical staff to a dietetic outpatient clinic.

Further reading

Ball M and Mann J (1988) *Lipids and Heart Disease, A practical Approach.* Oxford University Press, Oxford.

Cornett S and Watson J (1984) *Cardiac rehabilitation: An interdisciplinary team approach.* John Wiley, New York.

Department of Health (1991) *Dietary Reference Values for food, energy and nutrients in the United Kingdom.* Rep Hlth Soc Subj 41. HMSO, London.

DHSS *On the state of the public health for the year 1988.* HMSO, London.

Ewles L and Simnett I (1985) *Promoting health. A practical guide to health education.* John Wiley, Chichester.

Frohlich E (Ed) (1990) *Preventive aspects of coronary heart disease.* F A Davis, Philadelphia.

Leeds A, Judd P and Lewis B (Eds) (1990) *Nutrition matters for practice nurses.* John Libbey, London.

Royal College of Physicians (1984) *Coronary heart disease prevention. Plans for action.* Pitman, London.

Smith A and Jacobson B (1988) *The nation's health – a strategy for the 1990s.* Oxford University Press, Oxford.

Whitehead M (1988) *Inequalities in health: The Black Report and The Health Divide.* Penguin, London.

References

Anderson JW, Story L, Sieling B *et al* (1984) Hypocholesterolaemic effects of oat bran or bran intake for hypercholesterolaemic men. *Am J Clin Nutr* **40**, 1146.

Ashley FW and Kannel WB (1974) Relation of weight change to changes in atherogenic traits: The Framingham Study. *J Chron Dis* **27**, 103–14.

Baumgartner RN, Roche AF, Chumlea C *et al* (1987) Fatness and fat patterns: associations with plasma lipids and blood pressures in adults 18–57 years of age. *Am J Epidemiol* **126**, 614–28.

Black D (1988) In *Inequalities in Health. The Black Report and the Health Divide*, Whitehead M (Ed) Penguin, London.

Blankenhorn DH, Nessim SA, Johnson RI *et al* (1987) Beneficial effects of colestipol-niacin therapy on coronary atherosclerosis and coronary venous bypass grafts. *J Am Med Assoc* **257**, 3233–40.

Bonaa K, Arnesen E, Thellar DS *et al* (1988) Coffee and cholesterol: is it all in the brewing? The Tromso Study. *Br Med J* **297**, 1103–4.

British Cardiac Society (1987) *Report of British Cardiac Society Working Group on coronary disease prevention.* British Cardiac Society, London.

Burr ML, Fehily AM, Gilbert JF *et al* (1989) Effects of changes in fat, fish and fibre intakes on the frequency of myocardial reinfarctions: DART Study. *Lancet* **ii**, 757–62.

Castelli WP and Anderson K (1988) A population at risk: prevalence of high cholesterol levels in the Framingham Study. *Am J Med* **80**(Suppl 2A), 23–32.

Cornett SJ and Watson JE (1984) *Cardiac rehabilitation – an interdisciplinary team approach.* John Wiley, New York.

Coronary Prevention Group (1989) Guidelines for setting up and running a cardiac rehabilitation programme. Coronary Prevention Group, London.

Department of Health (1991) *Dietary Reference Values for food, energy and nutrients in the United Kingdom.* Rep Hlth Soc Subj 41. HMSO, London.

Donohue RD, Abbott E, Bloom DM *et al* (1987) Central obesity and coronary heart disease in men. *Lancet* **1**, 821–4.

Dyerberg J and Bang HO (1979) Haemostatic function and platelet polyunsaturated fatty acids in Eskimos. *Lancet* **ii**, 433–5.

Dyerberg J (1981) Platelet – vessel wall interaction: influence of diet. *Philos Trans R Soc London* **B294**: 373–87.

Dyerberg J and Bang HO (1982) A hypothesis on the development of acute myocardial infarction in Greenlanders. *Scand J Clin Lab Invest* **42**, 7–13.

European Atherosclerosis Society (1987) Strategies for the prevention of coronary heart disease. *Eur Heart J* **8**, 77–88.

Evans A, McCrum E and Patterson CC (1990) *The Change of Heart baseline clinical survey.* A report to the N I Health Promotion Unit by Belfast MONICA Project, Dept Epidemiology and Public Health, Royal Victoria Hospital, Belfast.

Exler J and Weihrauch J (1969) Comprehensive evaluation of fatty acids in foods. *J Am Dietet Assoc* **69**, 243–8.

Feher MD and Lant AF (1991) Management choices for hypertension with coexistent hypercholesterolaemia. *J Roy Soc Med* **84**, 203–205.

Fehily AM, Phillips KM and Yarnell JWG (1984) Diet, smoking, social class and body mass index in the Caerphilly Heart Disease Study. *Am J Clin Nutr* **40**, 827–33.

Francis J, Roche M, Mant D *et al* (1989) Would primary health care workers give appropriate dietary advice after cholesterol screening? *Br Med J* **298**, 1620–22.

Frick MH, Elo O, Haapa K *et al* (1987) Helsinki Heart Study: primary prevention trail with gemfibrozil in middle aged men with dyslipidaemia. *N Engl J Med* **317**, 1237–45.

Fulton M, Thomson M, Elton RA, Wood DA and Oliver MF (1988) Cigarette smoking, social class and nutrient intake. Relevance to coronary heart disease. *Eur J Clin Nutr* **42**, 797–803.

Gey KF, Stahelin HB, Puska P *et al* (1987) Relationship of plasma level of vitamin C to mortality from ischaemic heart disease. *Ann NY Acad Sci* **498**, 110–23.

Glomset JA (1985) Fish, fatty acids and human health. *N Engl J Med* **312**(19), 1253–4.

Gurr M (Ed) (1991) Polyunsaturates, their role in health and nutrition. The Butter Council.

Health Education Authority (1990) *Health update: Coronary heart disease.* HEA, London.

Herbert PW, Bernier DN, Cullinane EM *et al* (1984) High density lipoprotein metabolism in runners and sedentary men. *J Am Med Assoc* **252**(8), 1034–37.

Herold PM and Kinsella JE (1986) Fish oil consumption and decreased risk of cardiovascular disease: a comparison of findings from animal and human feeding trials. *Am J Clin Nutr* **43**, 566–98.

Hirai A, Hamazaki T, Terano T *et al* (1980) Eicosapentaenoic acid and platelet function in Japanese. *Lancet* **ii**, 1132–3.

Hjermann I, Velve Byre K, Holme I *et al* (1981) Effect of diet and smoking intervention on the incidence of coronary heart disease. Report from the Oslo group of a randomised trial of healthy men. *Lancet* **ii**, 1303–10.

Hopkins PW and Williams RR (1981) A survey of 246 suggested coronary risk factors. *Atherosclerosis* **40**, 1–52.

Jarrett RJ (1986) Is there an ideal body weight? *Br Med J* **293**, 493–5.

Kagawa Y, Nishizawa M, Suzuki M *et al* (1982) Eicosapolyenoic acid of serum lipids of Japanese islanders with low incidence of cardiovascular disease. *J Nutri Sci Vitaminal* (Tokyo) **28**, 441–53.

Kesaniemi YA and Grundy S (1983) Increased low density lipoprotein production associated with obesity. *Atherosclerosis* **3**, 170–77.

Khaw KT and Barrett-Connor E (1987) Dietary fiber and reduced ischaemic heart disease mortality rates in men and women: a 12 year prospective study. *Am J Epidemiol* **126**, 1093–102.

Kris Etherton PM, Krummel D, Russell ME *et al* (1988) National Cholesterol Education Programme – The effects of diet on plasma lipids, lipoproteins and coronary heart disease. *J Am Diet Assoc* **88**, 1373–400.

Kromhout D, Bosschieter EB and Coulander C de L (1982) Dietary fibre and 10 year mortality from coronary heart disease, cancer and all causes. The Zutphen Study. *Lancet* **1**, 518–22.

Kromhout D, Bosschieter EB and Coulander C de L (1985) The inverse relation between fish consumption and 20 year mortality from coronary heart disease. *N Engl J Med* **312**, 1205–9.

Kushi LH, Lew RA, Stare FJ *et al* (1985) Diet and 20 year mortality from coronary heart disease. *N Engl J Med* **312**, 811–18.

La Porte RE, Brenes G, Dearwater S *et al* (1983) HDL cholesterol across a spectrum of physical activity from quadraplegia to marathon running. *Lancet* **i**, 1212–13.

Larsson B, Sverdsudd K, Welin L *et al* (1984) Abdominal adipose tissue distribution, obesity and risk of cardiovascular disease and death: 13 year follow up of participants in the study of men born in 1913. *Br Med J* **288**, 1401–4.

Lee TH, Hoover RL, Williams JD *et al* (1985) Effect of dietary eicosapentaenoic and docohexaenoic acids on *in vitro* neutrophil and monocyte leukotriene generation and neutrophil function. *N Engl J Med* **312**, 19, 1217–24.

Levy RI, Brensike JF, Epstein SE *et al* (1984) The influence of changes in lipid values induced by cholestyramine and diet on the progression of coronary artery disease. Results of the NHLBI Type II coronary intervention study. *Circulation* **69**, 325–37.

Lipid Research Clinics Program (1984) The Lipid Research Clinics Coronary Prevention Trial Results. Reduction in incidence of coronary heart disease. *J Am Med Assoc* **251**, 351–64.

Mann JI, Lewis B, Shepherd J *et al* (1988) Blood lipid concentrations and other cardiovascular risk factors: distribution, prevalence, and detection in Britain. *Br Med J* **296**, 1702–6.

Marmot MG, Syme SL, Kagen A *et al* (1975) Epidemiologic studies of coronary heart disease and stroke in Japanese men living in Japan, Hawaii and California: prevalence of coronary and hypertensive heart disease and associated risk factors. *Am J Epidemiol* **102**(6), 514–25.

Marmot MG, Rose G, Shipley M *et al* (1978) Employment grade and coronary heart disease in British civil servants. *J Epidemiol Community Hlth* **32**, 244–9.

Marmot MG, Davey Smith G, Stansfeld S *et al* (1991) Health inequalities among British civil servants: the Whitehall II study. *Lancet* **337**, 1387–93.

Meade TW (1985) Thrombosis and ischaemic heart disease. *Br Heart J* **53**, 473–6.

Miettinen M, Turpeinen O, Karvonen MJ *et al* (1972) Effect of cholesterol lowering diet on mortality from coronary heart disease and other causes, a twelve year clinical trial in men and women. *Lancet* **ii**, 835.

Miettinen TA and Tarpila S (1977) Effect of pectin on serum cholesterol, fecal bile acids, and biliary lipids in normolipidemic and hyperlipidemic individuals. *Clin Chim Acta* **70**, 471.

Miettinen TA (1987) Dietary fiber and blood lipids. *Am J Clin Nutr* **45**, 1237–42.

Morris JN (1983) Exercise, health and medicine. *Br Med J* **286**, 1597–8.

Muldoon MF, Manuck SB, Matthews KA (1990) Lowering cholesterol concentrations and mortality: a quantitative review of primary prevention trials. *Br Med J* **301**, 309–314.

Multiple Risk Factor Intervention Trial Research Group (MRFIT) (1982) Risk factor changes and mortality results. *J Am Med Assoc* **248**, 1464–77.

National Forum for Coronary Heart Disease Prevention (1988) Coronary Heart Disease Prevention: action in the UK 1984–87. Pub. by Health Education Authority, London.

Oliver MF (1989) Cigarette smoking, polyunsaturated fats, linoleic acid and coronary heart disease. *Lancet* **1**, 1241–3.

Oliver MF (1991) Might treatment of hypercholesterolaemia increase non-cardiac mortality? *Lancet* **337**, 1529–31.

Pocock SJ, Shaper AG, Cook DG *et al* (1987) Social class differences in ischaemic heart disease in British men. *Lancet* **ii**, 197–201.

Puska P, Nissinen A, Tuomilehto J *et al* (1985) The community based strategy to prevent coronary heart disease. Conclusions from the 10 years of the North Karelia Project. *Ann Rev Public Hlth* **6**, 147–93.

Riemersa RA, Oliver M, Elton RA *et al* (1990) Plasma anti-oxidants and coronary heart disease. Vitamins C and E and selenium. *Eur J Clin Nutr* **44**, 143–50.

Riemersa RA, Wood DA, Macintyre CCA *et al* (1991) Risk of angina pectoris and plasma concentrations of vitamins A, C, E and carotene. *Lancet* **337**, 1–5.

Rose G and Shipley M (1986) Plasma cholesterol concentration and death from coronary heart disease: 10 year results of the Whitehall study. *Br Med J* **293**, 306–307.

Royal College of Physicians (1983) Obesity. *J Roy Coll Phys London* **17**, 3–58.

Shaper AG (1988) *Coronary heart disease, risks and reasons.* Current Medical Literature, London.

Slattery ML, Jacobs DR and Nichamon NZ (1989) Leisure time physical activity and coronary heart disease: the US railroad study. *Circulation* **79**, 304–311.

Smith WCS, Tunstall-Pedoe H, Crombie IK *et al* (1989) Concomitants of excess coronary deaths – major risk factor and lifestyle findings from 10 359 men and women in the Scottish heart health study. *Scot Med J* **34**, 550–55.

Stasse-Wolthuis M, Albers HFF, Van Jeveren JW *et al* (1980) Influence of dietary fiber from fruit and vegetables, bran or citrus pectin on serum lipids, fecal lipids and caloric function. *Am J Clin Nutr* **33**, 1745.

Strong JP and Oalmann MC (1990) In *Preventive aspects of coronary heart disease.* Frohlich ED (Ed) FA Davis, Philadelphia.

The National Diet Heart Study Report (1968) General summary, conclusions and recommendations. *Circulation* **37**(Supp I), 11–126.

Thelle DS, Arnesen E and Forde OH (1983) The Tromso heart study. Does coffee raise serum cholesterol? *N Engl J Med* **308**, 1454–7.

Thelle DS (1991) Coffee, cholesterol and coronary heart disease. The secret is in the brewing. *Br Med J* **302**, 804.

Tunstall-Pedoe H, Smith WCS and Tavendale R (1989a) Coronary risk factor variation across Scotland: results from the Scottish Heart Health Study. *Scot Med J* **34**, 556–60.

Tunstall-Pedoe H, Smith WCS and Tavendale R (1989b) How often that high graphs of serum cholesterol: finding from the Scottish Heart Health and Scottish MONICA Studies. *Lancet* **1**, 540–42.

US Consensus Conference National Institute of Health (1985) Lowering blood cholesterol and heart disease. *J Am Med Assoc* **253**, 2080–90.

Van Horn LV, Liu K, Parker D *et al* (1986) Serum lipid response to oat product intake with a fat modified diet. *J Am Diet Assoc* **86**, 759.

Wells N (1987) Coronary heart disease – the need for action. Office of Health Economics, London.

Whichelow MJ, Erzinclioglu SW and Cox BD (1991) A comparison of the diets of non smokers and smokers. *Br J Addict* **86**(1), 71–81.

Whitehead M (1988) The health divide. In *Inequalities in health, the Black Report and the health divide.* Penguin, London.

WHO (1982) *Prevention of coronary heart disease.* Technical Report 678. World Health Organization, Geneva.

WHO (1988) *World Health Statistics Annual 1988.* World Health Organization, Geneva.

WHO European Collaborative Group (1983) Multifactorial trial in the prevention of coronary heart disease. Incidence and mortality results. *Eur Heart J* **4**, 141–7.

WHO European Collaborative Group (1986) European collaborative trial of multifactorial prevention of coronary heart disease: final report on

the 6 year results. *Lancet* i, 869–72.
Williamson DF, Madans J, Anda RF *et al* (1991) Smoking cessation and severity of weight gain in a national cohort. *N Engl J Med* **324**, 739–45.
Wood DA, Riemersa RA, Butler S *et al* (1987) Linoleic and eicosapentaenoic acids in adipose tissue and platelets and risk of coronary heart disease. *Lancet* **i**, 177–80.

4.21 Stroke

'A stroke involves rapidly developed clinical signs of focal (or global) disturbance of cerebral function, lasting more than 24 hours or leading to death, with no apparent cause other than a vascular origin' (WHO 1973).

Strokes are usually the result of either cerebral infarction or cerebral haemorrhage, the clinical sequelae of which are wide ranging, and can include disorders of balance, movement, touch sensation, speech, vision and swallowing. The exact disability or loss of function caused by a stroke is dependent on the site of damage in the central nervous system.

There is no single cause of stroke, but as is the case for cerebrovascular disease, there are many risk factors. The most important of these is hypertension and its association with the development of arteriosclerosis predisposing to cerebral haemorrhage and infarction. Other factors associated with stroke are smoking, hyperlipidaemia and pre-existing heart disease. Both the Whitehall and Framingham Studies (Wolf *et al* 1982; Fuller *et al* 1983) also showed increased mortality from stroke amongst people with diabetes mellitus where incidence appears to be related to blood glucose control. As these risk factors often co-exist with hypertension, it is difficult to isolate the true relationship between them and stroke. Risk is likely to be greater where more than one of the factors exist.

4.21.1 Nutritional problems after stroke

Following a stroke, 30% of patients have dysphagia (Barer 1989). For some this will resolve within a few days, but for others there will be more prolonged eating difficulties, ranging from severe dysphagia, where the patient is unable to swallow any type of food or fluid safely, to the more difficult to detect 'silent' aspiration of fluid into the lungs on swallowing.

Dysphagia after stroke involves a range of disorders of deglutition, including difficulties with lip seal, tongue and jaw movements (mastication), delayed or absent swallow reflex, and an ineffective cough reflex, resulting in inability to protect the airway i.e. difficulties with both the oral and pharyngeal phases of swallowing.

Assessment of dysphagia

The stages in the normal swallow are outlined in Table 4.60. If any difficulty with swallowing is suspected, the clinician should refer the patient for assessment by a speech and language therapist, who is trained in the assessment, treatment and management of dysphagic patients. Testing for presence of gag reflex alone gives insufficient evidence for the presence of a safe swallow, and absence of aspiration.

Videofluoroscopy

If the safety of the patient's swallow is unclear from bedside assessment of oral function, cough and swallow reflexes, and laryngeal function, the speech and language therapist may suggest referral for videofluoroscopy, where this service exists. This provides more accurate diagnosis and guidelines for management. Videofluoroscopy, or modified barium swallow, is a video-recorded radiological procedure, giving lateral and antero-posterior views of the oral, pharyngeal and oesophageal phases of swallowing. This allows identification of motility problems, assesses aspiration, and evaluates the cause of aspiration.

During the examination, different food consistencies are given in the form of $\frac{1}{3}$ teaspoon barium liquid, $\frac{1}{3}$ teaspoon barium paste, and $\frac{1}{4}$ biscuit coated in barium, and all phases of the swallow observed. This gives useful information for diagnosis, and also gives the opportunity to view the effectiveness of compensatory techniques e.g. for alleviation of unilateral disorders or to minimize poor oral control.

Treatment techniques

Where the swallow reflex is absent or delayed, treatment techniques are available for stimulating the swallow or teaching the patient to swallow more safely. Again the speech and language therapist should be involved in carrying out or teaching these techniques to nursing staff and patients.

Thermal stimulation

The swallow reflex is triggered at the base of the anterior faucal arches at the back of the mouth. Icing of these areas, using a cotton swab chilled in iced water, will help stimulate the swallow reflex, and may speed up a delayed reflex. This procedure must be carried out at least five times a day, and will not be effective immediately, but over a period of time.

Supraglottic swallow

This technique can sometimes be taught to patients to

Table 4.60 The normal swallow

The pattern followed in the process of normal swallowing comprises four stages	
1 *Pre-oral stage*	This stage is mainly under voluntary control, food/drink is transferred from the plate/cup to the mouth. Food is selected and lifted to the mouth. Saliva production is stimulated by the sight, smell and taste of food. The head comes forward to meet the hand, the tongue protrudes, the lips and jaws open in preparation. Food/drink is placed in the mouth and the lips and jaw close to seal the mouth.
2 *Oral stage*	This stage too is mainly under voluntary control: food is prepared for passage from the mouth into the pharynx. The time taken varies according to the consistency of the food. The tongue moves food and positions it between the teeth. Chewing (mastication) is both reflex and voluntary, and is achieved by up, down, and rotary movements of the jaw in order to grind the food which is mixed with saliva. The tongue forms a central groove to collect food, with its tip sealed against the hard palate. The resulting bolus is propelled backwards by the posterior movement of the tongue.
3 *Pharyngeal stage*	This stage is involuntary: the food bolus passes from the mouth through the pharynx and into the oesophagus. The airway is protected by closure of the larynx to prevent aspiration of food or fluid. Sensation of the bolus at the anterior faucal arch (towards the back of the mouth) stimulates the swallowing centre in the brainstem. The swallow response is elicited: • The soft palate elevates to seal off the nasopharynx • The larynx elevates and so forces the epiglottis down to cover the larynx • The vocal cords (within the larynx) close • Respiration stops momentarily Food passes through the pharynx mainly by peristalsis, i.e. the muscles of the pharynx contract and move the bolus through, although gravity has some effect. The crico-pharyngeal sphincter relaxes, and is opened by the upward pull of the larynx, the food bolus passes into the oesophagus. This stage takes 1 second or less.
4 *Oesophageal stage*	This stage too is involuntary: the food bolus passes down the oesophagus into the stomach by peristalsis and gravity, the cardiac sphincter relaxes and food enters the stomach. Transit through the oesophagus may take between 8–20 seconds.

enable a safe swallow, by improving closure of vocal cords, and therefore protection of the airway. The patient is taught how to close the vocal cords voluntarily by holding the breath while swallowing.

Feeding the dysphagic patient

Non-oral feeding

If assessment reveals that the patient is unable to swallow safely, or can only manage very small amounts of oral nutrition, then an alternative method of feeding is indicated. In the first instance this should be feeding via a finebore nasogastric tube. While the patient is receiving total nasogastric feeding, good oral hygiene is essential, and the oral cavity should be kept clean and moist with regular cleaning of the teeth and mouth toilet. Artificial saliva given via a small spray may help if the patient has a persistently dry mouth.

As the swallow reflex improves, so tube feeding should be *gradually* replaced by oral feeding. Initially, overnight nasogastric feeding may be appropriate to supplement oral intake, but also to allow development of appetite during waking hours.

In some cases, dysphagia after stroke resolves very slowly or not at all, and in this situation a longer period of enteral feeding is required. If this is likely to be greater than six weeks from the onset of stroke, then feeding via a gastrostomy tube rather than a nasogastric tube should be considered. The former is more comfortable, generally better accepted by the patient and easier to manage in the community. Gastrostomy tubes can now be easily inserted by percutaneous endoscopic techniques using local anaesthetic and intravenous sedation, rather than by general anaesthetic and laparotomy as previously required; this greatly diminishes the operative risk.

Oral feeding

Precautions and assistance Where the patient has dysphagia following stroke, oral feeding should be introduced with caution, under the supervision of the speech and language therapist who will continue to assess and monitor the patient and advise on the most appropriate food textures. If the patient is felt to be at risk from aspiration into an unprotected airway, a nurse or physiotherapist and suction machine should always be nearby in case of emergencies.

Positioning of the patient The patient should be seated upright, with feet flat on the ground, and the affected side well supported. The head should be tipped slightly forward to provide protection of the airway. Tipping the head backwards makes swallowing more difficult. The physiotherapist can offer further advice on positioning.

Types of foods Suitable foods for introduction of oral diet are those which are soft, as these require little mastication. The speech and language therapist may advise starting with *chilled* soft foods e.g. ice cream, jellies, smooth yoghurt, mousses, thick custard, supplement desserts such as Fortipudding (Cow & Gate), Formance (Abbott). Chilled foods stimulate the swallow reflex more easily than warm foods as there are more receptors for cold than for warm at the back of the mouth (faucal arches).

Once chilled soft foods can be swallowed safely, then there should be a progression to a wider range of soft, moist foods of different temperatures. More difficult foods, e.g. those of mixed consistency or foods with skins should not be tried until much later. It may be necessary in the earlier stages to give a purėed diet for a short period, particularly if there are difficulties in the oral phase of swallowing, but this is often not required, and in most cases would not be acceptable to the patient in appearance.

Food preferences should of course be determined beforehand; the patient must not be given something which is disliked, or avoided on cultural or religious grounds.

Helping the patient to eat Many patients with a hemiparesis or hemiplegia will need help with eating at first, although most will eventually be able to feed themselves. Some may eat very slowly and need prompting. Encouragement, and verbal reminders to chew food well and clear the mouth, by swallowing, more than once if necessary, before taking the next mouthful may be necessary. If the patient suffers from loss of visual field e.g. homonymous hemianopia it may be necessary to move the plate around during the meal so that one side is not repeatedly ignored.

Some patients with physical disabilities may benefit from the use of specially developed cutlery and crockery. The occupational therapist can give advice in this area.

Fluids Fluid is usually the most difficult consistency to swallow, and would not normally be introduced until the patient can safely swallow soft foods, as it requires much greater control at the oral stage.

Hot drinks will exaggerate any swallowing difficulties and may cause coughing. Therefore fluids should be given chilled at first, and may be offered on a teaspoon. Once slightly larger amounts can be tolerated, the patient should be encouraged to take sips from an ordinary cup, beaker or glass. The use of feeder beakers is discouraged as their use requires the patient to tip back the head which makes swallowing more difficult, and provides less protection for the airway. Also, a large volume of fluid may be accidently delivered to the back of the mouth on which the patient may choke and aspirate. Feeder beakers may be useful, however, where the main problem is with the oral phase (e.g. poor lip closure and tongue movements, but safe pharyngeal phase), as the beaker enables placement of fluid at the back of the mouth, minimizing dribbling.

Some patients, although able to take adequate amounts of soft diet, continue to have dysphagia for fluids. For some this will necessitate the continuing use of a nasogastric or gastrostomy tube as a route for hydration. However, in other cases, fluids may be better tolerated if slightly thickened, making them easier to control in the mouth, and reducing the risk of aspiration. Suitable thickening agents for cold fluids are: Thixo D (Cirrus Associates), a modified corn starch, and Instant Carobel (Cow & Gate Nutricia) which is a carob bean gum. For hot drinks and soups, arrow-root, cornflour or instant thickening granules can be used.

Maintaining nutritional status

Care should be taken to ensure that the dietary intake is sufficient to meet nutritional needs and, if necessary, appropriate supplements should be given or nasogastric feeding continued. Conversely it may be necessary to advise on weight reduction if the patient is obese, as this hampers rehabilitation.

When discharge from hospital is planned, discussions should be held with the patient and carers, about the type and quantity of food which will be needed.

The multidisciplinary approach

All patients presenting with dysphagic symptoms require a rapid and co-ordinated response from the multidisciplinary team. The successful management of *all* people who have had a stroke depends on good liaison between all the people involved in their care – both carers and health professionals.

4.21.2 Communication difficulties after stroke

Many people have difficulty communicating following a stroke. They should be referred to the speech and language therapist who can assess them and advise on appropriate ways of communicating with them.

Communications problems include the following.

Dysphasia

This disorder affects the production and understanding of language. People with dysphasia may:

1 Produce unrecognizable words (jargon).
2 Have difficulty finding the word they want.
3 Be unable to read or write as well as before their stroke.
4 Have difficulty putting words together grammatically.
5 Be unable to understand complex or abstract sentences.
6 Use yes and no inappropriately.

Dysarthria

This motor disorder results from weakness of the oral and laryngeal musculature. As a result a dysarthric person's speech may sound slurred, quiet, monotone, hoarse or nasal. The person may be hard to understand in noisy or distracting environments or when tired, or may be totally unintelligible.

The speech and language therapist may advise the family and carers to speak simply (but not childishly) or to use gesture to back up their speech when communicating with a dysphasic person. When communicating with such patients, one should ascertain how much they are able to understand by discussing them with the speech and language therapist. If in doubt, written information should be provided to the patient's carers to back up what has been said. Remember that difficulties with understanding are often disguised.

The speech and language therapist may introduce a communication aid for dysarthric patients; these range from pencil and paper or an alphabet chart up to sophisticated electronic equipment.

Useful address

The Stroke Association, CHSA House, Whitecross Street, London EC1Y 8JJ, Tel 071–490 7999. (There are local support groups of this association in many areas).

Further reading

Isaacs B (1985) *Understanding stroke illness*. Chest, Heart and Stroke Association, London.

Logemann J (1983) *Evaluation and treatment of swallowing disorders*. College Hill, San Diego.

Rose FC and Capildeo R (1981) *Stroke: the facts*. Oxford University Press, Oxford.

References

Barer DH (1989) The natural history and functional consequences of dysphagia after hemispheric stroke. *J Neurology Neurosurgery Psychiatry* **52**, 236–41.

Fuller JH, Shipley MJ, Rox G, Jarrett RJ and Keen H (1983) Mortality from coronary heart disease and stroke in relation to degree of glycaemia – the Whitehall Study. *Br Med J* **287**, 867–70.

Wolf P, Kannel W and Verter J (1983) *Neurologic clinics* **1**, 317–43.

World Health Organization (1973) Control of stroke in the community: Methological considerations and protocol of WHO stroke register CVD/S/73.6. WHO, Geneva.

4.22 Multiple Sclerosis

Multiple Sclerosis (MS) is a degenerative disease of the central nervous system which is notoriously difficult to diagnose. It presents in two ways, the chronic progressive form and the more common remitting relapsing type. It can present at any age but usually starts in young adulthood. Symptoms include paraesthesia, episodes of blindness and weakness in various limbs. Remission can be long term but more typically is a course of attack, disability and partial recovery.

Very often no advice or medical treatment is offered, but drug therapy can be helpful for incontinence, frequency and for muscle spasm.

Physiotherapy helps maintain muscle function. Most MS patients, and especially those recently diagnosed, are in need of considerable psychological support, both from friends and relatives and in some cases from trained counsellors.

4.22.1 The role of diet in the management of MS

The role of diet in the treatment of MS is poorly documented and controversial.

Epidemiological studies have suggested that there may be a relationship between the amount and nature of dietary fat and the incidence of MS. There is a higher prevalence of MS in Northern Europe in countries where the diet is commonly high in saturated fat than in countries such as Japan where the diet is based on fish and therefore high in polyunsaturated fat. The incidence of MS is also higher in the Shetlands than in the Faroes where the traditional fishing industry has been retained and fish consumption is higher.

Sixty per cent of the solid matter of the brain and 70% of the myelin sheath is comprised of lipid, hence the interest in essential fatty acid nutrition and this disease of the central nervous system. Low levels of essential fatty acids (efa) have been found in the serum of MS patients and this finding led to the double blind trial of linoleic acid supplementation in MS patients in Belfast and Newcastle (Bates *et al* 1977). This indicated a decrease in frequency and duration of relapse in the supplemented group (87 patients) compared with the control group (85 patients). During the study period of 28 months, 41 relapses occurred in the supplemented group, the majority being of short duration, 62 relapses occurred in the control group, most being for periods of 6–9 weeks or more than ten weeks. In addition, further reappraisal of this work (Dworkin *et al* 1984) has demonstrated that patients who had minimal or no disability and a shorter duration of illness benefited most from a diet high in linoleic acid.

In a follow-up study of 150 MS patients between 1949 and 1984, Swank and Grimsgaard (1988) reported that the rates of both neurological deterioration and mortality were lower in those consuming a diet extremely low in fat content. They suggest that MS patients are very sensitive to, or intolerant of, saturated fatty acids. However, most people would find it extremely difficult to adhere to, or meet their energy needs, on the restrictive diet used in this study.

A five-year trial of the use of fish oil supplements (Bates *et al* 1989) gave some indications that these resulted in a decrease in the duration, frequency and severity of relapses; however the results were not statistically significant. Since there are practical drawbacks to this method of supplementation in terms of cost and the numbers of capsules needed to be consumed each day (20×0.5 g), encouraging patients to increase their consumption of fatty fish may be a better alternative.

A longitudinal dietary intervention study was initiated by Action and Research for Multiple Sclerosis (ARMS) and is being continued by the Multiple Sclerosis Unit at the Central Middlesex Hospital. Patients are encouraged to increase dietary sources of both families of essential fatty acids while decreasing saturated fat intake. Six-monthly nutritional, neurological and physiotherapy assessments are made. A nutrient score is derived from the intake of fatty acids, vitamins C, E, and B group, zinc, iron and fibre. Preliminary results (Fitzgerald *et al* 1987) suggest that those who achieved a good nutrient score remained neurologically stable during a three-year period while those with poor scores declined in neurological status. However, further research is needed to confirm these findings.

4.22.2 Dietary treatment of MS patients

It must be remembered that the relationships between diet and the progression or remission of MS are, at the present time, only suggestive rather than conclusive. Much more research in this area is needed, in particular prolonged trials of a double blind nature. However, such trials are especially difficult to conduct with MS patients who are often unwilling to commit themselves to one long term course of dietary treatment preferring, in their desperation to find a cure, to try a variety of dietary strategies.

Owing to the lack of conclusive proof of benefit, very few

MS patients are prescribed a 'special' diet as part of their clinical care. Most clinicians feel that the only justifiable dietary measures are those which correct either an inappropriate energy intake or a diet of poor nutritional quality. Simple changes in diet may also help prevent constipation which, because of bowel spasticity, is a common problem.

However, for many MS patients these measures are not enough and large numbers of them will instigate their own dietary therapy in the hope of obtaining some remission from the disease. MS patients respond readily to any new suggestion, particularly from the media, that a particular diet may be of benefit and are inevitably very vulnerable to 'quack' diets.

At the present time, very few MS patients will receive any professional dietetic guidance. However, some MS patients may be referred to a dietitian at their own insistence and others will be referred either for general dietary assessment or for some disorder unconnected with the MS. In these instances, the dietitian can play a valuable role by answering queries about diet and MS, and putting the facts into perspective, and by ensuring that any self-imposed dietary regimen is at least nutritionally adequate. Dietitians should ensure that any changes in eating habits which are recommended should not cause the patient any more difficulty with regard to shopping or cooking than is already encountered; it is important that both stress and fatigue are avoided.

Some of the most common diets which the dietitian may either encounter or be asked about are outlined below. Support organisations (listed in the Useful addresses list at the end of this Chapter) may be able to help dietitians locate new research papers on the role of diet in the treatment of MS.

Diets and supplements commonly used by MS patients

Low fat diet

This derives from the work of Swank (1988) who recommended a diet low in animal fat with elimination of hydrogenated margarines and oils.

The 'ARMS' diet

This diet was formulated by Crawford (1979) and is a low saturated fat diet high in essential fatty acids (of the ω6 and ω3 types). In addition, wholegrain cereals, vegetables and fruit are consumed in sufficient quantities to provide the necessary vitamins and minerals for conversion and utilization of the efa. For example, trace elements such as zinc, copper and iron are components of the desaturase and cyclo-oxygenase systems responsible for the synthesis of long chain derivatives and prostaglandins. The B vitamins are important for chain elongation reactions and vitamins C and E are vital as antioxidants (Crawford 1979). The diet has a P/S ratio greater than 1 and a vitamin E content of approximately 0.6 mg/g polyunsaturated fat.

Gluten-free (GF) diet (either with or without animal fat restriction)

The Roger McDougall and Rita Greer diets are variations often followed by MS patients. There is no evidence to show they are beneficial; however many MS sufferers maintain they are helped by them.

A study of plasma samples of 36 MS patients showed only one with evidence of gluten antibodies and maintained that even this level did not justify a GF diet (Hunter *et al* 1984). Hewson (1984) studied 17 subjects on a GF diet and supported the view that there is no conclusive evidence that it is beneficial, but gives guidelines for dietitians dealing with MS patients who wish to follow such a diet.

'Allergy' diets

Many MS patients maintain that spasm is worsened by eating certain foods and, in desperation, some may undergo cytotoxic testing. This involves having a blood sample analysed for sensitivity to specific foods which may then be eliminated from the diet to see if symptoms improve. While these diets may be of benefit to those who have atopic symptoms, there is no evidence of a direct link between allergy and MS and this type of dietary manipulation may result in serious nutritional deficiencies.

Supplements

Evening primrose oil This is a source of gamma linolenic acid (GLA) which is not normally derived from food but by conversion of linolenic acid. It is expensive and not obtainable on prescription for MS. When taking EPO with the average British diet, the activity of GLA will be suppressed as a result of competition with non essential fatty acids. EPO is probably only useful in conjuction with a low saturated fat diet. An effective daily dose may be at a much higher level than that typically consumed by patients; however this is an area of debate and research.

Sunflower seed oil This oil is rich in linoleic acid and is often recommended to patients. The dosage is normally six 0.5 ml sunflower seed oil capsules daily or 30 ml oil twice a day. Patients with a weight problem taking these supplements must be advised how to reduce their energy intake without impairing the dietary P/S ratio.

Marine oil capsules These are rich in eicosapentaenoic acid (EPA) and often taken by MS patients. However, they are expensive. Eating fatty fish two or three times weekly will also supply significant amounts of EPA.

Table 4.61 Comparison of some oils and supplements
The two tables below give the linoleic acid and vitamin E content of some food oils and capsules. As most people seem to take six capsules per day, for comparison purposes all contents quoted are per six capsules

(a) Linoleic acid and vitamin E content of some oils

Food	Linoleic acid g/100 g	Vitamin E mg/100 g
Safflower oil	62	39
Wheatgerm oil	55	133
Corn oil	53	11
Sunflower oil	50	49
Soya oil	50	10
Olive oil	11	5

(b) Linoleic GLA and vitamin E content of some supplements

Supplement per 6 capsules	Linoleic acid g/6 capsules	GLA g/6 capsules	Vitamin E mg/6 capsules
Naudicelle Bio-oils Research Ltd)	2.6	0.33	45
Efamol 500 (Britannia Pharmaceuticals Ltd)	2.2	0.21	60

Cod liver oil Cod liver oil is an alternative source of fish oil but is also a concentrated source of retinol and may be contraindicated if other retinol-rich foods are also being eaten regularly.

The composition of some of the oils and supplements which may be used by MS patients are compared in Table 4.61.

Useful addresses

The Multiple Sclerosis Unit, Central Middlesex Hospital Trust, Acton Lane, London NW 10 7NS. Tel 081–453 2332/2337.

The charity Action and Research for Multiple Sclerosis (ARMS) is no longer functioning. Some of its work is being continued by the Central Middlesex Hospital Trust Multiple Sclerosis Unit which is also a resource centre for people with multiple sclerosis, their carers and health professionals.

The Multiple Sclerosis Society, 25 Effie Road, Fulham, London SW6 1EE.

This society also supports research projects and has groups and welfare officers throughout the country.

Further reading

DeSouza L (1990) *Multiple sclerosis; approaches to management*. Chapman & Hall, London.
Graham J (1987) *MS: A self help guide to its management*. Thorsons, Wellingborough.
Matthews B (1982) *MS – the facts* 2e. Oxford University Press, Oxford.

References

Bates D, Fawcett PR, Shaw DA and Weightman D (1977) Trial of polyunsaturated fatty acids in non relapsing multiple sclerosis. *Br Med J* **2**, 932–3.
Bates D, Cartlidge NEF, French JM, Jackson MJ, Nightingale S, Shaw DA, Smith S, Woo E, Hawkins SA, Miller JHD, Belin J, Conroy DM, Gill SK, Sidey M, Smith AD, Thompson RHS, Zilkha K, Gale M and Sinclair HM (1989) A double-blind controlled trial of long chain n-3 polyunsaturated fatty acids in the treatment of multiple sclerosis. *J Neurol Neurosurg and Psych* **52**, 18–22.
Crawford MA (1979) Dietary management in MS. *Proc Nutr Soc* **38**, 373–89.
Dworkin RH, Bates D, Miller JH and Paty DW (1984) Linoleic acid and multiple sclerosis: a re-analysis of three double blind trials. *Neurology (Cleveland)* **43**, 1441–5.
Fitzgerald G, Harbige LS, Forti and Crawford MA (1987) The effect of nutritional counselling on diet and plasma EFA status in multiple sclerosis over 3 years. *Hum Nutr: Appl Nutr* **41A**, 297–310.
Hewson DC (1984) Is there a role for GF diets in MS? *Hum Nutr* **38A**, 417–20.
Hunter L, Rees BWG and Jones LT (1984) Gluten antibodies in patients with MS. *J Hum Nutr* **38A**, 142–3.
Swank RL and Grimsgaard A (1988) Multiple sclerosis: the lipid relationship. *Am J Clin Nutr* **48**, 1387–93.

4.23 Mental illness

Mental illness should be distinguished from mental handicap (learning difficulties or learning disability). Mental handicap is a condition which has been present from birth or the perinatal period; although the condition may be caused by disease or infection it is not, of itself, a disease or illness.

Mental illness can develop at any age in a previously healthy individual. The aetiology of mental illness is multifactorial. The interaction of social, environmental and genetic factors may result in physical or mental illness, or a combination of both.

The division between health and illness is not as clear in psychiatry as in other branches of medicine. Many of the symptoms are behavioural. What is considered normal or acceptable behaviour will vary with the context in which the behaviour occurs.

A neurotic illness is one in which a normal emotional response becomes intensified to the extent that it interferes significantly with the sufferer's ability to function socially, professionally or personally or causes physical illness. In psychoneurosis, contact with reality is usually maintained; this is in contrast to psychotic conditions where sufferers often have no insight into the fact that many of their experiences are unreal.

The classification of mental illness is shown in Table 4.62. The nutritional effects of some common symptoms of the various conditions are shown in Table 4.63.

4.23.1 Psychoneuroses and functional psychoses

Mood disorders

Depression and mania are collectively known as *affective* or *mood disorders*. (Affect is the term used in psychiatry when the mood is a symptom of the illness). Disturbance of mood is the primary symptom of these illnesses which may be either neurotic or psychotic in origin.

Depression is characterized by *dysphoric* mood described as 'sad, hopeless, miserable or low'. Normal or premorbid mood is described as *euthymic*.

Mania is characterized by *euphoric* mood, described as elated, happy, excited, irritable or high.

In *unipolar* illness, the disturbance presents as depression or mania only. In *bipolar* illness, there are both manic and depressive episodes hence, *manic-depression psychosis*.

Hypomania is used to describe an elevated mood or slight degree of mania.

Types of depression

1 *Endogenous depression (functional psychosis)* There is no apparent external cause. It is thought to arise from genetic and biochemical internal causes. Anorexia, constipation, indigestion and fluid refusal are symptoms of nutritional importance in endogenous depression.

2 *Reactive, neurotic or secondary depression (Psychoneurosis)* This is far more common than the endogenous type and presents as a morbid sadness which relates to a stress or loss such as bereavement or unemployment. It may be secondary to other physical or mental illnesses. Anorexia, fluid refusal, indigestion, diarrhoea, constipation or excessive eating may be found.

Neurotic depression should be distinguished from *grief*, which is an appropriate healthy feeling of sadness in response to a personal loss.

3 *Post-partum depression* This has elements of both endogenous and reactive depression.

4 *Seasonal affective disorder (SAD)* This condition is characterized by depression in Autumn and Winter, alternating with non-depressed periods in Spring and Summer (Rosenthal *et al* 1984).

During the depression, symptoms of fatigue, overeating, carbohydrate craving and weight gain are amongst the usual symptoms. Consumption of carbohydrate is reported to have a stimulating effect in contrast to the sedating effect of carbohydrate in normal subjects.

5 *Pseudo-dementia* Depression may present with confusion-cognitive deficits mimicking dementia. There are no organic changes in the brain and treatment of the underlying depression resolves the dementing symptoms.

6 *Agitated depression* The illness presents as anxiety or agitation. The underlying mood disturbance is dysphoric.

Schizophrenia

Schizophrenia is the most severe form of functional psychosis producing the greatest disorganization of personality. In severe cases the patient is out of touch with reality to such an extent that his or her ideas and behaviour are bizarre.

The peak incidence occurs at 25–30 years of age, with

Table 4.62 Classification of mental illness

Mental illness		
Psychoneurosis	Psychosis	
For example	*Functional*	*Organic*
Depressive neurosis Anxiety neurosis Obsessional neurosis Phobic neurosis Hysteria Post-traumatic neurosis	No pathology can be demonstrated e.g. manic-depressive psychosis; schizophrenia	Demonstrable or inferred lesion is present e.g. acute confusional state; Alzheimer's disease (AD); senile dementia of the Alzheimer type (SDAT); multi-infarct dementia (MID)

Table 4.63 Nutritional effect of some symptoms of mental illness

Disorder	Symptom	Effect on nutrition
Depression	Apathy, loss of pleasure or interest in food Anorexia	Significant weight loss
Depression	Loss of thirst Fluid refusal	Dehydration
Anxiety depression	Guilt, worthlessness — 'I don't deserve food'	Poor food intake
Depression	Suicidal intention — 'I want to die'. Food and fluid refusal	Poor food intake and/or dehydration
Mania Depression Anxiety Schizophrenia	Dry mouth or altered taste (May be primary symptom or caused by drugs)	Difficulties in chewing and swallowing Loss of food flavour Decrease food intake
Mania Depression Schizophrenia	Increased appetite Carbohydrate craving (May be primary symptom or side-effect of drug)	Weight gain
Depression Anxiety Schizophrenia	Constipation; impacted faeces Abdominal or pelvic pain or discomfort Nausea (May be primary symptom or side-effect of drug)	Food refusal
Anxiety Mania	Frequent loose stools (Usually described as 'diarrhoea')	Selective food refusal
Depression Anxiety Obsessional neurosis	Hypochondriacal preoccupation with functioning of digestive tract Delusional beliefs e.g. 'My bowels are twisted', 'My stomach is eaten away'	Food and/or fluid refusal
Depression Anxiety Mania Alcoholism Drug abuse	High alcohol intake or drug abuse	Poor food intake with malabsorption of thiamine and folic acid in alcohol abuse Chaotic eating Weight gain and loss both seen
Depression Schizophrenia	Psychomotor retardation Hypersomnia Lethargy Stupor Withdrawal	Missed meals Inadequate food intake Inadequate fluid intake Eventually may require nasogastric feeding
Depression Anxiety Mania Obsessional states	Psychomotor agitation Physical restlessness	Increased energy expenditure, often with decreased food intake
Mania	Increased in physical activity — work, socially, sexually Distractibility Excitement	Increased energy expenditure Food intake erratic

an estimated occurrence of 0.5–1.0% in the general population. The diagnosis of schizophrenia relies on descriptions of the patient's behaviour, mental state and history. There are no diagnostic laboratory tests and there are international differences on diagnostic criteria.

The term schizophrenia does not imply a 'split personality', but rather the splitting or disruption of the mental process of the sufferer. The illness always involves a deterioration from a previous level of functioning – socially, occupationally and in self-care. Skills such as shopping and preparing meals are often lost resulting in poor dietary intake if the patient lives alone.

The symptomology involves both the *content* (what is thought) and the *form* (the way it is thought) of thought process.

Content of thought

Delusions Persecutory delusions may involve beliefs that certain foods or drinks are poisoned or otherwise harmful. Bizarre demands for 'special diets' and/or very restricted food intakes may result from delusional beliefs about food.

Dietitians should understand that a delusion cannot be changed by logical argument or scientific evidence!

Hallucinations These are sensory experiences occurring without external stimuli. Auditory hallucinations are common and the 'voices' may instruct the patient as to what to eat or drink. An acutely ill patient will pay attention to internal voices rather than to the dietitian.

Poverty of content The patient may speak fluently for some time before the listener realizes that little, if any, information has been conveyed.

Form of thought

There may be a loss of logical, rational thinking. Normal associations between words and ideas break down. There may be thought blocking, when thoughts stop abruptly, or an inability to think in abstract terms. When thought disorder is severe, speech becomes incomprehensible.

4.23.2 Diet histories in mental illness

During the acute phase of mental illness such as depression, mania or psychosis, or dementia the patient may be, to all practical purposes, as inaccessible as a physically ill unconscious patient.

Attempting to obtain the traditional dietary history from the patient, and using this as a basis for offering nutritional advice, may be distressing or disturbing to the patient whose thought processes, cognitive functions or mood are severely disturbed.

On receiving such a referral, the dietitian should tactfully ascertain from the ward staff if the patient is well enough to furnish a reliable history and has sufficient understanding and motivation to undertake personal responsibility for dietary modification.

Close scrutiny of medical and nursing notes often enables the dietitian to identify factors relevant to the patient's nutritional status, which may otherwise be overlooked. If energy or fluid intake are suspected to be problematic, the dietitian should ensure that patients are regularly weighed and their food and fluid intake monitored.

Patients who are refusing food and fluids will require practical and effective dietetic support. This may include the provision of a wide range of supplements (e.g. sweet and savoury, milk and juice based) and advice on vitamin or mineral supplementation or, sometimes, enteral feeding.

When the mental state of the patient improves, the following factors may need to be explored at dietary interview (Crammer 1983):

1 What was the childhood experience of food? Regular meals? Emphasis on particular foods? Emergence of food fads?

2 What changes occurred in the month before admission? Were they precipitated by psychiatric illness or a change of residence or employment?

3 What changes in the patient's personal life have brought about changes in food intake?

4 What ethical or religious factors influence food intake?

5 What drugs, especially laxatives, psychotropics or oral contraceptives, does the patient use habitually?

The assessment should aim to identify long term peculiarities and recent changes in the diet. A recent acute deficiency superimposed on a long milder chronic lack is most likely to precipitate frank nutritional deficiency.

Patients recovered from acute psychotic, manic or depressed episodes become accessible to individual or group therapy if they are sufficiently motivated to undertake change in their eating patterns.

4.23.3 Dietary management of non-organic mental illness

Dietetic advice to patients on psychotropic medication

People admitted to hospital are often underweight, dehydrated and suffering from vitamin deficiencies of various degrees (Reynolds *et al* 1970; Carney *et al* 1979; Hancock *et al* 1985). Food and fluid intakes will be replenished by ward care although, to achieve normal vitamin status, supplementation may be necessary (Hancock *et al* 1985; Mandal and Ray 1987).

Treatment with psychotropic drugs often has significant effects on food intake through their action on the neurotransmitters. Kinney Parker *et al* (1989) review the relationship between pharmacology and anorectic drugs, biochemistry and food intake. Some of the biochemical factors which affect food intake are outlined below.

Norepinephrine This increases total food intake and delays satiety. There is a proportional increase in carbohydrate intake, with protein and fat intake unchanged. Tricyclic antidepressants increase levels of norepinephrine in the brain.

5HT or serotonin This appears to affect the same satiety mechanisms as norepinephrine but in the opposite direction. Less food is eaten. The intake of carbohydrate decreases relative to protein and fats. 5HT re-uptake inhibitors (antidepressants) increase levels of serotonin in the brain.

Dopamine Dopamine affects hunger (rather than satiety) mechanisms. When dopamine levels are high, hunger and meal frequency decrease. Protein intake is decreased together with overall energy intake. Drugs such as amphetamines have an anorectic effect by means of increasing dopamine levels. Drugs such as chlorpromazine block the action of dopamine and often increase food intake and meal frequency whilst patients complain of intense feelings of hunger.

Cholecystokinin This is an intestinal hormone which is released when chyme enters the duodenum. It is present in large quantities in the brain and has the effect of reducing feeding in hungry animals and increasing the interval between meals (Gibbs *et al* 1973; Hsiao *et al* 1979).

Awad (1984) gives an excellent review of commonly used psychotropic drugs and their effects on nutrition and food intake. Changes in hunger, appetite, taste and bowel function may be caused by the primary psychiatric condition or as a side effect of medication (Table 4.64).

Patients may express the intention to discontinue their medication because of the side effects, particularly when distressed by apparently uncontrollable weight gain. It is vital to reinforce the importance of compliance with medication whilst offering dietary advice.

The dietitian and patient need a clear understanding that the difficulties encountered in complying to a restricted food intake cannot be seen as simply in terms of willpower or self-control. 'The control of human appetite has often to be inferred from animal studies. While the biochemistry is probably similar, the added dimension of psychological, cultural and emotional factors affecting human food intake cannot be ignored' (Awad 1984). Psychiatric patients often cite boredom and lack of structured activity as an important factor in their difficulty in following dietetic advice.

Dietary strategy for carbohydrate craving or intense hunger

This comprises three main stages: explanation and exploration; weight stabilization; and weight reduction.

Explanation and exploration

There should be discussion with the patient in order to ascertain the cause of the weight gain in terms of changes in appetite, food intake, and food choice. It is important to explain to the patient that medication does not 'turn to fat' but acts to increase weight by increasing food intake. A careful dietary history will form the basis of the next stage.

Weight stabilization

This enables the patient to regain control over his or her food intake and thus creates self-confidence. Identification of the times of maximum food intake (often the evening) is important. For many patients a three hour gap between eating is the maximum they can tolerate at this stage.

A 1200–1500 kcal regimen, *supplemented by regular snacks to achieve energy balance* and paying particular attention to times of maximum hunger, may stop weight gain within one or two weeks.

Weight reduction

The patient will often proceed to this stage independently. It involves identifying which snacks can be discontinued or modified to produce weight loss.

It is important to secure the co-operation and support of occupational therapists, physiotherapists, nursing staff and visitors for the patient undertaking weight reduction whilst on appetite stimulating drugs. Knox (1980) reported good results with a 1000 kcal regimen in patients on psychogeriatric and long-stay wards, but poor results with patients on acute wards.

Dietetic advice to patients taking lithium

There is an inverse relationship between dietary sodium intake and serum lithium levels. Any dietary modifications which significantly alter sodium intake may cause changes in the serum lithium level which has a narrow therapeutic range. If a patient with stable lithium levels makes drastic changes to his or her salt intake, the dietitian should alert the patient's doctor. Serum lithium levels should be closely monitored until the new dietary pattern is established.

Patients taking lithium often experience an increase in appetite and also in thirst. Weight gain is also common and there may be a positive correlation between the degree of thirst and weight gain (Vandsborg *et al* 1976). Patients taking lithium should not restrict their fluid intake and

Table 4.64 Centrally active drugs: possible effects on nutrition

Type	Examples	Use	Side effects or nutritional consequence
1 *Antidepressants*			
Tricyclic	Amitriptyline Imipramine Lofepramine Dothiepin Doxepin	Depressive illness	Dry mouth Sour metallic taste Constipation or rarely diarrhoea Nausea and vomiting, epigastric distress Increased appetite and weight gain by carbohydrate craving Rarely anorexia
5HT Re-uptake inhibitors	Fluoxetine Fluvoxamine Paroxetine Sertraline	Depressive illness	Anorexia Nausea and vomiting Weight loss Dry mouth Dyspepsia diarrhoea 'Serotonin syndrome' — restlessness with agitation and GI distress with tryptophan 1–4 g per day
MAOI	Phenelzine Tranylcypromine Isocarboxazid	Depressive illness Atypical depression Depression with phobic symptoms	Nausea and vomiting Dry mouth Constipation Increased appetite and weight gain Potentiation of action of insulin or oral hypoglycaemic with lowered blood glucose Hypertensive crisis if foods containing tyramine are ingested
2 *Antipsychotics or major tranquillizers*			
Phenothiazines	Chlorpromazine Thioridazine Trifluoperazine Fluphenazine	Psychoses Schizophrenia	Dry mouth Constipation Photosensitivity leading to low vitamin D levels Appetite increase and weight gain High doses reduce response to hypoglycaemic agents causing elevated blood glucose
Butyrophenones	Haloperidol Droperidol	Psychoses Mania Schizophenia	Nausea, dyspepsia Loss of appetite Less effect on appetite than phenothiazines
Thioxanthines	Flupenthixol decanoate Zuclopenthixol decanoate	Psychoses Schizophrenia	Increased appetite and weight gain Less commonly weight loss May affect diabetic control
Substituted Benzamides	Pimozide (Remoxipride) (Sulpiride) (less side) (effects)	Mania Psychoses Schizophrenia	Nausea, dyspepsia Abdominal pain, constipation Dry mouth Changes in body weight Glycosuria
Dibenzo-diazepines	Loxapine Clozapine	Schizophrenia Psychoses	GI disturbances Nausea and vomiting Weight gain or loss Dry mouth or hypersalivation Polydipsia
3 *Hypnotics and anxiolytics*			
Benzodiazepines	Diazepam Chlordiazepoxide Lorazepam	Short term anxiety Alcohol withdrawal	*These symptoms have been reported both before and up to 6 weeks after withdrawal:* GI upsets, nausea and vomiting Diarrhoea or constipation Appetite and weight changes Dry mouth, metallic taste Dysphagia
	Temazepam Nitrazepam	Short term sleep disturbance	As above

Table 4.64 contd.

Type	Examples	Use	Side effects or nutritional consequence
4 *Mood stabilizers*			
Lithium salts	Lithium carbonate Lithium citrate	1 Treatment of mania and hypomania 2 Prophylactic treatment of recurrent affective disorders	*Early side effects* Nausea, metallic taste Increased thirst, polyuria Loose stools *Later* Weight gain, mild oedema Polyuria Metallic taste Possible hypothyroidism *Toxicity* Loss of appetite Vomiting, diarrhoea See page 495 for information on the relationship between dietary sodium intake and lithium levels.
5 *Anticonvulsants*			
Benzodiazepines	Clonazepam Clobazam	All forms of epileptic seizure	See under 3 *Hypnotics and anxiolytics*: Benzodiazepines
	Carbamazepine	Temporal lobe, tonic/clonic and partial seizures. (Mood regulation as an alternative to lithium.)	Mimics action of ADH on kidney, causing water retention Nausea, loss of appetite, vomiting Diarrhoea or constipation (high dose) Dry mouth Lowered sodium levels in blood
	Sodium valproate	All types of seizures	Nausea and vomiting, anorexia, gastric irritation or increased appetite and weight gain
	Phenytoin	Tonic/clonic seizures Following head injury or surgery	*Early*: Nausea and vomiting *Later*: Decreased absorption of Vit D leading to osteomalacia Increased turn over and decreased absorption of folic acid leading to megaloblastic anaemias Gum hyperplasia and soreness, tooth decay
Barbiturates	Phenobarbitone Primidone (4/5 of its activity is phenobarbitone)	Grand mal and focal seizures	Decreased vitamin D levels Decreased folate levels Rarely, GI upsets

should be encouraged to consume beverages with a low energy content.

Dietary advice to alcoholics or other substance abusers

Alcoholism does not necessarily cause malnutrition, although unsatisfactory food intakes will often result from the social, financial, psychosocial and physical effects of the dependency. Poor appetite and chronic gastritis are commonly found in chronic alcoholics.

Many detoxified alcoholic or other drug abusers are receptive to advice on weight reduction (when appropriate), meal planning, budgeting, shopping and healthy eating as part of the rehabilitation process. Regular attendance at a food and health group run by the dietetic and/or occupational therapy departments may be effective for the nutritional education of past alcohol (or drug) abusers.

Schizophrenia and gluten

It has been suggested that there may be a link between schizophrenia and coeliac disease but this remains controversial (Vlissides *et al* 1986). Schizophrenia appears to be less common in societies who consume few cereal foods and it has been suggested that grain glutens may evoke schizophrenia in those with the appropriate genotype for the disease (Dohan 1966; 1980).

Peptides in gluten protein digests, particularly from the gliadin fraction, appear to have high opioid activity and to act at sites in the brain sensitive to narcotics such as morphine or endorphins (Huebner *et al* 1984). It is conceivable that, as a result of gluten-induced damage to the intestinal mucosa, these peptides could enter the circulatory system and induce behavioural change.

However examination of the effect of either a gluten-free diet or gluten challenge in small groups of schizophrenic patients have yielded conflicting results; some studies appear to show a deleterious effect of gluten (Dohan and Grasberger 1973; Singh and Kay 1976) while others have shown no effect (Potkin *et al* 1981; Storms *et al* 1982).

In situations where a gluten-free diet is essential (i.e. clinically diagnosed coeliac disease confirmed by biopsy) the dietitian needs to ensure:

1 That the catering department is able to provide appropriate dishes. In the absence of a specialist diet cook, this may entail constant reinforcement and checking the output of a large brigade of general cooks with possibly little or no formal training in the preparation of therapeutic diets.

2 That the ward staff, including the night staff and domestics, are able to discriminate between gluten-free and other foods and drinks prepared at ward level.

3 That family and all other visitors are aware of, and co-operating with, the diet.

Because a gluten-free diet affects the content of all the main meals, snacks and many beverages, it may be difficult to achieve in practice in a psychiatric hospital. Problems with compliance may also arise because the acute or chronically psychotic patient is unlikely to be able to comprehend or co-operate with the ramifications of a gluten-free regimen. The dietary restrictions necessary may be interpreted as some form of 'punishment' or 'persecution'. Any lapses, confirmed or suspected (from whatever cause), should be clearly recorded in the medical and nursing notes so that other members of the psychiatric team are aware of the actual level of compliance achieved.

After discharge, a visit to the patient's home may be necessary, particularly in situations where food is provided by caterers or hostel staff. The cost of maintaining a gluten-free diet may prove to be prohibitive to patients depending on state benefits. The same constraints apply to other 'free-from' regimens.

General dietary aspects

Dry mouth and thirst

Advice on low energy drinks and the provision of artificial sweeteners and low energy squashes on ward beverage trolleys may help to prevent excessive intakes of sugar via soft drinks. Some patients may need to be discouraged from consuming large amounts of milk to quench their thirst or moisten their mouths.

Constipation

High fluid intakes should be emphasized particularly on wards where patients are unable to help themselves to drinks. High fibre breakfast cereals, wholemeal and higher fibre white breads, digestive biscuits, tinned peas and baked beans are more acceptable to older patients than wholemeal pasta, brown rice and green lentils. If raw bran is used it should be restricted to younger patients with good appetites, satisfactory mineral status and good fluid intakes. When appetites are small or food and fluid intakes are compromised, raw bran may exacerbate nutritional problems.

Prescribed isphaghula husk may be useful in some patients who require a high fibre intake for conditions such as diverticulosis and who are unable for any reason to obtain sufficient non-starch polysaccharide (NSP) from the hospital food. Some older patients may find it easier to eat the preparation by spoon in a semi-solid state rather than attempting to swallow it down quickly as a solution before it gels.

4.23.4 Other nutrition-related aspects of mental illness

Disorders of water and sodium metabolism

Polydipsia

Polydipsia is common in long-stay inpatients and may give rise to water intoxication if renal function is impaired (Crammer 1991). In polydipsia, fluid retention may lead to weight gain up to 0.5 kg per hour along with a fall in plasma sodium. Treatment is normally by fluid restriction which should be instituted if the patient has gained 7% or more of early morning weight. Twenty-four hour fluid restriction will not be tolerated by water-seeking patients who will search out water from any source (e.g. flower vases) but who may agree to a shorter period of fluid restriction on a daily basis.

Hyponatraemia

This is sometimes associated with depressive symptoms and it has been suggested by some authors that the psychiatric symptoms are secondary to metabolic imbalance (serum sodium < 125 mmol/l) (Anderson and Dawson 1963; Brown *et al* 1982; MacMillan *et al* 1990).

Hypernatraemia

Hypernatraemic dehydration has been found to be significantly negatively correlated with mental test scores in elderly people admitted to hospital as medical emergencies (Seymour 1980 *et al*). Macdonald *et al* (1989) found that hypernatraemic dehydration was common in a large hospital for mentally and physically handicapped people and suggested that elderly mentally ill people cared for in large institutes may also be at risk. Himmelstein *et al* (1983) conclude that hypernatraemic dehydration in an institutionalized patient may be an indicator of inadequate care.

Vitamins and mental illness

Dietitians should be aware that the vitamin status of many psychiatric patients may be inadequate. Severe psychiatric illness almost inevitably results in poor food intake, and the nutritional quality of some institutional or hospital food may be insufficient to correct, and may even compound, dietary deficiencies.

The incidence of psychiatric illness caused as a direct result of vitamin deficiencies is likely to be only a small proportion of those admitted. Nevertheless it is obviously vital that such cases are identified and treated. The role of vitamin deficiencies in the aetiology of mental illness can be overlooked by other disciplines and a dietitian is uniquely placed to identify patients at risk of deficiency and alert colleagues to this possibility.

Vitamin C

Ascorbic acid is required by the enzyme dopamine-β-hydroxylase which catalyses the hydroxylation of dopamine to norepinephrine. It is also essential for the conversion of tryptophan to 5-hydroxytryptophan which is the first step in serotonin synthesis. In normal subjects the concentration of ascorbic acid is three times higher in the cerebrospinal fluid and brain than in the plasma.

Deficiency of vitamin C may have effects on mental function. Kinsman and Hood (1971) described personality changes corresponding to the 'neurotic triad' of hysteria, depression and hypochondriasis during vitamin C deprivation of five healthy volunteers. It has been suggested that ascorbic acid deficiency slows the hydroxylation of dopamine thus causing a deficiency of noradrenaline and consequent state of depression (Dixit 1979). Walker (1968) reported that a severe depressive state is a striking clinical feature of chronic scurvy, and that this disappears after a few days treatment with ascorbic acid. Dietary intakes of vitamin C, but not other nutritional parameters, have been shown to be significantly lower in suicidal women than a comparable control group (Kitahara 1987).

Psychiatric patients have been reported to have low serum ascorbic acid levels (Thomas *et al* 1982). This may result from a low dietary intake; long stay patients in psychiatric hospitals are particularly dependent on the nutritional content of the food which may be severely deficient in vitamin C (Thomas *et al* 1986). However, it has also been suggested that some psychiatric patients, particularly those with schizophrenia, may have elevated ascorbic acid requirements (Suboticancc *et al* 1986; 1990).

Hancock *et al* (1987) found that active supplementation with ascorbic acid was needed to restore plasma levels in psychiatric patients admitted with plasma vitamin C levels below the normal range: the hospital diet alone cannot be relied upon to improve the vitamin C status. The type of supplement chosen must also be easy to administer on a regular basis. Use, for example, of a vitamin C fortified drink may not be successful if lack of staff supervision results in it not being given regularly, not being made up correctly, left to stand in sunlight for long periods or if it is refused by patients on the grounds of palatability.

Thiamin

Links have been suggested between thiamin deficiency and symptoms such as anorexia, anxiety, irritability (Keys *et al* 1945) and post-operative confusion in elderly women (Dickerson and Older 1982). Thomas *et al* (1986) found that more than one third of patients with dementia had erythrocyte transketolase activity levels indicative of thiamin deficiency. Some of these patients had low thiamin intakes. However, it is also known that there are abnormalities of thiamin dependent enzymes in Alzheimer's disease (Shaw *et al* 1988; Gibson *et al* 1988). Thiamin deficiency may also be found in patients with schizophrenia or alcoholism (Carney *et al* 1982).

The thiamin intake of hospitalized psychiatric patients is at risk of being inadequate due to the combination of anorexia and diets of poor thiamin content. Thomas *et al* (1988) examined the vitamin B content of hospital meal choices available to patients on an acute geriatric ward and found that a quarter of the choices would provide less than the 1979 RDA of thiamin, even if all the food chosen was consumed.

The use of high carbohydrate supplements in a psychiatric ward can also impose an additional stress on the thiamin status of patients. Dietitians should be ensure that medical staff are aware of the need for thiamin supplementation in these circumstances.

In acute psychiatric wards frank thiamin deficiency is most likely to present as part of the alcoholic syndrome. This may partly result from poor dietary habits but also from the toxic effects of alcohol on thiamin absorption and metabolism (Iber *et al* 1982; Ferro-Luzzi *et al* 1988).

Thiamin deficiency may also result in the Wernicke-Korsakoff syndrome, characterized by oculomotor disturbances and ataxia along with clouding of consciousness and severe memory and learning deficit. Confabulation (inventing material to fill gaps in the memory) is common.

The Wernicke-Korsakoff syndrome is commonly associated with alcoholism, but alcohol may not solely be responsible for the thiamin deficiency. Other factors such as dietary peculiarities, prolonged gastrointestinal upset or vomiting, or chronic laxative abuse may precipitate the syndrome (Conference Report 1979).

The syndrome is normally treated with intravenous or intramuscular doses of water-soluble vitamins. When thiamin appears in the urine, oral supplementation of up to 1 mg per day is commenced. Chronic intakes of thiamin of more than 3 g day are toxic to adults (DoH 1991) and this should be borne in mind when reviewing vitamin supplementation of alcoholic patients at the time of discharge.

Riboflavin

Riboflavin deficiency, indicated by erythrocyte glutathione reductase activity, has been linked with affective illnesses (Carney *et al* 1982). Symptoms of ariboflavinosis have also been found in patients treated with phenothiazines and it has been suggested that these drugs may inhibit riboflavin metabolism and deplete body stores of the vitamin (Zaslove *et al* 1983). Patients with borderline lifestyles and poor nutritional status may therefore be at particular risk of riboflavin deficiency during phenothiazine treatment.

Nicotinic acid

The mental symptoms of mild nicotinic acid deficiency include anxiety, irritability, fatigue, poor sleep and depression. In severe deficiency, an acute brain syndrome (delirium) or agitated depression occurs. The condition may also present as stupor, schizophrenia or dementia. Sufferers may be admitted to psychiatric hospital because of the severity of the mental symptoms which may be mistaken for psychoneuroses (Crammer 1983).

Hoffer (1971), in a series of papers published from 1957 onwards, claims that megadoses of niacin (3 g/day) are of benefit in the treatment of schizophrenia resulting in reductions in drug dosage, minimization of drug related side effects and decreased re-admission rates which are also shortened in duration. However, these findings remain controversial and such treatment is unlikely to be encountered in traditional British psychiatric practice.

Folic acid and vitamin B_{12}

Neurological symptoms, depression, dementia and psychosis have been associated with deficiencies of folic acid and vitamin B_{12} (Abou-Saleh and Coppen 1986; Ghadirian *et al* 1980; Goggans 1984). However, Bell *et al* (1990) suggests that haematological status and neuropsychiatric status are not coupled in a predictable manner.

The potential effects of folate and vitamin B_{12} on mental function centre on their involvement in three metabolic pathways:

1 Synthesis of neurotransmitters such as serotonin and catecholamines through the hydroxylation of tyrosine and tryptophan.

2 DNA synthesis, e.g. the bone marrow production of erythrocytes.

3 Myelin maintenance and the methylation cycle, e.g. in the synthesis of methyl donor S-adenosylmethionine (SAM). This is the main methyl donor in the brain and has been shown to have antidepressant properties.

The 'methyl folate trap' hypothesizes that lower levels of either B_{12} or folate may disrupt the relative levels between the above pathways resulting in a relative deficiency of serotonin and other neurotransmitters (Scott and Weir 1981). There is some evidence that supplementation with methylfolate (Godfrey *et al* 1990) or B_{12} (Evans *et al* 1983) may improve the mental state of those showing biochemical or psychiatric evidence of deficiency.

Botez *et al* (1982) suggest that it is possible to distinguish between patients whose psychiatric symptoms primarily result from folate deficiency and those who are folate deficient but have a different cause of their psychiatric illness, by measuring levels of 5-hydroxyindoleacetic acid (5-HIAA) in cerebrospinal fluid. Levels of 5-HIAA are low in patients with neuropsychiatric symptoms due to folate or B_{12} deficiency, but normal in patients with primary disorders. Patients with low levels will respond to folic acid or vitamin B_{12} therapy whilst those with normal levels will not.

4.23.5 Organic psychoses

Acute organic reactions

The word 'organic' signifies that there is a transient or permanent dysfunction of brain tissue. It also signifies that the disturbance of cerebral function is the cause of cognitive impairment such as clouding of consciousness, disorientation or memory loss. Symptoms such as mood changes or hallucinations are secondary to the cognitive losses. (This is in contrast to functional illnesses such as schizophrenia where such personality changes are the main symptoms.) 'Acute' signifies that the symptoms are reversible rather than implying sudden onset. Confusion, toxic confusional state, delirium, acute or transient confusional state are sometimes used interchangeably to emphasize a particular clinical situation.

Some causes of acute organic reactions are listed in Table 4.65.

Dietary management of acute organic reactions

Diet therapy should correct fluid and electrolyte imbalances and be appropriate to any underlying medical condition such as diabetes or liver disease. B complex vitamins are prescribed for patients with delirium tremens (acute alcohol withdrawal syndrome). Nasogastric feeding is sometimes necessary to ensure adequate intakes in confused patients who cannot or will not voluntarily eat or drink sufficiently. Overnight feeding, with normal meals being encouraged in the daytime, is a useful strategy if the patient is willing to tolerate the nasogastric tube.

Dehydration and confusion

There appear to be close links between dehydration and impaired mental function. Seymour *et al* (1980) found that as many as one in six elderly patients admitted as

Table 4.65 Some causes of acute organic reactions

Alzheimer's or multi-infarct dementias
Dehydration or water intoxication
Cerebral tumours
Trauma following head injury
Hepatic encephalopathy
Epilepsy
Pyrexia caused by infection or toxin
Uraemia
Electrolyte disturbances
Alkalosis or acidosis
Hyper or hypoglycaemia (insulinoma)
Hyper or hypothyroidism
Wernicke's encephalopathy
Drug or alcohol abuse or withdrawal
Congestive cardiac failure
Thiamin, nicotinic acid, B_{12} or folate deficiencies

medical emergencies had an acute confusional state which was related to dehydration.

Maintenance of adequate fluid intakes on many continuing care wards can be problematic. Staff and patients may believe that withholding fluids will help to relieve urinary incontinence. In fact it has the opposite effect as constipation can cause urinary incontinence by means of pressure on the bladder. Concentrated urine is also likely to lead to urinary tract infections, a further cause of incontinence (Fig. 4.14).

There is evidence that in many psychiatric and mental handicap hospitals, the hydration status of patients may be compromised (Himmelstein *et al* 1983; Farley *et al* 1986). Increasing the fluid intake of patients on a psychogeriatric ward in Cardiff to 2 l/day was, according to nursing staff, accompanied by decreases in noise and disturbance, laxative use and urinary incontinence. Such a level of fluid

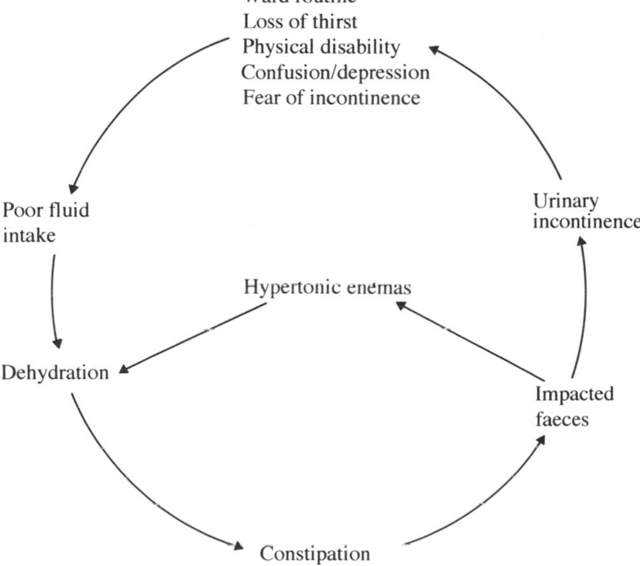

Fig. 4.14 The incontinence cycle

intake is difficult to achieve, particularly if patients are wholly dependent on staff for access to fluids. However, if nursing and catering staff can be convinced of the importance of adequate fluid provision, it can be done – for example, by offering two cups of fluid mid-morning and in mid-afternoon as well as a beverage after each main meal. Devising a fluid plan which details the quantity and frequency of drinks to be given to patients is helpful (Table 4.66). In order to maintain compliance, the dietitian will need to monitor the success of the plan and continue to motivate staff as necessary.

Chronic organic brain syndromes

In chronic organic brain syndromes it is the death of the brain tissue which gives rise to the symptoms (in contrast to acute states where symptoms are caused by cerebral dysfunction and are often reversible).

There are many symptoms common to both acute and chronic states, especially disorientation, short term memory loss, loss of cognitive function and deterioration in behaviour. It is possible for an acute state to be superimposed upon a chronic dementia process, for example in a series of cerebrovascular accidents (CVAs) during the course of multi-infarct dementia. Impacted faeces, dehydration and electrolyte imbalance, protein, energy or vitamin deficiencies may also occur in the demented patient and cause superimposed acute confusion. Dietetic intervention in the prevention of such hazards is important in maintaining the patient's general physical health and mental functioning at its optimum.

Dementia

Garland and Birkett (1983) have defined dementia as 'a cluster of conditions characterized by widespread loss of intellectual functions after they have matured, a strong tendency towards progressive deterioration and, usually, destructive pathological changes in the brain'.

The commonest forms of dementia are Alzheimer's disease, multi-infarct dementia and a combination of the two.

Types of dementia

Alzheimer's disease (AD) (SDAT) In 1907, the German physician Alzheimer first described the classic case of a 51 year old woman who exhibited cognitive and behavioural changes with the steady advance of mental regression, typical of the syndrome which now bears his name. Necroscopy revealed an atrophic brain with enlargement of the ventricles. Microscopy revealed senile plaques, neurofibrillary tangles and loss of neurones.

'Senility' and Alzheimer's pre-senile disease are generally considered to be the same degenerative process. The term senile dementia of the Alzheimer type (SDAT) is

Table 4.66 Suggested plan of fluid provision on psychiatric wards

Breakfast	Milk on cereal	150 ml
	Fruit juice	150 ml
	Choice of beverage 1 cup	150 ml
Mid-morning	Choice of beverage 2 cups	300 ml
Lunchtime	Gravy/custard	150 ml
	Water/squash	150 ml
	Choice of beverage 1 cup	150 ml
Teatime	Choice of beverage 2 cups	300 ml
Evening Meal	Soup or milk pudding	150 ml
	Water/squash	150 ml
	Choice of beverage 1 cup	150 ml
Bedtime	Choice of beverage 1 cup	150 ml
		2100 ml

The measure of 150 ml assumes that, in practice, ward cups are not filled to the brim or drained to the dregs. Many feeding cups are of smaller volume than the standard tea cups.

used to denote most of the patients who were formally designated as 'senile'.

Biochemical disturbances found in Alzheimer's disease include:

1 Reduced activity in the cholinergic systems due to a degeneration of cholinergic cells or their terminals. This is correlated with the degree of intellectual deterioration. Reduced conversion of choline to the neurotransmitter acetylcholine may impair memory performance (Bowden *et al* 1979). Attempts have been made to increase cholinergic activity via dietary supplements of choline but have met with little success (Bartus *et al* 1982).

2 Changes in serotonergic and dopaminergic systems. These neurotransmitters are important in the regulation of food intake (Reizine *et al* 1978).

3 Poor identification of smells. This is significantly worse in Alzheimer's disease than in other dementias. This may explain some of the changes found in eating patterns in SDAT.

4 Transketolase abnormalities and reduced activity of thiamin-dependent enzymes.

5 Changes in glucose metabolism.

6 Reduced levels of plasma tryptophan.

Multi-infarct or arteriosclerotic dementia (MID) Changes in the branches of the internal carotid and vertebral arteries, with the deposition of plaques of fatty material, may lead to infarction in the brain tissue. Infarction causes necrosis, liquefaction and eventually cavity formation. There is a relationship between the mental manifestations of cerebral thrombosis and neurological changes commonly known as a stroke.

Binswangers disease is a variant of MID when infarcts are found in the subcortical white matter. The condition is associated with hypertension.

The Hachinski Ischaemic score is used to distinguish between patients with multi-infarct and Alzheimer's dementia (Hachinski *et al* 1975). However, clinical diagnosis based on this and other tests has not always been shown to be correct at necropsy, and there may be a tendency towards overdiagnosis of Alzheimer's and under-diagnosis of cerebrovascular disease (Homer *et al* 1988).

Patients with multi-infarct dementia are more likely to have preserved their personality and to describe a sudden onset of symptoms, often with neurological evidence of a stroke. Sufferers from Alzheimer's disease are more severely demented, with greater physical mobility and a tendency to wander or pace incessantly.

Other causes of dementia

Creutzfeld-Jacob disease This is known to be transmissible between humans (by corneal grafts and possibly by pituitary gland extracts) and from humans to primates. It is caused by the infective agent responsible for scrapie in sheep and bovine spongiform encephalopathy (BSE). It presents as a rapidly progressing dementia with muscle wasting and extrapyramidal signs (i.e. abnormal involuntary movements, alterations in muscle tone, postural disturbances).

Dementia of frontal lobe type The average age of onset is 53–56 years with about an eight year survival span. Changes in personality and social behaviour are early clinical symptoms.

Picks disease This is a rare pre-senile dementia which resembles Alzheimer's disease, except that memory remains relatively intact and changes in personality and behaviour predominate. There is evidence of frontal lobe damage or atrophy.

Diogenes syndrome (senile breakdown) This is usually found in patients over the age of 70 years. There are signs of self-neglect in the absence of mental illness or cognitive decline. Often there is a history of heavy alcohol intake. All patients are of average to high IQ and tend to have a business or professional background. Symptoms of suspicion and aggression predominate and help is rejected until hospitalization is essential.

Other Other conditions in which dementia may occur include:
1 Parkinson's disease.
2 Huntingdon's chorea.
3 Multiple sclerosis.
4 Spino-cerebellar degeneration.
5 AIDS.
6 Chronic and repeated brain injuries ('punch drunk').
7 Neurosyphilis.
8 Normal pressure hydrocephalus.
9 Down's syndrome.

Aluminium and Alzheimer's disease

In recent years there has been speculation that aluminium may be involved in the aetiology of Alzheimer's disease. This has arisen from the following observations:
1 High levels of aluminium have been found in the cerebral cortex of some patients with Alzheimer's disease. This evidence has been reviewed by MacLachlan (1986). However some workers have been unable to substantiate these findings (Chafi *et al* 1991).
2 Some epidemiological studies have suggested that Alzheimer's disease is more common in areas with high concentrations of aluminium in the drinking water. However, methods of investigation have been criticised and results are contradictory (Simpson *et al* 1988; Martyn *et al* 1989).
3 Aluminium is known to be toxic to the brain and the cause of dialysis dementia. Encephalopathy can be induced experimentally in animals by injections of aluminium salts into the brain or other tissues. There are however important differences between Alzheimer's disease and dialysis dementia both clinically and histologically. The evidence is reviewed by Hamdy (1990) who concludes that Alzheimer's disease is not an aluminium neurotoxicity of the same type as dialysis encephalopathy.

It has been suggested that defective transport mechanisms may explain some of the associations seen between aluminium and Alzheimer's disease. Most aluminium is transported in blood bound to transferrin. Bound aluminium is unable to cross the blood-brain barrier but free aluminium is thought to be able to enter the central nervous system freely. There is some evidence that people with Alzheimer's disease (but not stroke dementia) may have defective aluminium-transferrin binding (Farrar *et al* 1990). Consequently, there is more free aluminium in the plasma which is able to enter the brain and exert a toxic effect.

Results from a recent two-year controlled trial suggest that administration of the aluminium bonding agent desferrioxamine may slow the rate of deterioration in Alzheimer's patients (McLachlan *et al* 1991).

Currently there is little evidence to suggest that dietetic measures to reduce aluminium intake are justified (Naylor *et al* 1990). Aluminium is a common element present in food, water, air and other substances such as toothpastes, cosmetics and medicinal preparations. The relative contribution of these sources to human intake has been the subject of research and speculation. Normal intakes of aluminium in Britain are estimated to be 5–10 mg per day (MAFF 1985; Graves *et al* 1990) but this is difficult to assess. The aluminium content of food is highly variable (Bjorksein *et al* 1988). There are also wide regional differences in the aluminium content of drinking water. In addition to this, the analytical content of aluminium may not reflect its bioavailability; in some circumstances, dietary aluminium may be unable to cross the gastrointestinal barrier (French *et al* 1989).

It is also possible that the amount of aluminium derived from toothpaste, antacid medications and antiperspirants may be greater than that obtained from food (Fleming *et al* 1989).

Concern has been expressed over the safety of aluminium cooking vessels. There is some evidence that aluminium can dissolve during cooking in the presence of organic acids, especially when oxalic acid containing foods such as rhubarb are boiled for a prolonged period (Flaten and Ødegard 1989).

Whether excessive aluminium is the cause or result of the neurological damage in Alzheimer's disease is not yet certain. Dietetic advice on maintenance of fluid intake and nutritional adequacy is probably of more practical benefit than attempts to manipulate the aluminium content of the diet.

General nutritional aspects of dementia

Energy balance Patients suffering from dementia are often underweight (Hancock *et al* 1985). However it is unclear whether this is the result of inadequate food intake, particularly in hospitals or homes, or a consequence of the disease itself (Bucht and Sandeman 1990). Some studies have suggested that people with dementia have a lower body weight than comparable controls despite a similar or even greater energy intake (Nes *et al* 1988; O'Neill *et al* 1990).

However the accuracy of the dietary assessment methods used in some of these studies can be questioned. In a more detailed investigation of weight-losing patients with advanced dementia, Sutherland *et al* (1990) suggest that a low energy intake is more likely to account for the weight loss observed. Prentice *et al* (1989) investigating severe wasting in elderly mental patients reported mean energy expenditures of 6 MJ/day with low BMRs of 4 MJ. Weight loss appeared to be an adaptation to the low energy content of the ward diet (6–8 MJ/day), patients being in energy balance at the time of the study. There was no evidence of excessive energy requirements except in those patients who were physically very active.

There are many reasons why low energy intakes are likely to occur. Staff may have insufficient time to feed patients, a problem compounded by very short intervals between meals, and there may be poor continuity of staff responsible for feeding an individual (Sandman *et al* 1987). The food intake of patients may be impaired by confusion, food refusal, paranoia and depression yet other factors resulting from the disease, such as agitation, may increase nutritional requirements (Litchfield and Wakefield 1987). Rheaume *et al* (1987) observed that constant walking (pacing) by patients with SDAT increased energy expenditure by 1600 kcal per day. The presence of infection will also increase nutritional requirements and increase the likelihood of malnutrition. This will in turn enhance the risk of infection so compounding the situation (Sandman *et al* 1987).

A number of strategies can be employed to optimize nutritional intake. Use of skilful feeding techniques, selection of foods with an appropriate consistency and the provision of adequate feeding time should be basic aspects of patient care. Nutritional supplements given, for example, via fortified beverages and/or puddings can make a significant contribution to overall energy and protein intake (Suski and Nielson 1989). It may also be possible to capitalise on the fact that food intake is usually better at breakfast and lunch (when cognitive abilities are at their peak) than at the evening meal.

Energy intakes upon admission to hospital may fall to levels significantly lower than those found amongst community living patients. Those admitted to hospital for long term care are the most dependent. It has been shown that dementia is the most common reason for patients living in nursing homes to be spoon fed (Bäckström *et al* 1987).

The dietitian advising on nutritional support will be faced with the problem of patients who are steadily losing weight while their carers are reporting 'good food intakes'.

Factors affecting food intake Vatassery and Maletta (1984) list a number of factors which may cause the food intake of dementia patients to deteriorate, and this in turn may cause deterioration of the nervous system because of lack of nutrients essential to its normal function.

1 Economic status.

2 Behavioural and depressive deterioration with loss of interest in food, especially following the death of a spouse.

3 Physical infirmity.

4 Loss of pleasure in eating because of physiological decline in sensory perception, especially smell and taste.

5 Mechanical problems in chewing.

6 Medications particularly those producing dry mouth and altered taste (e.g. antidepressants and antipsychotics).

The patient with dementia who lives alone During the early stages of dementia it is probable that the sufferer will be living at home. If there is a spouse or close relative to care for the patient, it is likely that food and nutrient intake at this stage will be satisfactory. Elderly men, who suddenly find themselves responsible for shopping and cooking for both themselves and their wife, may be particularly grateful for, and respond to, advice from a dietitian. The majority of elderly women suffering from dementia live alone (Nes *et al* 1988). In this situation the following problems may be encountered:

1 Food stores may contain rotting, out of date food or no food.

2 Food may be hidden, or stored in inappropriate locations.

3 Sufferers may be incapable of shopping for themselves and may either need to be accompanied to food shops or their shopping done for them by paid or voluntary helpers.

4 There must be an adequate supply of foods which do not require cooking and which can be opened easily, i.e. not canned or strongly packaged food. Examples of suitable foods are cheese, sliced ham, pork pies, bread and bananas.

5 Hot cooked meals may need to be provided by Meals on Wheels or other outside sources. It is important to ascertain that meals are actually eaten.

6 People with dementia may not experience thirst. A good supply of cold drinks is required if preparation of hot drinks is a problem. Prescribed supplements and milk are useful.

Common nutrition-related problems during the different phases of dementia

Early phase:

1 Difficulty in shopping, cooking and storing food.
2 Eating spoiled foods.
3 Forgetting to eat.
4 Forgetting having eaten.
5 Eating food which is too hot.
6 Changes in food choices (preferences for sweet, salty and spicy foods).
7 Unusual food choices (e.g. consuming a whole bottle of tomato ketchup).
8 Eating non-foods.
9 Gorging, particularly of sweets.
10 Patients with multi-infarct dementia may, in addition, exhibit the physical problems of stroke which will affect their feeding ability. Pseudo-bulbar palsy may be accompanied by weakness of facial and tongue movements, impaired co-ordination of chewing and swallowing and a hyperactive gag reflex.

During the middle phase:

1 Increased activity such as pacing or agitation.
2 Increased appetite but often inadequate intake.
3 Food is hoarded in mouth but not swallowed.

4 Food is not chewed sufficiently.
5 Ability to use cutlery is lost.

During the final phase:
1 Food is not recognized.
2 Patients refuse to open their mouths and turn away when food is offered.
3 Aphasia – the patient cannot ask for food or fluids.
4 Apraxia – the patient cannot initiate movement to open the mouth, cannot chew.
5 Dysphagia – the patient cannot swallow.

At the final stages of the illness, multidisciplinary decisions involving the family must be made concerning the use of enteral feeding or intravenous hydration. The ethical issues involved are discussed by Norberg *et al* (1987).

Improving the food intake of demented patients

1 There should be frequent provision of meals and snacks.
2 Present only one course at a time and have cutlery for only that course. The provision of extraneous objects such as flowers and cruets may cause extra confusion. However, in the institutional setting, the need for uncluttered tables must be balanced against the need to provide an attractive and homely eating environment.
3 If the patient can read, it may help to have eating instructions on the table or tray.
4 Avoid the use of covered containers; memory loss may make it difficult for the patient to find the food.
5 Minimize distractions such as a television on at meal times.
6 Serving foods such as casseroles and stews may minimize confusion, rather than having several foods on the plates.
7 Avoid tough, crunchy foods and particularly avoid mixed textures (e.g. peach slices in jelly or minestrone soup). Such items should be puréed to a smooth texture if the patient is likely to choke.
8 Friendly encouragement and a positive approach to mealtimes is important, with attention to individual likes and dislikes.
9 Portion sizes should be appropriate to the individual and second helpings available to patients who will take them.
10 The provision of plate guards and adapted utensils may encourage the patient to maintain independence.
11 If the patient has difficulty using utensils, the provision of finger foods is useful e.g. sandwiches, chips, hard boiled eggs, bananas, in addition to spoon feeding.
12 Liquids may be provided via jellies, puddings and sauces if choking is likely to be a problem.
13 Every patient needs to have a table and chair of a suitable height at which to dine. Encourage restless and wandering patients to finish their meals by choice of tables and chairs which are less easily vacated. This may be as effective as restraint and is less likely to frustrate the patient.
14 Plastic tablecloths are easily wiped after spillage. Plain colours may be less confusing than patterns.
15 Disposable napkins should be available and used to protect clothing. Avoid the use of 'geriatric' bibs.
16 Some patients eat better in groups and some alone. Patients with deteriorating table manners should be separated from others who may be distressed by their behaviour.
17 Plates should not be removed until it is certain that the patient has had enough and does not want a second helping.
18 Do not fill cups and glasses to the very top, allow for 'shaking' to avoid spillage.

Education of care staff

Care staff need to be educated on the importance of individual variations in the needs of patients, and the use and availability of high energy supplements for those with high energy expenditures. The importance of nutrition in the prevention of pressure sores and of adequate fluid intakes for all demented patients should be reinforced. Details of personal preferences and any religious or other cultural or medical factors affecting food choice should be recorded in care plans and integrated into meal service.

Useful addresses

Alzheimer's Disease Society, 158–160 Balham High Road, London SW12 9BN. Tel 081–675 6550/8/9.
MIND (National Association for Mental Health), 22 Harley Street, London W1N 2ED. Tel 071–637 0741.
National Schizophrenia Fellowship, 28 Castle Street, Kingston upon Thames, Surrey KT1 1SS. Tel 081–547 3937.

References

Abou-Saleh MT and Coppen A (1986) The biology of folate in depression: implications for nutritional hypotheses of the psychoses. *J Psych Res* **20**, 91–101.
Awad AG (1984) Diet and drug interactions in the treatment of mental illness – a review. *Can J Psych* **29**, 609–613.
Anderson WMcC and Dawson J (1963) Verbally retarded depression and sodium metabolism. *Br J Psych* **109**, 225–30.
Backstrom A, Norberg A and Norberg B (1987) Feeding difficulties in long-stay patients at nursing homes: caregiver turnover and caregivers assessment of duration and difficulty of assisted feeding and amount of food received by the patient. *Int J Nurs Studies* **24**, 69.
Bartus R, Dean R and Beer B (1982) The cholinergic hypothesis of geriatric memory dysfunction. *Science* **217**, 408–417.
Bell I, Edman JS, Marby DW, Saltlin A, Dreier T, Liptzin B and Cole J (1990) Vitamin B_{12} and folate status in acute geropsychiatric inpatients: Affective and cognitive characteristics of a vitamin non-deficient population. *Biol Psychiat* **27**, 125–37.
Bjorksein J, Yaeger LL and Wallace I (1988) Control of aluminium ingestion and its relation to longevity. *Int J Vit Nutr Res* **58**, 462–5.
Botez ML, Young SN, Bachevalier J *et al* (1982) Effect of folic acid and

vitamin B_{12} deficiencies on 5-hydroxyindoleacetic acid in human cerebrospinal fluid. *Am Neurol* **12**, 479–84.

Bowden D, White P, Spillane *et al* (1979) Accelerated aging or selected neuronal loss as an important cause of dementia? *Lancet* **1**, 11–14.

Brown RP, Kocsis JH and Cohen SK (1982) Delusional depression and inappropriate antidiuretic hormone secretion. *Biol Psychiatry* **18**, 1059–63.

Bucht G and Sandeman P (1990) Nutritional aspects of dementia, especially Alzheimer's disease. *Age and Aging* **19**, 532–36.

Carney MWP, Williams DG and Sheffield BF (1979) Thiamin and pyridoxin lack in newly admitted psychiatric patients. *Br J Psych* **135**, 249–54.

Carney MWP, Ravindran MG and Williams DG (1982) Thiamin, riboflavin and pyridoxin deficiency in psychiatric in-patients. *Br J Psych* **141**, 271–2.

Chafi AH, Havin J, Rancurel G, Berri J *et al* (1991) Absence of aluminium in Alzheimer's disease brain tissue: electron microprobe and ion microprobe studies. *Neuroscience Letters* **123**, 61–64.

Conference Report (1979) *Br Med J* **1**, 1768–72.

Crammer JL (1983) In *Handbook of psychiatry 2. Mental disorders and somatic illness* Lader MH (Ed) pp. 48–9. Cambridge University Press, Cambridge.

Crammer JL (1991) Drinking, thirst and water intoxication. *Br J Psych* **159**, 83–9.

Department of Health (1991) *Dietary Reference Values for food energy and nutrients for the United Kingdom*. Rep Hlth Soc Subj 41. HMSO, London.

Dickerson JWT and Older MWJ (1982) Thiamin and the elderly orthopaedic patient. *Age and Aging* **11**, 101–7.

Dixit VM (1979) Cause of depression in chronic scurvy. *Lancet* **2**, 1077.

Dohan FC (1966) Wartime changes in hospital admissions for schizophrenia and other syndromes in six countries in World War II. *Acta Psych* **42**, 1–22.

Dohan FC (1980) Hypothesis: Genes and neuroactive peptides from food as the cause of schizophrenia. In *Neural Peptides and Neuronal Communication*, Costa E and Trabucci M (Eds) Raven Press, New York.

Dohan FC and Grasberger JC (1973) Relapsed schizophrenics, earlier discharge from hospital after cereal-free, milk-free diet. *Am J Psych* **130**, 685–8.

Evans DE, Edelson GA and Goldan RN (1983) Organic psychosis without anaemia or spinal cord symptoms in patients with vitamin B_{12} deficiency. *Am J Psych* **140**, 218–21.

Farley PC, Lan KY and Suha S (1986) Severe hypernatraemia in a patient with psychiatric illness. *Arch Intern Med* **146**, 1214–5.

Farrar G, Altman P, Welch S *et al* (1990) Defective gallium transferrin binding in Alzheimer's disease and Down's syndrome; possible mechanism for accumulation of aluminium in the brain. *Lancet* **335**, 747–50.

Ferro-Luzzi A, Mobarhan S, Maiani G, Scaccini C and Nicastro A (1988) Habitual alcohol consumption and nutritional status of the elderly. *Eur J Clin Nutr* **42**, 5–13.

Flaten TP and Ødegard M (1989) Letter to the Editor. *Food Chem Toxic* **27**(7), 496–8.

Fleming LW, Prescott A, Stewart WK and Cargill RW (1989) Bioavailability of aluminium (letter) *Lancet* **i 298**, 433.

French P, Gradner MJ and Gunn (1989) Dietary aluminium and Alzheimer's disease (letter). *Food Chem Tox* **27**, 495–8.

Garland BJ and Birkett DP (1983) In *Handbook of psychiatry*, Vol 23. MH Lader (Ed) pp. 128. Cambridge University Press, Cambridge.

Ghadirion GE, Anath J and Englesmann F (1980) Folic acid deficiency and depression. *Psychosomatics* **21**, 929–9.

Gibbs J, Young RC and Smith GP (1973) Cholecystokinin reduces food intake in rats. *J Comp Psych* **84**, 488–95.

Gibson KF, Shaw R and Blass J (1988) Reduced activities of thiamin dependent enzymes in brains and peripheral tissues of patients with Alzheimer's disease. *Arch Neurol* **45**, 836–40.

Godfrey PSA, Toone BK, Carney MWP, Flynn TG *et al* (1990) Enhancement of recovery from psychiatric illness by methyl folate. *Lancet* **336**, 392–5.

Goggans FC (1984) A case of mania secondary to vitamin B_{12} deficiency. *Am J Psych* **141**, 300–310.

Graves AB, White E, Koepsell T *et al* (1990) The association between aluminium containing products and Alzheimers disease. *J Clin Epidemiol* **43**, 35–44.

Hancock MR, Hullen RP, Atlard PR, King JR and Morgan DB (1985) Nutritional state of elderly women on admission to mental hospital. *Br J Psych* **147**, 404–407.

Hancock MR, Mandal SK and Ray AK (1987) Vitamin C status of elderly patients on admittance into an assessment geriatric ward. *J Int Med Res* **15**, 95–8.

Hachinski VC, Linette D, Zilkha E *et al* (1975) Cerebral blood flow in dementia. *Arch Neurol* **32**, 632–7.

Hamdy RC (1990) Aluminium toxicity and Alzheimer's disease. Is there a connection? *Postgrad Med* **88**, 239–40.

Himmelstein DU, Jones AA and Woolhadly S (1983) Hypernatraemic dehydration in nursing home patients. An indicator of neglect. *Am Geriat Soc* **31**, 466–71.

Hoffer A (1971) Megavitamin B_3 therapy for schizophrenia. *J Canad Psych Assoc* **16**, 499–504.

Homer AC, Hanovar M, Lantos PL *et al* (1988) Diagnosing dementia: do we get it right? *Br Med J* **297**, 894–6.

Hsiao S, Wang CH and Scallert T (1979) Cholecystokinin, meal pattern and the inter-meal interval: can eating be stopped before it starts? *Physiolog Behav* **23**, 909–914.

Huebner FR, Weberman KW, Rubino RP and Wall JS (1984) Demonstration of high opioid like activity in isolated peptides from wheat protein hydrolysates. *Peptides* **5**, 1139–47.

Iber FL, Blass JP, Brun M and Leevy CM (1982) Thiamin in the elderly; relation to aloholism and degenerative diseases. *Am J Clin Nutr* **26**, 1067–82.

Keys A, Henschal A, Taylor HL, Mickelson O and Brozek J (1945) Experimental studies on man with a restricted intake of B vitamins. *Am J Physiol* **144**, 5–42.

Kinney-Parker J, Smith D and Ingle SF (1989) Fluoxetine and weight. Something lost, something gained? *Clin Pharmacol* **8**, 727–33.

Kinsman RA and Hood J (1971) Some behavioural effects of ascorbic acid deficiency. *Am J Clin Nutr* **24**, 455–64.

Kitahara M (1987) Insufficient ascorbic acid uptake from the diet and the tendency for suicide. *J Orthomol Med* **2**, 217–18.

Knox JM (1980) A study of weight reducing diets in psychiatric in-patients. *Br J Psych* **136**, 287–9.

Litchfield M and Wakefield L (1987) Nutrient intakes and energy expenditures of residents with senile edementia of the Alzheimer's type. *J Am Dietet Assoc* **87**, 211–13.

Macdonald NJ, NcConnell KN, Stephen MR and Dunnigan MG (1989) Hypernatraemic dehydration in patients in a large hospital for the mentally handicapped. *Br Med J* **299**, 1426–9.

MacMillan HL, Gibson JC and Steiner M (1990) Hyponatraemia and depression. *J Nerv Ment Dis* **178**, 720–22.

Mandal SK and Ray AK (1987) Vitamin C status of elderly patients on admission into an assessment geriatric ward. *J Internat Med Res* **15**, 96–8.

Martyn CN, Barker J, Osmond C *et al* (1989) Geographical relationship between Alzheimer's disease and aluminium in drinking water. *Lancet* **i**, 59–62.

McLachlan DRC (1986) Aluminium and Alzheimer's disease. *Neurobiology of Aging* **7**, 525–32.

McLachlan DRC, Dalton AJ, Pakruck T *et al* (1991) Intramuscular desferrioxamine in patients with Alzheimer's disease. *Lancet* **337**, 1304–8.

MAFF (1985) *Survey of aluminium, antimony, chromium, indium, nickel, thallium and tin in food.* The 15th Report of the steering group on food surveillance, the working party on the monitoring of foodstuffs for heavy metals. HMSO, London.

Naylor GJ, Sheped B, Irelining L *et al* (1990) Tissue aluminium concentration stability over time, relationship to age and dietary intake. *Biolog Psych* **2**, 884–90.

Nes M, Sem SW, Rousseau B *et al* (1988) Dietary intakes and nutritional status of old people living at home in Oslo. *Eur J Clin Nutr* **42**, 581–93.

Norberg A, Asplind K and Waxman H (1987) Withdrawing feeding and withholding artificial nutrition from severely demented patients, interviews with caregivers. *West J Nurs Res* **9**, 348–56.

O'Neill D, McKiernen M, Gibney M, Walsh JB and Coakley D (1990) Dietary and anthropometric measures in mild to moderate senile dementia of the Alzheimer's type (SDAT). *J Hum Nutr Dietet* **3**, 177–81.

Potkin SG, Weinberger D, Kleinenman J *et al* (1982) Wheat challenge in schizophrenia patients. *Am J Psych* **138**, 1208–221.

Prentice AM, Leavesley K, Murgatroyd PR, Coward WA, Schorah CJ, Bladon PT and Hullin RP (1989) Is severe wasting in elderly mental patients caused by an excessive energy requirement? *Age and Aging* **18**, 158–67.

Reizine T, Yamamura H, Bird E *et al* (1978) Pre- and post-synaptic neurochemical alterations in Alzheimer's disease. *Brain Res* **159**, 477–81.

Reynolds EH, Preece JM, Bailey J and Coppen A (1970) Folate deficiency in depressive illness. *Br J Psych* **117**, 287–92.

Rheaume Y, Riley M and Volicer L (1987) Meeting the nutritional needs of Alzheimer's patients who pace constantly. *J Nutr Elderly* **7**, 43–52.

Rosenthal NE, Sack DA, Gillin JC, Lewy AJ *et al* (1984) Seasonal affective disorder: a description of the syndrome and preliminary findings with light therapy. *Arch Gen Psych* **41**, 72–80.

Sandman P, Adolfson R, Nygren C *et al* (1987) Nutritional status and dietary intake in institutionalised patients with Alzheimer's disease and multi-infarct dementia. *J Am Geriat Soc* **35**, 31–8.

Scott JM and Weir DG (1981) The methyl folate trap. *Lancet* **2**, 337–340.

Seymour D, Cape R and Campbell A (1980) Acute confusional states and dementia in the elderly; the role of hydration, volume depletion, physical illness and age. *Age and Aging* **9**, 137–46.

Shaw KFR, Clarke DD and Kim YT (1988) Studies of transketolase abnormality in Alzheimer's disease. *Arch Neurol* **45**, 841–5.

Simpson AM, Sellars CJ and Perry RA (1988) European overview of aluminium in drinking water. Proceedings of the 2nd International Symposium on Geochemistry and Health, Northwood UK. *Science Rev* **15**, 44.

Singh MM and Kay SR (1976) Wheat gluten as a pathogenic factor in schizophrenia. *Science* **191**, 401–2.

Storms LH, Jamie M, Clopton MS *et al* (1982) Effects of gluten on schizophrenics. *Arch Gen Psych* **39**, 323–7.

Suboticanec K, Folnegovic-Small V, Turcin R, Mestrovic B and Buzina R (1986) Plasma levels and urinary vitamin C excretion in schizophrenic patients. *Hum Nutr: Clin Nutr* **40C**, 421–9.

Suboticanec K, Folnegovic-Small V, Korbar M, Mestrovic B and Buzina R (1990) Vitamin C status in chronic schizophrenia. *Biol Psych* **28**, 959–66.

Suski N and Nielson C (1989) Factors affecting food intake of women with Alzheimer's type dementia in long-term care. *J Am Dietet Assoc* **89**, 1770–73.

Sutherland R, Rucker J and Woolton S (1990) Energy intakes and weight loss in institutionalised psychiatric patients. *Proc Nutr Soc* **49**, 16A.

Thomas DE, Chung-A-On KO, Dickerson JWT, Tidmarsh SF and Shaw DM (1986) Tryptophan and the nutritional status of patients with senile dementia. *Psych Med* **16**, 297–305.

Thomas *et al* (1982) Risk of scurvy and osteomalacia in elderly long-stay psychiatric patients. *J Plant Foods* **4**, 191–7.

Thomas AJ, Finglas P and Bunker VW (1988) The B vitamin content of hospital meals and potential low intake by elderly in-patients. *J Hum Nutr Dietet* **1**, 309–320.

Vandsborg PB, Beck P and Rafaelsen O (1976) Lithium treatment and weight gain. *Acta Psych Scand* **53**, 139–47.

Vatassery GT and Maletta GJ (1984) Relationship between nutrition and dementia in the elderly. *Psych Med* **1**, 429–43.

Vlissides DN, Venulet A and Jenner FA (1986) A double-blind gluten-free/gluten-load controlled trial in a secure ward population. *Br J Psych* **148**, 447–52.

Walker A (1968) Chronic scurvy. *Br J Dermatol* **80**, 625–30.

Zaslove M, Silvero T and Minenna R (1983) Severe riboflavin deficiency: a previously undescribed side-effect of phenothiazines. *Orthomol Psych* **12**, 113–15.

4.24 Eating disorders

There is a very wide spectrum of people with eating disorders, from the emaciated, restricting anorexia nervosa sufferer, through the normal weight person with bulimia nervosa, to the overweight or obese binge eater (Freeman 1987). The first two groups are generally referred to psychiatrists, psychologists, or multidisciplinary eating disorder teams for treatment, but the overweight individual is likely to be referred to a dietitian without any psychological intervention. All three groups require a similar approach from dietitians to help them change the way in which they eat, and to help reduce their fears of change.

It is not the intention of this chapter to give a great deal of detail about the various treatment methods available for helping individuals with eating disorders, as these are well described elsewhere (Garner and Garfinkel 1985; Hsu 1986; Scott 1988). This section describes the prime features of eating disorders, highlights the opportunities for dietetic involvement, and describes the rationale for, and the methods of, dietetic interventions.

Ideally, this group of patients is best helped by an experienced multidisciplinary team, which includes a dietitian, but it is likely that not all dietitians using this Manual will be part of such a group. The following, therefore, concentrates on dietetic advice, and how this can best be integrated into whatever treatment regimen is used.

Dietitians must be well-informed regarding the underlying psychological disturbances present in people with eating disorders, and must be able to deal with them to enable effective dietary counselling. A number of particular communication skills (attentive listening, empathic responses, and verbal encouragement) have been identified as being essential for the dietitian working with those with anorexia nervosa (Omizo and Oda 1988), and these probably apply equally to all eating disorders. Omizo and Oda also stress the importance of encouraging self-decision making, and providing support and acceptance of thoughts, feelings, and actions.

There are a number of features common to all eating disordered individuals, in terms of underlying thoughts and feelings which drive the changes in behaviour, but a useful classification for defining these populations is that of the American Psychiatric Association (1987) (Table 4.67).

4.24.1 Anorexia nervosa

Features of anorexia nervosa

Patients are typically young and female, however there are significant numbers of older women (Szmukler 1985) and males (Fichter *et al* 1985) suffering from the disorder. It is often quoted that anorexia nervosa is a disorder of social class I and II families, but again there is an increasing awareness of a much wider social class range of occurrence (Szmukler *et al* 1986). Males still rarely suffer from the disorder, with females continuing to outnumber them by at least twenty to one (Hall and Hay 1991).

Due to the marked change in the physical health and appearance of the individual suffering from anorexia nervosa, it is difficult for the sufferer to hide the changes, and therefore the peak age of presentation to the psychiatric services with this disorder is close to the peak age of onset at 21.1 ± 7.4 years in men and 18.3 ± 5.6 years in women (Hall and Hay 1991).

It is frequently difficult in this group of patients to determine which features of their behaviour are primary features of the disorder, and which are features caused by lack of food intake. The state of starvation, both absolute and relative, has a number of physical and psychological effects which tend to reinforce anorexia nervosa (Table 4.68). In a large study in the USA, young male volunteers underwent controlled food deprivation and consequently weight loss (Keys *et al* 1950). The volunteers had had no periods of dieting, nor any history of psychiatric disorders, prior to the period of starvation, yet the range of changes the subjects experienced are classically reported as being features of anorexia nervosa. A number of these features of starvation make it very difficult at times for the patient to engage in treatment.

Treatment of anorexia nervosa

A large number of different forms of treatment have evolved, some focusing upon psychological input aimed at resolving personal or family conflicts, some on biological inputs aimed at weight restoration, but most combining these two. A combined approach is probably preferable, with early intervention in both areas.

When weight loss is very severe or very rapid, hospital admission may be required, generally due to deterioration of the physical state rather than due to weight loss *per se*. In such patients bradycardia, arrhythmias, hypotension (leading to increased risks of falls), and biochemical disturbances (most frequently hypokalaemia), are the main indications for hospital treatment. There are increasing moves towards more outpatient and day-patient treatment in the realization that in the absence of life-threatening physical compli-

Table 4.67 Classification of eating disorders (American Psychiatric Association 1987)

Anorexia nervosa	1	Refusal to maintain body weight over a minimum normal weight for age and height e.g. weight loss leading to maintenance of body weight, body weight 15% below that expected, or failure to make expected weight gain during a period of growth leading to body weight 15% below that expected
	2	Intense fear of gaining weight or becoming fat, even though underweight
	3	Disturbance in the way in which one's body weight, size or shape is experienced, e.g. the person who claims to 'feel fat' even when emaciated, believes one area of the body is 'too fat' when obviously underweight
	4	In females, the absence of at least three consecutive menstrual cycles when otherwise expected to occur (primary or secondary amenorrhoea)
Bulimia nervosa	1	Recurrent episodes of binge eating (rapid consumption of a large amount of food in a discrete period of time)
	2	A feeling of lack of control over eating behaviour during the eating binges
	3	The person regularly engages in either self-induced vomiting, use of laxatives or diuretics, strict dieting or fasting, or vigorous exercise in order to prevent weight gain
	4	A minimum average of two binge eating episodes per week for at least three months
	5	Persistent overconcern with body weight and shape

Reproduced with permission

Table 4.68 Symptoms of starvation

Preoccupation with food
Poor concentration
Irritability
Depression
Dreaming about food
Cutting food into small pieces and delaying meals
Ritualistic eating behaviours

cations, hospitalization is not necessary, and may even be counter productive (Crisp *et al* 1991; Freeman 1992).

The usual approach when treating sufferers as inpatients is a behavioural treatment programme, in which varying degrees of control of eating and other aspects of life are removed from the patient, and responsibilities are slowly given back as a reward for progress in treatment (usually measured as weight gain). The degree to which staff take control is agreed by the patient early in the admission, and is usually formalized by means of a written contract. These contracts are usually negotiated by medical or nursing staff, but is important that the dietary component is planned in consultation with the dietitian.

The approach to treatment of outpatients and day-patients has to be quite different, with the patient and therapist working together to tackle the problem by a process of education, and goal setting, with the individual retaining control of his or her eating. Because of the fears and anxieties regarding change, and the fact that individuals remain in control of their eating, there is often a need for an increased frequency of dietetic input in this group.

There are many criteria by which the effectiveness of treatment can be measured, including improvements in physical state and social function, increases in weight, and decreased weight/shape/food obsessions as measured by questionnaires – such as the Eating Attitudes Test (Garner and Garfinkel 1979) or the Eating Disorders Inventory (Garner *et al* 1983). A global assessment that looks at nutrition, menstruation, mental state, sexual adjustment and socioeconomic status (Morgan and Hayward 1988) is probably the best means of assessment.

Dietary intervention in anorexia nervosa

Dietetic input plays a very important part in the treatment of eating disorders, and its overall aims can be summarized as trying to help the individual to:

1 Correct abnormal attitudes towards food.
2 Reduce the fear of dietary change.
3 Establish normal patterns of meals.
4 Establish a normal range of foods consumed.

Although it has been suggested that patients with anorexia have a good level of nutritional knowledge, this has been disputed (Beumont *et al* 1981; Laessle *et al* 1988). It appears that they frequently have a detailed knowledge of energy contents of foods (Beumont *et al* 1981) but lack general nutritional knowledge that would enable them to plan appropriate dietary intakes after their fears of change have been reduced. Patients often have very strongly held beliefs regarding the 'healthiness' and 'unhealthiness' of particular foods. Information from a dietitian regarding how any foods can be included in a healthy overall dietary intake can be of great value. It has often been assumed that once the underlying psychological disturbances have been addressed by psychotherapy, then the individual would be able to resume normal eating, both in terms of quantity and quality. There is evidence (Hsu 1979) that this is not the case, and clearly there is a need to offer the individual advice to help in the process of normalization of eating.

Long term normalization of disturbed eating behaviour depends on both motivation and ability. Establishing the motivation to normalize eating behaviour is unlikely to be sufficient to maintain a nutritionally adequate diet, if knowledge and the ability to compose such a diet are lacking. In many cases, patients cannot respond to internal cues to regulate intake, even after months of treatment. They have to go through a period of structured and controlled eating which requires a high level of nutritional knowledge (Laessle *et al* 1988). This advice is best given by a dietitian with an understanding of the underlying thoughts and feelings of those with eating disorders.

When dealing with patients with anorexia nervosa it is

important to allow enough time to establish rapport and gather all relevant information on which to base advice. This is true of all dietetic consultations, but needs particular emphasis when considering eating-disordered patients due to their inherent fear of dietary change. The ideal time for dietetic input in this group seems to be when they have established rapport with their main therapist and are motivated to change eating, and are prepared for the effects upon their weight. Dietetic input will be of little benefit if the individual is resistant to making changes, but it is worth noting that appropriate information from a dietitian may help reduce this resistance by reducing fear of the consequences. Such patients, even once they have acknowledged the need to increase intake, will usually fear rapid uncontrolled weight gain. Discussion with a dietitian as detailed below, including information on changes in energy requirements with weight gain, the physiology of weight gain, and appropriate means of dietary regulation, should help to allay such fears.

Very variable methods of dietary restriction are used by anorexia nervosa patients, along with use of laxatives, vomiting, and exercise to promote weight loss. The stereotype of the calorie counting, fruit and vegetable eating, fat and sugar avoiding patient is not always experienced in clinical practice and studies of dietary patterns in anorexia nervosa have also revealed variations from this 'norm' (Huse and Lucas 1984). It is vital therefore to gain information from patients about their own patterns of eating, as well as about their underlying fears and concerns that drive these altered patterns, in order to individualize the dietary advice.

Due to fear of weight gain it can be beneficial, in order to help to establish rapport with the patient, to aim initially for dietary changes which improve the quality of the diet and pattern of eating, rather than to concentrate immediately on weight restoration. Such luxuries may not always be possible of course when dealing with very frail low weight patients. From this baseline, empirical dietary changes can be advised to promote weight gain with the emphasis on 'normal' foods. Despite common practice there is no need for very high levels of energy intake to facilitate weight gain, the combination of low weight, and starvation induced hypometabolism, enables weight gain to proceed on relatively low energy intakes (Huse and Lucas 1983; Vaisman *et al* 1988).

It is important to prepare the patient for the naturally occurring fluctuations in weight, and particularly for the initial disproportionate weight gain that may occur as a result of glycogen-obligated fluid in the first few days of dietary increase. Some preparation, and explanation of the changes occurring, can be very helpful in preventing panicky dietary restriction.

Most dietitians in the UK who work with eating-disordered individuals, use some method to help patients plan their food intake, and to help with the process of increasing intake. A variety of systems have evolved using food exchanges (Table 4.69) which have a number of benefits:

1 They enable the sufferer to retain a sense of control and consistency without the need for calorie counting, weighing of foods or rigid patterns of eating.
2 They encourage the introduction of difficult foods within a 'safe' framework.
3 They encourage appropriate variety and a nutritionally adequate range of foods.
4 They allow a structured, but non-rigid meal pattern.

4.24.2 Bulimia nervosa

Features of bulimia nervosa

The majority of those with this disorder are young and female. A survey of college students in the USA revealed that 19% of the women had bulimia compared to 5% of males (Halmi *et al* 1981). There can be a large gap between onset and presentation of the condition because the sufferer can conceal the presence of the behaviour. By definition, they maintain normal body weight and usually engage in vomiting and laxative use in a very private manner.

While some anorexic patients may sometimes binge eat and purge, the most distinguishing feature of bulimia nervosa is the regular frequent cycle of binge eating alternating with desperate attempts to counteract the effects of the binge. This purging behaviour can take the form of vomiting, starvation, laxative abuse, diuretic abuse and high levels of exercise. A bulimia sufferer may use any one of these behaviours or resort to a combination of them. The binge and purge cycle can occupy the sufferer for many hours of the day.

The underlying thoughts of the bulimic are very similar to those of the anorexic, namely, an obsession with food, distorted body image and loathing of their own bodies. There are clear vicious circles which develop, resulting in the maintenance of the bulimic condition (Fig. 4.15).

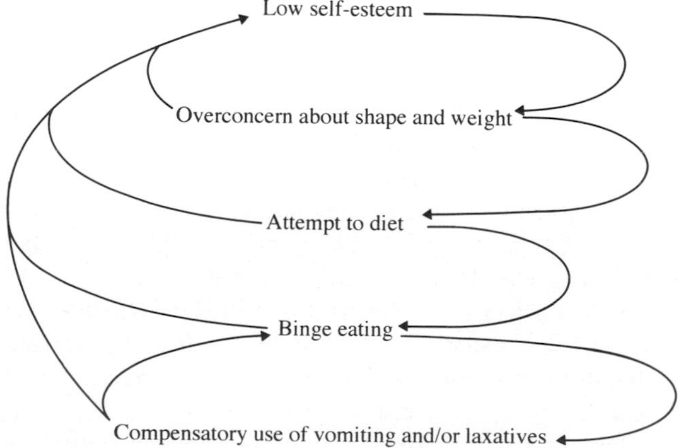

Fig. 4.15 Maintenance of the bulimic condition (Fairburn and Cooper 1989); Reproduced with permission from Oxford University Press.

Table 4.69 Dietary advice for patients with eating disorders

Establishing normal eating is an essential step to overcoming an eating disorder. Until the physical and psychological effects of dieting or chaotic eating are dealt with, it is difficult to benefit from other forms of eating.

People with eating disorders often have problems in knowing how much they should be eating. The following guidelines are a way of establishing how much you need to eat to maintain, increase or decrease your weight. They should enable you to eat a wide range of foods but still consume a consistent energy intake.

A system of food 'portions' is used to vary the overall level of food intake. These portions are basically what are usually termed carbohydrate foods and include bread, potato, fruit, crackers and biscuits, rice, cereals, pasta, cakes and puddings.

The following foods are counted as *one portion*:

1 slice of bread
2 plain biscuits
1 chocolate biscuit (digestive etc.)
2 oatcakes, crackers etc.
3 crispbreads etc.
1 bowl of porridge/breakfast cereal
1 piece of fruit
1 'diet' yoghurt
1 small potato or scoop of mashed potato
1 bowl of soup
2 tablespoons of rice
2 tablespoons of pasta
1 glass of fruit juice

The following foods count as *two portions*:

1 bread roll
1 pitta bread
1 large (e.g. baked) potato
1 scone, pancake etc.
1 croissant
1 fruit yoghurt
1 bag of crisps etc.
1 large chocolate biscuit (Club, Penguin etc.)
1 individual pudding (rice, custard tart, pie etc.)

These foods are of variable calorie content but, as long as you choose a variety of items each day, a consistent intake will result.

To start with, you should try to take __ portions per day.

It is important that these are spread throughout the day in order to avoid prolonged periods of hunger which may trigger binge eating, and also avoid over-fullness which may make the planned intake difficult to achieve.

For example:

Breakfast __ portions
Mid-morning __ portions
Midday __ portions
Mid-afternoon __ portions
Evening meal __ portions
Supper __ portions

Protein foods such as meat, fish, eggs, cheese and pulses are taken in fixed amounts. You should aim to include a helping of protein foods with your midday or evening meals (e.g. a sandwich at midday, part of the main course in the evening).

Vegetables, tea and coffee can be taken ad lib but avoid having them instead of carbohydrate portions.

Milk should be used in tea, coffee and with cereals.

When a regular pattern of meals has been established, adjustments can be made to the total number of portions in order to bring about controlled changes in your weight. These adjustments are best made infrequently (two weeks minimum) and will be discussed with you.

The purging behaviour is an ineffective means of weight control. Regular vomiting causes serious medical problems including bursting minor blood vessels in the eyes, swollen salivary glands and decaying teeth. Muscle weakness and palpitations can occur due to loss of body fluids and resulting hypokalaemia, especially if vomiting is used in conjunction with laxatives and diuretics.

The low self-esteem and depressive features can make intervention by the dietitian very difficult, the bingeing and purging behaviour often being mirrored in the way that these individuals handle relationships. They may eagerly seek information and advice, in the way that they grasp for food, only to reject the advice following even the smallest of failures.

Treatment of bulimia nervosa

The most widely recognized form of treatment for this disorder, and apparently the most successful, is cognitive behavioural therapy, the details of which have been described by Fairburn *et al* (1986). In summary, this involves the sufferer in close self-monitoring of their behaviours and of the underlying thoughts that drive them. Treatment combines encouraging changes in behaviour and examination and rationalization of automatic negative thoughts.

Treatment of bulimic patients is extremely effective in an outpatient setting and the use of group therapy increases the cost-effectiveness of the treatment (Freeman and Munro 1988). It is rare to have to hospitalize a bulimic patient and this is generally only necessary as a result of electrolyte disturbance or severely depressed mood.

Dietary intervention in bulimia nervosa

As with patients with anorexia nervosa, dietitians have an important role in the treatment of bulimia. The main features of dietary information are shown in Table 4.70. These can be successfully offered to a client who is following a cognitive/behavioural approach to their treatment.

Weight recording and nutritional advice and aimed at reducing the over-concern about shape and weight. Dietary advice and the establishment of regular eating, which is structured but not rigid, helps to reduce the urge to restrict intake. This in turn helps reduce the likelihood of binge eating being triggered.

Table 4.70 Features of dietary intervention in the management of bulimia nervosa

1 Weight monitoring and recording, to establish knowledge about fluctuations in body weight
2 Nutritional advice concerning metabolism and how the body works
3 Establishment of a regular eating pattern
4 Information about the links between dietary behaviour and feelings
5 Behavioural techniques to reduce binge eating

Dietitians may find exploring the link between feelings and dietary behaviour difficult to conduct on their own. As in the management of anorexia nervosa, the use of multidisciplinary teams in the treatment of bulimia nervosa is strongly recommended.

4.24.3 Compulsive eating syndrome

This is not a recognized psychiatric disorder although it is recognized as being an eating disorder (Lawrence and Dana 1990), and people with the condition are invited to belong to the Eating Disorders Association (EDA). This is a self-help group in the UK, which gives invaluable support to all those with an eating disorder. The characteristics of compulsive eating syndrome are given in Table 4.71.

Treatment of compulsive eating syndrome

Reducing diets are not helpful for this group. Diets are rooted in negative feelings about the person's self-image, for example 'If I were thinner then I would not feel so helpless'. These negative feelings are often reinforced by the negative feedback given by family and friends. This frequently leads to the dieting process breaking down, resulting in a self-perpetuating vicious circle (Fig. 4.16).

This cycle can and often does last a lifetime. People can follow both routes around this cycle. Those who repeatedly attempt to diet are more commonly the compulsive eaters of normal body weight, whereas the ones who more frequently binge rather than diet become overweight. Most diets have rigid rules which a person who is stressed will find difficult to adhere to. The rules are therefore broken and the failed dieters feel that they, rather than the over-rigid diet, are to blame. This lowers the self-esteem even further. Once the diet is broken dieters feel that they may as well continue eating all the forbidden foods and then recommence the diet tomorrow. The pleasure derived from eating forbidden foods results in distraction from current problems. However, failed dieters continually live with the spectre of guilt. Each guilty relapse episode is just more proof of failure. This failure is then one more stress that can provoke overeating.

Table 4.71 Characteristics of compulsive eating syndrome

1	The person has attempted to diet on a great number of occasions
2	The person is unable to sense true physical hunger and satiety
3	There is poor self image and often depressive personality traits
4	The sufferer is often thought to be addicted to food

Dietetic intervention in compulsive eating syndrome

To help people with compulsive eating syndrome, dietitians must recognize that diets do not work. This is a potentially threatening thing for a dietitian to do. However, once this hurdle is overcome, the person with compulsive eating syndrome can relax and the self-esteem rise.

Although the person with a compulsive eating problem may be overweight or obese, it is important to try and take the emphasis away from weight issues and not to weigh them on a regular basis.

The aim of dietetic treatment is to look at why the person turns to food, rather than what foods that person is eating. The use of self-monitoring is valuable as the sufferer can see what triggers their eating, and where and with whom they eat. Fig. 4.17 shows one style of a self-monitoring chart. Behavioural techniques can then be discussed and used.

It is important to help the person regain the knowledge of true hunger and satiety, showing them the difference between 'stomach' and 'mouth' hunger. This is then continued by establishing how satiety can be achieved by changes in the types and quantities of foods eaten. In dealing with hunger, the person must become aware of the 'need' for food, which is often interpreted as hunger, but more commonly is emotional 'need'.

By using the self-monitoring charts it is possible to see where and when overeating takes place. Guidelines to the compulsive eater are useful to ensure that food is eaten without distraction from other activities such as watching the television or eating automatically whilst serving food for others.

As with the other two eating disorders it is important that the patient addresses the problem of body image and the problems of being overweight in a 'fat phobic' society.

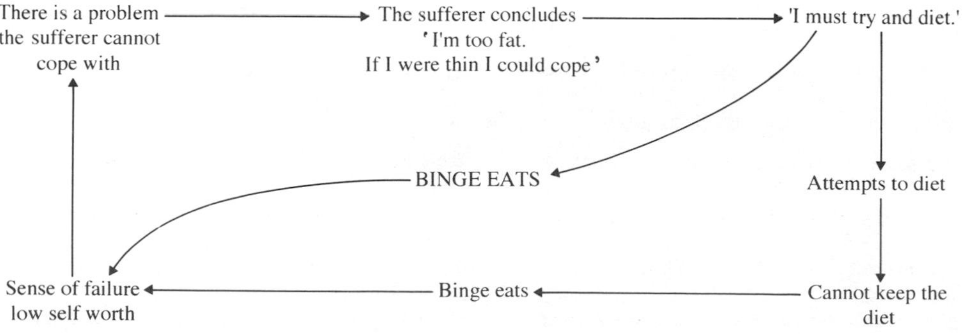

Fig. 4.16 Compulsive eating cycle.

Headings for Use in a Self Monitoring Chart for Compulsive Eating

Time	Food Eaten	Quantity	Who With	Where	Mood	Hunger

Fig. 4.17 Headings for use in a self-monitoring chart for compulsive eating.

As many compulsive eaters will only be seeing the dietitian and no other agency, it is appropriate that the dietitian looks at behavioural techniques and body image issues.

Useful addresses

Eating Disorders Association, Sackville Place, 44 Magdalen Street, Norwich, Norfolk. Tel 0603 621414.

The Women's Therapy Centre, 6 Manor Gardens, London N7.

Further reading

Agras WS (Ed) (1987) *Management of obesity, bulimia and anorexia nervosa.* Pergamon Press, Oxford.

Beumont PJV, O'Connor M, Touyz SW and Williams H (1987) Nutritional counselling in the treatment of anorexia and bulimia nervosa. In *Handbook of eating disorders Part 1*, Beumont, Burrows and Casper (Eds) Elsevier Science Publishers, Amsterdam.

Bowyer C (1988) Dietary factors in eating disorders. In *Anorexia and bulimia nervosa: practical approaches*, Scott D (Ed) Croom Helm, London.

Fairburn C (1985) Cognitive behavioural treatment of bulimia. In *Handbook of psychotherapy of anorexia and bulimia*, Garner DM and Garfinkel PE (Eds) Chapter 8. Guildford Press.

Gilbert S (1989) *Psychology of dieting.* Routledge, London.

Hirshmann and Munter C (1989) *Overcoming overeating.* Mandarin, London.

Orbach S (1978) *Fat is a feminist issue* Book 1. Hamlyn, London.

References

American Psychiatric Association (1987) *Diagnostic and statistical manual of mental disorders* 3e. Cambridge University Press, Cambridge.

Beumont PJV, Chambers TL, Rouse L and Abraham SF (1981) The diet composition and nutritional knowledge of patients with eating disorders. *J Hum Nutr* **35**(4), 265–73.

Crisp AH, Norton K, Gowers S, Halek C, Bowyer C, Yeldham D, Levett G and Bhat A (1991) A controlled study of the effect of therapies aimed at adolescent and family psychopathology in anorexia nervosa. *Br J Psych* **159**, 325–33.

Fairburn CG and Cooper PJ (1989) *Cognitive behavioural therapy for psychiatric problems – a practical guide*, Hawton, Salkavski, Kirk and Clark. Oxford University Press, Oxford.

Fairburn CG, Kirk J, O'Connor M and Cooper P (1986) A comparison of two psychological treatments for bulimia nervosa. *Behavioural Res and Therapy* **24**(6), 629–43.

Fichter MM, Daser C and Postpischil F (1985) Anorexic syndromes in the male. *J Psychiat Res* **19**, 305–313.

Freeman CP (1987) Eating disorders. *Medicine Int* 1846–50.

Freeman CP (1992) Day patient treatment for anorexia nervosa. *Br Rev Bulimia and Anorexia Nervosa* **6**(1), 3–8.

Freeman CPL and Munro JKM (1988) Drug and group treatment for bulimia/bulimia nervosa. *J Psychosomatic Res* **32**(6), 647–60.

Garner DM and Garfinkel PE (1979) The Eating Attitudes Test: an index of the symptoms of anorexia nervosa. *Psycholog Med* **9**, 273–9.

Garner DM and Garfinkel PE (Eds) (1985) *Handbook of psychotherapy for anorexia nervosa and bulimia.* Guildford Press.

Garner DM, Olmstead MP and Polivy J (1983) Development and validation of a multidimensional eating disorder inventory for anorexia nervosa and bulimia. *Int J Eating Dis* **2**, 15–34.

Hall A and Hay PJ (1991) Eating disorder referrals from a population region 1977–86. *Psycholog Med* **21**, 697–701.

Halmi K, Falk J and Schwartz E (1981) Binge eating and vomiting: a survey of a college population. *Psycholog Med* **11**, 697–706.

Hsu LKG (1979) Outcome of anorexia nervosa. *Lancet* **1**, 61–5.

Hsu LKG (1986) The treatment of anorexia nervosa. *Am J Psych* **143**(5), 573–81.

Huse DM and Lucas AR (1983) Dietary treatment of anorexia nervosa. *J Am Dietet Assoc* **83**(6), 687–90.

Huse DM and Lucas AR (1984) Dietary patterns in anorexia nervosa. *Am J Clin Nutr* **40**, 251–4.

Keys A, Brozek J, Henschel A, Mickelson O and Taylor HL (1950) *The Biology of Human Starvation.* University of Minnesota Press, Minneapolis.

Laessle RG, Schweiger U, Daute-Herold U, Schweiger M, Fichter MM and Pirke KM (1988) Nutritional knowledge in patients with eating disorders. *Int J Eating Dis* **7**, 1.

Lawrence M and Dana M (1990) What are eating disorders? In *Fighting Food.* Penguin Books, Harmondsworth.

Morgan HG and Hayward AE (1988) Clinical assessment of anorexia nervosa: The Morgan-Russell Outcome Assessment Schedule. *Br J Psych* **152**, 367–71.

Omizo A and Oda EA (1988) Anorexia nervosa: psychological considerations for nutrition counselling. *J Am Dietet Assoc* **88**, 49–51.

Scott D (Ed) (1988) *Anorexia and bulimia nervosa: practical approaches.* Croon Helm, London.

Szmukler GI (1985) The epidemiology of anorexia nervosa and bulimia. *J Psychiat Res* **129**, 143–53.

Szmukler G, McCance C, McCrone L and Hunter D (1986) Anorexia nervosa: a psychiatric case register study from Aberdeen. *Psycholog Med* **16**, 49–58.

Vaisman N, Rossi MF, Goldberg E, Dibden LJ, Wykes LJ and Pencharz PB (1988) Energy expenditure and body composition in patients with anorexia nervosa. *J Paediat* **113**, 919–24.

4.25 Prader-Willi Syndrome

The Prader-Willi Syndrome (PWS) was first described over 35 years-ago in Switzerland (Prader *et al* 1956) and in England five years later (Laurance 1961). It is characterized by severe hypotonia, poor weight gain and feeding difficulties in early life, accompanied by mental retardation, short stature and hypogonadism. A voracious appetite which develops can lead to severe obesity and occasionally diabetes mellitus follows. Other synonyms such as 'H2O' syndrome (indicating hypotonia, hypomentia and obesity) (Engel and Hogenhuis 1965) and 'HHHO' – adding hypogonadism (Zellweger and Schneider 1968) – are now not normally used.

4.25.1 Prevalence

Estimates of the prevalence differ. Holm *et al* (1981) suggested an incidence of 1 in 5000–10 000, an increase on an earlier figure of 1 in 170 000 (Spencer 1968). Laurance (1985) suggests 1 in 40 000 of the population is affected, but also surmises that greater awareness of the syndrome would result in increased diagnosis. According to Prader-Willi Syndrome Association (PWSA) (America) over 3000 cases have been identified throughout the world; more than 1000 individuals have been described in 160 reports.

The only data available in the UK is membership of the PWSA(UK); the current (1990) figure of over 400 (100% increase in five years) is clearly an underestimate.

4.25.2 Clinical features

Some patients display all of the described features, others fewer, but all are severely hypotonic at birth. If the mother has had a previous normal pregnancy she may recognize that fetal movements are less with the PWS pregnancy. The floppiness affects suckling to such an extent that nasogastric feeding is often essential. Nevertheless, artificial ventilation is never required and the absence of this feature helps to differentiate PWS from other causes of neonatal hypotonia such as Werdnig-Hoffman's disease. Although infants with PWS are grossly hypotonic there is potentially good underlying muscle power and they may be able to lift a limb against gravity, either in response to stimulation or spontaneously.

During the first 6–12 months, babies with PWS are often unresponsive – either to their own needs or to their environment – and may not cry when hungry or when disturbed by a loud noise, painful stimulus or frightening experience. The placid infant usually progresses to a naively charming child who occasionally has temper tantrums. (These may become worse in adulthood.) In addition, during the first 1–2 years of life, the infants fail to thrive. After the age of 2–4 years or sometimes earlier, there is a bizarre change in appetite (possibly as a result of hormonal changes affecting the appetite centre in the hypothalamus) so that the child becomes apparently insatiable. As a consequence, weight increases extremely rapidly and obesity becomes the major problem, unless energy intake is controlled. There is an indication (Laurance 1990) that weight increases in the latter half of the first year of life, before appetite increases, for reasons unknown.

Other features include small hands and feet, short stature (usually below the third centile), distinctive facial appearance (high forehead, almond shaped eyes, prominent nasal bridge and slightly open mouth), hypogonadism, scoliosis, strabismus and varying degrees of mental retardation. Occasionally there are dental deformities and saliva may be 'stickier' than normal. Skin-picking (which may be related to insensitivity to pain) and sleep disturbances (apnoea and daytime sleeping) often affect older individuals. Most people with PWS are warm, friendly and loving; occasionally they have uncontrollable short-lived temper tantrums or rages.

A child with PWS is rarely able to continue at a normal school for all education; some youngsters benefit from partial integration into such schools while others are better placed in special (ESN) schools. Boarding schools offering care for those with special needs may be appropriate. Subsequently most continue at training centres. Many individuals with PWS have gained one or more CSE/GCSE/City and Guilds certificates in either academic or artistic subjects. Sadly, for many, when statutory full-time education ceases, regular daily activity also stops. Individuals are then particularly vulnerable to rapid weight gain, primarily because of boredom, but also because supervision of dietary intake is more difficult.

4.25.3 Aetiology

Usually only one member of the family is affected; identical twins are known in the UK (Gellatly, personal communication). One source (Greenswag and Alexander 1988) summarizes the available literature of incidences of affected monozygote twins, cousins and siblings. Two families with several affected children are believed to have occurred as a result of an autosomal recessive trait.

Several sources have reported either translocation or

deletion of chromosome 15, but approximately half of affected individuals do not display the cytogenic deletion of the long arm of the parental chromosome 15, even when studied with advanced DNA molecular technology. Some sufferers with the deletion are found to lack many of the apparent clinical features; conversely some with many of the diagnostic features lack the deletion. It is suggested that a small and as yet undetectable chromosome deletion or the possibility of mosaicism could account for this. One study (Strakowski and Butler 1987) reports a significantly higher incidence of fathers' exposure to hydrocarbons at the time of conception. These results are reflected in a study in the UK (Gellatly 1989). The aetiology of the remainder is unknown. (NB Where there is a maternal deletion of chromosome 15, Angelman's syndrome results, not Prader-Willi Syndrome.)

The cause of PWS symptoms is not clear; the abnormalities observed possibly result from a localized primary disturbance in brain development above the spinal cord, e.g. a defect in the hypothalamic-pituitary axis (Gorlin *et al* 1976; Hanson 1981).

Deficiencies in fat metabolism (Afifi and Zellweger 1969; Tze *et al* 1981) or biochemical effects related to the level of lipoprotein lipase enzyme (Schwartz *et al* 1979) have also been suggested. The number and complexity of the alterations in body homeostatic functions strongly indicate that the hypothalamus is probably the site of major brain dysfunction in PWS. Increased levels of cholecystokinin have been found during the overeating period in a study of appetite control and the abnormalities in PWS (Holland 1991). Further investigation is needed to explain the observed failure to satiate.

4.25.4 Dietary management

PWS is clearly an eating rather than a weight disorder. The dietitian's involvement in treatment ranges from advice for the two extremes of the appetite problem of the syndrome: failure to thrive in infancy to hyperphagia (leading to gross obesity) in later years. The additional problems which individuals way have, e.g. physical, mental or learning difficulties, must also be considered and are discussed in general terms elsewhere – see Sections 3.3 (Infants), 3.12 (Learning disabilities), 3.11 (Physical disablement), 4.17 (Obesity) and 4.23 (Mental illness).

In infancy, once tube feeding is no longer required, it is important that energy intake should not be increased beyond the individual's requirements. By avoiding an increased food intake at this stage, there is less risk that the child will become accustomed to a higher one – undesirable in the gross appetite/obesity phase. Additionally dietitians must recognize that, due to parents' concern with preventing excessive weight gain, carers may be overzealous with dietary energy restriction.

There is evidence to suggest that children with PWS require a lower energy intake than the normal child; most gain appropriate weight on a daily intake of 10–11 kcal/cm height (Pipes and Holm 1973), and lose weight at any age on 7 kcal/cm. Energy requirements during exercise are reported to be similar to the non-PWS obese subject for the same level of work (Nelson *et al* 1973).

The importance of encouraging appropriate daily exercise from an early age must be emphasized; every opportunity should be taken to stimulate physical activity. Not only is it helpful in weight control, but it increases muscle tone. Individuals with PWS are naturally sedentary, but usually respond well to positive input from parents, e.g. family swimming sessions, bicycle rides, walks, or organized group activity such as discos, barn dances, club or school outings.

There is no evidence that extra energy supplements stimulate the release of growth hormone; such erroneous advice, which has been given in the past, is distressing to parents, many of whom understandably later lose confidence in their advisers. The use of growth hormone is controversial; an initial response may be encouraging but it is thought any benefit(s) may prove relatively transient. If treatment produces growth spurts, dietary intake requires appropriate energy adjustment.

Early diagnosis and intervention is essential for successful management before the hyperphagic phase leads to rapid weight gain. The literature on PWS generally describes grossly obese, retarded patients with early death from obesity-related diseases. If obesity can be controlled early death need not be the case. Crnic *et al* (1980) reported that early and comprehensive management can not only control obesity but also improve intellectual performance.

Regular and full recording of anthropometric measurements from a very early age is essential (Section 1.10.1). These data can be recorded on standard height/weight charts. Use of standard charts are not as helpful in the adolescent as in the young child; rarely is growth continued on the same centile. Attention is drawn to PWS-specific growth charts (reprinted as Appendix A in *Management of Prader-Willi Syndrome*, Greenswag and Alexander 1988) which take into account the lack of, or diminished, adolescent growth spurt. These specific charts therefore provide a means to detect deviant growth of individuals with PWS. A British study (Gellatly 1989) correlates with the American profiles of males and females. Use of height and weight measurements allows an appropriate diet to be designed including, if necessary, vitamin and/or mineral supplements.

Because of the hyperphagia, adherence to a strict dietary regimen is difficult but, if taught early enough, is not impossible. (It is extremely encouraging to note that the majority of UK children under 12 with PWS are controlling weight very satisfactorily, which contrasts significantly with those of similar age 10 years ago.) Dietitians should be aware of the lack of understanding of the hyperphagia and its associated problems by doctors, parents and indeed the older patients themselves. Ensuring awareness by all concerned avoids misunderstandings and is well worth the investment of the dietitian's time.

Many dietary regimens have been tried: strict energy control, an exchange system similar to that used in the treatment of diabetes, ketogenic diets or very low calorie diets. Some parents have attempted to use elimination type diets (dietary-linked behavioural problems have been reported in the USA), but if followed or attempted, energy restriction is also necessary, thus making the diet extremely difficult.

The regimen of choice is that which suits the individual and provides essential nutrients; the patient with PWS has to follow a diet for life so the nearer to normal the better.

Parents and patients must accept that diet control is vital; rules must be made and kept. Parents should be advised to weigh all food initially and not rely on guesswork when learning about the diet. Meals should be prepared so that they appear larger, visually, than they are (e.g. by using smaller, 8″ or 9″, plates in place of the usual 10″ size, cutting meat very thinly, or spreading the food out rather than piling it up).

Variety within the diet is essential as are occasional treats – perhaps as a reward or at Christmas or on a birthday, but the extra calories should be 'saved up' prior to the event – a surplus should not be allowed to accumulate. The subject of treats needs to be discussed with the parents – for example, should siblings have 'food' ones when the affected child is present or will low calorie treats be acceptable to the child with PWS as a substitute? Is a non-food item more appropriate for all the children?

Indeed many aspects of food provision for siblings must be discussed with parents. As with any diet, the PWS diet must fit in with family meals, and the dietary needs of the non-PWS members of the family, particularly other children, should not be overlooked. Parents and carers often need additional advice for these other family members, particularly when they are thin, very active and require high energy intakes.

The phenomen of food stealing is a major problem for many people with PWS. In one study (Page *et al* 1983) a behavioural approach reduced it successfully but only when the child was in a controlled setting. Any food left unguarded, including items normally accepted as unappetizing (e.g. food waste in dustbins, pet food, plants, berries, frozen products, packets of butter and margarine and plate waste) may be devoured. Pica (consumption of non-food items) may also be exhibited. For successful management, families must accept that they have to adopt extensive measures which upset their routine and conventional social behaviour. Food cupboards, freezers and refrigerators must be locked or made inaccessible. It may be easier to keep the kitchen locked which, although considered inconvenient, can soon become routine; the key(s) should be hidden carefully, and hiding places changed regularly. Other entries to the food storage areas or kitchens such as back doors, hatches and open windows must also be guarded. Siblings and other family members should be discouraged from keeping food in their rooms. Food should only be eaten at mealtimes – no crisps, sweets, fruit, etc. should be lying around. A meal being prepared in the kitchen should not be left unattended nor the table set with food unsupervized; at the end of a meal it should be cleared and dishes washed immediately. Individuals with PWS should not be left unsupervized at mealtimes. Problems are far fewer when dietary control has been taught early in life.

Friends, neighbours, relations, school and day centre staff need to have the condition explained so that they co-operate fully with the diet. As the child grows so do the problems – pocket money, collecting shopping, or attending youth groups and clubs where there is a 'tuck shop'. Wise parents usually limit the amount of spending money available to their children; PWS parents need even greater wisdom. Unfortunately there have been instances of shoplifting, money stealing or eating large meals in restaurants and cafés without the means to pay. It is important for others such as the police, local shopkeepers or assistants to understand the nature of the disorder and for all to remember how stressful these situations can be for both the individual and the family.

Hospital admissions can cause trauma and distress for all concerned, particularly if admission is to a busy ward. Other patients, nurses, domestics and porters must be made aware of the potential management problems of the patient with PWS. Volunteers who staff shops, trolleys and snack bars must be included in pre-admission inservice training. Unfortunately it is common for needs, other than that for which the patient is admitted, to be overlooked; for a syndrome sufferer this can mean a weight increase of several kilograms in two or three days unless dietary restrictions are strictly enforced.

It is imperative that medical advisers, including therapists and dietitians, as well as those caring for the patient (parents, social or voluntary service agencies), appreciate the necessity for dietary intervention, while at the same time recognizing mental or physical handicaps and behavioural disturbances. Many parents lose heart when their child is discharged from follow-up by the doctor or dietitian because there is little or no weight loss. This is especially so with the older child; doctors and others may lose patience with the child and parents/carers for perceived lack of effort.

The reasons for failing to lose weight are manifold – lack of compliance with a weight reducing regimen, too high an energy intake in the basic diet or, especially in the older child, the sheer physical impossibility of not eating because the appetite control centre has failed. Laurance (1985) suggests the child really can be kept to a reasonable weight without cruelty, but he also considers the battle is lost if dietary intervention is left too late, e.g. until 10–12 years. Dietitians need not be pessimistic; teenagers or older patients in a controlled environment (e.g. village or hostel for those with learning difficulties, or one-person flatlet with food sources strictly controlled) have achieved weight loss with an accompanying improvement in morale and the quality of life. These results, while rare, are regularly reported to PWSA(UK); fortunately good teamwork has resulted in more successful placements with better dietary control. The American model of homogenous group homes is extremely successful in overall management and at present unique to that country (PWSA 1987). Sweden plans to follow the role model with a five person home (Gellatly, personal communication) and one organization in the UK is currently considering transferring three adults with the syndrome to the one house (Gellatly, personal communication).

A sympathetic and supportive role is essential. For the person with PWS, obesity is only part of the problem; it is easy to overlook the slow development of the individual and complex behavioural management issues. Dietitians need to co-ordinate their work, not only with the parents but with all others caring for the child, e.g. physiotherapists, speech therapists, social workers, medical and nursing staff.

Non-dietetic measures such as the use of appetite suppressants e.g. fenfluramine and opiate antagonists, have been disappointingly ineffective. Surgical treatments such as intestinal bypass operations (both jejuno-ileal and gastric) have been tried, but such procedures are not readily acceptable to parents and are by no means always successful. However, in one reported case, a bypass operation not only produced a loss of 55 kg which aided mobility, but resulted in improvement in mental outlook. This allowed the individual to become more socially acceptable and to develop typing skills not previously thought possible (Gellatly, personal communication).

Jaw-wiring has been tried, but not in sufficient numbers of people to indicate whether this is a realistic option.

4.25.5 Independence

The life span of individuals with PWS is no longer only 20–30 years. With proper weight control individuals are living well into their 50s and even, though rarely, their 60s. Care in the community is therefore essential. Parents, particularly those with a handicapped dependent child, regardless of the disability, often find it very difficult to relinguish total control. Parents of teenagers/young adults with PWS find relinquishing responsibility particularly difficult when weight control has been successful in the home environment. As part of the preparation it is essential those planning care are fully conversant with all the potential problems and that appropriate long term arrangements are made. Too often inappropriate placements are/have been made with severe consequences – even death – which are totally preventable. The trauma to an individual whose placement breaks down must not be underestimated. 'Independence' must not include access, unsupervised, to food.

The community dietitian has a vital role to play during this transition period by providing nutritional support and continuity of care. The importance of a comprehensive understanding of the syndrome cannot be overstated.

The only 'treatment' at present is to establish a sheltered and regulated lifestyle in a loving and understanding environment; very few, if any, adults with PWS are ever able to achieve a fully independent lifestyle.

Useful addresses

Prader-Willi Syndrome Association (UK), 30 Follett Drive, Abbot's Langley, Herts WD5 0LP.

The PWSA(UK), a charitable organization, was constituted in 1981. It is run primarily by parents of people with PWS in conjunction with medical specialists. The organization aims to provide support for parents and carers, to promote knowledge and awareness of the syndrome amongst medical professionals as well as the public and to improve the quality of care given to people with PWS. Information leaflets and handbooks are readily available. The association actively promotes medical research by funding specific projects and seminars. Regional groups within the association work locally raising funds, spreading awareness of the syndrome and providing local support for individual members.

The annual subscription (in 1992) was £5.00 per Prader-Willi family. Interested professionals can become associate members for a reduced (£3.00) subscription. There are close links with the American counterpart (Prader-Willi Syndrome Association) which was established in 1975 regular contact with associations in Europe and liaison with Australia. In May 1991 an international organization was established with 14 member countries, 10 of which are European.

Further reading

Bray GA, Dahms WT, Swerdloff RS, Fiser RH, Atkinson RL and Carrel RE (1983) The Prader-Willi Syndrome: a study of 40 patients and a review of the literature. *Medicine* **62**(2), 59–79.

Caldwell ML and Taylor RL (1988) *Prader-Willi Syndrome. Selected research and management issues*. Springer-Verlag, New York.

Coplin SS, Hine JH and Gornican A (1976) Out-patient dietary management in the Prader-Willi Syndrome. *J Am Dietet Assoc* **68**, 330–34.

Greenswag LR and Alexander A (1988) *Management of Prader-Willi Syndrome*. Springer-Verlag, New York.

Holm VA and Pipes PL (1976) Food and children with Prader-Willi Syndrome. *Am J Dis Childh* **130**, 1063–7.

PWSA(UK) (1990) Prader-Willi Syndrome and the older person: a handbook for parents and professionals. PWSA, Herts.

References

Afifi AK and Zellweger H (1969) Pathology of muscular hypotonia in Prader-Willi Syndrome. *Am J Med Genetics* **28**, 889–95.

Crnic KA, Sulzbacher S, Snow J and Holm VA (1980) Preventing mental retardation associated with gross obesity in the Prader-Willi Syndrome. *Paediatrics* **66**, 787–9.

Engel WK and Hogenhuis LAH (1965) Genetically determined myopathies: conditions difficult to classify: H2O syndrome. *Clinical Orthop* **39**, 34–62.

Gellatly MSN (1989) Demography and nutritional support of Prader-Willi Syndrome in patients in the United Kingdom. PWSA 4th

Annual Conference. Abstract.

Gorlin RJ, Pindborg JJ and Cohen MM Jr (1976) Prader-Willi Syndrome. In *Syndromes of the head and neck* 2e. 618–21. McGraw-Hill, New York.

Greenswag LR and Alexander RC (1988) *Management of Prader-Willi Syndrome*. Springer-Verlag, New York.

Hanson J (1981) A view of etiology and pathogenesis of Prader-Willi Syndrome. In *The Prader-Willi Syndrome*, Holm VA, Sulzbacher SJ and Pipes PL (Eds) University Park Press, Baltimore.

Holland A (1991) Mechanisms of appetite control and their abnormality in Prader-Willi Syndrome. Prader-Willi Syndrome and other chromosome 15q deletion disorders, Scientific Workshop, Noordwijerhout, May 1991. Abstract.

Holm VA, Sulzbacher SJ and Pipes PL (Eds) (1981) *Prader-Willi Syndrome*, University Park Press, Baltimore.

Laurance BM (1961) Hypotonia, obesity, hypogonadism and mental retardation in children. *Arch Dis Childh* **36**, 690.

Laurance BM (1985) The Prader-Willi Syndrome. *Maternal and Child Health* **10**, 106–9.

Laurance BM (1990) Questionnaire re timing of weight and appetite increase. *PWSA(UK) Newsletter* **27**, 10.

Nelson RA, Anderson LF, Gastineau CF, Hayles AB and Stammes CL (1973) Physiology and natural history of obesity. *J Am Med Assoc* **223**(6), 627–30.

Page TJ, Finney JW, Parrish JM and Iwata BA (1983) Assessment and reduction of food stealing in Prader-Willi children. *Applied Res Mental Retardation* **4**, 219–28.

Pipes PL and Holm VA (1973) Weight control of children with Prader-Willi Syndrome. *J Am Diet Assoc* **62**, 520–24.

Prader A, Labhart A and Willi H (1956) Ein Syndrom von Adipositas, Kleinwuchs, Kryptorchismus, und Oligophrenie nach myatonieartigem Zustand im Neugeborenenalter. *Schweiz Med Wschr* **86**, 1260–61.

PWSA (1987) Development of proper placement for individuals with Prader-Willi Syndrome, Minneapolis. PWSA, USA.

Schwartz R, Brunzell J and Bierman E (1979) Elevated adipose tissue lipoprotein lipase in the pathogenesis of obesity in Prader-Willi Syndrome. *Clinical Res* **27**(2), 137–43.

Spencer DA (1968) Prader-Willi Syndrome. *Lancet* **ii**, 571.

Strakowski SM and Butler MG (1987) Parental hydrocarbon exposure in Prader-Willi Syndrome. *Lancet* **ii**, 1458.

Tze WJ, Dunn HG and Rothstein RL (1981) Endocrine profiles and metabolic aspects of Prader-Willi Syndrome. In *The Prader-Willi Syndrome* Holm VA, Sulzbacher SJ and Pipes PL (Eds) University Park Press, Baltimore.

Zellweger H and Schneider HJ (1968) Syndrome of hypotonia-hypomentia-hypogonadism-obesity (HHHO) or Prader-Willi Syndrome. *Am J Dis Childh* **115**, 558–98.

4.26 Diseases of the blood

4.26.1 Anaemias

Anaemia can be defined as a reduction in the concentration of haemoglobin in blood below the norm for the age and sex of the patient. The WHO (1970) recommends that anaemia exists when in adults the haemoglobin levels are below 13 g/dl (males) or 12 g/dl (females). Children aged six months to six years are considered anaemic at levels below 11 g/dl and those aged six to twelve years below 12 g/dl.

Classification

Two main classifications are in use:

1 The aetiological classification, based on the cause of the anaemia (Table 4.72).

2 The morphological classification based on the characteristics of the red cells. Two main criteria are used, the mean cell volume (MCV) and the mean cell haemoglobin concentration (MCHC). Three main morphological types of anaemia are recognized

- Normocytic anaemias, in which the MCV is within the normal range (76–96 fl). Most are also normochromic, that is, the MCHC is within the normal range (30–35 g/dl).
- Hypochromic microcytic anaemias, in which both the MCV and MCHC are reduced.
- Macrocytic anaemias, in which the MCV is increased. Most are normochromic. Some macrocytic anaemias are also megaloblastic, this being a term to describe distinctive cytological changes in red cells and their precursors due to impaired DNA synthesis.

These two classifications are complementary. The investigation of a patient with anaemia involves first, a decision on the morphological type (which often gives a pointer to the cause) and secondly, the determination of the cause of the anaemia (necessary to institute appropriate treatment). Those forms of anaemias in which dietary treatment is relevant are described below.

Iron deficiency anaemia

Iron deficiency anaemia is by far the most common form of anaemia encountered in clinical practice. It can occur at all ages but is commonest in women of child bearing age, in whom it is an important cause of chronic ill health. Morphologically it is a hypochromic, microcytic anaemia.

There are three major factors in its pathogenesis:

1. an increased physiological demand for iron
2. loss of blood by haemorrhage
3. inadequate iron intake.

The relative importance of these three factors varies with age and sex but blood loss, often from an occult source such as the gastrointestinal tract, is by far the commonest cause in adults in industrialized societies. The body cannot control its iron content by excretion as, once iron has been absorbed, only traces of it are lost, mainly in epithelial cells desquamated from skin and mucous membrane; iron in the faeces consists almost entirely of iron unabsorbed from food.

An increased physiological demand for iron occurs in infants and children during the period of growth and in women during their reproductive period of life. The normal full-term infant is born with a reserve of iron sufficient for the first four to six months of life, derived partly from the mother *in utero*, and partly from iron released by breakdown of red cells shortly after birth. Iron stores from the mother are laid down mainly in the third trimester of pregnancy so that premature infants are born with inadequate iron stores. Infants of iron-deficient mothers may also have inadequate iron stores at birth. Iron deficiency is less likely to occur in breast fed infants than in those who are fed with unmodified cow's milk (Saarinen and Siimes 1979).

During growth, which is maximal between 6 and 24 months, there is a progressive increase in blood volume and a resultant increase in demand for iron by the bone marrow. It is during this period, when iron reserves are depleted and the infant becomes dependent on dietary iron, that most cases of iron deficiency in infancy and childhood occur as a result of inadequate intake from faulty feeding. An infant should start being weaned between four and six months so that the increasing iron requirement will be met by a mixed diet by the time the iron stores are exhausted.

In females of childbearing age, menstruation, pregnancy, parturition and lactation all increase the physiological requirements for iron. Between 15–30 mg are lost each month through menstruation whilst 500–600 mg are needed for each pregnancy to satisfy the fetal requirement and compensate for the blood loss at childbirth.

During the past 50 years, improved standards of living, reduction in family size, better antenatal care and the availability of infant welfare services have done much to reduce the incidence of iron deficiency in industrialized countries, especially in adults. In addition, screening young children when they attend for immunization can be an

Table 4.72 Classification of anaemia by aetiology

Blood loss	Acute or chronic
Impaired red cell production	1 Deficiency of substances essential for red cell formation (erythropoeisis) e.g. Iron deficiency anaemia. Megaloblastic macrocytic anaemia due to vitamin B_{12} or folate deficiency. Anaemia in scurvy. Anaemia associated with protein malnutrition 2 Disturbed bone marrow function not due to the deficiency of an essential substance. e.g. aplastic anaemia, anaemia associated with infection, renal failure, collagen diseases, liver disease and disseminated malignancy. Anaemia associated with bone marrow infiltration, e.g. in leukaemia, lymphoma and myelosclerosis. Anaemia in endocrine gland dysfunction, e.g. myxoedema and hypopituitarism. Sideroblastic anaemia. Congenital disorders of haemoglobin structure and synthesis, e.g. sickle cell anaemia and thalassaemia
Increased red cell destruction	1 Haemolytic anaemia due to intrinsic red cell defect 2 Haemolytic anaemia due to extrinsic factors

Table 4.73 Main aetiological factors in iron deficiency anaemia

Population group	Aetiological factor
Infants and children	Defective diet Diminished iron stores at birth
Females of child bearing age	Menstruation Pregnancy Pathological blood loss Defective diet
Adult males and post-menopausal females	Pathological blood loss

acceptable and successful technique for identifying iron deficiency in deprived inner city communities (James *et al* 1989). Those most at risk are persons with a requirement above maintenance levels, such as young children and menstruating women, especially if they consume a vegetarian diet with a low citrus fruit content. Prevalence studies in women of childbearing age in Western Europe have found a frequency of iron deficiency anaemia of between 15–20% (Dresch 1970; Vellar 1970). Another group at risk are the elderly living on a nutritionally deficient diet, in whom the incidence has been found to be as high as 6% in men and 9% in women (McLennan *et al* 1973). In tropical countries iron deficiency anaemia is a major problem: this subject is discussed in detail by Cowan and Bharucha (1973).

Iron deficiency anaemia impairs the lives of over 700 million people worldwide. The development of primary health care in many countries now affords an opportunity to tackle the problem and the World Health Organization (1989) has published a book to assist in developing suitable control strategies.

The major aetiological factors in iron deficiency anaemia are listed in Table 4.73.

Dietary iron intake

Iron is found in a wide variety of animal and plant foods, usually in low concentration, and occurs in two main forms: haem compounds and ferric iron complexes. Iron contained in haem, released from food by gastric digestion, appears to enter the intestinal epithelium unchanged. Most of the available iron in food is in the form of ferric iron: before this can be absorbed it has to be released from the ferric complexes by the action of gastric acid, both hydrochloric acid and organic acids, and then reduced to the ferrous form at an acid pH by reducing agents in the food, e.g. ascorbic acid and the sulphydryl groups of proteins. The free ferrous ions are then absorbed, mainly in the duodenum and proximal jejunum, passing across the mucosal cell by an active metabolic process.

The two main factors which influence the amount of iron absorbed are the size of the iron stores and the rate of red cell formation. A decrease in iron stores increases absorption and an increase lessens absorption. In iron-deficient humans, the amount of iron absorbed from food is increased from the usual 5–10% to a level up to three times as great (Callender 1981). Stimulation of red cell formation by blood loss or red cell breakdown increases the absorption of iron. The actual controlling mechanism which determines the amount of iron absorbed is, however, unclear, though there have been recent advances in the knowledge of iron metabolism (Kühn 1991).

Iron is better absorbed from some foods than others and, in addition, some dietary constituents may impair or facilitate absorption. The iron in meat and fish is well absorbed and that in cereals and vegetables, except soya beans, less well so. Animal protein, however, will enhance iron absorption from vegetable sources and from haemoglobin. A high phosphorus diet impairs absorption by forming insoluble ferric phosphate, while conversely, a low phosphorus diet may result in increased absorption. Bread, cereals and milk are rich in phosphate. Phytic acid, present in some cereals, converts ferrous and ferric salts into insoluble phytates and may impair absorption. Ascorbic acid, because of its powerful reducing action, increases the conversion of ferric to ferrous iron and so increases absorption. These factors to some extent account for the difficulty in calculating the percentage of dietary iron which is likely to be absorbed.

The role of ascorbic acid in reducing dietary iron to its more absorbable ferrous form is particularly important in vegetarian diets, where all the dietary iron is derived from non-haem sources and the intake of phosphates and phytates, known to reduce iron absorption, is high. Seshadri *et al* (1985) showed that, over a 60 day period,

100 mg of ascorbic acid, given twice a day with lunch and dinner, significantly improved both the haemoglobin level and the appearance of the red cells in anaemic pre-school children consuming a purely vegetarian diet deficient in ascorbic acid. It has been shown that 100 ml of orange juice or 100 g of raw green pepper (presumably because of their high ascorbic acid content), will enhance the relatively poor absorption of non-haem iron from eggs and bread, though eggs reduce iron absorption from other non-haem iron-containing foods taken simultaneously (Dister *et al* 1975).

Dietary iron requirements, intake and bioavailability are discussed further in Section 2.8.2.

Megaloblastic anaemias

The megaloblastic anaemias are particular forms of macrocytic anaemia distinguished by distinctive cytological changes in red cells and their precursors. They were first described by Ehrlich in 1880 and are now known to be due to impaired DNA synthesis. They are deficiency diseases nearly always caused by lack of either vitamin B_{12} or folate, both of which are necessary for the normal development of red cells. Though less common than iron deficiency anaemia, megaloblastic anaemia is a significant cause of ill health worldwide. In Britain and other temperate countries, pernicious anaemia (vitamin B_{12} deficiency, resulting from a failure of secretion of intrinsic factor by the stomach), and folate deficiency (due to dietary lack or malabsorption) are both common, but in tropical countries most cases are caused by folate deficiency from a combination of low intake and malabsorption, vitamin B_{12} deficiency being much less prevalent. The megaloblastic anaemias are of particular clinical importance because of their excellent response to treatment. They are described in detail in the recent monograph by Chanarin (1990).

There are many similarities between the megaloblastic anaemias due to vitamin B_{12} and folate deficiency, especially in the clinical presentation and the morphological changes in the red cells. In addition to symptoms due to the anaemia, patients with both conditions often have a sore tongue and gastrointestinal upset, dyspepsia, anorexia, constipation or diarrhoea. Symptoms and signs due to degeneration of nerve tissue, in particular the spinal cord (subacute combined degeneration) and peripheral nerves, are, however, confined to those with vitamin B_{12} deficiency, in whom they may be the presenting feature.

The usual initial complaint is of parasthesiae, often numbness, tingling and pins and needles starting in the feet and spreading upwards. Weakness in the legs, unsteadiness of gait and clumsiness with fine movements are common. In severe cases impotence, loss of bladder and bowel control and even paraplegia are also present. It is important to make a firm diagnosis as to which deficiency is present because treating a patient with vitamin B_{12} deficiency with folate *per se* will often improve the anaemia but may cause a significant deterioration in the neurological state; serum assays of both substances are widely available. The main characteristics of vitamin B_{12} and folate are listed in Table 4.74.

Vitamin B_{12} deficiency anaemia

A mixed diet will provide about 30 μg vitamin B_{12} day but the vitamin is only present in foods of animal origin. The daily requirement for vitamin B_{12} is approximately 1–1.5 μg. It is a very stable vitamin, able to withstand heat and extremes of pH so little is lost in cooking. Dietary deficiency of vitamin B_{12} is therefore rare except in very strict vegetarians: the only B_{12} present in their diet will be by virtue of bacterial contamination. Many immigrants into Britain and other developed countries are strict vegetarians (Matthews and Wood 1984). The largest group of vegans are Hindus. Although more than 50% of vegans have low serum vitamin B_{12} levels (Wickramasinghe 1986), most vegans have normal haematological values and appear in good health. Some vegans do, however, develop a megaloblastic anaemia which responds to either oral or parenteral vitamin B_{12} therapy whilst breast fed infants of vegan mothers may develop vitamin B_{12} deficiency during the first year of life.

Most of the vitamin B_{12} in the diet is available for absorption. After release from foods by proteolytic enzymes it is bound to intrinsic factor, a glycoprotein secreted by the parietal cells of the gastric mucosa. The vitamin B_{12} – intrinsic factor complex, which is resistant to digestion, passes down to the terminal ileum where absorption takes place. The most common cause of vitamin B_{12} deficiency is a severe reduction or absence of intrinsic factor in the gastric secretion, secondary to atrophy of the gastric mucosa. Vitamin B_{12} present in the diet cannot therefore

Table 4.74 Characteristics of vitamin B_{12} and folate

	Vitamin B_{12}	Folate
Parent form	Cyanocobalamin	Pteroylglutamic acid (folic acid)
Food source	Animal origin only (liver, meat, fish and dairy produce)	Yeast, liver, green vegetables, nuts, cereals and fruit
Effect of cooking	10–30% loss	70–100% loss
Adult daily requirements	1–1.5 μg	100–200 μg
Adult daily intake	3–30 μg	100–500 μg
Site of absorption	Ileum	Duodenum and jejunum
Mechanism of absorption	Gastric intrinsic factor	Deconjugation, reduction and methylation
Body stores	3–5 mg (2–4 years' supply)	6–20 mg (4 months' supply)

be absorbed and pernicious anaemia develops. The disease is most common in people of Northern European extraction, in whom the prevalence approaches 10% after the age of 60 years. It is relatively uncommon in Africans and Asians. Treatment by regular subcutaneous injections of vitamin B_{12} is effective.

The great majority of other cases of acquired vitamin B_{12} deficiency are caused by disease of the gut. Surgical removal of part or whole of the stomach removes the source of intrinsic factor. However, the onset of megaloblastic anaemia following gastrectomy is often delayed for two years or more because of the high body stores of vitamin B_{12}.

Disease or surgical resection of the ileum will also affect the absorption of the vitamin. In particular, megaloblastic anaemia is present in many patients with coeliac or Crohn's disease and in 60–90% of patients with tropical sprue. About 90% of patients with tropical sprue malabsorb vitamin B_{12} and many also malabsorb folate. The absorption of vitamin B_{12} frequently returns to normal after a course of broad-spectrum antibiotics and in the early stages of the disease may improve following therapy with folic acid (Wickramasinghe 1986).

Another important cause of vitamin B_{12} deficiency is infestation with the fish tapeworm (*Diphyllobothrium latum*), which still occurs in Finland and the Commonwealth of Independent States (former Soviet Union). The tapeworm becomes attached to the lining of the small bowel and cause the deficiency by extracting vitamin B_{12} from the food as it passes down the bowel.

Malabsorption of vitamin B_{12} may also be drug-induced, e.g. by neomycin or paraminosalicylic acid (Jacobsen *et al* 1960; Heinivaara and Palva 1964) but in most cases the drug treatment is not continued for sufficiently long to produce clinical sequellae. The main causes of megaloblastic anaemia are listed in Table 4.75.

Folate deficiency anaemia

Folate compounds are present in all types of animal and vegetable foods. The richest sources are liver, yeast, green vegetables (especially spinach and Brussels sprouts), chocolate and nuts. In liver and other animal foods most of the folate is present as 5-methyltetrahydrofolate which is readily absorbed unaltered in the duodenum and jejunum. The folate content of an average mixed diet in Britain is between 100–500 μg/day (Gregory *et al* 1990). Some of this is present as polyglutamates which have to be hydrolysed into monoglutamates prior to absorption. Hydrolysis is carried out by the enzyme folate conjugase, probably in the lumen of the gut. The larger the number of glutamate residues in the polyglutamate chain, the less well the compound is absorbed (Baugh *et al* 1971). There is also a loss of folate in sweat, desquamated epithelial cells and urine.

The relatively large daily requirement means that folate stores may become depleted and folate-deficiency develop within three to four months of taking a folate depleted diet. The daily requirement of folate is 50–100 μg during the first two years of life (Chanarin 1978) and 200–300 μg during pregnancy. Folates are rapidly destroyed by heat and 30–90% may be lost during cooking, especially by methods which involve keeping food warm. As this is a regular practice in some hospitals it is not surprising that many elderly people in some long stay geriatric wards have been found to be folate deficient.

The main causes of folate deficiency anaemia are listed in Table 4.75. Megaloblastic anaemia due to dietary deficiency tends to occur in developed countries in the poor, the neglected elderly, the mentally disturbed, chronic alcoholics and infants fed almost exclusively on goats' milk, which contains little folate. A macrocytic anaemia is common in chronic alcoholism; in about 70% of cases this is associated with normoblastic erythropoiesis and may be a result of impairment of cell proliferation in the bone marrow by a direct effect of alcohol on red cell precursors. Folate deficiency is common however, more so in spirit than beer drinkers because beer is a significant source of folate. Herbert *et al* (1963) found normal folate values in only 7% of patient with chronic alcoholism.

Diseases affecting the upper small bowel, in particular coeliac disease, tropical sprue and Crohn's disease, often cause anaemia due to malabsorption of folate.

Folate requirements are increased in the following conditions.

1 In pregnancy due to the increase in maternal blood flow and the needs of the growing fetus.

2 In chronic haemolytic anaemias because of the increased red blood cell production.

Table 4.75 Causes of megaloblastic anaemia due to vitamin B_{12} and folate deficiency

Vitamin B_{12} deficiency	
Inadequate intake	Veganism
Gastric lesions	Pernicious anaemia, total or partial gastrectomy, congenital intrinsic factor deficiency.
Intestinal lesions	Crohn's disease, ileal resection, stagnant loop syndrome, coeliac disease, tropical sprue and fish tapeworm infestation
Folate deficiency	
Inadequate intake	Poverty, mental illness, alcoholism, infants fed on goat's milk, chronic illness, Kwashiorkor, etc.
Malabsorption	Coeliac disease, tropical sprue and jejunal resection
Increased requirement	Pregnancy and lactation, prematurity and infancy, haemolytic anaemia (e.g. sickle cell disease and thalassaemia), malignancy (e.g. carcinoma, leukaemia and lymphoma), chronic inflammatory diseases (e.g. rheumatoid arthritis, malaria and tuberculosis)
Drugs	Anticonvulsants, oral contraceptives, treatment with dihydrofolate reductase inhibitors (methotrexate, trimethoprim, pyrimethamine and triamterene)

3 In premature infants because of the rapid growth during the first two or three months.
4 In various malignant diseases, presumably in association with the increased production of tumour cells.

In all of these conditions this may result in megaloblastic anaemia, especially where the dietary intake is inadequate. In addition, folate deficiency in pregnancy can result in placental dysfunction and the premature birth of the infant. Before the use of folate supplements during pregnancy, megaloblastic red cells could be found in late pregnancy in up to 25% of women in the UK and up to 50% in southern India. However, the frequency of frank megaloblastic anaemia was then much lower, being 0.5–5.0% in the UK. It is still particularly common in twin pregnancies.

In patients with active chronic inflammation such as rheumatoid arthritis, three different mechanisms of folate deficiency may apply, 1. inadequate intake, 2. increased urinary loss and 3. increased demand to support the continued formation of chronic inflammatory cells.

About 80% of a 200 μg dose of folic acid is absorbed so that oral treatment of the anaemia is effective. Even where there is malabsorption a dose of 1 mg/day is usually sufficient. In many countries, folic acid supplements are given to pregnant women. Where poor intake has been a factor, it is, of course, necessary to emphasize to the patient that their diet has been deficient and should be changed. Where alcohol has been a factor both folate supplementation and abstinence from alcohol are usually required to achieve a normal blood profile. It must also be remembered that deficiency of both folate and vitamin B_{12} often co-exist so attention should be paid to ensuring an adequate intake of both.

Other deficiency anaemias

Anaemia in scurvy

The role of ascorbic acid in red cell formation is unclear. Nevertheless, anaemia is present in about 80% of patients with scurvy and usually responds to treatment with small doses of vitamin C on its own, or in a minority of cases, in combination with other haematinics. The anaemia is usually normochromic but may be hypochromic if there is associated iron deficiency.

Anaemia of protein deficiency

Anaemia is a common complication of severe protein malnutrition or ‘kwashiorkor’ and protein-energy malnutrition or ‘marasmus’. These conditions are most common in underdeveloped countries in the tropics, especially in young children and pregnant women, though they may occur at any age. Cases of protein malnutrition sometimes occur in industrialized societies in patients with gastrointestinal disease. The anaemia in uncomplicated cases is normocytic, of uncertain pathogenesis, and responds well to a high protein diet. Often, however, there are multiple associated deficiencies, especially of iron, folate, vitamin B_{12} and vitamin E and appropriate supplements to the diet are required.

4.26.2 Leukaemia

Leukaemia is a form of cancer of the blood-forming organs characterized by an uncontrolled, abnormal and widespread proliferation of leucocytes which infiltrate the bone marrow and body tissues, especially the liver, spleen and lymph nodes. This proliferation is usually accompanied by the appearance in the peripheral blood of immature leucocytes, many of which appear normal. In the past, leukaemia was invariably fatal. Now, with treatment, a significant number of patients with the acute form of the disease achieve remissions which may last for years and some are effectively cured. The aetiology is still uncertain but known precipitating factors are exposure to ionizing radiation, some toxic chemicals and cytototoxic drugs and certain viral infections. Leukaemia accounts for about 4% of all deaths from malignant disease.

Leukaemia occurs in a large number of forms, which differ in their clinical, pathological and haematological features. The two main criteria used in classification are the clinical course (acute or chronic) and the type and maturity of the dominant leukaemic cell. There are thus four main categories:

1 Acute lymphoblastic leukaemia.
2 Acute myeloid leukaemia.
3 Chronic lymphocytic leukaemia.
4 Chronic granulocytic leukaemia.

However, as the leukaemias arise from clonal proliferations, i.e. the leukaemic cell population arises from a single cell, a comprehensive classification is difficult to undertake. For example, there are probably at least five morphologically separate forms of chronic granulocytic leukaemia and several specific subvarieties, such as hairy cell leukaemia, have been described.

Acute lymphoblastic leukaemia is more common in children and, untreated, runs a shorter course than the other categories which occur typically in adults and are more prevalent. It responds well to modern treatment so that many patients may, in effect, be cured, i.e. their survival is the same as that of unaffected persons. Significant, and often lengthy remissions may be produced by treatment of patients affected by the other categories.

Treatment of leukaemia, based on chemotherapy and/or radiotherapy, with or without bone-marrow transplantation, is variable depending on the type, but all regimens tend to result in side effects which affect the nutrition of the patient. The most common problems are nausea and vomiting caused by chemotherapy, throat and mouth infections provoked by radiation therapy and an altered immune state, and loss or impairment of the sense of taste. These are discussed further in Section 4.34. Patients who are unable to eat sufficiently well to meet their nutritional requirements may require tube feeding using a suitable proprietary product or even total parenteral nutrition (see Sections 1.13 and 1.15).

The immunosuppression which results from radiotherapy or chemotherapy may necessitate the use of a 'sterile' diet (see Section 4.35). This usually becomes necessary when the patient's neutrophil count is less than 50% of the total white cell count. All foods which may contain or convey pathogens must be avoided; essentially these are foods which are either uncooked or have been exposed to the air (e.g. salads, raw fruit, ice cream, unwrapped cakes, filled biscuits, bottled sauces). Instead, food must be freshly prepared and served to the patient as soon as it has been cooked (either in a diet kitchen or in a microwave oven on the ward). A daily supply of fresh milk should be kept refrigerated on the ward for each patient. Patients should be seen daily to ensure that they are receiving food which they enjoy and which meets their nutritional requirements.

The preparation of diets for immunosuppressed patients is discussed in detail in Section 4.35.

4.26.3 Haemorrhagic disease of the newborn

Haemorrhagic disease of the newborn is due to a deficiency of vitamin K which exacerbates the low activity of the vitamin K-dependent coagulation factors in the neonate. The fall in activity is greater in the premature infant.

Bleeding, which can be severe, usually starts on the second or third day after birth and can be treated by injection of 0.5–1 mg of vitamin K (phylloquinone). It is routine practice in many hospitals however to give a single dose of vitamin K to infants immediately after birth. Thereafter the amount in human milk and modified milk feeds appears to be adequate (DHSS 1980).

References

Baugh CM, Krumdieck CL, Baker HJ and Butterworth CR Jr (1971) Studies on the absorption and metabolism of folic acid. *J Clin Invest* **50**, 2009–21.

Callender S (1981) Iron deficiency anaemia. In *Nutritional problems in modern society*. Howard AN (Ed). John Libbey, London.

Chanarin I (1978) Anaemias and coagulation disorders of nutritional origin. In *Nutrition in the clinical management of disease*. Dickerson JWT and Lee HA (Eds). Edward Arnold, London.

Chanarin I (1990) *The megaloblastic anaemias*, 3e. Blackwell Scientific Publications, Oxford.

Cowan B and Bharucha C (1973) Iron deficiency in the tropics. In *Clinics in haematology, Vol 2: Iron deficiency and iron overload*. Callender ST (Ed). WB Saunders, London.

Department of Health and Social Security (1980) *Artifical feeds for the young infant*. Rep Hlth Soc Subj 18. HMSO, London.

Dister PB, Lynch SR, Charlton RW, Torrance JD, Bothwell TH, Walker RB and Mayet F (1975) The effect of tea on iron absorption. *Gut* **16**, 193–200.

Dresch C (1970) Prevalence of iron deficiency in France. In *Iron deficiency*. Hallberg L, Harweth HG and Vannoth A (Eds) p. 423. Academic Press, London.

Gregory J, Foster K, Tyler H and Wiseman M (1990) *The dietary and nutritional survey of British adults*. HMSO, London.

Heinivaara O and Palva IP (1964) Malabsorption and deficiency of vitamin B_{12} caused by treatment with para aminosalicylic acid. *Acta Med Scand* **177**, 337–41.

Herbert V, Zalusky R and Davidson CS (1963) Correlation of folate deficiency with alcoholism and associated macrocytosis, anaemia and liver disease. *Ann Int Med* **58**, 977–88.

Jacobsen ED, Chodos RB and Faloon WW (1960) An experimental malabsorption syndrome induced by neomycin. *Am J Med* **28**, 524–33.

James J, Lawson P, Male P and Oakhill A (1989) Preventing iron deficiency in pre school children by implementing an eduational and screening programme in an inner city practice. *Br Med J* **299**, 838–40.

Kuhn LC (1991) mRNA-protein interactions regulate critical pathways in cellular iron metabolism. *Br J Haemat* **79**, 1–5.

Matthews JH and Wood JK (1984) Megaloblastic anaemia in vegetarian Asians. *Clin Lab Haematol* **6**, 1–7.

McLennan WJ, Andrews GR, Macleod C and Caird FI (1973) Iron deficiency in the elderly. *Quart J Med* **42**, 1.

Saarinen VM and Siimes MA (1979) Iron absorption from breast milk, cow's milk and iron supplemented formula: an opportunistic use of changes in total body iron determined by haemoglobin, ferritin and body weight in 132 infants. *Pediatr Res* **13**, 143–9.

Seshadri S, Shah A and Bhade S (1985) Haematological response of anaemic pre-school children to ascorbic acid supplementation. *Hum Nutr: Appl Nutr* **39A**, 151–4.

Vellar (1970) Prevalence of iron deficiency in Norway. In *Iron deficiency*. Hallberg L, Harweth HG and Vannotti A (Eds) p. 447. Academic Press, London.

Wickramasinghe SN (1986) *Systemic pathology: Vol 2: Blood and bone marrow*. Churchill Livingstone, Edinburgh.

World Health Organization (1970) *Requirements of ascorbic acid, vitamin D, vitamin B_{12}, folate and iron*. Technical Reports Series No 452. WHO, Geneva.

World Health Organization (1989) *Preventing and controlling iron deficiency through primary health care*. WHO, Geneva.

4.27 Rickets and osteomalacia

Rickets and osteomalacia are usually caused by dietary deficiency of vitamin D or a lack of sunlight exposure, and the consequent failure to absorb calcium from the gastrointestinal tract. Calcification of the bone matrix is deficient which results in softening of the bone. This is particularly likely to occur at times of increased growth and when nutritional requirements are increased such as during puberty and pregnancy. The elderly may have impaired vitamin D metabolism and calcium malabsorption leading to an increased risk of osteomalacia in those with poor diets. Dietary risk factors and ultraviolet radiation (UVR) deprivation co-exist in most cases of rickets and osteomalacia though in exceptional cases only one of these factors is responsible for the disease. In addition, rickets and osteomalacia can occur in circumstances where metabolism of vitamin D or absorption of calcium is impaired.

4.27.1 Vitamin D metabolism

Vitamin D status is dependent on both cutaneous production and dietary intake, so a deficiency is unlikely to occur unless the supply from both sources is defective or if there is an increased requirement for the vitamin. The vitamin D which is synthesized in the body is D_3 (cholecalciferol) and both D_2 (ergocalciferol) and D_3 are used therapeutically and for food fortification.

The metabolism of vitamin D has been clarified considerably (De Luca 1982). Although classed as a vitamin, the active metabolite 1,25 dihydroxycholecalciferol ($1,25(OH)D_3$)) may more properly be regarded as a hormone, and the dietary and endogenous precursors as prohormones (Fig. 4.18). Receptors for $1,25(OH)D_3$ have been found in a wide variety of tissues including stomach, parathyroid glands, gonads, brain, skeletal muscle, cardiac muscle, pancreas, activated T and B lymphocytes, skin and hair. The function of vitamin D receptors is to control cellular proliferation and differentiation, which may have implications for the role of vitamin D as an anti-cancer agent. Psoriasis has been successfully treated with vitamin D metabolites (Holick *et al* 1987) and a correlation between vitamin D status and concentration of humoral antibodies has been noted (Sedrani 1988).

4.27.2 Aetiology

Relative contribution from diet and sunlight

Vitamin D provision from synthesis in the skin is efficient and it has been suggested that this minimizes the need for dietary forms of the vitamin. The contribution to vitamin D status from sunlight is demonstrated by the seasonal variation in plasma 25(OH)D levels (Dunnigan 1977; Lawson *et al* 1979; Poskitt *et al* 1979). From October to March no ultraviolet (UV) light reaches the earth's surface in Britain, so synthesis in the skin is restricted to the rest of the year. Where solar exposure is inadequate, the dietary intake determines vitamin D status, though debate about their relative importance continues. The vitamin is not present in plentiful supply in food but evidence is accumulating to suggest that diet may play a role in the development of rickets and osteomalacia. In the presence of restricted UVR, a vegetarian diet substantially increases the risk of developing these conditions (see below).

Diet

Several dietary factors, singly or in combination, may contribute to the development of rickets and osteomalacia.

Vitamin D

Low dietary intakes of vitamin D have been suggested to be the sole cause of rickets and osteomalacia. Among Asians in Britain, some studies have shown dietary intakes to be lower than that of the indigenous population (Abraham 1983) but others (Dunnigan and Smith 1965) have found no difference, which suggests that a diet-UVR interaction is operating within this group. Among the elderly, low intakes of vitamin D may well be relevant (Nayal *et al* 1978; Sheltawy *et al* 1984).

Calcium

Rickets caused by low calcium intakes has been described in infants (Kooh *et al* 1977), in children on macrobiotic diets (Dagnelie *et al* 1989) and, despite relatively normal serum $25(OH)D_3$ levels, in South African children (Marie *et al* 1982). Inactivation of vitamin D in liver is increased by calcium deprivation in rats (Clements *et al* 1987), which represents a possible mechanism for rickets secondary to gastrointestinal disease, anticonvulsant therapy etc. This may explain the low plasma vitamin D levels seen in Crohn's disease with increased disease activity levels and the rapid disappearance of IV administered tritium labelled 25 hydroxyvitamin D (^3H $25(OH)D_3$) (Batchelor *et al* 1982).

Despite the considerably reduced absorption of calcium in the elderly, low calcium intakes do not appear to be causative or contributory.

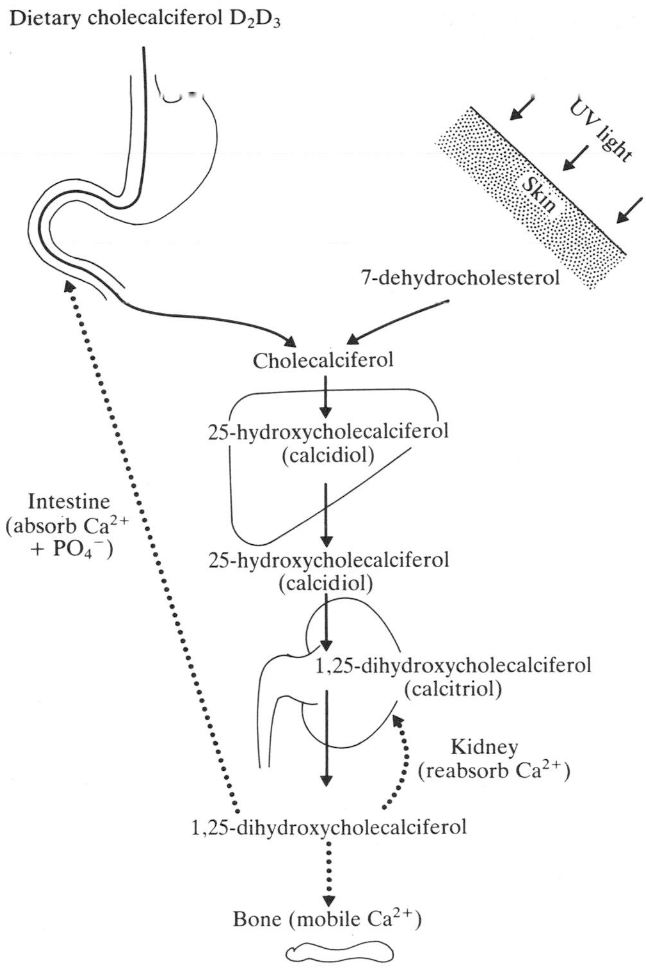

Fig. 4.18 Metabolism of vitamin D

Fibre and phytate

These act by binding calcium like other anions. (The interruption of the enterohepatic circulation of vitamin D metabolites by constituents of high extraction cereals and pulses now seems a less likely mechanism.) The increasing use of wholemeal products in the population may precipitate deficiency in those groups already at risk.

Fibre The role of high extraction flours in the aetiology of nutritional rickets was first suggested by Mellanby (1949) and has been reconsidered as a result of the prevalence of rickets and osteomalacia among Asians in the UK (Robertson *et al* 1982). Supportive evidence has been derived from the Irish National Nutrition Survey (1943–8) quoted by Robertson *et al* (1981), where a rise in the extraction rate of flour was believed to be responsible for the increased incidence in rickets in Dublin in 1942. In addition, the studies of rickets in Asian children in Glasgow have shown *high* fibre to be a significant risk factor.

Phytate Phytic acid can bind calcium and the presence of phytate in chapati flour has led to speculation that this may explain the increased incidence of rickets and osteomalacia in the Asian community. Healing of rickets has been reported following withdrawal of chapatis (Wills *et al* 1972), and Asian subjects have converted from negative to positive calcium balance on a chapati-free diet (Ford *et al* 1972). This hypothesis is unlikely to fully explain the higher incidence because the calcium intakes exceed the amounts likely to be bound by phytic acid.

Vegetarianism

Osteomalacia and rickets appeared in Austria and Germany at the end of the First World War during which people had reverted to a more vegetarian diet of bread and vegetables (Chick *et al* 1923). Epidemiological evidence from India and China support this link with vegetarianism. Mellanby in his early work on rachitic puppies noted that meat and suet were strongly anti-rachitic. In Glasgow, studies on privational rickets and osteomalacia among Asians have shown that a lactovegetarian diet as opposed to an omnivore diet was rachitogenic when UVR was restricted (Henderson *et al* 1987; Henderson *et al* 1990). Dietary fibre derived from high extraction rate wheat flour, fruit and pulses were the most important rachitogenic factors among children but fibre was not a significant risk factor among adults. Meat and fish were the most important protective foods in the children and in the adults osteomalacic risk was reduced by the consumption of eggs. There is preliminary evidence showing that meat contains metabolites of vitamin D and higher concentrations may occur as a result of over-fortification of animal feed (Kummerow *et al* 1976). This information has helped to clarify some of the earlier discrepancies in the diet hypothesis.

Sunlight

Sunlight exposure

Seasonal variations in plasma levels of 25 hydroxyvitamin D (25 OHD) and differences in 25(OH)D levels between indoor and outdoor workers (Neer *et al* 1977) demonstrate the relationship between vitamin D status and solar exposure. Calculations suggest that 1 cm of exposed skin could provide up to 380 iu D per day in midsummer if there were no loss processes in the skin (Beadle 1977). Badges of polysulphone film, worn on the lapel can be used to monitor exposure to UV radiation (Challoner *et al* 1976).

Though 90% of circulating 25 hydroxyvitamin D is in the cholecalciferol (rather than the ergocalciferol) form (Haddad and Hahn 1973), cutaneous synthesis cannot be regarded as a quantitatively more important source than diet in the adult because vitamin D3 is used for food fortification. The fact that rickets and osteomalacia remain important health problems in parts of Asia, the Middle East and Africa, areas with abundant sunshine, while it has virtually disappeared from Europe and North America suggest that the contribution from diet in the aetiology of these conditions is important.

Measurement of sunlight exposure has not been shown to differ between Asian children with and without rickets and their European peers (Dunnigan 1977); however, these results must be interpreted with caution as valid measurements of total body UV exposure are extremely difficult to obtain. Analysis of these data and that of adults point to dietary risk factors.

Skin pigmentation

Hess and Unger (1917) noted that black people in New York were more prone to develop osteomalacia than white people, but Stamp (1975) found no differences in the rise in serum 25 hydroxy vitamin D levels following UV radiation of white, Asian and West Indian subjects. If pigmentation is an important factor, rickets and osteomalacia would be expected to be much more common among West Indians and Africans in the UK but this is not the case.

4.27.3 High-risk groups

Groups at risk of developing rickets or osteomalacia fall into two main categories and are summarized in Table 4.76.

4.27.4 Clinical features

Rickets and osteomalacia are differentiated solely on epiphyseal fusion, so osteomalacia can be referred to as 'adult rickets'. Rickets is a developmental disease of bone in children which manifests itself in defects in calcification which, if unchecked, can lead to skeletal deformities such as knock-knees, bow legs and curvature of the spine. The symptoms of rickets depend on the age at which vitamin D deficiency occurs.

Table 4.76 Groups at risk of developing rickets and osteomalacia

1 Those on a rachitogenic diet with restricted UVR exposure:
   - Elderly people
   - Immigrants from India, Pakistan and Turkey (infancy/early childhood, adolescence and pregnancy are times of increased risk)
   - Food faddists, in particular those on macrobiotic diets and poor vegetarian diets

2 Those with conditions which interfere with the metabolism or absorption of vitamin D:
   - Malabsorption resulting from coeliac disease, gastric operations, bowel resection and bypass.
   - Cystic fibrosis
   - Renal disease – chronic renal failure, renal tubular disorders
   - Liver disease and alcoholism
   - Primary disorders of parathyroid function – hypoparathyroidism or hyperparathyroidism
   - Familial vitamin D resistant rickets
   - Prolonged use of drugs e.g. anticonvulsants
   - A high intake of aluminium

Infantile rickets

This is extremely rare in the indigenous population, though a mild rickets occurs in those children from the ethnic groups whose mothers practice late weaning and do not provide vitamin D supplements. At birth it presents as neonatal tetany and in infancy as craniotabes (unossified areas of the skull). Infants at risk include:

1 Those born to vitamin D deficient mothers.
2 Premature babies – this can be due to requirement of vitamin D being greater than met by parenteral nutrition or breast milk or due to lack of phosphate or calcium substrate.
3 Older babies on prolonged breast feeding and late weaning on to foods with low vitamin D content; particularly if no supplements are given.

Toddler rickets

Bow legs or knock-knees and 'rachitic rosary' (enlargement of the costochondral junction of the ribs) are classical signs. However, a milder form of rickets may be much more common and less easy to diagnose. This may be characterized by delays in mobility development (a child is slow to crawl, stand and walk), tooth eruption and closure of the anterior fontanelle.

Adolescent rickets

In adolescence, rickets presents with limb pains, usually involving the knees and thighs, a myopathic gait and in a few cases, genu valgum (knock-knees rickets). The growth spurt associated with puberty may precipitate this condition.

Osteomalacia

In the adult, the defective mineralization of the bone matrix (osteoid) is known as osteomalacia and can result in aching bone pain (often misdiagnosed as 'rheumatism' or even 'neurosis'). Muscular weakness caused by myopathy is common, and affects the proximal muscle groups. This may cause difficulty in rising from a chair, or climbing stairs. Spontaneous fractures are uncommon but pseudo-fractures may occasionally be seen on X-ray.

4.27.5 Diagnosis

In severe cases the presence of Looser's zones (pseudo-fractures) on X-ray, particularly of the long bones or pelvis, is diagnostic. In other patients the diagnosis can only be confirmed by bone biopsy. The essential histological criteria for osteomalacia are an increase in the volume and seam thickness of uncalcified bone (osteoid tissue), and reduction in calcification fronts at the surface of normal bone. These can be identified by the fluorescence caused by the antibiotic drug tetracycline, which is administered prior to bone biopsy for this purpose. In contrast to other bone diseases, osteomalacia affects the whole skeleton, but the iliac crest is the most convenient site to biopsy.

Ideally a diagnosis should be made before advanced clinical and radiological features occur, but the early symptoms are often subtle and non-specific. However, the alert clinician will always consider the possibility in those groups now recognized as being at high risk of vitamin D deficiency (see Table 4.76). In such patients a history of muscle or bone aches, or proximal muscle weakness (easily tested by seeing if they are capable of rising from a squatting position) should indicate the need for appropriate blood tests. Serum calcium and phosphate are often subnormal, depending on the secondary hyperparathyroidism present with an elevated alkaline phosphatase (of bone origin). However, in the elderly a raised alkaline phosphatase can be due to Paget's disease or occasionally osteoblastic metastases. The diagnosis can be confirmed by bone biopsy where radiology or biochemical testing is unhelpful.

4.27.6 Treatment

Primary deficiency

Simple nutritional rickets and osteomalacia usually respond rapidly to treatment with 2000–4000iu (50–100 μg) of vitamin D daily. It is unnecessary to use the newer metabolites of vitamin D and where there is doubt about compliance an intramuscular injection of 300 000–600 000 iu of vitamin D_2 is effective in a single dose. An oral supplement of calcium may help to restore the skeletal deficit more rapidly.

Secondary deficiency

Patients with osteomalacia caused by malabsorption syndromes can be given the newer metabolites (1,25(OH)D or 1α OHD). The advantage of these metabolites of vitamin D is that they have a shorter half-life and avoid the risk of overdosage. In patients with coeliac disease, a gluten-free diet may restore 'sensitivity' to oral vitamin D.

Vitamin D-resistant rickets for example caused by chronic renal failure, can be treated with daily oral doses of 1–4 μg of either 1α OHD or 1,25(OH)D. In these patients the plasma calcium and alkaline phosphatase should be monitored carefully. In all cases of secondary vitamin deficiency, the underlying cause must be treated wherever possible.

4.27.7 Prevention

Effective prophylaxis may be achieved by the provision of vitamin D supplements to groups at risk of developing nutritional rickets or osteomalacia. Attempts to increase the sunlight exposure and alter the diets have been futile. Foods rich in vitamin D such as margarine, butter, milk, Ovaltine and fortified cereals may be incorporated into the vegetarian diet but they will only make a small contribution so at risk groups should be given a supplement. Provision of a supplement to Asian women and children is endorsed in the recent Dietary Reference Value recommendations (DoH 1991) and the previous recommendation of 10 μg for older children and adolescents has been shown to be unnecessary. The suggestion that all those over 65 years should consume 10 μg vitamin D is one of the more controversial new recommendations.

References

Abraham R (1983) Ethnic and religious aspects of diet. In *Nutrition in pregnancy*, Campbell DM and Gillmer MDG (Eds) pp. 23–9. Royal College of Obstreticians and Gynaecologists, London.

Batchelor AJ, Watson G and Compston JE (1982) Changes in plasma half-life and clearance of ^{3}H-25-hydroxyvitamin D_3 in patients with intestinal malabsorption. *Gut* **23**, 1068–71.

Beadle PC (1977) Sunlight, ozone and vitamin D. *Br J Dermatol* **97**, 585–91.

Chick H, Dalyell EJ, Hume EM, Mackay HMM and Henderson Smith H (1923) *Studies of Rickets in Vienna 1919–1922*. Medical Research Council Special Report Series No 77 p. 122. HMSO, London.

Challoner AVJ, Corless D, Davies A, Deane GHW, Diffey BL, Gupta SP and Magnus IA (1976) Personnel monitoring of exposure to ultraviolet radiation. *Clin Exp Dermatol* **1**, 175–9.

Clements MR, Johnson L and Fraser DR (1987) A new mechanism for induced vitamin D deficiency in calcium deprivation. *Nature* **325**, 62–5.

Dagnelie PC, van Staveren WA, Verschuren SAJM and Hautvast JGAJ (1989) Nutritional status of infants aged 4–18 months on macrobiotic diets and matched omnivorous control infants: a population based mixed longitudinal study. 1 Weaning pattern, energy and nutrient intake. *Eur J Clin Nutr* **43**, 311–23.

De Luca HF (1982) New developments in the vitamin D endocrine system. *J Am Diet Assoc* **80**, 231–6.

Department of Health (1991) *Dietary Reference Values for food, energy and nutrients for the United Kingdom*. Rep Hlth Soc. Sub 41. HMSO, London.

Dunnigan MG and Smith GM (1965) The aetiology of late rickets in Pakistani children in Glasgow. Report of a diet survey. *Scot Med J* **10**, 1–9.

Dunnigan MG (1977) Asian rickets and osteomalacia in Britain. In *Child nutrition and its relation to mental and physical development*, pp. 43–70. Kellogg Company of Great Britain, Manchester.

Ford JA, Colhoun EM, McIntosh WB and Dunnigan MG (1972) Biochemical response of late rickets and osteomalacia to a chappathi-free diet. *Br Med J* **3**, 446–7.

Haddad JG and Hahn TJ (1973) Natural and synthetic sources of circulating 25 OHD in man. *Nature* **244**, 515–6.

Henderson JB, Dunnigan MG, McIntosh WB, Abdul-Motaal A, Gettingby G and Glekin BM (1987) The importance of limited exposure to ultraviolet radiation and dietary factors in the aetiology of Asian rickets: a risk factor model. *Q J Med* **24**, 413–25.

Henderson JB, Dunnigan MG, McIntosh WB, Abdul-Motaal A and Hole D (1990) Asian osteomalacia is determined by dietary factors when exposure to ultraviolet radiation is restricted: a risk factor model. *Q J Med* **76**, 923–34.

Hess AF and Unger LJ (1917) Prophylactic therapy for rickets in a negro community. *J Amer Med Assoc* **69**, 1583–6.

Holick MF, Smith E and Pincus S (1987) Skin as the site of vitamin D synthesis and target tissue for 1,25 dihydroxy vitamin D3. *Arch Dermatol* **123**, 1677–83.

Kooh SW, Fraser D, Reilly BJ, Hamilton JR, Gall DG and Bell L (1977) Rickets due to calcium deficiency. *N Eng J Med* **297**, 1264–6.

Kummerow FA, Cho BHS, Huang WY-T, Imai H, Kamio A, Deutsch MJ and Hooper WM (1976) Additive risk factors in atherosclerosis. *Am J Clin Nutr* **29**, 579–84.

Lawson DEM, Paul AA, Black AE, Cole TJ, Mande AR and Davie M (1979) Relative contributions of diet and sunlight to vitamin D state in the elderly. *Br Med J* **2**, 303–5.

Marie PJ, Pettifor JM, Ross P and Glorieux FH (1982) Histological osteomalacia due to dietary calcium deficiency. *N Eng J Med* **307**, 584–8.

Mellanby E (1949) The rickets-producing and anti-calcifying action of phytate. *J Physiol Lond* **109**, 488–533.

Nayal AS, MacLennan WJ, Hamilton JC, Rose P and Kong M (1978) 25 hydroxy vitamin D and sunlight exposure in patients admitted to a geriatric unit. *Gerontology* **24**, 117–22.

Neer R, Clark M, Friedman V, Belsey R, Sweeney M, Buouchristiani J and Potts J (1977) Environmental and nutritional influences on plasma 25 hydroxy vitamin D concentration and calcium metabolism in man. In *Vitamin D: biochemical and clinical aspects related to calcium metabolism*, Norman AW *et al* (Eds) pp. 595. Walter de Gruyter, Berlin.

Poskitt EM, Cole T and Lawson DEM (1979) Diet, sunlight and 25 OHD in healthy children and adults. *Br Med J* **1**, 221–3.

Robertson I, Ford JA, McIntosh WB and Dunnigan MG (1981) The role of cereals in the aetiology of nutritional rickets: the lesson of the Irish National Nutrition Survey 1943–8. *Br J Nutr* **45**, 17–22.

Robertson I, Glekin BM, Henderson JB, McIntosh WB, Lakhani A and Dunnigan MG (1982) Nutritional deficiencies among ethnic minorities in the UK. *Proc Nutr Soc* **41**(2), 243–56.

Sedrani SH (1988) Correlation between concentrations of humoral antibodies and vitamin D nutritional status: a survey study. *E J Clin Nutr* **42**, 243–48.

Sheltawy M, Newton H, Hay A, Morgan DB and Hullin RP (1984) The contribution of dietary vitamin D and sunlight to the plasma 25 OHD in the elderly. *Hum Nutr: Appl Nutr* **38C**, 191–4.

Stamp TCB (1975) Factors in human vitamin D nutrition and in the production and cure of classical rickets. *Proc Nutr Soc* **34**, 119–30.

Wills MR, Day RC, Phillips JB and Bateman EC (1972) Phytic acid and nutritional rickets in immigrants. *Lancet* **i**, 771–3.

4.28 Osteoporosis

4.28.1 Features and classification

Osteoporosis is a disease characterized by low bone mass, microarchitectural deterioration of bone tissue leading to enhanced bone fragility, and a consequent increase in fracture risk (Conference Report 1991)

Osteoporosis may be classified as follows:

1 *Juvenile*. This can occur, rarely, in children aged about 8–15 years.
2 *Young adult form*. This is rare and is sometimes seen in pregnancy.
3 *Postmenopausal (or Type 1)*: This occurs predominantly in women who have passed normally through the menopause, or in oophorectomized women.
4 *Senile (or Type II)*: This occurs in both men and women over the age of 75 years.
5 *Secondary*.

Idiopathic juvenile osteoporosis (IJO)

This is a rare condition described in 1965 (Dent and Friedman 1965). Typically bone pain develops 2–3 years prior to puberty and the severity of the disorder varies from mild vertebral osteoporosis to recurrent pathological fractures. Spontaneous remission usually follows the completion of puberty, but occasionally in severely affected children there may be permanent physical disability.

The cause of IJO is unknown. The bone becomes quiescent, unlike normal immature bone. Many patients show a negative calcium balance but not all, and no other metabolic abnormality is found. However, individual cases have been reported which appear to be linked with deficiency of calcitriol (1,25 dihydroxycholecalciferol) (Marder *et al* 1982) or calcitonin (Stevenson *et al* 1982; Alevizaki *et al* 1989) and which have responded to treatment with these substances. In another severe case, the bisphosphonate 3-amino-1-hydroxypropylidene (Pamidronate) caused a dramatic clinical and biochemical improvement (Hoekman *et al* 1985).

Osteoporosis in young adults and pregnancy

Transient osteoporosis of the hip may occur in both males and females, although this is commonly associated with pregnancy (Shifrin *et al* 1987), and can occur at other sites such as the feet and ankles.

Idiopathic spinal osteoporosis during pregnancy occurs rarely, and it is not known whether the association is accidental or causal. The patient presents with back pain and loss of height either in the last weeks of pregnancy or soon after delivery. In one study a few months after delivery, back pain ceased to be a problem and measured height increased. Osteoporosis and vertebral compression may not necessarily recur or worsen in subsequent pregnancies (Smith *et al* 1985a). Lowered levels of plasma 1,25 hydroxy vitamin D have been found in the osteoporosis of pregnancy (Smith *et al* 1985a).

Osteoporosis in pregnancy may occasionally be precipitated by the use of heparin anticoagulant therapy (Griffiths and Liu 1984). The maternal skeleton is thought to be protected from decalcification by a rise in production of calcitonin throughout pregnancy, and individuals with low levels of calcitonin during this period may be predisposed to skeletal demineralisation which is further aggravated by heparin therapy. Some success in prevention of this bone loss has been achieved with the use of ossein-hydroxyapatite which is a compound containing the components of the organic bone matrix (Ringe 1990).

Postmenopausal (Type I)

This may occur in postmenopausal women up to about the eight decade. A similar syndrome may occur in men who are deficient in testosterone. There is accelerated loss of trabecular bone leading, typically, to either collapsed or biconcave vertebrae or Colles' fracture of the wrist.

Senile (Type II)

This occurs in both men and women after the age of 75 years. There is a gradual general loss of both cortical and trabecular bone leading to fractures of the hip, or to wedge fractures of the vertebrae.

About 12% of women can expect to fracture their hip and rather more will suffer vertebral fracture(s) due to Type I or II osteoporosis during their lifetime.

Secondary osteoporosis

Osteoporosis may be found as a secondary condition and treatment will be aimed at resolving or stabilizing the primary condition (Table 4.77).

Table 4.77 Secondary causes of osteoporosis (Lindsay 1985)

Osteoporosis may be secondary to:	
Endocrine disorders	Cushings syndrome Diabetes mellitus Thyrotoxicosis Hypogonadism Acromegaly
Drug therapy	Glucocorticoids Thyroxine Heparin Diuretics Cytotoxic therapy
Immobilization	Bed rest Fracture immobilization

Osteoporosis may also be encountered in association with the following.

Osteoporosis associated with anorexia nervosa

Osteoporosis is a known consequence of anorexia nervosa (AN) in adults. In women this preferentially affects trabecular bone. Recent evidence suggests that AN which develops during adolescence and before the attainment of peak skeletal mass results in more bone loss than in adult-onset AN (Biller *et al* 1989). The severity of bone loss also appears to be related to the duration of amenorrhoea suggesting that gonadal steroid insufficiency plays a major role in the osteopenia of AN. Hypercortisolism may also contribute to trabecular bone loss (Biller *et al* 1989).

It has been suggested that the protective effect of weight-bearing activity is lost in AN patients (*Medical News & Perspective* 1987) although there is some evidence that people with AN who are more physically active have greater bone density than those who are less active (Rigotti *et al* 1984). If the strength of bone depends in part on the stress of supporting a certain body weight over time, some anorexic patients may not have sufficient weight to maintain adequate bone density.

It is not clear whether bone loss in adolescents reverses once feeding is reinstituted but results of one longitudinal study do not give grounds for optimism (Rigotti *et al* 1991). Anorectics would then be at risk of problems with osteoporosis at the menopause as they will have less bone density reserve to draw on (*Medical News & Perspectives* 1987).

Osteoporosis associated with Gaucher's disease

Gaucher's disease is a rare glycolipid storage disorder in which bone lesions are a major cause of morbidity in the adult form of the disease. Management of the bone complications has to date relied mainly on analgesia and orthopaedic procedures.

More recently some encouraging results have been gained from the use of oral aminohydroxypropylidene bisphosphonate (Pamidronate) (Harinck *et al* 1984). Possible mechanisms of action of the bisphosphonate have been discussed by Ostlere *et al* (1991).

Osteoporosis associated with rheumatoid arthritis

The osteoporosis that occurs in rheumatoid arthritis (RA) is generally considered to be of two types:

1 Localized juxta-articular osteoporosis of the involved joints, usually occurring early in the disease.

2 A generalized reduction in bone mass occurring more gradually (Sambrook and Reeve 1988).

A recent study on mostly postmenopausal women with rheumatoid arthritis showed no correlation between calcium intake (by questionnaire) and preservation of radial trabecular bone (Sambrook *et al* 1990). This is consistent with the results of other studies where supplements of calcium did not prevent bone loss in postmenopausal and senile osteoporosis in patients with RA (Sambrook and Reeve 1988).

Physical activity probably protects against bone loss in the spine and femoral neck in RA patients (Sambrook *et al* 1987).

Osteoporosis associated with Turner's syndrome

Bone demineralization may occur in gonadal dysgenesis, about 73% of subjects showing evidence of low bone mineral content. However, the absence of any decline in bone mineral content with age and no clear evidence of increase in frequency of fractures indicates that this condition is not comparable with postmenopausal osteoporosis and oestrogen therapy is not therefore indicated (Smith *et al* 1982). The osteopenia of Turner's syndrome may represent an independent effect of the chromosome constitution (Shore *et al* 1982).

4.28.2 Aetiology of osteoporosis

A number of dietary and non dietary factors may contribute to the development of osteoporosis and these have been reviewed in detail (Fehily 1989; Christiansen and Riis 1990; Griffin 1990).

Non-dietary factors which are associated with the development of osteoporosis are summarized in Table 4.78. Diet-related factors are discussed below.

Calcium

Overview

Opinion is divided over the question of whether dietary calcium can influence the development of osteoporosis and there are several detailed reviews of this subject (Black 1989; Fehily 1989; Griffin 1990). Kanis and Passmore (1989) argue that calcium deficiency is *not* a contributory factor to osteoporosis for the following reasons:

Table 4.78 Non-dietary risk factors for osteoporosis (Lindsay 1987)

Female sex
Caucasian or Asiatic ethnicity
Positive family history
Early menopause (or oophorectomy)
Sedentary lifestyle
Nulliparity
Cigarette smoking
Secondary causes (see Table 4.77)

1 Calcium requirements are based on balance studies which are flawed in design and interpretation and do not make allowances for man's ability to adapt to lower calcium intakes.
2 Genetic and environmental factors are more important than calcium intake for bone mass.
3 There are no controlled prospective studies which show that an increase in calcium intake increases peak skeletal mass independently of energy intake, or affects later fracture rate.
4 At the menopause, bone loss is the result of gonadal failure and supplying calcium will not necessarily offset calcium losses.

An alternative view in favour of a good calcium intake is put forward by Nordin and Heaney (1990) who:
1 Defend the balance studies done in young adults as indicating a daily allowance of 800–1000 mg calcium.
2 Consider that the increase in bone resorption at the menopause is in response to an increased excretion of calcium.
3 Comment that prospective studies in postmenopausal women do not take into account lifetime calcium intakes, the effect of other nutrients such as phosphorus, protein and sodium, and may be subject to errors in the diet histories.
4 Consider that although the results of calcium supplementation studies in postmenopausal women have not reached the level of statistical significance, they have shown a positive effect intermediate between no treatment and oestrogen treatment.

Calcium requirements

Recommended Daily Allowances for calcium vary widely between different countries. Those for the UK, USA and Australia have been summarized in Table 4.79.

Table 4.79 International Recommended Daily Amounts of Calcium (in mg)

	UK[1] RNI*	USA[2] RDA**	Australia[3] RNI*
Infants			
0–6 months	525	400	300 breast fed; 500 bottle fed
6–12 months	525	600	550
Children			
1–10 years	350–550	800	700–800 (*Female* 8–11 years, 900)
Adolescence			
Males 11–14 years	1000	1200	1200 (12–15 yrs)
15–18 years	1000	1200	1000 (16–18 yrs)
Females 11–14 years	800	1200	1000 (12–15 yrs)
15–18 years	800	1200	800 (16–18 yrs)
Early adulthood (19–24 years)			
Males	700	1200	800
Females	700	1200	800
Adults			
Males	700	800	800
Females	700	800	800
Elderly			
Males	700	800	800
Females	700	800	1000
Pregnancy	No increment	1200	+300
Lactation	+550	1200	+400

* Recommended nutrient intake
** Recommended daily allowance

[1] Department of Health (1991) *Dietary Reference Values for food energy and nutrients for the United Kingdom.* Rep Hlth Soc Subj 41 HMSO, London.
[2] National Research Council (1989) *Recommended Dietary Allowances* 10e. National Academy Press, Washington DC.
[3] Truswell AS (Ed) (1990) *Recommended Nutrient Intakes Australian Papers.* Australian Professional Publications, Sydney.

Discussions of calcium requirement in relation to osteoporosis can be divided into three life stages:

1 The growing years and early adulthood During childhood, linear growth of bone takes place and this is accelerated during the growth spurt of adolescence. Increased mineral deposition then takes place and the peak skeletal mass (PSM) is achieved in the third decade of life. This is determined by genetic and environmental factors and there is currently great interest in maximizing PSM and minimizing bone loss thereafter to maintain strong bones for old age. PSM is followed by a slow phase of bone loss between the age of 30 and the menopause, and the loss in women is accelerated after the menopause. Women start off with a smaller bone mass, and this in part makes them more susceptible to osteoporosis.

A few retrospective studies have attempted to link bone density in postmenopausal women with calcium intake in early life. Women were asked to recall their milk intake in childhood and adolescence and a significant effect on bone density has been described (Sandler *et al* 1985; Angus *et al* 1988). However, it is difficult to recall accurately dietary habits 30–40 years previously so, until this effect is demonstrated prospectively, it cannot be attributed solely to calcium.

In adolescence, it has been shown that calcium intake is one of the main determinants of calcium balance (Matkovic *et al* 1990). In addition, by collating results from 487 balances on normal healthy individuals from infancy to the age of 30, Matkovic (1991) has shown a significant positive relationship between calcium intake and body retention of calcium. Differences in bone density in young adults in two regions of former Yugoslavia have been attributed to calcium (Matkovic *et al* 1979). However, there were marked differences in the energy intake in these two regions which could reflect different levels of physical activity.

Preliminary results on supplementation with calcium of one of a pair of identical twins suggests that bone mass is improved (Slemenda *et al* 1991). Taken together the data does suggest that, in the growing years, calcium intake is an important determinant of bone mass.

The importance of physical exercise as well as calcium has been highlighted by Kanders *et al* (1988) and Halioua and Anderson (1989); their work suggests that the beneficial effect of a good calcium intake was dependent on adequate physical stresses on the skeleton. They suggest that regular weight-bearing activity such as walking should be an integral part of the daily lives of adult women.

A recent consensus conference (Conference Report 1991) has recommended a minimum intake of 800 mg calcium daily for all adults and higher intakes than this during childhood, adolescence, pregnancy and lactation.

2 The postmenopause Immediately postmenopausally there is an increase in urinary calcium excretion, a decrease in efficiency of intestinal calcium absorption and an increase in the rate of bone resorption. About 5–10 years after the menopause the rate of bone loss slows down. Balance studies (Heaney 1978) have suggested that postmenopausal women require 1500 mg of calcium daily to maintain zero calcium balance; those treated with hormone replacement require 1000 mg calcium daily.

Since the bone loss at this time is essentially the result of oestrogen deprivation the effectiveness of increasing dietary calcium at this time has been questioned. Studies which have attempted to correlate calcium intake with bone loss in postmenopausal women have shown equivocal results. (Dawson-Hughes *et al* 1987; Angus *et al* 1988; Stevenson *et al* 1988).

A number of studies have attempted to evaluate the value of calcium supplementation at this life stage (Horsman *et al* 1977; Recker and Heaney 1977; Lamke *et al* 1978; Polley *et al* 1987; Riis *et al* 1987; Smith *et al* 1989). Many can be criticized for their poor design but Cumming (1990) using the statistical technique of beta-analysis has shown that there is a consistent preventive effect of calcium supplements in tablet form on bone mass in postmenopausal women at all sites except the vertebrae. Subsequently, Dawson-Hughes *et al* (1990) have reported that supplements of calcium citrate malate prevented spinal bone loss in a group of women on habitually low calcium diets.

Further studies are needed to identify women at risk of developing postmenopausal osteoporosis and to identify the most effective measures to prevent bone loss at this age.

3 The elderly There is evidence of reduced efficiency of calcium absorption in the elderly (Avioli *et al* 1965; Bullamore *et al* 1970; Robinson 1986) and they may be unable to adapt to low calcium intake as a result of reduced kidney production of the active form of vitamin D (Slovik *et al* 1981). This, together with the lower dietary calcium intakes frequently seen in the elderly may predispose them to calcium deficiency and osteoporosis.

Below 75 years of age, reduced bone mass or osteoporosis appears to be a strong independent risk factor for hip fracture: over 75 years of age bone mass may be less important than neuromuscular protective responses (Cooper *et al* 1987).

A number of groups have studied hip fracture rates as a measure of the incidence of osteoporosis and related this to dietary calcium intake. Holbrook *et al* (1988), using the 24 hour dietary recall method, found an inverse relationship between fractured neck of femur and calcium intake in American Caucasians, independent of other factors such as smoking and alcohol intake, and exercise. Cooper *et al* (1988), using a food frequency and quantity questionnaire in British Caucasians, found that this inverse relationship held only in men consuming over 1 g calcium daily, but also found that, in both sexes, increased daily activity protected against fracture. A prospective study by Wickham *et al* (1989) concluded that reduced dietary calcium does not seem to be a risk factor for hip fracture. However, they found increased risk of hip fracture with decreasing mobility and concluded that physical activity in the elderly is protective. Differences in accuracy of assessing calcium intake may account for the different results from these studies.

Despite these seemingly equivocal results, a recent consensus conference (Conference Report 1991) has recommended a minimum daily intake of 800 mg for adults and higher amounts in old age. Active exercise is useful in the elderly to improve agility, muscular function and reduce the likelihood of falls.

Protein intake

It has been suggested that high protein intakes may contribute to osteoporosis as a result of detrimental effects on calcium balance. When dietary protein is increased experimentally as an isolated nutrient, urinary calcium increases (Johnson *et al* 1970; Walker and Linkswiler 1972; Anand and Linkswiler 1974; Schvette *et al* 1980), probably due to decreased renal tubular reabsorption of calcium (Allen *et al* 1979; Schuette *et al* 1980). If the protein increase is supplied as meat, the phosphorus content of meat may modify this calcuric effect, decreasing the calcium loss (Spencer *et al* 1978; Spencer *et al* 1983). However, phosphorus-rich, high protein diets based on non-meat protein still induce negative calcium balance (Johnson *et al* 1970; Walker and Linkswiler 1972; Hegsted *et al* 1981; Hegsted and Linkswiler 1981). Spencer *et al* (1983) have suggested that adaptation to high protein diets occurs with time. However, Allen *et al* (1979), from longer term studies using formula diets, conclude that even the consumption of high calcium diets is unlikely to prevent the negative calcium balance and probable bone loss induced by the consumption of high protein diets.

In a literature review, Kerstetter and Allen (1990) conclude that strong evidence links the intake of commonly consumed dietary proteins to urinary calcium and calcium balance at typical consumption levels of calcium and phosphorus. Protein intakes within the DRV are compatible with calcium equilibrium, but intakes above 75 g/day tend to result in negative calcium balance.

Lacto-ovo-vegetarian diets

A lacto-ovo-vegetarian (LOV) diet which contains milk, cheese, eggs, legumes and soya products but no meat or fish may have a protective effect on the skeleton, particularly in postmenopausal women. In one study, LOV women over 50 had a slower rate of bone loss than omnivores despite similar bone densities up until the age of 50 (Marsh *et al* 1980). Since the LOV subjects were Seventh Day Adventists, they may have had other favourable lifestyle variables such as not smoking and not drinking caffeinated beverages or alcohol. However, these lifestyle differences do not appear to have affected the two male groups in the same study, where bone densities between omnivores and LOV males were similar at all ages (Marsh *et al* 1983). Other work has shown that lacto-ovo-vegetarians of both sexes may be less prone to osteoporosis than omnivores (Ellis *et al* 1972).

Fibre intake

There have been few detailed studies on the effect of dietary fibre on mineral metabolism but those which have been done suggest that increasing dietary fibre significantly increases calcium excretion. It has been calculated by one group that an increase of fibre intake of 13 g/day increases calcium requirements by 75 mg/day (Heaney *et al* 1982). Similarly, Hallfrisch *et al* (1987) have suggested that high fibre diets increase the amount of dietary calcium required to maintain calcium balance.

Studies of high fibre diets containing either cereal or fruit/vegetable fibre have shown a trend towards negative calcium balance at high fibre intakes, despite increases of calcium with the additional fibre (Cummings 1978; Kelsay *et al* 1979). In the case of cereals, this may in part be due to the phytic acid content but it is possible that the fibre itself interferes with mineral absorption and metabolism (Cummings 1978). A recent study on young women has indicated that dietary fibre may lower plasma androgen concentrations and so lower peak trabecular bone density, but this observation needs further work (Leuenberger *et al* 1989).

Long term effects of high fibre intakes have not been studied and until it is established whether, over a course of weeks or months, humans are able to adapt and not lose calcium, it must be assumed that very high fibre intakes may be detrimental in terms of calcium absorption and metabolism.

Alcohol intake

Alcoholic patients with chronic liver disease have been shown to sustain more peripheral fractures than those with other liver disorders (Diamond *et al* 1990). In part this may be due to the increased likelihood of falls in this group, but there is also evidence that bone mineral content is decreased in alcoholics when compared to normal controls (Nilsson and Westlin 1973). Chronic alcohol abuse probably has a direct effect on bone remodelling (Bikle *et al* 1985; Feitelberg *et al* 1987) but there may be secondary effects on the bone due to liver damage and consequent disordered vitamin D metabolism (Lalor *et al* 1986) or parathyroid hormone metabolism (Feitelberg *et al* 1987). Poor nutrition may also be contributory, in particular inadequate vitamin D from either dietary sources or solar exposure (Lalor *et al* 1986; Feitelberg *et al* 1987).

The degree to which a moderate alcohol intake affects bone maintenance has not yet been established.

Sodium intake

An increase in salt intake causes an increase in urinary calcium excretion over a wide range of salt consumption, (Kleeman *et al* 1964, Meyer *et al* 1976; Breslau *et al* 1982; Zarkades *et al* 1989). In younger people there may be a compensatory increase in intestinal calcium absorption though increased 1,25 dihydroxy vitamin D synthesis, probably mediated by parathyroid hormone (Breslau *et al* 1982). As a result of this adaptive process, net calcium balance does not change (Meyer *et al* 1976). However, this compensatory rise in calcium absorption has been shown to be absent in elderly women (Parland *et al* 1989) possibly as a result of deficient production of active vitamin D in the kidney (Slovik *et al* 1981). Breslau *et al* (1982) hypothesize that, on a high sodium diet, failure to adapt to increased renal calcium losses by increased intestinal calcium absorption may be a contributory factor to the bone disease of elderly osteoporotics and individuals with pseudohypoparathyroidism.

Fluoride

Long term ingestion of fluoride leads to its accumulation in the skeleton owing to the conversion of hydroxyapatite to fluorapatite. This occurs in either treatment of osteoporosis with fluoride, or in the ingestion of drinking water with a high fluoride content (Meunier *et al* 1989). Whether the resulting bone is less prone to fracture is equivocal: fluoridic bone has increased crystallinity and may have decreased elasticity and be more brittle. Comparisons have been made between areas with either a high or low flouride content in drinking water but the conclusions are unclear. Some high fluoride areas show less evidence of osteoporosis (Bernstein *et al* 1966) or of fractured hip (Simonen and Laitinen 1985). Others have shown reduced bone mass in older women in a high fluoride community, but better bone mass in young women in a high fluoride community if they also consumed more than 800 mg calcium and 400 international units of vitamin D daily (Sowers *et al* 1986).

In subjects with renal impairment, habitual consumption of fluoride-rich mineral water could lead to skeletal fluorosis (Meunier *et al* 1989).

Boron, magnesium, zinc, manganese and copper

Boron is a mineral which is thought to have a close relationship with calcium metabolism. One small study (Nielson *et al* 1987) of supplementing postmenopausal women on low boron diets with 3 mg boron resulted in markedly elevated serum concentrations of 17 beta-oestradiol and testosterone particularly when dietary magnesium was low. These hormonal changes would be beneficial in preventing calcium loss and bone demineralization. However there is no other supporting evidence for this observation.

There has been little work with magnesium. There is a preliminary report of low serum magnesium in postmenopausal osteoporotics (Reginster *et al* 1989). This is probably not of dietary significance but low serum magnesium could be used as a diagnostic tool for identifying a subset of patients at risk of developing postmenopausal osteoporosis.

The concentration of zinc in bone is higher than in most other tissues and there is strong evidence that zinc has an active role in bone metabolism but the exact mechanism remains unknown (Calhoun *et al* 1974).

Manganese and copper are known to be required for bone growth but their role in the development of osteoporosis is not known (Heaney 1988).

Vitamin D

Although vitamin D is necessary for normal bone formation, osteoporosis is not considered to be a disorder of vitamin D deficiency. At all ages, adequate sunlight exposure should be encouraged so that normal skin production of vitamin can take place, but this is particularly important for the elderly, since skin capacity to produce vitamin D decreases with ageing (MacLaughlin and Holick 1985) and subclinical vitamin D deficiency may occur. In addition, with ageing, there is evidence of reduced kidney production of the active form of vitamin D, 1,25 dihydroxycholecalciferol (1,25 OHD). Low levels of 1,25 OHD have been found in postmenopausal women (Prince *et al* 1988), in elderly women (Tsai *et al* 1984) and in elderly osteoporotic patients (Slovik *et al* 1981). This may be one factor in the apparent rise in dietary requirement to maintain calcium balance in postmenopausal women. It would explain the reduced calcium absorption in the elderly, predisposing them to calcium deficiency at the low calcium intakes common in this age group.

Early reports indicate possible beneficial effects of vitamin D with calcium supplements in prevention of osteoporosis. Pouilles *et al* (1992) using 1-alpha dihydroxy vitamin D in postmenopausal women showed a reduction in vertebral bone loss. Using vitamin D3, Chapuy *et al* (1992) showed a reduction in the risk of hip fractures in elderly women. Although studies of the use of 1,25 dihydroxy vitamin D3 have given conflicting results concerning bone remodelling, this, or other vitamin D metabolites may have a role in the correction of calcium malabsorption (Lamberg-Allardt 1991).

Vitamin K

Vitamin K is required for the formation of a bone protein called osteocalcin but the function of osteocalcin is still uncertain (Nutrition Reviews 1979).

Low serum levels of vitamin K have been found in women with osteoporosis who have sustained either spinal crush-fractures or fractures of the neck of femur, but until more is known about the vitamin K content of foods, it is impossible to establish whether this is physiological or related to dietary deficiency.

Lactase deficiency

Lactase deficiency can affect calcium absorption. In normal adults, lactose (or its component sugars) may enhance jejunal calcium absorption in proportion to its effect on fluid absorption (King and Schuette 1988; Schuette *et al* 1989). However, in people with intestinal lactase deficiency, calcium absorption may be decreased in the presence of lactose (Condon *et al* 1970; Kocian *et al* 1973) although this reduction may not occur when smaller, more physiological loads of lactose are consumed (Smith *et al* 1985b; Tremaine *et al* 1986). Nevertheless, there is some evidence of increased incidence of osteoporosis in individuals with intolerance to lactose (Finkenstedt *et al* 1986) which may in part be the result of avoidance of milk and milk products and consequent fall in calcium intake (Birge *et al* 1967; Newcomer *et al* 1978; Horowitz *et al* 1987). It seems prudent to ensure that lactose-intolerant individuals include plenty of low lactose, high calcium foods in the diet such as enzyme treated milk and yoghurt, which is better digested by lactase deficient individuals (Kolars *et al* 1984) and hard cheese, which contains negligible amounts of lactose. Calcium supplements may sometimes be indicated.

Caffeine intake

Caffeine has been shown to increase calcium lost in the urine of healthy young women (Massey and Wise 1984) and to be associated with increased urinary calcium and intestinal calcium secretion in middle aged premenopausal women (Heaney and Recker 1982). This may contribute to a more negative calcium balance (Barger-Lux *et al* 1990), the significance of which is greater when combined with a low dietary calcium intake (Massey *et al* 1989). The effect may be quite small at lower intakes of caffeine, but may be significant at extreme intakes (above 1 g caffeine per day). 1 g caffeine would be obtained from about ten cups of percolated coffee or 15 cups of instant coffee daily, although this varies with brands and preparation methods (Bunker and McWilliams 1979; Scott *et al* 1989). Proprietary cold relief, pain relief or caffeine stimulant tablets provide further sources (Graham 1978).

Physical activity

Prolonged bed-rest leads to an increase in urinary and faecal calcium, with overall negative calcium balance and loss of bone mass (Krolner and Toft 1983). Reambulation will induce partial or complete remineralization of the skeleton (Donaldson *et al* 1970; Vogel and Whittle 1976; Krolner and Toft 1983).

The beneficial effect of exercise in the prevention of bone loss in postmenopausal women has been demonstrated in a number of controlled studies (Aloia *et al* 1978; Krolner *et al* 1983; Chow *et al* 1987). At the other extreme, strenuous athletic training in females can lead to low plasma oestrogen levels, amenorrhoea and reduced bone density. Weight-bearing activity increases the bone density of women with normal menses but does not enhance it in women with menstrual dysfunction (Howat *et al* 1989). Differences in calcium intake do not explain the reduced bone density associated with amenorrhoea, but there may be a link with negative energy balance which may be induced in athletes either by a reduced energy intake (Nelson *et al* 1986) or increased energy expenditure.

Body weight and smoking

Daniell (1976) noted a striking association between the early presence of osteoporosis and both cigarette smoking and lack of obesity in postmenopausal women. An association between low body weight and osteoporosis had already been noted, and it was suggested that fatty tissue may produce oestrogens in sufficient quantity to protect against the development of bone atrophy. Both smoking and low body weight tend to induce an earlier menopause which advances the development of osteoporosis by several years. However, more complex smoking-related phenomena other than an early menopause may be involved in the process.

4.28.3 Treatment of adult osteoporosis

Where osteoporosis is secondary to some other disorder such as malabsorption or hyperthyroidism, treatment is aimed at correction of the primary disorder, and the provision at the same time of an adequate calcium intake to enable the bones to heal. Where there is evidence of concomitant vitamin D deficiency, supplements should be given.

Adult osteoporosis is probably not a homogeneous disorder, and different sub-groups may respond to different treatments, but identification of these sub-groups is still in the research stage.

Many of the current treatments for postmenopausal osteoporosis are still in the investigational or experimental stage. (For useful reviews on the subject see Kanis 1986; Christianson and Riis 1990; *Lancet* 1990). Some of these treatments are outlined below.

Non-hormonal

Sodium fluoride with or without calcium or vitamin D

This has been used under research conditions for some

years but a recent randomized research trial in postmenopausal women has suggested that whereas the bone mass is increased by this treatment, it may not be increased in strength and so they may be no less prone to fractures (Riggs *et al* 1990). It is possible that at lower doses than used in Rigg's study, fluoride may still be a useful treatment but more research is needed in this area (Reeve *et al* 1990).

Bisphosphonates

Double-blind trials of the bisphosphonate Etidronate used for 2–3 years in women with postmenopausal osteoporosis have shown encouraging results (Storm *et al* 1990; Watts *et al* 1990). Those given the drug showed a moderate increase in vertebral bone density and reduction in fracture rates compare with controls. This is hopeful as an alternative for those women who cannot take hormone replacement (see below).

Hormonal

Calcitonin

In two year studies calcitonin has been shown to be successful in prevention (MacIntyre *et al* 1988) and treatment (Gruber *et al* 1984) of postmenopausal osteoporosis by reducing bone loss, but a reduction in fracture rates has not been demonstrated. Until recently synthetic human or synthetic salmon calcitonin was given by subcutaneous injection. Recent research studies have shown that administration of calcitonin by nasal sprays (Reginster *et al* 1987; Overgaard *et al* 1989) is effective and would be more universally acceptable to patients.

Synthetic parathyroid hormone

This has been researched for some years (Reeve *et al* 1976; 1980; 1989) and seems to stimulate the formation of new bone. Attempts to improve calcium absorption at the same time by the addition of 1,25 dihydroxycholecalciferol (Neer *et al* 1987) or oestrogens have shown early success (Reeve *et al* 1991). This is still a very expensive treatment which requires to be given by daily or frequent injections.

Oestrogen with or without gestagen

Oestrogen is known to prevent postmenopausal bone loss (Christiansen *et al* 1980; Stevenson and Whitehead 1982; Conference Report 1987), but does not increase bone mass (Christiansen and Riis 1990). Many gynaecologists consider the addition of a progestogen to the continuous oestrogen treatment is mandatory in women who have not had a hysterectomy, to prevent endometrial hyperplasia. This treatment is not suitable for all postmenopausal women, and the long term safety of hormone replacement therapy is not yet established. Current knowledge of short and long term risks have been discussed by Christiansen and Riis (1990).

Anabolic steroids

Anabolic steroids are synthetic derivatives of natural androgens. These include nandrolene decanoate and stanozolol which have for many years been used for the treatment of osteoporosis to stimulate bone formation (Christiansen and Riis 1990). They have not been shown to prevent bone fracture and their associated side effects may include fluid retention, virilization, hyperlipidaemia and cholestasis which limit their usefulness (Griffin 1990).

Monitoring treatment

Calcium balance studies may be used to monitor the progress of treatment (see Metabolic Balance diets, Section 6.1). The following factors should be noted when using this technique and interpreting results.

1 Level of activity. Immobilization leads to loss of calcium from the bones. During calcium balance studies patients should be encouraged to maintain their usual level of physical activity.

2 Weekly variations in calcium balance. There are week to week variations in calcium balance, both in normal subjects (Malm 1958) and in those with osteoporosis (Hesp *et al* 1979).

3 Seasonal variations in calcium balance. A seasonal cycle in calcium may occur in some subjects (Malm 1958).

4 Individual adaptation. Adaptation to the habitual diet may lead to a temporary negative balance if intake is reduced.

4.28.4 Prevention

Dietary aetiological risk factors for osteoporosis have been discussed above. The tendency for affluent Western societies to consume diets with high protein and relatively low calcium content, combined with increasing fibre intakes, may predispose to negative calcium balance and to enhanced bone loss. Increased dietary calcium intake may help to balance this loss.

The preservation of mobility may also be an important factor in reducing the rate of bone loss.

Postmenopausally, calcium supplements (discussed below) may help to slow down the rate of bone loss and, if instituted early enough in subjects at risk, could slow down the advent of fractures. However, it is an important research objective to develop simple means to identify clearly those individuals at risk of developing clinical osteoporosis with eventual fractures. For these patients, combination therapy (an oestrogen with a sequential gestagen) may be the only effective preventive measure (Christiansen *et al* 1980; Christiansen and Riis 1990).

Calcium supplementation

Calcium in tablet form may be required to boost calcium intake when dietary calcium cannot be increased or dairy products are excluded from the diet as part of treatment.

Many calcium supplements, such as gluconate, lactate and carbonate are commercially available. Calcium carbonate contains a higher percentage of calcium (40%) compared to calcium gluconate or lactate (10%) (Spencer and Kramer 1986). This means a smaller number of tablets are required and compliance is likely to be better.

Absorption studies on the various salts of calcium have shown similar absorptions from carbonate, acetate, lactate, gluconate and citrate salts in young healthy subjects (Sheikh *et al* 1987) but further studies are needed to determine the salts which are most suitable for older people. There is evidence that under fasting conditions, the absorption of calcium from calcium carbonate is reduced in subjects with achlorhydria. As achlorhydria is common in older persons a better alternative may be a soluble form of calcium such as a pH adjusted (5.8) citrate (Recker 1985). If calcium carbonate is used it would seem best to recommend that it is taken with a meal to facilitate normal absorption (Heaney *et al* 1989). However, one group has used an effervescent mixture of calcium gluconate, lactate and carbonate given in a single evening dose to ensure an adequate supply of calcium through the night, when there is no food intake and calcium continues to be lost from the body (Polley *et al* 1987).

Calcium supplements are contraindicated in patients who have or who have had calcium oxalate kidney stones but whether these supplements increase the risk of stone formation in the rest of the population is unknown (Waldron 1989). There is also some evidence to suggest that calcium supplements may inhibit the absorption of minerals, especially iron (Dawson-Hughes *et al* 1986; Cook *et al* 1991; Hallberg *et al* 1991). Further research is needed to establish whether this is likely to be a significant problem.

The topic of calcium supplements has recently been reviewed by Heaney (1991).

Useful addresses

The National Osteoporosis Society, PO Box 10, Radstock, Bath BA3 34B.

References

Alevizaki M, Stevenson JC, Girgis SI, MacIntyre I and Legon S (1989) Altered calcitonium gene in a young patient with osteoporosis. *Br Med J* **298**, 1215–16.

Allen LH, Oddoye EA and Margen S (1979) Protein induced hypercalciuria: a longer term study. *Am J Clin Nutr* **32**, 741–9.

Aloia JF, Cohn SH, Ostuni JA, Cane R and Ellis K (1978) Prevention of involutional bone loss by exercise. *Ann Intern Med* **89**, 356–8.

Anand CR and Linkswiler H (1974) Effect of protein intake on calcium balance of young men given 500 mg calcium daily. *J Nutr* **104**, 695–700.

Angus RM, Sambrook PM, Pocock NA and Eisman JA (1988) Dietary intake and bone mineral density. *Bone and Mineral* **4**, 265–77.

Avioli LV, McDonald JE and Lee SW (1965) The influence of age on the intestinal absorption of 47Ca in women and its relation to 47Ca absorption in postmenopausal osteoporosis. *J Clin Invest* **44**, 1960–67.

Barger-Lux MJ, Heaney Robert P and Stegman MR (1990) Effects of moderate caffeine intake on the calcium economy of premenopausal women. *Am J Clin Nutr* **52**, 722–5.

Bernstein DS, Sadowsky N, Hegsted DM, Guri CD and Stare FJ (1966) Prevalence of osteoporosis in high- and low-fluoride areas in North Dakota. *J Am Med Assoc* **198**, 85–90.

Bikle DD, Genant HK, Cann C, Recker RR, Halloran BP and Strewler GJ (1985) Bone disease in alcohol abuse. *Ann Intern Med* **103**, 42–8.

Biller BMK, Saxe V, Herzog DB, Rosenthal DI, Holzman S and Klibanski A (1989) Mechanisms of osteoporosis in adult and adolescent women with anorexia nervosa. *J Clin Endocrinol Metab* **65**(3), 548–52.

Birge SJ, Keutmann HT, Cuatrecasas P and Whedon GD (1967) Osteoporosis, intestinal lactase deficiency and low dietary calcium intake. *N Eng J Med* **276**, 445–8.

Black D (1989) *Calcium: the report of the British Nutrition Foundation's task force*. BNF, London.

Breslau NA, McGuire JL, Zerwekh JE and Pak CYC (1982) The role of dietary sodium on renal excretion and intestinal absorption of calcium and on vitamin D metabolism. *J Clin Endocrinol Metab* **55**, 369–73.

Bullamore JR, Gallagher JC, Wilkinson RY, Nordin BEC and Marshall DH (1970) Effect of age on calcium absorption. *Lancet* **ii**, 535–7.

Bunker ML and McWilliams M (1979) Caffeine content of common beverages. *J Am Dietet Assoc* **74**, 28–32.

Calhoun NR, Smith JC and Becker KL (1974) The role of zinc in bone metabolism. *Clin Orthop Rel Res* **103**, 212–34.

Chapuy MC, Arlot ME, Duboeuf F, Brun J, Crouzet MS, Arnaud S, Delmas PD, Meunier PJ (1992) Vitamin D3 and calcium to prevent hip fractures in elderly women *N Engl J Med* **327**, 1637–42.

Chow R, Harrison JE and Notarius C (1987) Effect of two randomised exercise programmes on bone mass of healthy postmenopausal women. *Br Med J* **295**, 1441–4.

Christiansen C, Christiansen MS, McNair P, Hagen C, Stocklund K and Transbol IB (1980) Prevention of early post-menopausal bone loss: controlled two year study in 315 normal females. *Eur J Clin Invest* **10**, 273–9.

Christiansen C and Riis BJ (1990) *The silent epidemic. Postmenopausal osteoporosis*. National Osteoporosis Society/European Foundation for Osteoporosis and Bone Disease.

Condon JR, Nassim JR, Millard FJC, Hilbe A and Stainthorpe EM (1970) Calcium and phosphorus metabolism in relation to lactose intolerance. *Lancet* **i**, 1027–9.

Conference Report (1991) Third International Symposium on Osteoporosis and Consensus Development, Copenhagen, Denmark, 14–20 October 1990. *Osteoporosis International* **1**(2), 114–17.

Conference Report (1987) Consensus development conference: prophylaxis and treatment of osteoporosis. *Br Med J* **295**, 914–15.

Cook JD, Dassenko SA and Whittaker P (1991) Calcium supplementation: effect on iron absorption. *Am J Clin Nutr* **53**, 106–111.

Cooper C, Barker DJP, Morris J and Briggs RSJ (1987) Osteoporosis, falls and age in fracture of the proximal femur *Br Med J* **295**, 13–15.

Cooper C, Barker DJP and Wickham C (1988) Physical activity, muscle strength and calcium intake in fracture of the proximal femur in Britain. *Br Med J* **297**, 1443–6.

Cumming RG (1990) Calcium intake and bone mass: A quantitative review of the evidence. *Calcif Tissue Int* **47**, 194–201.

Cummings JH (1978) Nutritional implications of dietary fiber. *Am J Clin Nutr* **31** (supplement), S21–S29.

Daniell HW (1976) Osteoporosis of the slender smoker. *Arch Intern Med* **136**, 298–304.

Dawson-Hughes B, Dallal GE, Krall EA, Sadowski L, Sahyoun N and Tannenbaum S (1990) A controlled trial of the effect of calcium supplementation on bone density in postmenopausal women. *N Engl J Med* **323**, 878–83.

Dawson-Hughes B, Jacques P and Shipp C (1987) Dietary calcium intake and bone loss from the spine in healthy postmenopausal women. *Am J Clin Nutr* **46**, 685–7.

Dawson-Hughes B, Seligson FH and Hughes VA (1986) Effects of calcium carbonate and hydroxyapatite on zinc and iron retention in postmenopausal women. *Am J Clin Nutr* **44**, 83–88.

Dent CE and Friedman M (1965) Idiopathic juvenile osteoporosis. *Quart J Med* **34**, 177–210.

Diamond T, Stiel D, Lunzer M, Wilkinson M, Roche J and Posen S (1990) Osteoporosis and skeletal fractures in chronic liver disease. *Gut* **31**, 82–7.

Donaldson CL, Hulley SB, Vogel JM, Hattner RS, Bayers JH and McMillan DE (1970) Effect of prolonged bed rest on bone mineral. *Metabolism* **19**, 1071–84.

Ellis FR, Holesh S and Ellis JW (1972) Incidence of osteoporosis in vegetarians and omnivores. *Am J Clin Nutr* **25**, 555–8.

Fehily AM (1989) Dietary determinants of bone mass and fracture risk: a review. *J Hum Nutr Dietet* **2**, 299–313.

Feitelberg S, Epstein S, Ismail F and D'Amanda C (1987) Deranged bone mineral metabolism in chronic alcoholism. *Metabolism* **36**, 322–66.

Finkenstedt G, Skrabal F, Gasser RW and Brausteiner H (1986) Lactose absorption, milk consumption, and fasting blood glucose concentration in women with idiopathic osteoporosis. *Br Med J* **292**, 161–2.

Graham DM (1978) Caffeine – its identity, dietary sources, intake and biological effects. *Nutr Rev* **36**, 97–102.

Griffiths HT and Liu DTY (1984) Severe heparin osteoporosis in pregnancy. *Postgrad Med J* **60**, 424–5.

Gruber HE, Ivey JL, Baylink DJ, Matthews M, Nelp WB, Sisom K and Chesnut CH (1984) Long-term Calcitonin therapy in postmenopausal osteoporosis. *Metabolism* **33**, 295–303.

Halioua L and Anderson JJB (1989) Lifetime calcium intake and physical activity habits: independent and combined effects on the radial bone of healthy premenopausal Caucasian women. *Am J Clin Nutr* **49**, 534–41.

Hallberg L, Brune M, Erlandsson M, Sandberg A and Rossander-Hulten L (1991) Calcium: effect of different amounts on nonheme and heme-iron absorption in humans. *Am J Clin Nutr* **53**, 112–19.

Hallfrisch J, Powell A, Carafelli C, Reiser S and Prather ES (1987) Mineral balances of men and women consuming high fibre diets with complex or simple carbohydrate. *J Nutr* **117**, 48–55.

Harinck HJ, Bijvoet OLM, Van de Meer JWH, Jones B and Onvlee GJ (1984) Regression of bone lesions in Gauchers disease during treatment with aminohydroxypropylidene bisphosphonate (letter). *Lancet* **ii**, 513.

Heaney RP (1988) Nutritional factors in causation of osteoporosis. *Ann Chir Gynaecol* **77**, 176–9.

Heaney RP (1991) Calcium supplements. Practical considerations. *Osteoporosis International* **1**(2), 65–71.

Heaney RP, Gallagher JC, Johnston CC, Neer R, Parfitt AM, Chir B and Whedon GD (1982) Calcium nutrition and bone health in the elderly. *Am J Clin Nutr* **36**, 986–1013.

Heaney RP and Recker RR (1982) Effects of nitrogen, phosphorus and caffeine on calcium balance in women. *J Lab Clin Med* **99**, 46–55.

Heaney RP, Recker RR and Saville PD (1978) Menopausal changes in calcium balance performance. *J Lab Clin Med* **92**(6), 953–63.

Heaney RP, Smith KT, Recker RR and Hinders SM (1989) Meal effects on calcium absorption. *Am J Clin Nutr* **49**, 372–6.

Hegsted M and Linkswiler HM (1981) Long term effects of level of protein intake on calcium metabolism in young adult women. *J Nutr* **111**, 244–51.

Hegsted M, Schuette SA, Zemel MB and Linkswiler HM (1981) Urinary calcium and calcium balance in young men as affected by level of protein and phosphorus intake. *J Nutr* **111**, 553–62.

Hesp R, Williams D, Rinsler M and Reeve J (1979) A comparison of chromium sesquioxide and 51Cr chromic chloride as inert markets in calcium balance studies. *Clin Sci* **57**, 89–92.

Hoekman K, Papapoulos SE, Peters ACB and Bijvoet OLM (1985) Characteristics and bisphosphate treatment of a patient with juvenile osteoporosis. *J Clin Endocrinol Metab* **61**, 952–6.

Holbrook TL, Barret-Connor E and Wingard DL (1988) Dietary calcium and risk of hip fracture: 14 year prospective population study. *Lancet* **ii**, 1046–9.

Horsman A, Gallagher JC, Simpson M and Nordin BEC (1977) Prospective trial of oestrogen and calcium in postmenopausal women. *Br Med J* **2**, 789–92.

Horowitz M, Wishart J, Mundy L and Nordin BEC (1987) Lactose and calcium absorption in postmenopausal osteoporosis. *Arch Intern Med* **147**, 534–6.

Howat PM, Carbo ML, Mills GQ and Wozniak P (1989) The influence of diet, body fat, menstrual cycling and activity upon the bone density of females. *J Am Dietet Assoc* **89**, 1305–7.

Johnson NE, Alcantara EN and Linkswiler H (1970) Effect of level of protein intake on urinary and faecal calcium and calcium retention of young adult males. *J Nutr* **100**, 1425–30.

Kanders B, Dempster DW and Lindsay R (1988) Interaction of calcium nutrition and physical activity on bone mass in young women. *J Bone Miner Res* **3**, 145–9.

Kanis JA (1986) Practical aspects of the management of osteoporosis. A round table discussion held at the Postgraduate Medical Centre, City Hospital, Nottingham 17th September 1986. Session III Treatment of Osteoporosis 19–21. *International Medicine Supplement* no 12.

Kanis JA and Passmore R (1989) Calcium supplementation of the diet. I. *Br Med J* **298**, 137–40. II. *Br Med J* **298**, 205–208.

Kelsay JL, Behall KM and Prather ES (1979) Effect of fiber from fruits and vegetables on metabolic responses of human subjects. II Calcium, magnesium, iron, and silicone balances. *Am J Clin Nutr* **32**, 1876–86.

Kerstetter JE and Allen LH (1990) Dietary protein increases urinary calcium. *J Nutr* **120**, 134–136.

King CM and Schuette SA (1988) The effect of lactose in milk on absorption of Ca by postmenopausal women. *Am J Clin Nutr* **47**, 788 (abstract).

Kleeman CR, Bohannan J, Bernstein D, Ling S and Maxwell MH (1964) Effect of variations in sodium intake on calcium excretion in normal humans. *Proc Soc Exp Biol* **115**, 29–32.

Kocian J, Skala I and Bakos K (1973) Calcium absorption from milk and lactose-free milk in healthy subjects and patients with lactose intolerance. *Digestion* **9**, 317–24.

Kolars JC, Levitt MD, Aouji M and Savaiano DA (1984) Yoghurt – an autodigesting source of lactose. *N Eng J Med* **310**, 1–3.

Krolner B and Toft B (1983) Vertebral bone loss: and un-heeded side effect of therapeutic bed rest. *Clin Sci* **64**, 537–40.

Krolner B, Toft B, Nielsen SP and Tondevold E (1983) Physical exercise as prophylaxis against involutional vertebral bone loss: a controlled trial. *Clin Sci* **64**, 541–6.

Lalor BC, France MW, Powell D, Adams PH and Counihan TB (1986) Bone and mineral metabolism in chronic alcohol abuse. *Quart J Med* **229**, 497–511.

Lamberg-Allardt C (1991) Is there a role for Vitamin D in Osteoporosis? *Calcif Tissue Int (Suppl)* **49**, S46–S49.

Lamke B, Sjoberg H and Sylven M (1978) Bone mineral content in women with Colles fractures: effect of calcium supplementation. *Acta Orthop Scand* **49**, 143–6.

Lancet (1990) Editorial. New treatments for osteoporosis *Lancet* **i**, 1065–6.

Leuenberger PK, Buchanan JR, Myers CA, Lloyd T and Demers LM

(1989) Determination of peak trabecular bone density: interplay of dietary fiber, carbohydrate, and androgens. *Am J Clin Nutr* **50**, 955–61.

Lindsay R (1985) The osteoporoses. *Medicine* **2**, 609–614.

Lindsay R (1987) Managing osteoporosis: current trends, future possibilities. *Geriatrics* **42**(3), 35–40.

MacIntyre I, Stevenson JC, Whitehead MI, Wimalawansa SJ, Banks LM and Healy MJR (1988) Calcitonin for prevention of postmenopausal bone loss. *Lancet* **i**, 900–901.

MacLaughlin J and Holick MF (1985) Aging decreases the capacity of human skin to produce vitamin D3. *J Clin Invest* **76**, 1536–8.

Mahalko JR, Stanstead HH, Johnson L and Milne DB (1983) Effect of a moderate increase in dietary protein on the retention and excretion of Ca, Cu, Fe, Mg, P and Zn by adult males. *Am J Clin Nutr* **37**, 8–14.

Malm OJ (1958) Calcium requirement and adaptation in adult man. *Scand J Clin Lab Invest* **10** (Suppl 36), 1–290.

Marder HK, Tsang RC, Hug G and Crawford AC (1982) Calcitriol deficiency in idiopathic juvenile osteoporosis. *Am J Dis Child* **136**, 914–17.

Marsh AG, Sanchez TV, Chaffee FL, Mayor GH and Mickelsen O (1983) Bone mineral mass in adult lacto-ovo-vegetarian and omniverous males. *Am J Clin Nutr* **37**, 453–6.

Marsh AG, Sanchez TV, Mickelsen O, Keiser J and Mayor G (1980) Cortical bone density of adult lact-ovo-vegetarian and omnivorous women. *J Am Dietet Assoc* **76**, 148–51.

Massey LK, Sherrard DJ and Bergman EA (1989) Dietary caffeine lowers ultrafiltrable calcium levels in women consuming low dietary calcium. *J Bone Mineral Res* **4**, S1–249 (abstr).

Massey LK and Wise KJ (1984) The effect of dietary caffeine on urinary excretion of calcium, magnesium, sodium and potassium in healthy young females. *Nut Res* **4**, 43–50.

Matkovik V (1991) Calcium metabolism and calcium requirements during skeletal modeling and consolidation of bone mass. *Am J Clin Nutr* **54** (Suppl), 245S–260S.

Matkovic V, Fontana D, Tominac C, Cedomil, Geol P and Chesnut CH (1990) Factors that influence peak bone mass formation: a study of calcium balance and the inheritance of bone mass in adolescent females. *Am J Clin Nutr* **52**, 873–88.

Matkovic V, Kostial K, Simonovic I, Buzina R, Brodarec A and Nordin BEC (1979) Bone status and fracture rates in two regions of Yugoslavia. *Am J Clin Nutr* **32**, 540–49.

Medical News & Perspective (1987) *J Am Med Assoc* **257**(24), 3324–5.

Meunier PJ, Femanias M, Dubeouf F, Chapuy MC and Delmas PD (1989) Increased vertebral bone density in heavy drinkers of mineral waters rich in fluoride (letter) *Lancet* **i**, 152.

Meyer WJ, Transbol I, Bartter FC and Delea C (1976) Control of calcium absorption: effect of sodium chloride loading and depletion. *Metabolism* **25**, 989–93.

Neer RM, Slovik D, Doppelt S, Daly M, Rosenthal D, Lo C and Potts JT Jr (1987) In (Editors) *Osteoporosis 1987* Christiansen *et al* p. 829. Osteopress ApS Copenhagen.

Nelson ME, Fisher EC, Catsos PD, Meredith CN, Turksoy RN and Evans WJ (1986) Diet and bone status in amenorrheic runners. *Am J Clin Nutr* **43**, 910–16.

Newcomer A, Hodgson SF, McGill DB and Thomas PJ (1978) Lactase deficiency: prevalence in osteoporosis. *Ann Intern Med* **89**, 219–20.

Nielsen FH, Hunt CD, Mullen LM and Hunt JR (1987) Effect of dietary boron on mineral, oestrogen, and testosterone metabolism in postmenopausal women. *Fed Amer Soc Exper Biol* **1**, 394–7.

Nilsson BE and Westlin NE (1973) Changes in bone mass in alcoholics. *Clin Orthop Rel Res* **90**, 229–32.

Nordin BEC and Heaney RP (1990) Calcium supplementation of the diet: justified by present evidence. *Br Med J* **300**, 1056–60.

Nutrition Reviews (1979) Osteocalcin: a vitamin K-dependent calcium-binding protein in bone. *Nutr Rev* **37**(2), 54–7.

Ostlere L, Warner T, Meunier PJ, Hulme P, Hesp R, Watts RWE and Reeve J (1991) Treatment of Type 1 Gaucher's disease affecting bone with aminohydroxypropylidene bisphosphonate (pamidronate). *Quart J Med* New Series 79, **290**, 503–15.

Overgaard K, Riis BJ, Christiansen C, Podenphant J and Johansen JS (1989) Nasal calcitonin for treatment of established osteoporosis. *Clin Endocrinol* **30**, 435–42.

Parland BE, Goulding A and Campbell AJ (1989) Dietary salt affects biochemical markers of resorption and formation of bone in elderly women. *Br Med J* **299**, 834–5.

Polley KJ, Nordin BEC, Baghurst PA, Walker CJ and Chatterton BE (1987) Effect of calcium supplementation on forearm bone mineral content in postmenopausal women: a prospective, sequential controlled trial. *J Nutr* **117** 1929–35.

Pouilles JM, Tremollieres F and Ribot C (1992) Prevention of post-menopausal bone loss with 1 alpha hydroxy vitamin D3. A three year prospective study. *Clin Rheumatol* **11(4)**, 492–7.

Prince R, Dick I, Boyd F, Kent N and Garcia-Webb P (1988) The effects of dietary calcium deprivation on serum calcitriol levels in premenopausal and postmenopausal women. *Metabolism* **37**, 727–31.

Recker RR (1985) Calcium absorption and achlorhydria. *N Engl J Med* **313**, 70–73.

Recker R and Heaney RP (1977) Effect of estrogens and calcium carbonate on bone loss in postmenopausal women. *Ann Intern Med* **87**, 649–55.

Reeve J, Bradbeer JN, Arlot M, Davies UM, Green JR, Hampton L, Edouard C, Hesp R, Hulme P, Ashby JP, Zanelli JM and Meunier PJ (1991) hPTH 1–34 treatment of osteoporosis with added hormone replacement therapy: biochemical, kinetic and histological responses. *Osteoporosis International* **1**(3), 162–70.

Reeve J, Davies UM, Hesp R, McNally E and Katz D (1990) Treatment of osteoporosis with human parathyroid peptide and observations on effect of sodium fluoride. *Br Med J* **301**, 314–18.

Reeve J, Hesp R, Williams D, Hulme P and Klenerman L (1976) Anabolic effect of low doses of a fragment of human parathpyroid hormone on the skeleton in postmenopausal osteoporosis. *Lancet* **i**, 1035–7.

Reeve J, Meunier PJ, Parsons JA, Bernat M, Bijvoet OLM, Courpron P, Edouard C, Klenerman L, Neer RM, Renier JC, Slovik D, Vismans FJFE and Potts JT (1980) Anabolic effect of human parathyroid fragment on trabecular bone in involutional osteoporosis: a multicentre trial. *Br Med J* **280**, 1340–44.

Reginster JY, Denis D, Albert A, Deroisy R, Lecart MP, Fontaine MA, Lambelin P and Franchimont P (1987) 1-year controlled randomised trial of prevention of early postmenopausal bone loss by intranasal calcitonins. *Lancet* **ii**, 1481–3.

Reginster JY, Strause L, Deroisy R, Lecart MP, Saltman P and Franchimont P (1989) Preliminary report of decreased serum magnesium in postmenopausal osteoporosis. *Magnesium* **8**, 106–9.

Rigotti NA, Neer RM, Skates SJ, Herzog DB and Nussbaum SR (1991) The clinical course of osteoporosis in anorexia nervosa. *J Am Med Assoc* **265**, 1133–8.

Rigotti N, Nussbaum SR, Herzog DB and Neer RM (1984) Osteoporosis in women with anorexia nervosa. *N Engl J Med* **311**, 1601–6.

Riggs BL, Hodgson SF, O'Fallon WM, Chao EYS, Wahner HW, Muhs JM, Cedel SL and Melton LJ (1990) Effect of fluoride treatment on the fracture rate in postmenopausal women with osteoporosis. *N Engl J Med* **322**, 802–9.

Riggs BL, Wahner HW, Melton LJ, Richelson LS, Judd HL and O'Fallon WM (1987) Dietary calcium intake and rates of bone loss in women. *J Clin Invest* **80**, 979–82.

Riis B, Thomsen K and Christiansen C (1987) Does Calcium supplementation prevent postmenopausal bone loss? *New Engl J Med* **316**, 173–7.

Ringe JD (1990) Prevention of heparin-induced osteoporosis during pregnancy by oral treatment with ossein-hydroxyapatite compound.

Third International Symposium on Osteoporosis 14–18 October 1990, Denmark 591 (Abstract)

Robinson CJ (1986) Practical aspects of the management of osteoporosis. A round table discussion held at the Postgraduate Medical Centre, City Hospital Nottingham, 17th Sept. 1986. Session IV Calcium and osteoporosis. *International Medicine Supplement* No 12.

Sambrook PN, Eisman JA, Champion GD, Yeates MG, Pocock NA and Eberl S (1987) Determinants of axial bone loss in rheumatoid arthritis. *Arthritis Rheum* **30**, 721–8.

Sambrook PN and Reeve J (1988) Bone disease in rheumatoid arthritis. *Clin Sci* **74**, 225–30.

Sambrook PN, Shawe D, Hesp R, Zanelli JM, Mitchell R, Katz D, Gumpel JM, Ansell BM and Reeve J (1990) Rapid periarticular bone loss in rheumatoid arthritis. *Arthritis Rheum* **33**, 615–22.

Sandler RB, Slemenda CW, LaPorte RE, Cauley JA, Schramm MM, Barresi ML, and Kriska AM (1985) Postmenopausal bone density and milk consumption in childhood and adolescence. *Am J Clin Nutr* **42**, 270–74.

Schvette SA, Knowles JB and Ford HE (1989) Effect of lactose or its component sugars on jejunal calcium absorption in adult man. *Am J Clin Nutr* **50**, 1084–7.

Schvette SA, Zemel MB and Linkswiler HM (1980) Studies on the mechanism of protein-induced hypercalciuria in older men and women. *J Nutr* **110** 305–15.

Scott NR, Chakraborty T and Marks V (1989) Caffeine consumption in the United Kingdom: a retrospective survey. *Food Sciences and Nutr* **42F**, 183–91.

Shore RM, Chesney RW, Mazess RB, Rose PG and Bargman GJ (1982) Skeletal demineralisation in Turners syndrome. *Calcif Tissue Int* **34**, 519–22.

Sheikh MS, Santa Ana CA, Nicar MJ, Schiller LR and Fordtran JS (1987) Gastrointestinal absorption of calcium from milk and calcium salts. *N Engl J Med* **317**, 532–6.

Shifrin LZ, Reis ND, Zinman H and Besser MI (1987) Idiopathic transient osteoporosis of the hip. *J Bone Joint Surg* **69B**(5), 769–73.

Simonen O and Laitinen O (1985) Does fluoridation of drinking-water prevent bone fragility and osteoporosis? *Lancet* **ii**, 432–4.

Slemenda C, Hui SL and Johnston CC (1991) Patterns of bone loss and physiologic growing: Prospects for prevention of osteoporosis by attainment of greater peak bone mass In *Osteoporosis 1990, Third International Symposium on Osteoporosis Copenhagen 1990.* (Eds) Christiansen C and Overgaard K.

Slovik DM, Adams JS, Neer RM, Holick MF and Potts JT (1981) Deficient production of 1,25 dihydroxyvitamin D in elderly osteoporotic patients. *N Engl J Med* **305**, 372–4.

Smith EL, Gilligan C, Smith PE and Sempas CT (1989) Calcium supplementation and bone loss in middle-aged women. *Am J Clin Nutr* **50**, 833–42.

Smith MA, Wilson J and Price WH (1982) Bone demineralisation in patients with Turners syndrome. *Journal of Medical Genetics*. **19**, 100–103.

Smith R, Stevenson JC, Winearls CG, Woods CG and Wordsworth BP (1985a) Osteoporosis of pregnancy. *Lancet* **i**, 1178–80.

Smith TM, Kolars JC, Savaiano DA and Levitt MD (1985b) Absorption of calcium from milk and yogurt. *Am J Clin Nutr* **42**, 1197–200.

Sowers M, Wallace RB and Lemke JH (1986) The relationship of bone mass and fracture history to fluoride and calcium intake: a study of three communities. *Am J Clin Nutr* **44**, 889–98.

Spencer H and Kramer L (1986) NIH Consensus Conference: Osteoporosis. Factors contributing to osteoporosis. *J Nutr* **116**, 316–19.

Spencer H, Kramer L, De Bartolo M, Norris C and Osis D (1983) Further studies of the effect of a high protein diet as meat on calcium absorption. *Am J Clin Nutr* **37**, 924–9.

Spencer H, Kramer L, Osis D and Norris C (1978) Effect of a high protein (meat) intake on calcium metabolism in man. *Am J Clin Nutr* **31**, 2167–80.

Stevenson JC, White MC, Joplin GF and MacIntyre I (1982) Osteoporosis and calcitonin deficiency. *Br Med J* **285**, 1010–11.

Stevenson JC and Whitehead MI (1982) Postmenopausal osteoporosis. *Br Med J* **285**, 585–8.

Stevenson JC, Whitehead MI, Padwick M, Endacott JA, Sutton C, Banks LM, Freemantle C, Spinks TJ and Hesp R (1988) Dietary intake of calcium and postmenopausal bone loss. *Br Med J* **297**, 15–17.

Storm T, Thamsborg G, Steiniche T, Genant HK and Sorensen OH (1990) Effect of intermittent cyclical etidronate therapy on bone mass and fracture rate in women with postmenopausal osteoporosis. *N Engl J Med* **332**, 1265–71.

Tremaine WJ, Newcomer AD, Riggs BL and McGill DB (1986) Calcium absorption from milk in Lactase-deficient and Lactase-sufficient adults. *Dig Dis Sci* **31**, 376–8.

Tsai K, Heath H, Kumar R and Riggs BL (1984) Impaired vitamin D metabolism with aging in women. *J Clin Invest* **73**, 1668–72.

Vogel JM and Whittle MW (1976) Bone mineral content changes in the skylab astronauts. *Am J Roentgenology Radium Ther Nucl Med* **126**, 1296–7.

Waldron O (1989) The relationship of dietary and supplemental calcium intake to bone loss and osteoporosis. *J Am Dietet Assoc* **89**, 397–400.

Walker RM and Linkswiler HM (1972) Calcium retention in the adult human male as affected by protein intake. *J Nutr* **102**, 1297–1302.

Watts NB, Harris ST, Genant HK, Wasnich RD, Miller PD, Jackson RD, Licata AA, Ross P, Woodson GC, Yanover MJ, Mysiw WJ, Kohse L, Rao MB, Steiger P, Richmond B and Chesnut C (1990) Intermittent cyclical etidronate treatment of postmenopausal osteoporosis. *N Engl J Med* **323**, 73–9.

Wickham CAC, Walsh K, Cooper C, Barker DJP, Margetts BM, Morris J and Bruce SA (1989) Dietary calcium, physical activity, and risk of hip fracture: a prospective study. *Br Med J* **299**, 889–92.

Zarkades M, Gougeon-Reyburn R, Marliss EB, Block E and Alton-Mackey M (1989) Sodium chloride and urinary calcium excretion in post-menopausal women. *Am J Clin Nutr* **50**, 1088–94.

4.29 Arthritis

Arthritis is not a new disease, fossil skeletons of apeman who lived two million years ago show evidence of osteoarthrosis. It is the largest cause of disability in Britain.

The term 'arthritis' means inflammation of a joint. There are several types of arthritis, the most common being osteoarthritis and rheumatoid arthritis. Other types include juvenile arthritis (Still's disease), ankylosing spondylitis and crystal arthritis (gout).

4.29.1 Osteoarthritis (osteoarthrosis)

Osteoarthritis is the most common form of arthritis, with up to 20% of the adult population in the UK showing radiological evidence of the disease (Swinson and Swinburn 1980). However, much of this is asymptomatic or of only minor clinical significance.

Osteoarthritis is more properly called osteoarthrosis because, whilst inflammation may occur in osteoarthritic joints, it is not a common feature of the disease. It is usually regarded as a degenerative condition and the incidence increases with age; however, it is not inevitable with increasing age, nor is it confined to the elderly.

Causes of osteoarthrosis

The following have been implicated as being important factors in the development of osteoarthrosis: trauma, congenital and development anomalies, other types of arthritis, metabolic causes, obesity age, climate, sex and heredity.

Characteristics and clinical features

Osteoarthrosis is characterized by the wearing away of joint cartilage and the production of new bone which appears beneath the worn cartilage and as outgrowths called osteophytes.

Osteoarthrosis may appear in joints which have been damaged in some way and this is termed *secondary osteoarthrosis*. In joints where no previous damage or disease can be found, the term *primary osteoarthrosis* is used.

Clinical features include pain which is generally felt on movement and which subsides with rest. There is mild early morning stiffness, reduced range of movement and deformity. Joints which are most susceptible to osteoarthrosis are the large joints of the body such as hips, knees and spine. (In contrast, rheumatoid arthritis affects the smaller more peripheral joints e.g. hands, wrists and feet).

Treatment of osteoarthrosis

Treatment consists chiefly of analgesics for relief of pain, or physical therapy using heat, cold or sound waves. Surgery may be required but is undertaken only where medical treatment has not controlled symptoms. Rehabilitation is heavily dependent upon physiotherapy and occupational therapy services.

Dietary management of osteoarthrosis

There is no 'special diet' for osteoarthrosis, however, a number of aspects should be considered, as discussed below.

Nutritional status

Food intake may be compromised as a result of mobility problems. The older person with chronic osteoarthrosis can be particularly at risk. Advice on good nutrition and simple easily prepared nourishing meals is invaluable (see Section 3.7.3). Meals on wheels provides a valuable service to those whose mobility is severely restricted.

Weight

Patients with osteoarthrosis may become overweight as a result of their decreased mobility and inappropriate dietary intake. Snacks of biscuits, cakes etc. are easier to eat than meals which require more preparation.

Osteoarthrosis commonly affects the load bearing joints such as the knee and hip and, since every step taken increases the load on the hip or knee joint by some 3–5 times body weight, excessive weight places on enormous stress on these joints. Weight reduction clearly is very important in order to minimize stress on the joint, to reduce pain and maintain or improve mobility.

For patients requiring surgery such as total hip or knee replacement, surgical intervention may well be delayed until a patient has achieved appropriate weight reduction.

When giving dietary guidelines for weight reduction, dietitians must consider the practicalities of any advice given in the light of any disabilities which the patient may have.

Fish oils

Since osteoarthrosis is not primarily an inflammatory disorder (unlike rheumatoid arthritis), it has been assumed that the anti-inflammatory effect of fish oils would be of little benefit to this group of patients. However, inflammation does occur in some cases of osteoarthrosis and a recent pilot study investigating the use of eicosapentaenoic acid (EPA) yielded results which, although not statistically significant, suggested that this aspect of treatment merits further investigation (Stammers *et al* 1989).

4.29.2 Rheumatoid arthritis

Rheumatoid arthritis (RA) is the most common type of inflammatory arthritis, affecting 1 in 100 of the population. It affects women two to three times more often than men. It is usually a disease of middle age but can affect children (Still's disease).

Causes of rheumatoid arthritis

The cause of rheumatoid arthritis is unclear but is thought to be a disease of the autoimmune system. Other factors that may have an influence include heredity, infection and trauma.

Presentation

The disease may be broadly divided into an early and a late phase. In the initial phase, symptoms are due to the active inflammation of the joints, whilst in the late phase symptoms are related to secondary osteoarthrosis and deformity.

The onset is often insidious, with swelling, pain and morning stiffness of hands, wrists and feet. The most constant and serious symptom is pain. Other symptoms include fatigue, muscle pain and general malaise. Excessive exercise has an adverse effect but gentle exercise can be beneficial in overcoming morning stiffness. The disease is characterized by remissions and relapses, with a slow and gradual progression.

Treatment of rheumatoid arthritis

Currently there is no cure for rheumatoid arthritis. Treatment is aimed at suppressing the disease where possible, reducing inflammation and pain, reducing joint destruction and avoiding deformities. Drug therapy includes the use of steroids, gold and non-steroidal anti-inflammatory drugs such as aspirin.

Dietary management of rheumatoid arthritis

The role of diet in the management of rheumatoid arthritis is unclear and remains controversial. Reports of successful dietary treatment tend to be anecdotal and subjective. Remission and relapses which are part of the normal course of the disease may be misinterpreted as dietary success. Well planned, double-blind studies making objective measurements have been sadly lacking. However a considerable amount of research into the relationship between diet and rheumatoid arthritis is currently being undertaken, particularly in the areas of food intolerance, dietary lipid modification (e.g. use of fish oils) and disturbance of gut flora.

Nutritional status

Patients with rheumatoid arthritis may be at risk of poor nutritional status; the disease activity itself can impair appetite and, in patients handicapped by immobility and deformity, there may be problems with the purchasing, preparing and consuming of food. In some patients, nutrient intake may be compromised as a result of following a 'self-help' regimen (see the paragraph on 'Food intolerance' below and Section 2.16).

Low dietary intake of folic acid, pyridoxine, zinc and magnesium have been reported in RA patients (Bigaouette *et al* 1987) and some medications may also interfere with the utilization of these nutrients. Kowsari *et al* (1983) found that many arthritis patients consumed diets which were at least marginally inadequate in a number of nutrients and they suggested that low intakes of vitamin E and zinc might affect the immunological events associated with the disease.

Anaemia This is a common feature of rheumatoid arthritis. It can result from a deficiency of iron, either as a result of poor dietary intake, or as a result of bleeding from the gastrointestinal tract. This may be unrelated to the disease or may be as a result of gastric erosion after taking non-steroidal anti-inflammatory drugs.

The anaemia may also result from the disease activity itself. Where systemic inflammation is present, production of haemoglobin is impaired. When treatment is successful and the inflammation subsides, haemoglobin levels usually rise.

Steroids These are commonly used in the treatment of rheumatoid arthritis. Long term, some are known to increase urinary excretion of zinc, calcium and nitrogen, thus affecting nutritional status (see also Section 2.10). Body proteins are also decreased leading to low serum albumen levels. Blood sugar levels, and body weight may increase, with some patients developing steroid-induced diabetes or obesity. Both conditions should be treated by conventional dietary advice.

Nutritional status can be improved if its importance is recognized. Nutritional counselling forms a valuable contribution to a comprehensive programme of care. Advice needs to be tailored to the individual's circumstances. Meals should be nutritionally balanced, easy to prepare and easy to eat. Small nourishing meals and snacks are often better tolerated than large meals. Nutrient-dense foods should be recommended.

Where physical feeding difficulties are present, an occupational therapist can advise on specially adapted feeding utensils (see Section 3.11.2). For those patients who are unable to manage an adequate food intake, supplementary drinks can help improve nutrient intake (see Section 1.13.3).

Dietary lipid modification

Dietary lipid modification may benefit some patients. The omega-3 series fatty acids such as eicosapentaenoic acid (EPA) and docosahexaenoic acid (DHA) found in marine oils appear to be less inflammatory than some omega-6 series fatty acids as a result of their effects on prostaglandin metabolism (see Section 2.3.2). A double-blind, placebo controlled trial by Kremer *et al* (1985) showed that an increase in dietary EPA content resulted in subjective improvement in patients with RA. After a 12 week study period, the experimental group had less morning stiffness and fewer tender joints. The patients relapsed on withdrawal.

Similar results have been demonstrated using evening primrose oil, a rich source of gamma-linolenic acid (GLA) (Belch *et al* 1988).

Food intolerance (see also Section 4.31)

In recent years, much interest has been shown in the idea that food intolerance may contribute to or exacerbate rheumatoid arthritis. However, in many of the dietary manipulations purporting to test this hypothesis, it is difficult to distinguish between effects which are attributable to food intolerance and those resulting from other factors such as weight loss, altered intake of substrates affecting prostaglandin production and the placebo effect. The possibility that symptom relief may be due to an episode of natural remission also has to be taken into account.

In a placebo-controlled blind study, Darlington *et al* (1986) found some evidence that an elimination diet resulted in improvement in some, but not all, of the experimental group. There appeared to be a better response in those with a family history of atopy.

Hicklin *et al* (1980) reported improvement in a third of rheumatoid patients treated with exclusion dieting. Panush *et al* (1983) investigating the Dong diet (free from additives, red meat, dairy produce, fruit and herbs) found no evidence of overall dietary benefit but suggested that individual dietary manipulations might be beneficial for selected rheumatoid patients.

4.29.3 Crystal arthritis (gout)

Gout is an inflammatory arthritis due to deposition of urate crystals within the joints. Symptoms include acute pain, swelling and intense irritation. For relevant dietary measures see Section 4.14.1.

4.29.4 Unproven and self-help remedies

(see also Section 2.16.2)

Many books have been written about unproven dietary treatments or even 'cures' for arthritis. These are the books which patients tend to read, and these are the diets which patients often follow. Dietitians should therefore be aware of what such books recommend. At best, their advice is harmless and may possibly produce a beneficial, if short lived, placebo effect. At worst, patients may follow a dietary regimen which is stringent, of doubtful value and which may be nutritionally unsound (Wolman 1987).

Long term adherence to such regimen can seriously

Table 4.80 Unproven diets popularly recommended for the treatment of arthritis

Diet	Rationale
Vegetarian diet	Meat causes arthritis
Vegetarian diet, no cooked or processed foods or grains except sprouted grains	Cleansing effect
Vegetarian diet, no cooked or processed foods. Coffee enemas plus diet supplements also advised	Cleansing effect
No meat, dairy products or additives	Allergy causes arthritis
Acid reducing diets	Acids cause arthritis
Only fish, brown rice and vegetables are permitted	Other foods cause arthritis
Whole milk before meals plus butter No margarine or skimmed milk	Lubricates joints
Fasting	Cleanses system of toxins and rests body
Fasting and enemas	Cleanses body of toxins and rests body

Table 4.81 Unproven supplements of foods, vitamins and minerals popularly recommended for the treatment of patients

Supplements	Cider vinegar Garlic Alfalfa Honey New Zealand green lipped mussel Kelp Devil's claw Ginseng
Minerals	Magnesium Zinc Selenium
Vitamins	A B_1 B_6 B_{12} Pantothenic acid Niacin C D E

undermine nutritional status. Table 4.80 lists some of the unproven dietary regimen found in popular books, while Table 4.81 lists foods and supplements which may be recommended.

A dietary history taken from patients with arthritis should include information about any 'special' diet followed, together with details of any nutritional supplements. Toxicity of high doses of vitamins and minerals should be considered and appropriate advice given. The dietitian should also ascertain whether fasting or the use of enemas form part of the dietary regimen.

Useful addresses

Arthritis Care, 5 Grosvenor Crescent, London SW1X 7ER. Tel 071–235 0902.

Arthritis and Rheumatism Council for Research, 41 Eagle Street, London WC1R 4AR. Tel 071–405 8672.

Further reading

Community Nutrition Group of the British Dietetic Association (1986) *Diet and arthritis*. Nutrition Group Information Sheet. BDA, London.

Swinson DR and Swinburn WR (1980) *Rheumatology*. Hodder and Stoughton, London.

References

Belch JJF, Ansell D, Madhock R, O'Dowd A and Sturrock RD (1988) The effects of altering dietary essential fatty acids as requirements for non-steroidal anti-inflammatory drugs in patients with rheumatoid arthritis: double blind placebo controlled study. *Ann Rheum Dis* **47**, 96–104.

Bigaouette J, Timchalk MA and Kremer J (1987) Nutritional adequacy of diet and supplements in patients with rheumatoid arthritis who take medications. *J Am Dietet Assoc* **87**, 1687–8.

Darlington LG, Ramsey NW and Mansfield JR (1986) Placebo controlled blind study of dietary manipulation therapy in rheumatoid arthritis. *Lancet* **1**, 236–8.

Hicklin JA, McEwen LM and Morgan JE (1980) The effect of diet in rheumatoid arthritis. *Clin Allergy* **10**, 463–7.

Kowsari B, Finnie SK, Carter RL, Love R, Katz P, Longley S and Panush RS (1983) Assessment of diet of patients with rheumatoid arthritis and osteoarthritis. *J Am Dietet Assoc* **82**, 657–9.

Kremer JM, Bigaouette J, Michalek AV, Timchalk MA, Liniger L, Rynes R *et al* (1985) Effects of manipulation of dietary fatty acids on clinical manifestations of rheumatoid arthritis. *Lancet* **1**, 184–7.

Panush RS, Carter RL, Katz P, Kowsari B, Longley S and Finnie S (1983) Diet therapy for rheumatoid arthritis. *Arthritis Rheum* **26**, 462–71.

Stammers T, Sibbald B and Freeling P (1989) Fish oil in osteoarthrosis (letter). *Lancet*, August 26, 503.

Swinson DR and Swinburn WR (1980) *Rheumatology*. Hodder & Stoughton, London.

Wolman PG (1987) Management of patients using unproven regimens for arthritis. *J Am Dietet Assoc* **87**, 1211–14.

4.30 Disorders of the skin

4.30.1 Atopic eczema (infantile eczema, dermatitis)

Eczema is one among several atopic diseases, including asthma, allergic rhinitis, allergic conjunctivitis, and urticaria. Those affected commonly have a genetic predisposition to develop hypersensitivity to foreign proteins and other macromolecules.

Symptoms

Symptoms are a reddening of the skin (erythema), accompanied by itching, scratching, and rubbing. Characteristic sites are the flexures, face, wrists, hands and legs, but lesions can occur anywhere. In most cases there is a varying degree of thickening of the skin, and scaliness, described as either icthyosis, or xeroderma. Many children with atopic eczema also have urticaria, and eventually develop asthma and allergic rhinitis. Some have unexplained short stature.

Onset and course of the disease

The onset of atopic eczema can be at any time, but it is most common before the age of six months. The disease fluctuates in its severity and there is a general trend towards spontaneous improvement (Atherton 1982; Devlin *et al* 1991a). However, the disease persists beyond early childhood in around 5% of cases and, for those who are severely affected, it can be a major handicap, physically and socially. Constant itching elicits scratching, which breaks the surface of the skin, causing bleeding, and weeping of serous fluid. Infection is common, principally with streptococci, staphylococci, or the virus herpes simplex. Children acquire nicknames, most commonly 'Scabby'. Passers-by in the street often mistake eczema for burns.

The itching and discomfort lead to countless nights without sleep for both the patient and parents, causing disruption to family life, tension and argument. Unsympathetic medical advice has been known to drive desperate parents to seek bizarre and scientifically unsound or dangerous treatment for their children (David 1985).

Treatment

Non-dietary treatment

Non-dietary measures which will improve symptoms and thus the quality of life for the patient, include the application of emollients and weak topical corticosteroids. The former are applied very liberally to the skin, as a means of keeping it moist, supple and unbroken. Infections are treated with topical antiseptics, or systemic antibiotics. Wool or man-made fibres in bed linen and clothing often have to be avoided, being replaced by pure cotton. Biological washing powders are best avoided.

House dust mite control measures, including removal of all fluffy toys, will help to improve symptoms for those who are sensitive to house dust mite. Finger nails need to be kept short by filing in order to reduce damage from scratching.

Dietary treatment

Dietary exclusion is part of the treatment for a minority of difficult cases. For those in whom dietary exclusion is necessary, the treatment will be incomplete, unless accompanied by all the above-mentioned measures.

All exclusion diets are difficult to implement and are often highly restrictive (see Section 4.31.6). It is always necessary to consider whether the diet is worse than the disease.

A careful and detailed history is essential. It will help to pinpoint individual foods to which the patient reacts. There are no reliable investigations, skin tests or blood tests which will diagnose food allergy with any accuracy or predict allergy to single foods (David 1983; Cant 1985).

The dietary treatment of atopic eczema ranges from simple exclusion of a single food, or a small number of foods, to the complete elimination of all foods, with nutritional intake maintained by an elemental formula, and followed by the reintroduction of foods one at a time. The prescription of a dietary regimen is a co-operative venture between clinician, dietitian and patient or the patient's parents.

Simple exclusion Dietary exclusion of cows' milk and eggs is advocated as a first step by some (Atherton *et al* 1978; Warner and Hathaway 1983), while others additionally exclude chicken, azo dyes and benzoate preservatives (Atherton 1985). (Details of exclusion diets are given in

Section 4.31.6 and Section 2.11). The patient must be seen by a dietitian who will take a comprehensive and detailed diet history in order to ascertain how the current diet needs to be altered. A diet sheet should be provided detailing the exclusions and emphasizing those foods which are permitted. For infants and children up to five years of age, a properly formulated milk substitute is essential, as whole cows' milk normally provides a major part of a child's intake of energy and protein, as well as other nutrients, especially calcium (Francis 1980). If the clinician has not already prescribed a cows' milk substitute, the dietitian should contact him or her in order to ascertain whether there is a reason for this. It should be recognized that infants will, with persuasion, take more readily to a milk substitute than will an older child who is used to the taste of cows' milk. Parents should be encouraged to report a child's refusal to drink the milk substitute so that a calcium and vitamin supplement can be prescribed. However, it is unsafe to assume that calcium requirements will be adequately provided by the prescription of a cows' milk substitute. A detailed diet history or survey is necessary to monitor dietary intake (Devlin *et al* 1989).

Further exclusions If the simple elimination diet fails to produce an improvement in the patient's eczema during a trial period of not less than two weeks (Warner and Hathaway 1983) and, ideally, eight weeks (Atherton 1982), compliance with the prescribed exclusion should be checked by a dietitian, and maintenance of topical treatment and other measures should be reviewed by the clinician. If all appears to be in order, trial of a more rigorous diet may be attempted. Careful consideration should be given to whether the family of the affected patient or child will be able to cope with the disruption of routine caused by a major revision of the eating habits of one person. The food choice of the whole family may have to change to fit in more easily with the constraints of the diet. Families relying heavily on processed or convenience foods may find the diet more difficult than continuing to live with the eczema. If the diet history indicates that this is a possibility, the dietitian should bring it to the attention of the clinician.

Diets may be prescribed individually on the basis already described, or a patient may be assigned to a multiple exclusion diet which eliminates a large number of common allergens or potentially provocative foods. Table 4.82 gives examples of some of the diets which have been used. Again, each patient should be seen by a dietitian who will explain how the diet may be best adhered to in the light of food preferences or meal pattern. A diet sheet must be provided for the patient. These multiple exclusion diets will probably include a milk substitute for a child under five years of age. After six weeks on such a diet a review will establish whether the diet has produced an improvement in the eczema and whether the improvement justifies

Table 4.82 Examples of multiple exclusion diets used in the treatment of eczema

Morgan (1980)	Warner and Hatthaway (1983)	Graham *et al* (1984)	Price (1984)	David (1989)
To be avoided Milk, cheese and egg	*To be avoided* Dairy products (milk) and eggs	*To be avoided* Milk, cheese and egg	*To be avoided* Milk, milk products and eggs	*To be avoided* Cows milk, egg Wheat
Pork, bacon, liver, all offal, fish and shellfish	Pork, offal, fish and shellfish	Pork, bacon, offal, fish and shellfish	Chicken	Fish Legumes (pea, bean, soya, lentil)
Nuts and pips	Nuts	Nuts and pips		Nuts
Fruit	Fruit (except rhubarb and bananas)	Fruit		Berries and currants Citrus fruit
Yeast Onions and garlic Honey Chewing gum	Vegetables Alcohol Herbs and spices	Yeasts Honey Sweets Gravy powder	Colouring in manufactured foods. Coloured drinks, sweets, jellies and instant puddings All foods with colouring added e.g. sausages, tinned fish, soups, baked beans and flavoured crisps	Food additives (azo-dyes, benzoates, and sulphites)
Allowed Carnation milk, tea, instant coffee, sugar, treacle, syrup salt, butter, lard, beef, lamb rabbit, green leafy vegetables celery, lettuce, carrot, potatoes mushrooms, bread, pastry, cakes and biscuits.				

the trouble taken over the diet. If the diet has not proved beneficial, then it may be abandoned or eliminated foods may be reintroduced one at a time, or, a yet more rigorous diet may be attempted.

If the diet is to continue, a diet survey should be conducted by the dietitian in order to monitor compliance and as a check on nutritional intake. Results should be forwarded to the clinician together with comments and recommendations for dietary modification or the prescription of vitamin and mineral supplements (David *et al* 1984). Although a diet may be theoretically adequate, individual food preference may well affect the nutritional intake.

An alternative course is to choose a diet consisting of a few rarely implicated or uncommon foods, a so called Few Food or oligo-antigenic diet (see also Section 4.31.6). Usually this consists of a meat protein food, a starchy food, a vegetable and a fruit. A trial period of up to six weeks may be necessary to observe whether it is to be of benefit. For children under the age of five years, a milk substitute is again essential in the long term as they are unlikely to be able to eat sufficient bulk of the permitted foods to satisfy energy and other nutritional requirements. Few Food diets are difficult to maintain in a domestic setting, and the lack of variety may lead to abandonment of the diet, before the trial period has elapsed. Although a third of patients may obtain no benefit, over half have been observed to obtain substantial improvement in the severity of the disease after six weeks (Devlin *et al* 1991a), and in another study 12 out of 66 children experienced prolonged and useful benefit (Pike *et al* 1989).

If the diet has resulted in remission of symptoms single foods may be reintroduced to the diet at weekly intervals. Examples of Few Food diets used in the treatment of eczema are given in Table 4.83.

Complete withdrawal of food/elemental formula diets For the more difficult cases, or when there is a long history of treatment as already outlined with little or no improvement in the condition, as a last resort it may be worth considering complete withdrawal of all food. It is of course, necessary to maintain an adequate nutritional intake and this may be attempted using an elemental formula such as those listed in Table 4.84.

Table 4.84 Elemental formulae used in the treatment of eczema

Product	Manufacturer
Elemental 028 (unflavoured)	Scientific Hospital Supplies
Neocate	Scientific Hospital Supplies
Flexical	Mead Johnson

This procedure is hazardous in young children and must only be undertaken during a hospital admission which may last for 8–10 weeks.

Several authors give details of the use of Vivonex (Norwich-Eaton) as the elemental formula in the treatment of severe eczema (Hill and Lynch 1982; David 1983; Devlin *et al* 1991b). However Vivonex has been unavailable since 1979. There is no published description of the use of other elemental formulae, although they may be suitable. Manufacturers' instructions regarding introduction, concentrations and quantities required should be followed. Practical details of the use of elemental diets are given in Section 4.31.6.

Although 5–20 days has been suggested as being sufficient for trial of an elemental diet (Goldsborough and Francis 1983), 3–4 weeks or more is usually required for extensive resolution of eczema to occur (David 1983; Devlin *et al* 1991b). Experienced clinical judgement must decide the degree of improvement obtained from a trial of the elemental regimen. The treatment of a total of 37 children with refractory widespread atopic eczema, and treated with an elemental formula, is described by Devlin *et al* (1991b). Improvement in the eczema was seen in three quarters of the patients. However 10 patients failed to

Table 4.83 Few Food diets used in the treatment of eczema

Morgan (1980)	Warner and Hatthaway (1983)	Graham *et al* (1984)	Atherton (1985)	David (1989)
Food allowed Lamb	*Food allowed* Lamb or rabbit	*Food allowed* Lamb	*Food allowed* Turkey or rabbit	*Food allowed* Lamb or turkey
Sago	Sago	Sago flour	Sago or rice or potato	Potato, rice and Rice Krispies
Fresh green leafy vegetables, carrots, celery and lettuce	Cabbage, carrots, celery lettuce and fresh rhubarb	Fresh green vegetables, celery and rhubarb	Cabbage or carrot or leek Rhubarb or stewed apple	Cauliflower, or cabbage or broccoli or sprouts Pear
Sugar, treacle and syrup	Sugar, treacle and syrup			
Water and tea	Water and tea (without milk)	Water and plain tea		
Salt	Tomor margarine	Kosher margarine	Tomor margarine, calcium, vitamins and sunflower seed oil	

respond to the regimen, or relapsed within 12 months. It must therefore be appreciated that despite the investment of a great deal of time and effort, failure is a possibility.

If the eczema has not improved significantly, the diet should be abandoned and a moderately restricted or normal diet resumed. If improvement has occurred single foods should be reintroduced along the guidelines given in Section 4.31.6. The choice of food will depend not only on the previous history of foods known to exacerbate the eczema, but also on the patient's food preference. It is pointless, for example, to suggest the introduction of cabbage to the diet if the patient dislikes it. Foods should be introduced singly, and at intervals of 5–7 days and, if the eczema worsens during that period, the food is withdrawn and then, when the skin has improved again, another food can be introduced.

Once the patient is on a diet of four or five foods the elemental formula may be replaced by a casein hydrolysate formula (e.g. Pregestimil) prior to discharge. A programme should be devised of foods to be introduced and tried at home, singly and at weekly intervals. While the diet consists of only a small number of foods, estimates of nutritional intake are necessary from time to time, and serious inadequacies should be corrected (David *et al* 1984a).

4.30.2 Urticaria (nettle rash)

Symptoms

Urticaria is an eruption on the skin of erythematous (red) and oedematous patches which may appear on any part of the body. The affected skin usually itches, and the episode may last from minutes (acute urticaria) to years (chronic urticaria).

Aetiology and treatment

In a large proportion of cases, no cause can be found. The most common triggers are viral infections, and foodstuffs – azo dyes, benzoate preservatives, salicylates, foods naturally containing salicylates, various other foods, some containing high levels of histamine, yeasts or foods containing yeasts, have all been implicated in the provocation of urticaria (August 1980), and are listed in Table 4.85.

Urticarial reactions may occur in children on contact with the food, in particular on the fingers, face or lips. Among adults, urticaria may be seen on the hands of those whose jobs involve the handling of foods.

Many people who have suffered an urticarial reaction to a food may never need to see a clinician in order to confirm the relationship between contact or ingestion and reaction. On taking a careful history the relationship may appear obvious, and no further advice is necessary other than to avoid the culprit food (Atherton 1985).

For chronic urticaria where no obvious relationship is manifest, a trial of an azo dye and preservative-free diet may be worthwhile (see Sections 2.11, 2.12 and 4.31). If no improvement occurs, a diet diary may help to pinpoint the cause, relating the occurrence of symptoms to food ingestion. The suspect food or foods can then be eliminated. If a diet is prescribed involving the exclusion of more than one or two important foods, the patient should be seen by a dietitian. A detailed diet history will show when the implicated foods are taken and how they can be avoided. In cases of multiple exclusion, a diet sheet individually produced for each patient may be necessary.

Table 4.85 Foods and food constituents implicated in the causation of urticaria

Food additives	*Azo dyes*	
	Tartrazine	(E102)
	Amaranth	(E123)
	Ponceau 4R/New coccine	(E124)
	Sunset yellow	(E110)
	Preservatives	
	Benzoic acid	(E210)
	Sodium benzoate	(E211)
	Sodium hydroxybenzoate	
	4-Hydroxy benzoic acid	
Salicylate-containing foods	Apples, blueberries, beer, cider, grapes, liquorice, plums, prunes, raspberries (and jam), red wine, sherry, rhubarb	
Other foods and yeast products	Milk, egg, nuts, fruits, cheese, fish, shellfish, pork, mutton, aldehydes in fried foods, gluten/wheat, menthol, brewer's yeast, marmite (yeast extract), yeast tablets, bread, rice, wines, beer, sausages	

4.30.3 Acrodermatitis enteropathica

Symptoms

The symptoms result from a severe zinc deficiency (Bleehan 1979) and include a characteristic eruption around mouth and anus, bullous or verrucous eruptions on the extremities, hair loss and severe diarrhoea.

Onset

Onset is usually in early infancy, or may be delayed until after weaning in breast fed babies. The condition is sometimes familial and it is likely that there is an inherited defect in the absorption of zinc from the gut. Serum zinc levels are invariably low, and may be well below the normal level of 10–18 μmol/l (Halsted and Smith 1970; David *et al* 1984b). The diagnosis is confirmed by a response to zinc supplements.

Treatment

There is no dietary treatment as such. Treatment is by zinc supplementation alone, and this is a life-long measure.

The supplement is zinc sulphate 25 mg, twice daily with meals (Bleehan 1979). The optimum level of supplementation is 75 mg, twice daily (Moynihan 1974). Zinc sulphate is a potential gastrointestinal irritant, although it is well tolerated if given with food. Alternative zinc salts such as the oxide, carbonate or acetate may be preferred. There is no risk of zinc toxicity with doses in the ranges given, but very much higher doses may interfere with iron and copper absorption, causing anaemia (Hambidge 1977). Control of serum zinc levels is especially important in early pregnancy, as zinc deficiency may be teratogenic.

4.30.4 Dermatitis herpetiformis

This is a rare, chronic, recurrent skin disease.

Symptoms

The skin lesions, which itch intensely, are erythematous, urticarial and symmetrical. The associated jejunal villous atrophy is present in most cases, and appears to be indistinguishable from that of coeliac disease (see Section 4.7).

Onset

Although the adult variety of the disease is seen occasionally in children, usually after the age of five years, the disease occurs mainly in adults between the ages of 20 and 55 years. The course of the disease is long term with many remissions and relapses. Relapse may be precipitated by acute infections and emotional disturbances (Sneddon 1979).

Treatment

Drug treatment is with dimethyl sulphone (Dapsone). Dietary treatment is with a gluten-free diet (see Section 2.14.1). It has been reported (Fry *et al* 1973) that 80% of patients who adhered to a gluten-free diet for more than one year, were able to stop or significantly reduce the dose of Dapsone required to control symptoms. The time taken to stop the drug treatment completely, while remaining on a gluten-free diet varied between eight months and four years.

In a study of ten highly motivated patients, a gluten-free diet allowed a reduction of Dapsone in all but one of the patients, and in six of the patients Dapsone was stopped completely within a year of starting the gluten-free diet (Harrington and Read 1977). Another study of patients with dermatitis herpetiformis showed that they have an increased risk of developing malignant tumours. However, those treated with a gluten-free diet had a reduced risk of malignancy compared with those taking a normal diet (Leonard *et al* 1983). Jejunal biopsies show improvement in the associated jejunal villous atrophy of those patients maintaining a gluten-free diet (Marks and Whittle 1969; Fry *et al* 1968).

Reports suggesting no benefit from a gluten-free diet have been criticised (Fry *et al* 1973) as being based on a small number of patients with only a short follow-up period. As the time on a strictly maintained gluten-free diet may be considerable before the level of Dapsone can be reduced without a relapse, patients need a great deal of encouragement with the diet, and frequent checks to ensure that elimination of gluten is complete.

Useful address

The National Eczema Society, Tavistock House North, Tavistock Square, London WC1H 9SR.

Further reading

Atherton DJ (1983) *Your child with eczema – a guide for parents*. Heinemann Medical, London.

Bleehan SS (1979) Acrodermatitis enteropathica. In *Textbook of dermatology* Vol II Rook A, Ebling FJG and Wilkinson DS (Eds). pp. 2086. Blackwell Scientific Publications, Oxford.

David TJ (1988) Food additives. *Arch Dis Childh* **63**, 582–3.

Denner WHB (1984) Colourings and preservatives in food. *Hum Nutr: Appl Nutr* **38A**(6), 435–49.

MacKie R (1983) *Eczema and dermatitis – how to cope with inflamed skin*. Martin Dunitz, London.

Supramanium G and Warner JO (1986) Artificial food additive intolerance in patients with angioedema and urticaria. *Lancet* **ii**, 907–9.

Workman E, Hunter J and Jones VA (1984) *The allergy diet – how to overcome your food intolerance*. Martin Dunitz, London.

Suitable reading for patients

Hanssen M (1987) *E for Additives*, Thorsons, Wellingborough.

Ministry of Agriculture, Fisheries and Food (1991) *Food additives – the balanced approach*. HMSO, London.

Workman E, Hunter J and Jones VA (1984) *The allergy diet: How to overcome your food intolerance*. Martin Dunitz, London.

References

Atherton DJ, Sewell M, Soothill JF, Wells RS and Chilvers CED (1978) A double blind crossover trial of an antigen avoidance diet in atopic eczema. *Lancet* **i**, 401–3.

Atherton DJ (1982) Atopic eczema. In *Clinics in Immunology and Allergy* **2**(1), 77. Brostoff J and Challacombe SJ (Eds) WB Saunders, Eastbourne.

Atherton DJ (1985) Skin disorders and food allergy. In *Food allergy in childhood*. David TJ and Dinwiddie R (Eds) *J Roy Soc Med* (Suppl) (5) **78**, 7.

August PJ (1980) Urticaria. In *Proceedings of the First Food Allergy Workshop* 76–81, MES Ltd, Oxford.

Cant AJ (1985) Food allergy in childhood. *Hum Nutr: Appl Nutr* **39A**, 277–93.

David TJ (1983) The investigation and treatment of severe childhood eczema. *Int Med* (Suppl) **6**, 19.

David TJ (1985) The overworked or fraudulent diagnosis of food allergy and food intolerance in children. In *Food allergy in childhood*, David TJ and Dinwiddie R (Eds) *J Roy Soc Med* (Suppl) (5) **78**, 21.

David TJ (1989) Dietary treatment of atopic eczema. *Arch Dis Childh* **64**, 1506–9.

David TJ, Waddington ER and Stanton RHJ (1984a) Nutritional hazards of elimination diets in children with atopic eczema. *Arch Dis Child* **59**(4), 323–5.

David TJ, Wells FE, Sharpe TC and Gibbs ACC (1984b) Low serum zinc in atopic eczema. *Br J Dermatol* **3**, 597–601.

Devlin J, Stanton RHJ and David TJ (1989) Calcium intake and cow's milk free diets. *Arch Dis Childh* **64**, 1183–4.

Devlin J, David TJ and Stanton RHJ (1991a) Six food diet for childhood atopic dermatitis. *Acta Derm Venereol (Stokh)* **71**, 20–24.

Devlin J, David TJ and Stanton RHJ (1991b) Elemental diet for refractory atopic eczema. *Arch Dis Childh* **66**, 93–9.

Francis DEM (1980) Dietary management. In *Proceedings of the First Food Allergy Workshop*, pp. 85–93, MES Ltd, Oxford.

Fry L, McMinn RMH, Cowan JD and Hoffbrand AV (1968) Effect of gluten-free diet on dermatological, intestinal and haematological manifestations of dermatitis herpetiformis. *Lancet* **i**, 557.

Fry L, Seah PP, Riches DJ and Hoffbrand AV (1973) Clearance of skin lesions in dermatitis herpetiforms after gluten withdrawal. *Lancet* **i**, 288–91.

Goldsborough J and Francis DEM (1983) Dietary management. In *Proceedings of the Second Fisons Food Allergy Workshop*. MES Ltd, Oxford.

Graham P, Hall-Smith SP, Harris JR and Price ML (1984) A study of hypo allergenic diets and oral sodium cromoglycate in the management of atopic eczema. *Br J Dermatol* **110**, 457–67.

Halsted JA and Smith JC (1970) Plasma zinc in health and disease. *Lancet* **i**, 322–4.

Hambidge KM (1977) The role of zinc and other trace metals in paediatric nutrition and health. *Paediatr Clin North Am* **24**(1), 100.

Harrington CI and Read NW (1977) Dermatitis herpetiformis: effect of gluten-free diet on skin IgA and jejunal structure and function. *Br Med J* **1**, 872.

Hill DJ and Lynch BC (1982) Elemental diet in the management of severe eczema in childhood. *Clin Allergy* **12**, 313–5.

Leonard JN, Tucker WF, Fry JS, Coulter CA, Boylston AW, McMinn RM, Haffenden GP, Swain AF and Fry L (1983) Increased incidence of malignancy in dermatitis herpetiformis. *Br Med J* **286**, 16–18.

Marks R and Whittle HW (1969) Results of treatment of dermatitis herpetiformis with a gluten-free diet after one year. *Br Med J* **iv**, 772.

Morgan JE (1980) In *Proceedings of the First Food Allergy Workshop*, pp. 93–4, MES Ltd, Oxford.

Moynihan EJ (1974) Acrodermatitis enteropathica – a lethal inherited human zinc deficiency disorder. *Lancet* **ii**, 399.

Pike MG, Carter CM, Boulton P, Turner MW, Soothill JF and Atherton DJ (1989) Few Food diets in the treatment of atopic eczema. *Arch Dis Childh* **64**, 1691–8.

Price ML (1984) The role of diet in the management of atopic eczema. *Hum Nutr* **38A**, 409–15.

Sneddon IB (1979) Dermatitis herpetiformis: In *Textbook of dermatology* Vol II. Rook A, Ebling FJG and Wilkinson DS (Eds) pp. 1467–8. Blackwell Scientific Publications, Oxford.

Warner JO and Hathaway MJ (1983) Dietary treatment of eczema due to food intolerance. In *Proceedings of the Second Fisons Food Allergy Workshop*, pp. 105–8, MES Ltd, Oxford.

4.31 Food allergy and food intolerance

The area of food allergy and food intolerance remains one of the more controversial subjects in modern medicine, with beliefs ranging from full, unconditional and uncritical support to total non-acceptance. It is likely that the truth lies somewhere between these extremes and fact must be sifted from fiction for a conclusion to be reached. Acceptance of a common terminology must form a foundation upon which an understanding of the mechanisms involved in this type of reaction can be built.

4.31.1 Terminology and definitions

The Joint Report of the Royal College of Physicians of London and the British Nutrition Foundation on Food Intolerance and Food Aversion (1984) offers the following definitions:

Food intolerance A reproducible, unpleasant (adverse), non-psychological reaction to a specific food or food ingredient.

Food allergy A form of food intolerance in which there is evidence of an abnormal immunological reaction to the food.

Food aversion which is subdivided into:

Psychological avoidance Avoidance of food for psychological reasons.

Psychological intolerance An unpleasant bodily reaction caused by emotions associated with the food.

The report gives examples of food intolerant reactions including pharmacological effects (e.g. those from caffeine) and enzyme deficiency (e.g. lactase) amongst others.

The report by the American Academy of Allergy (Metcalfe 1984) lists nine definitions to cover the same reactions, whilst Pearson (1987) offers no less than 25 possible terms to describe allergic and intolerant reactions.

For the purposes of this section, the terms described by the RCP/BNF report (1984) will be used.

4.31.2 Mechanisms of food allergy

Most of the food consumed by man is potentially allergenic. However, food preparation and cooking and the action of acid and enzymes in normal digestive processes destroys many of the likely allergens. The mucosa of the gastrointestinal tract contains cells with the capacity to produce all types of immunoglobulin (Ig) to form a defensive barrier. The responsible tissue is lymphatic in origin and may be located in nodules or as single cells, either lymphocytes or mast cells, which are widely scattered throughout the gut.

T-Lymphocytes recognize antigens and react by producing cytotoxic substances which act locally and directly with the antigen.

B-Lymphocytes when activated, give rise to plasma cells which synthesize and secrete immunoglobulins which are specific for each antigen.

Mast cells store mediators such as histamine in granules for later release and, when activated, can synthesize other agents such as prostaglandins and other leukotrienes. IgE attaches to the surface of mast cells and then forms complexes with antigens. These trigger the release of the mast cell mediators which cause the allergic reaction.

Histamine, the mediator released in the degranulation of mast cells, enters the circulation and causes contraction of smooth muscle, increased vascular permeability and stimulation of irritant receptors (causing itching). The increased vascular permeability can lead to a rapid reduction in blood volume and subsequent anaphylactic shock. Cramping is caused by gastrointestinal smooth muscle contraction. The essential fatty acids, arachidonic acid and gamma linoleic acid, are the precursors for other mast cell mediators including SRS-A (slow reacting substance of anaphylaxis), prostaglandins and other leukotrienes. SRS-A (a mixture of leukotrienes) is a more potent bronchoconstrictor than histamine and also induces increased vascular permeability and mucus production. It is therefore probably associated with asthma and has a slower but longer activity curve than histamine. The prostaglandins and leukotrienes act as secondary mediators which stimulate late inflammatory reactions.

Table 4.86 shows the different types of immunoglobulins and summarizes their functions.

4.31.3 Types of reaction

There are four basic types of allergic response.

Table 4.86 Immunoglobulin classes

IgG:	The most abundant Ig, it readily crosses the placenta and its main task is to combat bacteria and their toxins
IgA:	Appears in sero-mucous secretions defending external body surfaces including the gut
IgM:	Activates the complement system (a group of enzymes with cytolytic properties)
IgD:	A shortlived Ig whose function is not well understood
IgE:	Binds easily to mast cells and activates their degranulation so protecting external mucosal surfaces by triggering acute inflammatory responses.

Type i occurs within a few minutes of exposure to the antigen and is therefore termed an 'immediate' reaction. This classic anaphylactic response is triggered by the IgE-mast cell complex releasing chemical mediators. These cause the symptoms of rhinitis, asthma, vasodilation, oedema and bronchial smooth muscle contraction.

Type ii reactions are localized to cell membranes. They are known as cytotoxic reactions and also are immediate. The membrane is damaged due to interaction of the cell bound antigen with IgG. The subsequent activation of the complement system results in cell lysis.

Type iii responses occur some hours after exposure to the antigen so are termed 'late' reactions. The combination of IgG to circulating antigen results in activation of the complement system which triggers enzyme release. Typical reactions occur in the skin and bronchi.

Type iv or cellular immune reactions do not manifest until 24–48 hours after exposure and are termed 'delayed' reactions. The T-lymphocyte recognizes antigens bound to foreign cells and causes lysis. The sensitized T-cells can also release lymphokines which activate non sensitized cells to fight antigens.

Initial exposure to antigens leads to antibody production with subsequent memory storage in susceptible individuals. Further exposure causes production of more antibodies with an enhanced response. This process is known as sensitization and susceptible individuals are referred to as being *atopic*.

In the gastrointestinal tract, antigens combine with IgA to form a complex which is not readily absorbed. Any failure in the production of IgA can result in access to the circulatory system of the antigen. The presence of the antigen triggers IgE and IgG responses in the form of a Type i reaction as previously described.

4.31.4 Food intolerance

A wide range of reactions to foods which are not immunologically mediated fall into the category of food intolerance. The mechanisms involved in these responses are many and some are unexplained. It is often this lack of an explanation which causes the controversy commonly associated with intolerant reactions to food.

Non-allergic histamine release This causes signs which are indistinguishable from those associated with IgE triggered histamine release. Shellfish, strawberries and amine rich foods, when consumed in relatively large quantities, are known to cause this reaction.

Enzyme defects Enzyme defects, such as lactase deficiency or phenylalanine hydroxylase deficiency, result in adverse reactions which are resolved by the controlled intake of the associated foodstuffs.

Pharmacological reactions Pharmacological reactions to food components such as the vasoactive amines can be highly disturbing. The effects can include migraine, tremor, sweating and palpitations and can be triggered by relatively low intakes. As little as 200 mg of caffeine, a vasoactive amine found in coffee, tea, chocolate and cola drinks, can trigger a response in some individuals (Astrup *et al* 1990).

Histamine, serotonin, tryptamine and tyramine may also cause migraine and other reactions in susceptible individuals (Pachor *et al* 1989) and foods containing these substances should be avoided when monoamine oxidase inhibiting drugs are being taken (see Section 2.11.2).

Irritant effects Irritant effects on the gastrointestinal tract can be induced by foods such as curry and can be misconstrued as food allergy. *Kwok's* or the *Chinese restaurant syndrome* can follow the consumption of Chinese food containing monosodium glutamate (MSG). The response mimics the features of a myocardial infarction with chest pain radiating to both arms and the back and general weakness and palpitations. The mechanism is unknown. Asthma has also been reported as a reaction to MSG.

4.31.5 Diagnosis of food allergy

A number of tests for allergy exist which have a varying degree of accuracy, reliability and reproducibility.

RAST

The radioallergosorbent test (RAST) is a direct radioimmunoassay in which a specific allergen is exposed to patient serum allowing binding of antibody and antigen to occur. Then, a fixed amount of ^{125}I-labelled specific anti-IgE antibody is added which binds to the patient's IgE molecules bound to the allergen. The amount of bound activity is proportional to the amount of antigen-specific IgE in the patient serum (Fig. 4.19).

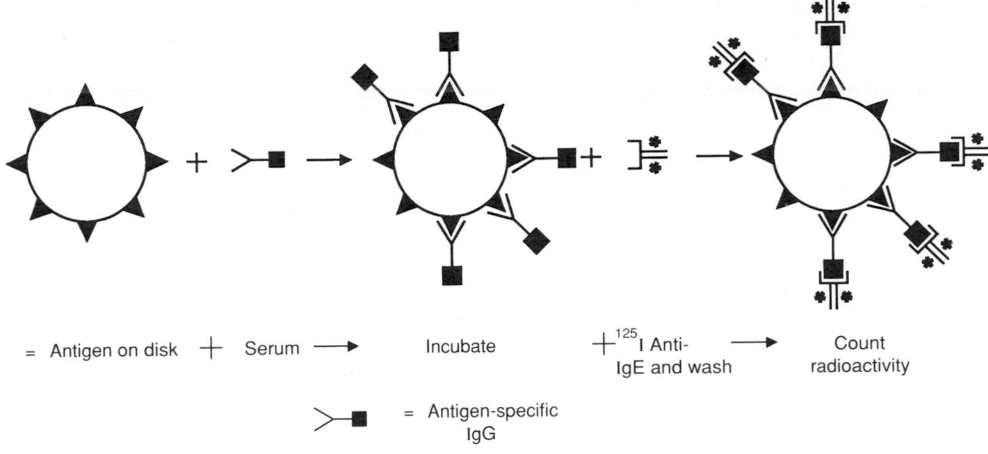

Fig. 4.19 The radioallergoasorbent test (RAST)

RAST is of variable accuracy and depends for example on the time lapse between the last exposure of the patient to the allergen and the performance of the test. This is because the half life of circulating IgE is only a few days. Only a limited range of allergen extracts for foods is available and their value is further affected by the possible chemical differences between the processed allergen and the 'natural' allergen in food.

Skin tests

A range of skin tests can be used to assess allergy including patch, prick, scratch, puncture and intradermal testing. These involve the exposure of the skin to the allergen for a period of time after which a local reaction may be identified by the presence of a weal and flare. The size of the reaction can be measured to give an indication of tissue fixed IgE antibodies. Skin tests may give a positive reaction to an allergen where a RAST test gives a negative response, as the half life of tissue bound IgE is greater than that of circulating IgE.

It should be noted that RAST and skin tests give both false positive and false negative results which may be misleading. The range of food allergens available for testing is not wide. These assays, therefore, may be of limited value in the identification of food allergy. They are not appropriate in the diagnosis of food intolerance which makes up about 80% of food related reactions.

Other more controversial tests which are less sensitive than previously mentioned techniques have been developed to diagnose allergy. They are not generally available on the NHS and their reproducibility has been shown to be very poor.

Other diagnostic tests

Cytotoxic food test

This procedure is founded on the premise that leucocytes lyse in the presence of allergens. Studies using a single blood sample, divided and sent for testing under two different names, have shown that the results for the samples of the same blood do not match (Lehman 1980). The blood from patients with known allergies has been sent for testing and the allergy has not been identified (Consumers Association 1987).

In any given sample, many foods may be claimed as allergens by the laboratories undertaking the testing but no advice is offered on how to manage a diet which excludes these foods. Nutritional inadequacy of the diet is therefore a potential sequel.

Hair and nail tests

Similar claims have been made for the evaluation of hair and nail samples. Whilst it is accepted that levels of minerals can be assayed in cases of poisoning, there is no evidence to suggest that such tests are of value in allergy testing.

Pulse testing

This test is based on the premise that the pulse rate rises after ingestion of a food allergen. The reliability of this test must be challenged on the grounds that a wide range of events cause changes in pulse rate, including stress.

Sublingual provocative testing

This technique involves the application of a few drops of extract of the supposed allergen under the tongue of an individual who has been deprived of that allergen for a short period. A reaction will indicate sensitivity. However, in some situations, the test can result in anaphylactic shock with rapid swelling of the tongue and pharynx leading to asphyxiation.

Many of the above tests were evaluated by the American Academy of Allergy whose report (1981) showed no evidence that the techniques were of value. In cases of delayed reactions to food and in most cases of food intolerance the assessment of the patient by dietary means seems to be the most reliable and effective technique.

4.31.6 Dietary investigation of food allergy and intolerance: diagnostic procedures

Since there are so few simple or reliable physiological tests for the diagnosis of food allergy, and virtually none for the diagnosis of food intolerance, dietary investigation remains the cornerstone of investigation and treatment.

However, manipulative dietary investigations should not be undertaken lightly. They are time-consuming procedures for both patients and professionals, and should only be attempted if the symptoms are sufficiently debilitating to justify the likely social disruption (Hathaway and Warner 1983), financial strain (Macdonald and Forsythe 1986) and periods of inadequate nutrient intake (Labib *et al* 1989). Furthermore there is no guarantee that the result will be relief from symptoms. Nevertheless, for some patients, successful dietary diagnosis and treatment can dramatically improve the quality of life.

Because of the problems associated with these diagnostic procedures and the potential hazards of anaphylaxis or other life-threatening symptoms which may result from the reintroduction of foods (David 1984; Egger *et al* 1989), all dietary investigations must be conducted in close collaboration with medical colleagues (BDA 1990).

Clinical history

The dietitian will need to build up a profile of the patient before deciding which dietary diagnostic procedure is appropriate. At the initial interview the following should be ascertained:

1 The symptoms and their frequency.

2 The clinical diagnosis and whether drug or other treatment has been, or is currently being, carried out.

3 Relevant anthropometric information e.g. height and weight in children.

4 Whether any foods are suspected of causing symptoms.

5 Whether any dietary measures have already been tried and with what result.

6 The general dietary history and current eating habits and meal patterns.

Dietary exclusion

Foods or food constituents which are suspected of causing allergy or intolerance are eliminated from the diet to see whether symptoms improve. There are four main ways in which this can be done.

1 Simple exclusion diets

A simple exclusion diet is one which excludes a single food or food constituent either because dietary enquiry suggests, or the patient has discovered, that symptoms are linked to this particular item. Although simple in name, these diets are not always simple in practice. While foods such as strawberries, chocolate and shellfish are easily eliminated, the sources of items such as wheat, milk, eggs or azo dyes are less obvious and their avoidance encompasses a wide range of foods. Patients will require clear but comprehensive information detailing which products must be avoided, and which products may need to be avoided and how this can be determined from labelling information. Patients may also require suggested alternatives to the excluded foods.

Considerable dietetic expertise may be needed to ensure that the nutritional requirements of children are met if foods which normally make a significant contribution to nutrient intake (such as milk and dairy products) are excluded. (Practical details of dietary regimens free from milk, egg, wheat etc. are given in Section 2.14).

2 Multiple food exclusion diet

A multiple exclusion diet excludes a number of foods which are commonly allergenic or potentially provocative. It is used when a dietary cause is suspected but cannot be identified. Since there is no standard elimination diet which is guaranteed to exclude all suspect foods for all patients, a multiple exclusion diet usually eliminates those foods to which food sensitive people most commonly react. In adults these are milk and dairy products, eggs, grains (especially wheat), and, to varying degrees, citrus fruits, nuts, coffee and chocolate (Lessof *et al* 1980; Alun Jones *et al* 1982; Wraith 1982; Carini *et al* 1984; Workman *et al* 1984; Nanda *et al* 1989; Blades 1990; Riordan *et al* 1990; Hawthorne *et al* 1991). Similar sensitivities occur in children and some may also be intolerant to fish and azo dyes (Hathaway and Warner 1983; Graham *et al* 1984; Carter *et al* 1985; Egger *et al* 1985; Supramaniam and Warner 1986; Wraith 1987; Egger *et al* 1989).

There is no universal consensus on the composition of a Multiple Exclusion diet but general guidelines are given in Table 4.87. (The Cambridge Exclusion diet used in the investigation of Irritable Bowel Syndrome can be found in Section 4.9.1). A multiple exclusion diet is usually followed for a period of 2–3 weeks but in conditions where there fluctuations in the disease pattern (for example, rheumatoid arthritis) it may be necessary to continue for up to six weeks.

An alternative multiple exclusion strategy which is sometimes used is to exclude foods or a food group singly for a period of 2–3 weeks but in a progressive manner – in effect, a series of simple exclusion diets which eventually become a multiple exclusion diet. In theory, the advantage

Table 4.87 General guidance for the composition of a Multiple Exclusion diet. (The choice of foods excluded depends on the symptoms being investigated and the dietary history)

Foods usually excluded	Milk and milk products Eggs Wheat Citrus fruit
Foods sometimes excluded	Pork, bacon, liver and offal Fish and shellfish Barley, oats, corn, rye Nuts and pips Yeasts Potatoes, tomatoes, onions and garlic Chocolate Coffee/tea Food colourings (especially azo dyes) Food preservatives (especially benzoates and sulphites) Soya
Foods usually permitted	Beef, lamb, turkey, rabbit Rice Sugar, treacle, syrup Lard Vegetables (except potatoes, tomatoes, onions and garlic) Fruit (except citrus fruit)

of this type of approach is that the offending food/foods may become readily apparent. However it has a number of disadvantages. Sensitivity may occur to several types of foods rather than one and improvement will not be complete unless all likely possibilities are removed simultaneously. Furthermore, since the procedure takes a long time, partial improvement in symptoms may lead to the patient abandoning the process before a complete diagnosis can be made.

If improvement occurs, foods then need to be appropriately reintroduced (see the section below on 'Food reintroduction') in order to establish which ones have provoked symptoms. If improvement does not occur, the dietitian must carefully review the patient's food intake to ascertain whether the procedure was followed correctly and, if so, must then decide whether other foods should be excluded or whether a food intolerance is unlikely to exist.

Non-dietary sources of substances which can provoke reactions may also need to be excluded. Colours or preservatives can be encountered via toothpastes, medicines, vitamin and mineral preparations, paints, chalk, crayons, and cosmetics. Play-doh contains gluten. Lactose, maize starch, wheat and yeast are present in many medicinal products; information on their content can usually be obtained from the hospital pharmacy or directly from the pharmaceutical manufacturers. The latter may be unwilling to provide a complete list of ingredients but are usually willing to state whether specific items are included. Any potential problems from medication should be discussed with the patient's physician who may be able to prescribe a product with a different excipient.

3 Few Food diets (also know as oligo-antigenic or hypoantigenic diets)

The Few Food diet is a much more restrictive regimen than the multiple exclusion diet. It is used when a multiple exclusion diet has failed to relieve symptoms but food intolerance is still suspected. It can also be useful for patients who present on a self-imposed restrictive dietary regimen but without having established any clear relationship with symptoms.

Unlike the Multiple Exclusion diet where a relatively small number of foods are excluded, Few Food diets are comprised solely of a small number of foods which rarely provoke sensitivity. Which foods should be permitted remains a matter of some debate and policy varies among treatment centres. Usually they comprise one or two meats, and a selection of starchy foods, vegetables and fruits (Table 4.88).

The choice of foods also depends on individual factors such as the acceptability and frequency of consumption of particular foods. For example, lamb is often recommended for inclusion but if this is already consumed frequently it may not be an appropriate choice; a less frequently consumed alternative such as turkey or rabbit may be a better alternative. Individual nutritional requirements, the likelihood of nutritional risk from a restricted diet and the nature of the disorder being investigated are also relevant considerations.

In infants and young children it is essential that a milk substitute is used according to individual needs. However, it should be borne in mind that approximately 50% of milk

Table 4.88 Example of a Few Food diet

2 meats or 1 meat and 1 fish	e.g. turkey and rabbit Plain meats except pork Fish if normally eaten infrequently and not implicated
2–3 vegetables	e.g. carrots; cauliflower; broccoli Any vegetables except onions, sweetcorn, tomatoes, soya and, in some centres, potatoes
2 starchy foods	e.g. rice/rice cakes/Kalo puffed rice; sweet potatoes Rice, tapioca, sago, buckwheat
2 fruits	e.g. pear; peach Any fruit except citrus
Oils and fat spreads	Sunflower, safflower, olive, rapeseed oils Milk-free margarine such as Tomor, Vitaquel, Suma or DP Pure
Water	Tap, mineral, soda water
Miscellaneous	Salt, sugar, syrup, treacle, honey Milk substitute for infants and young children

sensitive children also react to soya milk (Jenkins *et al* 1984). If older children do not use a milk substitute, daily calcium and vitamin supplements such as 6 × 600 mg calcium gluconate and 0.6 ml Abidec will be required.

If the first Few Food diet fails to relieve symptoms it may be necessary to construct a second diet using similar principles bearing no foods in common with the first. Vitamins, trace element and mineral preparations which may be suitable for use on this type of regimen are shown in Table 4.89.

This very restricted diet should not be continued for more than 2–3 weeks unless the symptoms are known to be delayed. If no improvement occurs the diet should be discontinued and the situation reassessed. Symptomatic relief should be followed by the reintroduction of single foods at appropriate intervals (see the section below on 'Food reintroduction').

4 Elemental and protein hydrolysate formula diets

A regimen which withdraws all food and replaces it with an elemental or formula diet may be used in cases where there is a long history of dietary treatment with very little improvement in the condition, or in infants and children before and while proceeding with a formal exclusion diet. These diets are unpalatable and monotonous and should only be used in those whose symptoms are sufficiently severe or debilitating to warrant such treatment. They have

Table 4.89 Vitamin, mineral and trace element supplements suitable for use in investigating food allergy/intolerance

Supplement	Content	Relevant excipients
Infants and children		
Paediatric Seravit (SHS)	Ca, P, Mg, Fe, Zn, I, Mn, Cu, Mo, Se, Cr Vitamins A, E, C, B_1, B_2, B_6, nic, pant, inositol, choline, D_3, B_{12}, folate, biotin, K	Maize Starch
Abidec (Warner & Lambert)	Vitamins A, D, B_1, B_2, nic, B_6, C	Sugar
Ketovite tablets (Paines & Byrne)	Vitamins B_1, B_2, B_6, nic, pant, C, E, inositol, K, biotin, folate	
Ketovite Liquid (Paines & Byrne)	Vitamins A, D, B_{12}, choline	Terpenless orange oil Methyl Hydroxy Benzoate
Adults		
Seravit Complete (SHS)	Na, K, Cl, Ca, P, Mg, Fe, Zn, I, Mn, Cu, Mo, Se, Cr, Vitamins A, E, C, B_1, B_2, B_6, nic, pant, inositol, choline, D_3, B_{12}, folate, biotin, K	Maize starch
Health Assurance (Healthcraft)	Ca, I, Fe, Mg, Zn, Vitamins A, B_1, B_2, B_6, B_{12}, nic, C, D, E, folate, biotin	Soya fibre Maize starch
Health Insurance Plus (Lamberts)	Ca, Cr, Fe, Mg, Mn, Mo, Se, Zn, I Vitamins A, D_3, B_1, B_2, B_6, B_{12}, C, E, biotin, pant, choline, folate, inositol, nic	(contains lemon bioflavinoids)
600 mg Calcium Gluconate Tablet (Evans)	54 mg Ca/tablet	Sucrose, theobroma (extract of cocoa)
Calcium gluconate ampoules 1 × 5 ml 1 × 10 ml (Evans)	 45 mg Ca/ampoule 90 mg Ca/ampoule	Calcium saccharate
Sandocal 400 Sandocal 1000 (Sandoz)	400 mg Ca/tab 1000 mg Ca/tab	Natural orange flavour Aspartame, citric acid
Calcium Sandoz syrup (Sandoz)	325 mg Ca/15 ml	Natural orange flavour Benzoic acid, sugar

Information correct as at February 1992

been particularly successful in the treatment of Crohn's disease and eczema in children.

Elemental and protein hydrolysate formula diets were primarily designed as a means of providing nutritional support in a readily absorbed form for children and adults with impaired gastrointestinal function. However, they have a use in the investigation of food allergy and intolerance because protein is supplied either in the form of amino acids or low molecular weight peptides which are less likely to be antigenic and provoke symptoms. Their use may also be preferable to a soya milk formula in the investigation of cows' milk intolerance (both immunological and non-immunological) in infants (Eastham 1987; Walker-Smith 1987; Witherly 1990). Available elemental and hydrolysate preparations are shown in Table 4.90. In deciding which formula to use, one needs to consider the source of each ingredient and its suitability for an individual patient; in most instances it may be preferable to commence treatment with an elemental preparation.

Elemental diets are hyperosmolar solutions and should be diluted 1 in 5 (using distilled or mineral water to eliminate the possibility of tap water intolerance). The volume needed to provide sufficient nutritional requirements can be over three litres per day. The quantity ingested should gradually be increased gradually to avoid hyperosmotic diarrhoea. Extra water can be taken but no other food or drink is permitted.

Some patients find elemental diets unpleasant to take but palatability can be improved by cooling the drink and using a covered container with a straw. Nausea and headaches may occur, particularly during the first few days. Once symptoms start to improve, patients usually find the diet more acceptable. If an elemental diet cannot be tolerated orally it can be administered by continuous nasogastric feeding over 24 hours.

During the period of an elemental diet, any medication is usually curtailed to ensure that symptom remission is related to food withdrawal and to prevent masking of any subsequent reaction when food reintroduction begins. If drugs are taken they should be in the form of capsules or tablets: capsules should be opened so that only their contents are administered and any surface colouring from tablets should be removed with running water. No toothpaste should be used; teeth should be cleaned with water.

The length of time patients should be allowed to remain on such a restricted regimen is a matter of debate but generally 2–3 weeks are sufficient to discern improvement. However, this will vary between patients and with the condition being investigated. If there is no improvement after this time, the normal diet should be resumed. If symptom remission has occurred, foods should be reintroduced singly and at intervals of a few days (see the section on 'Food reintroduction' below). If severe reaction occurs, patients should return to the elemental diet until better. During the first few weeks of testing, patients will need to take some elemental diet as a nutritional supplement.

Use of elemental diets in children Placing a child on an elemental diet is a hazardous procedure and should only be attempted as a last resort, for example in cases of severe eczema.

The volume of formula given should be based on fluid requirement for age and weight. No flavouring should be added and the initial use of low concentrations may help the patients become used to its unpleasant taste, but they make take as long as a week to do so.

Elemental formulae may be taken from a feeding bottle with a teat, from a covered feeding cup or from a covered beaker with a straw according to the patient's age and preference. It may also be frozen and consumed as either as 'ice lollies' or crushed and eaten with a spoon. The poor palatability of an unflavoured elemental formula may result in a child receiving less than the required amounts of energy and nutrients. However, no attempt should be made to force a particular volume on a patient with the aim of maximizing intake. Each child should be allowed to take as much or as little as he or she desires. No alternative drinks should be permitted, not even water as it tastes better than an elemental formula and will be taken in preference.

Daily consumption charts should be used to check the intake of formula. Weight should be recorded on alternate days and it is essential that serum electrolytes and protein are closely monitored. However, efforts must be made to draw the attention of parents away from their child's nutritional intake which may well be inadequate in the short term.

If symptom remission occurs, foods are reintroduced along the guidelines given below and in Table 4.93. A child may have an apparently unlimited appetite for a food after several weeks on an elemental formula and the first food to be reintroduced (e.g. lamb) may be demanded in large quantities. In order to avoid boredom after a few days, the food should be presented in a variety of ways to retain the child's interest. Lamb may be roasted and sliced, stewed or served as chops. It may be minced and turned into burgers, sausages or animal shapes. Lamb fat should be collected and retained for use in frying and roasting foods which are to be added to the diet later.

If the child is, as is most likely, an inpatient, close liaison will be required between dietitian and catering manager so that the latter understands the reason for an order of a large quantity of a single food for a single patient. It is also essential to have a diet bay with a competent and cooperative diet cook who understands the reasoning behind the apparently bizarre meals being requested.

Once four or five foods have been reintroduced, the elemental formula may be replaced by a protein hydrolysate formula (see Table 4.90) prior to discharge. A programme of foods to be introduced at home, singly and at weekly intervals, should be devised. While the diet consists of only a small number of foods, estimates of nutritional intake should be made at regular intervals and serious inad-

Table 4.90 Elemental and protein hydrolysate replacement formulae suitable for use in investigating food allergy/intolerance (Information as at February 1992)

	Products suitable for adults and older children	Protein source	Fat source	Carbohydrate source	Miscellaneous
ELEMENTAL FORMULAE	Elemental 028 (SHS)	Mixture of synthetic amino acids	Arachis oil (peanut)	Maltodextrin (maize)	
	Elemental 028 Flavoured (SHS)	Mixture of synthetic amino acids	Arachis oil (peanut)	Maltodextrin (maize) Sucrose	Orange flavour Colours: B carotene Beetroot red
	Flexical (MJ)	Hydrolysed casein L Tyrosine L Tryptophan L Methionine	Soya oil MCT oil	Glucose syrup solids Modified tapioca starch	
PROTEIN HYDROLYSATE FORMULAE	Pepdite 2+ (SHS)	Hydrolysed beef and soya plus amino acids	Maize oil Coconut oil	Maltodextrin (maize)	
	MCT peptide 2+ (SHS)	Hydrolysed beef and soya plus amino acids	Peanut oil Coconut oil Pork	Maltodextrin (maize)	
	PEPTI 2000 LF (Powder) (Cow & Gate)	Hydrolysed whey	MCT oil (coconut) Corn oil Lecithin	Maltodextrin (maize) Glucose syrup Tr Lactose	Vanilla flavour
	Peptamen (Clintec)	Hydrolysed whey	MCT oil (coconut) Lecithin Residual milk fat	Maltodextrin (maize) Corn starch	
	Product suitable for infants and young children	**Protein source**	**Fat source**	**Carbohydrate source**	
ELEMENTAL FORMULAE	Neocate (SHS)	Mixture of synthetic amino acids	Coconut oil Ground nut oil	Maltodextrin (Maize)	
PROTEIN HYDROLYSATE FORMULAE	Pregestimil (MJ)	Hydrolysed casein L Tyrosine L Cystine L Tryptophan	Corn oil MCT oil (coconut) Soya lecithin	Glucose syrup solid Modified corn starch	
	Nutramigen (MJ)	Hydrolysed casein	Corn oil	Glucose syrup solid Modified corn starch	
	Prejomin (Milupa)	Hydrolysed bovine collagen and whey plus amino acids	Palm oil Coconut oil Soya oil	Maltodextrin (maize) Corn starch Potato starch	
	Pepdite 0–2 (SHS)	Hydrolysed beef and soya plus amino acids	Coconut oil Ground nut oil Pork	Maltodextrin (maize)	
	MCT Peptide 0–2 (SHS)	Hydrolysed beef and soya plus amino acids	Coconut oil Sunflower oil	Maltodextrin (maize)	
	Alfare (Nestlé)	Hydrolysed whey	Corn oil MCT oil (coconut) Butter oil Soya lecithin	Maltodextrin (maize) Potato starch Tr Lactose	
	Pepti-junior (Cow & Gate)	Hydrolysed whey	Maize oil Coconut oil Lecithin	Glucose syrup Tr Lactose	

SHS = Scientific Hospital Supplies
MJ = Mead Johnson

equacies should be corrected (David 1984).

Infants may need to be maintained on a special formula for the first few months of life until weaning occurs. When foods are reintroduced, this should be done in small quantities and highly allergenic foods such as milk, wheat and eggs avoided until the age of 10–12 months.

Monitoring symptoms

Whichever type of dietary regimen is followed, the patient should be asked to keep a record of their symptoms on a daily basis. This may be done in either a graphical format or on a specially designed card where symptoms can recorded on a scale of increasing severity from 0–5 (Tables 4.91 and 4.92). This record should be completed twice daily, usually in the morning and evening. Ideally, recording should commence two weeks prior to commencing the diet and should continue throughout the elimination and reintroduction period so that alteration in symptoms can be related to any dietary change. If possible, an objective method of monitoring symptoms should be kept over the same period, for example, peak expiratory flow in asthmatics or grip strength in arthritics.

Table 4.91 Suggested format of combined symptom record and food diary

Name
Date
*New food**
Breakfast
Lunch
Evening
Symptoms
Vomiting
Headache
Diarrhoea
Constipation
Pain
Stress
x when the symptoms are present
xx when the symptoms are bad
xxx when the symptoms are very bad

* The Brand name should be included if appropriate, also the cooking method and quantity

Table 4.92 Suggested format of symptom record sheet for use in the investigation of food intolerance. Patients are asked to score twice daily how they feel

Date				
General well-being	am	−5	0	5
	pm	−5	0	5
		Unwell		Well
Bowels	am	−5	0	5
	pm	−5	0	5
		Diarrhoea	Normal	Constipation
....	am	−5	0	5
	pm	−5	0	5

Food reintroduction

After a period of exclusion, foods will need to be reintroduced. Foods are reintroduced singly and usually at intervals of a few days. The delay between the consumption of a food and the return of symptoms can vary from an immediate response to one week or more after daily ingestion of the suspect food (Lessof *et al* 1980; Wraith 1982).

There is no universally agreed order in which foods should be reintroduced. This will vary from patient to patient and according to the condition being treated. Foods which are most likely to cause problems are not tested until later and are interspersed with those which are unlikely to precipitate symptoms. A food reintroduction order should be devised for each patient based on considerations such as the original exclusion diet and individual needs.

The quantity of food reintroduced should be similar to the amount which may have created the problem in the first place. If this is difficult to assess then a larger intake is thought to be preferable because there is always a risk that too small a quantity of food will be insufficient to provoke symptoms. However, this is a matter of some debate and, in children and infants, because sensitivity may be increased after a period of exclusion, it may be desirable to introduce the suspect food gradually (David 1984). Francis (1987) provides a protocol for milk or food introduction for infants and children at risk of severe reaction.

It is important to give patients clear guidance on the form in which a food should be reintroduced. If testing wheat, for example, a sweet biscuit is an inappropriate source since it may contain other ingredients which may provoke symptoms. Table 4.93 lists the form in which some of the most commonly eliminated foods should be reintroduced. Foods should be fresh or frozen single items with no additions. Composite dishes, ready meals and other convenience foods should only be reintroduced into the diet when all the likely suspect ingredients have been tested separately. They should also be incorporated using the general principles of food reintroduction already described.

Dietary assessment should be carried out throughout this period to determine if any nutritional supplementation is required.

Table 4.93 Suggested form in which to reintroduce foods following exclusion

Food or food group	Test as
Wheat	Matzos, Puffed Wheat, Shredded Wheat, Cubs, wholemeal flour or unbleached white flour, semolina or pasta (free from colour or egg) If no reaction is seen to these then test wholemeal bread
Rye	Rye flour, original Ryvita (white packet)
Oats	Porridge oats, homemade muesli or flapjack, incorporating permitted ingredients
Corn (maize)	Cornflour, corn oil, sweetcorn, plain popcorn
Rice	Boiled rice, rice flour, rice cakes with or without salt only
Barley/malt	Pearl barley added to soups, casseroles. Malt extract, Rice Krispies or cornflakes if sugar/rice/corn are tolerated
Sugar	Beet (Silver Spoon) or cane (Tate & Lyle)
Cows' milk	Fresh pasteurized milk. If cows' milk is not tolerated goats' milk can be tried later
Dairy products	If milk is tolerated then test yoghurt, butter, cream
Cheese	If milk and dairy products are tolerated, test plain unprocessed cheese. If cheese is not tolerated, ewes' or goats' cheeses may be tried at a later date
Eggs	Fried, poached or boiled. (Some patients may tolerate small quantities of egg in cakes etc.)
Citrus fruit	Orange, grapefruit, lemon, lime, satsumas or tangerines — fresh fruit or freshly squeezed (home-made) juice
Chocolate	Ordinary plain or milk chocolate assuming other ingredients are permitted. Cocoa
Yeast	Crushed brewers yeast tablets, Marmite
Azo dyes	A few drops of artificial yellow or red food colouring added to food. If reaction is seen then it may be necessary to test each dye separately using specially prepared capsules
Sodium benzoate E211	Assuming sugar and citrus fruits are permitted choose a squash or fizzy drink which is free from artificial colour, but which contains sodium benzoate E211

The reintroduction process can be very slow, up to nine months in some cases. Patients need to be highly motivated and will require a lot of support from a dietitian. There is always a conflict between the desire to make the diet more acceptable to the patient and the need to ensure that foods are not introduced so quickly that no conclusions can be drawn. If carried out correctly, the potential rewards from these dietary manipulations are high; patients who have been chronically ill for years may be given a new lease of life. Conversely, patients who have undergone these procedures without identification of any food-related intolerance should be reassured that the investigation has not 'failed' but simply demonstrated that their symptoms are not diet-related.

Blind food challenge

Blind challenge — administering a food in a disguised form without the patient's knowledge — is a means of confirming a diagnosis of food intolerance. However it need not be carried out in every patient and should not be carried out if there is a clear history of major allergic symptoms following ingestion of a specific food, e.g. swelling of the lips, tongue or face, respiratory difficulties or anaphylaxis (Sampson *et al* 1987). Alternatively, the reaction to a food may be so obvious that the patient does not want to repeat it, or a food may have been taken by mistake and already identified by reaction.

The main reasons for using blind challenge are:

1 To confirm diagnosis.
2 If doubts still exist as to whether an intolerance exists.
3 To distinguish between food intolerance and food aversion.

Administering blind challenge

Blind challenge is not an easy procedure to carry out. There are three main ways in which can be given in a blind form but each method has its limitations:

1 By masking them with other foods.
2 By placement within an opaque gelatine capsule.
3 By administration via a nasogastric tube.

Masking with other foods Some suspect items can be disguised in soups, casseroles, fruit juices, puréed fruits or vegetables, bread, cakes or biscuits. These can be made up as required for in-patients; outpatients can be given previously prepared frozen products, some with and some without the test material, with instructions for use at home. As far as possible the suspect food should be given in a similar quantity and form to that which is normally consumed. The patient should not be able to distinguish, either by sight, smell or taste, which is the active and which is the placebo challenge. Suggestions for disguising some of the most commonly implicated foods are given in Table 4.94. For research studies, it may be possible to enlist the help of a food manufacturer to disguise foods in cans or baked products.

It is difficult to mask some of the stronger tasting foods such as cheese or fish. If these are not considered a nutritionally important part of the diet, their continued avoidance may have to be justified on the ground of open challenge only.

Nasogastric administration Delivery by nasogastric tube is an effective way of preventing identification of the food by the subject. It is also relatively easy to incorporate commonly suspected foods into products such as Elemental 028 (SHS) or Fortison Soya (Cow & Gate). However it is an invasive technique for the patient and cannot be justified

Table 4.94 Ways in which foods may be disguised for blind food challenge

Test food	Suitable base materials for disguise
Cows' milk	Soya milk, mashed potato, puréed lentils, soups, casseroles
Soya milk	Cows' milk, puréed lentils
Egg	Mashed potato, puréed lentils
Wheat	Puréed lentils, oatcakes, flapjacks, gluten-free foods
Corn	Oatcakes, flapjacks, soups, casseroles
Rye	Gluten-free bread, soups, casseroles
Oats	Soups, casseroles
Barley	Soups, casseroles
Orange juice	Carrot juice
Sugar	Carrot juice, 'Diet' drinks
Food colours	Carrot juice, orange juice
Preservatives	Orange juice

for either routine investigation or controlled studies. An additional criticism is that it bypasses the oral cavity where enzymic release of antigens and their absorption may occur.

Opaque gelatine capsules Encapsulation of foods may seem an ideal means of disguise but there are obvious limitations in terms of the type and amount of food which can be administered. Small quantities of food may be sufficient to trigger allergic reactions but not other types of food intolerance (RCP/BNF 1984). The problem of bypassing the oral cavity (see above) also applies.

The main advantage of this method is it can provide an 'off-the-shelf' range of readily available challenges, and is a particularly useful way of testing sensitivity to food additives. Pharmacy departments may be able to assist in the preparation of suitable test materials.

Challenge procedure

Whichever method is used, the patient should be observed for a period exceeding the time determined in the history between food ingestion and recurrence of symptoms. (Note: this isn't possible if patients take the test food home – see above under Masking). If no symptoms are produced by the test doses on a single occasion, the challenge should be repeated – this may need to be on a daily basis for 1–2 weeks (Lessof *et al* 1980).

After a period of avoidance from the offending food, response to challenge may be accentuated, possibly with anaphylaxis, but can also be diminished, particularly by prolonged abstinence. Suitable placebos to which the patient is known not to be sensitive must also be administered, ideally in a crossover format. Egger *et al* (1989) document a protocol used in investigation of children with epilepsy or migraine. An objective method of assessing results is required and it must be borne in mind that results can be affected by spontaneous fluctuations in disease severity, changing levels of sensitivity and the presence or absence of other precipitating factors such as environmental pollutants or emotional stress. Many symptoms need to be described by the patient so comparison of severity is subjective and depends on accurate and consistent reporting by the patient.

Interpretation of the results is easy if a patient consistently fails to react to the tested ingredient or has a high placebo response rate. Equally, consistent responses to the test material but not the placebo yield an obvious conclusion. Pearson (1987) has suggested that in order to be 95% certain that the correct conclusion is reached, at least eight provocations per allergen are required of which at least seven should be identified by the patient. However Duncan and Avery (1988) feel this is unrealistic and Warner (1987) feels that three independently elicited pieces of information, including one objective test, in relation to a single food may be sufficient to make a diagnosis.

Maintenance diets

Patients who are sensitive to a number of foods need considerable practical guidance and support to ensure that the diet is nutritionally adequate and as manageable as possible. Factors such as lifestyle, shopping facilities, cooking ability and meals consumed outside the home are all relevant.

Some patients with severe food allergies may benefit from mast cell stabilizing drugs such as sodium cromoglycate which inhibit degranulation of the mast cell and prevent the release of histamine and other mediators of the allergic response (Wraith *et al* 1979). These preparations are particularly useful as a prophylactic treatment enabling some patients to tolerate a food without total exclusion or to eat a meal which contains unknown ingredients (Lessof 1983).

Avoidance of a food may not necessarily be permanent. After six months to a year of avoidance, foods can often gradually be reintroduced without a return of symptoms. Children commonly grow out of their intolerance (Dannaeus and Inganas 1981).

Alternative diets used in the investigation and treatment of food allergy or intolerance

Rotation or rotary diets

These have been recommended as a way of diagnosing masked food allergy and also treating multiple food allergy (Radcliffe 1982).

Foods are divided into food 'families' based on botanical classification on the presumption that there may be some degree of cross-reaction from foods. The diet is arranged so that no closely related foods are eaten on consecutive days and thus exposure to each food family is rotated throughout a four or five day cycle. The practical relevance of cross-reaction to foods in the same family is debatable; there is no evidence that foods from the same botanical family trigger reactions other than in an independent way (Haworth 1991). Such a diet is socially very restricting and very expensive because non-seasonal foods often have to be purchased to ensure an adequate nutritional intake. There is little evidence of benefit from this rigorous regimen.

Feingold diet

See Sections 2.16.2 and 3.6.6.

Anti-candida diet

See Section 2.16.2.

Dong diet

See Section 4.29.2.

4.31.7 Prevention of food allergy in children

Atopic disorders such as eczema and asthma in children may be related to food sensitization either *in utero* or during infancy. It has been suggested that this can be reduced or prevented in children at high risk (e.g. those with a strong family history of the disease) by maternal or infant dietary modification during these periods (Shacks and Heiner 1982; Burr 1983; Cant 1984; Cant *et al* 1986; Chandra *et al* 1986; Eastham 1987).

The long term benefit of early avoidance of cows' milk has not yet been established. Breast feeding certainly appears to offer some protection (Burr 1983; Miskelly *et al* 1988) although Atherton (1988) points out that the incidence of atopic eczema in the UK has continued to increase despite an increased prevalence of breastfeeding.

The maternal diet during lactation may also be relevant. In a study of the development of atopic eczema in high risk children, Chandra *et al* (1989) recommended that breast feeding mothers of such children should avoid allergenic foods such as milk and dairy products, eggs, fish, peanuts and soya beans.

In children who are not breast fed, there is little evidence that use of a soya milk is less likely to provoke allergenic disease than cows' milk (Miskelly *et al* 1988), a view supported by Witherly (1990). Chandra *et al* (1989) recommend that infants at high risk of developing eczema whose mothers choose not to breast feed should be given a hydrolysate formula rather than a cows' milk or soya based one.

There is evidence (Cant 1984) that delaying the introduction of highly allergenic foods until at least the age of 8 months may benefit children at risk of atopic disease. Details of such a programme which is both hypoallergenic and nutritionally adequate have been given by Cant and Bailes (1984).

4.31.8 Role of the dietitian in the management of food allergy and intolerance

The dietitian has a vital role to play in the successful diagnosis and management of a food-related allergy or intolerance. If patients are not given sufficiently detailed guidance on how to avoid or reintroduce foods, there is a strong likelihood of a missed or incorrect diagnosis. A dietitian can also provide practical suggestions on dietary substitutions or variations which are essential if patients are to persevere with what can be a protracted and difficult dietary regimen. A dietitian is also well placed to detect at an early stage the nutritional inadequacies which may develop after prolonged periods of dietary investigation, particularly in children.

A summary of the dietitian's role in the investigation and

Table 4.95 The role of the dietitian in the investigation and management of food allergy or intolerance

1	Elicit a symptomatic and dietary profile of the patient as a baseline for diagnostic procedures
2	Decide, in conjunction with medical colleagues, the most appropriate strategy for dietary investigation
3	Explain the purpose of the diet to the patient
4	Provide up-to-date written advice appropriate for the patient's clinical and practical needs e.g. lists of foods to be either included or excluded
5	Provide other support material which may help patients follow the prescribed regimen e.g. recipes, guidance for adaptation of recipes, use of alternative foods and where these may be purchased.
6	Discuss and give practical guidance on the social problems of adhering to an exclusion diet e.g. cheating, hunger, boredom, entertaining, eating away from home (at work, at school, on holiday, etc.) It may be necessary to postpone commencement of the diet to a more convenient time
7	Discuss the cost implications of the diet. Advise on eligibility for receiving special products on prescription and make the appropriate arrangements
8	If necessary, discuss the need and use of special supplements such as vitamins and minerals
9	Check usage of medicines for implicated agents and discuss the need for any changes with the patient's physician
10	Explain how symptoms are to be recorded and monitored by means of a simple score system
11	Make follow-up arrangements with the patient
12	Encourage the patient/parent to make contact by phone in case of any doubt or difficulty
13	Provide written advice on food reintroduction i.e. which foods, how frequently and in what quantity
14	Monitor the nutritional adequacy of the diet; maintain growth charts for children
15	If the elimination and reintroduction procedures result in the identification or one or more suspect foods, provide the patient with long-term guidance on its/their avoidance. A follow-up visit should be arranged to check that this is being done correctly and appears to be beneficial

management of food allergy or intolerance is given in Table 4.95.

Cross-references

The role of food allergy and intolerance in some specific disorders can be found in:

Oro-facial granulomatosis (Section 4.1.4, p. 349)
Crohn's and inflammatory bowel disease (Section 4.8, p. 384)
Irritable bowel syndrome (Section 4.9.1, p. 390)
Coeliac disease (Section 4.7, p. 378)
Rheumatoid arthritis (Section 4.29.2, p. 545)
Eczema (Section 4.30.1, p. 547)

Useful addresses

Action Against Allergy, 43 The Downs, London SW20 8HS.

Asthma Society and Friends of the Asthma Research Council, St Thomas' Hospital, Lambeth Palace Road, London SE1 7EH.

Hyperactive Children's Support Group, c/o 59 Meadowside, Angmering, West Sussex BN14 4BW.

Migraine Trust, 45 Great Ormond Street, London WC1N 3HD.

National Association for Colitis and Crohns Disease, 98A London Road, St Albans, Herts AL1 1NX.

National Society for Research into Allergy, PO Box 45, Hinckley, Leicestershire.

Further reading

Brostoff J and Challacombe S (1982) *Food allergy*. WB Saunders, London.

Brostoff J and Challacombe S (1987) *Food Allergy and intolerance*. Baillière Tindall, London.

Chiaramonte LT, Schneider AT and Liftshitz F (1988) *Food allergy*. Marcel Dekker, New York.

Dobbing J (Ed) (1987) *Food intolerance*. Baillière Tindall, London.

Francis D (1987) Food intolerance and allergy. In *Diets for sick children*, 4e, pp. 77–127. Blackwell Scientific Publications, Oxford.

Human Nutrition: Applied Nutrition Vol 38A, (No 6) (1984). Contains a number of articles of interest.

Joint Report of the Royal College of Physicians and the British Nutrition Foundation. (1984) *Food intolerance and food aversion. J Roy Coll Phys* **18**, 83–123.

Lessof MH (Ed) (1983) *Clinical reactions to food*. John Wiley, Chichester.

Sells S (1987) *Basic immunology*. Elsevier, New York.

References

Alun Jones V, McLaughlan P, Shorthouse M, Workman E and Hunter JO (1982) Food intolerance: a major factor in the pathogenesis of irritable bowel syndrome. *Lancet* **ii**, 1115–7.

American Academy of Allergy (1981) Position statement on controversial techniques. *Allergy and Clin Allergy* **67**(5), 332–8.

Astrup A, Toubro S, Cannon S, Hein P, Breum L and Madsen J (1990) Caffeine: a double-blind, placebo-controlled study of its thermogenic, metabolic and cardiovascular effects in healthy volunteers. *Am J Clin Nutr* **51**(5), 759–67.

Atherton DJ (1988) Diet and atopic eczema. *Clin Allergy* **18**, 215–28.

Blades M (1990) A review of patients attending a dietetic out-patient clinic for patients with food sensitivity. *J Hum Nutr Diet* **3**(5), 368.

British Dietetic Association (1990) *Policy Statement: Food allergy and intolerance*. BDA, Birmingham.

Burr ML (1983) Does infant feeding affect the risk of allergy? *Arch Dis Childh* **58**, 561–3.

Cant AJ (1984) Diet and the prevention of childhood allergic disease. *Hum Nutr: Appl Nutr* **38A**(6), 455–68.

Cant AJ and Bailes JA (1984) How should we feed the potentially allergic infant? *Hum Nutr: Appl Nutr* **38A**(6), 474–6.

Cant AJ, Bailes JA, Marsden RA and Hewitt D (1986) Effect of maternal exclusion on breast fed infants with eczema: two controlled studies. *Br Med J* **293**, 321–3.

Carini C, Brostoff J and Wraith DG (1984) Food allergy as a cause of arthralgia. *Immunol Clin Sper* **III**(1), 31–9.

Carter CM, Egger J and Soothill JF (1985) A dietary management of severe childhood migraine. *Hum Nutr: Apply Nutr* **39A**(4), 294–303.

Chandra RK, Puri S, Suraiya C and Cheema PS (1986) Influence of maternal food antigen avoidance during pregnancy and lactation on incidence of atopic eczema in infants. *Clin Allergy* **16**, 563–9.

Chandra RK, Puri S and Hamid A (1989) Influence of maternal diet during lactation and use of formula feeds on development of atopic eczema in high risk infants. *Br Med J* **299**, 228–30.

Consumers' Association (1987) Allergies to food. *Which? Magazine* Jan, 6–8.

Dannaeus A and Inganas M (1981) A follow up study of children with food allergy. Clinical course in relation to serum IgE and IgG antibody levels to mild, egg and fish. *Clin Allergy* **11**, 533–9.

David TJ (1984) Anaphylatic shock during elimination diets for severe atopic eczema. *Arch Dis Childh* **59**, 983–6.

Duncan P and Avery J (1988) Investigation for possible error in food elimination and challenge testing. In *Dietetics in the 90s. Role of dietitian/nutritionist*, Moyal MF (Ed) pp. 197–201. John Libby Eurotext Ltd, London.

Eastham EJ (1987) Soya formulae: Development and drawbacks. In *Food intolerance*, Dobbing J, (Ed) pp. 112–26. Baillière Tindall, London.

Egger J, Carter CM, Graham PJ, Gumley D and Soothill JF (1985) A controlled trial of oligoantigenic diet treatment in the hyperkinetic syndrome. *Lancet* **i**, 940–45.

Egger J, Carter CM, Soothill JF and Wilson J (1989) Oligoantigenic diet treatment of children with epilepsy and migraine. *J Paediatr* **114**, 51–8.

Francis D (1987) Food intolerance and allergy. In *Diets for sick children*, 4e. pp. 77–127. Blackwell Scientific Publications, Oxford.

Graham P, Hall-Smith SP, Harris JR and Price ML (1984) A study of hypoallergenic diets and oral sodium cromoglycate in the management of atopic eczema. *Br J Dermat* **110**, 457–67.

Hathaway MJ and Warner JO (1983) Compliance problems in the dietary management of eczema. *Arch Dis Childh* **59**, 151–6.

Haworth RJP (1991) Food intolerance in oro-facial granulomatosis. M. Phil thesis, The Queen's College, Glasgow.

Hawthorne B, Lambert S, Scott D and Scott B (1991) Food intolerance and the irritable bowel syndrome. *J Hum Nutr Dietet* **3**, 19–23.

Jenkins HR, Pincott JR, Soothill JF, Milla PJ and Harries JT (1984) Food allergy: the major cause of infantile colitis. *Arch Dis Childh* **59**, 326–9.

Joint Committee of the Royal College of Physicians of London and the British Nutrition Foundation (1984) Food intolerance and food aversion. *J Roy Coll Physicians Lond* **18**, 83–123.

Labib M, Gama R, Wright J, Marks V and Robins D (1989) Dietary maladvice as a cause of hypothroidism and short stature. *Brit Med J* **298**, 232–3.

Lehman CW (1980) The leucocytic food allergy test: a study of its reliability and reproducibility. *Ann Allergy* **45**, 150–158.

Lessof MH (1983) Food intolerance and allergy – a review. *Quart J Med* **206**, 111–19.

Lessof MH, Wraith DG, Merrett TG, Merrett J and Buisseret PD (1980) Food allergy and intolerance in 100 patients: Local and systemic effects. *Quart J Med* **49**, 259–71.

Macdonald A and Forsythe WI (1986) The cost of nutrition and diet therapy for low income families. *Hum Nutr: Appl Nutr* **40A**(2), 87–96.

Metcalfe DD (1984) Food hypersensitivity. *J Allergy Clin Immunology* **73**, 749–62.

Miskelly FG, Burr ML, Vaughan Williams E, Fehily AM, Butland BK and Merrett TG (1988) Infant feeding and allergy. *Arch Dis Childh* **63**, 388–93.

Nanda R, James R, Smith H, Dudley CRK and Jewell DP (1989) Food intolerance and irritable bowel syndrome. *Gut* **30**, 1099–1104.

Pachor ML, Nicolis F, Cortina P, Peroli P, Venturini G, Andri L, Corroher R and Lunardi C (1989) Migraine and food. *Recenti Prog Med* **80**(2), 53–5.

Pearson DJ (1987) Problems with terminology and with study design in food sensitivity. In *Food intolerance*, Dobbing J (Ed) pp. 1–23. Baillière Tindall, London.

Radcliffe MJ (1982) Clinical methods for diagnosis. In *Food Allergy*, Brostoff J and Challacombe SJ (Eds) pp 205–20, WB Saunders, London.

Riordan AR, Cotterell JC, Pickersgill CS, Workman EM and Hunter JO (1990) Evaluating an exclusion diet in the treatment of patients with irritable bowel syndrome. *J Hum Nutr Dietet* **3**(5), 362–3.

Sampson HA, Hatcher Buckley R and Metcalf DD (1987) Food allergy. *J Am Med Assoc*, 2886–90.

Shacks SJ and Heiner DC (1982) Allergy to breast milk. In *Food allergy*, Brostoff J and Challacombe SJ (Eds) pp. 121–36. WB Saunders, London.

Supramaniam G and Warner JO (1986) Artificial food additive intolerance in patients with angio-oedema and urticaria. *Lancet* **ii**, 907–9.

Walker-Smith JA (1987) Gastrointestinal food allergy in children. In *Food intolerance* Dobbing J (Ed) pp. 87–95. Baillière Tindall, London.

Warner JO (1987) Artificial food additive intolerance: fact or fiction? In *Food intolerance*, Dobbing J (Ed) pp. 133–47. Baillière Tindall, London.

Witherley S (1990) Soya formulas are not hypoallergenic. *Am J Clin Nutr* **51**, 705–6.

Workman EM, Alun Jones V, Wilson AJ and Hunter JO (1984) Diet in the management of Crohn's disease. *Hum Nutr: Appl Nutr* **38A**(6), 469–73.

Wraith DG (1982) Asthma and rhinitis. *Clin Immunol Allergy* **2**, 101–12.

Wraith DG (1987) Asthma. In *Food allergy and intolerance*, Brostoff J and Challacombe S (Eds) pp. 486–97. Baillière Tindall, London.

Wraith DG, Young GVW and Lee TH (1979) The management of food allergy with diet and Nalcrom. In *The mast cell*, Pepys J and Edwards AM (Eds) pp. 443. Pitman Medical, London.

4.32 AIDS and HIV disease

The acquired immunodeficiency syndrome (AIDS) is a disorder resulting in a profound immunosuppression that renders the body highly susceptible to life-threatening opportunistic infections and tumours (Raiten 1991). AIDS is caused by infection with the human immunodeficiency virus (HIV).

4.32.1 Prevalence of AIDS/HIV disease

The first cases of AIDS were reported in June 1981. By the beginning of January 1992, 446 681 cases of AIDS had been reported worldwide (WHO 1992). Under-diagnosing and under-reporting means that this figure represents only the minimum number of people affected. Furthermore, the number of AIDS cases is considerably less than the number of people estimated to be infected with HIV. It is not known whether everyone infected with HIV will go on to develop AIDS. Current data suggests that approximately 50% of those infected with HIV will have developed AIDS after 10 years of infection (Anderson 1990). This period is much shorter for perinatally infected children and elderly people.

Worldwide the most common mode of transmission is sexual with heterosexual transmission the most frequent route of spread. Homosexual and bisexual men still comprise the group most affected by HIV disease in the UK but intravenous drug users, their sexual partners and their children represent an increasing proportion of cases (Table 4.96).

Trends in reported cases of infection suggest significant declines in the incidence of new infections in homosexual/bisexual men and intravenous drug users. However, the trend for heterosexuals suggests a pattern of continued transmission with no significant decline in new reports (Anderson 1990). The World Health Organization estimates that if no effective vaccine or treatment becomes widely available, about three times as many people will contract HIV worldwide in the 1990s as did in the 1980s. By the year 2000, as many as 6 million people may have developed AIDS (AIDS-UK 1990).

Table 4.96 Number of reported cases of AIDS in the UK and USA in 1985 and 1991 (Communicable Disease Report Weekly 1992; Centers for Disease Control 1991)

Number of cases reported in the UK stratified by risk group	1985	1991
Homosexual	227 (93%)	4297 (79%)
Heterosexual	9	443
Intravenous drug use	7	245
Total number of reported cases in UK*	259	5451
Total number of reported cases in USA*	32 985**	196 161***

* Other cases include blood transfusion and tissue recipients, vertical transmission from mother to infant and those of undetermined origin

** Before September 1986

*** To end of December 1991

4.32.2 Immunology

Immunological aspects of AIDS/HIV

An understanding of the immune system is important in understanding the effects of HIV and the role of nutrition in this disease.

The body has two lines of defence against invading antigens: non-specific and specific immunity. The non-specific immune response relies on the physical barrier of the skin in combination with protective chemicals such as lysozyme in tears and saliva, and hydrochloric acid in gastric juice. The formation of a clot by the activated complement system and the phagocytic capacity of the blood also form effective barriers to the entry of foreign antigens.

If an antigen manages to break through these barriers, a second line of defence is provided by specific immune responses. The main components of the specific immune system are the white cells of the blood and in particular the lymphocytes. When lymphocytes of the immune system meet an antigen, a series of events occurs resulting in the production of activated T-lymphocytes and antibodies (Fig. 4.20). If successful, these eliminate the antigen. This is known as the cell-mediated immune response.

HIV is a retrovirus which has an affinity for a particular subset of lymphocytes, the T-helper/inducer cells. HIV enters the target cell by binding to a protein receptor (CD4) on the cell surface. The virus then replicates by transcribing its RNA genome to double-stranded DNA (with the aid of an enzyme reverse transcriptase) (Fig. 4.21). This DNA is then integrated into the cell and replicated with it.

CD4 receptors are also found on the surface of monocytes/macrophages, which can thus also be infected with HIV. This is important as they are transported to other sites of the body which may explain some of the diverse effects seen in this disease.

The immune response is influenced by genetic potential,

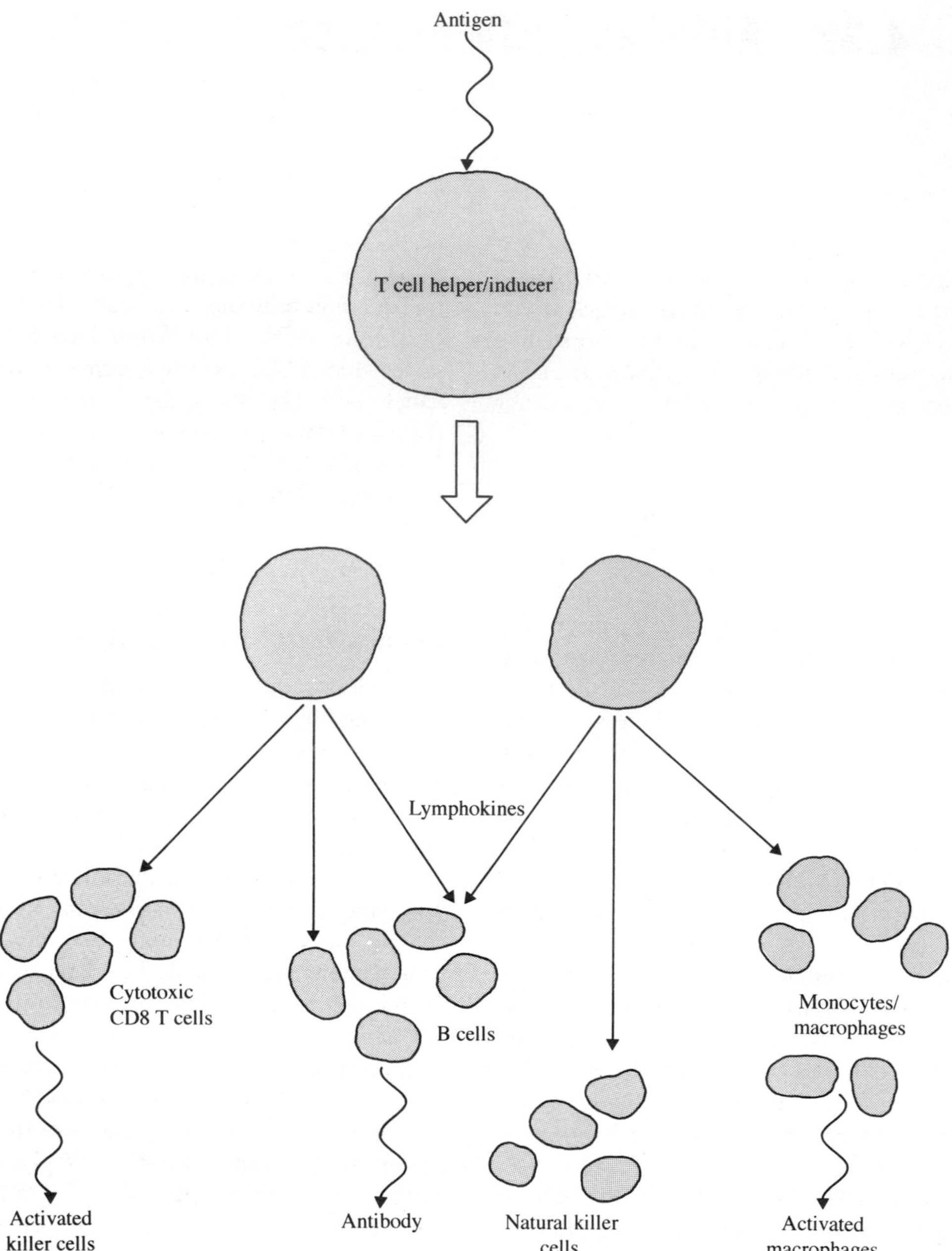

Fig. 4.20 The T-cell mediated immune response
From ABC of AIDS (British Medical Journal); reproduced with permission

age, number of T- and B-lymphocytes and macrophages, the presence of infection and the nature of the antigen (Chandra 1984). In addition, it has been established that nutrition is an important determinant of immune response (Chandra 1984).

Undernutrition has its most profound effects on the cell-mediated immune response. All of the lymphoid organs are atrophied and depleted of lymphocytes and the proportion and absolute number of T-cells are decreased (Chandra 1981a). Secondary to the impaired cell-mediated immunity are reductions in complement function, bactericidal activity, reduced secretion of IgA and impaired cutaneous sensitivity reactions (Chandra 1981a) (Fig. 4.22).

HIV has its most profound effects on the T-cell mediated immune responses, resulting in the immune system failing to function effectively even though it remains largely intact. This very selective destruction of particular cells within the immune system accounts for the fact that certain rare infections cause problems in people who are HIV positive.

Although individuals may be HIV antibody positive and healthy for long periods, the disease is characterized by a progressive and inexorable fall in the number of T-helper/inducer CD4 positive cells. The measurement of CD4 positive cell numbers or the ratio of helper (T4) to

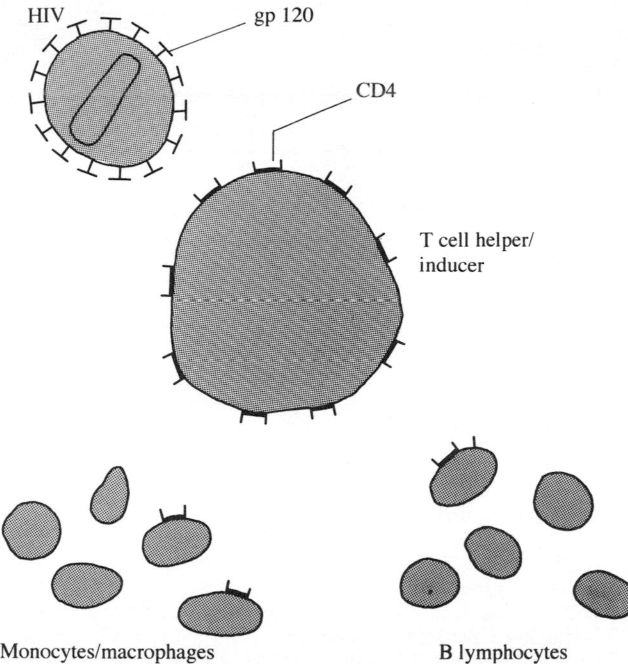

Fig. 4.21 The binding of HIV to a T-cell
From Adler (1987) ABC of AIDS (British Medical Journal); reproduced with permission

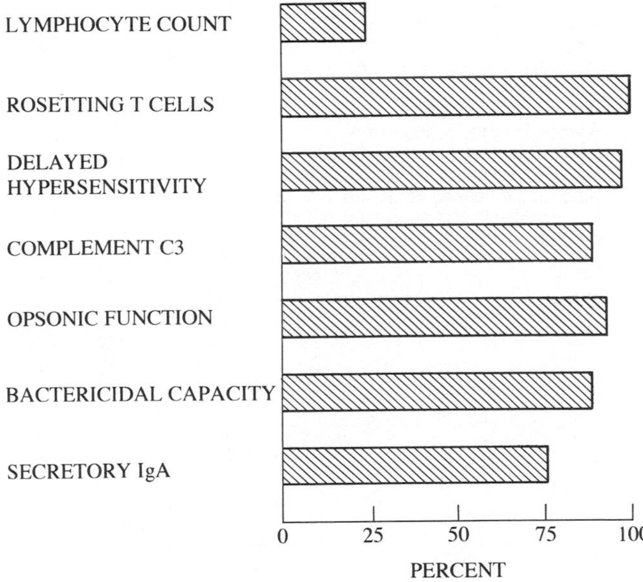

Fig. 4.22 Immunological changes associated with severe protein-energy malnutrition
From Chandra (1981a); reproduced with permission

suppressor (T8) lymphocytes is considered a useful indicator of immune status during HIV infection. The normal ratio is 2:1, this ratio changes in HIV disease.

Nutrition and immune function

Human malnutrition is not just deficiency of a single nutrient but is composed of multiple nutrient deficiencies. It is therefore important to examine the influence of individual nutrients on the immune system. This subject has received wide attention in the literature (Cunningham-Rundles 1982; Moseson *et al* 1989). Furthermore, nutritional deficiencies can impair gastrointestinal function while infectious diseases can influence nutrient requirements by altering the efficiency of absorption and rate of tissue metabolism (Moseson *et al* 1989).

The immunological abnormalities seen in HIV disease and AIDS are very similar to those seen in various nutritional deficiency states. It has been suggested that dietary manipulations might diminish the immune defects seen in HIV infection and enhance resistance to opportunistic infections (Jain and Chandra 1984; Moseson *et al* 1989). Adverse effects of supplementation have been reported (Beisel *et al* 1981; Chandra 1984; Moseson *et al* 1989). Further studies are needed before specific recommendations can be made.

4.32.3 Classification of HIV disease

It is usual to view HIV disease along a spectrum, from infection with HIV to AIDS. The clinical course and timescale of the disease varies considerably from individual to individual. It is not yet known whether every HIV positive individual will develop AIDS.

Following infection, patients may experience a glandular fever-like or seroconversion illness lasting about two weeks, after which they become asymptomatic or are left with persistent generalized lymphadenopathy. After some time, a variety of symptoms may occur such as persistent lymphadenopathy, recurrent fevers or night sweats, unintentional weight loss, intermittent diarrhoea, lethargy and fatigue. Viral infections such as *Herpes simplex*, warts and *Molluscum contagiosum* may occur more frequently and at unusual sites. The occurrence of *Candida* (thrush) in the mouth, oral hairy leukoplakia and multidermatomal shingles (*Herpes zoster*) are commonly described as the AIDS Related Complex (ARC). The advanced stage of disease is characterized by marked weight loss and major opportunistic infections and neoplasms, although people diagnosed as having AIDS on clinical criteria can be physically very well and often enjoy active and productive lives.

The Centers of Disease Control (CDC) in America have devised a classification system for HIV disease which recognizes four stages (Fig. 4.23). It is only once a person is diagnosed with conditions from group IV that they are considered to have AIDS.

4.32.4 Modes of transmission

HIV has been isolated from semen, cervical secretions, lymphocytes, cell-free plasma, cerebrospinal fluid, tears, saliva, urine and breast milk. This does not mean however that all these fluids transmit infection since the concen-

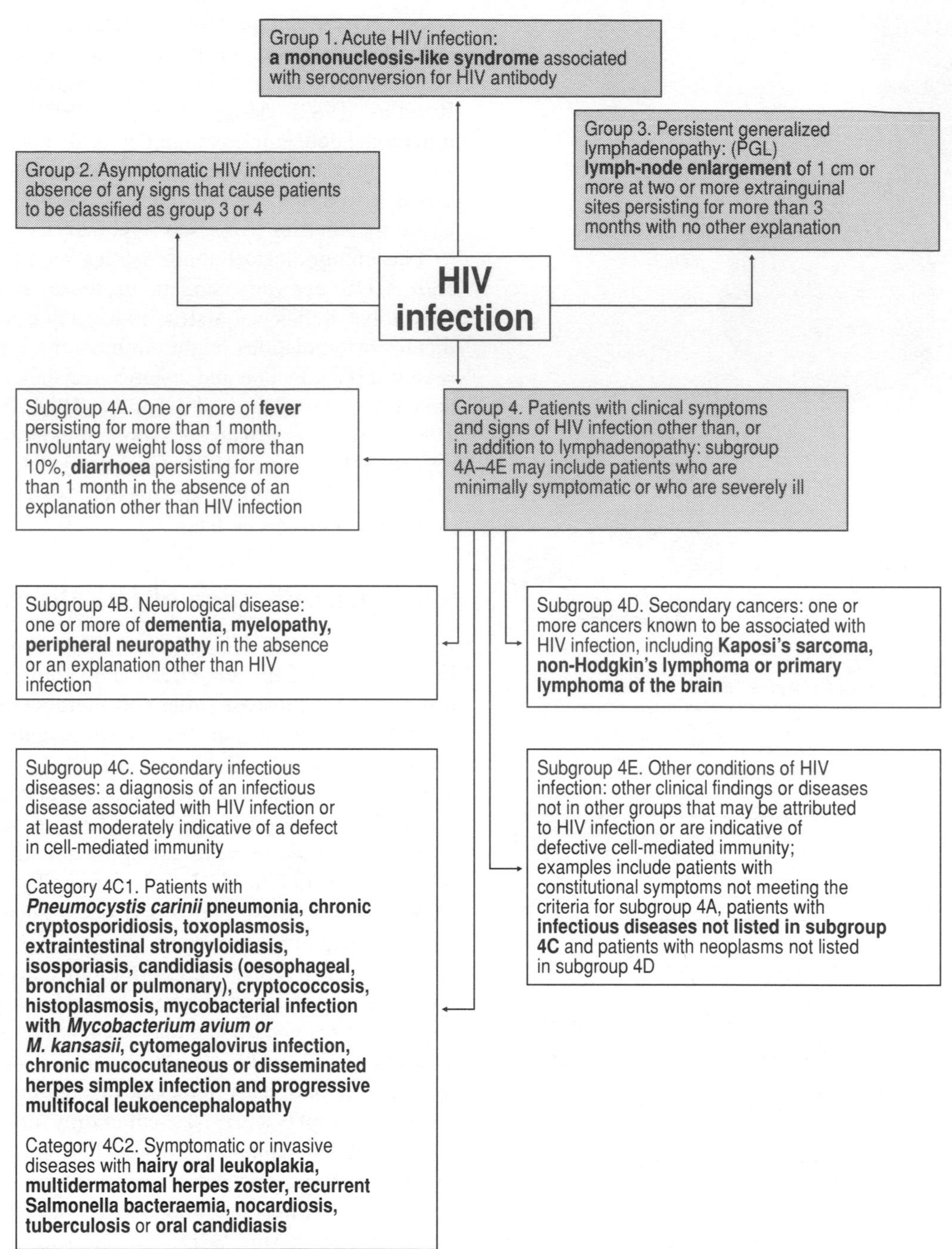

Fig. 4.23 Staging of HIV infection based on criteria set by the American Communicable Diseases Center, 1988. Aspects of the staging that have an infection-related aetiology (or a suspected infection-related aetiology) are shown in bold (Peck and Johnson 1990). Reproduced with permission

tration of virus in them varies considerably (Adler 1987).

HIV is known to be transmitted by:

1 Sexual intercourse, both vaginal and anal.

2 The receipt of infected blood products via transfusion or contaminated needles.

3 From mother to child in utero and delivery, and during breast feeding.

4 Via organ/tissue donation.

In the UK, HIV positive mothers are currently advised against breast feeding (DHSS 1988). The World Health Organization has advised that breast feeding may still be preferable, irrespective of the mother's HIV status, if safe and effective use of alternatives is not possible as may be the case in developing countries where contaminated water supplies, lack of sterilization facilities and inadequate supplies of artificial milks may result in increased morbidity and mortality.

Infection with the virus can be detected by a test for a

specific antibody in the blood which is usually detectable from 2–12 weeks after infection; in some people this may be longer. Viral components (P24 antigen) may be detected prior to the development of antibodies at the seroconversion.

4.32.5 Nutritional aspects of asymptomatic HIV disease

Being diagnosed as having a life-threatening disease often leaves people feeling out of control. Following the initial shock, people often seek strategies for maintaining and promoting health. Food choice is a facet of management in which a person can exert control. Dietary advice should not threaten that control but seek to optimize food intake and achieve nutritional adequacy within the limits of personal choice and social circumstances.

The rationale for giving nutritional advice in asymptomatic HIV disease is based on avoiding deficiencies which may have an impact on immune function, and preventing weight loss which is often difficult to reverse. The relationship between nutrition and the immune system is well documented (Chandra 1983). Malnutrition in an HIV positive person may be a cofactor in disease progression (Kotler 1987). Significant weight loss and malnutrition is common in advancing HIV disease (Garcia *et al* 1987; Hickey and Weaver 1988). Early nutritional assessment and advice may minimize complications seen in late stages of disease.

The optimum time for nutrition intervention to begin is as soon as possible after a person has been diagnosed as HIV positive. For many people this will be early in the course of their disease when they are asymptomatic but it is important to remember that some people are diagnosed late in disease when there may already have been considerable depletion of nutrient reserves.

For the asymptomatic person, advice is aimed at preserving lean body mass, preventing nutrient deficiencies and optimizing nutritional stores (Task Force 1989). A baseline nutritional assessment should include a thorough diet history in combination with measurement of height, weight, body mass index and anthropometric and biochemical measures. Dietary advice should promote a regular, balanced intake of protein, fat, carbohydrate, vitamins and minerals so that the recommendations set out in the Dietary Reference Values (DoH 1991) are met. There is no evidence to suggest that energy and protein requirements are increased in the asymptomatic person. Precise vitamin and mineral requirements in HIV disease are not known. There is some evidence that blood levels of many vitamins and minerals are below normal in the later stages of disease (Chandra 1984). A modest supplement of 1–2 tablets of a complete vitamin and mineral supplement daily is probably appropriate in all patients to cover increased needs and is clearly indicated when food intake is compromised. Although the use of vitamin and mineral supplements containing 100% of the DRV for all micronutrients is acceptable to ensure sufficiency, there is no evidence that megadoses of any vitamin or mineral will alter the course of the disease or further improve nutritional status of patients (Task Force 1989).

The use of food groups with an indication of number of choices from each group, and ideas on putting together meals and snacks, is a useful way of teaching balanced nutrition. The healthy eating guidelines proposed by the National Advisory Committee on Nutrition Education (NACNE 1983) are designed for the general population and are inappropriate in this group of people who are at risk of weight loss and malnutrition. This may need to be reviewed in the future because people with HIV disease are living longer.

For the uncomplicated asymptomatic patient, dietetic review should coincide with medical review, probably 3–6 monthly. More frequent review may be necessary in some cases.

People with HIV disease represent all segments of society with varying socioeconomic circumstances and varying amounts of nutrition knowledge. Food choice may be complicated by factors such as lack of money, lack of skills, lack of energy and motivation, and lack of facilities. Advice must be flexible and practical to accommodate people's varying lifestyles; for example, advice on appropriate choice of takeaway foods may be most useful to the homeless HIV positive drug user (Peck and Johnson 1989).

4.32.6 Nutritional aspects of symptomatic HIV disease (AIDS)

Malnutrition is a predominant feature of symptomatic HIV disease, sometimes termed AIDS related complex (ARC), and AIDS (Chelluri and Jastremski 1989). An average weight loss of 16% from pre-illness weight to death has been observed (Hickey and Weaver 1988). Furthermore, malnutrition is a major source of morbidity in HIV seropositive individuals independent of immune deficiency (Kotler *et al* 1989a), and reduces quality of life experienced by this group. The cause of malnutrition is multifactorial and reflects the variety of symptoms and infections that these individuals may suffer (Summerbell *et al* 1993b). Whatever the cause, the correct diagnosis and treatment of any underlying disease is of prime importance in reversing the malnutrition (Grunfeld and Kotler 1991). The main factors precipitating malnutrition in symptomatic HIV disease are:

1 Reduced food intake.
2 Altered metabolic requirements.
3 Malabsorption.

The weight loss experienced in HIV infection reflects a depletion of lean body mass (LBM), body fat and intracellular water (Hecker and Kotler 1990). The loss of LBM resembles that of a stressed or injured state, rather than simple starvation (Kotler *et al* 1985) (see Section 5.1). On refeeding, stressed patients tend to deposit fat rather than muscle (Streat *et al* 1987). However, recent work in people with AIDS suggests that where malabsorption is the major factor causing the weight loss, an increase in LBM may be achieved (Kotler *et al* 1990a).

To date, there is no evidence that reversing this malnourished state alters the course of the disease (Raiten 1990). However, the deleterious effect of malnutrition on immune function is well documented in non-AIDS patients (Chandra 1981b) and therefore it must be prudent to avoid compromising the immune system further. This nutritional support should be highly individualized to correct for nutritional deficiencies as much as possible in line with patient acceptability, tolerance and socioeconomic circumstances (Summerbell *et al* 1993a). To this end, it is important that other members of the care team are aware of the importance of nutritional support in HIV infected patients.

The aims of nutritional support in symptomatic HIV infection are:

1 To preserve or increase lean body mass.
2 To provide adequate levels of all nutrients.
3 To achieve/maintain ideal body weight.
4 To provide symptomatic relief.

Basic dietetic principles for nutritional intervention apply (see Section 1.13) and an assessment of nutritional status should be made initially (see Section 1.11) and repeated at regular intervals. Nutritional requirements of the patient may be altered and can be assessed using standard methods (see Section 1.12). Vitamin and mineral intake should be 100% of the DRV and in cases of malabsorption it is recommended that a supplement equivalent to this should be given daily (Winick *et al* 1989). The benefit of micronutrient doses above the DRV is unproven.

The composition of the diet and most effective route of administration is dependent on the nutritional status, presenting symptoms and stage of disease of the patient. Bear in mind that the multifactorial nature of AIDS can produce a different combination of symptoms in each individual (Winick *et al* 1989). Patients often have periods of relative well-being between infections. Such remission time should be used to optimize nutritional repletion.

4.32.7 Nutritional problems associated with symptomatic HIV disease

The manifestations of the acquired immune deficiency syndrome are numerous and diverse, and reflect the most prevalent pathogens in the local population. The presenting symptoms which arise and their treatments can have a potent effect on nutritional status (Table 4.97).

Commonly seen nutritional problems are described below and strategies for their management are summarized in Table 4.98.

Table 4.97 Common manifestations of AIDS and associated nutritional problems

AIDS-related infections and cancers	Associated nutritional problems
Opportunistic infections	
Fungal:	
Candida	
Oral	Sore mouth, altered taste perception, anorexia, reduced saliva production
Oesophageal	Dysphagia
Cryptococcus	
Meningitis	Pyrexia, nausea and vomiting
Protozoan:	
Toxoplasmosis	Pyrexia, lethargy, confusion
Pneumocystis carinii Pneumonia (PCP)	Pyrexia, dyspnoea, anorexia and weight loss, tiredness and lethargy
Bacterial:	
Myobacterium Avium-Intracellular (MAI)	Pyrexia, anorexia and weight loss, diarrhoea and malabsorption
Viral:	
Cytomegalovirus (CMV)	Pyrexia, diarrhoea and malabsorption
Herpes simplex (Oral)	Dysphagia
Human immunodeficiency virus (HIV)	Pyrexia, diarrhoea and weight loss
Parasitic:	
Cryptosporidium	Diarrhoea and malabsorption, anorexia, weight loss, nausea and vomiting, pyrexia
Cancers:	
Kaposi's sarcoma (gastrointestinal)	Dysphagia, sore mouth, anorexia, abdominal discomfort and obstruction, diarrhoea and malabsorption
Non-Hodgkins Lymphoma	Anorexia, weight loss, dysphagia, and diarrhoea
Other:	
AIDS enteropathy	Diarrhoea and malabsorption, weight loss
AIDS encephalitis	Confusion, dementia, lethargy

Anorexia

Loss of appetite is a common problem in individuals with symptomatic HIV disease and AIDS and may result from fever, infection, gastrointestinal symptoms, medication side effects and emotional issues (Resler 1988). As in other chronic diseases, once the downward cycle of anorexia has started, it may be self-perpetuating, especially if coupled with protein-energy malnutrition (PEM), dehydration or infection (Ghiron *et al* 1989). Eating may also be self-limited by early satiety and fear of pain or diarrhoea (Winick *et al* 1989).

Nausea and vomiting

In most cases nausea and vomiting are temporary, intermittent symptoms. Often these symptoms are a side effect of drug therapy (see the section below on 'Drugs used in HIV disease'). Organic causes, such as development of Kaposi's sarcoma lesions along the gastrointestinal tract,

Table 4.98 Dietary management of common nutritional problems associated with AIDS

Symptom	Management
Anorexia	High energy, high protein diet; nutrient-dense supplements; eat little and often; encourage favourite foods; flexible timing of meals; nutritious snacks and convenience foods; appetite stimulant (e.g. megestrol acetate); check other drug interactions and change medication times if indicated; nasogastric or gastrostomy feeding
Nausea and vomiting	Use antiemetics and/or alter timings of emetic medication; small frequent meals; drink plenty of fluids; avoid drinking with meals; avoid cooking smells; avoid rich, fatty and spicy foods; try plain, dry or salty foods; have food cool or cold rather than hot; encourage nutrient-dense supplements; relax when eating; do not lie down after eating
Neurological problems	Close monitoring and encouragement of patient; help at mealtimes; involve family, friends, carers; may need home help or meals on wheels; involve voluntary organizations if appropriate; in case of motor impairment provide modified texture diet and/or consider special utensils
Tiredness and depression	Involve friends, family, other carers; support through volunteers, home help, meals on wheels, day centres; advice on nutritious convenience and snack foods; encourage supplements
Altered metabolism	Drink plenty of fluids; encourage high calorie, high protein diet; use nutrient-dense supplements
Diarrhoea and malabsorption	Small, frequent meals; low fat, low lactose, low residue diet; low lactose nutrient dense supplements; warm food rather than extremes of hot or cold; elemental or peptide feeding; TPN may be indicated
Sore mouth	Modify texture to suit individual – soft, semi-solid or fluid; moist foods may be easier to manage; avoid spicy, salty, acidic or rough foods; take fluids through a straw; avoid extremes of temperature, cold or warm foods are more soothing and taste better; use nutritionally complete liquids; good oral hygiene is important; may need to consider nasogastric feeding if prolonged
Dry mouth	Frequent drinks, especially sips of fizzy drinks; avoid too much salt and salty foods; make foods moist with gravies and sauces; try saliva stimulating pastilles or an artificial saliva spray; keep lips moist with vaseline or lip balm
Taste changes	Provide a variety of textures; use strong smelling foods; use more herbs and spices; cold foods may taste better than hot; use alternative protein sources, marinading meat may make it taste better; encourage good oral hygiene
Swallowing problems	Modify texture to individual tolerance – smooth, thick consistency is often best; encourage nutritionally complete supplements; may need to consider nasogastric or gastrostomy feed if dysphagia very bad
Night fevers and sweats	Replace fluids and salts
Blindness	Appropriate management and utensils

may also lead to nausea and vomiting (Hyman and Kaufman 1989).

Initiation of aggressive nutritional support depends on the cause and duration of the nausea and vomiting, nutritional status and predicted length of drug therapy.

Diarrhoea and malabsorption

These symptoms are caused by gastrointestinal micro-organisms, antibiotic therapy, AIDS enteropathy or malnutrition itself (Ghiron *et al* 1989).

Some infections of the GI tract such as Candida, Herpes Simplex virus and Salmonella can be effectively treated (Resler 1988). Other opportunistic infections such as *Cryptosporidium* are more resistant to treatment and result in profuse diarrhoea which limits absorption and causes rapid weight loss. Dietary treatment is aimed at relieving symptoms and improving nutritional status where possible. In all cases increased fluid intake should be encouraged to maintain hydration.

A low fat, low lactose diet may be useful if steatorrhoea is present (MCTs may be better absorbed – see Section 4.6), or a low fibre diet if there is gastrointestinal inflammation or ulceration (King *et al* 1989). However, in many cases dietary restrictions may be of little benefit.

If malabsorption is present the use of an elemental or peptide feed should be considered either as a supplement or as a source of total nutrition (Hickey and Weaver 1988). TPN may be used if bowel rest would relieve symptoms (see Section 1.15).

Disorders of the upper gastrointestinal tract

Oral and oesophageal complications of AIDS are common, and result in chewing and swallowing problems and altered taste perception. Causes include infective or malignant lesions of the mouth or oesophagus (e.g. candidiasis, cytomegalovirus, Kaposi's sarcoma) and treatment (e.g. radiotherapy). In one study, 94% of people with AIDS had oral candidiasis (Barr and Torosian 1986) causing sore mouth and reduced saliva secretion. Effective treatments are available for most of these problems so dietary modification is necessary only until symptoms subside.

Altered metabolism

The literature on altered metabolism in HIV disease is conflicting. Kotler found that clinically stable patients with symptomatic disease and AIDS did not appear to have a raised metabolic rate, and indeed adapted to a lower body weight (Kotler *et al* 1990b). Conversely, other studies have shown that a similar group of patients exhibited a raised metabolic rate (Hommes *et al* 1990; Hommes *et al* 1991; Melchior *et al* 1991).

Neurological problems

Central nervous system involvement in AIDS ranges from psychomotor retardation to severe dementia (Winick *et al* 1989), with the latter affecting 60% of AIDS patients (Hyman and Kaufman 1989). Encephalopathy may be caused by the HIV virus itself or opportunistic infections such as toxoplasmosis or cytomegalovirus encephalitis. Symptoms include memory difficulties, apathy, short concentration span and impaired motor ability such as tremor and dysphagia (Resler 1988). All these factors further reduce the individual's capacity to maintain an adequate nutritional intake.

Tiredness and depression

Some people may be too tired or unmotivated to shop or cook for themselves. The effect of this on nutritional intake is significant and should not be underestimated.

Night sweats and fevers

Night fevers and sweats are a common feature of HIV disease although their cause is unknown. However, these symptoms have nutritional implications in terms of replacing fluids and salts.

Blindness

The cytomegalovirus may cause retinitis leading to diminished vision. Appropriate care should be offered in such cases.

4.32.8 Nutritional support in patients with symptomatic HIV disease

Currently there is very little published data on the efficacy, in terms of improvement in weight, LBM and immune function, of enteral/parenteral therapy in HIV disease. In the USA, one group concluded that enteral nutritional therapy can promote body mass repletion in AIDS, though this was not shown to be obviously beneficial to immune function (Ferraro *et al* 1989). Other workers have shown that enteral feeding or total parenteral nutrition (TPN) is an effective way to reverse the wasting syndrome particularly when malabsorption is the main feature in the absence of systemic infection (Janson and Feasley 1989; Singer *et al* 1989; Kotler *et al* 1990a; Kotler *et al* 1991).

Enteral feeding

Sip feeds

Where patients cannot achieve adequate nourishment using normal foods, intake should be supplemented with or replaced by nourishing fluids taken at regular intervals. Commercially manufactured protein and energy supplements are very useful (see Appendix 6, Tables 7.44–7.46). Where possible offer a range of products/flavours to avoid taste fatigue.

Tube feeding

If a patient fails to achieve adequate intake orally, nasogastric feeding should be initiated (see Section 1.13.4). This may be difficult if the patient has nausea and vomiting or has a severe Candida overgrowth of the oesophagus. For gastrointestinal complications and/or malabsorption states, e.g. cytomegalovirus (CMV) pancreatitis/colitis, elemental feeds which are generally low in fats (e.g. Elemental 028, Cow & Gate) may be best tolerated. Alternatively digestive enzyme replacement capsules may be helpful in such cases.

For long term feeding a gastrostomy may be considered (Kelson *et al* 1991). This has the advantage of being more socially acceptable for the individual in terms of self image, although care must be taken in minimising infection risk in this immunocompromised patient group. Ideally, enteral feeds should be:

- Low lactose;
- Low residue;
- Low fat, if steatorrhoea is present;
- Elemental, if malabsorption is severe (e.g. total small bowel enteropathy).

Total parenteral nutrition (TPN)

Parenteral nutrition should be reserved for cases when the gastrointestinal tract cannot be used, e.g. total small bowel disease, cryptosporidiosis or CMV inflammation, which gives rise to uncontrolled diarrhoea and malabsorption. In the USA, central parenteral nutrition (CPN) and peripheral parenteral nutrition (PPN) are much more frequently used to manage HIV wasting syndrome than in the UK. PPN is used for short term feeding (7–10 days). For more prolonged feeding a central line is indicated. Home TPN is used at some centres in the USA and at least one centre in London is also involved in a home TPN scheme (Peck *et al* 1991).

(*Note*: Many HIV infected patients obtain advice/treatment solely from Sexually Transmitted Disease/HIV clinics and may not have a GP or may choose not to involve their GP. Also, patients may travel a long way to centres for treatment. This raises the question of who prescribes/supplies the product. Hospital prescriptions must be endorsed to be valid outside the hospital pharmacy and home deliveries need a financial code from a hospital source. Dietitians should check with their pharmacy for the correct procedure.)

4.32.9 Terminal care

The role of nutritional support in late HIV disease/AIDS is similar to that in terminal oncology patients (see Section 4.36). It is sometimes assumed that nutritional support in this group is of little importance and whereas this may be true for some patients, it is not true for all and the potential positive benefits to psychological status should not be forgotten (Peck *et al* 1991).

The difference for people with AIDS is that they may suddenly succumb to a debilitating, life-threatening infection after previously being well or even unaware of their HIV positive status. This rapid onset of end stage HIV disease may leave a person with little time to tackle personal goals, e.g. coming to terms with death; seeing loved ones for the last time; making a will; the wish to die at home.

Nutritional support in this context may be used not to increase weight but to stabilize and control symptoms. The result is the extension of effective life so that some of the remaining goals may be realized.

4.32.10 Nutrition in children with HIV disease

Background information

AIDS was first described in children in 1982 and, by the end of 1990, 2120 cases had been reported to the Centers for Disease Control in the United States and from 31 European countries, half of whom were Romanian children (Mok 1991). These figures are small when compared to those calculated by WHO who predict by the end of 1992 over one million children worldwide will be infected with HIV, half of whom will have AIDS (Mok 1991). Indeed, in the USA, HIV disease is already among the ten leading causes of death in infants, young children and adolescents, and is likely to be among the top five causes by 1992 (Pizzo 1990).

Mode of transmission

There are several ways in which a child can become HIV positive. These are by vertical transmission from mother to child *in utero*, during breast feeding (Oxtoby 1988), from transfusion with infected blood and blood products, and by sexual abuse. Vertical transmission accounts for about 80% of HIV infected children and is therefore the most common route (Cowan *et al* 1984). Current evidence suggests that this occurs transplacentally and possibly early in pregnancy, perhaps during the first or second trimester (Marion *et al* 1989). Some studies suggest that about one third of infants born to HIV infected mothers will be infected themselves (Blanche *et al* 1989). However the most recent data suggests a lower figure of about 13% (European Collaborative Study 1991).

HIV can be cultured from breast milk although the significance of this route of transmission has not been proven. In the UK at present the general recommendation is that HIV positive mothers should be discouraged from breast feeding (DHSS 1988). However this must remain a subject of debate as breast feeding confers many advantages, both nutritional and immunological, to a newborn baby. WHO advises that breast feeding should continue in developing countries where malnutrition presents a greater risk of morbidity and mortality than HIV infection.

Infection from transfused blood and blood products should lessen in developed countries with routine screening of blood donors and the treatment of blood products.

Diagnosis

A clear diagnosis before the age of 18 months is complicated by the presence of maternal antibodies. Therefore diagnosis is either a positive presence of abnormal immune function or clinical evidence of the disease. Children with the highest risk for AIDS are those with a parent belonging to a high risk group. New methods of testing are being evaluated.

Clinical findings

The classification of paediatric HIV infection (Centers for Disease Control 1987) is shown in Table 4.99.

Where sophisticated diagnostic methods are not available, a clinical case definition has been proposed by WHO (1986) (Table 4.100). Paediatric AIDS is suspected in a child presenting with at least two of the major signs, associated with at least two of the minor signs, in the

Table 4.99 Centers for Disease Control classification for paediatric HIV infection

Indeterminate infection		
Asymptomatic infection:		
	A	Normal immune function
	B	Abnormal immune function
	C	Immune function not studied
Symptomatic infection:		
	A	Non-specific signs and symptoms
	B	Progressive neurological disease
	C	Lymphocytic interstitial pneumonitis
	D	Secondary infectious diseases
	E	Secondary cancers
	F	Other diseases possibly due to HIV

Source: Centers for Disease Control (1987)

Table 4.100 World Health Organization clinical case definition for paediatric HIV infection

Major signs:	Weight loss or failure to thrive Persistent diarrhoea Recurrent unexplained fever
Minor signs:	Generalized lymphadenopathy Oropharyngeal candidiasis Repeated common infections Persistent cough Generalized dermatitis Confirmed maternal HIV infection

Source: World Health Organization (1986)

absence of known causes of immunosuppression, such as cancer or severe malnutrition (Lambert and Friesen 1989).

The clinical presentation in infants and children often differs from that in adults. Recurrent bacterial infections are more common in children whereas certain opportunistic infections (e.g. toxoplasmosis and cryptococcal meningitis) are infrequent. Kaposi's sarcoma (KS) is also uncommon in children and AIDS-associated malignancies (e.g. lymphomas) are relatively rare compared with adults (Pizzo 1990).

The mean age of diagnosis of AIDS in children is six months. Older children often present with milder disease symptoms. The prognosis for children with AIDS is poor (European Collaborative Study 1988). Currently it appears that the prognosis of HIV-infected infants is adversely affected by the diagnosis of either *Pneumocystis carinii* pneumonia (PCP) (Bernstein *et al* 1989) or encephalopathy, whereas children whose predominant symptom is lymphocytic interstitial pneumonitis have a more favourable prognosis. Little is known about the outcome of the much larger proportion of HIV infected children with less severe or no symptoms.

Early disease often manifests in a non-specific way with symptoms including:

- Failure to thrive;
- Recurrent respiratory infections;
- Candidiasis;
- Persistant diarrhoea;
- Unexplained fever;
- General lymphadenopathy.

These children experience normal development which therefore means that general practitioners and paediatricians need to have a high degree of suspicion particularly in urban areas with a high seroprevalence of HIV amongst women (e.g. Edinburgh, UK and New York, Newark, Miami and urban areas of Texas and California USA) (Pizzo 1990).

Respiratory symptoms are frequently seen and range from recurrent minor infections to opportunistic infection with *Pneumocystis carinii* (PCP). Encephalopathy may affect 50–90% of children with AIDS meaning that they may not attain normal milestones, or lose previously acquired skills.

The gastrointestinal tract is also involved, commonly with Candida infection affecting both the mouth and oesophagus. Other organisms which cause infectious enterocolitis include cytomegalovirus (CMV), atypical mycobacteria, Salmonella and Cryptosporidium. Malabsorption can also occur as a direct result of HIV infection and non-specific villous atrophy has been found on biopsy. The end result is severe wasting which is seen when the disease is terminal.

Management

The infant or young child with AIDS presents especially difficult clinical and social problems (Shannon and Ammann 1985). Whilst there is as yet no cure for AIDS, good nutrition will help strengthen the immune system and help the child fight infection.

As with adults, nutritional support and intervention is generally based on symptomatic approach whilst bearing in mind that children are still growing and nutritional support must allow for this. There has been very little documented about this subject to date particularly from this country. Some work has been published from the USA (Bentler and Stanish 1987; Fennoy and Leung 1990).

Nutritional support is very important from the time of diagnosis onwards (Mok 1990). Ideally the dietitian should work closely with other members of the multidisciplinary team. Nutritional advice must be geared towards the capabilities of the individual family or carer of the child taking into account social and financial circumstances, and health of other members of the family. In the case of intravenous drug users (IVDUs) the mother herself is likely to be HIV infected and so may other siblings. Often HIV is yet another problem that affected families have to deal with in the midst of inadequate housing, poverty, unemployment, imprisonment and continuing drug abuse (Mok 1990).

Guidelines on nutritional management

The overall aim is to provide a well balanced nutritionally adequate diet in an appropriate way for the child to manage. Most children with AIDS have difficulty gaining weight and lose weight very easily. Poor appetite is common.

In the USA, the energy requirements for the catabolic child are determined as follows (Bentler and Stanish 1987):

Minimum: Weight (kg) at 50th percentile for actual height × calories per kg based on age.

Maximum: Weight (kg) for age at 50th percentile × calories per kg based on age.

Protein requirements are based on the DRV for age and increased by 50–100% to compensate for increased needs and nitrogen losses when these arise. Supplementation of vitamins and minerals to a level which does not exceed 1–2 × the DRV may be beneficial during active stages of infection.

In the UK, nutrient guidelines for catabolic infants are provided by Francis (1987).

Interestingly, Fennoy and Leung (1990) document the case of four children with HIV related failure to thrive who all gained weight on energy intakes well within the normal range of DRVs.

The most pressing dietetic problems are:

- Fever;
- Weight loss;

- Persistent diarrhoea;
- Oral thrush;
- Nausea;
- Anorexia;
- Dyspnoea;
- Fatigue.

Table 4.101 outlines the nutritional management of these problems (adapted from Bentler and Stanish 1987).

4.32.11 Food and water safety and hygiene in relation to HIV disease

Intestinal infectious diseases and resulting systemic infections can be threatening to people with HIV disease (Archer 1989). Food is an important vector for many infectious diseases which manifest as acute gastrointestinal disturbances, but which can progress to septicaemia, specific organ infection and death (Archer 1989). The risk of adverse outcome is greater for those whose immune systems are compromised.

People with HIV disease suffer from a wide variety of fungal, protozoal, bacterial, viral and amoebic infections (Archer and Glinsmann 1985; Smith *et al* 1988). The general population acquires most gastrointestinal infections via the faecal-oral route, by consuming contaminated food and water, and this is probably true for people with HIV disease (Archer 1989). Sexual practices may further contribute to transmission of infection by this route.

The body's response to invasion by infectious micro-organisms requires an intact T-cell mediated immune system; it is not surprising therefore that advancing HIV disease is associated with an increased incidence of some foodborne infectious diseases. One report noted a twenty-fold increase in the incidence of salmonella infections in men with AIDS compared with men with early HIV infection (Celum *et al* 1987).

The incidence of *Listeria monocytogenes* infection in the UK is increasing and, although it is an unusual manifestation of HIV disease, people with HIV disease are at greater risk of acquiring this infection than the general population (Mascola *et al* 1988; Coffey *et al* 1989).

Foodborne infections can be prevented by following simple rules on hygiene. Patients should be given information on the safe handling and cooking of food as well as general good hygiene practices. Raw milk and improperly pasteurized dairy products have been linked to the development of brucellosis, campylobacteriosis, salmonellosis and possibly listeriosis. Patients with AIDS should probably be advised against consuming these products. In addition, AIDS patients should wash all raw fruits and vegetables thoroughly to avoid soil contamination (Mascola *et al* 1988).

Cryptosporidium has been isolated from tap water. It has been suggested that people with HIV disease use only boiled tap water for drinking but this remains an area of controversy; tap water is only one of numerous possible sources of infection and some people do not have the facilities to boil all drinking water. However it is a potential safeguard for those able to do so. Further information is needed on this subject.

Table 4.101 Plan for nutrition intervention in the paediatric patient with AIDS

Problem	Approach
Poor oral intake (e.g. due to anorexia, nausea, dyspnoea, fatigue)	Evaluate food preferences. High energy, nutrient dense small meals or formula feeds for infants. For infants aim to provide 80–100 kcal/100 ml by addition of carbohydrate and/or fat. Frequent 'snacks'. Nutritional supplements when appropriate. Multivitamin supplement. — Enteral feeding, as supplement or total diet — Parenteral nutrition
Oral lesions (e.g. due to Candida or herpes infections)	Soft, non-irritating foods served cold or at room temperature. Cold drinks or ice lollies may help to numb the mouth and oesophagus if there is pain on swallowing. Non acidic juices e.g. apple. Small frequent meals/feeds
Infection/pneumonia	Increase energy and protein. Multivatimin supplement
Diarrhoea/malabsorption	If the diarrhoea is acute, oral rehydration therapy for 24 hours followed by reintroduction of milk/liquids and solids For chronic diarrhoea, lactose restriction may be beneficial (adjusted to the individual child's tolerance) — Elemental diet — Enteral feeding — Parenteral feeding (as a short term measure to maintain or improve nutritional status). At all times ensure good liquid and potassium intake NB: Risk of catheter sepsis in the immunocompromised child
Developmental problems/ neurological impairment	Bottle feed or spoon feed as necessary. Liaise with speech therapist, and other members of the multidisciplinary team as appropriate

Adapted from Bentler and Stanish (1987)

4.32.12 Drugs used in HIV disease

There are many drugs currently used in the management of HIV disease (Tuazon and Labriola 1987; Erskine 1990). It is important to note that the choice of drug treatment in the management of HIV disease varies between hospitals and over time as results from research trials become available. Those drugs which may have nutritional consequences are listed in Table 4.102.

Routine antiemetics, antidiarrhoeal drugs and appetite stimulants are commonly prescribed in the management of HIV infection. Recently, a synthetic progesterone called megestrol acetate routinely used in the treatment of breast

Table 4.102 Potential nutritional consequences associated with drugs used in the management of HIV disease

Aids related infections	Drug treatments	Potential nutritional consequences
Viral:		
HIV	Zidovudine (AZT)	Nausea, vomiting
	Dideoxyinosine (DDI)	Nausea, vomiting, diarrhoea, raised blood glucose, Steven Johnson's syndrome
Herpes simplex	Acyclovir	Nausea, vomiting, diarrhoea
Cytomegalovirus (CMV)	Ganciclovir	Nausea, vomiting
	Foscarnet	Anaemia, nausea, vomiting, nephrotoxic
	Acyclovir	(As above)
Fungal infections:		
Candida	Ketoconazole	These three drugs may cause mild nausea, diarrhoea and/or vomiting
	Itraconazole	
	Fluconazole	
	Nystatin lozenges	These lozenges cause negligible side effects
	Amphotericin lozenges	
Protozoan:		
Pneumocystis carinii pneumonia (PCP)	Pentamidine	Diarrhoea
	FansidarR (Roche)	Mild nausea after eating
	Dapsone	Mild nausea
	Co-trimoxazole	Nausea, diarrhoea, Steven Johnson's syndrome
Toxoplasmosis	FansidarR (Roche)	(As above)
Bacterial:		
Mycobacterium avium intacellulare (MAI)	Rifabutin	Nausea, diarrhoea
	Clofazimine	Nausea
Parasitic:		
Cryptosporidium	Azithromycin	Nausea, diarrhoea
	Erythromycin	Nausea
	Spiramycin	Nausea
Cancers:		
Kaposi's sarcoma	Chemotherapy (e.g. vinblastine/ vincristine)	Nausea, vomiting
	Radiotherapy	Depends on site of radiotherapy (see Section 4.34.2)

cancer, has been used as an appetite stimulant in the management of weight loss in HIV infection. Initial studies show promising results (Von Roenn *et al* 1989; Chen *et al* 1990).

Beneficial side effects, in terms of weight gain, have been reported with the use of certain antiviral agents, e.g. AZT (Fischl *et al* 1987), DHPG (Kotler *et al* 1986) and Gancyclovir (Kotler *et al* 1989b).

Many patients with HIV infection may be prescribed a combination of those drugs described above. The nutritional consequences of these drug combinations are less clear.

4.32.13 Unproven diet therapies

There is currently no cure for AIDS. Faced with this, many people seek to take control of their treatment and this often includes the use of diet therapies which claim to prevent the progression of, or cure, disease. There can be tremendous psychological benefit from following a particular treatment and people should not be discouraged from following a regimen of their choice but helped to evaluate and adjust their chosen eating habits in order to meet nutritional goals (Resler 1988). It is important that eating remains an enjoyable experience and that people do not subject their food choice to unnecessarily rigid rules that may detract from enjoyment.

The following considerations may be helpful in evaluating a self-chosen dietary regimen (Pike 1988):

1 It should not contain substances in amounts that may be physically harmful.

2 It should not completely replace health care that is generally regarded as effective.

3 It should provide an adequate energy and protein intake along with a variety of foods.

4 It should not incur unnecessary expense.

Some commonly used regimens are discussed below.

Macrobiotics

This diet is based on oriental philosophy and is designed to restore the balance and harmony between yin and yang forces and thereby ameliorate disease (Muramoto 1988).

In an extreme form, a macrobiotic diet may result in many nutritional deficiencies, most notably protein, energy, calcium, iron and vitamin B_{12} (Pike 1988). A modified diet meeting nutritional requirements may be used as part of an holistic approach to health.

Marharishi Aurveda

This way of eating is based on mind body type (doshas). It is thought that when the doshas are in balance the individual enjoys good health and well-being; imbalance of the doshas leads to disease. The dietary principles are designed to promote the necessary balance and include advice on atmosphere, speed and quantity of food eaten as well as specific foods and food combinations to be avoided.

These 'principles of healthy eating' do not take into account the wide variety of needs of HIV positive people, do not describe how a balanced food intake is to be achieved and do not appear to be based on scientific fact. The vague advice may lead to poor nutrition and confusion.

AL 721

AL 721 is made from three lipids derived from egg yolks. AL stands for active lipid and 721 is the ratio of the components. It is thought to reduce the rate at which HIV can infect cells by extracting cholesterol from cell membranes, making it harder for the virus to attach to receptor sites.

An open label dose-ranging trial of AL 721 in 40 patients with mid-stage disease found very little toxicity but few consistent improvements in disease parameters (Mildvan *et al* 1989). A recent study in the UK failed to show any clinical or laboratory evidence of benefit with the use of AL 721 and suggested that it is ineffective in people with AIDS Related Complex (ARC) and AIDS (Peters *et al* 1990).

There are some hazards associated with the use of AL 721. As this substance is derived from egg yolk, a number of home-made recipes have been devised and these are of concern in relation to salmonella contamination of raw eggs (Peck and Johnson 1989). In addition, the advice that food should not be taken either three hours before or after taking AL 721 may seriously reduce the quantity of food which a person can eat and hence impair dietary adequacy.

Anti-Candida diet

An overgrowth of *Candida albicans*, both oral and oesophageal, is common in people who are HIV positive. It has been suggested that a diet excluding carbohydrate-rich and yeast-containing foods will prevent candidiasis by depriving the opportunistic organism of a suitable environment for growth (Crook 1985). Such a diet avoids foods containing sugar or yeast; alcoholic beverages; malt products; condiments; sauces; processed and smoked meats; dried and candied fruits; fruit juices that are canned, bottled or frozen; coffee and tea; melons; mushrooms; cheese, peanuts; vinegar-containing foods; vitamin and mineral tablets (unless free from sugar and yeast); and antibiotics.

The underlying theory has been characterized as speculative by the American Academy of Allergy and Immunology (Pike 1988). As with any restricted diet, undernutrition is possible.

Herbal remedies

It has been suggested that a number of herbs, both English and Chinese, can regenerate the immune system but there have been few controlled studies to investigate this assertion.

Garlic is thought to have anti-viral and anti-parasitic characteristics and is used in Chinese medicine in the treatment of cryptococcal meningitis (Raiten 1991). A twelve week trial of garlic extract on a small number of HIV positive people showed some improvement in T4:T8 cell ratio and an increase in natural killer cell activity (Abdullah *et al* 1989).

Glycyrrhizin, a compound found in liquorice, is thought to inhibit viral activity (Hattori *et al* 1989; Ikegami *et al* 1989). Long term use of excessive amounts may result in a syndrome resembling aldosteronism, with high blood pressure and water retention.

Hypericin, an extract from the plant St John's wort, is a recognized herbal medicine. It has been shown to work well in the laboratory but as yet has only been used in low doses in a small number of human subjects.

Compound Q is a purified protein extract from the root of a Chinese cucumber plant. There can be serious side effects to this drug so it must be used under medical supervision but early trials have shown interesting results (Raiten 1991).

Megadoses of vitamins and minerals

Those most commonly taken are vitamins A, C, E and B_{12} and selenium and zinc. In large doses, these nutrients have been reported to restore cell-mediated immunity by increasing T-cell number and activity, but efficacy has not been established. Abnormally low blood levels of some vitamins and minerals have been noted in early HIV infection (Beach *et al* 1989). In one study, 35% of subjects had vitamin B_{12} levels considered to represent overt deficiency, and zinc, copper and selenium levels were marginal in a number of people (Fordyce-Baum *et al* 1989).

The use of massive doses of vitamin C (up to 200 g daily) has been reported to suppress disease and reduce the rate of secondary infections (Fordyce-Baum *et al* 1989). The methods used to assess benefit can be questioned; patients' symptoms were assessed subjectively and there was no control group. Although adequate vitamin C is necessary for some aspects of immune response, more research is needed to determine the effectiveness of high doses in immunocompromised people who are HIV positive (Cathcart 1984).

An uncontrolled trial of the administration of zinc gluconate to immunocompromised patients suggested some degree of immunorestoration (Mathe *et al* 1986). However, one study showed that doses in excess of 300–400 mg per day can actually impair immune function (Chandra 1985; Fosmire 1990). Zinc intake of 10–12 times the Dietary Reference Value (15 mg/day) may impair lymphocyte function and cause vomiting, abdominal cramps and diarrhoea (Pike 1988).

Toxicity is associated with chronic intakes of vitamin A in excess of 50 000 iu per day (Raiten 1991). Beta-carotene has not been shown to be toxic even in large doses. One study reports an increase in the number of cells with natural killer activity after three months of treatment with 30 mg per day of beta-carotene (Watson *et al* 1989).

Germanium has been promoted for use in a variety of non-specific complaints and has been used by people who are HIV positive. Germanium is associated with nephropathy, in some case leading to renal failure and death, cardiomyopathy and peripheral myopathy. Pathological changes have been shown in people taking doses of 50–250 mg/day for between four and eighteen months. In October 1989, the Department of Health issued a warning against the use of germanium supplements (Acheson 1989).

The critical level of intake for specific vitamins and minerals in people who are HIV positive is not known. A supplement may be necessary when a person is eating poorly, when medication has caused a deficiency, or in vomiting and diarrhoea. There is not enough evidence to support the use of megadoses of vitamins and minerals and there is a need for clinical trials to be established to clarify the issue.

4.32.14 Community care of the HIV patient

The scope of nutrition in the care of HIV positive people in the community is enormous and embraces a wide range of different areas.

Working with non-statutory organizations

A number of support services exist for people who are HIV positive, in addition to health and social service provision (see the 'Useful addresses' list at the end of this chapter). Nutritionists can be involved in a number of ways; contributing to advice leaflets and newsletters, training sessions with staff and volunteers, providing workshops and one-to-one advice sessions.

Outreach projects and the voluntary sector

There is a great need for nutrition incentives and advice in HIV-related projects e.g. street drug agencies, needle exchange schemes and health improvement services for the street population.

Nutritional advice needs to be interpreted to meet the needs of people who may be homeless, suffering financial hardship and who give little priority to food, and this may take the form of literature and information, education of other workers and individual advice sessions. In providing services to people with HIV-related illness on a community level, sometimes the most basic need of people in crisis – the need for food – is forgotten (Korda and Hall 1989). The USA has set an example in setting up a variety of food assistance programmes (Table 4.103). Some local projects have begun in the UK but there is a great need for more.

Respite, terminal care and convalescent services

Such services are most usually provided by the hospice movement and are not part of the NHS but part of the voluntary sector. Many of them have clauses in their constitutions which limit them to accepting only people with cancer for terminal care, but this is changing and,

Table 4.103 Food assistance programmes used in the USA

Food bank	A distribution system for large amounts of surplus or donated food obtained from industry, growers and manufacturers
Food pantries	A distribution system for food that has been donated by individuals or groups from the community or obtained from food banks directly to clients for home preparation and consumption
Voucher systems	Setting up of accounts with local retailers where clients may purchase some specified amount of food and the purchase is billed to an AIDS service organization account
Hot meals programs	Provision of meals prepared in advance and served in a common eating space
Home meal delivery	Delivery of meals that are donated by local restaurants or prepared at designated kitchen facilities
Equipment loan	Provision of microwave ovens or other cooking equipment to individuals for use in their homes

increasingly, non-specialized hospices are accepting people with AIDS. There are a small number of hospices dedicated to caring for people with HIV and more are planned.

There is a need to work with staff and carers to ensure that people receive good nutritional care.

Home care teams

Many centres offering treatment to people who are HIV positive have established multidisciplinary teams able to provide 24-hour care for people who are no longer able to attend hospital and who wish to remain in their homes.

It may be necessary to provide nutritional support in the home in the form of high energy, high protein supplements, nastrogastric feeding and total parenteral nutrition. It is advisable to have policies to cover such provision should the situation arise (Peck and Johnson 1990).

4.32.15 Role of the dietitian in the care of people with HIV disease

HIV disease and AIDS have posed a unique challenge for health care professionals and have necessitated a re-examination of attitudes and practice in many areas (Peck 1990).

Care of the HIV positive person extends far beyond the treatment of a medical problem. People who are HIV positive are primarily young adults who are frequently well-informed about their condition and want to be involved in decisions about their care. They are facing periods of poor health, physical changes and premature death all of which have an impact on different areas of their life which may range from work, finance and housing to family and social support and their ability to feed and care for themselves. A variety of expertise working in co-operation with one another is essential in helping people to understand their options and make decisions.

Maintaining a good food intake is important throughout the course of the disease. There may be many factors influencing what a person is able to eat and dietary advice must be given in the context of individual circumstances. A multidisciplinary team approach to management draws together and co-ordinates all the service possibilities that can help a person achieve nutritional goals.

There is still considerable stigma attached to being HIV positive. People who are affected by HIV need to be cared for in a safe and non-judgmental environment. People working in this field, including dietitians, must address their own attitudes towards such issues as homosexuality and drug use, as well as death and dying. An ability to assess one's own feelings, knowledge and experience, and good personal support is essential for any dietitian working in this area (Adler 1987).

Useful addresses

Some of the non-statutory organizations working with people who are HIV positive are listed below. More details are available in the National AIDS Manual (see 'Further reading').

Terrence Higgins Trust, 52–54 Grays Inn Road, London WC1X 8JU. Tel 071–831 0330.
A charity set up to inform, advise and help with AIDS related conditions. Its objectives are to:
- Provide welfare, legal and counselling help and support;
- Disseminate accurate information to the public, media and policy makers;
- Provide health education;
- Support research into the causes and treatment of HIV disease.

FACTS (Foundation for AIDS Counselling Treatment and Support) 23 and 25 Weston Park, Crouch End, London N8 9SY. Tel 081–348 9195.
An organization aiming to promote the highest standards of health care for people with HIV disease. It offers:
- Training and support to health professionals;
- Help to individuals on how get the best from their GP and nationwide GP referral service;
- GP-type care to people in their area;
- Medical studies and trials of anti-HIV drugs.

The Landmark, 47a Tulse Hill, London SW2. Tel 081–678 6686.
A 'walk-in' centre offering a wide range of support services and practical help, meals, laundry facilities and a number of complementary therapies.

The London Lighthouse, 111–117 Lancaster Road, London W11 1QT. Tel 071–792 1200.
A major centre for people affected by HIV/AIDS offering a wide range of integrated services and including a 24-bedded residential unit.

National AIDS Helpline, Tel 0800–567123.
A free and confidential phoneline.

Body Positive, 51b Philbeach Gardens, Earls Court, London SW5 9EB. Tel 071–835 1045.
A centre offering a wide range of facilities including meals, laundry facilities, recreational space, social events and advice and information.

Mainliners, Mainliners Ltd, PO Box 125, London SW9 8EF.
An agency which promotes self-help and provides a range of services for all those affected by HIV and drugs. Publishes a monthly newsletter.

Blackliners Helpline, PO Box 1274, London SW9 8EZ. Tel 071–738 5274.
A counselling and support service for people affected by HIV/AIDS from Africa, the Caribbean and Asia. Also provides education and practical help.

Positively Women, 5 Sebastian Street, London EC1V 0ME. Tel 071–490 5515.
Provides a range of free and confidential counselling support and practical help to women with HIV/AIDS.

ACET (AIDS, Care, Education and Training), PO Box 1323, London W5 5TF. Tel 081–840 7879.
A Christian AIDS charity aiming to provide services to people irrespective of background, sexuality, ethnic origin or lifestyle. Provides an excellent home care service.

AIDS/HIV support services in Scotland

ACET (see above), PO Box 151, Edinburgh EH8 9NY. Tel 031–667 1978.

Body Positive (see above), 37–39 Montrose Terrace, Edinburgh EH7 5DJ. Tel 031–652 0754.

City Wide Family Support Group, 43 Groathill Road North, Edinburgh EH4 2RS. Tel 031–332 9279.
A 24-hour advice helpline for those with HIV/AIDS and drug-related problems.

EAST (Ecumenical AIDS Support Team), 3 Hamilton Terrace, Edinburgh EH13 1NB. Tel 0968 60253.
Practical help and support for anyone with, or affected by, HIV/AIDS.

HIV/AIDS and Drugs Team, Lothian Health Board, Northern General Hospital, Ferry Road, Edinburgh EH5 3DQ. Tel 031–332 2525.
A team involved in planning and co-ordinating all aspects of Lothian Health Board's response to HIV/AIDS.

HIV/AIDS Back-up Service, Health Education Department, 61 Grange Loan, Edinburgh EH9 2ER. Tel 031–447 6271.
Supports health promotion, education and training in Lothian. Offers training, resources, information and networking.

HIV Counselling Clinic, Ward 14, City Hospital, 51 Greenbank Drive, Edinburgh EH10 5SB. Tel 031–447 1001; Advice line: 031–447 0411.
Offers confidential counselling and support and HIV testing.

Lothian Community Project (The Salvation Army), 77 Bread Street, Edinburgh. Tel 031–228 5351.
Drop-in facility and support for those with HIV or AIDS.

Milestone House, (Waverley Care – an AIDS Trust), 113 Oxgangs Road North, Edinburgh EH14 1EB. Tel 031–441 6989.
Convalescent, respite and terminal care.

SAM (Scottish AIDS Monitor), 64 Broughton Street, Edinburgh EH1 3SA. Tel 031–557 3885.
Information and support.

Further reading

Adler MW (Ed) (1987) *ABC of AIDS*. British Medical Journal, London.

Scott P (1981) *National AIDS Manual*. Vol 1: *Topics*. Vol 2: *Directory*. NAM Publications Limited, London.

Scientific American (1988) October Issue.

Kotler DP (Ed) (1991) *Gastrointestinal and nutritional manifestations of the Acquired Immunodeficiency Syndrome*. Raven Press, New York.

Youle M, Clarbour J, Wade P and Farthing C (1988) *AIDS – Therapeutics in HIV disease*. Churchill Livingstone, Edinburgh.

References

Abdullah T, Kirkpatrick DV, Williams L and Carter J (1989) Garlic as an antimicrobial and immune modulator in AIDS (abstract). *Proceedings of the Fifth International Conference on AIDS, June 4–9, Montreal*. p. 466.

Acheson D (1989) *Germanium-containing dietary supplements*. PL/CMO (1989) 9. Department of Health. HMSO, London.

Adler MW (1987) *ABC of AIDS*. British Medical Journal, London.

AIDS-UK (1990) A quarterly epidemiological briefing on AIDS/HIV in the United Kingdom. Issue 9, p. 2. Health Education Authority and Public Health Laboratory Service AIDS Centre, London.

Anderson R (1990) Prospects for the UK. The AIDS epidemic in the UK; past trends and future predictions. In *HIV and AIDS – An assessment of current and future spread in the UK*. Report of a symposium held on 24 November 1989. UK Health Departments/Health Education Authority, London.

Archer DL (1989) Food counselling for persons infected with HIV: Strategy for defensive living. *Public Health Reports* **104**(2), 196–8.

Archer DL and Glinsmann WH (1985) Enteric infections and other cofactors in AIDS. *Immunol Today* **6**, 292–5.

Barr CE and Torosian JP (1986) Oral manifestations in patients with AIDS or AIDS related complex. *Lancet* **2**, 288.

Beach RS, Mantero-Atienza E, Van-Riel F, Morgan R and Fordyce-Baum MK (1989) Nutritional abnormalities in early HIV-1 infection. 1. Plasma vitamin levels (abstract). In *Proceedings of the Fifth International Conference on AIDS, June 4–9, Montreal*. p. 218.

Beisel WR, Edelman R, Nauss K and Suskind RM (1981) Single nutrient effects on immunological functions. *J Am Med Assoc* **245**(1), 53–8.

Bentler MA and Stanish M (1987) Nutritional support of the paediatric patient with AIDS. *J Am Diet Assoc* **87**, 488–91.

Bernstein LJ, Bye MR and Rubinstein A (1989) Prognostic factors and life expectancy in children with acquired immunodeficiency syndrome. *Am J Dis Childh* **143**, 775–8.

Blanche S, Rouzioux C, Moscato MLG, Veber F, Mayaux MJ, Jacomet C, Triocoire J, Deville A, Vial M, Firtion G, de Crepy A, Douard D, Robin M, Courpotin C, Ciraru-Vigneron N, le Deist F and Griscelli C (1989) A prospective study of infants born to women seropositive for human immunodeficiency virus type I. *New Engl J Med* **320**, 1643–8.

Cathcart RF (1984) Vitamin C in the treatment of the acquired immune deficiency syndrome (AIDS) *Med Hypotheses* **14**, 423–33.

Celum CL, Chaisson RE, Rutherford GW *et al* (1987) Incidence of Salmonellosis in patients with AIDS. *J Infectious Dis* **156**(6), 998–1002.

Centers for Disease Control. Update: acquired immunodeficiency syndrome – USA (1987) Mortality and morbidity weekly report (MWWR). Classification system for HIV infection in children under thirteen years of age. *MWWR* **36**, 225–30.

Centers for Disease Control (1991) *HIV/AIDS Surveillance Report*. December 1991, 1–18.

Chandra RK (1981a) Immunodeficiency in undernutrition and overnutrition. *Nutr Rev* **39**(6), 225–31.

Chandra RK (1981b) Immunocompetence as a functional index of nutritional status. *Brit Med Bull* **37**(1), 89–94.

Chandra RK (1983) Nutrition, immunity and infection: present knowledge and future directions. *Lancet* **1**, 688–91.

Chandra RK (1984) Nutrition and immunology: from basic observations to clinical applications. *Recent Advances in Clin Nutr* **11**, 221–5.

Chandra RK (1985) Megadose zinc intakes impair immune responses. *Nutr Rev* **43**, 141–3.

Chelluri L and Jastremski MS (1989) Incidence of malnutrition inpatients with acquired immunodeficiency syndrome. *Nutr Clin Prac* **4**, 16–18.

Chen W, Brown S, Gazzard B and Howard L (1990) A retrospective study on the effect of megace on body weight in HIV infected patients who had lost more than 5% body weight (abstract). In *Proceedings of the Sixth International Conference on AIDS, San Francisco*. p. Th.B 209.

Coffey T, Nelson M, Bower M and Gazzard BE (1989) Listeria monocytogenes meningitis in an HIV infected patients. *AIDS* **3**(9), 614–15.

Communicable Disease Report Weekly (1992) Volume 2 (4). Public Health Laboratory Service, Colindale, UK.

Cowan M, Hellman D, Chudwin D, Wara DW, Chang RS and Amman AJ (1984) Maternal transmission of AIDS. *Paediatrics* **73**, 382.

Crook WG (1985) *The yeast connection: a medical breakthrough*. Professional Books/Future Health Inc, Jackson, Tennessee.

Cunningham-Rundles S (1982) The effects of nutritional status on immunological function. *Am J Clin Nutr* **35**, 1202–10.

Department of Health (1991) *Dietary Reference Values for food energy and nutrients for the United Kingdom*. Rep Hlth Soc Subj 41. HMSO, London.

Department of Health and Social Security (1988) *HIV infection, breast-feeding and human milk banking*. PL/CMO (1988) 13 and PL/CNO (1988) 7. HMSO, London.

Erskine D (1990) The use of drugs in patients with gastrointestinal manifestations of AIDS. *Baillière's Clinical Gastroenterology* **4**(2), 563–83.

The European Collaborative Study (1988) Mother-to-child transmission of HIV Infection. *Lancet* **ii**, 1039–42.

The European Collaborative Study (1991) Children born to women with HIV I infection: natural history and risk of transmission. *Lancet* **337**, 253–60.

Fennoy I and Leung J (1990) Refeeding and subsequent growth in the child with AIDS. *Nutr Clin Prac* **5**, 54–8.

Ferraro R, Kotler DP, Cuff P, Tierney AR, Smith R and Hamsfield S (1989) Effect of enteral nutritional therapy on body cell mass in AIDS. (abstract). In *Proceedings of the Fifth International Conference on AIDS, June 4–9, Montreal*. p. Th.B 312.

Fischl MA, Richman DD, Grieco MH, Gottlieb MS, Volberding PA, Laskin OL, Leedom JM, Groopman JE, Mildvan D, Schooley RT, Jackson GG, Durack DT and King D (1987) The efficacy of azidothymidine (AZT) in the treatment of patients with AIDS and AIDS related complex. A double blind placebo controlled trial. *New Eng J Med* **317**, 185–91.

Fordyce-Baum MK, Mantero-Ationza E, Crass R, Morgan R and Beach RS (1989) Nutritional Abnormalities in early HIV-1 infection. 11 Trace Elements (abstract). In *Proceedings of the Fifth International Conference on AIDS, June 4–9, Montreal*. p. 467.

Fosmire GJ (1990) Zinc toxicity. *Am J Clin Nutr* **51**, 225–7.

Francis DEM (1987) Gastrointestinal disorders. *Diets for sick children* 4e. Blackwell Scientific Publications, Oxford. p. 33.

Garcia ME, Collins CL and Mansell PWA (1987) The acquired immunodeficiency syndrome: nutritional complications and assessment of body weight status. *Nutr Clin Pract* **2**, 108.

Ghiron E, Dwyer LJ and Stollman LB (1989) Nutrition support of the HIV Positive, ARC and AIDS patient. *Clin Nutr* **8**, 103–13.

Grunfeld C and Kotler DP (1991) The wasting syndrome and nutritional support in AIDS. *Seminars in Gastrointestinal Disease* **2**(1), 25–36.

Hattori T, Ikematsu S, Koito A, Matsushita S, Maeda Y, Hada M, Fujimaki M and Takatsuki K (1989) Preliminary evidence for inhibitory effect of glycyrrhizin on HIV replication in patients with AIDS. *Antiviral Res* **11**, 255–62.

Hecker LM and Kotler DP (1990) Malnutrition in patients with AIDS. *Nutr Rev* **48**, 11.

Hickey MS and Weaver KE (1988) Nutritional management of patients with ARC or AIDS. *Gastroenterol Clin N Am* **17**(3), 545–61.

Hommes MJT, Romijin JA, Godfried MH, Weftinck Schattenker JKM, Buurman WA, Endert E and Sauerwein HP (1990) Increased resting energy expenditure in human immunodeficiency virus-infected men. *Metabolism* **39**(11), 1186–90.

Hommes MJT, Romijin JA, Endert E and Sauerwein HP (1991) Resting energy expenditure and substrate oxidation in human immunodeficiency virus (HIV) infected asymptomatic men: HIV affects host metabolism in the early asymptomatic stage. *Am J Clin Nutr* **54**, 311–15.

Hyman C and Kaufman S (1989) Nutritional impact of acquired immune deficiency syndrome: a unique counselling opportunity. *J Am Diet Assoc* **89**, 520–24.

Ikegami N, Yoshioka K and Akatani K (1989) Clinical evaluation of glycyrrhizin on HIV-infected asymptomatic haemophiliac patients in Japan (abstract). In *Proceedings of the Fifth International Conference on AIDS, June 4–9, Montreal*. p. 401.

Jain VK and Chandra RK (1984) Does nutritional deficiency predispose to acquired immune deficiency syndrome? *Nutr Res* **4**, 537–43.

Janson DD and Feasley KM (1989) Parenteral nutrition in the management of gastrointestinal Kaposi's sarcoma in a patient with AIDS. *Clin Phar* **8**, 536–44.

Kelson K, Malcolm J, Brantsma A and Sutherland DC (1991) Percutaneous endoscopic gastrostomy feeding in AIDS (abstract). In *Proceedings of the Seventh International Conference on AIDS*, Florence. p. MB 2414.

King AB, McMillan G, St Arnaud J and Ward TT (1989) Less diarrhoea in HIV patients on a low fat, elemental diet (abstract). In *Proceedings of the Fifth International Conference on AIDS, June 4–9, Montreal*. p. Th.B 300.

Korda H and Hall CS (1989) *Food programs: assessing and developing community based nutritional support programs for people with HIV-related illness*. NAN Technical Assistance Series. National AIDS Network, Washington.

Kotler DP (1987) Why study nutrition in AIDS? *Nutr Clin Prac* **1**, 94–5.

Kotler DP, Culpepper-Morgan JA, Tierney AR and Klien EB (1986) Treatment of disseminated cytomegalovirus infection with 9-(1,3 dihydroxy-2-propoxymethyl) guanine: evidence of prolonged survival in patients with AIDS. *AIDS Res* **2**(4), 299–307.

Kotler DP, Tierney AR, Wang J and Pierson RN (1989a) Magnitude of body cell mass depletion and the timing of death from wasting in AIDS. *Am J Clin Nutr* **50**, 444–7.

Kotler DP, Tierney AR, Altilio D, Wang J and Pierson RN (1989b) Body mass repletion during ganciclovir treatment of cytomegalovirus infections in patients with AIDS. *Arch Intern Med* **149**, 90–5.

Kotler DP, Tierney AR, Culpepper-Morgan JA, Wang J and Pierson RN (1990a) Effect of home total parenteral nutrition on body composition in patients with acquired immunodeficiency syndrome. *JPEN* **14**(5), 454–8.

Kotler DP, Tierney AR, Bremer SK, Couture S, Wang J and Pierson RN (1990b) Preservation of short term energy balance in clinically stable patients with AIDS. *Am J Clin Nutr* **51**(1), 7–13.

Kotler DP, Tierney AR, Ferraro R, Cuff P, Wang J, Pierson RN and Heymsfeild (1991) Enteral alimentation and repletion of body cell mass in malnourished patients with acquired immunodeficiency syndrome. *Am J Clin Nutr* **53**, 149–54.

Kotler DP, Wang J and Pierson RN (1985) Body composition studies in patients with the acquired immunodeficiency syndrome. *Am J Clin Nutr* **43**, 1255–65.

Lambert HJ and Friesen H (1989) Clinical features of paediatric AIDS in Uganda. *Annals of Tropical Paediatrics* **9**, 1–5.

Marion RW, Wiznia AA, Hutcheon RG and Rubinstein A (1989) Human T-cell lymphotropic virus type III (HTLV-III) embryopathy: a new dysmorphic syndrome associated with intrauterine HTLV-III infection. *Am J Dis Chldh* **140**, 638–40.

Mascola L, Lieb L, Chiu J, Fannin SL and Linnan MJ (1988) Listeriosis: an uncommon opportunistic infection in patients with acquired immunodeficiency syndrome. *Am J Med* **84**, 162–4.

Mathe G, Misset JL, Gil-Delgado M, Musset M, Reizenstein P and Canon C (1986) A phase II trial of immunorestoration with zinc gluconate in immunodepressed cancer patients. *Biomed Pharmacother* **40**, 383–5.

Melchior JC, Salmon D, Rigaud D, Leport C, Bouvet E, Detruchis P, Vilde JL, Vachon F, Coulaud JP and Apfelbaum M (1991) Resting energy expenditure is increased in stable, malnourished HIV infected patients. *Am J Clin Nutr* **53**, 437–41.

Mildvan D, Armstrong D, Antoniskis D, Sacks H, Balfour H, Buzas J and Perrinelli C (1989) An open label dose-ranging trial of AL721 in PGL and ARC (abstract). In *Proceedings of the Fifth International Conference on AIDS, June 4–9, Montreal*. p. 404.

Mok JYQ (1990) Paediatric AIDS. *Maternal and Child Health* November, 349–52.

Mok JYQ (1991) HIV infection in children. *Brit Med J* **302**, 921–2.

Moseson M, Zeleniuch-Jacquote A, Belsito DV, Shore RE, Marmor M and Pasternack B (1989) The potential role of nutritional factors in the induction of immunological abnormalities in HIV positive homosexual men. *J Acquired Immune Deficiency Syndrome* **2**, 235–47.

Muramoto NB (1988) Natural immunity and insights on diet and AIDS. George Ohsawa Macrobiotic Foundation, California.

NACNE (1983) *A discussion paper on proposals for nutritional guidelines for health education in Britain*. Health Education Council, London.

Oxtoby MJ (1988) Human immunodeficiency virus and other viruses in human milk: placing the issues in broader perspective. *Paediatr Infect Dis J* **7**, 825–35.

Peck K (1990) Nutritional support in late stage HIV infection. *Clinical Nutr Update* **1**(9), 8.

Peck K, Howes G, Robinson V and George R (1991) Total parenteral nutrition in palliation of AIDS (abstract). In *Proceedings of the Seventh*

International Conference on AIDS, Florence. p. MD 4182.
Peck K and Johnson S (1990) The role of nutrition in HIV infection. *J Hum Nutr Diet* **3**(3), 147–57.
Peters BS, Bennett J, Jeffries DJ, Knox K, Koisis A and Pinching AJ (1990) Ineffectiveness of AL721 in HIV disease. *Lancet* **335**, 545–6.
Pike JT (1988) Alternative nutritional therapies – where is the evidence? *AIDS Patient Care* February, 31–3.
Pizzo PA (1990) Paediatric AIDS: problems within problems. *J Inf Dis* **161**, 316–25.
Raiten DJ (1990) *Nutrition and HIV infection*. Prepared for the Center for Food Safety and Applied Nutrition Food and Drug Administration Department of the Health and Human Services, Washington DC. 20204 PDA Contract 223–88–2124.
Raiten DJ (1991) Nutrition and HIV infection: a review and evaluation of the extant knowledge of the relationship between nutrition and HIV infection. *Nutrition in Clinical Practice* **6**(3) June (Suppl).
Resler SS (1988) Nutrition care of AIDS patients. *J Am Dietet Assoc* **88**(7), 828–32.
Shannon KM and Ammann AJ (1985) Acquired immune deficiency syndrome in childhood. *J Paed* **106**, 332–42.
Singer P, Rothkops MM, Kvetan V, Gaare S, Mellow L and Askanazi S (1989) Nutrition, the gastrointestinal tract and the acquired immune deficiency syndrome. Facts and perspective. *Clin Nutr* **8**, 281–7.
Smith PD, Lane HC, Gill VJ, Minischowitz JF, Quinnan GV, Fauci AS and Masur H (1988) Intestinal infections in patients with the acquired immunodeficiency syndrome (AIDS). *Ann Intern Med* **108**, 328–33.
Streat SJ, Beddoe AH and Hill GL (1987) Aggressive nutritional support does not prevent protein loss despite fat gain in septic intensive care patients. *J Trauma* **27**(3), 262.
Summerbell CD, Catalan J and Gazzard BG (1993a) A comparison of the nutritional beliefs of human immunodeficiency virus (HIV) seropositive and seronegative homosexual men. *J Hum Nutr Dietet* **6**, 23–7.
Summerbell CD, Perret J and Gazzard BG (1993b) Causes of weight loss in human immunodeficiency virus infection. *Int J STD & AIDS* (in press).
Task Force on Nutrition Support in AIDS (1989) Guidelines for nutrition support in AIDS. *Nutrition* **5**(1), 39–46.
Tuazon CU and Labriola AM (1987) Management of infections and immunological complications of AIDS: Current and future prospects. *Drugs* **33**, 66–84.
Von Roenn J, Murphy R, Williams L and Weitzman S (1989) Magesterol acetate in the treatment of HIV related cachexia (abstract). In *Proceedings of the Fifth International Conference on AIDS, June 4–9, Montreal*. p. Th.B 309.
Watson RR, Garewal HS, Ampel NM, Prabhala RM, Allen V, Dols C and Hichs MJ (1989) Immunostimulatory effects of beta carotene on T-cell activation markers and NK cells in HIV infected patients (abstract). In *Proceedings of the Fifth International conference on AIDS, June 4–9, Montreal*. p. 663.
Winick M, Andrassy RJ, Armstrong D, Bryan MA, Chandra RK, Kotler DP, Neary CA, Norton JA, Rodriguez K, Rosenberg IH and Weaver KE (1989) Task Force on Nutrition Support in AIDS. *Nutrition* **5**(1), 39–46.
World Health Organization (1986) Acquired immunodeficiency syndrome: WHO/CDC case definition for AIDS. *Wkly Epidemiol Rec* **61**, 69–73.
World Health Organization (1992) *Wkly Epidemiol Rec* **67**(3), 10.

4.33 Cancer: diet and causation

4.33.1 Incidence

Cancer is second only to heart disease as a cause of death in Westernized countries. In Britain it accounts for 23% of all deaths and with few exceptions the risk of it increases with age. For example, rates for colon cancer in men are 7 per 100 000 at age 40–45, rising to 60 at age 60–65, and to 240 at age 80–85 (Muir *et al* 1987). Age-standardized rates for stomach cancer in men and women in Britain are declining but increasing for cancer of the skin and bladder. In women, breast cancer incidence is increasing, as is cancer of the lung. In men, rates for cancer of the prostate, colon and oesophagus are increasing.

4.33.2 Environment and diet

A number of observations strongly suggest that environment can influence cancer risk. First, there are widely differing rates for cancers of different organs in different parts of the world. Cancers of the lung, breast and large bowel are commonest in developed countries, and cancer of the cervix, stomach and mouth are most frequent in developing countries. These different rates could be due to racial factors, but studies of the cancer patterns of migrants suggest that there are other factors. The Japanese, for example, used to have low rates of breast and large bowel cancer and high rates of stomach cancer. However, Japanese who migrated to the USA have taken on the same pattern as their host country, that is high rates of large bowel cancer, and low rates for stomach cancer. These rates changed within one generation for the stomach and large bowel, and within two generations for cancer of the breast. Furthermore, there have been striking changes in incidence within populations, for example the recent rise in lung cancer in women in the UK, and a six-fold increase in colon cancer incidence in Japan over the past 20 years (Muir *et al* 1987).

Of the many possible environmental factors, exposure to sunlight and tobacco are well known causes of cancer of the skin and lung respectively. There is now also consistent evidence from animal, epidemiological and other studies of a role for alcohol in cancer of the oral cavity, pharynx, larynx, oesophagus and liver (IARC 1987). There is a marked multiplicative effect of alcohol with cigarette smoking. In countries with high levels of consumption, alcohol-related cancers contribute a substantial proportion to the total. In Britain, these cancers are less common with present levels of alcohol consumption.

Many other factors in diet have also been implicated in either the causation of, or more frequently, protection against, cancer (Armstrong and Doll 1975). To date, information from a number of epidemiological and experimental studies is awaited before either the mechanisms, or precise estimates of risk from diet are known. However, one estimate of the proportion of all cancers attributable to diet ranges from 10–70%, with an overall average of 35%. This compares with 25–40% from tobacco and 2–8% from occupational exposure. At less than 1%, food additives are estimated to contribute virtually no risk and some may be protective (Doll and Peto 1981).

4.33.3 Dietary factors and cancer causation

Cancers represent a collection of different abnormalities which occur when the process of cell division during growth and renewal goes out of control. Cells rapidly divide (proliferate) in an uncontrolled way, independent of the normal growth control factors, and do not form themselves (differentiate) into specialized tissues. Cancer development is thought to be a several stage process of initiation, followed by promotion. The initiation step is brought about by carcinogens which are widespread in the environment and which cause changes in the DNA of cells. Before malignancy develops, another stage, promotion, is necessary. In general, diet is thought to be particularly important in the promotion of cancer and in protection against the effects of carcinogens, rather than as a carrier of carcinogens themselves.

It is to be expected that the causes of cancers in different organs of the body would be different, but the way in which diet is thought to be involved is often uncertain. In addition, several sites have a dietary constituent in common. Those that have been implicated in either promotion of or protection against cancer are shown in Table 4.104 (NRC 1982; DHHS 1988). For more detailed discussion of the evidence relating these items to cancer, and the suggested ways in which they might be involved, see Bingham (1990b).

Fat, cholesterol and obesity

High fat diets increase the number of tumours initiated by a variety of chemical carcinogens in virtually all animal models of breast, bowel, pancreas and prostate cancer provided that the diets fed supply sufficient of the essential n-6 polyunsaturate, linoleic acid, for which there is a tumour requirement of approximately 10% of total energy

Table 4.104 Dietary factors implicated in the promotion of, or protection against, cancer

Possible initiators and promoters of cancer	Fat Cholesterol Obesity Protein and meat Sodium (salt) Nitrate and nitrite N-nitroso compounds Mycotoxins Other naturally occurring carcinogens and contaminants Alcohol
Possible protective constituents of food against cancer	Non-starch polysaccharides (dietary 'fibre') and starch Vitamin A and carotene Vitamins C and E Vitamin D Selenium Calcium Other minerals and vitamins Fruit and vegetables

(Ip 1987). The current level of polyunsaturated fatty acids in the British diet is about 6% of total energy. Incidence is approximately doubled in animals fed 40% energy as fat compared with those fed 20%. Present levels of fat in the UK diet are about 40% of total energy. Recent evidence suggests that the other group of essential ω3 polyunsaturates from alpha-linolenic acid, found in fish oils, tend to suppress tumour promotion, in contrast to the effects of the linoleic group of fatty acids.

So far, however, there is only limited evidence of these associations in humans. In the largest and most accurate prospective study of diet and cancer risk, no associations between total fat and breast cancer were shown, although the risk for bowel cancer was increased in individuals who had consumed a higher total fat diet than others (Willett *et al* 1987a; 1990). Results are awaited from other prospective studies to confirm these effects of total fat, and of the relative roles of different types of fat, at different cancer sites.

The evidence relating cholesterol to cancer risk is conflicting. Animals fed cholesterol in conjunction with a chemical carcinogen have shown an increased incidence of bowel tumours, and it is possible that there is an increased tumour requirement for cholesterol.

In contrast, a number of studies have reported that a low serum cholesterol is associated with increased risk of cancer (inverse association). Some of these studies were small and the increased risk was usually shown for lung cancer which is primarily related to cigarette smoking. In a report of 1500 individuals in Scotland for example, there was a strong negative association in men between serum cholesterol and lung cancer but there was no such association in the few patients who developed colon cancer, nor in women who developed breast cancer (Isles *et al* 1990). The evidence for any relationship between blood cholesterol levels and cancer is therefore inconclusive and controversial.

Animal studies which suggest an effect of fat in the promotion of cancer can largely be explained by the fact that over-feeding had a definite and marked effect on the progression of cancers of the large bowel, breast, and probably pancreas. However, a marked energy restriction of approximately 20% is needed to overcome the effect of fat in animal studies. There is no evidence that this level of energy restriction alters cancer risk in humans. Risks of mortality from, or development of, post-menopausal breast cancer and cancer of the endometrium are probably increased with increasing obesity, but may be decreased in pre-menopausal breast cancer (Willett *et al* 1987).

Protein and meat

International correlation studies between food consumption and cancer incidence have shown relationships between cancer of the large bowel, breast, kidney and pancreas that are at least as good with meat and animal protein as they are with fat (Armstrong and Doll 1975).

Meat also contains heterocyclic amines which are produced during cooking at relatively low temperatures. They are carcinogenic in animal feeding studies, although at levels several orders of magnitude greater than found in food (Bingham 1990b).

Vegetarians are at reduced risk of colon cancer, and some case-control studies and one prospective study have indicated an increased risk of colon cancer in high meat consumers (Willet *et al* 1990). More information is required to confirm these findings.

Sodium, nitrate, N-nitroso compounds

Internationally, populations at high risk for stomach cancer are also at high risk for stroke and hypertension, and it has been suggested that salt is the causative factor in both. This suggestion has prompted work showing abnormal divisions in cells of the stomach mucosa in association with high levels of salt. However, elevated risks for both these diseases are not always seen within countries and comparisons of total sodium intake (from 24 hour urine analysis) have shown increased levels in areas at high risk of stomach cancer compared with areas at low risk in some studies, but not in others.

Case-control studies generally suggest that consumption of foods preserved in salt, which may also be pickled and smoked, and heavy salting of food is associated with an increased risk of stomach cancer. In general, however, relative risks are more consistent, and of a greater magnitude, for a protective effect of vegetables and fruit. Any reported elevated risk in stomach cancer may therefore be due to the absence of vegetables, fruit and vitamin C rather than an independent effect of salt.

Nitrate and nitrite are present naturally in food, the level depending on fertilizer use (both organic and inorganic). The major sources are vegetables, which supply 70–90% of the total, and water which supplies 5–20%. Less than 3% of the total is supplied by added nitrite and nitrate used to preserve foods such as ham, bacon and corned beef.

Added nitrate is metabolized in the body to nitrite which is also produced in the body by white blood cells in response to infection and inflammation. Under certain conditions, nitrite can combine with nitrogen-containing substances to form N-nitroso compounds, most of which are known to be potent carcinogens. There is however, no consistent epidemiological evidence to suggest that individuals consuming more nitrate or nitrite are at greater risk than those consuming less, rather the reverse. In Britain, mortality from stomach cancer is lowest in areas where exposure to nitrate is highest, for example in East Anglia (Forman *et al* 1985).

Vegetables contain vitamin C, which is known to inhibit N-nitroso compound formation, and there is accumulating evidence that vegetables are protective in many cancers including stomach cancer, with which nitrate is particularly associated.

Mycotoxins and other naturally occurring carcinogens and contaminants

One of the most well known toxins produced by moulds contaminating foods is aflatoxin B_1, a potent carcinogen inducing cancer of the liver in many animal species. In Western countries such as Britain, aflatoxin contamination is very low, as are liver cancer levels.

Numerous other naturally occurring carcinogens and contaminants occur in food, such as alkaloids found in ragwort and comfrey, benzene derivatives in tarragon, cycasin in cycad nuts and urethane particularly in stone fruit brandies.

Polycyclic hydrocarbons are formed on smoked and barbecued food in addition to contaminating vegetables, fats and grains, and are particularly implicated in cancer of the upper digestive tract tissues which would be in direct contact with them. The associations with smoked food in gastric cancer are less strong than the protective effect of vegetables.

As with nitroso compounds, the risks of polycyclic hydrocarbons in food are small compared with those from tobacco, but it is recommended that smoked and barbecued food consumption should not increase above current low levels.

Alcohol

The case for alcohol being involved in the causation of cancer is much stronger than for other items of diet, and a recent expert body has found sufficient evidence to classify alcoholic beverages as carcinogenic to humans.

Dose responses to alcohol have been found in cancer of the oral cavity, pharynx, larynx, oesophagus and liver. These cancers are less common in Britain compared with communities with a high level of alcohol consumption, such as France, where incidence rates are higher, and contribute a substantial proportion to the total cancer burden. An elevated risk, by about 20%, is evident with only moderate alcohol consumption of 10 g/day and there is a multiplicative effect with smoking. Heavy smokers (40 per day) and drinkers (40 g/day) have a relative risk of the order of 15 for cancer of the oral cavity and pharynx, whereas heavy drinkers alone have a relative risk of 2.

There is also suggestive evidence from both case-control and prospective studies that alcohol elevates relative risk for breast cancer by up to 1.5 to 2 for 40 grams of alcohol, particularly in young women.

Studies with pure ethanol have not yielded evidence that alcohol is a direct carcinogen, but acetaldehyde is also found in alcoholic drinks and is the main metabolic product from alcohol in humans, particularly in chronic consumers. Acetaldehyde is a known carcinogen for animals and causes chromosomal damage in test systems (IARC 1987).

Non-starch polysaccharides (dietary 'fibre') and starch

NSP and starch surviving digestion in the small gut is fermented by the bacterial flora in the large gut. Fermentation leads to an increase in bacterial mass which together with unfermented NSP (particularly from bran) increases faecal weight, dilutes the contents of the large gut and shortens transit time. This leads to a reduction in the amount of time for which possible carcinogens are in contact with the large bowel mucosa. Populations with a high faecal weight and shorter transit time are known to be at reduced risk of bowel cancer. In addition, one of the end products of fermentation, butyrate, may be important in reducing the rate at which mucosal cells proliferate.

In general, fibre from bran and cellulose seems to be protective against the effect of chemical carcinogens in animal studies. In humans, the majority of studies of healthy controls compared with cases of bowel cancer since 1975 have shown a reduction in risk, but usually as a result of increased vegetable consumption, rather than cereal fibre (Bingham 1990a). In two large studies which attempted to measure starch consumption, cases were shown to be consuming fewer starch containing foods. However, no effect of fibre or vegetables was shown in one prospective study of American nurses (Willett *et al* 1990) and further results are awaited in order that a consensus view may be formed.

Vitamins A, E, C, carotene and selenium

All of these vitamins and carotenoids, including beta-carotene, are part of the antioxidant defence system of the body. Oxidant damage may be important in the initiation of cancer at all sites, and vitamin C in addition inhibits the formation of nitrosamines. Retinol is also well known to control cellular differentiation and proliferation. However vitamin A is toxic in excess and levels in excess of the DRVs are not recommended.

In general, case control studies have tended to show that patients with cancers at several sites reported eating less of all these items than healthy controls, mainly because patients reported eating fewer vegetables than controls (Wald 1987).

More than a dozen prospective intervention trials using high doses (15–50 mg) of beta-carotene are now in progress to determine whether or not participants experience lower risks of cancer of the skin, lung, cervix, oral cavity, uterus and colon in particular. Vitamin C and other antioxidant carotenoids may however be as important (Thurnham 1990).

Selenium, via the antioxidant properties of glutathione peroxidase, a selenium containing enzyme, has also been proposed as important in cancer protection. However this generally has not been supported by epidemiological studies. A plateau value in glutathione peroxidase activity is reached beyond a certain selenium concentration in food or drinking water, and no relationship has been shown in recent experiments relating glutathione peroxidase to excessive levels of oxidized fats, lack of selenium, and occurrence of tumours in animal studies.

Vitamin D and calcium

Vitamin D is classically associated with calcium homeostasis but a more fundamental role in controlling cell growth and differentiation has recently emerged. Nearly all tissues so far examined have been found to have vitamin D receptors, as do most malignant tissues including breast, colon, cervix and pancreas. Some, but not all, animal studies suggest that the active form of vitamin D (1,25 dihydroxy cholecalciferol) may inhibit tumour growth and there has been one report of an anti-tumour effect in lymphoma. These studies indicate that vitamin D analogues might be useful in the treatment of cancer as is the case with vitamin A. As with vitamin A, large dietary doses of vitamin D are toxic.

Calcium has been implicated in protecting against cancer of the large bowel, following the suggestion that its presence in the large bowel would counteract the irritating effects of free fatty acids or bile acids arising from a high fat diet. Supplements of calcium carbonate have been shown to reduce cell proliferation in the large bowel in both animals and humans at high risk of colon cancer, although calcium has been viewed in general as an enhancer rather than an inhibitor in various test systems of chemical carcinogens.

Calcium intakes tend to be elevated in areas at high risk of colon cancer, such as Britain and New Zealand, although in some prospective studies and a number of case-control studies within populations the majority suggest that calcium may be protective. The results of further prospective studies are awaited.

Other minerals and vitamins

Magnesium, zinc, iron, copper, iodine, molybdenum, B vitamins and choline have all been considered mainly as protective against cancer particularly at levels sufficient to prevent deficiency. For example, iodine deficiency is associated with increased risk for thyroid cancer and riboflavin deficiency with increased risk for oesophageal cancer. However, there are insufficient or contradictory findings from animal and epidemiological studies allowing no conclusions concerning their relevance to human cancer.

Fruit and vegetables

In addition to vitamins C, E, beta-carotene and NSP, discussed above, vegetables contain numerous colouring and flavouring substances including flavonoids, tannins, isothiocyanates, indoles and phenols. Isothiocyanates are released from cabbage and other vegetables on cutting and are responsible for their pungency. Many of these substances are pharmacologically active so that when large amounts are fed in animal experiments, the metabolism of some chemical carcinogens is increased, and in others blocked (Wattenburg 1985).

Despite uncertainties regarding the active ingredient, a clear picture is emerging from case-control studies showing a protective effect for fruit and vegetables, particularly in stomach and large bowel cancer. Colon cancer patients in studies in the USA, Scandinavia, France, Australia, Belgium, Greece and Singapore have all been found to have reported a lower consumption of vegetables than their matched controls. Decreased vegetable and fruit consumption has also been reported in case-control studies of breast, lung and oesophageal cancer. For these and other reasons (see Section 1.1) vegetable consumption should be doubled.

References

Armstrong B and Doll R (1975) Environmental factors and cancer incidence in different countries with special reference to dietary practices. *Int J Cancer* **15**, 617–31.

Bingham S (1990a) NSP and starch and large bowel cancer. *Proc Nut Soc* **49**, 153–71.

Bingham S (1990b) *Diet and cancer*. Health Education Authority, London.

Department of Health and Human Services (1988) *The Surgeon General's report on nutrition and health*. DHHS Publication No 88–502–10, Washington, DC.

Doll R and Peto R (1981) The causes of cancer; quantitative estimates of avoidable risks of cancer in the United States today. *J Nat Cancer Inst* **66**, 1192–308.

Forman D, Dabbagh SA and Doll R (1985) Nitrates, nitrites and gastric cancer in Great Britain. *Nature* **313**, 620–25.

IARC (1987) *Monographs on the evaluation of carcinogenic risk to humans*:

44. Alcohol drinking. IARC, Lyon, France.

Ip C (1987) Fat and essential fatty acids in mammary carcinogenesis. *Am J Clin Nutr* **45**(Suppl 1), 218–24.

Isles CG, Hole JH, Gillis CR, Hawthorne VM and Lever AF (1990) Plasma cholesterol, CHD and cancer in the Renfrew and Paisley survey. *Br Med J* **298**, 920–24.

Muir C, Waterhouse J, Mack T, Powell J and Whelan F (Eds) (1987) Cancer incidence in five continents, Vol 5. IARC Scientific Publication No 88. IARC, Lyon, France.

National Research Council (1982) *Diet, nutrition and cancer.* National Academic Press, Washington DC.

Thurnham DI (1990) Antioxidant vitamins and cancer prevention. *J Micro Anal* **7**, 279–99.

Wald NJ (1987) β-carotene and cancer. *Cancer Surveys* **6**, 635–52.

Wattenburg LW (1985) Chemo-prevention of cancer. *Cancer Research* **45**, 1–8.

Willett WC (1987) Implications of total energy intake for epidemiologic studies of breast and bowel cancer. *Am J Clin Nutr* **45**(Suppl), 354–60.

Willett WC, Meir J, Stampfer MD and Graham A (1987) Dietary fat and the risk of breast cancer. *N Engl J Med* **316**, 22–8.

Willett WC, Stampfer MD, Colditz GA, Rosner BA & Speizer MD (1990) Meat, fat and fiber and the risk of colon cancer in a prospective study amongst women. *N Engl J Med* **323**, 1664–72.

4.34 Cancer: dietary management

4.34.1 General aspects of dietary management

Nutrition plays an important role in the care of the person with cancer, from diagnosis onwards. Provision of adequate nutrition makes a major contribution toward the clinical, biochemical and psychological status of the cancer patient in the face of the disease process (Shils 1979). Nutritional support may also help to reduce the incidence and severity of undesirable, adverse effects of treatment and so improve outcome (Von-Meyenfeldt *et al* 1988).

A majority of cancer patients will experience eating difficulties and weight loss, to a greater or lesser extent, during their disease or its treatment. Between 3–38% of patients have been reported to show signs of severe malnutrition, and up to 80% may be mildly malnourished (Von-Meyenfeldt *et al* 1988). The presence of malnutrition has been associated with decreased performance status, increased complication rates of cancer treatment and decreased survival (De Wys *et al* 1980; De Wys 1986; Bonadonna *et al* 1986; Muller *et al* 1986). However, some patients do not experience problems with appetite or weight maintenance, or are able to return to normal eating once treatment is complete. The nutritional care of this latter group of patients is also important. Some patients may be tempted to follow one of the 'alternative' or 'complementary' dietary regimens which are often targeted at people with cancer. People who do so may need expert nutritional advice and their nutritional intake and status should be closely monitored.

The nutritional advice and support needed by people with cancer will range, therefore, from general healthy eating, through overcoming eating difficulties to intensive enteral or parenteral nutritional support methods.

Patients without nutritional problems

Some patients will present at diagnosis without any deterioration in their ability to eat or in their nutritional status. The same may apply to some patients receiving treatment or to those whose treatment is completed. These patients should be given general advice to follow a healthy, well-balanced diet in order to maintain optimum nutritional status. They should be advised to seek further help as soon as any eating difficulties arise.

Patients with nutritional problems

Patients may present at diagnosis with nutritional problems or these may develop during the course of their treatment or beyond. Nutritional support for these patients should be instigated as soon as possible. The aim of nutritional support in these patients is to restore them to their optimum nutritional status as soon as possible. Patients with advanced disease need particular care and support and this is discussed in Section 4.36.

4.34.2 Cancer treatments

The various cancer treatment modalities and their nutritional effects are outlined below followed by the suggested dietary advice for the most common of these effects.

Radiotherapy

On average, a course of radiotherapy consists of five treatments per week for six weeks. Nutritional problems may arise depending on the location and size of the treatment field. Radiation to the head and neck area, particularly to the tongue, palate and nasopharynx, causes many nutritional problems. Reactions include a burning sensation to the throat, loss of appetite, taste alterations and soreness of the mouth. Dry mouth is a common problem with patients receiving radiotherapy to the area including the salivary glands. This then causes problems with swallowing due to lack of saliva (see also Section 4.2.2).

Decreased tolerance to foods can result from radiation to the upper abdomen which frequently causes cramping, malabsorption and diarrhoea.

Chemotherapy

The number of drugs used singly or in combination in the treatment of cancer is rapidly increasing. Most regimens involve several drugs given over a period of weeks. Nausea and vomiting are the common side effects affecting the patient's ability to eat. Depending on the dose and duration of treatment, other side effects can occur, such as taste changes (mouth blindness), stomatitis, mucositis, oesophagitis and malabsorption. These effects also severely affect the patient's food intake.

Surgery

As well as the general metabolic effects of surgery (see Section 5.5) patients undergoing surgery for treatment of cancer have further specific nutritional problems:

1 Surgical removal of any tumour may frequently involve removal of considerable amounts of neighbouring tissue to reduce the likelihood of the malignancy spreading. Major surgery to any area of the gastrointestinal tract will lead to problems affecting the patient's ability to eat and possibly lead to malabsorption.

2 Surgical removal of head and neck tumours may involve long term enteral feeding and the possibility of soft and/or liquid feeds permanently.

3 An oesophagectomy, total or partial gastrectomy or colostomy can create its own specific problem (see Sections 4.2.2, 4.3.2, 4.10).

The suggested dietary treatment of common nutritional problems related to cancer and its treatment are summarized in Table 4.105.

4.34.3 Alternative or complementary diets

The terms 'alternative' or 'complementary' diet refer to any modification of a normal diet which claim to cure or treat a disease such as cancer. These dietary therapies may be advocated for use in conjunction with, or instead of, conventional anti-cancer treatments. The severity of the diets, and the range of claims made for them, are varied and often contradictory. This has led them to be received with scepticism by the dietetic and medical professions. Despite this, they have become popular with patients.

Most of these dietary therapies, such as Macrobiotics or the Gerson therapy, share the same common principles. These are:

1 Vegetarian or vegan diet.
2 Large amounts of raw food.
3 Sugar free.
4 Low salt.

These principles often result in diets which contain no

Table 4.105 Nutritional problems related to cancer and its treatment – suggested dietary management

Problem	Cause	Suggested dietary management
Anorexia	Disease state Radiotherapy Chemotherapy	Small attractive nourishing meals Snacks and/or nourishing drinks between meals. Use of energy and protein supplements, e.g. Maxijul/Caloreen, Fortical/Hycal, Maxipro/Casilan. Meals to be eaten slowly in a relaxed manner. Use of appetite stimulants, e.g. alcohol, prednisolone
Severe anorexia	As above	Tube feeding may be necessary
Inability to prepare meals due to tiredness or weakness	Disease state Treatment in general	Make use of store cupboard of convenience foods, tinned soups, tinned fruits and puddings, packet instant desserts, tinned meals, tinned snacks, etc. Arrange meals on wheels, home help it appropriate. Use meal replacements, e.g. Complan, Build Up
Sense of fullness	Disease state Radiotherapy to upper abdominal area	Small frequent meals. Reduction of fatty foods may help Avoidance of drinks with meals (to be taken $\frac{1}{2}$ hour before or after) Use of nourishing drinks, e.g. milk shakes, (fortified if necessary with energy or protein supplements) Build-up, Complan, Ensure, Fortisip, etc.
Nausea	Disease state Radiation to upper gastrointestinal tract Chemotherapy	Small frequent meals Keep patient away from cooking smells if possible. Suggest a short walk before meals to get some fresh air. For early morning nausea try unbuttered toast, cream crackers or plain biscuits Give dry meals with drinks before or after. Reduce very sweet or very greasy foods Try cold foods; these have less smell than cooked foods. Use of fizzy drinks, e.g. ginger ale may help
Severe nausea	As above	As above. Consult doctor regarding appropriate antiemetics
Severe vomiting	As above	Total parenteral nutrition may be necessary
Metallic taste in mouth	Certain types of chemotherapy	Elimination of foods accentuating this taste according to patient's individual tolerance
Loss of taste (mouth blindness)	Certain types of chemotherapy Radiotherapy to mouth and throat	Emphasis on aroma of food. Marinate food to enhance flavour, use stronger seasonings and herbs. Avoid very hot foods, these often taste better at room temperature

Table 4.105 *contd.*

Problem	Cause	Suggested dietary management	
Dry mouth	Radiotherapy to mouth and throat	Frequent drinks. Give ice cubes to suck. Give fruit drops, boiled sweets to suck. Regular mouthwashes. Lemon and glycerine mouth swabs. Avoidance of very dry foods. Artificial saliva — Salivex tablets are available on prescription. Hospital pharmacy may produce its own artificial saliva. Spray saliva, Glandosane (Fresenius), is also available	
Sore mouth/throat (stomatitis, mucositis)	Certain types of chemotherapy Radiation to mouth and throat	Soft, moist foods. Use nourishing drinks. Avoidance of very salty or spicy foods. Cold foods are often soothing. Avoidance of very hot foods — allow to cool a little. Give drinks through a straw if necessary. Avoidance of rough or very dry foods	
General difficulties with chewing and swallowing	Radiotherapy to mouth and throat Oral surgery Oesophageal carcinoma, Insertion of palliative oesophageal tubes	Soft, semi-solid or liquid diet. Small frequent meals. Use of nourishing drinks. Use of fizzy drinks to clear oesophageal tubes	
Severe difficulties in chewing and swallowing	As above	Tube feeding	
Intestinal cramping, abdominal pain	Radiotherapy to lower abdomen Certain types of chemotherapy	Try low fibre diet	
Diarrhoea	As above	Low fibre diet with high fluid intake	
Severe diarrhoea	As above	Use of antidiarrhoeal agents	
Intermittent constipation	Certain types of chemotherapy	High fibre, diet, plenty of fluids	
Severe constipation	As above	Possible use of laxatives	
Malabsorption	Radiotherapy to lower gastrointestinal tract Surgery to gastrointestinal tract	Low fat diet Low fibre diet Lactose-free diet Enteral feeds e.g. Ensure, Isocal, etc. Total parenteral nutrition	As appropriate for the type of malabsorption problem

animal or dairy products, little protein, a low energy value and high bulk. These therapies may also recommend the use of megadose vitamin and mineral supplements and other unusual treatments such as the use of coffee enemas and pancreatic enzymes.

The dietary constraints imposed can cause many problems for cancer patients, especially those already experiencing nutritional difficulties. These problems include difficulty in food preparation, low palatability, high cost and weight loss and deterioration in nutritional status. The harm that can, and does, result from these regimens far outweighs any physical benefit (Hunter 1988). However, these dietary therapies do seem to help a small number of cancer patients. The reason for this is unclear but is likely to be associated with the psychological support offered by these diets and the other holistic therapies often associated with them, such as visualization, relaxation etc. By following such a therapy the patients feel that they are doing something positive for themselves and thereby have some control over their disease and its treatment (Hunter 1991).

In view of the serious potential nutritional problems these diets inflict, they cannot be openly recommended for cancer patients. The psychological role of these diets, however, must not be underestimated. Patients following, or seeking to follow such, need careful dietary counselling. The advantages and disadvantages of the diets must be discussed fully and openly with the patient. It may be possible to integrate some aspects of the diet that interests them into an individual well balanced nutritional programme. The patient may decide to remain strictly on a particular diet despite it being of poor nutritional value. This choice must be made by the patient, though it is the responsibility of the dietitian to ensure that it is an informed one.

All patients following any alternative dietary therapy

should have their nutritional intake and status monitored on a regular basis together with careful dietary counselling to ensure that they maintain their optimum nutritional status and quality of life.

Useful addresses

BACUP (British Association for Cancer United Patients and their families and friends), 121/123 Charterhouse Street, London EC1M 6AA. Cancer Information Service 071–608 1661.
This registered charity provides advice and information on all aspects of cancer as well as emotional support for cancer patients and their families. Several useful booklets are available.

Cancer Relief Macmillan Fund, Anchor House, 15/19 Britten Street, London SW3 3TZ. Tel 071–351 7811.
Provides Macmillan Home Care Nurses, and continuing day care and specialist inpatient facilities. Financial grants are also available for cancer patients and their families.

The Ulster Cancer Foundation, 40–42 Eglantine Avenue, Belfast BT9 6DX. Tel 0232 663281.
Provides information over the phone about all aspects of cancer.

Tak Tent, 132 Hill Street, Glasgow. Tel 041–332 3639.
Provides training courses for people setting up self-help groups; produces written material.

Tenovus Cancer Information Centre, 11 Whitchurch Road, Cardiff CF3 3JN. Tel 0222 619846.
Provides a counselling and information service personally or over the telephone.

Cancer Link, 46 Pentonville Road, London N1. Tel 071–833 2451.
Resource centre for cancer self-help and support groups throughout Britain and a telephone information service on all aspects of cancer.

Further reading

Aihara H (1985) *Basic macrobiotics*. Japan Publications Inc, Tokyo.

De Wys WD and Hillenbrand HS (1977) Oral feeding in the nutritional management of the cancer patient. *Cancer Research* **37**, 2429–31.

Dornan V (1985) Diet in Terminal illness. *Nursing Mirror* **160**(8), 39–41.

Gerson M (1977) *A cancer therapy – results of 50 cases*. Totality Books, California.

Hill GL (Ed) (1981) *Nutrition and the surgical patient*. Churchill Livingstone, Edinburgh.

Kushi M (1984) *The cancer prevention diet*. Thorsons, Wellingborough.

Kushi M (1985) *The macrobiotic way*. Avery, New Jersey.

Royal Marsden Hospital (1989) *Overcoming eating difficulties – a guide for cancer patients*. Patient Information Series No 9. Royal Marsden Hospital, London.

Shaw C and Hunter M (1991) *Special diet cookbook: cancer*. Thorsons, London.

Soukop M and Calman KC (1977) Nutrition support in patients with malignant disease. Nutrition and cancer 5. *J Hum Nutr* **33**, 179–88.

Tiffany R (Ed) (1988) *Oncology for nurses and health care professionals*. Vols I and II. Harper & Row, London.

Tresillian M (1971) *Does diet cure cancer?* Thorsons, Wellingborough.

References

Bonadonna G, Valagussa P and Santoro A (1986) Alternating non-cross-resistant combination chemotherapy or MOPP in stage IV Hodgkin's disease: a report of 8-year results. *Annals of Internal Medicine* **104**, 739–46.

De Wys WD, Begg C, Lavin PT *et al* (1980) Prognostic effect of weight loss prior to chemotherapy in cancer patients. *American Journal of Medicine* **69**, 491–7.

De Wys WD (1986) Weight loss and nutritional abnormalities in cancer patients: incidence, severity and significance. *Clinics in Oncology* **5**, 251–61.

Hunter M (1988) Unproven dietary methods of treatment in oncology patients. In *Supportive care in cancer patients II. Recent results in cancer research*, Vol 108, Senn HJ, Glaus A and Schmid L (Eds) pp. 235–8. Springer-Verlag, Berlin.

Hunter M (1991) Alternative dietary therapies in cancer patients. In *Supportive care in cancer patients II. Recent results in cancer research*, Vol 121, Senn HJ and Glaus A (Eds) pp. 293–5. Springer-Verlag, Berlin.

Muller JM, Keller HW, Brenner U, Walter M and Holzmuller W (1986) Indications and effects of preoperative parenteral nutrition. *World Journal of Surgery* **10**, 53–63.

Shils ME (1979) Principles of nutritional therapy. *Cancer* **43**, 2093–2102.

Von-Meyenfeldt MF, Fredrix EWHM, Haagh WAJJM, Van Der Aalst ACMJ and Soeters PB (1988) The aetiology and management of weight loss and malnutrition in cancer patients. *Baillière's Clinical Gastroenterology*, Vol 2, Part 4, pp. 869–85.

4.35 Diets for immunosuppressed patients

Patients who have had their natural immunity to infection reduced by chemotherapy or radiation therapy may be at risk of microbiological contamination from the food eaten.

However, it is important to clarify that only those with *no* functioning bone marrow (i.e. bone marrow transplant patients) require 'sterile' or 'very clean' food. Other organ transplant patients and those undergoing chemotherapy or radiotherapy for other disease states (e.g. leukaemia) do not require such a strict regimen although it is prudent for there to be a high standard of food hygiene.

Many foods which we eat contain small and usually insignificant numbers of micro-organisms, but for patients who are immunocompromised, even minute amounts of these micro-organisms could prove to be harmful. It is therefore necessary to minimize microbiological contamination in the diet.

Other precautions which may be taken are the use of Laminar Air Flow (LAF) cubicles and administration of oral non-absorbable antibiotics. Use of food with a low microbe content and oral non-absorbable antibiotics can together achieve acceptable gut sterilization of patients in LAF environments. This has not been tested without LAF, and use of oral non-absorbable antibiotics without sterile or very clean food may not be adequate because of the possible development of resistant micro-organisms (Driedger and Burstall 1987).

Surveys of food preparation and service to bone marrow patients, both in this country and in the USA, reveal little or no uniformity (Aker and Cheney 1983; Beckles-Willson, personal communication). Each unit has developed its own protocol for oral feeding often based on custom and practice, individual judgement and local facilities. Despite the importance of nutrition for these patients, there has been little study to determine the safest food service procedures and much more research is needed (Dezenhall *et al* 1987). This section describes the procedures adopted in one of the leading UK centres for bone marrow transplantation.

4.35.1 General nutritional aspects of diets for immunosuppressed patients

Oral feeding of patients who are so ill is a difficult challenge. In many, enteral feeding (whether oral or nasogastric) is not viable for at least part of the treatment period, and TPN is essential. As the patient improves, oral feeding is gradually resumed; the goal of all those involved should be to encourage and assist the patient's oral intake so that the need for TPN is kept to a minimum.

Factors which should be considered in order to improve appetite are:

1 Palatability: there may be altered taste perception, increased sensitivity to the smell of food, nausea, vomiting and anorexia.

2 Texture: chewing and swallowing may be difficult because of mucositis, oesophagitis. Dysgeusia (loss of or change in taste perception) may also be a temporary side-effect of total body irradiation and some drugs.

3 Individual food preference, ethnic or religious requirements.

General nutritional factors to be considered include:

1 The psychological importance of food in an isolated, controlled environment.

2 Increased nutritional requirements, because of the effects of treatment on the metabolism of certain nutrients.

3 Dietary manipulation to treat organ dysfunction e.g. drug side effects on cardiopulmonary, hepatic and renal function.

4 The contribution of potentially pathogenic organisms from food e.g. *Klebsiella* and *Pseudomonas* (Pizzo *et al* 1982).

5 Graft-versus-host disease (GVHD) of the gastrointestinal tract leading to temporary lactose and/or gluten intolerance, with resultant diarrhoea or steatorrhoea and malabsorption (in the bone marrow transplant patient) (Gauvreau *et al* 1981). GVHD occurs when immunologically competent cells from the donor marrow recognize the host tissues as 'foreign' and mount an attack against them. This is most likely to occur in the first three months post-transplant and may be acute (usually affecting skin, liver or the gastrointestinal tract) or chronic (when it is insidious and may attack additional organs). GVHD reduces immunological capability and increases susceptibility to infection.

4.35.2 Dietary regimens for immunosuppressed patients

Diets for immunosuppressed patients can be divided into four types according to their degree of sterility:

1 Sterile Food Regimen.

2 Very Clean Food ('Low Microbe') Regimen.

3 Clean Food Regimen/modified ward diet.

4 Post-hospitalization Clean Food Regimen.

Foods suitable for each of these regimens are summarized in Table 4.106.

Table 4.106 Suitable food sources for immunosuppressed patients

* Food	'Sterile' food	Very Clean Food As 'sterile' plus the following:	Clean Food modified ward diet As 'Very Clean Food' plus the following:	Home As 'modified ward diet' plus the following:
Water	Boiled, bottled sterile, canned mineral water			Run tap for 2 minutes after any period without use (e.g. every morning)
Milk + Cream	Sterilized or UHT, refrigerated once opened and used within 24 hours. Tinned evaporated/ condensed milk. Tinned cream			Fresh, pasteurized milk daily
Drinks	Coffee — individual sachets Tea — gamma irradiated Teabags (using boiling water) Canned/bottled fizzy drinks Fortical/Hycal (useful if fluid restricted)	Fruit juice — small tetra-packs Fruit squash — use within 72 hours	Coffee and tea, freshly made. Fruit juice	Fruit juice from carton — freshly opened every 24 hours
Tube feeds supplements	Commercially-prepared where possible, rather than 'home-made' tube feeds			
Butter margarine	Individual portions Keep refrigerated		Own supply in cubicle Use well within 'sell by' date	
Bread	Gamma irradiated Served toasted	Not irradiated, but toasted to kill surface yeasts. Use wrapped loaf. On opening, portion (2 slices), package and date for freezing. Use within 2 weeks. Serve toasted only. Chapatis and pitta bread can be treated similarly	Fresh bread, used within 24 hours. (or freeze to extend shelf life)	Fresh daily
Eggs	Unsuitable	Cooked until yolk and white set. Or use pasteurized egg	Only suitable if cooked until yolk and white set	
Main meals	Canned meat/fish/veg/fruit/ puddings	Frozen meals from reputable manufacturers	Served immediately from ward trolley/kitchen	Freshly cooked, home-made foods avoiding reheated foods
Cheese	Unsuitable	Acceptable only when well-cooked or as cheese-spread 'triangles'		Vacuum-wrapped hard cheese and processed cheeses. NOT Brie or blue cheese types
Vegetables	Canned	Frozen	Fresh and frozen, served hot, straight from trolley/kitchen	
Fruit	Canned	Frozen; cooked by a suitable method	Peeled fruit	
Dried foodstuffs	Breakfast cereals, biscuits, sugar are gamma irradiated then individual packets opened and served on cubicles	Individual packs, where possible. Dried milk puddings, cornflour, custard, packet soup, rice and pasta, should be well-cooked, preferably in a pressure cooker or individual steamer	Large packets can be used and contents discarded after 5 days	Used within 'sell-by' date
Cake	Gamma irradiated	Doubled-wrapped and well within 'sell-by' date from good manufacturer, or freshly baked, covered cooked and eaten within 24 hours		

Table 4.106 *contd.*

* Food	'Sterile' food	Very Clean Food As 'sterile' plus the following:	Clean Food modified ward diet As 'Very Clean Food' plus the following:	Home As 'modified ward diet' plus the following:
Sweets, chocolates and crisps	Gamma irradiated	Doubled-wrapped, well within the 'sell-by' date from a reputable manufacturer		
Infant feeding	Ready-to-feed formulae. Proprietary jars and cans of baby foods	Make up using sterile equipment in very clean environment	Dried baby foods may be opened in the cubicle and made up with boiling water or milk	
Salt	Individual sachets, gamma irradiated	Individual sachets, not gamma irradiated		Family salt pot
Pepper and other spices	Gamma irradiated as they contain many fungal spores not otherwise destroyed by cooking temperatures			In cooked dishes only

* Once opened, all items should be refrigerated and used within 24 hours unless otherwise stated

Sterile food regimen

Complete sterilization of food is difficult, expensive and results in an extremely limited and unpalatable diet. It can be achieved by canning, prolonged oven-baking, autoclaving or gamma-irradiation. Obviously it requires special kitchen facilities and is labour-intensive (Aker and Cheney 1983). Flavour, texture, colour and acceptability of the food are all affected.

Some specialist units prepare 'commercially sterile' foods. This means that the food is not totally sterile but that it has an extremely low level of contamination. This level of 'sterility' is achieved by using gamma-irradiated and canned foods only. In some units the food is prepared in a Laminar Air-Flow cabinet. Canned foods, for example, are opened and warmed in the cabinet, then placed in special foil-closed containers, double-wrapped in sterile paper bags and taken straight to the patients. Increasingly, units are finding that this level of 'sterility' confers no practical advantage in terms of the incidence of food-related infection and a Very Clean Food regimen is becoming more common.

Very clean regimen or 'low microbe diet'

This may be a more practical alternative. It aims to provide a nutritionally adequate, palatable diet comprised of foods which are either well-cooked or have a minimum number of potential pathogen-forming units and which therefore minimize the risk to the patient (Pizzo *et al* 1982).

Ideally, food preparation and service should be carried out in a kitchen within the ward or unit where patients are treated. This has several advantages (Gauvreau-Stern *et al* 1989):

1 An 'a la carte' restaurant service without fixed meal times can be provided and this encourages more frequent food and drink consumption by the patient.

2 Food intake is more easily monitored.

3 Food preparation is more easily controlled and hence there is less risk of food contamination.

4 It promotes better communication between patients, families, cooks, dietitian, medical and nursing staff. The role of the cook is extended as a result of close interaction with patients and their families, particularly when there are ethnic preferences or requirements.

Suitable foods for a Very Clean Food regimen

These are summarized in Table 4.106. General points to remember are:

1 Raw foods must not be served.

2 Frozen foods should be obtained from a supplier who will deliver from the source of manufacture with minimum delay so that foods have a long 'use-by' date. There must be no risk of rise in temperature during storage and transport. Frozen entrées should be single portion servings from a reputable manufacturer.

3 Hot foods must be served hot; they may be kept hot for a maximum of 15 minutes before service. After this they must be discarded.

4 All foods and drinks should be eaten or drunk within half an hour of service. Anything not consumed within this time must be discarded.

5 Because of the above constraints on temperature and holding time, foods prepared in the home by the families of bone marrow transplant patients are unsuitable. Families wishing to bring additional foods from outside as 'treats' must first discuss their suitability with the dietitian. Generally, items must:

- Be a reputable brand;

- Be double-wrapped (e.g. bags of 'fun-size' Mars, Smarties etc., or multi-packs of crisps containing a number of individual bags);
- Be bought from a shop with fast turnover and good storage facilities;
- Have a long 'use-by' date.

Cooking methods for a Very Clean Food regimen

Suitable cooking methods The following equipment is suitable:

1 Conventional cooker, either gas or electric.
2 Pressure cooker or hospital/industrial steamer.

Conventional gas or electric cooker: oven cooking This method of cooking may be used but certain precautions should be taken. The oven should always be pre-heated to minimize the time when the food will be 'warm'. The aim is to ensure that the heat has thoroughly penetrated the food; minimum acceptable core temperature of the food is 70°C. The core temperature of the food can be checked using a thermometer with a probe on a *duplicate* food sample; the probe must not be used on the foods to be eaten by the patient.

Boiling on the hob Food should always be put into rapidly boiling water, and brought back to boiling point as soon as possible. Once again the minimum acceptable core temperature of the food is 70°C and can be checked (on duplicate food samples) with a probe thermometer.

Some examples of appropriate cooking times using either a conventional oven or hob are given in Table 4.107.

Pressure cooking/steaming Pressure cooking is an excellent way of preparing meals for the immunosuppressed patient and is the method of choice in many hospitals. A domestic-sized pressure cooker or large scale catering steamer may be used. It may then be possible for the patient to choose main meals from the general hospital menu and for these meals to be cooked under pressure. Case must be taken in transporting meals to the patient because, once the food has been cooked, any subsequent contamination could put the immunosuppressed paticnt at risk. Food must be thoroughly cooked, plated and covered immediately, kept hot (above 70°C) and served to the patient with the minimum delay. The cover must not be removed until the food is served to the patient.

Unsuitable cooking methods The following methods should NOT be used for the preparation of Very Clean food:

1 Microwave ovens.
2 Cook-chill systems.

Table 4.107 Cooking food for immunosuppressed patients — some examples

Food	Method of cooking	Cooking temperature	Cooking time	Core temperature of food after cooking
Lamb chops	Oven	200°C	35 min	80°C
Faggots in gravy	Oven	230°C	40 min	92°C
Fish fingers	Oven	200°C	10 min	90°C
Fish cakes	Oven	200°C	15 min	88°C
Minced beef/ onion pie	Oven	220°C	35 min	99°C
Sausages	Oven	220°C	20 min	97°C
Oven chips	Oven	200°C	10 min	82°C
Chicken portion	Oven	200°C	25 min	87°C
Cod in batter	Oven	200°C	15 min	64°C
Chicken and mushroom casserole	Boil in the bag		15 min from water reboiling	90°C
Cod in parsley sauce	Boil in the bag		20 min from water reboiling	85°C
Roast beef in gravy	Boil in the bag		15 min from water reboiling	76°C

Microwave ovens Although convenient, these may not be as efficient at killing micro-organisms as a conventional cooking method. The rapid rise in temperature in food cooked in a microwave oven does not kill bacteria as efficiently as a conventional oven with its high temperature over a longer period (Fruin and Gutherz 1982). Much depends on the size and power of the oven, volume of the food (its uniformity of shape and thickness), the nature of the food (water, fat and ion content) (Dealler and Lacey 1990) and observation of the oven manufacturers' recommendations on 'standing times' after cooking. The use of microwave ovens has become accepted practice in many units but because there are so many variables, it is best to avoid their use except for heating 'sterile' canned or frozen foods. They should not be used to cook food in its raw state.

Cook-chill systems Methods of cooking, chilling, storage and re-heating involve unsuitable temperatures, an unacceptable amount of food handling and consequently, too many opportunities for contamination to make this a safe system for use for patients with no natural immunity.

Preparation and service of food for a Very Clean Food regimen

Where possible, premises should have a 'Very Clean kitchen' for the cooking and serving of food and a separate ward kitchen for disposal of all waste and washing of utensils prior to autoclaving.

All preparation of raw food should also take place in the ward kitchen; raw food must not go into the 'Very Clean kitchen' unless in a closed, sealed pressure cooker. Furthermore, the outside of the pressure cooker must be wiped with 'Alcowipes' before it is taken into the 'Very Clean kitchen' and the lid of the pressure cooker must not be removed until the food has been cooked.

Carefully defined procedures should be followed when preparing and serving food. These include:

1 Food should be prepared for only one patient at a time.

2 Hands must be washed with 'Hibiscrub' or equivalent.

3 Rubber gloves, hat, mask and apron (all disposable) must be worn and changed before preparing food for another patient.

4 All working surfaces, the outsides of all tins and packets, serving trays, plates, covers, saucepans etc. should be cleaned with 'Alcowipes', 'Hibiscrub' or 'Dispray'.

5 Disposable crockery and cutlery (in sealed packets) or cutlery which has been autoclaved should be used for food service.

6 All food to be served should be covered immediately it is cooked and portioned, before leaving the kitchen.

7 All waste and used cutlery etc. must be taken to the ward kitchen and not returned to the 'Very Clean kitchen'.

8 Cooking utensils (such as saucepans) must be washed thoroughly and autoclaved before being used again.

9 The cooker, work surfaces and floor must be thoroughly cleaned at the end of each period of food preparation.

10 There should be a list of daily, weekly and monthly duties for cooks. This should include cleaning, ordering and rotation of stock and discarding of all food which has exceeded its expiry date for a Very Clean Food regimen. These foods should be used on other wards or in the main catering department.

Shelf life of processed foods

Canned foods can be stored for a very long time (Table 4.108). Even after the times suggested, the food should be microbiologically safe for immunosuppressed patients but there may be a slight change in colour, texture or flavour.

Stored cans should be marked with the date they are received and used in rotation. They should always be stored in a cool, dry place. All dried, frozen foods should be used well within the manufacturers' 'use by' date.

The recommended storage life of some types of canned foods are given in Table 4.108.

Table 4.108 Recommended storage times of canned foods for use by immunosuppressed patients

Canned food item	Recommended storage time
Milk products e.g. Cream, Evaporated milk, Milk puddings	1 year
Rhubarb	9 months
Fruit juice	1 year
Prunes	1 year
Blackberries, blackcurrants, gooseberries, raspberries, and strawberries	18 months
Other fruits	2 years
Vegetables (except new potatoes)	2 years
New potatoes	18 months
Baked beans	2 years
Pasta products e.g. canned macaroni	2 years
Soups	2 years
Fruit sauce	2 years
Solid pack, cold meat products, e.g. ham, corned beef	5 years
Fish in oil	5 years

Clean Food regimen/modified ward diet

The provision of Very Clean Food regimen is possible only on those units with appropriate facilities. Where a patient is treated in a cubicle on an ordinary ward, it is possible to provide a Clean Food regimen using a modified ward diet. Suitable foods are listed in Table 4.106. Microwave ovens must not be used to heat/re-heat food items (see Microwave ovens above).

The following points should also be observed:

1 Hot food must be served hot (over 70°C). Food must be plated, served and eaten immediately after cooking.

2 Disposable or plastic cutlery should be used and kept in Milton solution within the patient's cubicle.

3 Food should be transferred to disposable plates or to crockery kept in Milton solution in the patient's cubicle, and served on a tray kept inside the cubicle.

4 Utensils used on the ward to produce snacks and drinks should be washed *before* as well as after use.

Post-hospitalization Clean Food regimen

When the previously immunosuppressed patient's white cell count has increased to a level where he or she can come out of isolation, usually a neutrophil count of 1×10^9/l (normal range $2.5-5 \times 10^9$/l), a more relaxed diet can be followed.

For at least three months following discharge from

hospital, the following precautionary measures should be taken:

1 Food should be served immediately it is cooked.

2 Food should not be kept or re-heated.

3 A microwave oven should not be used for cooking or re-heating.

4 The 'use-by' date on all foods should be checked and packets or cans which are damaged or dented should be avoided.

5 All foods should be purchased from a reputable source with a fast turnover and good storage facilities. Unpackaged 'loose' foods should not be used other than meat, fruit and vegetables which are to be cooked.

6 No take away food or meals eaten outside the home should be consumed for at least three months. After this time, any such food must be freshly cooked and served hot; not kept hot and served from a heated display cabinet. No cold foods should be eaten.

Further reading

Aker SN and Lenssen P (1988) *A guide to good nutrition during and after chemotherapy and radiation*. Fred Hutchinson Cancer Research Center, Seattle.

Baldwin RE (1983) Microwave cooking: an overview. *J Food Protection* **46**(3), 266–9.

Crespo FL *et al* (1977) Effect of conventional microwave heating on *Pseudomonas putrefaciens*, *Streptococcus faecalis* and *Lactobacillus plantorum* in meat tissue. *J Food Protection* **40**(9), 588–91.

Cunningham FE (1980) Influence of microwave radiation on psychotrophic bacteria. *J Food Protection* **43**(8), 651–5.

Dahl CA *et al* (1980) Fate of *Staphylococcus aureus* in beef loaf, potatoes and frozen and canned green beans after microwave heating in a simulated cook/chill hospital food service system. *J Food Protection* **43**(12), 916–23.

Dreyfuss MS and Chipley JR (1980) Comparison of effects of sublethal microwave radiation and conventional heating on the metabolic activity of Staphylococcus aureus. *Appl Environ Microbiol* **39**(1), 13–6.

Good RA (1986) Bone marrow transplantation. In *Fundamentals of immunology and allergy*, Lockey R and Bukantz S (Eds) WB Saunders, New York.

Lenssen P and Aker SN (Eds) (1985) *Nutritional assessment and management during marrow transplantation – a resource manual*. Fred Hutchinson Cancer Research Center, Washington.

Page W and Martin WG (1978) Survival of microbial films in the microwave oven. *Can J Microbiol* **24**(11), 1431–3.

Szeluga DJ, Stuart RK, Brookmeyer R, Utermohlen V and Santos GW (1987) Nutritional support of bone marrow transplant recipients: a prospective, randomized clinical trial comparing total parenteral nutrition to an enteral feeding programme. *Cancer Res* **47**, 3309.

Vela CR and Wu JF (1979) Mechanism of lethal action of 2450 MHz radiation on micro-organisms. *Appl Environ Microbiol* **37**(3), 550–3.

References

Aker SN and Cheney CL (1983) The use of sterile and low microbial diets in ultra-isolation environments. *JPEN* **7**, 390.

Dealler SF and Lacey RW (1990) Superficial microwave heating. (Letter) *Nature* **344**, 496.

Dezenhall A, Curry-Bartley K, Blackburn SA, De Lamerens S and Khan AR (1987) Food and nutrition services in bone marrow transplantation centers. *J Am Dietet Assoc* **87**(10), 1351–3.

Driedger L and Burstall CD (1987) Bone marrow transplantation: dietitians' experience and perspective. *J Am Dietet Assoc* **87**(10), 1387–8.

Fruin J and Guthertz L (1982) Survival of bacteria in food cooked by microwave oven, conventional oven and slow cookers. *J Food Protection* **45**(8), 695–8.

Gauvreau JM, Lenssen P, Cheney CL, Aker SN, Hutchinson ML and Barale KV (1981) Nutritional management of patients with intestinal graft-versus-host disease. *J Am Dietet Assoc* **79**, 673.

Gauvreau-Stern JM, Cheney CL, Aker SN and Lenssen P (1989) Food intake patterns and food-service requirements on a marrow transplant unit. *J Am Dietet Assoc* **89**(3), 367–72.

Pizzo PA, Purvis DS and Waters C (1982) Microbiological evaluation of food items. *J Am Dietet Assoc* **81**, 272.

4.36 Care of the terminally ill

Terminal care is defined as the management of a patient for whom the event of death does not seem far off, and for whom care has turned from curative to palliative. Nutrition in terminal care is concerned with helping to maximize the quality of life of an individual. The patient should be encouraged and enabled to be in control of his or her own food intake for as long as possible. This involves the skills of careful listening, discussion, then providing nourishment in the most appropriate form.

4.36.1 Hospices

Hospices or palliative care units provide support and specialist care to patients with terminal cancer. Some also accept people with motor neurone disease and other disorders. New hospices have been opened to care for AIDS patients (see Section 4.32).

Palliative medicine has been recognized as a speciality by the Royal College of Physicians. Effective palliation is multidisciplinary and ranges from inpatient assessment and relief of symptoms to the training and support of district nurses who visit the patient at home.

Care teams require to recognize the needs of the patients' families and carers as well (Higginson *et al* 1990). The giving and receiving of food can reflect love and affection, so rejection of carefully prepared meals can induce strong feelings of hurt. Carers often put undue emphasis on food intake which can lead to anxiety on both sides.

4.36.2 Symptoms affecting food intake

Pain

Food intake can rarely be satisfactory in the presence of pain. Combination therapies for pain relief can often be arranged in relation to timing of meals.

Dry mouth

This can be caused by a diminished secretion of saliva due to oral cancer and its treatment. Diuretics, antispasmodics and some other drugs may also have this effect. Mouth breathing leads to excessive evaporation of fluid. Poor fluid intake which causes dehydration also has to be considered (Regnard and Fitton 1989).

When dehydration is the primary problem, frequent and regular offering of preferred fluids in easily handled containers is required. The enthusiastic provision of sip feeds such as Complan or Build-up can lead to hyperosmolar dehydration if only small quantities of clear fluids are taken as well.

Once the causes of dry mouth have been established, treatment will include frequent mouth care. Glycerine-based mouthwashes moisten a dry mouth and artificial saliva may prove useful. Dietary assistance can include provision of strongly flavoured sweets such as peppermints and fruit-flavoured boiled sweets which may give temporary relief. Small portions of sorbets or crushed ice flavoured with fruit juices or flavoured syrups can also ease discomfort.

Painful mouth or throat

This can be due to candidiasis, aphthous ulcers, side effects of drug therapy, palliative radiotherapy or prolonged malnutrition leading to stomatitis.

Until relief is obtained by appropriate treatment, all acidic foods and drinks must be avoided as they can cause acute pain. These include citrus fruit and fruit juices, most cola and flavoured fizzy drinks, tomato soups and pickles. Non-carbonated apple and pear juices are usually well tolerated, particularly if taken through a wide bore flexi-straw. Salty or spicy foods and curries are also likely to cause discomfort. The texture of foods provided may need to be soft or even liquidized for a time. Cool foods and drinks are tolerated better than hot or very cold ones (Regnard 1990).

Dysphagia and its treatment are discussed in Section 4.2.2.

Altered taste acuity

Around half of all patients with cancer experience a change in their sensation of taste. This can present as a dislike of the brand of tea on offer, and may lead to considerable distress. The causes are unclear but is thought to be associated with the state of catabolism. There is usually a low threshold for bitterness while the sensation of sweetness can be increased or decreased. Red meats – particularly if hot and aromatic – can be especially distasteful, whereas cold ham, chicken, eggs and dairy products are normally well tolerated. If the mouth is not painful then highly flavoured foods such as kippers and strong cheese can be appreciated, while pickles or sauces make cold foods and sandwiches more tasty. Lemon tea usually tastes more refreshing than tea with milk. Regular mouth care is particularly important and there will usually be a local mouth care policy for nursing staff to implement.

Constipation

This is often a major unrecognized problem and is the most common cause of abdominal pain, nausea and vomiting in advanced malignancy.

Difficulty in passing infrequent bowel movements can have many causes. These include dehydration, a reduced volume of food intake, inactivity, weak musculature and an inability to reach the toilet at the time of the urge to defaecate. Constipation is a known side effect of opiate drugs which are usually prescribed along with a stool softener.

Relief of constipation by medical means should be followed by prevention of its recurrence. This will usually involve a combination of drug treatment, bulk softeners and colonic stimulation. An adequate fluid intake is the most important dietary measure. If some of this can include citrus juices for their laxative effect so much the better. Soups containing peas, lentils or other pulses can also help as long as they do not cause flatulence. Porridge is often appreciated as a meal at any time of the day. Unprocessed bran should not be used unless a good fluid intake is established, otherwise this can worsen the constipation and lead to impaction.

Diarrhoea

This can have many causes in terminal cancer (Regnard and Mannix 1990) and treatment will be based on the underlying pathology. When this is related to malabsorption of lipids, appropriate dietary supplements may be required (see Section 1.13.3 and Appendix 6). Radiotherapy of the lower gastrointestinal tract can lead to lactase deficiency so a reduction or exclusion of milk can be helpful (see Section 2.14.4). Manipulation of the dietary fibre content may be beneficial in some instances.

4.36.3 Alleviating poor food intake

General aspects

All the symptoms previously referred to will adversely affect enjoyment of food and thus its intake. There are many other reasons for lack of interest in food which can be identified and improved as well. Control of unpleasant odours can be particularly important. Fatigue can lessen intake, so care should be taken to ensure that the patient has plenty of rest. Small portions presented on tea plates are more appetizing than large helpings. These can be supplemented by a variety of snacks and drinks between mealtimes. A feeling of fullness can be reduced if fluids are taken after, rather than with, meals.

Pre-packed foods such as individual marmalade portions can be difficult to open, so assistance should be given.

Anxiety is understandable and can be lessened by discussion and counselling. The use of alcohol as an appetite stimulant can be considered.

Provision of fluid and food should be discussed with carers, so that they become aware of the factors limiting and enabling intake. Most require reassurance that the patient's diminished intake is no reflection on their ability or care.

Tube feeding

This is normally not indicated in terminal care. It can provide a means of prolonging life when there is an obstruction of the upper gastrointestinal tract.

Tube feeding can be managed at home (Taylor *et al* 1989). The nasogastric route may be used and lightweight tubes are available which will last for several weeks (see Section 1.13.4).

Gastrostomy or jejunostomy feeding is less distressing for both patient and carers and may be considered when the risks associated with this minor surgical procedure are acceptable.

Supplementary oral feeding

Several ready-to-use proprietary products are available for patients with cancer-related cachexia. These can be found in the borderline substances section of the Monthly Index of Medical Specialities (MIMS). Some products are available in savoury flavours, as are Complan and Build-up which are available from retail chemists.

4.36.4 Role of the dietitian in the care of the terminally ill

Palliative care involves a number of disciplines. The dietitian can be most effective as a source of information on nutrition and dietetics, a teacher of staff in hospital and community and a provider of appropriate literature.

Working liaison should be established with all members of the palliative care team who include medical staff, hospice/ward nurses, liaison sisters, Macmillan nurses, nurse tutors, occupational therapists and physiotherapists, speech and language therapists, social workers and day care staff.

Good food provision depends on sound working relationships between the caterer and ward sister/nursing officer, both of whom should have ready access to the dietitian. Good quality crockery in small sizes, double handed soup bowls or mugs, dishes which keep liquidized meals at a suitable temperature, all help to maintain standards consistent with good household practice. Ward/hospice liquidizers and microwave ovens allow for flexibility of texture, temperature and timing of meals and drinks. Clear guidelines for their use should conform to environmental health standards (DHSS 1986). Dietary care (as opposed to treatment) can do much to maintain the morale of the terminally ill person and his or her carers.

Useful addresses

BACUP (British Association for Cancer United Patients and their families and friends), 121/123 Charterhouse Street, London EC1M 6AA. Cancer Information Service 071–608 1661.
This registered charity provides advice and information on all aspects of cancer as well as emotional support for cancer patients and their families. Several useful booklets are available.

Cancer Relief Macmillan Fund, Anchor House, 15/19 Britten Street, London SW3 3TZ. Tel 071–351 7811.
Provides Macmillan Home Care Nurses, and continuing day care and specialist in-patient facilities. Financial grants are also available for cancer patients and their families.

Details of other support organizations can be found in the sections on Cancer (4.34) and AIDS/HIV (4.32).

Further reading

Saunders C (1990) *Hospice and palliative care – an interdisciplinary approach*. Edward Arnold, Sevenoaks.

Lewis M (1989) *Tears and smiles – the hospice handbook*. Michael O'Mara Books.

Scott M and Findlay IG (1984) *Care of the dying: a clinical handbook*. Churchill Livingstone, Edinburgh.

Waine C (Ed) (1989) *Terminal care*. Royal College of General Practitioners, London.

Twycross, RG and Lack S (1990) *Therapeutics in terminal cancer*. Churchill Livingstone, Edinburgh.

References

DHSS (1986) *Health service catering hygiene*. HMSO, London.

Higginson I, Wade A and McCarthy M (1990) *Palliative care: views of patients and their families*. *Br Med J* **301**, 227–81.

Regnard C and Fitton S (1989) Mouth care: a flow diagram. *Palliative Medicine* 3, 67–9.

Regnard C (1990) Managing dysphagia in advanced cancer: a flow diagram. *Palliative Medicine* 4, 215–18.

Regnard C and Mannix K (1990) The control of diarrhoea in advanced cancer: a flow diagram. *Palliative Medicine* 4, 139–42.

Taylor M, Moran BJ and Jackson A (1989) Nutritional problems and care of patients with far-advanced disease. *Palliative Medicine* 3, 31–8.

Section 5 **Dietetic management of acute trauma**

5.1 Metabolic consequences of injury

5.1.1 Differences between the effects of starvation and injury

Starvation

Starvation, particularly for long periods, should not occur under medical supervision, but patients requiring complex examinations, particularly for investigation of gastrointestinal disease, often undergo repeated periods of starvation prior to medical or surgical treatment. Patients with a defective gastrointestinal tract may endure prolonged periods of undernutrition before seeking medical advice.

The changes in metabolism which occur during starvation aim to conserve body tissue, in particular body protein. This is achieved mainly by reducing metabolic rate and nitrogen losses.

Injury

The changes which occur following injury are different, being designed to mobilize tissues for defence and repair. The metabolic response to injury has three phases:

1 The 'ebb' phase.
2 The catabolic or 'flow' phase.
3 The anabolic phase.

The *ebb phase* lasts only a few hours; there is a depression of metabolic function and a reduction of energy expenditure.

The *flow phase* soon follows; metabolic rate increases, energy reserves from fat are mobilized, and body protein reserves – mainly from muscle, are broken down to provide energy by gluconeogenesis. The negative nitrogen balance which occurs at this time may reflect reduced protein synthesis in addition to the increase in protein breakdown (O'Keefe *et al* 1974). Large nitrogen losses may be encountered and it is not always practical or necessary to replace the total amount of nitrogen lost per day. It is during this flow or catabolic phase that rapid weight losses occur. Nutritional therapy during this phase must be defensive. It should aim to reduce catabolism, minimize losses and the wasting of important tissues.

Eventually catabolism declines and the flow phase passes into the *anabolic phase*. This is usually coupled with an increase in appetite and ambulation. The nutritional therapy should now aim to restore muscle mass and increase protein synthesis.

The metabolic changes after injury are proportional to the severity of the injury and are most extreme following burn injuries (Wilmore 1978) (see Section 5.4.3 and Fig. 5.5).

Comparative effects of injury and starvation

The major effects of starvation and injury are summarized in Table 5.1. Seldom do patients simply fall into one category or the other. They may be injured after a period of undernutrition or underfed for some time after an injury. Combinations of both situations complicate the clinical picture and increase the metabolic response.

5.1.2 Nutritional implications of the effects of injury

The application of current knowledge of nutritional pharmacology and effective pain relief can modify the metabolic response and reduce the clinical consequences.

Glutamine efflux from muscle may form part of the response to trauma and sepsis, and help to maintain the integrity of the gut (Souba *et al* 1985), and improve immune function (Newsholme *et al* 1987).

Recent research has suggested that cytokines released at the site of infection or injury may be important mediators of the change in metabolism. Interleukin 1 (IL1), Interleukin 6 (IL6) and Tumour Necrosis Factor (TNF) appear to mimic many of the responses to injury and infection (Grimbel 1989).

The ornithine salt of α-ketoglutarate has been shown to improve nitrogen balance in catabolic states (Cynober *et al* 1984; Leander *et al* 1985).

Lipids also are of clinical interest. The inclusion of MCTs in enteral feeds has been shown to improve body mass, mucosal mass and liver and protein synthesis (Schwartz *et al* 1987). Polyunsaturated fatty acids (PUFA) – namely omega-6 and omega-3 – may be clinically significant (Wau and Grimble 1987). ω3 may have an anti-inflammatory role and omega-6 may decrease the immune response (Alexander *et al* 1986).

Even food itself can minimize the effects of catabolism by maintaining gut integrity and the barrier function of the gut. In consequence, the translocation of micro-organisms from the lumen of the gut into the lymph system, which may occur after injury, can be reversed by enteral feeding (Inoue *et al* 1988).

Further research into the inclusion of these substrates in products formulated for nutritional support is required before they gain widespread acceptance in clinical nutrition.

Table 5.1 Comparison of the effects of starvation and injury (Woolfson 1978)

	Starvation	Injury
Metabolic rate	Decreased	Increased
Weight	Slow loss, almost all from fat stores	Rapid loss, 80% from fat stores. Remainder from body protein
Nitrogen	Losses reduced	Losses increased
Hormones	Early small increases in catecholamines, cortisol, hGH. Then slow fall. Insulin decreased	Increases in catecholamines, glucagon, cortisol, hGH. Insulin increased but relative insulin deficiency
Water and sodium	Initial loss Late retention	Retention

References

Alexander JW, Saito H, Trocki O *et al* (1986) The importance of lipid type in the diet following burn injury. *Ann Surg* **204**, 1–8.

Cynober L, Vaubaurdolle M, Dore A and Giboudeau J (1984) Kinetics and metabolic effects of orally administered ornithine-ketoglutarate in healthy subjects fed with a standardized regimen. *Am J Clin Nutr* **39**, 514–19.

Grimble RF (1989) Cytokines: their relevance to nutrition. *Eur J Clin Nutr* **43**, 217–30.

Inoue S, Epstein M, Alexander JW and Trocki O (1988) Prevention of yeast translocation across the gut by a single enteral feeding after burn injury. *J Parent Ent Nutr* **12**, 55.

Leander V, Furst P, Vesterberg K and Vinnars E (1985) Nitrogen sparing effect of Ornicetil in the immediate postoperative state: clinical biochemistry and nitrogen balance. *Clin Nutr* **4**, 43–51.

Newsholme EA, Newsholme P and Curi R (1987) The role of the citric acid cycle in cells of the immune system and its importance in sepsis, trauma and burns. *Bioch Soc Symp* **54**, 145–61.

O'Keefe SJD, Sender PM and James WPT (1974) 'Catabolic' loss of body nitrogen in response to surgery. *Lancet* **2**, 1035–8.

Schwartz S, Farriol M, Garcia E, Afonso JJ and Rodriguez R (1987) Influence of MCT/LCT ratio in enteral nutrition on liver and jejunal mucosa protein synthesis in post surgical stress. *J Clin Nutr Gastroenterol* **2**, 31–7.

Souba WW, Scott TE and Wilmore DW (1985) Intestinal consumption of intravenously administered fuels. *J Parent Ent Nutr* **9**, 18–22.

Wau JM and Grimble RF (1987) Effect of dietary linoleate content on the metabolic response of rats to *Escherichia coli* endotoxin. *Clin Sci* **72**, 383–5.

Wilmore DW (1978) *Metabolic management of the critically ill.* Plenum Press, New York.

Woolfson AMJ (1978) Metabolic considerations in nutritional support. In Johnson IDFA and Lee HA (Eds) *Developments in clinical nutrition.* Proceedings of a Symposium held at the Royal College of Physicians, London, October 1978. pp. 35–47. MCS Consultants, Tunbridge Wells.

5.2 Intensive therapy units

The intensive therapy unit (ITU) is a relatively recent development of medicine primarily concerned with the management of patients with acute life-threatening disorders. The immediate objective of care is to preserve life and to prevent, minimize or reverse damage to vital organs. The objectives of nutritional support are the same.

Department of Health guidelines suggest that 1–2% of acute beds in a general hospital should be designated ITU beds and that this number be greater when there are specialist units e.g. cardiac, major vascular or neurosurgery. Most patients on ITU have more than one organ system failure. Nursing ITU patients involves total patient care, with a patient: nurse ratio of at least 1:1. Mortality risk is highly variable, dependent on clinical condition.

Common causes for admission to an ITU include:

1 Major trauma including head injury, road traffic accidents.

2 Post-operative care – cardiac, abdominal, transplantation or major vascular surgery.

3 Respiratory failure.

4 Post cardiopulmonary resuscitation.

5 Drug overdose.

6 Pre-operative stabilization termed 'optimalization'.

Scoring systems are used on ITU to predict the severity of illness and the chance of survival. The most commonly utilized score is the APACHE II (Acute Physiology and Chronic Health Evaluation) score. Age, the Glasgow Coma Scale score, 12 current physiological variables, and chronic health status are used to stratify acutely ill patients into prognostic mortality risk categories, but it is not meant to assist in the making of individual treatment decisions (Knaus *et al* 1986). Although there is a strong correlation between severity of illness and mortality probability, the APACHE II score has poor outcome predictors and so is of limited use in predicting outcomes between scores of 10–25; below 10 there are few deaths, beyond 25 there are few survivors. A further modification – APACHE III – is currently on trial.

ITU patients suffer from severe multi-system derangement with frequent alterations in metabolic processes and fuel utilization (Goldstein and Elwyn 1989) and rarely manage an adequate nutritional intake via the oral route. Detailed verbal or written dietary advice is inappropriate at this time as patients remember little of their stay on ITU (Turner *et al* 1990).

5.2.1 How to review ITU data

Information regarding the patient on an ITU is to be found in a variety of locations. The general clinical notes provide the usual background health evaluation, and indicate the current reason for admission. Doctors' notes written during the ITU stay may be kept in this folder or in a separate folder at the patient's bed.

Unlike general wards where blood pressure, temperature and fluids are kept on separate sheets, the ITU patient will have a daily record sheet for temperature, respiratory and cardiac monitoring, fluid balance and serum electrolytes on which values for fluid balance and cardiac monitoring may be computed hourly. Drug therapy is recorded on a usual drug chart, but also on the daily record sheet – especially IV drugs. Separate information is also kept on the mode and type of ventilation. Daily blood results are recorded on an accumulative 'flow chart'. Twenty four hours is a long time in ITU, and so blood results from three days ago may be of little help in assessing the current picture (Runcie and Dougall 1990).

Biochemical, haematological data, and the introduction of nutritional support should be reviewed in the context of the clinical picture. Serial results are used to interpret the clinical condition and treatment progress. Clinical condition, drug treatment and iatrogenic causes interfere with nutrition therapy. The treatment schedule and daily plan of action for that patient will indicate any particular nutrition restrictions relevant to the choice of feed.

5.2.2 ITU equipment

Each piece of equipment surrounding the ITU patient is there to support one failing organ only. A brief review of equipment not usually found on a general ward is discussed below.

Artificial ventilator (life support machine)

The artificial ventilator is used to control the breathing pattern of patients who have acute breathing problems (respiratory failure with worsening blood gases, neuromuscular problems e.g. Guillain-Barré syndrome), or to prevent hypercarbia and localized hypoxaemia in head injured patients (refer to Table 5.2). The ventilator can deliver a controlled inspired oxygen supply varying from 20% oxygen (room air) to 100% oxygen as necessary.

The use of a positive (i.e. greater than atmospheric)

Table 5.2 Arterial blood gas measurements breathing room air

	Normal values	Acute respiratory failure
$PaCO_2$	4.7–6.0 kPa (35–45 mmHg)	>6.0 kPa (>45 mmHg)
PaO_2	9.3–14.0 kPa (70–100 mmHg)	<8.0 kPa (<60 mmHg)
	Saturation: 95–100%	

pressure throughout the expiratory phase of the respiratory cycle may be used to prevent the collapse of peripheral airways and improve gas exchange. This is termed Positive End-Expiratory Pressure (PEEP). Increasing pressure of PEEP will improve arterial oxygenation but compromise venous drainage, which is dependent on a negative pressure in the chest wall (Campbell and Cone 1991). Fluid and sodium imbalance can develop secondary to the resulting impaired renal perfusion, and cause renal insufficiency. This undesirable effect can be offset in part by the use of a renal vasodilator (e.g. renal doses of dopamine) or diuretic therapy. An energy-dense feed may also be required.

High fat feeds reduce carbon dioxide production because of their effect on the respiratory quotient (RQ) and are of most benefit in patients with previously good lung function who are hypercapnic, or patients with chronic obstructive airways disease (COAD) who have an arterial carbon dioxide ($PaCO_2$) above tolerable levels (Al-Saady *et al* 1989). Overfeeding negates any beneficial response to high fat feeds, as the conversion of energy to body fat involves a disproportionately large production of CO_2 (Larca and Greenbaum 1982).

The patient is ventilated via an endotracheal (ET) tube passed through the mouth, or sometimes the nose, into the trachea. Tracheostomy is considered if long term ventilatory support appears likely. A 'cuffed' endotracheal tube or tracheostomy may be a risk factor for the insertion of a fine bore feeding tube, as the ET tube may keep the glottis partially opened, or may inadvertantly act as a guide for the feeding tube to track downwards into the lung.

All nasogastric feeding tubes may predispose the patient to nasal and maxillary sinus inflammation but this is less likely in the ventilated or tracheostomy patient because air does not flow across the nasal turbinates (Desmond *et al* 1991). A wide bore tube is chosen for ease of gastric aspiration.

The presence of an ET tube for any length of time causes problems with temporary dysphagia and inability to co-ordinate swallowing (especially with liquids) once oral diet is recommended. The presence of a gag reflex does not necessarily confer protection against aspiration of pharyngeal contents (DeVita and Spierer-Rundback 1990).

Intra-aortic balloon pump (IABP)

This controls cardiac function in the presence of a failing heart. It acts synergistically with the failing heart to provide cardiac support post-operatively, or to maintain the patient with severe heart failure awaiting transplantation (Holzum 1990). Patients may experience fluid retention, electrolyte abnormalities, and progressive renal failure associated more with poor cardiac function rather than intervention therapy. Anti-clotting therapy is required, although this is usually achieved with heparin rather than warfarin.

Swan-Ganz or pulmonary artery catheters (PAC)

It is difficult to determine cardiac output (CO) and pulmonary artery pressures in patients with rapidly changing haemodynamics, especially in those with impaired myocardial function or respiratory disease.

These double or triple lumen catheters are advanced via a central vein through the right atrium, right ventricle and into the pulmonary artery, where the tip of the catheter rests. Catheters to measure CO incorporate a thermistor near the catheter tip, and a hub for connection to a cardiac monitor. Cardiac output is calculated by thermodilution, which involves the injection of 10 ml of ice-cold 5% dextrose through the CVP lumen, and the subsequent measurement of the blood cooling curve obtained in the pulmonary artery. The fluid requirement for CO measurement is unlikely to exceed 50 ml per day.

The inflatable balloon at the tip of the Swan-Ganz catheter can be temporarily inflated in the pulmonary artery to measure the ('wedge') pressure of blood leaving the heart which will indicate both cardiac function and fluid balance.

Air fluidized beds

These are designed to reduce the incidence of pressure sores and enhance the healing process. The 'Clinitron' model is 2 metres long, a metre wide, and 45 cm deep, and filled with 700 kg of silicon-coated glass microspheres covered by a polyester sheet to allow free air flow. The alkaline environment (pH 7–11) of the beads is bacteriostatic.

Air is drawn in through the base of the bed, warmed, filtered and then passes through the bead mattress to the patient. The minimum temperature differential is 6°C above room temperature, but this can be varied from 28–36°C; humidity is fixed at 35–40%.

Conversely, losses from diarrhoea, wound drainage and fistulae drain into the mattress, forming clumps with the beads which sink into a collection chamber and are emptied by the company's own personnel. Increased skin losses from nursing at a higher ambient temperature, together with the inability accurately to measure body fluids lost into the bed, often causes the patient to develop a negative fluid balance. The effect of ambient temperature on patients' protein and energy balance reduces nitrogen turnover in ITU patients (Ryan and Clague 1990).

Continuous arteriovenous haemodiafiltration (CAVHD)

Acute renal failure is a common problem in the ITU patient, occurring in isolation or combined with other organ dysfunction or multi-organ failure. CAVHD allows for clearances of small molecular weight solutes and large volumes of water without aggravating haemodynamic instability, and allows almost unrestricted use of nutrition support and fluid administration in critically ill patients.

Dialysing against a 1.5% glucose dialysate flowing at a rate of 1 litre/hour leads to the delivery of 6 g glucose/hour to the patient. An increase in flow rate or dialysate glucose concentration increases the glucose delivery. As 50% of dialysate glucose can potentially be extracted from a flat-plate dialyser during CAVHD, nutritional support should be tailored accordingly. Nitrogen losses can amount to 24 g per day, with a mean negative nitrogen balance during feeding of 3.6 g N/24 hours. Urea N comprises 60–70% of total urinary excretion, the remaining being non-urea nitrogen. Lipid homeostasis is unaffected by CAVHD (Bellomo *et al* 1991).

5.2.3 Nutritional requirements

General considerations

Feeding schedules should include information on the choice of feed, its composition (electrolyte concentrations of sodium, potassium, and calcium) and, if the patient is ventilated, phosphate levels as well. An introduction regimen, optimum feeding rate and total fluid volume at full rate should also be noted, along with any potential drug interactions. Hyperglycaemic patients should have the carbohydrate load from the feed indicated as grams/hour.

Energy requirements

Patients can be broadly distinguished into two categories – nutritionally depleted patients with resolving medical problems who can safely be fed to repletion levels, and stressed/unstable patients who derive most benefit from 'maintenance' support (to avoid further compromise of the pre-existing organ failure) until the clinical condition is stabilized (Apovian *et al* 1990). The latter form the majority of ITU patients.

Energy supply is the most important factor in feeding the ITU patient, and the provision of adequate non-nitrogen calories maintains nitrogen balance whilst avoiding excessive amounts of dietary nitrogen which may compromise renal function.

Resting energy expenditure (REE) of the ITU patient is variable, influenced by the impact of the illness and its treatment (Cortes and Nelson 1989). Factors influencing REE are summarized in Table 5.3.

Table 5.3 Factors influencing REE

Factors increasing REE	Factors reducing REE
Severe stress/injury	Anaesthesia
Sepsis	Hypothermia
Pyrexia	High ambient temperature
Discomfort and pain	Pain control
Overfeeding	Sedation
Physiotherapy	Sleep
Drugs stimulating sympathetic drive (e.g. adrenalin, dopamine)	Starvation
	Continuous feeding techniques

Sources: Weissman *et al* (1984); Heymsfield *et al* (1987); Swinamer *et al* (1987); Ryan and Clague (1990)

The normal cyclical diurnal variation in basal energy expenditure present in healthy individuals is abolished in ventilated patients (van Lanschot *et al* 1988), and so there are few metabolic problems associated with virtually continuous enteral feeding. Accurate prediction of the REE in the critically ill is difficult because of the diversity of clinical conditions. Recent authors have attempted to define energy requirements from the indirect calorimetry technique. This method has been utilized in both general situations (Table 5.4), and specific disease states (Tables 5.5a, 5.5b and 5.5c).

Non-feed energy sources should be included in calculations so that overfeeding is avoided. Vaso-irritant drugs (such as the anaesthetic Propofol, and the benzodiazepines) are administered in a lipid base (Intralipid) which contributes 1 kcal/ml. Dextrose saline 5% provides 200 kcal/l, and additional glucose is provided from the dialysate during haemodiafiltration (see the paragraph on CAVHD in Section 5.2.2, ITU equipment).

Hyperglycaemia is a neuroendocrine response in both diabetic and non-diabetic ITU patients, primarily from the synergistic effects of high levels of insulin antagonists e.g. noradrenalin, adrenalin, cortisol and glucagon. Chronic sepsis lowers the proportion of mitochondrial pyruvate dehydrogenase complex, which converts pyruvate into acetyl CoA, and thus limits the oxidation of glucose (Seigal *et al* 1989).

Insulin resistance and hyperglycaemia are well documented in sepsis (Jeevanandam *et al* 1990a), with the preferential utilization of fatty acids and MCTs as alternative energy sources (Klein *et al* 1991). Injured or burned patients also oxidize less glucose, preferring fat as a primary energy source (Goldstein and Elwyn 1989).

Hyperglycaemia may delay wound healing, increase fibrinogen levels, and reduce erythrocyte lifespan and total lymphocyte count (Schumann 1990). Maximum glucose utilization is approximately 3–5 g/kg/day. Sliding scale insulin is standard treatment and it may be of benefit to consider a feed with a higher fat profile. Some 100–130 g carbohydrate is essential per day as a primary fuel source for the brain as ketone body production is suppressed with

Table 5.4 Estimated energy requirements in general situations

Requirements kcal/kg/day	Group	Author(s)
22	Healthy young men at rest	Jeevanandam 1990a
24	Septic patients, ITU	
35	'Flow' phase of severe trauma	Jeevanandam 1990b
25–35	General requirements	Cerra 1987 Hunter *et al* 1988
30 ± 5	Multi-organ failure	Forsberg *et al* 1991
57 ± 14	Non-paralysed children	Chwals *et al* 1988
43 ± 17	Paralysed children (mean age 14 months)	

Table 5.5a Estimated energy requirements in specific situations: Brain injury (Ott *et al* 1990)

Type of patient	Measured EE kcal/day
Brain dead	980–1200
Head injury (acute)	1900–2300
Posturing	3700–4400
Musculoskeletal blocking drugs	1200–1400

Table 5.5b Estimated energy requirements in specific situations: Liver failure and transplantation (DiCecco *et al* 1991)

Type of patient (n = 8)	Measured EE kcal/day
Estimate from Harris-Benedict Equation	1384 ± 193
Chronic disease	1570 ± 298
Post-transplant	
day 1	1500 ± 96
day 3	1344 ± 245
days 5–7	1680 ± 398
day 14	1576 ± 407

Energy expenditure on a basis of weight is inappropriate in view of ascites

Table 5.5c Estimated energy requirements in specific situations: Pancreatitis (Dickerson *et al* 1991)

Type of patient	REE kcal/kg/day
Acute	25.6 ± 3.9
Chronic	24.9 ± 4.4
Sepsis	26.4 ± 4.4

Energy expenditure is influenced by the degree of sepsis, rather than pancreatitis *per se*

trauma or sepsis. Dietary fat sources can provide up to 60% of non-nitrogen calories, which paradoxically prevent the development of fatty liver secondary to hypertriglyceridaemia associated with excessive glucose administration (Hawker 1991).

Nitrogen requirement

This is estimated from the amount of nitrogen and energy required to create a positive nitrogen balance, but few patients achieve this whilst critically ill. Protein dynamics in surgical stress are influenced by both severity of surgical trauma, and underlying nutritional status. With mild injury such as elective surgery, there is a normal or slightly depressed rate of protein synthesis but, with severe injury, the rates of both protein synthesis and breakdown are increased (Tashiro *et al* 1991). This may be a teleological response to mobilize amino acids from skeletal muscle to the plasma, for utilization by the liver and other tissues (Pittiruti *et al* 1989; Fischer and Hasselgren 1991).

Aggressive nutritional support cannot reverse the negative nitrogen balance of septic intensive care patients, despite a gain in body fat stores (Seigal *et al* 1989). Similarly, acute phase protein synthesis is increased at the expense of serum albumin maintenance during stress situations, therefore the usual 'nutritional protein markers' are invalid, and are more likely to indicate the severity of illness rather than nutritional status.

Nitrogen balance – the difference between nitrogen output and nitrogen input – is used to estimate the protein status in an individual. Absolute nitrogen output measurement requires the collection and analysis of all body fluids excreted, which is usually determined by measurement of urinary urea nitrogen and the assumption that this represents 80% of total urinary nitrogen excretion. However, urinary urea nitrogen may be too insensitive for calculating nitrogen balance studies in the post-operative ITU patient. Urea production is influenced by liver failure, sepsis, starvation or stress, thus urinary urea nitrogen is insensitive as a consistent and reliable measure of nitrogen loss in clinically unstable patients, is often inaccurate and reflects a lag in response time to changes in therapy. The ratio of total urea nitrogen: urinary urea nitrogen is not constant, varying with the degree of stress, course of an illness, or with different disease states (Konstantinides *et al* 1991).

However, in a study of clinically stable patients receiving a continuous infusion of parenteral nutrition, a 12 hour collection period from midnight to midday, when doubled, gave a satisfactory estimate of 24 hour urinary urea excretion (Candio *et al* 1991) within a much shorter time period. This finding is of limited use in the majority of unstable cases on ITU. Approximate protein requirements derived from studies on ITU patients are summarized in Table 5.6.

Table 5.6 Protein requirements

Clinical condition	g protein/kg body weight/day
Head injury (acute)	1.5–2.5
Post-liver transplant	1.7
General requirements	1.0–2.5

Hypoalbuminaemia may result from many causes, including the metabolic response to injury and infection, and malnutrition in the ITU patient (Rothschild *et al* 1988; Bistrian 1990; Klein 1990). Albumin and other serum measurements appear low if the patient is fluid overloaded. A fall in plasma albumin and transferrin post-trauma is associated with a consecutive rise in the acute phase proteins e.g. C-reactive protein (CRP), haptoglobulin, ceruloplasmin and fibrinogen. The acute-phase protein response is non-specific, and is mediated in part by Interleukin-1. CRP levels can be used to differentiate the hypoalbuminaemia of malnutrition from the response to injury or trauma. A low albumin with normal or low CRP indicates malnutrition; a low albumin with raised CRP levels indicates active disease e.g. trauma or sepsis without necessarily malnutrition.

Hypoalbuminaemia may be a teleological situation, reflecting the relative unimportance of albumin in the stressed, infective or traumatized patient. Albumin synthesis may be elevated, but increased rates of turnover, together with increased transcapillary escape (10–15% per hour compared with the normal 5% per hour) because of increased vascular permeability will reduce serum levels (Rothschild *et al* 1988). Replacement of serum albumin in critically ill patients has no clinical benefit in reducing mortality or the complication rate (Blackburn and Driscoll 1992).

Fluid requirements

Normal fluid requirements in the adult patient are 20–50 ml/kg/day. Patients in renal and respiratory failure may require fluid restriction, and critically ill patients are easily fluid overloaded. Urine output is influenced by diuretic therapy, renal perfusion adequacy and the use of peripheral vasodilators e.g. renal doses of dopamine.

Patients nursed on air-fluidized beds have increased skin losses due to nursing at a higher ambient temperature. Body fluids lost into the bed cannot be recovered and so patients often appear to be in positive fluid balance. Allow an additional 500 ml fluid daily to compensate for increased dermal losses.

Humidified gases used in ventilated patients will reduce by 50% (or some 500–900 ml) normal insensible water losses through the lungs. Ventilated patients requiring PEEP (or its equivalent CPAP when the patient is breathing spontaneously) greater than 10 cm H_2O pressure may require fluid restriction of 1.5 l of feed per day maximum.

Patients with head injury are often fluid restricted and given IV mannitol in an attempt to reduce cerebral swelling and prevent further brain damage. A normal-to-high arterial CO_2 can also influence vasodilation, and thus many head-injured patients are electively ventilated to keep arterial CO_2 artificially low, even though they could breathe spontaneously if allowed. An energy-dense, high fat feed is the optimal feed for such patients, provided that sodium content of such feeds does not compromise their use.

Fluid balance is recorded hourly, and records of the previous 2–3 days are useful to establish fluid balance. The drug chart/daily spread sheet will indicate the minimum fluid contribution from drugs and IV line flushing. Fluid balance may reflect the use of drugs such as renal vasodilators or diuretics rather than the normal physiological reaction to fluid overload.

Due to cardiac and haemodynamic instability, a large intermittent bolus of feed or fluid will adversely affect organ function. Additional fluid can be added to the feed as sterile water, which will present a constant nutritional and fluid load to be utilized by the patient. Factors increasing fluid requirements are outlined in Table 5.7.

Sodium requirements

Sodium is an extracellular ion, with levels of around 140 mmol/l in extracellular fluid, compared with 5 mmol/l in intracellular fluid. Normal requirements are 70–120 mmol per day. Salt and water overload should be avoided in patients in the early stages of refeeding who suffer from cardiopulmonary disorders.

Hypernatraemia is a common occurrence in the critically ill patient, caused by excessive sodium administration, inadequate water intake, excessive water loss, or a combination of these factors (Oh and Carroll 1992).

Sodium retention may occur in acute renal failure, or as stress related secondary hyperaldosteronism with active retention of urinary sodium. A 24 hour urine collection for urinary urea, electrolytes and osmolality should define the cause of hypernatraemia. Low or negligible urinary sodium excretion indicates a metabolic response which is unlikely to be corrected solely by the use of a low sodium feed.

Hypernatraemia with a raised urinary sodium excretion indicates sodium overload. This is difficult to achieve by enteral feed alone, but may be caused by high levels of sodium in TPN, the use of normal saline (containing 150 mmol/l) instead of dextrose saline (30 mmol/l), magnesium-containing antacids, sodium salts of antibiotics (e.g. ampicillin), Gaviscon (6 mmol per 10 ml) or administration of excessive sodium as 8.4% sodium bicarbonate to correct a metabolic acidosis. If the primary source of

Table 5.7 Factors increasing fluid requirements

Diarrhoea
Fistulae drainage
Sweating/pyrexia
Hyperventilation with inadequate humidity
Diuretic therapy
Osmotic diuresis (hyperglycaemia)
Diabetes insipidus (head injury)
Ambient temperature

sodium is drug related and now halted, it may not be necessary to introduce a low sodium feed. The use of a low sodium feed, alone or in combination with a standard feed may be of benefit if sodium input from non-feed sources is high.

Hyponatraemia is caused by water intoxication or depletion of total body sodium. Causes include diuretic therapy, renal disease, or loss of fluid from the gastrointestinal tract and intra-abdominal drains (Arieff 1991). Significant sodium depletion will stimulate aldosterone release through the loss of intravascular volume which will cause loss of potassium in the urine whilst retaining sodium.

Potassium requirements

Potassium is mainly an intracellular cation, at concentrations in the ICF of around 140 mmol/l. Dietary requirements will be in the region of 80–120 mmol/day.

Hyperkalaemia may be iatrogenic, associated with excessive use of potassium sparing diuretics, potassium supplements (often administered IV), catabolic states, or the metabolic acidosis of progressive renal failure.

Hypokalaemia is associated with the use of steroids, diuretics, continuous haemofiltration or haemodialysis. Anabolic states may deplete potassium, phosphate and magnesium as these minerals are incorporated into body cells – a process termed 'cellular steal' or 'refeeding syndrome'. The fall in serum potassium levels is most dramatic 2–3 days after initiation of feeding following a period of starvation. Hypokalaemia can result from the cellular uptake of glucose, which is more pronounced with insulin therapy. The body has no known potassium-retaining hormone, so increased urinary or GI losses may also induce hypokalaemia. Around 3 mmol of potassium is required for each gram of nitrogen retained.

Magnesium requirements

Hypokalaemia is an associated risk factor for hypomagnesaemia: 60–65% of surgical ITU patients have low serum magnesium (Chernow *et al* 1989; Ryzen 1989). Clinical conditions which will reduce serum magnesium include hypothermia, burns, and increased gastrointestinal and renal losses. Drugs which will reduce serum magnesium include aminoglycosides, mannitol, diuretics, digitalis, cisplatin, cyclosporin, and chelation therapy. Clinical consequences of deficiency include cardiac dysrrhythmias and neurotoxicity (muscle weakness). Requirements are in the region of 15–20 mmol per day. Hypophosphataemic patients are usually magnesium deficient.

Phosphate requirements

Hypophosphataemia (<0.08 mmol/l) is a common occurrence on ITU, leading to respiratory insufficiency, muscle weakness and anorexia. Ventilated patients are prone to develop hypophosphataemia, the net effect of which is to reduce oxygen transport by diminishing both red blood cell 2,3 diphosphoglycerate (inhibits the affinity of oxygen to haemoglobin, causing tissue hypoxia), and tissue ATP (a major phosphate compound required for cell function). Hypophosphataemia will impair skeletal muscle strength and delay weaning the ventilated patient (Conti *et al* 1990).

Negative phosphate balance may be associated with increased renal excretion and GI losses, respiratory alkalosis, excessive use of aluminium containing antacids, provision of glucose calories alone in TPN solutions, and is compounded by the 'refeeding syndrome'. Administration of 0.5 mmol phosphate/kg body weight/day will prevent a fall in the serum level (Daily *et al* 1990). Daily requirements are 14–16 mmol.

Calcium requirements

Hypocalcaemia is a common occurrence in ITU patients, with multi-factorial causes including sepsis, hypomagnesaemia, rhabdomyolysis, renal disease, and primary or secondary hypoparathyroidism. Most patients with a ionized calcium concentration >0.8 mmol/l are asymptomatic, and do not require intervention unless they become symptomatic. Conservative treatment is preferred as calcium supplementation can be harmful during ischaemic and septic states. If necessary, calcium repletion is usually commenced with IV calcium, and once the serum levels have stabilized, the enteral route can be used. Most patients require 1–4 g per day, administered as a continuous infusion or in divided doses (Zaloga 1992).

Additions of electrolytes to enteral feeds

These can be added to feeds if serum levels are subnormal to provide a constant infusion to a non-stable patient. Ampoules of electrolytes intended for injection are physically compatible with enteral feeds and provide a defined dose in a small volume. Suitable ampoules to use include:

NaCl 30% w/v = 50 mmol/10 ml
KCl 20% w/v = 27 mmol/10 ml
$CaCl_2$ = 5 mmol/10 ml

The decision of how much supplementary electrolytes to add enterally can be estimated from the previous day's drug chart. Rapid electrolyte replacement is administered intravenously, and will have been written up on the drug chart. Add 1–2 × 10 ml ampoule(s) per 10–12 hours of feed (usually around 1 litre of feed) initially, and titre according to the blood results. Alternatively, check the quantity of the previous day's intravenous infusion and add this amount back to the current feed regimen. Large quantities of electrolytes are well tolerated (Hamill *et al* 1991).

Vitamin and mineral requirements

Mineral requirements are difficult to determine in the ITU patient because the impact of the clinical disease and its treatment will often influence markers, such as plasma protein carriers (Singh *et al* 1991).

Ferritin level in plasma is often used to reflect iron stores but is unreliable in patients with inflammation and liver disease. Transferrin saturation that determines the flow of iron to tissues is reduced in the presence of inflammation. Haemoglobin levels reflect recent blood transfusion, or anaemia secondary to acute or chronic blood loss. Caeruloplasmin – an indicator of copper status – is an acute-phase protein and so will be increased in the presence of any metabolic or stress situation.

Zinc deficiency will alter protein synthesis and directly affect cellular immunity, wound healing rates, and plasma protein synthesis. Increased losses in the ITU patient may occur from diarrhoea, stoma or fistulae losses, or increased urinary excretion from hypermetabolism and the administration of amino acid infusions.

The RNI should be the minimum aim, bearing in mind that excessive amounts of trace elements may compromise the response to infection, etc. If considered necessary, trace elements and vitamins can be added e.g. Seravit (SHS) which will supplement the feed without an additional load of sodium or potassium.

5.2.4 Feeding considerations

When and how to feed

Should ITU patients be fed? Among patients with similar APACHE II scores, a 73% survival rate was demonstrated in those with an adequate energy intake, compared to 43% of those with an inadequate intake (Kresowick *et al* 1985), although early APACHE II scoring cannot identify patients who would benefit most from nutritional support (Hopefl *et al* 1989). A higher mortality rate has been demonstrated in post-surgical patients with a cumulative energy deficit of >10 000 kcal – equivalent to 3–6 days semi-starvation (Bartlett *et al* 1982), and nutritional support has also been associated with earlier weaning from artificial ventilation (Larca and Greenbaum 1982).

Choice of feeding method

Over the last 10 years, research has demonstrated the importance of using the GI tract whenever possible, and most ITUs are now preferentially attempting to feed patients enterally before considering TPN. Enteral nutrition can prevent stress ulceration (Ephgrave *et al* 1990) and maintain gut integrity.

It has been hypothesized that the inability to provide enteral nutrition is a significant risk factor for sepsis (Lowe and Puyana 1991). Bacterial invasion (translocation) from the intestine occurs when there is altered permeability of the intestinal mucosa, and is potentiated by the presence of malnutrition and gut atrophy associated with starvation. Enteral nutrition maintains gut integrity and trophism, enhances biliary immunoglobulin A secretion, and reduces the production of acute-phase proteins (Kemper *et al* 1992). The presence of glutamine in enteral feeds may also be an advantage (see Section 5.1.2).

With the exception of the risk of aspiration, enteral feeding carries less risk of complications. The major problems with TPN are the complications associated with catheter insertion and the potential complications of both catheter and distant focus sepsis (Chuang and Chuang 1991). It is possible to use a triple lumen or pulmonary artery catheter already *in situ* to monitor haemodynamics (Horowitz *et al* 1990). TPN is discussed in greater detail in Section 1.15. The remaining text in this section is concerned with the use of enteral feeding in the critically ill patient.

Feed introduction

Feed should be introduced at full strength and in a small volume. Additional IV fluid will maintain fluid balance until feeding is established. The feeding rate should be reviewed by four-hourly aspirations and the feed rate increased if aspirate and GI tolerance is acceptable. Once sterile water is tolerated, feeding can be commenced at 50 ml full strength hourly, and increased four-hourly in increments of 25 ml, until the desired volume is achieved. This ensures that optimal feeding regimen is reached within 24 hours. (See also the text below on Gastric emptying and Feed aspiration).

Continuous feeding versus intermittent bolus techniques

Continuous feeding techniques have a clinical advantage over intermittent bolus methods by minimizing potentially adverse metabolic effects on cardiac, respiratory and renal function. Twenty-four hour continuous feeding at 30 kcal/kg/day (equivalent to 1.4–1.8 × resting metabolic rate) has been shown to increase lean body mass and reduce extracellular fluid in patients with congestive heart failure without compromising cardiac function (Heymsfield and Casper 1989). Continuous feeding diminishes the thermogenic response compared with intermittent feeding techniques by some 10–15% of total daily REE (Heymsfield *et al* 1987). Continuous feeding for 20 out of 24 hours at estimated requirements has little influence on dietary induced thermogenesis, and allows time for assessment of gastric emptying.

It is common on ITUs to suppress gastric acid production prophylactically in an attempt to prevent stress ulceration. Continuous intragastric feeding may abolish the need for treatment as this has been demonstrated to prevent the occurrence of stress ulcers. It is unknown whether this is a function of raised intragastric pH, or the cytoprotective effect of specific components of food (Kleibeuker and Ek 1991). Continuous nasogastric feeding raises pH more effectively than intraduodenal feeding (Valentine *et al* 1986).

Feeding tubes

Fine bore enteral feeding tubes are impractical in the ITU setting as many medications are administered nasogastrically, and mechanical obstruction of such tubes often follows administration of crushed tablets or drug suspensions (Abernathy *et al* 1989). Fine bore feeding tubes offer little benefit in preventing aspiration (Sands 1991), and tend to reduce checking of residual gastric volumes (Metheny *et al* 1986). Rapid decompression of the stomach to prevent aspiration also necessitates the use of a wider bore tube.

The use of a larger bore feeding tube may be beneficial for use in those patients considered at high risk of pneumothorax (Carey and Holcombe 1991). Once the patient is more alert, the larger bore feeding tube can be used as an introducer for a fine bore feeding tube, without the risk of pulmonary complications (Harris and Huseby 1989).

Interruptions to feed

Feeding time is rarely lost through ITU patients having investigative procedures elsewhere. With the exception of whole body or CAT scanners, diagnostic procedures come to the patient. Very little aggressive physiotherapy is performed on the ITU patient and feeding is often continued throughout the procedure. If it is considered necessary for the feed to be stopped, a 10 minute period is considered sufficient before physiotherapy commences.

Gastric emptying

Anaesthesia, sedatives and muscle relaxants can all affect small bowel motility, thus restricting the ability to feed enterally. Enteral nutrition of ITU patients is often delayed if paralytic ileus is thought to be present although the absence of bowel sounds alone is not a contraindication to enteral feeding.

Jejunostomy feeding at full strength but low volume, and started immediately post-surgery is well tolerated in head injured patients, despite the presence of a clinically silent abdomen (Grahm *et al* 1989). Despite the early return of post-gastric motility, few ITU patients return from theatre with a nasojejunal or jejunostomy feeding tube *in situ*, and their clinical instability often precludes their return to theatre or for endoscopy to have one placed.

Gastric emptying rates during the first eight hours of feeding are variable, with maximum gastric residues for both whole protein and pre-digested formulas, infused at a constant rate, occurring around two hours post-feed commencement (Kleibeuker and Ek 1991), thus aspiration to check gastric emptying rates should be delayed until this peak has passed. Hyperosmolar solutions and solutions containing a high proportion of LCT (Paraskevopoulos *et al* 1988) may also retard gastric emptying.

Gastric stasis can be overcome by the regular administration of drugs which enhance gastric emptying, e.g. Cisapride (Rowbotham 1988). Patients with persistent hypomotility problems are candidates for TPN, until such gastrointestinal problems resolve.

Feed aspiration

Feed aspiration (dePaso 1991) (i.e. feed entering the lungs) is a serious development and a major complication of enteral feeding, leading to respiratory distress, respiratory arrest and subsequent ischaemic cardiac arrest if not promptly corrected. The presence of an ET tube or tracheostomy is no guarantee of a protected airway because feed can easily leak around the high volume low pressure tracheal cuff (Elpern *et al* 1987). However, as in many ITU situations, there is a paradox of treatment. The presence of feed in the stomach will raise intragastric pH and may prevent stress ulcers, yet a persistently raised gastric pH (>3.5) supports bacterial growth in more than 50% of continuously fed patients. Bacterial overgrowth may enhance the retrograde movement of gut bacteria which, together with aspiration of contaminated nasopharyngeal secretions, is considered the most likely cause of nosocomial pneumonia in the ITU patient (Jacobs *et al* 1990).

Recent authors have disputed this claim however and suggest that ischaemic gut mucosal injury and subsequent translocation of enteric bacteria and toxins are more important in the pathogenesis of ITU pneumonia (Fiddian-Green and Baker 1991). A rest period of 3–4 hours per 24 hour period to allow gastric pH to fall may be advisable in patients at risk of pneumonia.

Subclinical aspiration of feed and subsequent development of aspiration pneumonia has been demonstrated to occur in 20% of all ventilated patients (Kingston *et al* 1991). Testing endotracheal aspirates twice daily for the presence of glucose (from the enteral feed) using a glucose oxidase reagent strip can help identify those at risk of aspiration pneumonia (Kingston *et al* 1991).

Preventative measures to minimize the risk include elevation of the head of the bed, the use of gastric motility agents, and the frequent checking of residual gastric volumes. A single, high residual volume (>200 ml) should not cause immediate cessation of an enteral feed, as subsequent residual volumes may well decrease (McClave *et al* 1992).

Continuous feeding, post-pyloric tube placements and PEGs are recommended, but unproven, techniques to reduce feed aspiration (dePaso 1991). However, the risk of aspiration in the ITU patient is small compared with the ward situation – with a probability of 0.9%, compared with 4.9% on medical/surgical wards (Mullan *et al* 1992).

Diarrhoea

This is a frequent occurrence. Individual tolerance to enteral feed is unpredictable, but malabsorption, faecal impaction or hypoalbuminaemia do not appear to be risk factors for the development of diarrhoea (Patterson *et al* 1990). Hypertonic feeds administered to critically ill patients have little influence on intolerance (Pesola *et al* 1990), but elixir drugs with a sorbitol content of 10–20 g per day can induce diarrhoea (Edes *et al* 1990).

The cause of the diarrhoea should be determined and treated before the feed is stopped. Check that the patient is not continuing to receive laxative therapy or magnesium-containing antacids (Fine *et al* 1991), both of which are likely to cause diarrhoea. Long term antibiotics are also associated with pseudomembranous colitis or decimation of commensile gut flora, and the subsequent colonization by antibiotic resistant bowel pathogens. Stool cultures should be taken to exclude the gut pathogen *Clostridium difficile* (McFarland *et al* 1990).

Soy polysaccharide containing feeds to increase faecal bulk are of little clinical benefit in alleviating diarrhoea in the ITU patient (Dobb and Towler 1990), although the use of live yoghurt administered at regular intervals during the feeding period may help to recolonize the gut following antibiotic therapy (Siitonen *et al* 1990).

Pre-digested feeds should be considered if malabsorption is suspected, and are worth a trial before referral for TPN.

Interaction between nutrition support and drug therapy

In the early days of enteral feeding, high levels of vitamin K were associated with pronounced warfarin antagonism. Most enteral feeds now contain between 70–300 micrograms or less of vitamin K and yet 70 micrograms has been associated with an antagonistic response to warfarin therapy (Martin and Lutomski 1989). Clinicians should be made aware of the potential interaction, especially with patients stabilized on warfarin prior to commencement of enteral feed. Prothrombin time should be regularly monitored during feeding. If feeding is halted for interventive therapy (e.g. if the patient is to have a tracheostomy) it may be necessary to reduce the warfarin dose, otherwise surgery may be delayed because the clotting time is prolonged. Heparin may also be used as an anticoagulant and is not affected by the enteral feed.

Physical incompatibility of medications with enteral feeds has been demonstrated with non-aqueous preparations (such as theophylline elixirs and effervescent potassium) and those with a pH < 4.0 (Cutie *et al* 1983), although incidence of incompatibility is reduced if elemental rather than whole protein feeds are given (Burns *et al* 1988).

Several reports have documented a fall in plasma phenytoin levels below the serum therapeutic range when the oral form of the drug is given concurrently with feeds, although this can be overcome by increasing the amount of phenytoin administered, halting the enteral feed for one hour prior and three hours post drug administration or by the use of the IV form (Holtz *et al* 1987; Fleisher *et al* 1990).

Nutritional pharmacology

Current nutritional support techniques aim to influence morbidity and mortality by preventing generalized or specific nutrient deficiency. However, specific components to the diet can influence organ specific functions, and nutrients are now considered to have as much potential for modifying the immune response as pharmacological agents (Haw *et al* 1991).

Dietary fat

A major component of cell membranes are polyunsaturated fats. These are responsible for the structural and functional integrity of the cell, and influence the production and release of membrane eicosanoids. Omega-6 fatty acids are the precursors of the dienoic series of arachidonic acid metabolites. High doses are associated with reduced cell mediated immunity, reduced phagocytosis, and increased production of macrophage-derived dienoic prostaglandins (such as prostaglandin E2) and cytokines such as Interleukin-1 (IL-1), Interleukin-6 (IL-6) and Tumour Necrosing Factor (TNF), released locally to potentiate the inflammatory response to trauma and sepsis.

Omega-3 PUFAs can preferentially replace their omega-6 counterparts in the cell membrane, with a resultant alteration in membrane fluidity, and eicosanoid, Interleukin and TNF release. Omega-3 fatty acids form the trienoic series of prostaglandins and leukotrienes, which tend to reduce thrombogenesis and blunt the inflammatory response.

As the two metabolic pathways are mutually competitive, it may be possible to modify the inflammatory response by nutritional means (Kinsella and Lokesh 1990). Reduction of the inflammatory response is beneficial in that the localized and gradually diffuse tissue damage which occurs in progressive organ failure is blunted, and tissue viability is maintained (Cerra 1991). It appears that the critically ill patient may be unable to metabolize long chain fats effectively, and so feeds containing the precursor fat linoleic acid have little evidence of clinical efficacy. Modified feeds which also contain fish oil (EPA) have been demonstrated in initial studies to be of clinical advantage over a standard feed.

Recent research has suggested that overfeeding high fat formulations rich in omega-6 PUFA may be detrimental. Corn oil is the most common fat source used in enteral feeds, of which 51% of its fatty acid composition are omega-6 PUFA. High fat feeds are used with ventilated patients – a group at high risk of sepsis and multi-organ failure syndrome (MOFS), a term for the sequential failure of the respiratory, renal and hepatic systems, with an overall high mortality. It would appear prudent to ensure that overfeeding does not occur in this group. Maximum level of omega-6 PUFA of 1 g/kg/day is considered acceptable (Cerra 1991).

Glutamine

This is a non-essential amino acid found in large quantities in the bloodsteam. It can be used as a protein or energy source. Enterocytes contain a large quantity of glutaminase enzyme to utilize luminal sources and circulating glutamine from the mesenteries as an energy source.

During prolonged stress and inadequate enteral nutritional support, plasma glutamine levels are reduced, and atrophy of the gut mucosa occurs. Starvation, immunosuppression, chemotherapy, injury, infection, and the use of TPN in the presence of bowel rest are also associated with a breakdown in the barrier function of the gut (Souba *et al* 1990). Difficulty in the reintroduction of nutrients to the gastrointestinal tract following a period of TPN may be partly due to the lack of glutamine in TPN solutions (as it is an unstable amino acid), and gut atrophy that has occurred as a consequence of bowel rest.

Translocation of enteric bacteria through the gut mucosa may initiate the septicaemia which can progress to MOFS. Enteral nutrition support may prevent this sequelae by maintaining the gut function and providing glutamine from the feed (Wilmore *et al* 1988), but it cannot influence MOFS once sepsis is established (Cerra *et al* 1988).

Arginine

This is classed as a semi-essential amino acid required for growth and in post-traumatic states, but supplementation (of 25 g L-arginine per day) may enhance or preserve immune function in high risk surgical patients and theoretically improve the host's resistance to infection (Daly *et al* 1990).

Summary

Nutritional intervention in patients with organ failure can influence outcome. Dietitians working in the field of critical care should take time to familiarize themselves with the equipment and treatment procedures if appropriate dietary advice is to be given.

A shortcut in clinical appraisal is rather like writing a pocket reference on dismantling bombs – cutting corners can be disastrous! Nutritional support should be carefully tailored to the patient's clinical condition and treatment schedules, and should be based on current dietary principles. Current developments may herald the development of a new discipline in dietetics related to nutrition pharmacology.

Further reading

Hinds CJ (1988) *Intensive care: a concise textbook*. Baillière-Tindall, London.
Park GR and Manara AR (1988) *Intensive care – pocket reference*. Castle House Publications, Tunbridge Wells.

Journals

Critical Care Medicine, Williams and Wilkins.
Intensive Care Medicine, Springer-Verlag.

References

Abernathy GB, Heizer WD, Holcombe BJ *et al* (1989) Efficacy of tube feeding in supplying energy requirements of hospitalized patients. *J Parent Ent Nutr* **13**, 387–91.
Al-Saady NM, Blackmore CM and Bennett ED (1989) High fat, low carbohydrate enteral feeding lowers $PaCO_2$ and reduces the period of ventilation in artificially ventilated patients. *Crit Care Med* **15**, 290–95.
Apovian CM, McMahon M and Bistrian B (1990) Guidelines for refeeding the marasmic patient. *Crit Care Med* **18**, 1030–33.
Arieff AI (1991) Treatment of symptomatic hyponatremia. *Crit Care Med* **19**, 748–51.
Bartlett RH, Dechert RE, Mault JR *et al* (1982) Measurement of metabolism in multiple organ failure. *Surgery* **92**, 771–8.
Bellomo R, Martin H, Parkin G *et al* (1991) Continuous arteriovenous haemodiafiltration in the critically ill: influence on major nutrient balance. *Int Care Med* **17**, 399–402.
Bistrian BR (1990) Recent advances in parenteral and enteral nutrition: a personal perspective. *JPEN* **14**, 329–34.
Blackburn GL and Driscoll DF (1992) Time to abandon routine albumin supplementation. *Crit Care Med* **20**, 157–8.
Burns PE, McCall L and Wirsching R (1988) Physical compatability of enteral formulas with various common medications. *JADA* **88**, 1094–6.
Campbell GS and Cone JB (1991) Adult respiratory distress syndrome. *Am J Surg* **161**, 239–42.
Candio JA, Hoffman MJ and Lucke JF (1991) Estimation of nitrogen excretion based on abbreviated urinary collections in patients on continuous parenteral nutrition. *J Parent Ent Nutr* **15**, 148–51.
Carey TS and Holcombe BJ (1991) Endotracheal intubation as a risk factor for the complications of nasoenteric tube insertion. *Crit Care Med* **19**, 427–9.
Cerra FB (1987) Hypermetabolism, organ failure and metabolic support. *Surgery* **101**, 1–8.
Cerra FB (1991) Nutrient modulation of inflammatory and immune function. *Am J Surg* **161**, 230–34.
Cerra FB, McPherson JP, Konstantinides FN *et al* (1988) Enteral nutrition does not prevent multiple organ failure syndrome (MOFS) after sepsis. *Surgery* **104**, 727–33.
Chernow B, Bamberger S, Stoiko M *et al* (1989) Hypomagnesemia in patients in post operative intensive care. *Chest* **95**, 391–7.
Chuang JH and Chuang S-F (1991) Implication of a distant septic focus in parenteral nutrition. *J Parent Ent Nutr* **15**, 173–5.
Chwals WJ, Lally KP, Woolley MM and Mahour GH (1988) Measured energy expenditure in critically ill infants and young children. *J Surg Res* **44**, 467–72.
Conti G, Rocco M and Gasparetto A (1990) Acute hypophosphataemia. Update in *Intensive Care and Emergency Medicine* **10**, 792–7. Springer-Verlag, Vienna.
Cortes V and Nelson LD (1989) Errors in estimating energy expenditure in critically ill surgical patients. *Arch Surg* **124**, 287–90.
Cutie AJ, Altman E and Lenkel L (1983) Compatability of enteral products with commonly employed drug additives. *J Parent Ent Nutr* **7**, 186–91.

Daily WH, Tonneson AS and Allen SJ (1990) Hypophosphatemia – incidence, etiology and prevention in the trauma patient. *Crit Care Med* **18**(11), 1210–14.

Daly JM, Reynolds J, Sigal *et al* (1990) Effect of dietary protein and amino acids on immune function. *Crit Care Med* **18**, S86–93.

DePaso WJ (1991) Aspiration pneumonia. *Clin in Chest Med* **12**, 269–84.

Desmond P, Raman R and Idikula J (1991) Effect of nasogastric tubes on the nose and maxillary sinus. *Crit Care Med* **19**, 509–11.

DeVita MA and Spierer-Rundbeck L (1990) Swallowing disorders in patients with prolonged orotracheal intubation or tracheostomy tubes. *Crit Care Med* **18**, 1328–30.

DiCecco SR, Plevak D, Weisner R *et al* (1991) Poster discussion: Do we accurately estimate caloric and nitrogen requirements in the liver transplant patient? *Crit Care Med* **19**, S55.

Dickerson RN, Vehe KL, Mullen JL and Feurer ID (1991) Resting energy expenditure in patients with pancreatitis. *Crit Care Med* **1**, 484–90.

Dobb GJ and Towler SC (1990) Diarrhoea during enteral feeding in the critically ill: a comparison of feeds with and without fibre. *Int Care Med* **16**, 252–5.

Edes TE, Walk BE and Austin JL (1990) Diarrhea in tube fed patients: feeding formula not necessarily the cause. *Am J Med* **88**, 91–3.

Elpern EH, Jacobs ER and Bone RC (1987) Incidence of aspiration in tracheally intubated adults. *Heart Lung* **16**, 527–31.

Ephgrave KS, Kleiman-Wexler RL and Adair CG (1990) Enteral nutrients prevent stress ulceration and increase intragastric volume. *Crit Care Med* **18**, 621–4.

Fiddian-Green RG and Baker S (1991) Nosocomial pneumonia in the critically ill: product of aspiration or translocation? *Crit Care Med* **19**, 763–9.

Fine KD, Santa Ana CA and Fordtran JS (1991) Diagnosis of magnesium-induced diarrhoea. *New Engl J Med* **324**, 1012–17.

Fischer JE and Hasselgren P-O (1991) Cytokines and glucocorticoids in the regulation of the 'Hepato-skeletal muscle axis' in sepsis. *Am J Surg* **161**, 266–71.

Fleisher D, Sheth N and Kou JH (1990) Phenytoin interactions with enteral feedings administered through nasogastric tubes. *J Parent Ent Nutr* **14**, 513–16.

Forsberg E, Soop M and Thorne A (1991) Energy expenditure and outcome in patients with multiple organ failure following abdominal surgery. *Int Care Med* **17**, 403–9.

Goldstein SA and Elwyn DH (1989) The effects of injury and sepsis on fuel utilization. *Ann Rev Nutr* **9**, 445–73.

Grahm TW, Zadrozny RN and Harrington T (1989) The benefits of early jejunal hyperalimentation in the head-injured patient. *Neurosurgery* **25**, 729–35.

Hamill RJ, Robinson LM, Wexler HR and Moote C (1991) Efficacy and safety of potassium infusion therapy in hypokalaemic critically ill patients. *Crit Care Med* **19**, 694–9.

Harris MR and Huseby JS (1989) Pulmonary complications from naso-enteral feeding tube insertion in an intensive care unit: incidence and prevention. *Crit Care Med* **17**, 917–19.

Haw MP, Bell SJ and Blackburn GL (1991) Potential of parenteral and enteral nutrition in inflammation and immune dysfunction: a new challenge for dietitians. *JADA* **91**, 701–6.

Hawker F (1991) Liver dysfunction in critical illness. *Anaesth Intens Care* **19**, 165–81.

Heymsfield SB and Casper K (1989) Congestive heart failure: clinical management by use of continuous nasoenteric feeding. *Am J Clin Nutr* **50**, 539–44.

Heymsfield SB, Casper K and Grossman GD (1987) Bioenergetic and metabolic response to continuous intermittent nasoenteric feeding. *Metabolism* **36**, 570–75.

Holtz L, Milton J and Sturek JK (1987) Compatability of medications with enteral feedings. *J Parent Ent Nutr* **11**, 183–6.

Holzum D (1990) Intrapulmonary artery balloon pumping after CABG surgery. *Crit Care Nurse* **10**, 48–53.

Hopefl AW, Taaffe CL and Herrmann VM (1989) Failure of APACHE II alone as a predictor of mortality in patients receiving total parenteral nutrition. *Crit Care Med* **17**, 414–17.

Horowitz HW, Dworkin BM, Savino JA *et al* (1990) Central catheter-related infections: comparison of pulmonary artery catheters and triple lumen catheters in a critical care setting. *JPEN* **14**, 588–92.

Hunter DC, Jaksic T, Lewis D *et al* (1988) Resting energy expenditure in the critically ill: estimations versus measurement. *Br J Surg* **75**, 875–8.

Jacobs S, Chang RWS, Lee B and Bartlett FW (1990) Continuous enteral feeding: a major cause of pneumonia amongst ventilated intensive care unit patients. *J Parent Ent Nutr* **14**, 353–6.

Jeevanandam M, Grote-Holman E, Chikenji T *et al* (1990a) Effects of glucose on fuel utilization and glycerol turnover in normal and injured man. *Crit Care Med* **18**, 125–37.

Jeevanandam M, Young DH and Schiller WR (1990b) Influence of parenteral nutrition on rates of net substrate oxidation in severe trauma patients. *Crit Care Med* **18**, 467–73.

Kemper M, Weissman C and Hyman AI (1992) Caloric requirements and supply in critically ill surgical patients. *Crit Care Med* **20**, 344–8.

Kingston GW, Phang PT and Leathley MJ (1991) Increased incidence of nosocomial pneumonia in mechanically ventilated patients with sub-clinical aspiration. *Am J Surg* **161**, 589–92.

Kinsella JE and Lokesh B (1990) Dietary lipids, eicosanoids, and the immune system. *Crit Care Med* **18**, S94–S113.

Kleibeuker JH and Ek B-V (1991) Acute effects of continuous nasogastric tube feeding on gastric function: comparison of a polymeric and a non-polymeric formula. *J Parent Ent Nutr* **15**, 80–84.

Klein S (1990) The myth of serum albumin as a measure of nutritional status. *Gastroenterol* **99**, 1845–6.

Klein S, Peters EJ, Shangraw RE and Wolfe RR (1991) Lipolytic response to metabolic stress in critically ill patients. *Crit Care Med* **19**, 776–9.

Knaus WA, Draper EA, Wagner DP and Zimmerman JE (1986) An evaluation of outcome from intensive care in major medical centers. *Ann Int Med* **104**, 410–18.

Konstantinides FN, Konstantinides NN, Li JC *et al* (1991) Urinary urea nitrogen: too insensitive for calculating nitrogen balance studies in surgical clinical nutrition. *J Parent Ent Nutr* **15**, 189–93.

Kresowick TF, Dechert RE, Mault JR *et al* (1985) Does nutritional support affect survival in critically ill patients? *Surg Forum* **35**, 108.

Larca L and Greenbaum DM (1982) Effectiveness of intensive nutritional regimens in patients who fail to wean from mechanical ventilation. *Crit Care Med* **10**, 297–300.

Lowe DK and Puyana JC (1991) Nutritional support in the intensive care unit. *Curr Opin Gastroenterol* **7**, 290–98.

Martin JE and Lutomski DM (1989) Warfarin resistance and enteral feedings. *J Parent Ent Nutr* **13**, 206–8.

McClave SA, Snider HL, Lowen CC *et al* (1992) Use of residual volume as a marker for enteral feeding intolerance: prospective blinded comparison with physical examination and radiographic findings. *J Parent Ent Nutr* **16**, 99–105.

McFarland LV, Surawicz CM and Stamm WE (1990) Risk factors of *C. Difficile* carriage and *C. Difficile* associated diarrhoea in a cohort of hospitalized patients. *J Infect Dis* **162**, 678–84.

Metheny NA, Eisenberg P and Spies M (1986) Aspiration pneumonia in patients fed through nasoenteral tubes. *Heart Lung* **15**, 256–61.

Mullan H, Roubenoff RA and Roubenoff R (1992) Risk of pulmonary aspiration among patients receiving enteral nutrition support. *JPEN* **16**, 160–64.

Oh MS and Carroll HJ (1992) Disorders of sodium metabolism: hyper-natremia and hyponatremia. *Crit Care Med* **20**, 94–103.

Ott L, Young B, Phillips R and McClain C (1990) Brain injury and nutrition. *Nutr in Clin Pract* **5**, 68–73.

Paraskevopoulos JA, Houghton LA, Eyre-Brooke I *et al* (1988) Effect of composition of gastric contents on resistance to emptying of liquids from stomach in humans. *Dig Dis and Sci* **33**, 914–18.

Patterson ML, Dominguez JM, Lyman B *et al* (1990) Enteral feeding in the hypoalbuminemic patient. *J Parent Ent Nutr* **14**, 362–5.

Pesola GR, Hogg JE, Eissa N *et al* (1990) Hypertonic nasogastric tube feedings: do they cause diarrhea? *Crit Care Med* **18**, 1378–82.

Pittiruti M, Siegal JH, Sganga *et al* (1989) Determinants of urea nitrogen production in sepsis. *Arch Surg* **124**, 362–72.

Rothschild MA, Oratz M and Schreiber SS (1988) Serum albumin. *Hepatology* **8**, 385–401.

Rowbotham DJ (1988) Comparison of the effects of cisapride and metaclopramide on morphine-induced delay in gastric emptying. *Br J Clin Pharmacol* **26**, 741–6.

Runcie CJ and Dougall JR (1990) Assessment of the critically ill patient. *Br J Hosp Med* **43**, 74–6.

Ryan DW and Clague MB (1990) Nitrogen sparing and the catabolic hormones in patients nursed at an ambient temperature following major surgery. *Int Care Med* **16**, 287–90.

Ryzen E (1989) Magnesium homeostasis in critically ill patients. *Magnesium* **8**, 201–212.

Sands JA (1991) Incidence of pulmonary aspiration in intubated patients receiving enteral nutrition through wide- and narrow-bore nasogastric feeding tubes. *Heart and Lung* **20**, 75–80.

Schumann D (1990) Post-operative hyperglycaemia: clinical benefits of insulin therapy. *Heart Lung* **19**, 165–73.

Seigal JH, Vary TC, Rivkind A *et al* (1989) Abnormal metabolic control in the septic multiple organ failure syndrome: pharmacotherapy for altered fuel control mechanisms. *Second Vienna Shock Forum*, 535–54.

Siitonen S, Vapaatalo H, Salminen S *et al* (1990) Effect of *Lactobacillus GG* yoghurt in prevention of antibiotic associated diarrhoea. *Ann Med* **22**, 57–9.

Singh A, Smoak B, Patterson KY *et al* (1991) Biochemical indices of selected trace elements in man: effect of stress. *Am J Clin Nutr* **53**, 126–31.

Souba WW, Klimberg S, Plumley DA *et al* (1990) Current research review: The role of glutamine in maintaining a healthy gut and supporting the metabolic response to injury and infection. *J Surg Res* **48**, 383–91.

Swinamer DL, Phang PT, Jones RL *et al* (1987) Twenty four hour energy expenditure in critically ill patients. *Crit Care Med* **15**, 637–43.

Tashiro T, Mashima Y, Yamamori H *et al* (1991) Alteration of whole-body protein kinetics according to severity of surgical trauma in patients receiving total parenteral nutrition. *JPEN* **15**, 169–72.

Turner JS, Briggs SJ, Springhorn HE and Potgeiter PD (1990) Patients' recollection of intensive care unit experience. *Crit Care Med* **18**, 966–68.

Valentine RJ, Turner WW, Borman KR and Weigelt JA (1986) Does nasoenteral feeding afford adequate gastroduodenal stress prophylaxis? *Crit Care Med* **14**, 599–601.

Van Lanschot JJB, Feenstra B, Vermeij CG and Bruining HA (1988) Accuracy of intermittent metabolic gas exchange recordings extrapolated for diurnal variation. *Crit Care Med* **16**, 737–42.

Weissman C, Kemper M, Damask MC *et al* (1984) Effect of routine intensive care interactions on metabolic rate. *Chest* **86**, 815–18.

Wilmore DW, Smith RJ, O'Dwyer ST *et al* (1988) The gut: a central organ after surgical stress. *Surgery* **104**, 917–23.

Zaloga GP (1992) Hypocalcemia in critically ill patients. *Crit Care Med* **20**, 251–62.

5.3 Spinal cord and brain injury

5.3.1 Spinal injuries

Prevalence and general aspects of management

The UK has eleven spinal injury units with a total of over 400 beds for the rehabilitation of patients who have a spinal injury (Fig. 5.1). The first UK unit was opened in 1944 (Stoke Mandeville) and the newest unit was opened in 1992 (Glasgow).

About 500 people each year sustain an injury sufficiently serious to require admission to a spinal unit in the UK. Most patients are young and male; 55% of injuries are as a result of road traffic accidents, 30% industrial/domestic, and 18% are sports injuries (Burke and Murray 1988). Other injuries such as head and chest injury may complicate management and rehabilitation.

A questionnaire survey of the UK units (Steven 1985) revealed that only seven units have as much as a weekly service from their local dietetic department and nine units are unable to weigh their patients. A working party report (RCS 1984) failed to recognize the existence of dietitians working in this area. The appointment of the first dietitian specifically designated to a spinal injury unit in 1989 (Senior I, Stoke Mandeville) was long overdue. The newly created Scottish Spinal Injury Unit has the best ratio of dietitians to spinal cord injury (SCI) patients within the UK (Edmonds 1992).

The First Symposium on Nutrition in Spinal Injury Units 1989, held at Edenhall, was the first opportunity for dietitians and other health professionals to consider the provision of nutrition and dietetic services to SCI patients.

The metabolic response to injury is well documented (see Section 5.1) and the prevalence of malnutrition and its effect on the SCI patients have long been recognized. Hippocrates, in 400 BC, described a method of nutritionally supporting SCI patients who were unable to feed themselves. He advocated a large fluid intake consisting of four to nine pints of ass milk, honey and mild white Mendes wine; a nutritionally complete liquid diet (Guttmann 1973).

Prior to World War II few SCI patients survived more than two years. Today the mortality rate is 10–20% greater than for the able-bodied population.

Potential consequences of spinal cord injury

The effects of SCI depend on which segments of the spinal cord (Fig. 5.2) are damaged. Fig. 5.3 shows the likely consequences of spinal injury on sensory dermatomes (areas of skin supplied with afferent nerve fibres by a single posterior spinal root).

Paraplegia

Paraplegia describes the condition where the SCI patient has lost function of the lower limbs resulting from damage to the thoracic, lumbar or, to a lesser extent, sacral cord segments.

Quadriplegia

Quadriplegia (tetraplegia) results from damage to cervical segments and these patients have lost function of all four limbs. In both conditions there is impairment of autonomic function, including bladder and bowel control.

Muscle wasting

Muscle mass above the level of injury has the potential to be entirely normal. At the level of the lesion there is a band of denervation and consequent muscle atrophy. Although loss of muscle is observed above and below the lesion, it is difficult to assess how much is due to denervation or malnutrition. Post injury muscle wasting results in a reduction of lean body mass and in the longer term a sedentary lifestyle encourages an increase in total body fat (Greenway *et al* 1970; Shizgal *et al* 1986; Rasmann Nuhlicek *et al* 1988).

Dietetic management during the initial post-injury period (e.g. within one week of injury)

The newly injured patient, usually cared for in the intensive therapy unit (ITU), may have a paralytic ileus lasting one week or longer. Paralytic ileus is described as paralysis of the smooth muscle of the small intestine. It leads to abdominal distension and is a contraindication to enteral feeding. Early introduction of enteral feeding can be life-threatening if the patient aspirates feed which has accumulated in the stomach having failed to be transported by peristalsis through the small intestine.

The initial nutritional needs of SCI patients are far from clear and some studies have shown energy requirements to be as low as 1500 kcal/6.25 MJ per day while others suggest that requirements may exceed those of burns patients (Clarke 1966; Kearns *et al* 1982; Cox *et al* 1985; Kaufman *et al* 1985; Mollinger *et al* 1985). Priorities in

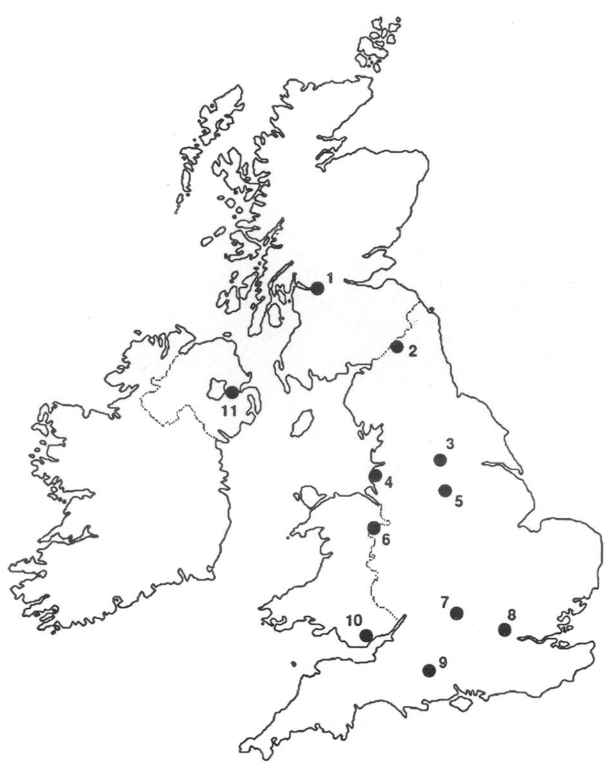

1	Scottish Spinal Injury Unit Southern General Hospital, Glasgow	(48)
2	Hexham	(30)
3	Pinderfields, Wakefield	(30)
4	Fornby District General NHS Trust, Southport	(35)
5	Lodge Moor, Sheffield	(64)*
6	The Midland, Oswestry	(46)
7	National Centre Stoke Mandeville, Aylesbury	(120)
8	Royal National Orthopaedic Hospital, Stanmore	(24)
9	Odstock, Salisbury	(48)
10	Rockwood, Cardiff	(20)
11	Musgrave Park, Belfast	(20)

* Northern General Hospital, Sheffield (60)
Planned change in service: 1994

Fig. 5.1 Map of UK spinal injury units with bed complement

clinical care may result in neglect of nutritional requirements; weighing the patient is often impossible and interpretation of anthropometry difficult. It is not unusual therefore for SCI patients to transfer from general hospital into spinal injury units having had no nutritional assessment or support. Nutritional status in spinal cord injury patients has been discussed by Cliff-Peace (1991).

Dietetic management during the subsequent post-injury period (e.g. within 12 weeks of injury)

All patients with SCI are transferred as soon as possible to one of the UK spinal injury units. In these units early assessment of oral intake and introduction of naso-gastric feeding is increasingly recognized. Where there are contraindications to using the enteral route (and there are few at this stage), units are evaluating peripheral intravenous nutrition.

It is essential that dietitians working in this area have a clear understanding of the extent of the patient's injuries (see Figs. 5.2 and 5.3), the profound psychological effects of those injuries and the practical difficulties of nutritional assessment and support.

Nutritional risk factors for SCI patients and guidelines for weighing SCI patients are summarized in Tables 5.8 and 5.9. Dietitians should be cautious of using reference ranges or nutritional assessment equations based on the healthy able-bodied population. However, it is well accepted that nutritional status is adversely affected by SCI, particularly during the first 2–4 weeks (Laven *et al* 1989), and this remains a challenge for dietitians in terms of treatment and evaluation.

Table 5.8 Nutritional risk factors for spinal cord injury patients

1	Nutrient depletion as a result of the initial metabolic response to trauma, particularly if no nutritional support has been given
2	Nausea e.g. due to antibiotic therapy or postural hypotension
3	Vomiting e.g. due to infection, constipation or more rarely hypercalcaemia
4	Inability to eat — confinement to bed, lying prone, paralysis. Patients may object to being fed by nursing staff/relatives and yet unable to feed themselves, relying on soups and puddings
5	Refusing to eat/drink — depression, anger or attention-seeking behaviour. Emotional problems relating to the injury or isolation from home and relatives. Intake should be monitored
6	Concurrent infection e.g. urinary tract/bladder infections, infected pressure sores, chest infection
7	Weight loss — visible but not always recorded. The inability to weigh patients puts them more at risk
8	Pressure sores — caused by loss of sensation, ischaemia of skin, obesity, patients' inability to change position in bed or wheelchair
9	Total plasma proteins — repeated levels dropping below normal range
10	Plasma albumin — repeated levels dropping below normal range

During this phase the dietitian should assess the patient with whatever data are available, for example the following.

Anthropometric Pre-morbid height and weight, current weight if available, visual weight loss. The difficulties

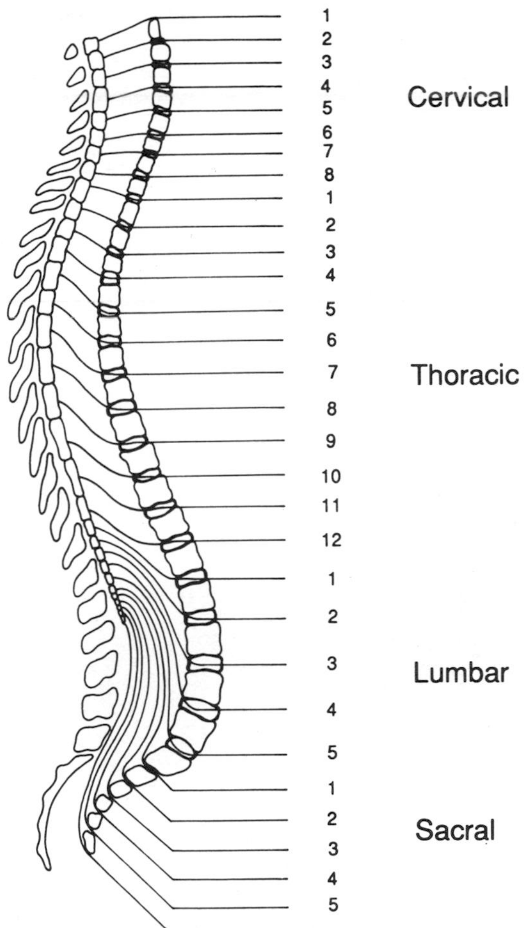

Fig. 5.2 The spinal cord

involved in weighing the patient, unless in a bed with integral scales, are acknowledged. Visual weight loss assessment may be complicated by loss of muscle mass resulting from the injury rather than from nutritional deficiency.

Food intake Current intake charted by ward staff, trends in appetite, pre-morbid intake and nutritional status (liaise with family and friends if appropriate).

Biochemical data Trends in serum albumin, transferrin, total leucocyte count etc, urinary nitrogen losses etc. Urinary protein losses may also indicate muscle wasting caused by spinal cord injury and not necessarily nutritional intake deficiencies. Further work is necessary in this area where 'marker proteins' can be isolated to determine the nutritional deficiency.

Dynamometry Absolute or trends in grip strength and/or muscle strength (liaise with occupational therapy and physiotherapy). Dynamometry is inappropriate in those quadriplegic patients who have little or no arm function due to the injury.

Table 5.9 Guide to weighing patients

Type of patient	Suitable weighing method
1 Fully mobile patient:	
(a) with good balance	Standing scales, i.e. platform/bathroom type
(b) with poor balance	Chair scales, e.g. Avery
2 Wheelchair dependent patient:	
(a) able to transfer and can hold legs free from the floor	Chair scales, e.g. Avery
(b) unable/inconvenient to transfer in wheelchair	Platform scales plus ramp, e.g. Kelgray Electronic Scales, Marsden Wheelchair Ramp or weighbridge sited near or in the unit, e.g. Avery
(c) able to transfer but cannot hold legs free from the chair	Platform scales plus ramp or weighbridge
3 Patient in or on bed/trolley and patient can be lifted by hoist	Hoist scale with sling or stretcher attachment, e.g. Mecanaid electronic box on hoist
4 Patient bed-bound and bed can be moved easily	Weighbridge sited in or near unit e.g. Avery
5 Patient bed-bound, bed cannot be moved	Electronic scales with jack that can raise bed on to sensitive weighing pads, e.g. Seca
6 Patient bed-bound, bed has internal weighing device or it can be attached	The Egerton Paragon 9000 Turning Bed. Clinitron Low Flow Therapy Unit with scale attachment

Address for manufacturers of this equipment are given in the Useful addresses list at the end of this section

Symptomatic Bowel sounds present, abdominal distension, flatus, bowels open. Anorexia, nausea, vomiting or diarrhoea.

Cognitive Chat to the patient and find out what he or she feels able to eat or drink. (It is very difficult to eat or drink while lying flat.) Does the patient know why these are important?

Presentation Identify the most appropriate route or combination of routes to deliver the nutrient requirement and monitor its delivery and effect.

Dietetic management in rehabilitation and continuing care

The aim of rehabilitation is to enable patients to develop the maximum potential possible for their disability. For the patient who has lost weight during the acute post-injury period, the nutritional repletion during rehabilitation becomes much more pertinent. The patient's inability

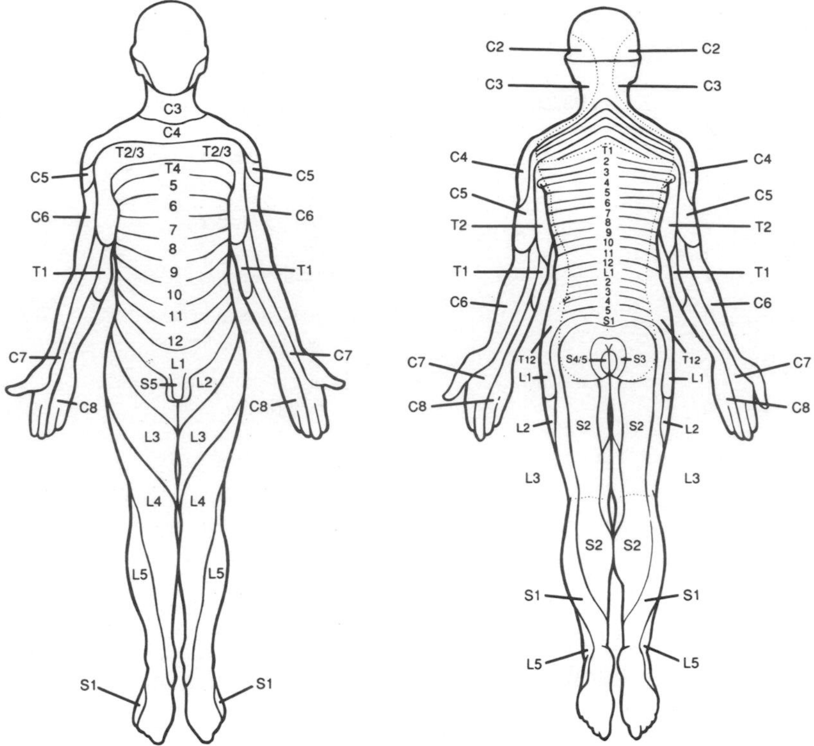

Fig. 5.3 Sensory dermatomes

to participate in physiotherapy and occupational therapy sessions due to lack of muscle strength is undoubtedly a motivating factor to improving nutritional intake. The dietitian working in the therapy team can encourage the use of ready-made nutritionally complete, high energy drinks and snacks, particularly between occupational therapy and physiotherapy sessions. Where patients are still unable to meet their needs by oral intake alone, overnight nasogastric feeding is indicated. There are two advantages to this method of nutritional support:

1 It does not upset their busy daytime therapy sessions.
2 Additional nutrients are supplied passively allowing the patient to improve their oral intake at regular mealtimes (Baugh 1985).

Early assessment of the patient's weight, height and percentage weight loss should be made and a realistic target weight set. It is important that dietitians understand the practical problems involved in making these measurements and setting targets. Height cannot be measured by staediometer when the patient is unable to stand; the best method is measuring the patient's length lying flat in bed or arm span. A guide for weighing is useful for SCI units (Table 5.9). Those units with platform scales encourage patients to record the weight of their wheelchair and cushions so that future weight checks indicate actual body weight.

Pfeiffer *et al* (1981) recommended acceptable weights for paraplegic and tetraplegic patients of between 10–15 lbs below the Metropolitan Life Insurance tables for paraplegic patients and 15–20 lbs below for tetraplegic patients. However, these were derived from only 18 patients. Greenway *et al* (1970) found that in a group of six patients with tetraplegia, the average lean body mass was 6.5 kg (14 lbs) less than in a control group. Suitable weight targets for SCI patients may therefore be about 4.5–6.5 kg below comparable able-bodied people. A recent study of over 200 SCI patients >3 months post-injury (Steven *et al* 1990) concluded that, based on these acceptable ranges, the prevalence of obesity (BMI >25) would be 48%. In the long term, SCI patients will be at risk from obesity, and nutrition education during rehabilitation should therefore be directed at prevention. The dietitian's role needs to change from therapist to health promoter. There are no specifically appropriate nutrition education leaflets available for use in SCI units; literature is often unsuitable featuring able-bodied people exercising or being weighed. A working party formed at The Second Nutrition and Spinal Injury Symposium 1990 in Odstock, Salisbury has the remit of preparing suitable dietary literature for SCI patients.

Dietitians can also become involved in the nutritional assessment and treatment of outpatients at spinal injury units. SCI patients have a greater tendency to formation of renal calculi, primarily as a result of recurrent bladder infections and immobility. Dietary restriction of calcium is not indicated.

'Old' injury patients admitted to units frequently present with pressure sores and concomitant malnutrition. Pressure sores increase nutritional requirements as they expose tissue to infection and leak exudate which is protein-rich. Antibiotic treatment can cause nausea and reduce patients' oral intake. The incidence of pressure sores is increased if the patient is either underweight or overweight. They are caused by the loss of sensation of pressure, ischaemia of the skin, incontinence and patient's inability/reluctance to change position. Pressure sores may need prolonged hospitalization with surgery and patients are frequently nursed on air filled beds, e.g. Clinitron. The dietitian's role in nursing in-service education can do much to improve the implementation of nutritional support for such patients. By high-lighting the nutritional risk factors as in Table 5.8, the dietitian is prompting standard nursing procedures for assessment of those patients at risk and encouraging the early medical referral of appropriate patients for diet therapy. There is a dilemma when an obese patient is admitted for treatment of pressure sores. It is preferable to treat obesity after the sores have healed.

The prevention and management of pressure sores is discussed in more detail in Section 5.6.

5.3.2 Brain injury

Prevalence and general aspects of management

Brain injury is defined as damage to living brain tissue which is caused by an external mechanical force. It is usually characterized by a period of altered consciousness (amnesia or coma) which can be brief (minutes) or exceedingly long (months/indefinitely). The resulting tissue damage impairs an individual's physical, mental or psychological activities.

Brain injury is one of the most common causes of serious disability in young adults. The newly brain-injured patient is commonly male and young (15–35 years). The most common cause of injury is a road traffic accident (RTA): 50% of brain injuries are RTA related. However, there is an additional peak of incidence among the elderly.

Survivable brain injury does not usually reduce life expectancy; young brain injured patients can therefore face years of survival in a physically and/or mentally disabled state (Rosenthal *et al* 1983). As a result of this and the prolonged duration of the recovery process, the prevalence of people with brain injury related disability is approximately 100–150 per 100 000 of the UK population. This means that a health authority with an average population of 250 000 will contain between 250–375 survivors of brain injury at any one time. Each year, approximately 20 people within this area will suffer severe brain injuries and 44 will sustain moderately severe injuries. Six months after injury, about five of these will still have severe disabilities and five will have moderate disabilities.

Brain injured patients may be cared for by a hospital disability team or a community disability team.

The hospital disability team This is responsible for the assessment and treatment of disabled people. It is normally led by a consultant and includes a clinical psychologist, nurse, occupational therapist, physiotherapist, social worker, speech therapist and others as appropriate.

The community disability team This is the community equivalent of a hospital team, often led by a general practitioner but in some teams by a social worker or therapist.

Despite the fact that brain injury is 10 times more frequent than spinal injury in the UK (and 40 times more frequent in the USA), there is much less chance that a victim of a brain injury will be fortunate enough to find a coherent and expertly conceived rehabilitation programme (Vogenthaler 1987). Rehabilitation in the UK is patchy and many neurologists agree that there is a need to set up specialist units as in the case of the spinal injury service. A recent document from the Scottish Office NHS (1992) specifically mentions the important role of the dietitian in the assessment and rehabilitation of patients with post-traumatic injury. A review article on the nutritional management of head injury has been published in America by Brooke *et al* (1989), but further dietetic evaluation is badly needed.

Classification of brain injury

The main classifications of brain injury are detailed in Table 5.10. The Glasgow Coma Scale (GCS) (Teasdale and Jennett 1974) is the measurement used to assess the degree of damage soon after the initial insult. Once the patient has regained consciousness, a more accurate assessment of severity can be achieved by defining the duration of post-traumatic amnesia (PTA) i.e. when the patient is unable to recollect where he or she is or know what time it is, and is likely to forget previously well-known names. Some definitions associated with brain injury are summarized in Table 5.11.

Dietetic management in the acute post-injury period

Dietitians need to have knowledge and understanding in order to provided effective dietary treatment for brain-injured patients.

The overall aim of treatment in this period is to prevent complications resulting from the injury i.e. increased intracranial pressure (ICP) and infection. Severely injured patients have been shown to have a metabolic response similar to that reported for patients with burns of 20–40% of the body surface (Clifton *et al* 1984). Careful monitoring of electrolyte balance to prevent hyponatraemia (serum sodium <120 mmol/l) is essential. The early intolerance of nutritional support via the enteral route along with the preceding factors often indicate the need for total parenteral nutrition (TPN). When clinically feasible, the

Table 5.10 Classification and characteristics of brain injury

Glasgow Coma Scale[1]	Degree of damage	Length of time in coma	Outcome
<8	Severe brain damage	True coma lasting weeks/months. Vegetative state emerges; 17% of patients in coma >15 days	Permanent brain damage, occasionally obeying very simple commands. Totally dependent on others for feeding. Usually transferred to long term care
8–13	Moderate severe brain damage	>1 day 51% recover in <7 days	Commonly there are degrees of cognitive, behavioural, physical and emotional problems. Few return to work. Require rehabilitation
12–14	Moderate brain damage	1–24 hours	May have physical and cognitive problems. Recovery time 6–12 months. May be unable to return to work at previous level
14–15	Mild brain damage	<20 minutes	No obvious neurological signs initially but may present with post-concussive syndrome

[1] Note: The Glasgow Coma Scale can change with time, and some patients with an initial scale of 8 may have moderate (8–12) to mild (13–15) disability eventually

careful introduction of enteral feeding by a nasogastric tube which can be aspirated, i.e. not fine bore, is preferred. Brain injured patients, even without the effects of opioid drugs, have a tendency towards delayed gastric emptying. The residual volume of gastric contents varies from 50–100 ml. Bolus feeding, following by checking the volume of aspirate is standard nursing practice for the first few days. Checking gastric emptying is vital when there is risk of gastric reflux and aspiration. Twyman *et al* (1985) reported that in severely brain-injured patients, delayed gastric emptying meant that full strength, full rate feedings were not possible until 10 days post-injury, thereafter necessitating the use of high nitrogen regimens to achieve positive nitrogen balance. Turner (1985) recognizes that increased nutritional requirements are the typical sequellae of brain injury and that enteral nutrition offers significant economic and physiological benefits over parenteral nutrition. Increasing attention is being focussed on newer techniques of enteral access, namely percutaneous endoscopic gastrostomies (PEG) which achieve improved feeding tolerance and reduce the risk of tracheobronchial aspiration. PEG feeding can be beneficial both in the acute stage of brain injury and in the long term (Haynes 1989). Gastro-oesophageal reflux (GER) is a common problem associated with gastrostomy and nasogastric feeding, and is of particular concern in the neurologically impaired brain-injury patients with depressed levels of consciousness (Podell 1989).

Dietetic management in rehabilitation of the brain-injured patient

Following a brain injury, individuals may experience decreased physical abilities, decreased cognitive abilities and/or changes in behaviour and emotional control. Those of particular relevance affecting nutritional status are as follows:

Physical

1 Loss of smell.
2 Problems with taste perception.
3 Loss of bowel control.
4 Inability to use cutlery or feed themselves.

Cognitive

1 Difficulty in remembering meal times.
2 Taking a long time to finish meal/food.
3 Playing with food rather than eating it.

Behavioural

Depression/withdrawal.
Poor social interaction e.g. poor table manners.

Advice for carers may include:
1 Providing food that can be chewed easily.
2 Encouraging drinking between mouthfuls.
3 Keeping a daily activity schedule as a memory aid for patients who may forget about meals.
4 Discouraging the patient from taking alcohol, as after brain injury the effects are greater. A list of low alcohol drinks and advice on their use may be helpful.

Reduced physical activity may lead to obesity, although there are no specific reports in the literature. Dietitians

Table 5.11 Definitions associated with brain injury

Traumatic brain injury	Brain injury caused by trauma to the head (including the effects upon the brain of other possible complications of injury notably hypoxaemia and hypotension, and intracerebral haematoma)
Minor brain injury	An injury causing unconsciousness for 15 mins or less
Moderate brain injury	An injury causing unconsciousness for more than 15 mins but less than 6 hours, and a PTA (post-traumatic amnesia) of less than 24 hours
Severe brain injury	An injury causing unconsciousness for 6 hours or more, or a post-traumatic amnesia (PTA) of 24 hours or more. (This category includes very severe head injury)
Very severe brain injury	An injury causing unconsciousness for 48 hours or more or a post-traumatic amnesia of 7 days or more
Post-traumatic amnesia (PTA)	The time interval between the injury and the reinstatement of continuous day-to-day memory, as assessed clinically. (NB This is not the same as the interval between the injury and the first remembered event after the injury)
Unconsciousness	A state of unconsciousness scoring 9 points or less on the Glasgow Coma Scale
Rehabilitation	An active process by which those disabled by injury achieve a full recovery, or if full recovery is not possible, realise their optimal physical, mental and social potential and are integrated into their most appropriate environment

(Medical Disability Society 1988) Reproduced with Permission

involved in rehabilitation will find that patients and their relatives need to be advised on maintaining an acceptable healthy weight.

Communicating with brain injured patients

Difficulties in communication may result from:

1 Physical difficulties
- Visual
- Aural
- Speech.

2 Cognitive difficulties
- Reduced attention span
- Poor memory
- Slower thought process.

3 Behavioural difficulties
- Anger
- Aggression
- Verbal abuse
- Apathy.

Effective communication nearly always requires involvement of relatives/carers.

Useful addresses

National Head Injuries Association HEADWAY, 200 Mansfield Road, Nottingham NG1 3HX.
Spinal Injuries Association (UK) 76 St James Lane, London N10 3DF.
Scottish Spinal Cord Injury Association (SSCIA), Unit 22, 100 Elderpark Street, Glasgow G51 3TR.

Spinal Injury Units in the UK

1 Scottish Spinal Injury Unit, Southern General Hospital, 1345 Govan Road, Glasgow, G51 4TF.
2 Hexham General Hospital, Hexham, Northumberland NE46 1QJ.
3 Pinderfields General Hospital, Aberford Road, Wakefield WF1 4DG.
4 Promenade Hospital, Leicester Street, Southport PR9 0HY.
5 Lodge Moor Hospital, Sheffield S10 4LH.
6 The Midland SIU, The Robert Jones and Agnes Hunt Orthopaedic Hospital, Oswestry, Shopshire SY10 7AG.
7 National Spinal Injuries Centre, Stoke Mandeville Hospital, Mandeville Road, Aylesbury, Bucks HP21 8AL.
8 Stanmore SIU, Royal National Orthopaedic Hospital, Brockley Hill, Stanmore, Middlesex HA7 4LP.
9 Odstock SIU, Odstock Hospital, Salisbury SP2 8BJ.
10 SIU/Rehabilitation Unit, Rockwood Hospital, Fairwater Road, Cardiff CF5 2YN.
11 Belfast SIU, Musgrave Park Hospital, Stockman's Lane, Balmoral, Belfast BT9 7JB.

Addresses for manufacturers of weighing equipment (see Table 5.9)

Avery Ltd, Foundry Lane, Smethwick, Warley, West Midlands B66 2LP. Tel 021–558 1112/2161.
Egerton Hospital Equipment Ltd, Farwig Lane, Bromley, Kent BR1 3TU.
Kelgray Marketing Ltd, Kelgray House, Spindleway, Crawley RH10 1TH. Tel 0293–518 733.
Marsden Weighing Machine Group Ltd, 187 Cross Street, Sale, Manchester M33 1JG. Tel 061–962 1562.
Mecanaid Ltd, St Catherine's Street, Gloucester. Tel 0452–500 200.
Seca Ltd, Seca House, 40 Barn Street, Digbeth, Birmingham B5 5QB.
SSI Medical Services, Clinitron House, Ruddington Lane, Nottingham. Tel 0602 455355.

Further reading

Burke DC and Murray DD (1988) *Handbook of spinal cord medicine.* Macmillan Education, London.
Guttmann L (1973) *Spinal cord injuries: comprehensive management and research.* Blackwell Scientific Publications, Oxford.
Rosenthal M, Griffith ER, Bond R and Miller JD (1983) *Rehabilitation of the head injured adult.* FA Davis, Philadelphia.
Spinal Injuries Association (1980) *People with spinal injuries, treatment and care Vol 1.* Spinal Injuries Association, London.

References

Baugh E (1985) Actions to improve nutrition care on a general rehabilitation unit. *JADA* 85(20), 1632–4.

Brooke *et al* (1989) Nutritional status during rehabilitation after head injury. *J Neuro Rehab* **3**, 27–33.

Burke DC and Murray DD (1988) *Handbook of spinal cord medicine.* Macmillan Education, London.

Clarke KS (1966) Caloric costs of activity in paraplegic persons. *Arch Phys Med Rehab* **47**, 427–35.

Cliff-Peace L (1991) Nutritional status in spinal cord injury patients. In *Proceedings of the International Medical Society of Paraplegia.* To be published in *Paraplegia.*

Clifton GL, Roberton CS, Grossman RG, Hodge S, Foltz R and Garza C (1984) Enteral hyperalimentation in head injury. *J Neurosurg* **60**(4), 687–96.

Cox SAR, Weiss SM, Posuniak EA, Worthington P, Prioleau M and Heffley G (1985) Energy expenditure after spinal cord injury: an evaluation of stable rehabilitating patients. *J Trauma* **25**, 419–23.

Edmonds P (1992) Spinal injury in Scotland. *Paraplegia* **30**, 35–6.

Greenway RM, Houser H, Lindan O and Weir DR (1970) Long term changes in gross body composition of paraplegic and quadriplegic patients. *Paraplegia* **7**, 301–318.

Guttmann L (1973) *Spinal cord injuries: comprehensive management and research.* Blackwell Scientific Publications, Oxford.

Haynes M (1989) Taking a short cut to health. *Clin Nutr Update* **2**(7), 5.

Kaufman H, Rowlands BJ, Stein DK, Kopaniky DR and Gildenberg PL (1985) General metabolism in patients with acute paraplegia and quadriplegia. *Neurosurgery* **16**, 309–313.

Kearns PJ, Pipp TL, Quirk M and Campolo M (1982) Nutritional requirements in quadriplegics. *J Parent Ent Nutr* **6**(6), 577.

Laven GT, Huang CT, DeVivo MJ, Stover SL, Kuhlemeier KV and Fine PR (1989) Nutritional status during the acute stage of spinal cord injury. *Arch Phys Med Rehab* **70**, 277–82.

Medical Disability Society (1988) *The management of traumatic brain injury.* Medical Disability Society, London.

Mollinger LA, Spurr GB, ElGhatit AZ, Barboriak JJ and Rooney CB (1985) Daily energy expenditure and basal metabolic rates of patients with spinal cord injury. *Arch Phys Med Rehab* **66**(7), 420–26.

Pfeiffer SC, Blust P and Leyson JFJ (1981) Nutritional assessment of the spinal cord injured patient. *Perspectives in Practice* **78**, 501–5.

Podell SK (1989) Intermittent tube feedings and gastroesophageal reflux control in head injured patients. *JADA* **89**(1), 102–102.

Rasmann Nuhlicek DN, Spurr GB, Barboriak JJ, Rooney CB, Elghatit AZ and Bangard RD (1988) Body composition of patients with spinal cord injury. *Eur J Clin Nutr* **42**, 765–73.

Rosenthal M, Griffith ER, Bond R and Miller JD (1990) *Rehabilitation of the adult and child with traumatic brain injury,* 2e. FA Davis, Philadelphia.

Royal College of Surgeons of England Commission on the Provision of Surgical Services (1984) *Report of the Working Party on Spinal Injury Units.* RCS, London.

Scottish Office NHS (1992) *National Specialist Services — Rehabilitation services for patients with brain injury.* NHS Management Executive Document 20.

Shizgal HM, Roza A, Leduc B, Drouien G, Villemure JG and Yaffe C (1986) Body composition in quadriplegic patients. *J Parent Ent Nutr* **10**(4), 364–8.

Spinal Injuries Association (1980) *People with spinal injuries, treatment and care Vol 1.* Galliard Printers, Great Britain.

Steven FG (1985) Results of questionnaire to assess the dietetic services in UK spinal injury units. Unpublished.

Steven FG, Greasey GH and Couser AE (1990) Nutritional status of a Scottish spinal injury population. *J Hum Nutr Dietet* **3**(5), 371–2.

Teasdale G and Jennett B (1974) Assessment of coma and impaired consciousness: a practical scale. *Lancet* **2**, 81–6.

Turner WW (1985) Nutritional considerations in the patient with disabling brain disease. *Neurosurgery* **16**(5), 707–713.

Twyman D, Young AB and Ott L (1985) High protein enteral feedings: a means of achieving positive nitrogen balance in head injured patients. *J Parent Ent Nutr* **9**(6), 679–84.

Vogenthaler DR (1987) An overview of head injury: its consequences and rehabilitation. *Brain Injury* **1**(1), 113–27.

5.4 Burn injury

Extensive thermal injury elicits the most pronounced response to stress that the human body is capable of generating. Resting metabolic expenditure (RME) increases as hormone-induced breakdown of body protein and fat occurs at greatly accelerated rates. Weight loss of 1.5 kg/day is possible. The patient is almost certain to die if weight loss approaches 30% of the pre-burn weight (Davenport 1979).

Nutritional therapy must provide sufficient nutrients to prevent weight loss, or in practice to restrict weight loss to less than 10%. The aim is to preserve lean body mass, thereby ensuring that wound healing and the 'taking' of skin grafts proceed at maximal rates and immunocompetence is maintained. In order to maintain or restore lean body mass, Molnar *et al* (1983) recommend that aggressive nutritional therapy is undertaken in burn patients with the following features or complications:

1 >20% burn.
2 Pre-injury malnutrition.
3 Septic complications.
4 Associated injury including pulmonary.
5 Threat of >10% weight loss.

5.4.1 Fatal burn injuries

As a 'rule of thumb', a patient with a percentage body surface area burn (Fig. 5.4) and an age which when totalled together exceeds 100 is unlikely to survive, e.g. 86 year old with 30% burn = 116 − survival unlikely; 13 year old with 55% burn = 68 − survival likely. This formula does not apply to children less than ten years old. More complicated formulae also exist for predicting mortality (Tobiasen *et al* 1982).

In cases of non-survivable injury, the patient should be kept well hydrated and given adequate pain relief, but no nutritional therapy is attempted; the patient usually succumbs to the injury within a few days.

5.4.2 Minor burn injuries

Small percentage burn injuries (i.e. <15% in adults, <10% in children) do not require resuscitation with intravenous fluids. RME is not elevated to any great extent. Weight can usually be maintained on a high protein, high energy diet supplemented with *palatable* high energy and/or high protein drinks (see Section 1.13.3 and Appendix 6). Glucose polymers can be added to drinking water although the concentrated solutions designed for renal patients are best avoided because their high osmolarity can cause diarrhoea or dehydration. However, food intake may be low for various reasons. 'Nil by mouth' regimens for change of dressings or theatre procedures which require anaesthesia, lead to reduced intakes of food and fluids. Fear, pain or foul smelling dressings may reduce appetite. Patients cannot be made to eat to order, so flexibility in the catering arrangements is an advantage.

5.4.3 Major burn injuries

Ebb phase

Immediately post-burn, fluid moves from the circulation into the tissues. Plasma and other fluids are given parenterally to preserve blood volume and urine output. Burn patients become hypercatabolic within hours of injury. However traditional clinical teaching restricts oral and enteral feeding at this time because of decreased blood flow to the gut and the risk of paralytic ileus (non-peristalsis).

Nonetheless research has shown that feeding within several hours of burn injury can prevent gut vasoconstriction (Inoue *et al* 1989), preventing atrophy of gut mucosal cells and blunting the hypermetabolic response (Mochizuki *et al* 1984). Some UK burn units now feed nasogastrically within six hours of injury with a low incidence of paralytic ileus. Nasoduodenal feeding early post-burn may have some advantages over nasogastric feeding since ileus may not affect the duodenum and feeding into the duodenum may reduce the incidence of bloating, aspiration and nausea.

Flow phase

This will be well underway by the end of the resuscitation period and its duration will be determined by the depth of the burn (Table 5.12) and the time taken to achieve skin coverage, along with inevitable episodes of septicaemia. Increased production of catabolic hormones (adrenaline, noradrenaline, glucagon and the corticosteroids) leads to hypermetabolism, accelerated protein and fat breakdown and altered carbohydrate metabolism (Fig 5.5). The abnormalities of carbohydrate metabolism include elevated glucose levels, increased gluconeogenesis, altered insulin levels and profound insulin resistance. All are attributable to the hormonal imbalance which suppresses the influence of insulin on peripheral tissues (Davies 1977; Richards 1977; Wilmore and McDougal 1977).

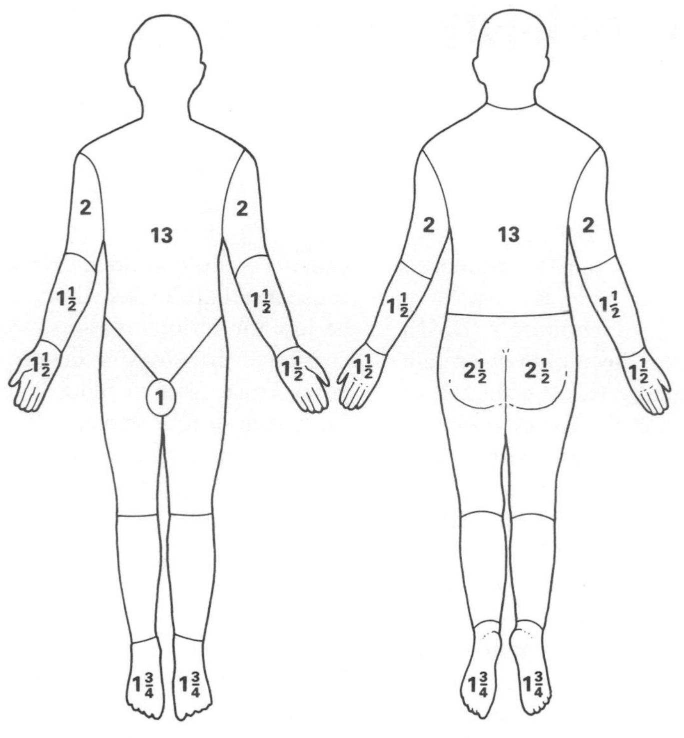

Age	Age (years)					
	0	1	5	10	15	Adult
Head and neck	21	19	15	13	11	9
Thigh	$5\frac{1}{2}$	$6\frac{1}{2}$	8	9	9	$9\frac{1}{2}$
Calf	5	5	$5\frac{1}{2}$	6	$6\frac{1}{2}$	7

Fig. 5.4 Percentage of different parts of the body at various ages. Harvey Kemble and Lamb (1984). Reproduced with permission.

Septicaemia will further accentuate post-injury glucose intolerance necessitating large doses of insulin, but this requirement drops rapidly if treatment of sepsis is successful (Woolfson *et al* 1977). Insulin resistance occurs in severe trauma or infection, hence the name 'stress diabetes' or 'diabetes of trauma'. However the patient seldom exhibits ketoacidosis so it is sometimes called 'pseudodiabetes'. More insulin, and not a reduction in nutrient intake, is required to treat the hyperglycaemia, but it may be worth rechecking calculations to see whether an overestimation of energy requirement has been made (was the correct weight used?)

Maximum catabolic response usually occurs 5–10 days post-burn. Thereafter healing of partial thickness burns and early excision and grafting of deep burns reduce wound size and thus the exogenous demand for nutrients.

Anabolic phase

Provided no weight loss has occurred, intakes can return to normal levels as healing progresses. Soroff *et al* (1961) showed that patients with major burn injuries were entering an 'anabolic' phase by 30 days post-burn. However synthesis of lean body mass may require extra vitamin and mineral supplementation. Burn contractures of the lips

Table 5.12 Burn wounds

	Superficial	Partial thickness	Full thickness
Depth of burn	Epidermis only	Some of dermis	All of dermis
Healing time	3–10 days	10–14 days	Many months or never
Scarring	No	Deep burns likely to produce scarring and contractures	Contractures unless grafted
Skin grafting	No	Deep burns may need grafting	Large areas need grafting

Pressure or infection may convert a partial thickness burn into a full thickness burn

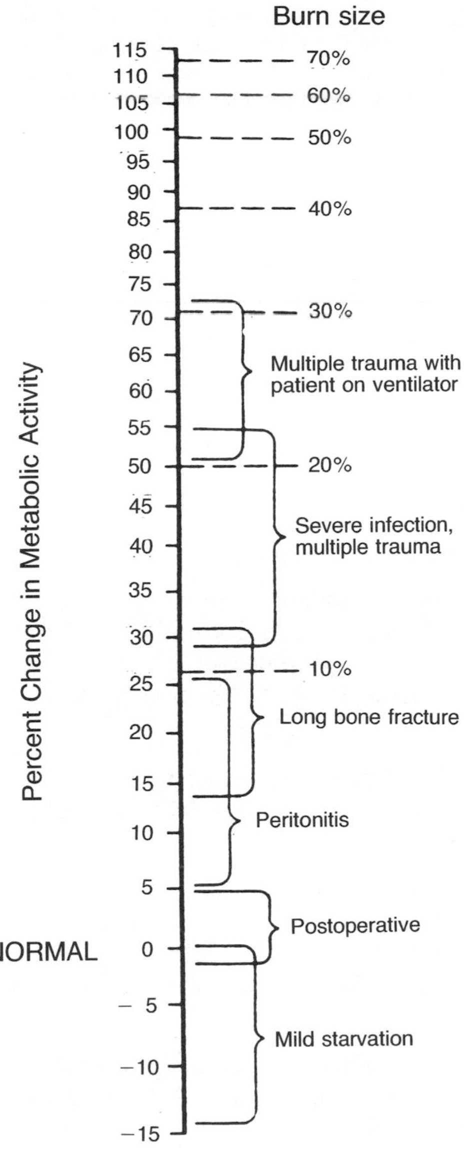

Fig. 5.5 Increase in metabolic activity following injury or infection. Wilmore and McDougal (1977). Reproduced with permission.

may make the wearing of dentures impossible, or hypertrophic scarring of the cheeks may cause discomfort by rubbing against dentures.

Water and nutrient losses

Urine

Increased urinary urea is the principal route of nitrogen loss. Other non-urea nitrogen compounds are also increased in the urine.

Exudate

Fluid loss from a burn wound may be considerable and may contain 4–6 g protein/100 ml representing 25–50% of total nitrogen loss (Molnar *et al* 1983). Exudate losses vary in a patient from day to day. This loss cannot be measured routinely in burn units so it has to be estimated. Davies (1977) has reviewed the literature and suggests a figure of 0.2 g N/% burn/day for the first week post-burn. Subsequently the losses decrease as healing progresses. The exudate nitrogen loss from partial thickness burns rapidly decreases to 0.1 g N/% burn/day. When the burns are extensive and full thickness so that virtually no healing occurs, the exudate losses continue at 0.2 g N/% burn/day until the eschar (burned layer of skin) separates to reveal granulating tissue.

Evaporation

Burn patients lack the water impermeable barrier of the skin over large areas of their body. Evaporation losses are therefore high, despite attempts to reduce energy losses as heat by nursing in a warm, dry environment. Wilmore and McDougal (1977) estimate the evaporative water loss using the formula: (25 + % burn) × body surface area in m^2 = ml water lost/hour. This formula is in agreement with the finding of Micheels and Sorenson (1983) that a healthy non-burned volunteer on a Clinitron (air fluidized) bed lost 63.5 ml/hour/m^2. With burn injury the loss may be increased to 3 litres/day.

Faecal

Nitrogen losses via the faecal route are 1–3 g N/day (Davies 1977) and relatively small compared to urine and exudate losses. They will increase if the patient suffers from diarrhoea.

Vitamins and minerals

With loss of skin tissue, increased muscle breakdown and increased fluid throughput, vitamin and mineral losses are likely to exceed the DRV for non-stressed individuals. However there are no firm recommendations for replacement in burn patients (Molnar *et al* 1983). The following should be borne in mind:

1 Vitamin C has a known role in collagen synthesis. Recommendations suggest total daily intakes of 300–1000 mg/day.

2 High intakes of energy, either enterally or parenterally, lead to an proportionally increased demand for B vitamins.

3 Vitamin A deficiency may play a role in causing stress ulcers due to thinning of the gut epithelium (Molnar *et al* 1983; Gottschlich 1989).

4 Iron supplements are often given in an attempt to increase haemoglobin levels.

5 Twenty per cent of body zinc is found in skin so burns inevitably cause zinc loss. Zinc losses in urine are also increased as a result of muscle breakdown. Zinc is a

constituent of many metalloenzymes and important in DNA/RNA synthesis (Kay 1981).

The Burn Interest Group of the BDA recommends giving twice the DRV of the remaining vitamins and minerals to avoid any potential problems with overdosage. Most enteral feeds suitable for major burn patients provide approximately this level in two litres of feed and often contain more than twice the DRV of the nutrients listed above. The Burn Interest Group considers that, with the possible exception of vitamin C, additional supplementation is unnecessary and results in an unbalanced intake which potentially interferes with the absorption of other nutrients (e.g. Zn/Cu interaction).

For minor burn and convalescence patients, the DRVs for an adult can be provided by 4 Ensure Plus (1200 kcal, 50 g protein) or 5 Fortimel (1000 kcal, 100 g protein) per day.

Estimating nutritional requirements

Many formulae have been devised to assess the energy and protein required to prevent weight loss in burns (Davies 1977). None take into account all the factors which affect requirements – weight, sex, height, percentage burn, percentage deep burn, respiratory involvement, activity level, infection and other injuries. Estimates of requirements must be regarded only as guidelines for intake which must be tailored for each individual patient.

However even with massive burns it is rare for a patient's resting metabolic expenditure (RME) to exceed twice basal metabolic rate (BMR) as this seems to be the limit set by the cardiovascular and respiratory systems (Fig. 5.6). Molnar *et al* (1983) suggest giving energy at BMR × 2 (Burke's formula) to minimize weight loss irrespective of burn size. This formula depends on knowing the patient's body surface area (see Appendix 4, Fig. 7.3) and age and uses a table to determine BMR. A pocket computer is now available which can calculate BMR (Colley *et al* 1985). As no account is taken of burn size, the formula may overestimate requirements for small burns, however Molnar *et al* (1983) argue that there is an inverse relationship between physical activity and burn size which makes the formula valid for smaller burns. They base BMR on ideal weight for height to allow for malnourished patients who would otherwise be underfed and obese patients who likewise would be overfed.

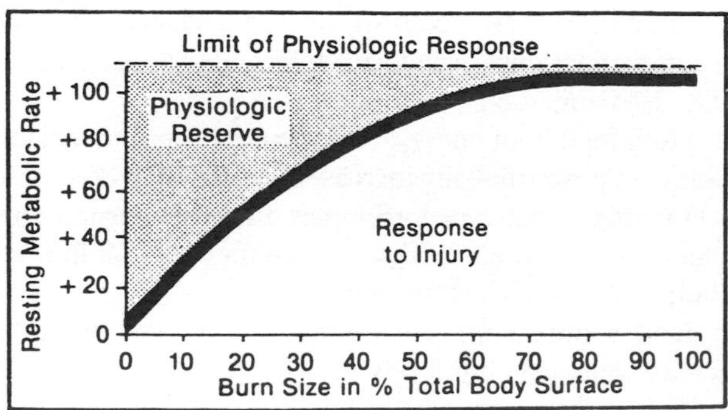

Fig. 5.6 Response to burn injury as a function of injury severity (Wilmore 1976). Reproduced with permission.

Example using Burke's formula:

70 kg male, 5′10″, 25 yrs, 30% burn
BMR = 1664 kcal BMR × 2 = 3328 kcal

60 kg female, 5′6″, 25 yrs, 30% burn
BMR = 1371 kcal BMR × 2 = 2742 kcal

The Sutherland formula (1987) is widely used:

Energy requirement = 20 kcal (84 kJ)/kg + 50 kcal (210 kJ) per % burn
Protein requirement = 1 g/kg + 2 g per % burn.

Example using Sutherland formula:

For 70 kg patient with 30% burn
Energy requirement = (20 × 70) + (50 × 30)
= 2900 kcal
Protein requirement = (1 × 70) + (2 × 30)
= 130 g

Other formulae depend on adding various activity and injury factors on to BMR e.g. Elia (1982), Schofield (1985) (Tables 5.13, 14 and 15).

E.g. 70 kg male, 30% burn, 25 yrs:
18–30 yrs 15 × 70 kg + 690 = 1740 kcal = BMR
Adjust BMR for 'stress': 1740 + 50% = 2610 kcal
Adjust for being 'bedbound but mobile': 2610 + 30% = 3393 kcal.

However actual measurements of energy expenditure (by indirect calorimetry) usually show a lower total than that derived from formulae.

Nasoenteric feeding of burn patients

The majority of burn units in the UK use either Clinifeed Extra or Fresubin 750 MCT for hypercatabolic patients. Both feeds are near isotonic but do require additional water be given to the patient (especially if the patient is ventilated) to fulfil water requirements as they are energy-

Table 5.13 Basal metabolic rate in the adult

Age (yrs)	Basal metabolic rate (kcal) Male	Female
15–18	17.6 × wt (kg) + 656	13.3 × wt (kg) + 690
18–30	15 × wt (kg) + 690	14.8 × wt (kg) + 485
30–60	11.4 × wt (kg) + 870	8.1 × wt (kg) + 842
>60	11.7 × wt (kg) + 585	9 × wt (kg) + 656

After Schofield (1985)

Table 5.14 Increase in metabolic rate with size of burn

Burn size (% BSA)	% increase in metabolic rate	'Equivalent injuries'
10	20	Long bone fracture Moderate infection
20	40	Multiple injuries Severe infection
30	50	Multiple injuries/
40	60	severe infection with
50	70	patient on ventilator
60	80	
70	90	

From Elia (1982). Reproduced with permission from Churchill Livingstone

Table 5.15 Estimation of energy requirements in the adult

1 Determine basal metabolic rate
2 Adjust basal metabolic rate for stress
3 Adjust metabolic rate (stress) for 24 h energy expenditure:
  (a) 'Immobile' +20%
  (b) Bed bound but mobile +30%
  (c) Mobile in ward +40%

Modified from Elia (1982). Reproduced with permision from Churchill Livingstone

dense (>1 kcal/ml) and contain 80% water. Water can be given orally, nasoentericaliy or parenterally (as 5% dextrose).

Protein

Whole protein is more advantageous than either parenteral/enteral amino acid based or peptide based feeds, as well as considerably cheaper (Alexander and Gottschlich 1990). There is no place for routine use of elemental feeds in burn therapy (Wilmore and McDougal 1977). Some amino acids added to whole protein may improve the response to nutrition, such as arginine, histidine and cysteine (Alexander and Gottschlich 1990) or leucine (King and Power 1990). Burn patients use protein to provide around 20% of their energy expenditure so a suitable feed must provide this high protein: energy ratio (NPE:N of 100:1).

Lipid

The lipid component is often supplied by either corn or sunflower oil, both high in linoleic acid which is an essential fatty acid (EFA) of the omega-6 family. However many burn feeds now contain medium chain triglycerides (MCTs) in substantial quantities because of advantages such as preferential usage in stress-adapted metabolism (Cerra *et al* 1980). Recent research (Alexander *et al* 1986) points to the use of fish oil (eicosapentaenoic acid, an EFA of the omega-3 family) as being capable of reducing the hypermetabolic response and boosting immunocompetence, omega-6 EFA being possibly immunosuppressive. Artificially 'structured' lipids of MCT/fish oil appear to reduce the metabolic response compared with conventional lipid (Teo *et al* 1989), as do MCT/LCT structured lipids (DeMichele *et al* 1989) and future burn feed formulations may include such lipids.

Carbohydrate

Glucose polymers form a smaller proportion of the energy content of burn feeds than standard feeds because of the inability of burn patients to oxidize large amounts of glucose. Lipid is increased to make good this energy shortfall so burn feeds contain approximately 45% carbohydrate, 35% lipid and 20% protein. The lower carbohydrate content reduces the osmolarity of these energy-dense feeds to close to isotonicity.

Further considerations

Diluting the feed does not reduce the incidence of nausea and diarrhoea but does reduce nutrient intake at a vital time. Diarrhoea is associated with the use of antibiotics during enteral feeding (Keohane *et al* 1984). Hopefully drugs causing the problem can be stopped or alternatives prescribed. The feed is usually started at less than full rate (i.e. 50 ml/h for several hours) although this obviously leads to a reduced intake over that day.

Enteral pumps enable volumes exceeding 3 l/day to be given via a 1.5 mm internal diameter enteric tube. Even patients with severe facial burns can tolerate these tubes. Enteral feeding should continue until only small areas of burn are left to heal. If problems such as extensive weight loss, poorly healing wounds or graft rejection occur, enteral feeding should continue.

Constipation may occur due to side effects of analgesia or lack of dietary fibre in a milk-based feed. Long term enteral feeding with no oral intake of dietary fibre can lead to diarrhoea, constipation or faecal impaction with 'overflow' diarrhoea. Use of a feed containing soya bran may alleviate these problems.

Feeding gastrostomies have been described for burn patients (Kahn *et al* 1984).

Parenteral feeding (see Section 1.15)

Despite the risk of septicaemia, in the case of prolonged paralytic ileus there may be no choice other than to feed parenterally. The same nutritional principles should apply to total parental nutrition (TPN) as to enteral feeding. Total nitrogen input should, if possible, exceed total nitrogen output.

Fat-free regimens should be discouraged as the burns patient cannot oxidize glucose at as great a rate as healthy individuals. If glucose intake exceeds the maximal oxidation rate (Table 5.16), fat is synthesized. This is an energy-

Table 5.16 Maximal glucose oxidation rate for 70 kg male

	Rate (mg/kg/minute)	Maximum amount of glucose which can be metabolized in 24 hours
Non-burned	7	706 g
Burned	5	504 g

consuming process and large volumes of CO_2 are produced raising the respiratory quotient which may be dangerous to patients with pulmonary insufficiency. Overfeeding is known to increase metabolic rates in both normal and hypermetabolic humans. It is possible that extremely high energy intakes of 8–10 000 kcal (33–42 MJ)/day given to burns patients in the past may have contributed in part to the high measured metabolic rates (Molnar *et al* 1983). Synthesis of inappropriate quantities of fat from glucose can lead to fatty liver which in the past was thought to be caused by intravenously administered fat. In fact Intralipid has been used for many years in burns patients without apparent ill effect. Apart from supplying essential fatty acids one litre of Intralipid (20%) supplies 2000 kcal (8.4 MJ) and can be given peripherally (Davies 1977).

Many intravenous regimens have too high a NPE:N ratio for burns patients. Vitamin and mineral preparations often provide only basal requirements for healthy adults, not catabolic patients.

Monitoring progress

Morath *et al* (1983) reviewed the problems of monitoring nutritional therapy in burns patients and concluded that no single parameter indicates short term nutritional status but that regular repeated measurements can indicate trends (Table 5.17).

Body weight

Oedema during the resuscitation period increases body weight by at least 10%. 'Dry weight' occurs some 14 days post-burn so weight measured before 14 days is distorted by oedema. Thereafter accurate repeated measurements of body weight help to assess nutritional therapy. Exudate soaked dressings invalidate daily weighing so the patient is weighed in dressings before the dressings are changed.

Table 5.17 Post-burn nutritional monitoring

Test	Frequency
24-hour urine collection	Daily
Maximum body temperature	Daily
Nutrient record	Daily
Body weight	When dressings are changed
Serum urea and electrolytes	Twice weekly
Serum transferrin	Twice weekly
Liver function tests	Twice monthly

Discarded dressings are collected in a plastic bag and weighed to give an accurate body weight.

Nutrient intake

Food and drink consumed should be recorded by nursing staff. Total intake can be calculated from oral, enteral and parenteral records and compared to predicted requirements. Administered blood products are not usually included in nutrient totals.

Serum proteins

Serum albumin decreases very quickly post-burn and is slow to reflect improvement in nutritional status due to its long half life (20 days). Transferrin has a shorter high life (eight days) and may be a more sensitive short term indicator of nutritional status. Ogle and Alexander (1982) have found that transferrin levels of less than 2 g/litre are associated with an increased incidence of bacteraemia in burns.

Urinary urea

Urinary urea is the yardstick used to estimate stress. Twenty-four hour urinary urea nitrogen indicates internal nitrogen metabolism (Lee and Hartley 1975). However, nitrogen output depends on both nitrogen intake and nitrogen retention, and the latter is influenced by the magnitude of catabolic stress. The catabolic index (Bistrian 1979) indicates the magnitude of this stress.

Catabolic index: urinary urea nitrogen − (0.5 × dietary nitrogen + 3 g)
A value of <0 indicates no stress
0–5 indicates moderate stress
>5 indicates severe stress.

This assumes that 50% of ingested protein is catabolized via gluconeogenesis. The constant (3 g) added for non-urea nitrogen loss will almost always underestimate true losses in burns due to exudation, nonetheless the catabolic index usefully indicates the change from stressed to non-stressed status.

Daily maximum body temperature

All the above tests give results retrospectively. A test is needed which is more immediately and freely available to all burn units. Body temperature indicates the extent of hypermetabolism at any given time. Each 1°C above normal produces a 10–12% rise in BMR.

5.4.4 Electrical burns

Care must be taken with the nutrition of patients with high voltage electrical injury. In addition to surface burn injury

Table 5.18 Energy and nitrogen requirements in the burned child

Age (yrs)	kcal/kg.		Nitrogen*/kg.	
	<20% burn	>20% burn	<20% burn	>20% burn
0–1	125	150	0.45	0.5
1–8	100	125	0.3	0.45
8–15	75	100	0.25	0.3

From Grotte *et al* (1982). Reproduced with permission from Churchill Livingstone
* Multiply nitrogen figure by 6.25 to obtain grams of protein

(entry and exit points) conduction through the body causes destruction of the underlying nerves, blood vessels, muscles, bones, tendons and visceral coverings. The more resistant the tissue, the more heat is generated as current flows through it (Diamond *et al* 1982) thus muscle close to bone may be necrosed. A high urinary urea output in these patients indicates that severe damage has occurred (Balogh and Bauer 1982). Burns feeding formulae based on percentage burn will underestimate the amount of nutrients required by these patients.

5.4.5 Burn injury in children

Children have a higher BMR than adults and a greater requirement for protein per kg body weight. Burn injury does not raise RME proportionally as much in children as in adults and when normally active children are confined to bed by burn injury, this saving in energy output partially offsets the increase in RME. If on average the EAR for a non-burned child can be achieved, weight loss can, in theory, be curtailed. For example:

2 yr female, 30% scald, 12.5 kg (50th percentile)
EAR for energy = (95 kcal × 12.5) = 1180 kcal
RNI for protein = (1.1 × 12.5) = 13.8 g protein.

This will provide 4.6% energy from protein.

However the increase in catabolism in these patients suggests that more energy and protein is required, and that protein should provide a greater proportion of the energy. The formula proposed by Grotte *et al* (1982) provides a convenient method of calculating requirements in the burned child (Table 5.18). Using the above example the Grotte formula gives 1563 kcal and 35.2 g protein (providing 9% of energy).

Alternatively, feeding a child with extensive burns who is on the 50th centile for weight and height as though she or he is on the 97th centile requires even less calculation:

50th centile 12.5 kg child = 1180 kcal
97th centile 15.0 kg child = 1425 kcal.

In the past the formula of Sutherland and Batchelor (1968) has provided a useful guideline for feeding burned children under 10 years old:

Energy = 60 kcal (252 kJ) per kg + 35 kcal (147 kJ) per % burn
Protein = 3 g per kg + 1 g per % burn.

This gives 1800 kcal, 67.5 g protein = 15% energy from protein using the above example.

Enteral feeding of children aged 1–6 years with large burns can be successfully carried out using Paediasure (Ross) or Nutrison Paediatric (Cow & Gate Nutricia). Protein supplies approximately 12% of the energy content, whereas some authorities recommend up to 23% (Alexander *et al* 1980).

Enteral feeding can often be avoided in burned children provided they will drink milky supplements. Milk can be fortified with dried milk powder (30 g to 500 ml). Alternatively Build Up reconstituted with milk can be given, provided it is diluted with an equal quantity of water to reduce the osmolarity. Both will boost protein intakes in burned children.

References

Alexander JW and Gottschlich MM (1990) Nutritional immunomodulation in burn patients. *Crit Care Med* **18**(2), S149–153.

Alexander JW, Macmillan BG, Stinnet JD, Ogle CK, Bozian RC, Fischer JF, Oakes JB, Morris MJ and Krummel R (1980) Beneficial effects of aggressive protein feeding in severely burned children. *Ann Surg* **193**(4), 505–16.

Alexander JW, Saito H, Ogle CK and Trocki O (1986) The importance of lipid type in the diet after burn injury. *Ann Surg* **204**(1), 1–8.

Balogh D and Bauer M (1982) Determination of catabolism in the burns patient. *Chir Plastica* **7**, 67–74.

Bistrian BR (1979) A simple technique to estimate the severity of stress. *Surg Gynaecol Obstet* **148**, 675–8.

Cerra FB, Siegel JH, Coleman B, Border MD & McMenamy RR (1980) Septic autocannibalism. A failure to provide exogenous nutritional support. *Ann Surg* **192**(4), 570–79.

Colley CM, Fleck A and Howard JP (1985) The pocket computer – a new aid to nutritional support. *Br Med J* **290**, 1403–6.

Davenport PJ (1979) Nutritional support in severe burns. *Res Clin Forums* **1**(1), 79–82.

Davies JWL (1977) The nutrition of patients with burns. In *Nutritional aspects of care of the critically ill*, Richards JR and Kinney JM (Eds) pp. 595–623. Churchill Livingstone, Edinburgh.

DeMichele SJ, Karlstaad MD, Bistrian BR, Istafan N, Babayan VK and Blackburn GL (1989) Enteral nutrition with structured lipids: effect on protein metabolism in thermal injury. *Am J Clin Nutr* **50**, 1295–302.

Diamond TH, Twomey A and Myburgh DF (1982) High voltage electrical injury. *S A Med J* **27**, 318–21.

Elia M (1982) Effect of nitrogen and energy intake on the metabolism of normal, depleted and injured man. *Clin Nutr* **1**, 173.

Gottschlich MM (1989) Micronutrients. In *Dietitian's handbook of enteral and parenteral nutrition*, Slipper A (Ed), ASPEN Publishers Inc, New York.

Grotte G, Meurling S and Wretling A (1982) Parenteral nutrition. In *Textbook of paediatric nutrition* McClaren DS and Burman D (Eds) pp. 228–58. Churchill Livingstone, Edinburgh.

Harvey Kemble JV and Lamb BE (1984) *Plastic surgical and burns nursing (current nursing practice)*. pp. 236. Baillière Tindall, Eastborne.

Inoue S, Lukes S, Alexander JW, Trocki O and Silberstein EB (1989) Increased gut blood flow with early enteral feeding in burned guinea-pigs. *J Burn Care Rehab* **10**(4), 300–308.

Kahn AM, Kross ME and Geller FM (1984) Feeding gastrostomy for the severely burned patient. *Arch Surg* **119**, 1316–17.

Kay RG (1981) Zinc and copper in human nutrition. *J Hum Nutr* **35**(1), 25–36.

Keohane PP, Attrill H, Love M, Frost P and Silk DBA (1984) Relation between osmolarity of diet and gastrointestinal side effects in enteral nutrition. *Br Med J* **288**, 678–80.

King P and Power DM (1990) Branched chain amino/keto acid supplementation following severe burn injury: a preliminary report. *Clin Nutr* **9**, 226–30.

Lee HA and Hartley TF (1975) A method of determining daily nitrogen requirements. *Postgrad Med J* **51**, 441–5.

Micheels J & Sorensen B (1983) The physiology of a healthy normal person in the air-fluidised bed. *Burns* **9**, 158–68.

Mochizuki H, Trocki O, Dominoni L, Brackett KA, Joffe SN and Alexander JW (1984) Mechanism of prevention of postburn hypermetabolism and catabolism by early enteral feeding. *Ann Surg* **200**(3), 297–308.

Molnar JA, Wolfe RR and Burke JF (1983) Burns: metabolism and nutritional therapy in thermal injury. In *Nutritional support of medical practice* Schneider HA, Anderson CE and Cousin DB (Eds) 2e. pp. 260–81. Harper & Row, Philadelphia.

Morath MA, Miller SF, Finley RK and Jones LM (1983) Interpretation of nutritional parameters in burns patients. *J Burn Care Rehab* **4**(5), 361–6.

Ogle CK and Alexander JW (1982) The relationship between bacteremia to levels of transferrin and total serum protein in burns patients. *Burns* **8**, 32–8.

Richards JR (1977) Metabolic responses to injury and starvation. An overview. In *Nutritional aspects of care in the critically ill*, Richards JR and Kinney JM (Eds) pp. 273–302. Churchill Livingstone, Edinburgh.

Schofield WN (1985) Predicting basal metabolic rate, new standards and review of previous work. *Hum Nutr Clin Nutr* **39** (Supp 1), 5.

Soroff HS, Pearson E and Artz CP (1961) An estimation of the nitrogen requirements for equilibrium in burned patients. *Surg Gynae Obstet* **112**, 159–72.

Sutherland AB (1987) Nutrition of the burn patient. *Clinical Anaesthesiology* **1**(3), 663–71.

Sutherland AB and Batchelor ADC (1968) Nitrogen balance in burned children. *Ann NY Academy of Sciences* **150**, 700.

Teo TC, DeMichele SJ, Selleck KM, Babayan VK, Blackburn GL and Bistrian BR (1989) Administration of structural lipid composed of MCT and fish oil reduces net protein catabolism in enterally fed burned rats. *Ann Surg* **210**(1), 100–107.

Tobiason J, Hiebert JM and Edlich RF (1982) A practical burn severity index. *J Burn Care Rehab* **3**(4), 229–32.

Wilmore DW (1976) Hormonal responses and their effect on metabolism. *Surg Clin N Am*, **56**(5), 999–1018.

Wilmore DW (1977) *Metabolic management of the critically ill*, 3e. Plenum, New York.

Wilmore DW and McDougal WS (1977) Nutrition in burns. In *Nutritional aspects of care in the critically ill*, Richards JR and Kinney JM (Eds) pp. 583–94. Churchill Livingstone, Edinburgh.

Woolfson AMJ, Heatley RV and Allison SP (1977) Significance of insulin in the metabolic response to injury. In *Nutritional aspects of care in the critically ill*, Richards JR and Kinney JM (Eds) pp. 367–88. Churchill Livingstone, Edinburgh.

5.5 Surgery

5.5.1 Pre- and post-operative malnutrition

The term protein-energy malnutrition is usually associated with victims of starvation in underdeveloped countries and in particular, with malnourished children. However, it has been shown (Bistrian *et al* 1974; Hill *et al* 1977) that 40–50% of surgical patients in British and American hospitals have signs of protein-energy malnutrition after one week or more following surgery.

The following hypothetical example demonstrates how rapidly an energy deficit can build up in a patient who is not eating if the nutritional needs are ignored.

Female, age 35 yrs, weight 58 kg, maintained on 2 litres 5% dextrose daily for seven days after operation

Energy input	= 100 g dextrose		
	× 3.75 kcal		
	× 7 days	=	2625 kcal
Energy output	= 1315 kcal (Schofield BMR)		
	× 1.2 activity factor		
	× 1.2 injury factor		
	× 7 days	=	13 225 kcal

The deficit of nearly 10 600 kcal represents around 1.2 kg of adipose tissue or 10 kg of lean tissue.

The most fundamental nutritional requirement of the body is for energy. In surgical patients, energy requirement is usually above the normal range whereas their energy intake frequently falls below it.

Most surgical patients are anxious and unsure about the surgical procedure they are to undergo. Suddenly their surroundings have changed, friends and relatives are absent and the foods offered and methods of meal service are all very different. In addition, many patients need to be 'nil by mouth' for some periods of time due to peri-operative investigations. Physical difficulty with eating, pain, nausea and diarrhoea all affect a patient's ability to consume an adequate diet. Malnutrition can occur both pre- and post-operatively.

Pre-operative malnutrition

This may be due to a number of causes, e.g. poor appetite, dysphagia, prolonged malabsorption, malignancy or inflammatory bowel disease, and repeated pre-operative investigations.

Post-operative malnutrition

This is not a risk in all surgical patients and many patients can withstand a short stay in hospital for minor surgery with an inadequate intake of protein and calories and the consequent weight loss without becoming wasted. If major surgery is undertaken, malnutrition is more likely to occur if:

1 Pre-operative malnutrition existed.
2 Oral intake is withheld or refused post-operatively for more than 5–7 days.
3 Post-operative complications occur, e.g. sepsis, wound breakdown, ileus.

From a nutritional point of view, malnourished surgical patients may be classified into four groups and their nutritional requirements must be assessed accordingly (Elwyn 1980):

1 Depleted.
2 Hypercatabolic.
3 Hypercatabolic and depleted.
4 Chronic malabsorption.

5.5.2 The significance of undernutrition in surgical patients

The objectives of nutritional support in surgical patients are:

1 To enhance wound healing.
2 To reduce post-operative complications.
3 To reduce the period of convalescence.
4 To prevent further deterioration of the nutritional state.

Some controversy exists regarding the benefit of pre- and post-operative nutritional support and its effect on morbidity and mortality. However, protein-energy malnutrition in hospital patients has been associated with impaired cell-mediated immunity (Bistrian *et al* 1975) and prolonged post-operative recovery (Goode and Hawkins 1978). It may also reduce pulmonary function and increase the risk of the surgical procedure itself.

Peri-operative nutritional support has been shown to reduce significantly the incidence of wound infections (Williams *et al* 1977) and to improve the rate of wound healing (Moghissi *et al* 1977). Jeejeebhoy (1985) demonstrated that nutritional support improved muscle function and Bastow *et al* (1985) clearly showed that overnight nasogastric feeding of malnourished patients with a fractured femur improved their mobility and rehabilitation, increased their voluntary food intake and reduced their period of hospitalization.

5.5.3 Identification of patients at risk

Early identification of those patients with existing malnutrition and those likely to become malnourished is most important.

Routine pre-operative nutritional assessment and monitoring should be undertaken on all surgical patients by nursing and dietetic staff and include at least the following observations

1 Record of body weight – both on admission and regularly thereafter. Any recent marked loss of body weight should be noted.

2 Diet history – to include a brief account of any eating problems and loss of appetite.

3 Supervision of meal choice and assistance with eating if required.

4 Observation of food and fluids consumed – keeping an accurate record of nutritional intake if requested.

These simple measures, together with routine biochemical and haematological tests, and an understanding of the underlying medical conditional and surgical procedure can help to identify at an early stage those patients in need of nutritional support.

5.5.4 Methods of improving the nutritional status of surgical patients

Enteral and parenteral nutritional support techniques are discussed in detail in Sections 1.13 and 1.15.

Introduction of post-operative oral fluids and diet

After a general anaesthetic, gastric motility is reduced and emptying is delayed. If gastrointestinal surgery has been undertaken, normal gut function may be slow to return. Oral fluids and food are usually withheld until the surgeon feels that gastric emptying and gut function are returning. Initially, the patient may only be offered sips of water. Small volumes, e.g. 15 ml and 30 ml may then be given hourly and if tolerated the volume is increased gradually over a few days. During this stage, fluid requirements but not nutritional requirements are met by intravenous infusion of saline and/or dextrose (2 litres of 5% dextrose provides a mere 400 kcal). Once the patient is taking fluids freely throughout the day, intravenous fluids can be reduced or discontinued and the patient can progress via soup and light sweet at lunch and supper to a light diet plus nutritional supplements if indicated. Throughout this time an accurate daily record of fluid balance should be kept.

Following other types of surgery, oral diet may well be given on the first post-operative day. However, Manners (1974) and Walesby *et al* (1979) reported very low energy and protein intakes in patients following cardiopulmonary bypass surgery, and post-operative anorexia is frequently seen on general surgical wards.

Monitoring

Regular monitoring of the patient's fluid intake and output, body weight, haematology, and serum and urinary biochemistry should be carried out throughout the hospital stay. This is discussed in detail in Section 1.11.

Most patients are discharged home before their natural appetite fully returns and dietetic advice and supervision should continue in the community and at follow-up clinics whenever possible.

Obesity and surgery

Gross obesity is associated with increased surgical risks in the case of elective surgery, severe obesity should be remedied beforehand by planned weight reduction over a period of time, rather than by short term crash dieting.

Obesity can mask underlying malnutrition and should not be used as a reason for withholding nutritional support in surgical patients if post-operative complications exist or if anthropometric and biochemical nutritional indices show evidence of deficiencies and malnutrition. The obesity should be treated at a later stage when the patient has fully recovered.

References

Bastow MD, Rawlings J and Allison SP (1985) Overnight nasogastric tube feeding. *Clin Nutr* **4**, 7–11.

Bistrian BR, Blackburn GL, Hallowell E and Heddle R (1974) Protein status of general surgical patients. *J Am Med Assoc* **230**, 858–60.

Bistrian BR, Blackburn GL, Scrimshaw NS and Flatt J (1975) Cellular immunity in semi-starved states in hospitalized adults. *Am J Clin Nutr* **28**, 1148–55.

Elwyn DH (1980) Nutritional requirements of adult surgical patients. *Crit Care Med* **8**, 9–20.

Goode AW and Hawkins T (1978) In *Advances in parenteral nutrition*, Johnston IDA (Ed) p. 557. MTP Press, Lancaster.

Hill GL, Blackett RL, Pickford I, Burkinshaw L, Young GA, Warren JV, Schorah CJ and Morgan DB (1977) Malnutrition in surgical patients: an unrecognized problem. *Lancet* **i**, 689–92.

Jeejeebhoy KN (1985) Changes in body composition and muscle function and effect of nutritional support. *Proceedings of the 4th World Congress on Intensive Critical Care Medicine*. p. 161.

Manners JM (1974) Nutrition after cardiac surgery. *Anaesthesia* **29**, 675–88.

Moghissi K, Hornshaw J, Teasdale PR and Dawes EA (1977) Parenteral nutrition in carcinoma of the oesophagus treated by surgery: nitrogen balance and clinical studies. *Br J Surg* **64**, 125–8.

Walesby RK, Goode AW, Spinks TJ, Herring A, Ranicar AS and Bentall HH (1979) Nutritional status of patients requiring cardiac surgery. *J Thorac Cardiovasc Surg* **77**, 570–76.

Williams RHP, Heatley RV, Lewis MH and Hughes LE (1977) In *Clinical parenteral nutrition*, Baxter DH and Jackson GM (Eds) p. 52. Geistlich Education, Chester.

5.6 Pressure sores

Pressure sores are a serious and costly problem (*Lancet* 1982). They can cause great pain and distress to the patient, may significantly extend the length of a hospital stay and, if severe, may lead to life-threatening complications such as septicaemia.

5.6.1 Aetiology of pressure sores

Pressure sores or decubitus ulcers are primarily caused by unrelieved pressure. Sustained pressure, without periodic relief, causes damage to the local micro-circulation leading to hypoxia and tissue necrosis (Fig. 5.7). Other factors, predominantly shearing forces, friction and moisture, contribute to sore development by providing indirect pressure, increased friction and breakdown of the skin's integrity. A number of secondary factors have also been identified (Table 5.19); the contribution each makes to the development of sores will vary according to individual circumstances.

Areas of the body where skin lies over a bony prominence, and which are not adapted for weight-bearing over prolonged periods, are most susceptible to pressure sore development. These include the back of the head, the spines of the scapulae, the sides of the ankles (malleoli), the great trochanters, elbows, heels and the lower sacrum (Fig. 5.8).

Individuals who are particularly at risk are those who are unconscious and/or immobile, e.g. head and spinal injury patients, orthopaedic patients, those with a physical handicap, the elderly and the chronically ill.

Pressure sores can be classified into five grades according to their developmental stage (Waterlow 1977) (Table 5.20).

5.6.2 Nutritional aspects of pressure sore development

Nutrition has an important role in both the prevention and treatment of pressure sores. Malnutrition and specific nutrient deficiencies compromise the body's wound healing process while the overall effects of poor nutritional intake may increase an individual's susceptibility to pressure sore development.

Energy

Fat stores provide cushioning against pressure. Weight loss and muscle atrophy, resulting from an inadequate energy intake, reduce the effectiveness of the subcutaneous tissue as a mechanical padding between bones and skin and hence increase the likelihood of pressure sores.

Malnutrition also impairs the immune system and increases the likelihood of pressure sore development and risk of infection (Higgs 1987). If pyrexia and anorexia result, nutritional status may deteriorate further thus exacerbating this situation.

An adequate energy intake is also essential in order to prevent dietary and tissue protein being used as a source of energy.

Protein

Protein depletion states adversely affect the wound healing process (Mullholland *et al* 1943). Protein synthesis is reduced affecting the maturation of connective tissue and decreasing the wound's tensile strength.

The presence of oedema, particularly where oedematous tissue extends through the wound opening, may aggravate protein losses. A large wound may lose 90–100 g protein per day in this way.

During wound healing, protein requirements may rise to between 1.2–2.0 g per kg body weight per day in order to provide the protein necessary for protein synthesis and to achieve a positive nitrogen balance. Calculations should be based on actual body weight and exclude any weight increase due to the presence of oedema.

Fatty acids

Fatty acids are an essential component of cell membranes and dietary deficiency will inhibit tissue repair and wound healing.

Vitamins

The major vitamin implicated in the healing process is vitamin C. This is vital for collagen synthesis as it is an essential co-factor in the hydroxylation of proline.

When dietary intake of vitamin C is unrestricted and tissue levels are normal, wounds heal quite rapidly. Mega doses have little effect in accelerating wound healing and indeed may trigger a rebound deficiency causing breakdown of the initial sore when supplementation is discontinued (Tyrrell 1974).

Vitamins A and the B complex may also be important. Vitamin A, a co-factor in collagen synthesis, promotes epithelialization and granulation of healing wounds. The B

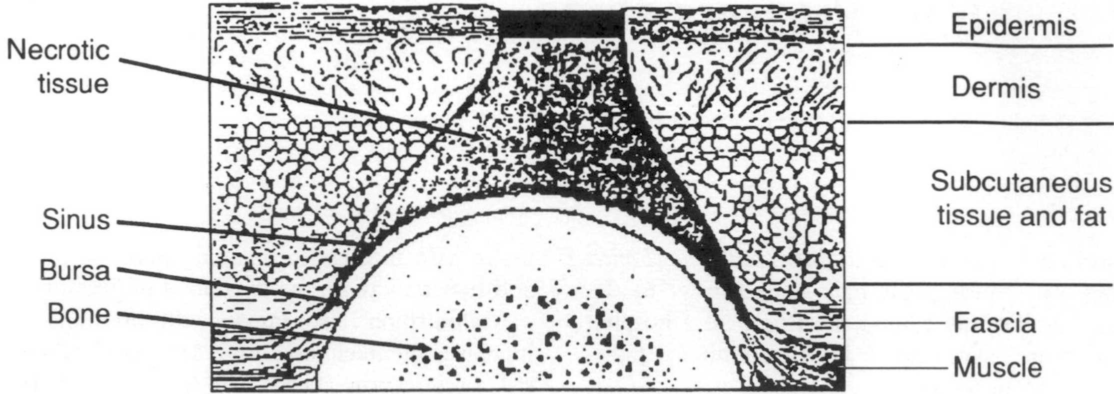

Fig. 5.7 Diagram of a necrotic pressure sore showing deep tissue destruction.

Supine

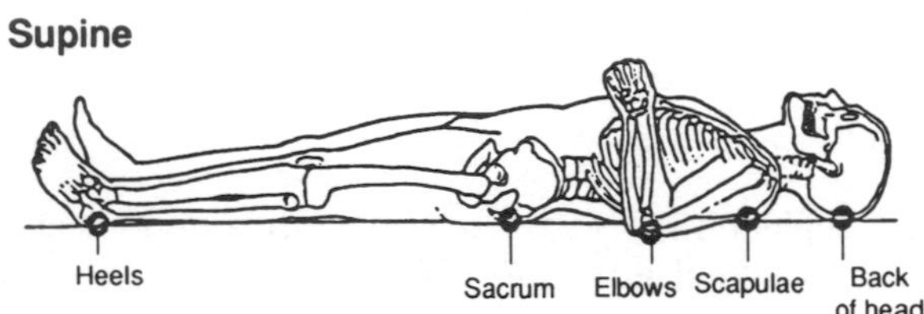

Side lying

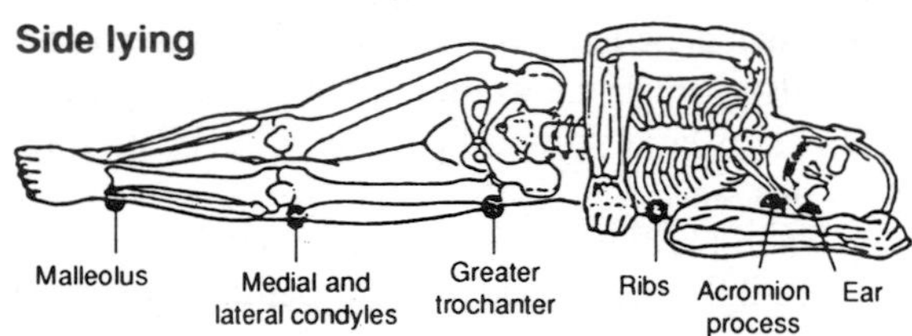

Prone

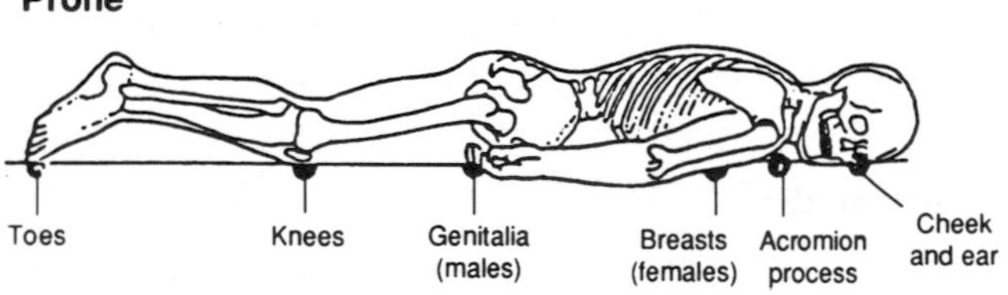

Fig. 5.8 Pressure points in various positions from Gruis and Innes (1976) Assessment essential to prevent pressure sores. *American Journal of Nursing*, November. Reproduced with permission.

vitamins affect enzyme activity in the metabolism of protein, fat and carbohydrate and may have a role in cellular immunity (Bobel 1987).

Minerals

Zinc deficiency inhibits wound repair by reducing the rate of epithelialization and cellular proliferation. The mineral is an essential co-factor in many enzyme systems. Low zinc levels have been directly associated with poor wound healing and inadequate tissue repair, and supplementation has promoted the healing process (Pories *et al* 1967; Hallbrook and Lanner 1972). However this effect has only been seen in those individuals who are biochemically zinc deficient (Weisman 1980).

Low haemoglobin levels are always seen in those with established pressure sores. Healing cannot occur until this is corrected since an adequate blood flow is essential at

Table 5.19 Factors involved in the aetiology of pressure sores

Primary	Secondary
Pressure	Immobility, and its duration
Shearing forces	Body weight
Friction	Infection
Moisture	Pyrexia
	Nutritional status
	Anaemia
	Neurological changes (e.g. loss of pain sensation)
	Medication
	Dehydration
	Age
	Chronic illness
	Iatrogenic (e.g. poor lifting technique, hard surfaces)

Table 5.20 Classification of pressure sores (Waterlow 1977)

Stage 1	Discolouration of skin with persistent erythema after pressure is released. (Blanching with light finger pressure indicates that the microcirculation is still intact.) A blister may be forming
Stage 2	Oedema, blistering, epidermal skin loss, with exposure of the dermis. Pain is present. Abrasions can cause this pressure sore
Stage 3	Loss of tissue through the dermis. The edge of the pressure sore is distinct and is surrounded by erythema and induration
Stage 4	Lesions extend into the subcutaneous tissue and may penetrate into the deep fascia and muscle. This presents initially as an area of bluish-black discolouration which turns into a black scar. After a few days this separates to reveal an underlying cavity formed by pressure destruction of deep tissue
Stage 5	Joints and body cavities may become involved, multiple sores may merge together. Infection and septicaemia can occur

Fig. 5.9 Examples of Pressure Sore Risk Assessment cards
(a) (left) Douglas pressure sore indicator.
(b) (below left) Waterlow pressure sore prevention/treatment policy.
(c) (bottom of page) Norton scale.

The Douglas Pressure Sore Risk Calculator

Score 18 or less = "At Risk"

Nutritional Status	
Well Balanced Diet	4
Inadequate Diet	3
Fluids only	2
Peripheral-parenteral feeding	1
Low Haemoglobin (<10)	1

Activity	
Fully mobile	4
Walk with difficulty	3
Chairbound	2
Bedfast	1

Incontinence	
Continent	4
Occasionally	3
Urine	2
Doubly	1

Pain	
Pain Free	4
Fear of pain	3
Periodic	2
Pain on movement	1
Continual Discomfort	0

Skin State	
Intact	4
Dry/red/thin	3
Superficial break	2
Full tissue thickness/cavity	1

Mental State	
Alert	4
Apathetic	3
Stuporous	2
Unco-operative	1
Comatose	0

Special risks: Deduct 2 for each of the following:-
Steroid therapy, diabetes, cytotoxic therapy, dyspnoea

WATERLOW RISK ASSESSMENT CARD

RING SCORES IN TABLE, ADD TOTAL
SEVERAL SCORES PER CATEGORY CAN BE USED

BUILD / WEIGHT FOR HEIGHT	•
AVERAGE	0
ABOVE AVERAGE	1
OBESE	2
BELOW AVERAGE	3
CONTINENCE	•
COMPLETE/CATHETERIZED	0
OCCASION INCONT.	1
CATH/INCONTINENT OF FAECES	2
DOUBLY INCONT.	3

RISK AREAS VISUAL SKIN TYPE	•
HEALTHY	0
TISSUE PAPER	1
DRY	2
OEDEMATOUS	3
CLAMMY T ⇑	4
DISCOLOURED	5
BROKEN/SPOT	6
MOBILITY	•
FULLY	1
RESTLESS/FIDGITY	2
APATHETIC	3
RESTRICTED	4
INERT/TRACTION BOUND	5
CHAIRBOUND	6

SEX AGE	•
MALE	1
FEMALE	2
14-49	1
50-64	2
65-74	3
75-80	4
81 +	5
APPETITE	•
AVERAGE	0
POOR	1
N.G. TUBE / FLUIDS	2
NBM / ANOREXIC	3

SPECIAL RISKS	•
TISSUE MALNUTRITION	•
EG: TERMINAL CACHEXIA	8
CARDIAC FAILURE	5
PERIPHERAL VASCULAR FAILURE	5
ANAEMIA	2
SMOKING	1
NEUROLOGICAL DEFICIT	•
EG: DIABETES, CVA, M.S., PARAPLEGIA, MOTOR SENSORY	4-6
MAJOR SURGERY/TRAUMA	•
ORTHOPAEDIC - BELOW WAIST, SPINAL	5
ON TABLE > 2 HOURS	5
MEDICATION	•
STERIOIDS, CYTOTOXICS, ANTI-INFLAMITORY	4

SCORE: 10 + AT RISK 15 + HIGH RISK 20 + VERY HIGH RISK

NORTON SCALE

(score of 14 or below - "at risk")

A		B		C		D		E	
Physical Condition *		**Mental**		**Activity**		**Mobility**		**Incontinence**	
Good	4	Alert	4	Walks	4	Full	4	Does not have	4
Fair	3	Apathetic	3	Walks with help	3	Slightly limited	3	Has occasionally	3
Poor	2	Confused	2	Chairbound	2	Very limited	2	Usually urinary	2
Very Bad	1	Stuporous	1	Bedfast	1	Immobile	1	Double	1

*General Status, not degree of disease or prognosis

the wound site (McClemont *et al* 1984). Blood transfusions may be indicated, particularly when surgery is contemplated; otherwise, iron supplements should be given.

Fluid

Dehydrated skin becomes inelastic, fragile and more susceptible to breakdown. The fluid intake of at risk patients should therefore be an important consideration. Older debilitated patients are particularly vulnerable to dehydration and hence pressure sore formation (Natow 1983).

5.6.3 Nutritional treatment of pressure sores

Nutritional support should follow an individualised treatment plan aimed at the specific needs of the patient. Assessment of a patient's requirements should consider the following factors:

Age
Body weight/weight loss
Reason for admission/underlying clinical condition
Grade of pressure sore
Losses from wound site
Pyrexia
Mobility
Pain
Nutritional intake.

Fortification of foods with energy and/or protein supplements can enhance the quality of the diet. Supplementary drinks and sip feeds provide an additional source of nutrients. If nutritional intake remains inadequate, total or overnight nasogastric feeding should be considered. Methods of calculating individual nutritional requirements and details on the provision of nutritional support are given in Sections 1.12 and 1.13 respectively.

A minimum of 60 mg vitamin C should be supplied daily, preferably via dietary sources and/or with the use of additional drinks such as fresh fruit juice or fortified blackcurrant drinks. Multivitamin preparations may be useful if requirements cannot be met by diet alone and in some hospitals are given routinely to all patients with, or at-risk from, pressure sores. Ascorbic acid supplements, ranging from 200 mg to one gram per day, may be considered in those with high grade or poorly healing sores (Taylor *et al* 1974).

Biochemical zinc levels are rarely available and are not a reliable indicator of zinc status. The decision to give zinc supplements is therefore largely based on the current dietary intake, physical manifestations of zinc deficiency and the clinical response to supplementation. It is primarily a clinical decision but should always be a consideration in patients with severe sores or those which are slow to heal. When necessary, supplements of 200–220 mg zinc sulphate are usually administered one to three times per day.

Clinical anaemia is usually treated with 200 mg ferrous sulphate, two to three times daily. Blood haemoglobin levels lower than 8 g/100 ml invariably require one or more units of transfused blood.

Over-supplementation of any one mineral should be avoided since this may affect absorptive or metabolic interactions between zinc, iron and copper and impair nutritional status.

5.6.4 Prevention of pressure sores

The early identification of at risk patients is vital for the prevention of pressure sores. A variety of risk assessment charts are available for identifying such patients at an early stage (Fig. 5.9). One of these assessments should ideally be carried out by nursing staff within one hour of a patient's admission. Reassessment should occur whenever there is a significant change in the patient's condition e.g. the level of consciousness or degree of mobility.

While the importance of some factors such as good skin care are usually recognized by the health care team, the benefits of good nutritional status are often overlooked. Educational programmes, aimed at reducing the incidence of pressure sores, should ensure that staff are aware of the vital role of nutrition and know how to identify individuals with nutritional difficulties. The primary aim should be to increase awareness at ward level and prompt early referral of patients to the dietitian, ideally before the development of sores. The provision of nutritional assessment charts, such as that shown in Table 5.21, which enable nursing staff to assess dietary adequacy and identify those who may benefit from dietetic advice, are a useful way of achieving this.

Further reading

Barton A and Barton M (1981) *The management and prevention of pressure sores*. Faber & Faber, London.
Waterlow JA (1991) A policy that protects. *Professional Nurse* **6**, 258–64.

References

Bobel LM (1987) Nutritional implications in the patient with pressure sores. *Nursing Clinics of North America* **22**, 379–80.
Hallbrook T and Lanner E (1972) Serum zinc and healing of various leg ulcers. *Lancet* **2**, 780–82.
Higgs JD (1987) Pressure sores: is there a place for nutritional support? *Physiotherapy* **73**, 457–9.
Lancet (1982) Editorial: The cost of pressure sores. *Lancet* **2**, 1150–52.
McClemont EJW, Archibald RM and Ramsay BM (1984) Pressure sores. *Nursing* Supplement, Series 2(21), 1046.
Mullholland J, Tui G, Wright AM *et al* (1943) Protein metabolism and bedsores. *Ann Surgery* **118**, 1015–23.
Natow AB (1983) Nutrition in the prevention and treatment of decubitus ulcers. *Topics Clin Nurs* **5**, 39–44.

Table 5.21 Nutritional risk assessment chart

NUTRITIONAL ASSESSMENT: **Pressure sore healing**

Scoring:

Ward ....

Minimal risk	22–28
Moderate risk	21–17
High risk	below 17

Weight	Age	Ability to eat	Energy	Protein/Zinc	Vitamin C	Supplements
4	4	4	4	4	4	4
Normal	Below 60	Able to eat independently	Good – clears plate	Meat/Fish Milk/Eggs Daily in Portions	Fresh Citrus Fruit/Juice Blackcurrant drink daily	Build Up/ Fortisip 2–3 times per day
2	3	3	3	3	3	3
Underweight recent loss of up to 10% or currently losing weight	60–70 yrs	Requires help with eating	Poor – eats only small amounts	Meat/Fish *or* Milk/Eggs taken 2–3 times a week in restricted amounts	Fresh citrus fruit/juice Blackcurrant drink 2–3 times a week	Build-up/ Fortisip once daily
3	2	2	2	2	2	2
Up to 10% overweight	70–80 yrs	Needs to be fed	Refuses food/ drink	Meat/Fish/Milk/ Eggs less than twice a week *or* 'Picks' at Protein foods	Fresh citrus fruit/juice Blackcurrant drink less than twice a week	Build-up/ Fortisip 2–3 times a week
1	1	1	3	4	4	1
Cachetic (Skeletal)	Over 80 yrs	Unable to take food orally e.g. dysphagia	Reducing diet	Supplementary zinc sulphate 220 mg once daily	Supplementary vitamin C 250 mg (ascorbic acid)	Build-up/ Fortisip never

Action

Moderate risk

1. Observe patients eating
2. Assist with food choice
3. Record daily food and fluid taken refer to dietitian for assessment
4. Review weekly
5. Document nursing process

High risk

1. Refer to dietitian for Assessment
2. Record daily food/fluid intake
3. Assist with food choice and eating
4. Review
5. Document nursing process

NUTRITIONAL ASSESSMENT SCORE

DATE	SCORE	DIETITIAN REFERRAL

Pories WJ, Henzel JH, Rob CG and Strain WH (1967) Acceleration of wound healing in man with zinc sulphate given by mouth. *Lancet* **1**, 121–4.

Taylor TW, Rimmer S, Dais B, Butcher J and Dymock IW (1974) Ascorbic acid supplementation in the treatment of pressure sores. *Lancet* **ii**, 544–6.

Tyrrell DAJ (1974) Vitamin C and the common cold. *Prescribers J* **14**, 21–4.

Waterlow JA (1985) A risk assessment card. *Nursing Times* **89**(27), 49–51.

Waterlow J (1977) Waterlow card for prevention and management of pressure sores – towards a pocket policy. *Care Science and Practitioner* **6**, 80–86.

Weisman K (1980) Zinc metabolism in the skin. In *Recent advances in dermatology 5*, Rock A and Savin JA (Eds) pp. 109–129. Churchill Livingstone, Edinburgh.

Section 6 **Investigative procedures**

6.1 Metabolic balance diets

The aim of a metabolic balance is to compare the amount of a nutrient or other chemical which enters the body with the amount which leaves it. An individual is said to be in positive balance when output is less than intake, or in negative balance when output exceeds intake.

Nutrients can enter the body both orally, via the diet and medications, and parentally. The routes by which unwanted metabolites are excreted from the body are through faeces, urine, lungs, skin, and in special cases by dialysis. Accuracy of measurement of intake and excretion is crucial to the success of the investigation.

A major limitation of metabolic balance studies is that they indicate only total net change of a substance in the body. They do not provide information about internal body distribution, turnover rates, pool sizes or the amounts of endogenous substances excreted by urine or faeces (Torun 1984). To gain such information requires the use of more sophisticated techniques such as kinetic studies using stable isotopes.

A *balance* diet, such as a calcium/phosphorus/magnesium balance, provides a constant daily intake of the specified nutrients, which is very carefully controlled and usually adhered to for a relatively lengthy period of time. Collections of both stools and urine are usually made.

A *constant* diet, such as a constant calcium diet, is less restricted in terms of the degree of accuracy, the number of nutrients and/or the time period involved. Collections are usually made of urine only, and not of stools.

6.1.1 Facilities required for balance studies

Because of the need for accuracy, the preparation of food for dietary balance studies should be undertaken by a trained diet cook or diet technician, in a specially equipped metabolic diet kitchen. A dietitian's office, diet store, food freezer and fridge should be located nearby. In addition to the usual ward facilities there should be dry toilets with refrigerated storage space for urine and faeces. Nursing staff must be trained in the accurate collection of urine stools and any other metabolic products required. Phlebotomy and laboratory services must be available.

6.1.2 Planning balance studies

The planning of the metabolic balance study is co-ordinated by a team of specialists consisting of physician, nursing staff, dietitian and laboratory staff. Figure 6.1 shows the involvement of these specialists during a typical calcium balance, and includes other departments whose help will be required. The specialist team plan the patient's protocol and at regular intervals monitor the progress of the study and resolve any problems. The protocol is the central source of information for all involved and will show:

1 The type of balance study which is being undertaken, the nutrients being measured and any additional restriction in the diet, e.g. low protein for a patient with renal bone disease.

2 The timing of the 24-hour day for urine and stool collections, e.g. 8AM–8AM or 10AM–10AM. (*Note*: there will be less likelihood of error if the collection period commences in the working day and not at midnight.)

3 The type of urine/stool/sweat, etc. collections which will be required, e.g. 24-hour urine collections for calcium measurement collected in boric acid preservative.

4 The length of the equilibration period, sometimes termed the 'run-in', and the length of the balance period.

5 All tests to be undertaken on the patient during the balance period which may require medical, dietetic, phlebotomy or clinical chemistry involvement.

Table 6.1 gives details of aspects to be considered when planning metabolic dietary studies.

6.1.3 Organizing the metabolic diet

Foods used in balance diets and their preparation

Food included in the menus for metabolic balance studies should vary as little as possible in compositional analysis and should be kept simple in type and number to limit the variation inherent in foods. Regular availability, cost, storage properties, ease of preparation, palatability and acceptability of the foods must be considered. Foods should be bought in bulk for the period of the balance, including the stabilization period, and duplicate meals prepared for analysis (Reifenstein *et al* 1945; Isaksson and Sjorgen 1965). Foods such as meat can be prepared, cooked, weighed into portions, labelled and frozen before the balance commences. Likewise, dry goods can be weighed in advance. Tables 6.2 and 6.3 give details of foods suitable for metabolic dietary studies. Methods of cooking should be standardized and where possible foods should be served in the container in which they were cooked (Heaney *et al* 1977). Pressure cooking, casserole cooking and foil-wrap baking are all suitable cooking methods for preserving nutrient content.

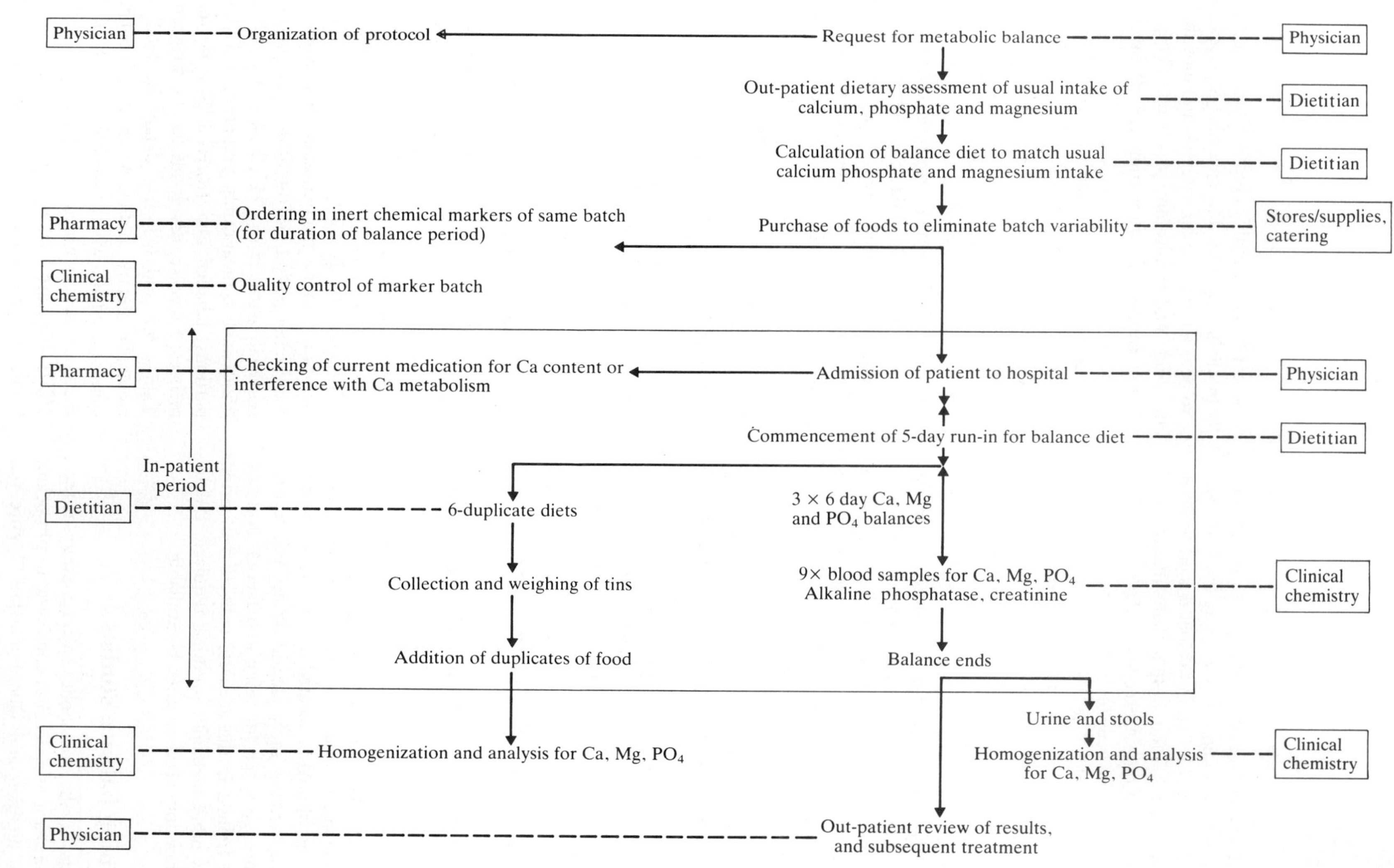

Fig. 6.1 Flow chart for a typical calcium balance — interaction with other departments.

Table 6.1 Aspects to be considered when planning metabolic balance studies

Type of study	Water	Food choice	Menu rotation	Length of run-in period	Length of balance periods	Types of collection	Markers	Duplicate diets	Toothpastes, medicaments and miscellaneous
Calcium, magnesium phosphorus	Distilled or deionized for cooking and all beverages	Constant source, batched for entire study	1, 2 or 3 daily menus rotated. Matched for minerals being studied	Balances 5–8 days Constant diets 2–5 days	May be 4 days × 4 5 days × 3 6 days × 3	*Balances* 24-hour urines in boric acid Daily stool Blood as necessary *Constant diets* 24-hour urines in boric acid	Continuous faecal markers	Essential for balance diets. 1 per balance period or 1 of each menu per balance period Not required for constant diets	Calcium-free toothpaste: use those with a silica abrasive
Sodium potassium	Distilled or deionized for cooking and all beverages	Constant source, batched for entire study Sodium – avoid high sodium foods Potassium – avoid leaf tea and substitute instant tea.	1, 2 or 3 daily menus rotated	2–3 days. For large dietary changes allow longer run-in	Variable	*Balances* 24-hour urines in boric acid. Daily stool. Blood as necessary *Constant diets* 24-hour urines in boric acid	Not usually required	Essential for balance diets	May require use of salt-free toothpaste
Nitrogen	Tap water for cooking and all beverages	Constant source; batched for entire study	1, 2 or 3 daily menus rotated	2–6 days	Variable	*Balances* 24-hour urines in boric acid. Daily stool. Sometimes skin losses *Constant diets* 24-hour urines in boric acid	Faecal or urinary	Essential for balance diets	Avoid use of all ointments, powder, purgatives and toothpaste unless authorized by clinician
Purine-free	Tap water for cooking and all beverages	See Table 6.3. Not necessary to batch foods. Fresh foods may be used daily	Single menu	5 days	3 days	24-hour urines in boric acid. Blood for uric acid creatinine	Not required	Not required	Not restricted

The type of water (i.e whether distilled, deionized or tap water) which should be used for cooking, drinking and in beverages in each type of study is indicated in Table 6.1.

The metabolic diet is prepared by a trained diet cook or diet technician using menu plans drawn up by the dietitian.

Planning the menu

The menu to be used during the balance period may be based on:

1 A standard diet used by the metabolic unit.

2 A basic diet with selected increments to achieve the required intake.

3 Simulation of the patient's usual home intake of particular nutrient(s).

It may be necessary to keep patients in their current equilibrium, or steady state, for one or more nutrients. This steady state needs to be maintained where adaptation to different intakes of nutrients may take months, e.g. calcium (Isaksson and Sjorgen 1967; Lentner *et al* 1975). In this case a detailed dietary history of a typical week's food intake at home will be needed. With the help of the dietitian, the patient chooses the foods to be consumed during the balance period. The nutrient content of the chosen diet is calculated from standard food tables and adjusted to meet the required level of the nutrients to be investigated (see previous section on foods used in balance diets). Care should be taken to see that the choice provides a palatable, nutritious and attractive menu. The metabolic balance procedure is a demanding discipline for the patient,

Table 6.2 Description of foods used in metabolic studies, their preparation and storage

Food group	Comments
Cereals	
Breakfast cereals	From the same batch, weighed out into airtight containers before the study commences. Puffed Wheat, Shredded Wheat, Cornflakes, Rice Krispies, Weetabix, All Bran. Special K and porridge are all commonly used.
Bread	From the same batch. Wholemeal or white, weighed out before the study commences, crusts removed, trimmed to correct weight, packed appropriately and frozen. Alternatively, 'home made' bread may be baked to a standard recipe using ingredients of known, constant composition
Biscuits	From the same batch; only biscuits of uniform composition should be used, e.g. Rich Tea, Marie, digestives, cream crackers, Ryvita, scraped to correct weight and wrapped in cling film
Puddings	Sago, rice, tapioca, semolina or custard, cooked in a pyrex dish in a microwave oven or bain-marie and served directly to the patient in this dish
Dairy products, eggs and fats	
Milk	Fresh milk, homogenized to provide an even distribution of fat, Dried skimmed milk or whitener are alternatives
Butter	Unsalted or salted can be used depending on whether or not constant sodium is required. Always obtain from the same batch and freeze beforehand if necessary
Cheese	From the same batch, analysed by laboratory if necessary and frozen until required. Processed cheese may be more homogenous than hard cheeses. Avoid cheese in sodium-controlled studies
Eggs	Either homogenize eggs and use a constant quantity of homogenate or weigh eggs, e.g. 57 g egg provides 50 g whole egg and 7 g shell. Egg may be boiled, poached, scrambled or as omelette
Margarine	Margarine may be used in preference to butter.
Vegetable oil	May be used in weighed quantities
Meats	All meat used must be completely lean and be bone, skin and rind free. It must be cooked without salt before the balance commences, portioned, wrapped and frozen. It is advisable to use beef – topside or rump; lamb – leg; pork – loin; and chicken breast. Ham may be included if the diet is not sodium-controlled
Fish	Fish is not generally used in metabolic studies because of storage difficulties and variations in water lost. If used, care must be taken to ensure that the fish is free of bones
Vegetables	
Salad vegetables	Fresh salad vegetables may be used, e.g. lettuce, tomato, cucumber, pepper, celery and cress. These must be very well washed in distilled water and dried before use
Frozen vegetables	Frozen vegetables are preferable to fresh. Bought in batches before the balance commences. e.g. cauliflower, peas, runner beans, brussels sprouts and carrots. These are cooked in distilled water or deionized water, drained in sieve, then weighed
Tinned vegetables	Should be avoided in sodium-controlled studies
Potatoes	Instant potato flakes or powder reconstituted with distilled water are the most accurate. If fresh potatoes are used these should be steamed, or roasted in a weighed quantity of cooking oil
Fruit	
Tinned fruit	From the same batch. Can be weighed into small containers with a measured quantity of fruit and syrup then frozen until required. Tinned grapefruit, mandarins, pears, peaches, pineapple and apricots, are all suitable
Fresh fruit	All fresh fruit must be peeled, cored and flesh weighed as required
Fruit juice	From the same batch. May be weighed and frozen prior to the balance study.
Beverages	
Tea	A standard brew is made using tea bags or leaf tea. If potassium is being assessed instant tea should be used. In studies involving diuretic drugs use decaffeinated tea
Coffee	Instant coffee is suitable. It can be weighed into small pots before the study commences. In studies involving diuretic drugs, decaffeinated should be used
Bedtime drinks	Horlicks, drinking chocolate, cocoa and Ovaltine are all suitable
Miscellaneous	
Ice cream	From the same batch
Jelly	From the same batch, made up to a standard recipe
Fruit squash	Each portion of undiluted squash must be be weighed
Preserves	From the same batch, marmalade, seedless jam and honey are all suitable
Sugar	Weighed quantities in beverages if the patient requires it
Boiled sweets, chocolate	Use, if required, in weighed quantities
Salad cream	Use in weighed quantities
Vinegar	Use in weighed quantities

Table 6.3 List of food choices for purine-free constant diets

Foods to be avoided	Foods allowed
All meat, poultry, fish, offal, meat extracts, wholegrain cereals, potatoes peas, beans, lentils, spinach, asparagus, celery, onion, radishes, mushrooms, chocolate, drinking chocolate, Ovaltine, Bournvita, tea, coffee and alcohol	Eggs, cheese (cheddar or processed cheese spread) Milk (homogenized) Cereals – white bread, plain biscuits, e.g. marie, rich tea, morning coffee. Cornflakes, custard powder, rice and semolina Vegetables – cauliflower, carrots, lettuce, tomatoes and cucumber Fruit (fresh) – apples and bananas Fruit (tinned) – peaches, pears, pineapple, apricots, mandarins and grapefruit. Fruit (juice) – grapefruit, orange and pineapple Fats – butter and oils Beverages – fruit squashes Miscellaneous – jams, marmalade, honey, sugar and boiled sweets

and the dietitian is responsible for providing a diet which is acceptable, while at the same time fulfilling the requirements of the dietary investigation.

Patient training

The dietitian is responsible for explaining to the patient:

1 The purpose of the dietary procedure.

2 The necessity to consume all food and fluid provided.

3 How to clear all plates with either a small portion of bread included in the diet for this purpose or a flexible spatula (Reifenstein *et al* 1945).

4 How to rinse all drink containers with distilled water and to consume the rinsing water.

5 The importance of not taking any food or fluid other than those prescribed in the diet.

6 Where necessary, the restriction of toothpaste and talcum powder.

The physician should advise the patient on the desirable level of physical activity, for example, avoiding excessive sweating during sodium balances but keeping reasonable levels of physical activity during calcium balances.

Menu rotation

Constant or balance diets are planned on a one, two or three-day rotating menu. The single-day form has the advantage of ensuring greater constancy of nutrient intake. Two or three-day rotating menus calculated to provide an identical intake of nutrients are less monotonous but inevitably introduce greater daily variability of nutrient intake in practice. If rotating menus are used, each balance period must comprise the same number of each alternating menu. For constant nitrogen studies it is often useful to make exchanges of meals of similar nitrogen composition, with meats, cereals and vegetables grouped into separate exchange lists making three or four week menu cycles possible. This is important for compliance in studies which continue for several weeks.

Other considerations

Drugs

Any drugs which the patient is taking must be checked for relevant mineral content or possible interference with the balance study. When preparing duplicate diets for analysis (see below), it may be desirable to include duplicate doses of any drugs taken which contain significant quantities of the mineral being measured.

If it is necessary to give a high sodium intake this may be achieved by giving weighed amounts of sodium chloride to be added to food and additional 'slow sodium' tablets if necessary. Similarly, an increase in potassium intake may be effected using 'slow potassium' tablets.

Toothpastes

For calcium studies a low calcium toothpaste should be used by patients who have their own teeth; suitable toothpastes contain a silica abrasive (rather than a calcium or aluminium abrasive) and are low in calcium and phosphorus.

Examples, currently, are Signal, SR, Macleans Sensitive and Sensodyne Original and Mint, but the manufacturers should be contacted to confirm that no major formulation changes have been made.

Denture users should be taught to rinse their dentures thoroughly with distilled water after cleaning.

Sodium studies may require the use of salt-free toothpaste (made up by the pharmacy). A suitable formulation is given in Table 6.4.

The use of toothpaste may be restricted in nitrogen studies at the discretion of the physician in charge.

Ointments and powders

In nitrogen studies, ointments and powders should not be used unless authorized by the physician in charge as they may directly or indirectly affect the nitrogen balance (for example, cortisol-based creams).

6.1.4 Stabilization or run-in period

Prior to commencing the balance study, the patient has a run-in period, which is a trial of the balance diet, and covers the period of time necessary for the patient's adaptation to the constant diet. This leads into the balance period. During the run-in period the patient becomes accustomed to the idea of being on a balance diet and learns the procedures required of him for the completion of the diet and for urine and stool collections (although no collections are made during this period). It is also a time when any problems over the diet are sorted out so that the final diet for the balance period can be tailored to suit the patient in both type and quantity of foods. The length of time of the run-in period will vary according to the type of balance and length of adaptation needed.

For calcium balances the run-in is 5–6 days and changes in the balance diet should not be made after about day 4. For gelatin-free diets for hydroxyproline excretion studies, 24 hours only are required (Gasser *et al* 1979).

Table 6.4 Sodium-free toothpaste (Courtesy of the Glasgow Dental Hospital and School of Dentistry)

10 ml gum acacia
50 ml boiling water
10 ml glycerol
80 mg calcium carbonate
5 drops of carvone to flavour
5 drops of methylene blue to colour

This formulation contains no preservative so it should be kept refrigerated

For sodium and potassium balances the run-in may only be 2–3 days if the dietary change is not great, as adaptation to different intakes of these minerals is rapid. When signficant increases or decreases of dietary nutrients are made, a run-in of five days may be required (for example, a 350 mmol sodium diet).

For purine-free diets, a five day run-in is necessary during which time dietary sources of uric acid are eliminated from the body.

During the run-in, the internal markers for the balance period will be given so that these have reached equilibrium in the gut by the time the balance starts (see below).

6.1.5 Balance study procedures

Balance periods

The length of balance will vary considerably according to the information required. Points to consider are:

1 For minerals, longer studies give greater precision (Lentner *et al* 1975).

2 Where treatment changes are made during balance periods, a transitional period will occur before a new equilibrium is reached. Effectively another run-in period is required during this time before the balance can continue in the new equilibrium (for example in electrolyte studies).

3 There should be at least two metabolic periods for each regimen otherwise any trend creeping in due to unforeseen variables may be missed.

4 Balance periods longer than six days will involve volumes of faecal collections too large to be handled with ease (Reifenstein *et al* 1945).

Types of collection

Most balances require 24-hour urine and daily faecal collections. Daily faecal collections may be analysed individually or subsequently pooled for aliquot analysis. For constant diets (such as sodium and calcium) 24-hour urine collections are made without faecal collections.

Blood samples are often necessary, depending on the individual study, and sometimes measurements of skin losses are made during nitrogen, sodium or potassium balances (Isaksson and Sjorgen 1967) (see Table 6.1). This is a time-consuming task (Calloway *et al* 1971) and correction factors are more likely to be used.

Markers – faecal and urinary

Faecal markers

For balance studies an inert faecal marker is necessary to correct for incomplete stool collections and variations in faecal output and transit time. There are two types of marker, intermittent and continuous.

Intermittent or visual markers

Intermittent markers are visible after transit through the gut, so that if markers are given at known times, stool collections can be made between the appearance of these markers.

Carmine is the most commonly used intermittent marker (Rose 1964; Pak *et al* 1980).

Continuous markers

Continuous markers ar given in known quantities throughout the run-in and balance periods. Since they remain totally unabsorbed during transit through the intestine, the quantity appearing in the stool can be used to correct for incomplete stool collections. Continuous markers are:

1 Chromium sesquioxide (Cr_2O_3) (Rose 1964; Fisher *et al* 1972; Lentner *et al* 1975; Branch and Cummings 1978; Pak *et al* 1980). This marker can be a hazard during the analysis of faeces when chromium is oxidized to chromate with perchlorate; dry perchlorate salts may explode, and the material should be handled only in a fume cupboard with non-absorbent surfaces (Hesp *et al* 1979).

2 [^{51}Cr] chromic chloride (Hesp *et al* 1979).

3 Radio-opaque pellets (Branch and Cummings 1978).

4 Polyethylene glycol (4000–PEG) (Soergel 1968; Wilkinson 1971; Lentner *et al* 1975; Pak *et al* 1980).

Other substances sometimes used as markers in balance studies have disadvantages which limit their usefulness. For example, barium sulphate ($BaSO_4$) is time-consuming to analyse by the gravimetric method, and using flame photometry the method is insensitive and other elements interfere (Bacon 1980). Copper thiocyanate (CuSCN) may interfere with thyroid uptake of iodine. (Ingbar and Woeber 1968). However, the choice of marker is a matter of individual preference (Bacon 1980). Further merits and problems with markers have been discussed in some detail by Morgan (1986).

Intermittent and continuous markers may be used concurrently (Pak *et al* 1980). The use of faecal markers may be invalid in gastrointestinal disease (Soergel 1968).

Urinary markers

Urine creatinine has been used as a measure of completeness of urine collections. Since creatinine excretion is related to lean body mass, it was assumed to be constant from day to day in any individual. However, urinary creatinine is also affected by diet, particularly meat consumption. Limited calorimetric studies have shown that even on a constant diet, day to day variations in urinary creatinine are quite large. It is advisable therefore to use a urine marker to check for completeness of urine collections.

Para-amino benzoic acid (in a dose of one 80 mg capsule three times daily) has a high percentage of recovery in urine. Collections containing less than 85% of the administered para-amino benzoic acid are probably incomplete (Bingham and Cummings 1983). These markers may be given combined with a faecal marker.

Duplicate diets

A duplicate diet consists of a 24-hour food intake, identical to the balance diet, which is submitted to the laboratory for analysis. This technique is employed as a measurement of the patient's actual food intake as opposed to the theoretical intake calculated from standard food tables.

A duplicate day's menu is prepared, cooked and sent to the laboratory for homogenization and analysis of an aliquot. Some food may be omitted, e.g. butter (because of its tendency to float to the top causing an unrepresentative aliquot to be taken), or tea infusions (where capacity of the homogenizing equipment is limited). The theoretical values for these omitted foods are added to the analysed values to give the true totals.

The total number of duplicates analysed varies with the number of menus and balance periods. If periods are short, with one menu, one duplicate should be prepared for each period; for alternating menus, one duplicate of each menu should be prepared for each balance period.

The precision of estimating true dietary intake increases with the number of duplicate diets analysed. For example, in the case of calcium, if one duplicate diet estimates the true dietary intake of calcium with a precision of 1.53 mmol (= 60 mg calcium), for six duplicate diets this figure is divided by $\sqrt{n}$, i.e.

$$\frac{1.53}{\sqrt{6}} = 25\,\text{mg}.$$

Duplicate diets are not usually required for constant diets.

Verification

The dietitian is responsible for checking all food which leaves the metabolic kitchen, for appearance, temperature and accuracy. Spot checks for weight error may at times be necessary. All trays from patients on metabolic balance diets should be returned to the metabolic kitchen to be checked for rejections.

Rejected food

This is kept to a minimum by patient co-operation. Where minor rejects occur, these should be analysed either individually or added to the stool pot for analysis with the faeces of the same date as the rejects. Rejections should be charted in a book kept in the metabolic kitchen. In some studies it may be necessary to make up the nutrient loss by replacing with alternative foods (for example, in fat balances). If it becomes apparent that rejections are so great as to invalidate the balance results, the possibility of terminating the balance study must be considered. In the event of a temporary illness it may be necessary to stop collections until the patient is well again, then allow a new run-in period before balance collections recommence.

Coding

In all metabolic wards a considerable amount of staff time is spent teaching the patient dietary and toilet regimens. In order to minimize possible errors, a system of coding (colour or letter) of equipment may be used. Each metabolic patient has his own colour or code and all equipment pertaining to his bedroom and toilet is labelled with his colour or code. All cooking dishes and crockery may be similarly coded.

Records

Throughout the study accurate records must be kept. These may include calculated dietary intakes of nutrients, fluid charts, prescription charts to show times that markers are given, and urine and stool charts.

References

Bacon S (1980) Faecal markers in metabolic balance studies. *J Hum Nutr* 34, 445–9.

Bingham SA, Cummings JH (1983) The use of 4-aminobenzoic acid as a marker to validate the completeness of 24-hour urine collections in man. *Clin Sci* **64**, 629–35.

Branch WJ and Cummings JH (1978) Comparison of radio-opaque pellets and chromium sesquioxide markers in studies requiring accurate faecal collections. *Gut* **19**, 371–6.

Calloway DH *et al* (1971) Sweat and miscellaneous nitrogen losses in human balance studies. *J Nutr* **101**, 775–86.

Fisher MT, Atkins PR and Joplin GF (1972) A method for measuring faecal chromium and its use as a marker in human metabolic balances. *Clin Chim Acta* **41**, 109–22.

Gasser A, Celada A, Courvoisier B, Depierre D, Hulme PM, Rinsler M, Williams D and Wootton R (1979) The clinical measurement of urinary total hydroxyproline excretion. *Clin Chim Acta* **95**, 487–91.

Heaney RP, Recker RR and Saville PD (1977) Calcium balance and calcium requirements in middle-aged women. *Am J Clin Nutr* **30**, 1603–11.

Hesp R, Williams D, Rinsler M and Reeve J (1979) A comparison of chromium sesquioxide and [^{51}Cr] chromic chloride as inert markers in calcium balance studies. *Clin Sci* **57**, 89–92.

Ingbar SH and Woeber KA (1968) *Textbook of endocrinology*, Williams RH (Ed) p. 105. WB Saunders, Philadelphia.

Isaksson B and Sjorgen B (1965) On the concept 'constant diet' in metabolic balance studies. *Nutritio Dieta* **7**, 175–85.

Isaksson B and Sjorgen B (1967) A critical evaluation of the mineral and nitrogen balances in man. *Proc Nutr Soc* **26**, 106–16.

Lentner C, Lauffenburger T, Guncaga J, Dambacher MA and Haas HG (1975) The metabolic balance technique: a critical reappraisal. *Metabolism* **24**, 461–71.

Morgan JB (1986) Use of non-absorbable markers in studies of human nutrient absorption. *Hum Nutr: Appl Nutr* **40A**, 399–411.

Pak CYC, Stewart A, Rasin P and Galosy RA (1980) A simple and reliable method for calcium balance using combined period and continuous faecal markers. *Metabolism* **29**, 793–6.

Reifenstein EC, Albright F and Wells SL (1945) The accumulation, interpretation and presentation of data pertaining to metabolic balances, notably those of calcium, phosphorus and nitrogen. *J Clin Endocrinol* 5, 367–95.

Rose GA (1964) Experiences with the use of interrupted carmine red and continuous chromium sesquioxide marking of human faeces with reference to calcium, phosphorus and magnesium. *Gut* 5, 274–9.

Soergel KH (1968) Inert markers. *Gastroenterology* 54, 449–52.

Torun B (1984) In *Genetic factors in nutrition. International Workshop on Genetic Factors in Nutrition 1982 (San Juan Teotihuac án Mexico)*, Velasquez A and Bourges H (Eds) Academic Press, New York.

Wilkinson R (1971) Polyethylene glycol 4000 as a continuously administered non-absorbable faecal marker for metabolic balance studies in human subjects. *Gut* 12, 654–60.

6.2 Diagnostic tests

6.2.1 Fat malabsorption — total faecal fat estimation

Dietary manipulation may be required to ensure that adequate fat (see below) is ingested for at least two days prior to the beginning of the test and for the duration of the test.

Many patients requiring this test have a poor fat tolerance and achieving an adequate fat intake can be a problem, causing further steatorrhoea and nausea.

An adequate fat intake is between 50–150 g fat/day for adults; 100 g fat daily is commonly used. A minimum of 40 g fat daily is recommended for a child. In infants, the actual fat content of the current feeding regimen is calculated and will be adequate unless steps have been taken to reduce the fat content. In hospital, the normal hospital diet, plus a regimen of fat supplements, can ensure a minimum daily fat intake of 100 g.

For example:

5 butter/margarine portions (7 g each)	=	28 g fat
1 pint whole milk	=	21 g fat
50 g hard cheese	=	16 g fat
50 g chocolate (milk)	=	15 g fat
30 g peanuts	=	15 g fat
30 g double cream	=	15 g fat
	=	110 g fat

A record should be kept of food and fat supplements eaten during the two days prior to the test and for the duration of the tests (three or five days) so that the validity of the test can be checked. The patient may be well enough to keep the record (Tietz 1983). Normal faecal fat range = <7 g/day or < 24 mmol/24 hours.

6.2.2 Gluten challenge

It is usual to confirm the diagnosis of coeliac disease (see Section 4.7) by the reintroduction of gluten for a period of three months. This is followed by a jejunal biopsy to examine the villi of the intestinal mucosa. The challenge may be in a child or an adult. The method by which this is done varies from unit to unit but is based on (1) the use of gluten-containing foods or (2) the use of pure gluten powder. Whichever method is used, it is important to ensure that an adequate quantity of gluten is being ingested to constitute a challenge to the gut.

Gluten challenge using gluten-containing foods

An intake of at least 10 g wheat protein daily is recommended (Francis 1974) for children and 15–20 g wheat protein daily for teenagers and adults. This can be calculated using the protein content of foods whose protein source is wheat. For example, 10 g wheat protein can be provided by four large, thin slices of ordinary bread, brown or white, *or* four Weetabix, *or* 60 g raw spaghetti, *or* 100 g digestive biscuits.

The introduction of foods which have previously been forbidden to the coeliac patient, especially if a child, may lead to problems of dietary compliance in the future if the challenge confirms the diagnosis of coeliac disease.

Gluten challenge using pure gluten powder

Gluten powder is added to foods which make up the gluten free diet. The powder is very fine and has a strong taste. It does not mix with liquid but mixes well with thicker foods such as mashed potato, yogurt or rice pudding. It can also be taken mixed with jam or other preserves as a 'medicine'. Children should be given 20 g twice a day; teenagers or adults should consume 20–40 g twice a day.

If during the challenge, unpleasant symptoms occur, the patient undergoes a jejunal biopsy before the three month period is completed. (Alderhay Children's Hospital, Dietetic Department, personal communication).

6.2.3 Glucose tolerance test

It is unlikely that the dietitian will be involved in the procedure for a glucose tolerance test. However, dietitians should be aware that the patient should not be placed on a diet which restricts carbohydrate intake prior to this diagnostic test being carried out as this can impair the results.

The World Health Organization (1985) has laid down diagnostic criteria and a classification of diagnosis based on the results of an oral glucose tolerance test comprised of 75 g glucose in 250–300 ml of water, drunk over 10 minutes, for adults, or 1.75 g glucose/kg body weight (to a maximum of 75 g glucose) for children. The test is carried out after an overnight (6–8 hour) fast with the person at rest and not smoking.

Diagnostic criteria are given in Appendix 2, Section 7.2.5.

6.2.4 Vanillylmandelic acid (VMA) test (for phaeochromocytoma)

Phaeochromocytoma is a rare syndrome caused by overactivity of the adrenal medulla, usually due to a benign adrenal medullary tumour.

The disease is characterized by increased amounts of catecholamine metabolites such as vanillylmandelic acid (VMA) in the urine. Formerly, methods of measuring VMA also detected other phenolic acids so this test needed to be preceded by a diet free of tea, coffee, chocolate, nuts, bananas, vanilla essence, custard, blancmange, sponges, cakes, biscuits and sweets (except boiled).

Aspirin, or aspirin containing preparations, sympathomimetic agents and MAO inhibitors also had to be avoided during the test period. The diet was usually maintained for 72 hours and a urine collection obtained during the last 24 hours. However, the development of highly specific liquid chromatography estimation methods means that dietary restriction should no longer be necessary.

Normal values: up to 9 mg VMA in urine over 24 hours.

Further reading

Amery A and Conway J (1967) A critical review of diagnostic tests for phaeochromocytoma. *Am Heart J* **73**, 129.

British Dietetic Association (1984) *Handbook of Metabolic Dietetics*. BDA, Birmingham.

References

Francis DEM (1986) *Diets for sick children* 4e. Blackwell Scientific Publications, Oxford.

Tietz NW (1983) *Clinical guide to laboratory tests*, p. 188. WB Saunders, Philadelphia.

World Health Organization (1985) *Second report of the Expert Committee on Diabetes Mellitus*. WHO Tech Rep Ser 727. WHO, Geneva.

6.3 Preparation of the bowel for investigative procedures and surgery

Adequate preparation of the bowel is essential for double contrast examination of the large bowel (Dickie *et al* 1970) as it improves interpretation and the chances of a single diagnostic study. The preparation should result in a clean bowel with no residual faecal matter. Preparation of the bowel for surgery should also result in a clean, empty bowel, particularly if a bowel resection is to be performed. If a total colectomy is planned, e.g. for ulcerative colitis, it may not be necessary to thoroughly cleanse and empty the bowel.

A number of procedures have been advocated and the procedure of choice varies from one centre to another. Consideration should be given to the effects of the evacuant on the patient's mental, physical and metabolic state. Side effects should be minimal and the preparation be easily administered, preferably by the oral route.

Bowel preparation procedures

Whole gut irrigation

This is now seldom used. This procedure involved the administration of a large volume (10–15 litres) of normal saline into the gut by rapid, continuous drip via a nasogastric tube, until the anal effluent was clear. This would take a number of hours to complete and left the patient feeling weakened and exhausted.

Purgatives

The oral intake of 500 ml of 10% mannitol solution (flavoured with lemon or orange juice) and followed by 2 litres of clear fluids is a more acceptable, quicker and effective method of cleansing the bowel. Solutions of 25% magnesium sulphate are also used to purge and cleanse the bowel.

Excellent results have been reported using Picolax® (sodium picosulphate/magnesium citrate) (De Lacey *et al* 1980, 1982). Picolax® is presented in unit dose sachets containing 16.3 g of powder and administered orally. On the day prior to investigation two sachets of Picolax® are taken: one before breakfast and one before the evening meal. A light, low residue diet may be taken during the day and patients are encouraged to drink as much clear fluid as possible. A diet sheet is incorporated into the instructions (Table 6.5) although this may be modified to meet home or hospital catering arrangements (Table 6.6). The dietary instructions for patients taking Picolax® prior to colonoscopy may be modified further (Table 6.6).

Rapid cleansing of the bowel with or without colonic lavage may result in a low blood sugar. Consideration of this must be given to patients with diabetes who require bowel preparation. Insulin dependent diabetics should undergo the procedure with hospital supervision and will require intravenous dextrose and regular blood glucose monitoring. Diabetic patients controlled by hypoglycaemic agents should also be carefully monitored to maintain acceptable blood glucose levels. It may be appropriate to omit their tablets on both the day of preparation and the day of investigation. In any event these diabetics should take glucose-containing clear fluids at regular intervals throughout the day.

Low residue diets in bowel preparation

Low residue diets may be used to prepare the bowel for surgery. Unless food is passing very rapidly through the gut it will take a number of days to prepare the bowel by this method. If patients are already established on a low residue diet as part of the management of inflammatory

Table 6.5 Dietary advice for patients taking Picolax® (Nordic)
During this treatment carefully follow any instructions given by the hospital, the following *may* be allowed on the day before the examination. *Throughout the treatment drink as much water as desired*

Meal	Food allowed
Breakfast (8–9am) (After the first dose has been taken)	1 boiled/poached egg 1 slice white bread + honey (not jam or marmalade) 1 cup tea/coffee with sugar and milk if desired
Mid-morning (10.30am)	1 cup tea/coffee without milk. Sugar if liked. No food
Lunch (12–1.30pm)	Small portion grilled/poached fish or chicken Small portion boiled potato or white bread, clear jelly 1 cup tea/coffee without milk
Afternoon	No food but drink plenty of water
Supper (7–9pm)	Clear soup or meat extract drinks but no food, clear jelly

No further food is allowed until after the examination but fluids may be taken as desired

[Table] 6.6 Example of modified dietary instructions to prepare the bowel for barium enema and colonoscopy using Picolax®

Investigation	Timing	Method	Precautions
Barium enema	Day before investigation	2 sachets Picolax®: 1 before breakfast, 1 before evening meal Diet – light, very low residue diet or high protein, high calorie fluids plus 3 litres clear fluids	Careful blood glucose monitoring in patients with diabetes
	Day of examination	Clear fluids only	
Colonoscopy		May use modified Picolax® preparation	Elderly patients may need preparation of bowel in hospital
	Day 4 before investigation	Mild laxative at night	Careful glucose monitoring in patients with diabetes, particularly on the day prior to and the day of examination
	Days 2 and 3 before investigation	Low residue diet	
	Day 1 before investigation	2 sachets Picolax®: 1 early morning, 1 late afternoon Diet – clear fluids, clear soups, plain jelly, very little milk in 1 or 2 cups of tea. 3 litres clear fluids	
	Day of examination	Clear fluids only	

bowel disease, they may continue with the diet prior to surgery. Such patients are likely to have diarrhoea which obviously would result in regular emptying of the bowel and therefore the low residue diet may be quite adequate and no further dietary modification be required. Immediately prior to surgery or investigation, the bowel will need to be cleansed by bowel washout or enema.

Proprietary enteral feeds – use in bowel preparation

Low residue enteral feeds alone are not an effective method of bowel preparation and bowel cleansing will also usually be necessary. However, deterioration of nutritional status in the pre-operative period may be prevented by sip feeding with enteral feeds. Elemental enteral feeds have been recommended for bowel preparation as they are absorbed mainly in the upper small bowel and leave a minimal residue in the large bowel, although clinicians disagree over the value of such products for this purpose (Keohane and Silk 1982). Elemental enteral feeds are hyperosmolar, unpleasant to take and more expensive than liquid whole protein foods. Provided that pancreatic, biliary and small intestinal absorption are not impaired, liquid whole protein enteral feeds result in a comparatively low residue in the large bowel (Jones *et al* 1983; Russell and Evans 1984) and may be equally as suitable as elemental enteral feeds.

In the preparation of the bowel for surgery or investigation it is probably more important to encourage the drinking of at least 3 litres of clear fluids per day rather than to assess the advantages or disadvantages of a predigested enteral feed over a whole protein enteral feed requiring normal digestion.

The preparation used to evacuate the bowel should result in a clean, residue-free bowel without causing undue distress to the patient or requiring unnecessary nursing time for lavage. The patient's metabolic state and general sense of well-being should be maintained and time spent in hospital ward and X-ray department kept to a minimum.

References

De Lacey G, Benson M, Wilkins R, Spencer J and Cramer B (1980) Colon preparation for double contrast enemas: a comparison of four regimens. Paper presented at Spring Meeting of British Society of Gastroenterologists and Association of Surgeons, Bournemouth, 1980.

De Lacey G, Benson M, Wilkins R, Spencer J and Cramer B (1982) Routine colonic lavage is unnecessary for double contrast barium enema in outpatients. *Br Med J* **284**, 1021–1022.

Dickie J, James WB, Hume R and Robertson D (1970) A comparison of three substances used for bowel preparation prior to radiological examination. *Clin Radiol* **21**, 201–202.

Jones BJM, Lees R, Andrews J, Frost P and Silk DBA (1983) Comparison of an elemental and polymeric diet in patients with normal gastro-intestinal function. *Gut* **24**, 78–84.

Keohane P and Silk DBA (1982) Low residue enteral diets and bowel preparation. *Nursing* **5**, 136–7.

Russell CA and Evans SJ (1984) A comparison of the absorption from 'chemically-defined elemental' and 'whole protein' enteral feeds by the human small bowel. *Proc Nutr Soc* **43**, 123A.

6.4 Dietetic research

Dietetic research can take many forms. It can evaluate the effectiveness of existing dietetic practices (e.g. in terms of patient compliance or response to treatment) or it may investigate the effects of a new type of treatment or a new way of administering an existing one. Studies can be based on individuals or different sized groups of people. They may take the form of case histories, direct measurements or controlled trials. They may require data reported by the participant, clinical measurements, biochemical measurements or measurements of food intakes. They may involve one-to-one interviews, questions or group interviews.

Whatever the type of research being undertaken the ultimate aim should be to improve dietetic practice and nutrition education (Table 6.7).

Research does not have to be complex in order to be useful. Relatively simple studies conducted by one person can yield valuable information. However, all good research, whether large or small scale, does require careful planning in advance.

Research is also more likely to be successful and enjoyable if it has the interest and support of all members of the department, especially the most senior. Regular discussions about each other's work and observations and formal allocation of time for all dietitians to read journals and published work are vital if an environment conducive to self-appraisal and advancement of knowledge is to be fostered.

6.4.1 General principles of research

There are a number of general principles which apply to all types of evaluative research. These are outlined below and described in detail by Calnan (1976). Table 6.8 summarizes the main steps.

The hypothesis

In order to conduct any research there must be a hypothesis. The hypothesis should be a very basic statement which clearly defines what is to be assessed. It should:

1 Summarize the relevant known facts or close observations.
2 Be consistent with the known facts or observations.
3 Be as simple and straightforward as possible.
4 Explain what it is designed to do.
5 Be able to be verified or refuted, i.e. tested.

Literature search

Before any planning is undertaken it is very important and useful to look at previous research into similar hypotheses. Previous knowledge of faults, useful tips and tested methodologies can save a great deal of time and money. Locating a comprehensive review article is a good starting point. This should be followed by a search in the appropriate subject section of *Index Medicus* which is published monthly in the UK. A summary of the content of many nutritional papers can be found in *Nutrition Abstracts and Reviews*, also published monthly. The full text of any particularly relevant papers should then be read in detail.

Planning

All research must be well thought out and planned before it is begun. The aims and objectives must be absolutely clear in the researcher's mind. The primary objectives should be narrowed to two or three simple but important questions. Secondary objectives can answer other less important but, nevertheless, interesting questions.

Table 6.9 gives guidelines for drawing up a 'Project Planning Form' (Calnan 1976). No more than two sheets of A4 paper should be used and the plan should be as concise as possible.

Table 6.7 The advantages of research

It improves the effectiveness of the dietitian's work
It widens the horizons of the work
It forces reading of relevant literature and other studies which have been undertaken
It enforces disciplined thinking and a more organised approach

Table 6.8 The main steps of a study

1	Make an observation about your work as accurately as possible
2	Try to repeat the observation. Be as objective and dispassionate as possible
3	Try to connect the conditions which explain your observations
4	Propose a hypothesis
5	Test the hypothesis
6	Think about the results — do they stand-up? Do they fit in with current knowledge? Do they contest current knowledge? Are they some completely new findings?
7	Draw your conclusions. Can a new hypothesis be formed?
8	Discuss the results with other people
9	Publish your work for the benefit of others

Table 6.9 Project Planning Form

1	Name and date
2	Proposed work
3	Expected findings
4	Clinical significance or application of findings
5	Work previously done on the subject by others (two to four references)
6	Criticism of work done by others
7	Reasons for undertaking
8	Treatment/diet to be used
9	Methods of the experiment – experimental design and experimental technique
10	Duration of the experiment
11	Special technical assistance required
12	Other assistance required
13	Whether Ethical Committee permission is needed

The protocol

When the outline plan is clear, a full protocol can then be prepared. Writing a protocol helps the researcher to think all his/her ideas through clearly and discuss them with others in an organized way. It is a detailed written statement for everyone likely to be involved, e.g. the Ethical Committee and for those funding the project or giving other kinds of back-up and support. Table 6.10 outlines the basic structure of a useful protocol.

Ethics

All proposed research projects should be submitted to the local Ethical Committee. Permission to proceed will usually be granted if there is *no doubt* about the safety of the diet or treatment being tested. However, particularly strict rules apply to research with children and the handicapped. Also, if a research programme seems to be giving no useful results it may be judged more ethical to terminate it prematurely. Since Ethical Committees are usually comprised of people with a lot of research experience, their evaluation of proposed research projects often yields valuable comments and suggestions in addition to their opinion of its ethical nature.

The sample

The number of participants involved in the study will depend primarily on the aims of the study. For studies hoping to show changes in behaviour or some other measurable factor, the sample size needed to show significant changes depends on the degree of change anticipated; the smaller the expected change the larger the number of participants required in the study to give meaningful results (Kirkwood 1988). It is always best to ask a statistician's advice about sample size before embarking on any study since the required sample size is assessed by complicated mathematical formulae.

The type of participants to be studied should be clearly defined beforehand. There should be strict criteria about age, sex, social class, ethnic group, and type of patient (e.g. insulin dependent and/or non-insulin dependent diabetics).

If only a proportion of a group is being studied (e.g. one-fifth of the clinic population) selection of those people must be done on a random basis. This excludes the researcher's own preferences and bias and enables more balanced judgements to be made. Systematic or stratified sampling techniques can also be used. Simple statistics books explain these methods but the advice of a statistician is often a wise precaution.

Table 6.10 Protocol outline

Title	Title of project and names of all researchers (separate page)
Introduction	Outline why the study is being undertaken and any relevant previous research findings
Aims	Give a short, clear statement of the hypothesis and how it is to be tested. (One or two sentences only)
Outline of study	Give details of the hypothesis to be tested and describe the overall plan of the study
Method	Give details of the exact methods to be used. For example: the sample to be tested, the treatment or diet, the measurement and assessment techniques to be used, the details of control populations, the duration of the study, etc.
Phases of the study	Give a simple step-by-step list of each phase and what it is hoped will be achieved at each stage
Evaluation and interpretation	Give a detailed account of how all the data collected will be analysed and the statistical procedures to be used. Define the criteria for success or failure
Applications of findings	Describe the expected benefits and uses of the findings
Proposed time-scale	Give a timetable of the length of each phase of the study and when publication of results can be expected
Facilities to be used	Give a brief description of what facilities are already available, what support and backing will be used and from whom
Budget	If extra funds will be needed, draw up a budget for each phase of the study. This should include costs of extra staff, travel, equipment, computer analyses, extra stationery and postage
Flow Chart	Give a simple diagrammatic summary of all the stages in the research
Appendices	These should include questionnaires, coding methods, data processing methods and other information which is an integral part of the study

The methodology

The methods of the study must be worked out in detail.

Criteria

The criteria to be measured must be clearly defined. For example, if the study is to measure dietary compliance, the exact definitions of 'compliance' and 'non-compliance' must be clarified.

Methods

It is important to work out in advance:

1 Details of all the materials and equipment which will be required, e.g. questionnaires, diet history sheets, food diaries, scales and laboratory tests.

2 The exact procedures to be followed, e.g. questionnaire distribution, type of interview, presence of a control population, types of measurement to be made – indirect (e.g. interviews, impressions, or state of health of participant) or direct (e.g. blood tests, urine tests, weights or skinfold thickness).

3 How observations will be made and how they will be presented.

4 The calculations and statistics to be used.

Control groups

Not all studies will involve control groups but for those which do, the controls should be monitored at the same time as the treated group. They should also be matched for age, sex, social class, ethnic group and any other relevant factors.

Pilot studies

Pilot studies are designed to check the techniques to be used in the study – the data handling methods; whether there will be sufficient data from which to draw conclusions; whether the budget is realistic and whether completion of the project will be possible. They are carried out on a small number of people, similar to those who will be studied. The pilot study should identify any potential difficulties, enabling them to be eliminated before the main study. All questionnaires, survey methods and interview techniques *must* be piloted.

Communication

The language used must avoid jargon and be suitable for the population being studied. Attention should be paid to the needs of multi-ethnic populations and different literacy and language levels generally.

Questionnaires must be valid and reliable. They should be fully understood and stimulate replies. Before writing them, the questions they are designed to answer must be clear and they must be designed to find the answers to those questions. They should give the respondent the minimum amount of work but provide all the information needed (Bennett and Ritchie 1975; Oppenheim 1966).

Computers

Computers can relieve the researcher of many of the time-consuming and difficult aspects of nutritional and statistical analysis. Care must be taken to comply with the requirements of the Data Protection Act (1984) which places conditions on the storage of, for example, the names and addresses of individuals (see Section 1.5).

The results

The main stages in the analysis of results are outlined in Table 6.11. Results should be presented so they can be written up including tables, diagrams and simple statistics. Simple statistical techniques are described in many books (Swinscow 1978; Perry 1979; Greer 1980) but professional statistical guidance will help the inexperienced.

The conclusions

Once the data has been analysed there are three possibilities. The conclusions may agree with and reinforce what is already known, or they may sustain ideas and views suspected to be true but as yet unsubstantiated, or they may be entirely new. If the third option is the case they may need to be confirmed and tested by others.

There is another possible, but less welcome, outcome which is that the results may be too inconclusive either to support or refute a hypothesis. This situation is highly undesirable since it means that the study has largely been a waste of time. It is precisely to avoid this outcome

Table 6.11 Analysing results

Type of analysis	Purpose
Quantitative analysis	Sorting out material, editing, categorizing, coding and tabulating
Qualitative analysis	People's views and impressions. (More difficult to analyse because bias can occur)
Investigating bias	Bias may occur in the sample source, the questions asked or method used, or the analysis
Testing for significance	Are any apparent effects, changes or differences found likely to be 'real' effects in statistical terms, or could they have arisen by chance?
Interpretation of facts	Bridging the gap between what has been discovered and what this means for the future
Recommendations	These may support or refute the original hypothesis and may raise new questions to be answered

that careful planning in the early stages of a study is so important.

All conclusions must be justified by comparing them with theoretical knowledge and other people's results, by questioning the appropriateness of the methods used, by looking for the possibility of human error and any distorting environmental factors and by judging their relevance to the situation.

It is often possible for 'fallacies of logic' to occur. For example 'three men went into three pubs; at the first they drank whisky and water, at the second brandy and water, at the third vodka and water. Next morning they came to the conclusion that the cause of their hangover was from drinking water! Moreover, a modern hospital measuring the output of urine would have supported this hypothesis' (Calnan 1976). All results and conclusions should be widely discussed with colleagues and other interested people before anything is published. Dangers can occur in:

1 Ambiguity of words.
2 Taking statements or events out of context.
3 Arguing from a position of power even if there is no evidence.
4 Constructing arguments based on feelings rather than facts.
5 Accepting lack of contradictory evidence as proof of the hypothesis.
6 Drawing conclusions on the basis of partial truths.
7 Misuse of statistics.
8 Forming irrelevant conclusions.

It is important to remember that in many aspects of nutrition or dietetic research absolute proof is not possible. Conclusions and recommendations have to be made on the basis of probabilities.

Reappraisal

At the end of the study it is important to assess how successful the study has been in order to pinpoint any weaknesses which could be avoided in future investigations. Table 6.12 suggests some of the ways in which this can be done.

Publication and presentation

Publication of research findings is essential if dietitians are to improve the service offered throughout the country. Negative findings are just as interesting and useful as positive findings and all should be shared. Information gleaned in one department may save time and money for many departments but unless it is published few will know about it.

Table 6.13 gives guidelines for writing up research work. Authors must, however, check with specific journals for details of presentation as these differ. Public presentation of results is extremely important for raising relevant issues among interested individuals and for stimulating discussion. Presentation at departmental meetings and local hospital groups is excellent experience and should be encouraged by all departments.

Table 6.12 Self-assessment for the researcher

Methods	Were they reliable and accurate? Were they acceptable to the subjects? Were there any inherent errors? Were the methods up to date? Had the methods previously been tested and found to be competent? Would it have been possible to use any better methods?
Materials	Was the sample tested representative of the group under discussion? Was the control group matched? Were any comparisons justifiably made?
Conclusions	Are they supported by the evidence? Are they reliable? Are they feasible? Are they important?

Table 6.13 Guidelines for writing-up research findings

Title and authors	The title of the project The names of all the researchers. These may be in alphabetical order of surname or with the main workers first The name of the department undertaking the research
Summary	A brief description of the time of the research, the sample, the method and the main conclusions. (Usually not more than about 500 words)
Introduction	Details of the background to the study, previous research and the need for the study
Materials	Description of the subjects and any relevant advice they received
Methods	Details of all the phases of the research including techniques for sampling, measuring, assessment and analysis
Results	The main findings of the survey presented mainly in a textual format but with tables to illustrate points where necessary
Discussion	Interpretation of the results in the light of current knowledge and the implications for the future
Conclusion	Details of what exactly the study has shown or not shown
Acknowledgements	Thanks to all people who have been involved with the research but are not included in the list of authors
References	A list of all papers and publications referred to or used as background to the research. They should give enough detail to enable readers to find the articles from libraries with ease
Appendices	In some instances further material which supports the body of the paper (e.g. diet sheets or questionnaires used) may be appended

6.4.2 Research methodology

Randomized controlled clinical trials

This type of major research project will probably be undertaken less frequently than other forms of research. Controlled clinical trials are likely to be larger studies involving considerable amounts of time and manpower and the implications will be very important. They may be used, for example, to test the efficacy of treatments which are new or already in use. The methodology can be complicated and controlled trials need to be carried out meticulously if useful results are to be achieved. There are a number of books available describing this type of research in detail (Schwartz *et al* 1980; Friedman *et al* 1981; Bulpitt 1983).

Controlled trials are prospective and are usually undertaken if:

1 There is genuine doubt about the usefulness of a diet or treatment for a specific condition.

2 There is a new treatment which may be more effective than the one already in use.

3 There is a need to find out more about how the health problem responds to the dietary change.

Clinical trials need very careful planning and well thought out protocols. The problem being treated and the diet or treatment to be advised need to be very clearly defined. There must also be a properly matched control group and the inexperienced should seek advice on how to obtain such a group. The main principles of a controlled clinical trial are outlined in Table 6.14.

Table 6.14 Principles of a controlled clinical trial

1 Aim to give a definitive answer to one or two precise questions
2 Select the participants according to specific criteria
3 Ensure the sample size is sufficient to show positive results if there are any to be found
4 Randomly allocate participants to the control and intervention groups
5 Ensure the control group will remain 'uncontaminated' by the advice given to the intervention group
6 Make all observations in a systematic way
7 Where relevant the study should be conducted 'blind', i.e. neither the dietitian nor the participant should know who is in the control group and who is in the intervention group (but make sure that somebody knows!)
8 If the control group becomes 'contaminated' accept that they are not a true control and that the results of the trial may not be conclusive

Other methods

Research methods in general practice have been described by Howie (1979). The role of evaluation in nutrition education has been described by Wolf (1980) and Rodwell-Williams (1978). A course 'Learning about methods of research' has been offered in the past by the Open University (Jupp 1981). This course covered social surveys and sampling questionnaires, ethnography (putting emphasis on the collection of data in natural situations) and methodology (initial formulation of ideas, research design, data collection, analyses, presentation and reporting results).

Further reading

Epidemiology for nutritionists. A series of articles in *Human Nutrition: Applied Nutrition* (1983/4):

Burr ML (1983)	1 Some general principles. **37A**, 259–64.
Elwood PC (1983)	2 Sampling. **37A**, 265–9.
Burr ML (1983)	3 The design of studies. **37A**, 339–47.
Fehily AM (1983)	4 Survey methods. **37A**, 419–25.
Sweetnam PM (1984)	5 Some statistical aspects. **38A**, 215–22.
Burr ML (1984)	6 The interpretation of data. **38A**, 324–30.

BDA Research Committee *Getting started on research*. Available from the British Dietetic Association, Birmingham.

References

Bennett AE and Ritchie K (1975) *Questionnaires in medicine – a guide to their design and use*. Oxford University Press, London.

Bulpitt CJ (1983) *Randomized controlled clinical trials*. Martinus Nijhoff Publishers, The Hague.

Calnan J (1976) *One way to do research – the A–Z for those who must*. Heinemann Medical, London.

Friedman LM, Furberg CD and De Mets DL (1981) *Fundamentals of clinical trials*. John Wright, Bristol.

Greer A (1980) *A first course in statistics*. Stanley Thornes, Cheltenham.

Howie JGR (1979) *Research in general practice*. Croom Helm, London.

Jupp V (1981) Learning about methods of research with the Open University. *Nursing Times* **77**(2nd Sept), 1559.

Kirkwood B (1988) *Essentials of medical statistics*. Blackwell Scientific Publications, Oxford.

Oppenheim AN (1966) *Questionnaire design and attitude measurement*. Heinemann, London.

Perry FE (1979) *Statistics revision cards* 4e. Michael Benn, Wetherby.

Rodwell-Williams S (1978) *Essentials of nutrition and diet therapy* 2e. Chapter 11, p. 143. CV Mosby, St Louis.

Schwartz D, Flamant R and Lellouch J (1980) *Clinical trials*. Academic Press, London.

Swinscow TDV (1978) *Statistics at square one*. British Medical Association, London.

Wolf R (1980) The role of evaluation in nutrition education. In *World nutrition and nutrition education*, Sinclair HM and Howat GR (Eds) Chapter 13, p. 109. Oxford University Press, Oxford.

Section 7 **Appendices**

7.1 Appendix 1: Conversion factors and formulae

7.1.1 General

Length/height

Table 7.1

1 inch	=	2.54 cm
1 foot	=	30.48 cm
1 yard	=	91.44 cm
1 cm	=	0.394 inch
1 m	=	39.37 inches

Height conversion tables

Table 7.2 Centimetres/inches

Inches to centimetres		Centimetres to inches	
Inches	cm	cm	Inches
1	2.54	1	0.39
2	5.08	2	0.79
3	7.62	3	1.18
4	10.16	4	1.57
5	12.70	5	1.97
6	15.25	6	2.36
7	17.78	7	2.76
8	20.32	8	3.15
9	22.86	9	3.54
10	25.40	10	3.94
20	50.80	20	7.87
30	76.20	30	11.81
40	101.60	40	15.75
50	127.00	50	19.69
60	152.40	60	23.62
70	177.80	70	27.56
80	203.20	80	31.50
90	228.60	90	35.43
100	254.0	100	39.37
200	508.0	200	78.74
300	762.0	300	118.11
400	1016.0	400	157.48
500	1270.0	500	196.85
600	1524.0	600	236.22
700	1778.0	700	275.59
800	2032.0	800	314.96
900	2286.0	900	354.33
1000	2540.0	1000	393.70

Mass/weight

Table 7.3 Imperial/metric weights

1 ounce	=	28.35 g
1 pound	=	454 g or 0.45 kg
1 g		0.0352 ounces
1 kg		2.203 pounds

Weight conversion tables

Table 7.4 Grams/ounces

Grams to ounces		Ounces to grams	
g	oz	oz	g
1	0.04	1	28.35
2	0.07	2	56.70
3	0.11	3	85.05
4	0.14	4	113.40
5	0.18	5	141.75
6	0.21	6	170.10
7	0.25	7	198.45
8	0.28	8	226.80
9	0.32	9	255.15
10	0.35	10	283.50
15	0.50	11	311.85
20	0.71	12	340.20
30	1.06	13	368.55
40	1.41	14	396.90
50	1.76	15	425.25
60	2.12	16	453.60
70	2.47		
80	2.82		
90	3.17		
100	3.53		

Table 7.5 Kilograms/pounds

Kilograms to pounds			Pounds to kilograms	
kg	lb	oz	lb	kg
0.2	0	7	1	0.453
0.3	0	11	2	0.907
0.4	0	14	3	1.361
0.5	1	2	4	1.814
0.6	1	5	5	2.268
0.7	1	9	6	2.272
0.8	1	13	7	3.175
0.9	2	0	8	3.629
1	2	3	9	4.082
2	4	7	10	4.536
3	6	10	20	9.072
4	8	13	30	13.608
5	11	0	40	18.144
6	13	3	50	22.680
7	15	7	60	27.215
8	17	10	70	31.752
9	19	13	80	36.287
10	22	1	90	40.823
20	44	1	100	45.359
30	66	2	200	90.718
40	88	3	300	136.077
50	110	4	400	181.436
60	132	4	500	226.795
70	154	5		
80	176	6		
90	198	7		
100	220	7		
200	440	15		

Table 7.6 Stones/pounds

Stones to pounds	
Stones	lb
1	14
2	28
3	42
4	56
5	70
6	84
7	98
8	122
9	126
10	140
11	154
12	168
13	182
14	196
15	210
16	224
17	238
18	252
19	266
20	280

Obesity

Table 7.7 Body Mass Index (BMI)

$$\text{BMI} = \frac{\text{Weight (kg)}}{\text{Height (m)}^2}$$

<20 = Long term hazard to health
20–24.9 = Desirable range
25–29.9 = Moderate obesity
>30 = Severe obesity

Volume

Table 7.8 Pints/litres

1 pint = 568 ml or 0.568 l
1 litre = 1.76 pints

7.1.2 Dietary conversion factors

Dietary energy

Table 7.9 SI conversion factors for energy*

Unit	Conversion factor
1 kilocalorie (kcal)	= 4.184 kilojoules (kJ)
	= 0.004184 megajoules (MJ)
1000 kilocalories (kcal)	= 4184 kilojoules (kJ)
	= 4.184 megajoules (MJ)
1 kilojoule (kJ)	= 0.239 kilocalories (kcal)
1 megajoule (MJ)	= 1000 kilojoules (kJ)
	= 239 kilocalories (kcal)

* For interconverting the total energy content of diets of normal composition, a conversion factor of 1 kcal = 4.2 kJ can be used.

To convert:

1 Kilocalories to kilojoules: $\text{kJ} = \text{kcal} \times 4.184$

2 Kilojoules to kilocalories: $\text{kcal} = \dfrac{\text{kJ}}{4.184}$

3 Kilocalories to megajoules: $\text{MJ} = \text{kcal} \times 0.0042$ (or $\text{kcal} \div 239$)

4 Megajoules to kilocalories: $\text{kcal} = \text{MJ} \times 239$

Table 7.10 Nutrient energy yields

Nutrient	Energy yield	
1 g protein provides	4 kcal	(17 kJ)
1 g fat provides	9 kcal	(37 kJ)
1 g carbohydrate provides	3.75 kcal	(16 kJ)
1 g alcohol provides	7 kcal	(29 kJ)
1 g medium chain triglyceride (MCT) provides	8.4 kcal	(35 kJ)

Protein/nitrogen

Dietary protein/dietary nitrogen

Dietary protein (g) = Dietary nitrogen (g) × 6.25*
Dietary nitrogen (g) = Dietary protein (g) ÷ 6.25*

Nitrogen excretion from 24-hour urinary urea

$$\text{Nitrogen excretion (g)} = \text{g urinary urea excreted in 24 hours} \times \frac{28^{\dagger}}{60} \times \frac{6^{\S}}{5}$$

For practical purposes, this formula can be condensed to:

$$\text{Nitrogen excretion (g)} = \frac{\text{mmol urinary urea excreted in 24 hours}}{30}$$

Protein excretion from 24-hour urinary urea

Protein lost in 24 hours (g) = mmol urinary urea lost in 24 hours × 0.212

Correction factor for nitrogen excreted according to changes in plasma urea levels

$$N(g) = (\text{Urea } 2 - \text{Urea } 1) \times W \times 0.6 \times 0.028$$

where Urea 1 = plasma urea (mmol/l) at start of period; Urea 2 = plasma urea (mmol/l) at end of period; 0.6 = factor to estimate body water and W = body weight in kg and 0.028 is the factor to convert mmol to grams.

In anuric patient or renal failure:

$$[(\text{Urea } 2 - \text{Urea } 1) \times W \times 0.6 + (W\ \text{gain} \times \text{Urea } 2)] \times 0.028$$

Calculation of nitrogen balance

1 Nitrogen input (g) = g protein taken in 24 hours ÷ 6.25
2 Nitrogen output (g) = g nitrogen lost in urine + 2–4 g (obligatory nitrogen losses in skin and faeces) + correction for rise in blood urea (subtracted if urea falls)** + nitrogen lost as protein in body fluids††
3 Nitrogen balance = nitrogen input − nitrogen output

Vitamin A

The active vitamin A content of a diet is usually expressed in retinol equivalents.

1 μg retinol equivalent = 1 μg retinol or 6 μg β carotene

$$\therefore \mu\text{g retinol equivalents} = \mu\text{g retinol} + \frac{\mu\text{g } \beta \text{ carotene}}{6}$$

Occasionally, the vitamin A content of foods is still expressed in international units (i.u.).

1 i.u. vitamin A = 0.3 μg retinol or 0.6 μg β carotene.

To convert i.u. to μg retinol equivalents:

μg retinol equivalents = i.u. vitamin A × 0.3 in animal foods (retinol)
or i.u. vitamin A × 0.1 in plant foods (β carotene).

Vitamin D

1 μg vitamin D = 40 i.u.

To convert i.u. to μg

$$\mu\text{g vitamin D} = \frac{\text{i.u.}}{40}$$

Nicotinic acid/tryptophan

Tryptophan can be converted to nicotinic acid.

60 mg tryptophan are required to produce 1 mg nicotinic acid.

1 mg nicotinic acid equivalent = 1 mg available nicotinic acid or 60 mg tryptophan.

$$\text{Nicotinic acid content of a diet in mg equivalents} = \text{nicotinic acid (mg)} + \frac{\left(\text{tryptophan (mg)}\right)}{60}$$

---

*This conversion factor is only appropriate for a mixture of foods. For milk or cereals alone, the factors 6.4 or 5.7 respectively should be used
†The molecular weight of urea is 60, of which 28 parts are nitrogen
§Approximately 80% of the total urinary nitrogen is urea
**If applicable, e.g. in renal failure. For calculation of correction factor see calculation above
††If applicable, e.g. exudate losses from burns or fistulae

7.1.3 Biochemical conversion factors

Millimoles, milligrams and milliequivalents

1 1 millimole (mmol) = atomic weight in mg

To convert mg to mmol

$$\text{mmol} = \text{mg} \div \text{atomic weight.}$$

To convert mmol to mg

$$\text{mg} = \text{mmol} \times \text{atomic weight.}$$

2 1 milliequivalent (mEq) = atomic weight in mg divided by the valency.
To convert mg to mEq

$$\text{mEq} = \frac{\text{mg} \times \text{valency}}{\text{atomic weight}}$$

To convert mEq to mg

$$\text{mg} = \frac{\text{mEq} \times \text{atomic weight}}{\text{valency.}}$$

For minerals with a valency of 1, mEq = mmol; for minerals with a valency of 2, mEq = mmol × 2. Table 7.11 lists the atomic weights and valencies of some minerals and trace elements.

Table 7.11 Atomic weights and valencies of some minerals and trace elements

Mineral	Atomic weight	Valency
Sodium	23.0	1
Potassium	39.0	1
Phosphorus	31.0	2
Calcium	40.0	2
Magnesium	24.3	2
Chlorine	35.4	1
Sulphur	32.0	2
Zinc	65.4	2

Table 7.13 Mineral content of compounds and solutions

Solution/compound	Mineral content	
1 g sodium chloride	393 mg Na	(17.1 mmol Na^+)
1 g sodium bicarbonate	274 mg Na	(12 mmol Na^+)
1 g potassium bicarbonate	390 mg K	(10 mmol K^+)
1 g calcium chloride (dihydrate)	273 mg Ca	(6.8 mmol Ca^{2+})
1 g calcium carbonate	400 mg Ca	(10 mmol Ca^{2+})
1 g calcium gluconate	89 mg Ca	(2.2 mmol Ca^{2+})
1 litre normal saline	3450 mg Na	(150 mmol Na^+)

Table 7.12 Conversion tables: Mmol/mg mEq conversion factors for minerals

Mineral	mg/mmol		mg/mEq		mmol/mEq	
	mg =	mmol =	mg =	mEq =	mmol =	mEq =
Sodium	mmol × 23	mg ÷ 23	mEq × 23	mg ÷ 23	mEq	mmol
Potassium	mmol × 39	mg ÷ 39	mEq × 39	mg ÷ 39	mEq	mmol
Phosphorus	mmol × 31	mg ÷ 31	mEq × 15.5	mg ÷ 15.5	mEq ÷ 2	mmol × 2
Calcium	mmol × 40	mg ÷ 40	mEq × 20	mg ÷ 20	mEq ÷ 2	mmol × 2
Magnesium	mmol × 24.3	mg ÷ 24.3	mEq × 12.15	mg ÷ 12.15	mEq ÷ 2	mmol × 2
Chlorine	mmol × 35.4	mg ÷ 35.4	mEq × 35.4	mg ÷ 35.4	mEq	mmol
Sulphur	mmol × 32	mg ÷ 32	mEq × 16	mg ÷ 16	mEq ÷ 2	mmol × 2
Zinc	mmol × 65.4	mg ÷ 65.4	mEq × 32.7	mg ÷ 32.7	mEq ÷ 2	mmol × 2

Correction of serum calcium for low albumin

$$\begin{array}{l}\text{Corrected serum calcium}\\ \text{level (mmol/l)}\end{array} = \begin{array}{l}\text{Measured serum}\\ \text{calcium}\\ \text{(mmol/l)}\end{array} + \left(\frac{40 - \text{measured albumin}}{40}\right)$$

An alternative (and possibly more accurate) formula is:

$$\begin{array}{l}\text{Corrected serum calcium}\\ \text{level (mmol/l)}\end{array} = \begin{array}{l}\text{Measured serum}\\ \text{calcium}\\ \text{(mmol/l)}\end{array} + \left[\left(40 - \begin{array}{c}\text{measured}\\ \text{albumin}\end{array}\right) \times 0.02\right]$$

To be even more accurate, the serum protein level should be considered as well

$$\begin{array}{l}\text{Corrected serum calcium}\\ \text{level (mmol/l)}\end{array} = \begin{array}{l}\text{Measured serum}\\ \text{calcium}\\ \text{(mmol/l)}\end{array} + \left[\left(72 - \begin{array}{c}\text{measured}\\ \text{protein}\end{array}\right) \times 0.02\right]$$

This corrected calcium value should be added to that obtained from the correction for low albumin, and a mean of the two levels obtained, calculated to two decimal places.

Table 7.14 SI Conversion factors for biochemical constituents

Biochemical constituent	SI to traditional	Traditional to SI
Albumin	g/l × 0.1 = g/dl	g/dl × 10 = g/l
Bicarbonate	mmol/l = mEq/l	mEq/l = mmol/l
Bilirubin	μmol/l × 0.058 = mg/dl	mg/dl × 17 = μmol/l
pCO_2	kPa × 7.5 = mm Hg	mm Hg × 0.133 = kPa
pO_2	kPa × 7.5 = mm Hg	mm Hg × 0.133 = kPa
Calcium	mmol/l × 4 = mg/dl	mg/dl × 0.25 = mmol/l
Chloride	mmol/l = mEq/l	mEq/l = mmol/l
Cholesterol	mmol/l × 39 = mg/dl	mg/dl × 0.0259 = mmol/l
Cortisol	mmol/l × 0.036 = μg/dl	μg/dl × 27.6 = mmol/l
Creatinine	μmol/l × 0.11 = mg/dl	mg/dl × 88.4 = μmol/l
Glucose	mmol/l × 18 = mg/dl	mg/dl × 0.055 = mmol/l
Iron	μmol/l × 5.6 = μg/dl	μg/dl × 0.179 = μmol/l
TIBC	μmol/l × 5.6 = μg/dl	μg/dl × 0.179 = μmol/l
Magnesium	mmol/l × 2.43 = mg/dl	mg/dl × 0.411 = mmol/l
Osmolality	mmol/kg = mosmol/kg	mosmol/kg = mmol/kg
Protein	g/l × 0.1 = g/dl	g/dl × 10 = g/l
Urate	mmol/l × 17 = mg/dl	mg/dl × 0.0595 = mmol/l
Urea	mmol/l × 6 = mg/dl	mg/dl × 0.166 = mmol/l
Potassium	mmol/l = mEq/l	mEq/l = mmol/l
Sodium	mmol/l = mEq/l	mEq/l = mmol/l
Triglyceride	mmol/l × 88.5 = mg/dl	mg/dl × 0.0113 = mmol/l
Calcium (urine)	mmol/24 h × 40 = mg/24 h	mg/24 h × 0.025 = mmol/24 h
Creatinine (urine)	mmol/24 h × 113 = mg/24 h	mg/24 h × 0.0088 = mmol/24 h
Phosphate (urine)	mmol/24 h × 31 = mg/24 h	mg/24 h × 0.032 = mmol/24 h
Urate (urine)	mmol/24 h × 168 = mg/24 h	mg/24 h × 0.0059 = mmol/24 h
Urea (urine)	mmol/24 h × 0.06 = g/24 h	g/24 h × 16.66 = mmol/24 h
Faecal fat	mmol/l × 0.3 = g/24 h	g/24 h × 3.33 = mmol/l

SI units

The International System of Unit (Système International SI) was accepted in 1960 as a logical and coherent system for measurements. This system has been adopted by most laboratories in the UK. Table 7.14 contains the factor necessary to convert some clinical biochemistry constituents from SI units to traditional units and vice versa (Baron *et al* 1974).

Osmolality and osmolarity

Osmolality is the number of osmotically active particles (milliosmoles) in a *kilogram* of *solvent*. Osmolarity is the number of osmotically active particles in a *litre* of *solution* (i.e. solvent + solute).

In body fluids, there is only a small difference between the two. However, in commercially prepared feeds, osmolality is always much higher than osmolarity. Osmolality is therefore the preferred term for comparing the potential hypertonic effect of liquid diets (although in practice, it is often osmolarity which is stated).

The osmolality of a liquid feed is considerably influenced by the content of amino acids and electrolytes such as sodium and potassium. Carbohydrates with a small particle size (e.g. simple sugars) increase osmolality more than complex carbohydrates with a higher molecular weight. Fats do not increase the osmolality of solutions because of their insolubility in water.

The osmolality of blood plasma is normally in the range of 280–300 mosmol/kg and the body attempts to keep the osmolality of the contents of the stomach and intestine at an isotonic level. It does this by producing intestinal secretions which dilute a concentrated meal or drink. If enteral feeds with a high osmolality are administered, large quantities of intestinal secretions will be produced rapidly in order to reduce the osmolality. In order to avoid diarrhoea, it is therefore important to administer such feeds slowly; the number of mosmoles given per unit of time is more important than the number of mosmoles per unit of volume.

Reference

Baron DN, Broughton PMG, Cohen M, Lansley TS, Lewis SM and Shinton NK (1974) The use of SI units in reporting results obtained in hospital laboratories. *J Clin Path* **27**, 590–7.

7.2 Appendix 2: Biochemical and haematological reference ranges

The results of laboratory tests are interpreted by comparison to reference or normal ranges. These are usually defined as the mean ±2 SD (standard deviation) this assumes a Gaussian or Normal (symmetrical) type distribution (Fig. 7.1). Unfortunately most biological data have a skewed rather than a symmetrical distribution and more complex statistical calculations are required to define the reference ranges.

The reference ranges as defined usually include approximately 95% of the normal 'healthy' population, consequently 5% of this population will have values outside the reference range but cannot be said to be abnormal. The use of reference ranges may be illustrated by taking the reference range for blood urea as 3.3–6.7 mmol/l. Approximately 95% of the normal 'healthy' population would come within these limits. However, it would be wrong to interpret a value of 6.4 mmol/l as normal while assuming a value of 7.0 mmol/l to be abnormal. Nature 'abhors abrupt transitions', consequently there is no clear-cut division between 'normal' and 'abnormal', this applies equally well to body weight and height and also to measurements undertaken in the laboratory.

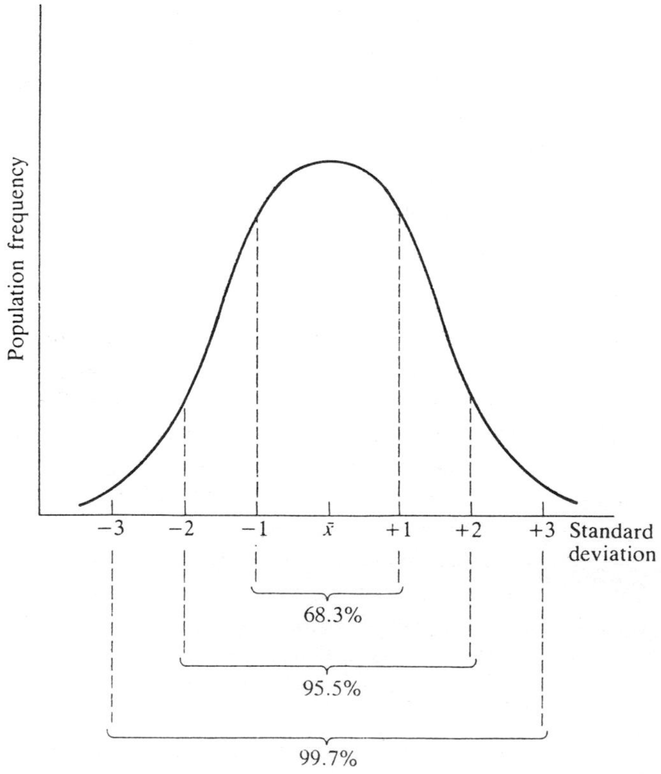

The majority of the normal 'healthy' population will have results close to the mean value for the population as a whole and all values will be distributed around that mean. Consequently the probability that a value is abnormal increases the further it is from the mean value (Fig. 7.2).

A variety of factors can cause variation in the biochemical and haematological constituents present within the blood. These can be conveniently divided into factors which cause variation within an individual and those causing variation between groups of individuals.

Fig. 7.1 Normal or Gaussian distribution curve

7.2.1 Variations within individuals

The following factors can cause significant variation in clinical biochemical and haematological data and should be considered when interpreting individual results.

Diet

Variation in diet can affect the levels of triglycerides, cholesterol, glucose, urea and other blood constituents.

Drugs

These can have significant effects on a number of biochemical determinations, often resulting from secondary

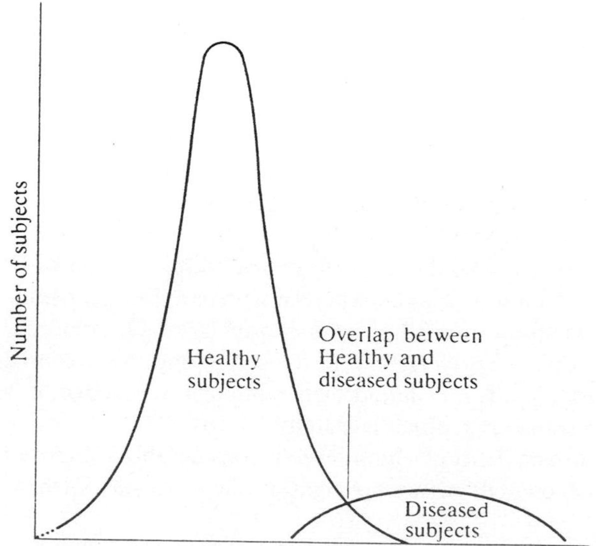

Fig. 7.2 Theoretical distribution of results from healthy and diseased subjects

effects on sensitive organs, e.g. liver, kidney and endocrine glands. Steroids, including oral contraceptives, can cause variations in a number of biochemical and haematological parameters including a reduction in albumin, increases in several carrier proteins, e.g. transcortin, thyroxine binding globulin, caeruloplasmin and transferrin, as well as increases in coagulation factors, e.g. fibrinogen, Factor VII and Factor X.

Menstrual cycle

Several biochemical constituents show marked variations with the phase of the cycle; these include the pituitary gonadotrophins, ovarian steroids and their metabolites. There is also a marked fall in plasma iron just prior to and during menstruation. This is probably produced by hormonal changes rather than blood loss.

Muscular exercise

Moderate exercise can cause increases in levels of potassium, together with a number of enzymes including aspartate transferase, lactate dehydrogenase, creatine kinase and hydroxybutyrate dehydrogenase.

Posture

Significant differences in the concentration of many blood constituents may be obtained by collecting blood samples from ambulant as compared to recumbent individuals. The red cell and white cell counts together with the concentration of proteins (albumin, immunoglobulins, etc.) and protein bound substances (e.g. calcium, cholesterol, T4, cortisol, etc.) may decrease by up to 15% following 30 min recumbency. This is probably due to fluid redistribution within the body. Hospitalized patients usually have their blood samples collected early in the morning following overnight recumbency and consequently have significantly lower values than the normal ambulant (outpatient) population.

Stress

Both emotional and physical stress can alter circulating biochemical constituents causing increases in the levels of pituitary hormones (ACTH, prolactin, growth hormone, etc.) and adrenal steroids (cortisol).

Time of day

Some substances exhibit a marked circadian (diurnal) variation which is independent of meals or other activities, e.g. serum cortisol, iron and the amino acids tyrosine, phenylalanine and tryptophan. Cortisol levels are at their highest in the morning (9AM) and at their lowest levels at midnight while iron concentration may decrease by 50% between the morning and evening. Plasma phenylalanine levels are at their lowest after midnight and reach their highest concentrations between 8.30–10.30AM.

7.2.2 Variation between groups of individuals

A number of factors influence the reference values quoted for individuals. These include age, sex and race.

Age

The blood levels of many biochemical and haematological constituents are age related, these include haemoglobin, total leucocyte count, creatinine, urea, inorganic phosphate and many enzymes, e.g. alkaline phosphatase, creatine kinase and γ-glutamyl transferase. Haemoglobin levels and total leucocyte counts are highest in the newborn and gradually decrease through childhood reaching the adult reference range at puberty. As creatinine is related to muscle mass, paediatric reference ranges are lower than those of adults. Urea levels rise slightly with age but this may well indicate impaired renal function. Alkaline phosphatase activity and inorganic phosphate levels are at their highest during childhood, reaching peak levels at puberty.

Sex

Many biochemical and haematological parameters show concentration differences which are sex dependent including creatinine, iron, urate, urea and of course the various sex hormones. Ferritin, haemoglobin and red cell counts are slightly higher in males than in females. Creatinine and urea levels are 15–20% lower in premenopausal females than in males. Premenopausal females also have lower serum iron levels than males, but after the menopause iron levels are similar in both sexes.

Race

Racial differences have been reported in some biochemical constituents, including cholesterol and protein. The reference ranges for cholesterol are higher in Europeans than in similar groups of Japanese. Similarly the Bantu Africans have higher serum globulins than corresponding Europeans. African and Middle-Eastern individuals have lower total leucocyte and neutrophil counts than other races. Some of these racial differences are probably genetic in origin, although the environment and diet may also be contributory.

7.2.3 Laboratory variations

Methods of analysis and standardizations vary considerably from laboratory to laboratory. These differences will influence the quoted reference ranges, and consequently readers are advised to use only those quoted by their local laboratory. Local reference ranges may be at variance with the levels quoted in the following sections.

7.2.4 Clinical biochemistry reference ranges

Table 7.15 Serum/plasma levels — general biochemistry

Blood constituent	Sex	Range	Units
Albumin		35–45	g/l
Bicarbonate		22–32	mmol/l
Bilirubin		<17	μmol/l
Calcium		2.25–2.65	mmol/l
Chloride		95–105	mmol/l
Cholesterol (desirable)		2.5–5.5	mmol/l
Creatinine		40–130	μmol/l
Glucose (fasting)		3.0–5.0	mmol/l
Inorganic phosphate		0.8–1.4	mmol/l
Magnesium		0.7–1.0	mmol/l
Osmolality		278–305	mosmol/kg
Potassium		3.5–5.0	mmol/l
Sodium		135–150	mmol/l
Total protein		60–80	g/l
Triglycerides		0.5–2.2	mmol/l
Urate	Male	0.25–0.45	mmol/l
	Female	0.15–0.35	mmol/l
Urea		3.3–6.7	mmol/l

Table 7.16 Serum/plasma lipid fractions

Lipid fraction	Sex	Range	Units
HDL cholesterol	Male	0.61–1.57	mmol/l
	Female	0.89–2.05	mmol/l
LDL cholesterol	Male	1.46–5.54	mmol/l
	Female	1.7–5.62	mmol/l
VLDL triglycerides	Male	0.3–2.32	mmol/l
	Female	0.1–0.76	mmol/l

Table 7.17 Serum/plasma enzyme levels

Enzyme	Sex	Range	Units
Acid phosphatase		<8	i.u./l
Alanine transaminase		<35	i.u./l
Alkaline phosphatase		90–300	i.u./l
Amylase		<300	i.u./l
Aspartate transaminase		10–40	i.u./l
Creatinine kinase	Male	<220	i.u./l
	Female	<150	i.u./l
Gamma glutamyl transferase	Male	<43	i.u./l
	Female	<28	i.u./l
Hydroxybutyrate dehydrogenase		<150	i.u./l

Table 7.18 Serum/plasma hormone levels

Hormone	Sex	Time	Range	Units
ACTH			<10–80	ng/l
Cortisol		am	280–700	nmol/l
		pm	140–280	nmol/l
Cortisol (urinary free)			<280	nmol/24 h
Follicle Stimulating Hormone (FSH)			2–8	U/l
Gastrin			<40	pmol/l
Growth Hormone			<20	mU/l
Insulin (fasting)			<15	mU/l
LH			2–8	U/l
17 β Oestradiol	Male		<150	pmol/l
	Female			
	follicular		80–250	pmol/l
	mid cycle		1000–1800	pmol/l
	luteal		400–900	pmol/l
	post-menopausal		<85	pmol/l
Parathormone			<0.73	μg/l
Progesterone	Male		<5	nmol/l
	Female		15–77	nmol/l
Prolactin	Male		<450	U/l
	Female		<600	U/l
TBG			7–17	mg/l
Testosterone	Male		10–30	nmol/l
	Female		0.8–2.8	nmol/l
Thyroxine (T4)			70–140	nmol/l
Tri-iodothyronine (T3)			1.2–3.0	nmol/l
Free Thyroxine			9–22	pmol/l
TSH			<6	mU/l

Table 7.19 Serum protein levels

Protein	Range	Units
∞ 1–antitrypsin	1.8–3.0	g/l
Albumin	35–45	g/l
B2–microglobulin	1.1–2.4	mg/l
C Reactive protein	<10	mg/l
C3 complement	0.7–1.3	g/l
C4 complement	0.12–0.27	g/l
Caeruloplasmin	0.3–0.6	g/l
Fibrinogen (in plasma)	2.0–4.0	g/l
Globulin	19–33	g/l
Haemoglobin A1c	5–8	%
Haptoglobin	0.3–2.0	g/l
Immunoglobulins IgA	0.9–3.4	g/l
Immunoglobulins IgG	5.4–16.1	g/l
Immunoglobulins IgM	0.5–2.0	g/l
Orosomucoid	0.5–1.0	g/l
Prealbumin	200–400	mg/l
Retinol binding protein (RBP)	30–65	mg/l
Thyroxine binding prealbumin (TBPA)	200–400	mg/l
Total protein	60–80	g/l
Transferrin	2.2–3.8	g/l

Table 7.20 Whole blood gases

Gas	Range	Units
pH	7.35–7.45	
Arterial carbon dioxide	4.7–6.0	kPa
Arterial oxygen	>10.6	kPa

Table 7.21 Serum/plasma vitamin levels

Vitamin	Range	Units
Ascorbate	34–68	μmol/l
β carotene	0.9–5.6	μmol/l
Folate	3.0–15.0	μg/l
Red cell folate	160–640	μg/l
Pyridoxine (B_6)	>178	nmol/l
Riboflavin (B_2)	Free <21.3	nmol/l
Riboflavin (B_2)	Total <85.0	nmol/l
Thiamin (B_1)	>40	nmol/l
Vitamin A	0.7–1.7	μmol/l
Vitamin B_{12}	160–925	ng/l
Vitamin D	24–111	nmol/l

Table 7.22 Urine constituents

Constituent	Range	Units
Calcium	<7.5	mmol/24 h
Creatinine	9–18	mmol/24 h
Inorganic phosphate	15–50	mmol/24 h
Osmolality	50–1500	mosmol/24 h
Potassium	40–120	mmol/24 h
Protein	<0.50	g/24 h
Sodium	100–250	mmol/24 h
Urate	<3.0	mmol/24 h
Urea	250–600	mmol/24 h

Table 7.23 Serum/plasma trace element and metal levels

Element		Range	Units
Cadmium (whole blood)		27–480	nmol/l
Calcium		2.25–2.65	mmol/l
Chloride		95–105	mmol/l
Chromium		94–183	nmol/l
Cobalt		8.8–7.3	nmol/l
Copper		10–20	μmol/l
Gold		20–203	pmol/l
Iron	Male	14–31	μmol/l
	Female	11–30	μmol/l
Lead (whole blood)	Adult	<1.8	μmol/l
Magnesium		0.7–1.0	mmol/l
Manganese (whole blood)		100–200	nmol/l
Potassium		3.5–5.0	mmol/l
Selenium*	Child	0.4–1.1	μmol/l
	Adult	1.1–1.9	μmol/l
Sodium		135–150	mmol/l
Zinc		10–18	μmol/l

* Erythrocyte Glutathione peroxidase levels are a good indicator of long term selenium status; for reference ranges contact the laboratory

Table 7.24 Cerebrospinal fluid (CSF) constituents

Constituent	Range	Units
Glucose	2.5–5.0	mmol/l
Protein	0.15–0.45	g/l

Table 7.25 Faeces constituents

Constituent	Range	Units
Faecal fat	<18	mmol/24 h
Nitrogen	70–140	mmol/24 h

7.2.5 Plasma glucose levels in diabetes mellitus

A clinical diagnosis of diabetes mellitus (DM) should not be made on one biochemical result or set of results. Even glucose tolerance tests should be confirmed as there are considerable individual variations.

Any one of the following may be considered as biochemically indicative of diabetes:

1 Presence of the classic symptoms of diabetes namely polyuria, polydipsia, ketonuria and rapid weight loss and unequivocal hyperglycaemia.

2 A subject without obvious symptoms having plasma glucose greater than 8.0 mmol on more than one occasion.

Blood glucose levels

Sample	Excludes DM	Equivocal Repeat with GGT	Diagnostic of DM
Fasting	<5.6	6.0–8.0	>8.0
Random	<8.0	8.0–11.0	>11.0

Glucose tolerance tests

Currently most laboratories in the UK use a 75 g glucose tolerance test and follow the WHO criteria for classification. Samples are collected fasting and at 30, 60, 90 and 120 minutes after a 75 g glucose load. Diagnostic values for venous plasma are as follows:

	Normal response	Impaired glucose tolerance	Diabetes mellitus
Fasting level	<6.5 mmol/l	<7.8 mmol/l	>7.8 mmol/l
Two hour level	<7.8 mmol/l	7.8–11.1 mmol/l	>11.1 mmol/l
All samples	<11.0 mmol/l	one level above 11.1 mmol/l	all levels above 11.1 mmol/l

The responses of individual patients to repeated GTTs under standard conditions over a year vary considerably. It is therefore obligatory to demonstrate a diabetic response to a GTT on more than one occasion before making the diagnosis, with all its social and economic implications.

7.2.6 Haematological reference ranges

Table 7.26 Red cells

Parameter	Age/Sex	Range	Units
Haemoglobin	Male	13.5–17.5	g/dl
	Female	11.5–15.5	g/dl
	Newborn	15–21	g/dl
	3 Months	9.5–12.5	g/dl
Haematocrit (PCV)	Male	40–52	%
	Female	36–48	%
Red cell count	Male	4.5–6.3	10^{12}/l
	Female	4.2–5.4	10^{12}/l
Mean cell haemoglobin (MCH)		27–32	pg
Mean cell volume (MCV)		80–95	fl
Mean cell haemoglobin concentration (MCHC)		32–36	g/dl

Table 7.27 White cells

Cells	Range	Units
White blood count (WBC)	4.0–11.0	10^9/l
Neutrophils	2.5–7.5	10^9/l
Eosinophils	0.04–0.4	10^9/l
Monocytes	0.2–0.8	10^9/l
Basophils	0.01–0.1	10^9/l
Lymphocytes	1.5–3.5	10^9/l
Platelets	150–350	10^9/l

Table 7.28 General haematological values

Parameter	Age/sex	Range	Units
Erythrocyte Sedimentation Rate (ESR)	Male	3–5	mm/h
	Female	4–7	mm/h
Ferritin	Male	40–340	μg/l
	Female	14–148	μg/l
	Children	7–142	μg/l
Serum B12		160–925	ngram/l
Serum folate		3.0–15.0	μg/l
Red cell folate		160–640	μg/l
Prothrombin time (PT)		10–14	seconds
Activated partial thromboplastin time (APTT)		30–40	seconds
Thrombin time (TT)		10–12	seconds

7.2.7 Interpretation of biochemical and haematological data

It is suggested that readers can find further information on the interpretation of biochemical and haematological data from the references at the end of this section. The books by Hoffbrand and Pettit, Walmsley and White and Zilva and Pannall are particularly recommended as giving concise guidelines on interpretation.

References and further reading

Giles AM and Ross BD (1987) Normal or reference values for biochemical data. In *Oxford textbook of medicine*, Weatherall DJ, Ledingham JGC and Worrell DA (Eds) pp. 29.1–29.9. Oxford University Press. Oxford.

Hoffbrand AV and Pettit JE (1980) *Essential haematology*. Blackwell Scientific Publications, Oxford.

Tietz NW (1987) *Fundamentals of clinical chemistry*. WB Saunders, Philadelphia.

Walmsey RN and White GH (1985) *A guide to diagnostic clinical chemistry*. Blackwell Scientific Publications, Oxford.

Whitby LG, Percy-Robb IW and Smith AF (1984) *Lecture notes on clinical chemistry*. Blackwell Scientific Publications, Oxford.

Wilding P and Bailey A (1978) The normal range. In *Scientific foundation of clinical biochemistry Vol 1. Analytical aspects*. Williams DL, Nunn RF and Marks V (Eds) Heinemann Medical, London.

Zilva JF and Pannall PR (1988) *Clinical chemistry in diagnosis and treatment*. Lloyd-Luke, London.

7.3 Appendix 3: Height, weight and skinfold standards

7.3.1 Height and weight standards

Infants and children

Weight and height attained

Many height and weight tables have been compiled for children. One well known set were derived from the combined data of Stuart (Boston) and Meredith (Iowa). Published in Nelson's *Textbook of paediatrics* they gained worldwide use and were also the basis for the WHO standards (Jelliffe 1966). These have been superseded for international use by the US National Center for Health Statistics (NCHS) Standards; these are derived from a very large body of data gathered in the US in the late 1960s and early 1970s. The sample, the construction of the standards, charts and how the data may be used are described by Hamill *et al* (1979), who provide a full list of background references, and NCHS (1977). Tables 7.29 and 7.30 give the recumbent length and weight of children aged 0–3 years, and Tables 7.31 and 7.32 the standing height and weights of children aged 2–18 years.

The British Standards for many years were those of Tanner *et al* (1966a, b). For ages 0–5 years, these were based on about 80 London children of each sex followed longitudinally and 250 Oxford children of each sex at each age. For ages 5–16 years they were based on approximately 24 000 London schoolchildren and from 16–18, on approximately 30 adolescents followed longitudinally.

In 1993 these were superseded by new UK standards based on some 26 000 children aged 0–18 years. The data derive from several large regional and national studies. A5 and A4 charts are available for weight-for-age and height-for-age for 0–18 years and head circumference for 0–12 months. Enquiries should be addressed to the Child Growth Foundation, 2 Mayfield Avenue, Chiswick, London W4 1PW.

There is evidence that growth of infants peaked in the 1960s. Australian studies conducted between 1920 and 1980 show similar birth weights, but median weights at 3, 6, 9 and 12 months rising from 1920 and peaking in 1964, with the 1980 values being similar to those found in the 1930s (Hitchcock *et al* 1981; Gracey and Hitchcock 1985). Studies of breast fed infants in Western countries in the

Table 7.29 Smoothed percentiles of recumbent length (in cm) by sex and age: statistics from NCHS and data from Fels Research Institute, birth to 36 months (NCHS 1977; Hamill *et al* 1979). Reproduced with permission from the National Center for Health Statistics

Sex and age	Smoothed percentile						
	5th	10th	25th	50th	75th	90th	95th
	Recumbent length (cm)						
Male							
Birth	46.4	47.5	49.0	50.5	51.8	53.5	54.4
1 month	50.4	51.3	53.0	54.6	56.2	57.7	58.6
3 months	56.7	57.7	59.4	61.1	63.0	64.5	65.4
6 months	63.4	64.4	66.1	67.8	69.7	71.3	72.3
9 months	68.0	69.1	70.6	72.3	74.0	75.9	77.1
12 months	71.7	72.8	74.3	76.1	77.7	79.8	81.2
18 months	77.5	78.7	80.5	82.4	84.3	86.6	88.1
24 months	82.3	83.5	85.6	87.6	89.9	92.2	93.8
30 months	87.0	88.2	90.1	92.3	94.6	97.0	98.7
36 months	91.6	92.4	94.2	96.5	98.9	101.4	103.1
Female							
Birth	45.4	46.4	48.2	49.9	51.0	52.0	52.9
1 month	49.2	50.2	51.9	53.5	54.9	56.1	56.9
3 months	55.4	56.2	57.8	59.5	61.2	62.7	63.4
6 months	61.8	62.6	64.2	65.9	67.8	69.4	70.2
9 months	66.1	67.0	68.7	70.4	72.4	74.0	75.0
12 months	69.8	70.8	72.4	74.3	76.3	78.0	79.1
18 months	76.0	77.2	78.8	80.9	83.0	85.0	86.1
24 months	81.3	82.5	84.2	86.5	88.7	90.8	92.0
30 months	86.0	87.0	88.9	91.3	93.7	95.6	96.9
36 months	90.0	91.0	93.1	95.6	98.1	100.0	101.5

Table 7.30 Smoothed percentiles of weight (in kg) by sex and age: statistics from NCHS and data from Fels Research Institute, birth to 36 months (NCHS 1977; Hamill *et al* 1979). Reproduced with permission from the National Center for Health Statistics

Sex and age	Smoothed percentile						
	5th	10th	25th	50th	75th	90th	95th
Male				Weight (kg)			
Birth	2.54	2.78	3.00	3.27	3.64	3.82	4.15
1 month	3.16	3.43	3.82	4.29	4.75	5.14	5.38
3 months	4.43	4.78	5.32	5.98	6.56	7.14	7.37
6 months	6.20	6.61	7.20	7.85	8.49	9.10	9.46
9 months	7.52	7.95	8.56	9.18	9.88	10.49	10.93
12 months	8.43	8.84	9.49	10.15	10.91	11.54	11.99
18 months	9.59	9.92	10.67	11.47	12.31	13.05	13.44
24 months	10.54	10.85	11.65	12.59	13.44	14.29	14.70
30 months	11.44	11.80	12.63	13.67	14.51	15.47	15.97
36 months	12.26	12.69	13.58	14.69	15.59	16.66	17.28
Female							
Birth	2.36	2.58	2.93	3.23	3.52	3.64	3.81
1 month	2.97	3.22	3.59	3.98	4.36	4.65	4.92
3 months	4.18	4.47	4.88	5.40	5.90	6.39	6.74
6 months	5.79	6.12	6.60	7.21	7.83	8.38	8.73
9 months	7.00	7.34	7.89	8.56	9.24	9.83	10.17
12 months	7.84	8.19	8.81	9.53	10.23	10.87	11.24
18 months	8.92	9.30	10.04	10.82	11.55	12.30	12.76
24 months	9.87	10.26	11.10	11.90	12.74	13.57	14.08
30 months	10.78	11.21	12.11	12.93	13.93	14.81	15.35
36 months	11.60	12.07	12.99	13.93	15.03	15.97	16.54

Table 7.31 Smoothed percentiles of stature (in cm), by sex and age: Data and statistics from National Center for Health Statistics, 2 to 18 years (From NCHS 1977; Hamill *et al* 1979). Reproduced with permission from the National Center for Health Statistics

Sex and age	Smoothed percentile						
	5th	10th	25th	50th	75th	90th	95th
Male				Stature (cm)			
2.0 years[1]	82.5	83.5	85.3	86.8	89.2	92.0	94.4
2.5 years	85.4	86.5	88.5	90.4	92.9	95.6	97.8
3.0 years	89.0	90.3	92.6	94.9	97.5	100.1	102.0
3.5 years	92.5	93.9	96.4	99.1	101.7	104.3	106.1
4.0 years	95.8	97.3	100.0	102.9	105.7	108.2	109.9
4.5 years	98.9	100.6	103.4	106.6	109.4	111.9	113.5
5.0 years	102.0	103.7	106.5	109.9	112.8	115.4	117.0
5.5 years	104.9	106.7	109.6	113.1	116.1	118.7	120.3
6.0 years	107.7	109.6	112.5	116.1	119.2	121.9	123.5
6.5 years	110.4	112.3	115.3	119.0	122.2	124.9	126.6
7.0 years	113.0	115.0	118.0	121.7	125.0	127.9	129.7
7.5 years	115.6	117.6	120.6	124.4	127.8	130.8	132.7
8.0 years	118.1	120.2	123.2	127.0	130.5	133.6	135.7
8.5 years	120.5	122.7	125.7	129.6	133.2	136.5	138.8
9.0 years	122.9	125.2	128.2	132.2	136.0	139.4	141.8
9.5 years	125.3	127.6	130.8	134.8	138.8	142.4	144.9
10.0 years	127.7	130.1	133.4	137.5	141.6	145.5	148.1
10.5 years	130.1	132.6	136.0	140.3	144.6	148.7	151.5
11.0 years	132.6	135.1	138.7	143.3	147.8	152.1	154.9
11.5 years	135.0	137.7	141.5	146.4	151.1	155.6	158.5
12.0 years	137.6	140.3	144.4	149.7	154.6	159.4	162.3
12.5 years	140.2	143.0	147.4	153.0	158.2	163.2	166.1
13.0 years	142.9	145.8	150.5	156.5	161.8	167.0	169.8
13.5 years	145.7	148.7	153.6	159.9	165.3	170.5	173.4
14.0 years	148.8	151.8	156.9	163.1	168.5	173.8	176.7
14.5 years	152.0	155.0	160.1	166.2	171.5	176.6	179.5
15.0 years	155.2	158.2	163.3	169.0	174.1	178.9	181.9
15.5 years	158.3	161.2	166.2	171.5	176.3	180.8	183.9
16.0 years	161.1	163.9	168.7	173.5	178.1	182.4	185.4

contd.

Table 7.31 *contd.*

Sex and age	Smoothed percentile						
	5th	10th	25th	50th	75th	90th	95th
16.5 years	163.4	166.1	170.6	175.2	179.5	183.6	186.6
17.0 years	164.9	167.7	171.9	176.2	180.5	184.4	187.3
17.5 years	165.6	168.5	172.4	176.7	181.0	185.0	187.6
18.0 years	165.7	168.7	172.3	176.8	181.2	185.3	187.6
Female							
2.0 years	81.6	82.1	84.0	86.8	89.3	92.0	93.6
2.5 years	84.6	85.3	87.3	90.0	92.5	95.0	96.6
3.0 years	88.3	89.3	91.4	94.1	96.6	99.0	100.6
3.5 years	91.7	93.0	95.2	97.9	100.5	102.8	104.5
4.0 years	95.0	96.4	98.8	101.6	104.3	106.6	108.3
4.5 years	98.1	99.7	102.2	105.0	107.9	110.2	112.0
5.0 years	101.1	102.7	105.4	108.4	111.4	113.8	115.6
5.5 years	103.9	105.6	108.4	111.6	114.8	117.4	119.2
6.0 years	106.6	108.4	111.3	114.6	118.1	120.8	122.7
6.5 years	109.2	111.0	114.1	117.6	121.3	124.2	126.1
7.0 years	111.8	113.6	116.8	120.6	124.4	127.6	129.5
7.5 years	114.4	116.2	119.5	123.5	127.5	130.9	132.9
8.0 years	116.9	118.7	122.2	126.4	130.6	134.2	136.2
8.5 years	119.5	121.3	124.9	129.3	133.6	137.4	139.6
9.0 years	122.1	123.9	127.7	132.2	136.7	140.7	142.9
9.5 years	124.8	126.6	130.6	135.2	139.8	143.9	146.2
10.0 years	127.5	129.5	133.6	138.3	142.9	147.2	149.5
10.5 years	130.4	132.5	136.7	141.5	146.1	150.4	152.8
11.0 years	133.5	135.6	140.0	144.8	149.3	153.7	156.2
11.5 years	136.6	139.0	143.5	148.2	152.6	156.9	159.5
12.0 years	139.8	142.3	147.0	151.5	155.8	160.0	162.7
12.5 years	142.7	145.4	150.1	154.6	158.8	162.9	165.6
13.0 years	145.2	148.0	152.8	157.1	161.3	165.3	168.1
13.5 years	147.2	150.0	154.7	159.0	163.2	167.3	170.0
14.0 years	148.7	151.5	155.9	160.4	164.6	168.7	171.3
14.5 years	149.7	152.5	156.8	161.2	165.6	169.8	172.2
15.0 years	150.5	153.2	157.2	161.8	166.3	170.5	172.8
15.5 years	151.1	153.6	157.5	162.1	166.7	170.9	173.1
16.0 years	151.6	154.1	157.8	162.4	166.9	171.1	173.3
16.5 years	152.2	154.6	158.2	162.7	167.1	171.2	173.4
17.0 years	152.7	155.1	158.7	163.1	167.3	171.2	173.5
17.5 years	153.2	155.6	159.1	163.4	167.5	171.1	173.5
18.0 years	153.6	156.0	159.6	163.7	167.6	171.0	173.6

[1] Because of a logistic problem the percentiles of stature for children under 2.5 years are not highly reliable. The age interval represented is 2.00–2.25 years

late 1970s and early 1980s show mean weights and heights close to the 50th NCHS centile until about six months and then falling close to the 25th centile (Whitehead and Paul 1985). No studies have yet continued beyond two or three years, and more work needs to be done to determine the normal pattern of growth for breast fed infants and young children. Smoothed centile charts may be disguising the true natural history of growth.

Weight-for-height standards

The NCHS standards include a table of weight-for-height. However it has two disadvantages (a) it only goes up to 11 years and (b) it is unsound for the assessment of weight-for-height in very tall or very short children – just those for whom clinical assessments are most likely to be needed (Cole 1985).

A good measurement of adiposity should be independent of height and highly correlated with weight and with body fat. Cole *et al* (1981) and Rolland-Cachera *et al* (1982, 1984) have argued for the use of W/H^2. However, because the proportions of fat to lean body mass in the individual and the distribution of degrees of adiposity vary with age, the index has to be age standardized. There is a rapid increase in weight for height until about 12 months, a progressive fall to around six years, and a progressive rise to adulthood.

Cole (1979) and Cole *et al* (1981) have devised a hand slide-rule which gives the Tanner height- and weight-for-age standards for boys and girls, and also has a scale which

Table 7.32 Smoothed percentiles of weight (in kilograms), by sex and age: Data and statistics from National Center for Health Statistics, 1.5 to 18 years (From NCHS 1977; Hamill *et al* 1979) Reproduced with permission from the National Center for Health Statistics

Sex and age	Smoothed percentile						
	5th	10th	25th	50th	75th	90th	95th
Male				Weight (kg)			
1.5 years	9.72	10.18	10.51	11.09	12.02	12.95	14.42
2.0 years	10.49	10.96	11.55	12.34	13.36	14.38	15.50
2.5 years	11.27	11.77	12.55	13.52	14.61	15.71	16.61
3.0 years	12.05	12.58	13.52	14.62	15.78	16.95	17.77
3.5 years	12.84	13.41	14.46	15.68	16.90	18.15	18.98
4.0 years	13.64	14.24	15.39	16.69	17.99	19.32	20.27
4.5 years	14.45	15.10	16.30	17.69	19.06	20.50	21.63
5.0 years	15.27	15.96	17.22	18.67	20.14	21.70	23.09
5.5 years	16.09	16.83	18.14	19.67	21.25	22.96	24.66
6.0 years	16.93	17.72	19.07	20.69	22.40	24.31	26.34
6.5 years	17.78	18.62	20.02	21.74	23.62	25.76	28.16
7.0 years	18.64	19.53	21.00	22.85	24.94	27.36	30.12
7.5 years	19.52	20.45	22.02	24.03	26.36	29.11	32.73
8.0 years	20.40	21.39	23.09	25.30	27.91	31.06	34.51
8.5 years	21.31	22.34	24.21	26.66	29.61	33.22	36.96
9.0 years	22.25	23.33	25.40	28.13	31.46	35.57	39.58
9.5 years	23.25	24.38	26.68	29.73	33.46	38.11	42.35
10.0 years	24.33	25.52	28.07	31.44	35.61	40.80	45.27
10.5 years	25.51	26.78	29.59	33.30	37.92	43.63	48.31
11.0 years	26.80	28.17	31.25	35.30	40.38	46.57	51.47
11.5 years	28.24	29.72	33.08	37.46	43.00	49.61	54.73
12.0 years	29.85	31.46	35.09	39.78	45.77	52.73	58.09
12.5 years	31.64	33.41	37.31	42.27	48.70	55.91	61.52
13.0 years	33.64	35.60	39.74	44.95	51.79	59.12	65.02
13.5 years	35.85	38.03	42.40	47.81	55.02	62.35	68.51
14.0 years	38.22	40.64	45.21	50.77	58.31	65.57	72.13
14.5 years	40.66	43.34	48.08	53.76	61.58	68.76	75.66
15.0 years	43.11	46.06	50.92	56.71	64.72	71.91	79.12
15.5 years	45.50	48.69	53.64	59.51	67.64	74.98	82.45
16.0 years	47.74	51.16	56.16	62.10	70.26	77.97	85.62
16.5 years	49.76	53.39	58.38	64.39	72.46	80.84	88.59
17.0 years	51.50	55.28	60.22	66.31	74.17	83.58	91.31
17.5 years	52.89	56.78	61.61	67.78	75.32	86.14	93.73
18.0 years	53.97	57.89	62.61	68.88	76.04	88.41	95.76
Female							
1.5 years	9.02	9.16	9.61	10.38	10.94	11.75	12.36
2.0 years	9.95	10.32	10.96	11.80	12.73	13.58	14.15
2.5 years	10.80	11.35	12.11	13.03	14.23	15.16	15.76
3.0 years	11.61	12.26	13.11	14.10	15.50	16.54	17.22
3.5 years	12.37	13.08	14.00	15.07	16.59	17.77	18.59
4.0 years	13.11	13.84	14.80	15.96	17.56	18.93	19.91
4.5 years	13.83	14.56	15.55	16.81	18.48	20.06	21.24
5.0 years	14.55	15.26	16.29	17.66	19.39	21.23	22.62
5.5 years	15.29	15.97	17.05	18.56	20.36	22.48	24.11
6.0 years	16.05	16.72	17.86	19.52	21.44	23.89	25.75
6.5 years	16.85	17.51	18.76	20.61	22.68	25.50	27.59
7.0 years	17.71	18.39	19.78	21.84	24.16	27.39	29.68
7.5 years	18.62	19.37	20.95	23.26	25.90	29.57	32.07
8.0 years	19.62	20.45	22.26	24.84	27.88	32.04	34.71
8.5 years	20.68	21.64	23.70	26.58	30.08	34.73	37.58
9.0 years	21.82	22.92	25.27	28.46	32.44	37.60	40.64
9.5 years	23.05	24.29	26.94	30.45	34.94	40.61	43.85
10.0 years	24.36	25.76	28.71	32.55	37.53	43.70	47.17
10.5 years	25.75	27.32	30,57	34.72	40.17	46.84	50.57
11.0 years	27.24	28.97	32.49	36.95	42.84	49.96	54.00
11.5 years	28.83	30.71	34.48	39.23	45.48	53.03	57.42
12.0 years	30.52	32.53	36.52	41.53	48.07	55.99	60.81
12.5 years	32.30	34.42	38.59	43.84	50.56	58.81	64.12
13.0 years	34.14	36.35	40.65	46.10	52.91	61.45	67.30
13.5 years	35.98	38.26	42.65	48.26	55.11	63.87	70.30

contd.

Table 7.32 *contd.*

Sex and age	Smoothed percentile						
	5th	10th	25th	50th	75th	90th	95th
14.0 years	37.76	40.11	44.54	50.28	57.09	66.04	73.08
14.5 years	39.45	41.83	46.28	52.10	58.84	67.95	75.59
15.0 years	40.99	43.38	47.82	53.68	60.32	69.54	77.78
15.5 years	42.32	44.72	49.10	54.96	61.48	70.79	79.59
16.0 years	43.41	45.78	50.09	55.89	62.29	71.68	80.99
16.5 years	44.20	46.54	50.75	56.44	62.75	72.18	81.93
17.0 years	44.74	47.04	51.14	56.69	62.91	72.38	82.46
17.5 years	45.08	47.33	51.33	56.71	62.89	72.37	82.62
18.0 years	45.26	47.47	51.39	56.62	62.78	72.25	82.47

Table 7.33 1983 Metropolitan height and weight tables for men and women on metric basis. According to frame, ages 25–59 (Metropolitan Life Insurance Co 1983). Reproduced courtesy of the Statistical Bulletin, Metropolitan Life Insurance Company

Men Weight in kg (in indoor clothing)*					Women Weight in kg (in indoor clothing)*				
Height (in shoes)† (cm)	Small frame	Medium frame	Mid point	Large frame	Height (in shoes)† (cm)	Small frame	Medium frame	Mid point	Large frame
158	58.3–61.0	59.6–64.2	61.9	62.8–68.3	148	46.4–50.6	49.6–55.1	52.4	53.7–59.8
159	58.6–61.3	59.9–64.5	62.2	63.1–68.8	149	46.6–51.0	50.0–55.5	52.3	54.1–60.3
160	59.0–61.7	60.3–64.9	62.6	63.5–69.4	150	46.7–51.3	50.3–55.9	53.1	54.4–60.9
161	59.3–62.0	60.6–65.2	62.9	63.8–69.9	151	46.9–51.7	50.7–56.4	53.6	54.8–61.4
162	59.7–62.4	61.0–65.6	63.3	64.2–70.5	152	47.1–52.1	51.1–57.0	54.1	55.2–61.9
163	60.0–62.7	61.3–66.0	63.7	64.5–71.1	153	47.4–52.5	51.5–57.5	54.5	55.6–62.4
164	60.4–63.1	61.7–66.5	64.1	64.9–71.8	154	47.8–53.0	51.9–58.0	55.0	56.2–63.0
165	60.8–63.5	62.1–67.0	64.6	65.3–72.5	155	48.1–53.6	52.2–58.6	55.4	56.8–63.6
166	61.1–63.8	62.4–67.6	65.0	65.6–73.2	156	48.5–54.1	52.7–59.1	55.9	57.3–64.1
167	61.5–64.2	62.8–68.2	65.5	66.0–74.0	157	48.8–54.6	53.2–59.6	56.4	57.8–64.6
168	61.8–64.6	63.2–68.7	66.0	66.4–74.7	158	49.3–55.2	53.8–60.2	57.0	58.4–65.3
169	62.2–65.2	63.8–69.3	66.6	67.0–75.4	159	49.8–55.7	54.3–60.7	57.5	58.9–66.0
170	62.5–65.7	64.3–69.8	67.1	67.5–76.1	160	50.3–56.2	54.9–61.2	58.1	59.4–66.7
171	62.9–66.2	64.8–70.3	67.6	68.0–76.8	161	50.8–56.7	55.4–61.7	58.6	59.9–67.4
172	63.2–66.7	65.4–70.8	68.1	68.5–77.5	162	51.4–57.3	55.9–62.3	59.1	60.5–68.1
173	63.6–67.3	65.9–71.4	68.7	69.1–78.2	163	51.9–57.8	56.4–62.8	59.6	61.0–68.8
174	63.9–67.8	66.4–71.9	69.2	69.6–78.9	164	52.5–58.4	57.0–63.4	60.2	61.5–69.5
175	64.3–68.3	66.9–72.4	69.7	70.1–79.6	165	53.0–58.9	57.5–63.9	60.7	62.0–70.2
176	64.7–68.9	67.5–73.0	70.3	70.7–80.3	166	53.6–59.5	58.1–64.5	61.3	62.6–70.9
177	65.0–69.5	68.1–73.5	70.8	71.3–81.0	167	54.1–60.0	58.7–65.0	61.9	63.2–71.7
178	65.4–70.0	68.6–74.0	71.3	71.8–81.8	168	54.6–60.5	59.2–65.5	62.4	63.7–72.4
179	65.7–70.5	69.2–74.6	71.9	72.3–82.5	169	55.2–61.1	59.7–66.1	62.9	64.3–73.1
180	66.1–71.0	69.7–75.1	72.4	72.8–83.3	170	55.7–61.6	60.2–66.6	63.4	64.8–73.8
181	66.6–71.6	70.2–75.8	73.0	73.4–84.0	171	56.2–62.1	60.7–67.1	63.9	65.3–74.5
182	67.1–72.1	70.7–76.5	73.6	73.9–84.7	172	56.8–62.6	61.3–67.6	64.5	65.8–75.2
183	67.7–72.7	71.3–77.2	74.3	74.5–85.4	173	57.3–63.2	61.8–68.2	65.0	66.4–75.9
184	68.2–73.4	71.8–77.9	74.9	75.2–86.1	174	57.8–63.7	62.3–68.7	65.5	66.9–76.4
185	68.7–74.1	72.4–78.6	75.5	75.9–86.8	175	58.3–64.2	62.8–69.2	66.0	67.4–76.9
186	69.2–74.8	73.0–79.3	76.2	76.6–87.6	176	58.9–64.8	63.4–69.8	66.6	68.0–77.5
187	69.8–75.5	73.7–80.0	76.9	77.3–88.5	177	59.5–65.4	64.0–70.4	67.2	68.5–78.1
188	70.3–76.2	74.4–80.7	77.6	78.0–89.4	178	60.0–65.9	64.5–70.9	67.7	69.0–78.6
189	70.9–76.9	74.9–81.5	78.2	78.7–90.3	179	60.5–66.4	65.1–71.4	68.3	69.6–79.1
190	71.4–77.6	75.4–82.2	78.8	79.4–91.2	180	61.0–66.9	65.6–71.9	68.8	70.1–79.6
191	72.1–78.4	76.1–83.0	79.6	80.3–92.1	181	61.6–67.5	66.1–72.5	69.3	70.7–80.2
192	72.8–79.1	76.8–83.9	80.4	81.2–93.0	182	62.1–68.0	66.6–73.0	69.8	71.2–80.7
193	73.5–79.8	77.6–84.8	81.2	82.1–93.9	183	62.6–68.5	67.1–73.5	70.3	71.7–81.2

* Indoor clothing weighing 2.3 kilograms for men and 1.4 kilograms for women

† Shoes with 2.5 cm heels

Source of basic data *Build Study 1979.* Society of Actuaries and Association of Life Insurance Medical Directors of America assesses weight-for-height (W/H^2) on an age standardized basis. It is obtainable from Castlemead Publications, Swains Mill, 4A Crane Mead, Ware, Herts SG12 9PY.

Rolland-Cachera and her colleagues (1982, 1984) have produced charts for clinical records which show the distribution of W/H^2 from birth to 21 years. These can be obtained from Marie-Françoise Rolland-Cachera, ISTNA, CNAM 2-rue Conté, F-75003 Paris, France.

Adults

Relative weight

The tables used for many years to judge the weight of adults are those of the Metropolitan Life Insurance Co. of New York (Metropolitan Life 1959). These have recently been updated (Metropolitan Life 1983) giving slightly higher weights. The tables represent the heights and weights at the time of taking out insurance policies of men and women in apparently good health who subsequently had the best mortality experience, i.e. lived longest. The 1959 tables refer to policies taken out during 1935–54, and 1983 tables to policies of 1954–72. The tables give desirable weights for small, medium and large 'frames'. Table 7.33 gives the 1983 values.

Frame size

Frisancho and Flegal (1983) have suggested that elbow breadth can be used as a measure of frame size, and this concept has been incorporated into the Metropolitan Life Insurance tables. 'The frame designations were developed from elbow breadth measurements taken from the National Health and Nutrition Examination Survey 1971–5 and were devised so that 50% of the population falls within the medium frame and 25% each falls within the small and large frames.'

To make a simple approximation of frame size, extend the arm of the subject and bend the forearm upwards at a 90° angle. Keep the fingers straight and turn the inside of the wrist toward the body. With calipers, measure the distance between the two prominent bones on either side of the elbow.

Table 7.34 lists the elbow measurements for men and women of medium frame at various heights. Measurements lower than those listed indicate a small frame while higher measurements indicate a large frame.

Table 7.34 Determination of body frame by elbow breadth. Reproduced courtesy of the Statistical Bulletin, Metropolitan Life Insurance Co. (Metropolitan Life 1983)

Height (in 1-in heels)	Elbow breadth (in)	Height (in 2.5 cm heels)	Elbow breadth (cm)
Men			
5′2″–5′3″	$2\frac{1}{2}$–$2\frac{7}{8}$″	158–161	6.4–7.2
5′4″–5′7″	$2\frac{5}{8}$–$2\frac{7}{8}$″	162–171	6.7–7.4
5′8″–5′11″	$2\frac{3}{4}$–3″	172–181	6.9–7.6
6′0″–6′3″	$2\frac{3}{4}$–$3\frac{1}{8}$″	182–191	7.1–7.8
6′4″	$2\frac{7}{8}$–$3\frac{1}{4}$″	192–193	7.4–8.1
Women			
4′10″–4′11″	$2\frac{1}{4}$–$2\frac{1}{2}$″	148–151	5.6–6.4
5′0″–5′3″	$2\frac{1}{4}$–$2\frac{1}{2}$″	152–161	5.8–6.5
5′4″–5′7″	$2\frac{3}{8}$–$2\frac{5}{8}$″	162–171	5.9–6.6
5′8″–5′11″	$2\frac{3}{8}$–$2\frac{5}{8}$″	172–181	6.1–6.8
6′0″	$2\frac{1}{2}$–$2\frac{3}{4}$″	182–183	6.2–6.9

Source of basic data. Data tape HANES 1-Anthropometry goniometry skeletal age bone density and cortical thickness, ages 1–74. National Health and Nutrition Examination Survey 1971–75. National Center for Health Statistics. Copyright 1983 Metropolitan Life Insurance Company

7.3.2 Skinfold standards

(Note: The practicalities of measuring skinfold thickness are discussed in Section 1.10.1).

Infancy

Skinfold measurements (like those of adiposity) increase from birth to until they plateau at around 6–9 months of age; they then decrease during early childhood.

The secular trend in infant growth discussed in Section 7.3.1 is also reflected in skinfold measurements. This is illustrated in Table 7.35 which shows the 50th centile values at six and 12 months as reported from studies conducted over the past 25 years.

The three studies conducted in the 1950s and 1960s (Karlberg *et al* 1968; Hutchinson-Smith 1970; Corbier 1980) gave significantly higher values than the three studies conducted since 1974 (Schlüter *et al* 1976; Boulton 1981;

Table 7.35 50th centile value for triceps skinfolds in infants aged 6–12 months as measured in different studies (mm)

Author	Place	Year	Sex	Triceps skinfold	
				6 months	12 months
Corbier (1980)	Brussels	1955–8	Boys	10.3	10.4
			Girls	10.6	11.0
Karlberg *et al* (1968)	Solna, Sweden	1955–8	Boys	9.7	10.4
			Girls	9.8	9.8
Hutchinson-Smith (1970)	Bakewell, Derby, UK	1966–7	Boys	12.0	11.8
			Girls	10.8	11.7
Schluter *et al* (1976)	W. Berlin	1974–5	Boys + Girls	8.5	8.2
Boulton (1981)	Australia	1976–8	Boys	9.0	8.8
			Girls	8.9	9.0
Whitehead and Paul (1985)	Cambridge	1978–9	Boys	7.8	8.0
			Girls	7.5	8.5

Whitehead and Paul 1985). It has been suggested that this reflects the changeover from a high incidence of bottle feeding using unmodified formulae, to the much greater frequency of breast feeding and the use of modified formulae for bottle feeding.

In the UK, Tanner and Whitehouse (1962, 1975) have published two sets of centile charts for triceps and subscapular skinfolds in children. The data for the age-range one month to two years in the 1962 charts are those of Corbicr (1980) from the years 1955–58 and in the 1975 charts they are those of Hutchinson-Smith (1970) from the years 1966–67; they are almost certainly no longer appropriate standards. The values from the post 1974 studies tend to cluster round the 10th centile of the Tanner and Whitehouse 1975 charts.

Table 7.36 gives the values from the Australian studies of Boulton (1981). Studies in progress in Cambridge should provide better UK standards in the near future.

Childhood

Information on skinfold measurements in children of 2–18 years is limited. For 2–5 year olds, the Tanner and Whitehouse charts (1962 and 1975) are based on data from the Longitudinal Growth Study of the Institute of Child Health during the 1950s. For 6–16 year olds, the 1962 charts were based on data from a London County Council survey of school children in 1959, and the 1975 charts on an ILEA survey of 1966. Both studies measured approximately 1000 children of each sex at each age. The latter represent children born between 1950 and 1960.

More recent data are those from the USA National Center of Health Statistics. Preliminary charts of centiles for triceps and subscapular skinfold thicknesses in 2–18 year olds have been published (Owen 1982). These are based on measurements of some 20 000 children in 1963–74. No secular trend was found in this data over the period of time studied. Owen (1982) describes the sample on which the NCHS charts are based and also discusses the limitations on their use.

The 1975 Tanner & Whitehouse charts and the NCHS charts are similar, both in the median (50th centile) and range of values. The major differences are:

1 For the subscapular skinfold in boys, the NCHS chart has lower values at the upper extreme end of the range at all ages.

2 For the subscapular skinfold in girls, the NCHS 50th centile lies on the Tanner and Whitehouse 25th centile.

Table 7.36a–d Percentile values for skinfold thicknesses. Reproduced with permission from Boulton (1981)

a) Triceps skinfold thickness (mm)

Age group (years)		Percentiles 3	10	25	50	75	90	97
0.25	Boys	4.5	5.9	6.9	8.1	9.3	10.5	11.5
	Girls	5.1	5.9	6.7	7.7	8.8	10.3	11.5
0.50	Boys	6.3	6.9	8.1	9.0	10.4	11.5	12.7
	Girls	5.5	5.6	7.6	8.9	10.2	11.4	12.5
1	Boys		6.4	7.5	8.8	10.3	11.5	13.0
	Girls	5.3	6.1	7.4	9.0	10.6	11.8	13.0
2	Boys	5.8	7.2	8.2	9.7	11.2	12.9	14.6
	Girls	5.9	6.9	7.8	9.9	11.9	12.9	14.1
4	Boys	4.0	4.8	6.0	7.7	9.5	11.7	14.0
	Girls	4.5	5.3	6.5	8.6	10.5	12.6	16.0

b) Subscapular skinfold thickness (mm)

Age group (years)		Percentiles 3	10	25	50	75	90	97
0.25	Boys	4.5	5.3	6.1	7.1	8.3	10.6	11.0
	Girls	4.7	5.4	6.3	7.2	8.4	9.5	10.5
0.50	Boys		5.3	6.1	7.2	8.5	9.5	11.5
	Girls		5.4	6.3	7.4	8.6	9.7	11.0
1	Boys		5.2	5.9	7.0	8.5	9.8	10.8
	Girls		5.1	6.1	7.5	8.9	11.1	12.5
2	Boys	4.7	5.3	5.9	6.8	8.0	9.0	11.0
	Girls	5.2	5.7	6.2	7.6	8.9	10.1	12.1

c) Biceps skinfold thickness (mm)

Age group (years)		Percentiles 3	10	25	50	75	90	97
0.25	Boys		4.3	4.9	5.7	7.8	8.0	9.0
	Girls	3.2	3.9	4.7	5.6	6.7	7.8	8.8
0.50	Boys		4.8	5.5	6.3	8.3	9.5	10.5
	Girls	4.0	4.6	5.4	6.4	7.4	8.7	10.5
1	Boys	4.0	4.4	5.1	5.9	6.9	7.9	10.0
	Girls		4.3	5.1	6.2	7.2	8.5	9.2
2	Boys	3.9	4.8	5.3	5.9	7.0	8.4	10.2
	Girls	4.0	4.7	5.5	6.3	7.3	8.5	9.8

d) Supra-iliac skinfold thickness (mm)

Age group (years)		Percentiles 3	10	25	50	75	90	97
0.25	Boys	4.6	5.8	7.3	9.3	11.3	13.8	16.8
	Girls	5.0	6.1	7.3	9.1	11.8	14.7	15.9
0.50	Boys	5.2	6.5	7.8	9.5	11.5	13.5	15.5
	Girls	5.1	6.3	7.8	8.8	11.8	13.8	16.6
1	Boys	4.3	5.3	6.5	8.3	10.7	12.9	16.9
	Girls	4.5	5.6	7.2	9.5	11.6	13.7	15.5
2	Boys	4.0	5.1	5.9	7.7	9.7	11.0	14.8
	Girls	4.9	5.9	7.0	9.1	10.7	13.3	16.0

Table 7.37a–c Age- and sex-specific reference values for upper arm anthropometric measurements of American men. (Developed from the data collected during the NHANES Survey of 1971–4.) Bishop, Bowen and Ritchey (1981). Reproduced with permission from the *Am J Clin Nutr*

a) Triceps skinfold thickness (mm)

Age group (years)	Sample size	Mean (mm)	Percentile						
			5th	10th	25th	50th	75th	90th	95th
18–74	5261	12.0	4.5	6.0	8.0	11.0	15.0	20.0	23.0
18–24	773	11.2	4.0	5.0	7.0	9.5	14.0	20.0	23.0
25–34	804	12.6	4.5	5.5	8.0	12.0	16.0	21.5	24.0
35–44	664	12.4	5.0	6.0	8.5	12.0	15.5	20.0	23.0
45–54	765	12.4	5.0	6.0	8.0	11.0	15.0	20.0	25.5
55–64	598	11.6	5.0	6.0	8.0	11.0	14.0	18.0	21.5
65–74	1657	11.8	4.5	5.5	8.0	11.0	15.0	19.0	22.0

b) Mid upper arm circumference (cm)

Age group (years)	Sample size	Mean (cm)	Percentile						
			5th	10th	25th	50th	75th	90th	95th
18–74	5261	31.8	26.4	27.6	29.6	31.7	33.9	36.0	37.3
18–24	773	30.9	25.7	27.1	28.7	30.7	32.9	35.5	37.4
25–34	804	32.3	27.0	28.2	30.0	32.0	34.4	36.5	37.6
35–44	664	32.7	27.8	28.7	30.7	32.7	34.8	36.3	37.1
45–54	765	32.1	26.7	27.8	30.0	32.0	34.2	36.2	37.6
55–64	598	31.5	25.6	27.3	29.6	31.7	33.4	35.2	36.6
65–74	1657	30.5	25.3	26.5	28.5	30.7	32.4	34.4	35.5

c) Mid upper arm muscle circumference (cm)

Age group (years)	Sample size	Mean (cm)	Percentile						
			5th	10th	25th	50th	75th	90th	95th
18–74	5261	28.0	23.8	24.8	26.3	27.9	29.6	31.4	32.5
18–24	773	27.4	23.5	24.4	25.8	27.2	28.9	30.8	32.3
25–34	804	28.3	24.2	25.3	26.5	28.0	30.0	31.7	32.9
35–44	664	28.8	25.0	25.6	27.1	28.7	30.3	32.1	33.0
45–54	765	28.2	24.0	24.9	26.5	28.1	29.8	31.5	32.6
55–64	598	27.8	22.8	24.4	26.2	27.9	29.6	31.0	31.8
65–74	1657	26.8	22.5	23.7	25.3	26.9	28.5	29.9	30.7

Adults

Skinfolds and mid upper arm circumference in the clinical assessment of malnutrition (see also Chapter 1.11)

Jelliffe (1966) published standards for triceps skinfold, the mid upper arm circumference (MUAC) and the mid arm muscle circumference (MAMC), which consisted of a single figure for each measurement for each sex. These figures have been widely used in the assessment of malnutrition. For lack of better data at the time, these standards were derived from a survey of military personnel in Turkey, Greece and Italy in 1960–1 for the design of protective clothing, and a survey among an unspecified sample of American women in 1939–40, to improve garment and pattern construction, and thus are not highly relevant to whole populations in the 1980s.

Burgert and Anderson (1979) and Bishop and Ritchey (1984) have discussed the limitations of these figures and their use in assessing nutritional status. It is recommended that those concerned in the clinical assessment of nutritional status read these papers for the full discussion. A brief summary follows.

1 The Jelliffe standards were derived from different populations, at different times and by different observers. Neither survey took a random population sample. The precise way in which the standards were derived from the published data is unclear.

2 In 1979 Burgert and Anderson reported an anthropometric study of 77 healthy American adults all within 15% of ideal body weight. The median triceps skinfold thickness, MUAC and MAMC were significantly different from the Jelliffe standards, but not significantly different from measurements obtained in the USA in the Ten State

Table 7.38a–c Age- and sex-specific reference values for the upper arm anthropometric measurements of American women. (Developed from data collected during the NHANES Survey of 1971–4.) Bishop, Bowen and Ritchey (1981). Reproduced with permission from the *Am J Clin Nutr* **34**

a) Triceps skinfold thickness (mm)

Age group (years)	Sample size	Mean (mm)	Percentile 5th	10th	25th	50th	75th	90th	95th
18–74	8410	23.0	11.0	13.0	17.0	22.0	28.0	34.0	37.5
18–24	1523	19.4	9.4	11.0	14.0	18.0	24.0	30.0	34.0
25–34	1896	21.9	10.5	12.0	16.0	21.0	26.5	33.5	37.0
35–44	1664	24.0	12.0	14.0	18.0	23.0	29.5	35.5	39.0
45–54	836	25.4	13.0	15.0	20.0	25.0	30.0	36.0	40.0
55–64	669	24.9	11.0	14.0	19.0	25.0	30.5	35.0	39.0
65–74	1822	23.3	11.5	14.0	18.0	23.0	28.0	33.0	36.0

b) Mid upper arm circumference (cm)

Age group (years)	Sample size	Mean (cm)	Percentile 5th	10th	25th	50th	75th	90th	95th
18–74	8410	29.4	23.2	24.3	26.2	28.7	31.9	35.2	37.8
18–24	1523	27.0	22.1	23.0	24.5	26.4	28.8	31.7	34.3
25–34	1896	28.6	23.3	24.2	25.7	27.8	30.4	34.1	37.2
35–44	1664	30.0	24.1	25.2	26.8	29.2	32.2	36.2	38.5
45–54	836	30.7	24.3	25.7	27.5	30.3	32.9	36.8	39.3
55–64	669	30.7	23.9	25.1	27.7	30.2	33.3	36.3	38.2
65–74	1822	30.1	23.8	25.2	27.4	29.9	32.5	35.3	37.2

c) Mid upper arm muscle circumference (cm)

Age group (years)	Sample size	Mean (cm)	Percentile 5th	10th	25th	50th	75th	90th	95th
18–74	8410	22.2	18.4	19.0	20.2	21.8	23.6	25.8	27.4
18–24	1523	20.9	17.7	18.5	19.4	20.6	22.1	23.6	24.9
25–34	1896	21.7	18.3	18.9	20.0	21.4	22.9	24.9	26.6
35–44	1664	22.5	18.5	19.2	20.6	22.0	24.0	26.1	27.4
45–54	836	22.7	18.8	19.5	20.7	22.2	24.3	26.6	27.8
55–64	669	22.8	18.6	19.5	20.8	22.6	24.4	26.3	28.1
65–74	1822	22.8	18.6	19.5	20.8	22.5	24.4	26.5	28.1

Nutrition Survey (Frisancho 1974). This suggested that the 'standards' were not appropriate to the US population of the early 1970s.

3 The Jelliffe standards are sex-specific, but not age-specific. However these measurements, particularly in women, increase in middle-age and decline in old age. Thus, if a single figure standard is used at different ages widely varying proportions of the population will be defined as 'malnourished'.

4 Severity of nutritional depletion was defined by Jelliffe as a percentage of the standard without identifying the normal distribution of this measurement in the population. Thus, since the patterns of distribution are not the same for triceps skinfold thickness, MUAC and MAMC, a different proportion of the population will be defined as depleted (say less than 60% of the standard) depending on which measurement is under consideration.

The requirement of a standard is that it should reflect the distribution of that measurement in the population under consideration. Such figures do not exist for the UK, but several sets of age-sex specific centiles for upper arm anthropometry have been published for the USA.

Such centiles are available from the Ten State Nutrition Survey (TSNS) of 1968–70 (Frisancho 1974) and the National Health and Nutrition Examination Survey 1971–4 (NHANES I) (Frisancho 1981; Bishop *et al* 1981) and also NHANES II (Frisancho 1984). Tables 7.37 and 7.38 give the values published by Bishop, Bowen and Ritchey (1981). These were chosen for several reasons:

1 Frisancho (1981) gives data from the TSNS, which was biased towards low income groups, and gives values only to age 44.

2 Frisancho (1984) is based on the largest body of data (NHANES I and II), but gives tables which are over-complicated for routine clinical practice, being broken down into both sexes, two broad age groups, three frame

sizes and height in twelve increments of one inch. In addition, while he gives subscapular as well as triceps skinfolds, he does not give MUAC, a direct measurement, but instead gives the derived value 'bone-free arm muscle area'.

3 Bishop *et al* (1981) give data derived from NHANES I only, but this nevertheless represents 5261 men and 8410 women, and the data are corrected to allow for over-representation among the poor. The authors give the triceps skinfold thickness (TST), MUAC and also the more simply derived mid arm muscle circumference (MAMC), which is calculated as

$$\text{MAMC} = \text{MUAC (cm)} - 0.3142\ \text{TST (mm)}.$$

In the interpretation of upper arm anthropometry, perhaps the precise value or values used as standards are of minor importance, since each clinical team will develop its own criteria of malnutrition based on their own experience. However, it is useful to have a generally accepted yardstick, if only to facilitate communications between different groups of workers. The figures in Table 7.37 and 7.38 are put forward as the most appropriate at the time of writing.

Gray and Gray (1979) have suggested that measurements below the 5th percentile be considered as evidence of depletion, and that measurements below the 10th, 15th or other arbitrarily chosen percentile as evidence of marginal depletion.

References

Bishop CW, Bowen PE and Ritchey SJ (1981) Norms for nutritional assessment of American adults by upper arm anthropometry. *Am J Clin Nutr* **34**, 2530–9.

Bishop CW and Ritchey SJ (1984) Evaluating upper arm anthropometric measurements. *J Am Diet Assoc* **84**, 330–5.

Boulton J (1981) Nutrition in childhood and its relationship to early somatic growth, body fat, blood pressure and physical fitness, *Act Paediatr Scand* Suppl 284.

Burgert SL and Anderson CF (1979) An evaluation of upper arm measurements used in nutritional assessment. *Am J Clin Nutr* **32**, 2136–42.

Cole TJ (1979) A method for assessing age standardized weight-for-height in children seen cross-sectionally. *Ann Hum Biol* **6**, 249–68.

Cole TJ (1985) A critique of the NCHS weight for height standard. *Hum Biol* **57**, 183–96.

Cole TJ, Donnet ML and Stanfield JP (1981) Weight-for-height indices to assess nutritional status – a new index on a slide-rule. *Am J Clin Nutr* **34**, 1935–43.

Corbier J (1980) L'evolution de l'epaisseur du tissu cellulaire souscutane chez l'enfant normal, de la naissance a 3 ans. *Courrier* **30**, 40–53.

Frisancho AR (1974) Triceps skinfold and upper arm muscle size norms for assessment of nutritional status. *Am J Clin Nutr* **27**, 1052–8.

Frisancho AR (1981) New norms of upper limb fat and muscle areas for assessment of nutritional status. *Am J Clin Nutr* **34**, 2540–5.

Frisancho AR (1984) New standards of weight and body composition by frame size and height for assessment of nutritional status of adults and the elderly. *Am J Clin Nutr* **40**, 808–19.

Frisancho AR and Flegel PN (1983) Elbow breadth as a measure of frame size for US males and females. *Am J Clin Nutr* **37**, 311–4.

Gairdner D and Pearson J (1971) A growth chart for premature and other infants. *Arch Dis Childh* **46**, 783–7.

Gracey M and Hitchcock NE (1985) Studies of growth of Australian infants. In *Nutritional needs and assessment of normal growth*. Nestlé Nutrition Workshop Series No 7, Gracey M and Falkner F (Eds) Raven Press, New York.

Gray GE and Gray LK (1979) Validity of anthropometric norms used in the assessment of hospitalized patients. *J Parent Ent Nutr* **3**, 366.

Hamill PVV, Drizd TA, Johnson CL, Reed RB, Roche AF and Moore WM (1979) Physical growth: National Center for Health Statistics percentiles. *Am J Clin Nutr* **32**, 607–29.

Hitchcock NE, Owles EN and Gracey M (1981) Breast feeding and growth of healthy infants. *Med J Aust* **2**, 536–7.

Hutchinson-Smith B (1970) The relationship between the weight of an infant and lower respiratory infection. *Med Officer* **May 8**, 257–62.

Hutchinson-Smith B (1973) Skinfold thickness in infancy in relation to birth weight. *Dev Med Child Neurol* **15**, 628–34.

Jelliffe DB (1966) *The assessment of the nutritional status of the community*. World Health Organization, Geneva.

Karlberg P, Klackenberg G, Engstrom I, Klackenberg-Larsson I, Lichtenstein H, Stensson J and Svennberg I (1968) The development of children in a Swedish urban community. A prospective longitudinal study. *Acta Paediatr Scand* Suppl 187.

Metropolitan Life (1959) Metropolitan Life Insurance Company Statistical Bulletin **40** (Nov–Dec).

Metropolitan Life (1983) Metropolitan Life Insurance Company Statistical Bulletin **64**, 1–9.

National Center for Health Statistics (1977) *NCHS growth curves for children 0–18 years, United States*. Vital and health statistics Series 11, No 165, Health Resources Administration. Government Printing Office, Washington DC.

Owen GM (1982) Measurement, recording and assessment of skinfold thickness in childhood and adolescence: report of a small meeting. *Am J Clin Nutr* **35**, 629–38.

Rolland-Cachera MF, Deheeger M, Bellisle F, Sempé M, Guilloud-Bataille M and Patois E (1984) Adiposity rebound in children: a simple indicator for predicting obesity. *Am J Clin Nutr* **39**, 129–35.

Rolland-Cachera MF, Sempe M, Gilloud-Bataille M, Patois E, Pequignot-Guggenbuhl F and Fautrad V (1982) Adiposity indices in children. *Am J Clin Nutr* **36**, 178–84.

Schluter K, Funfack W, Pachaly J and Weber B (1976) Development of subcutaneous fat in infancy. Standards for tricipital, subscapular and supra-iliac skinfolds in German infants. *Europ J Pediatr* **123**, 255–67.

Tanner JM and Whitehouse RH (1962) Standards for subcutaneous fat in British children. Percentiles for thickness of skinfolds over triceps and below scapula. *Br Med J* **1**, 446–50.

Tanner JM and Whitehouse RH (1975) Revised standards for triceps and subscapular skinfolds in British children. *Arch Dis Childh* **50**, 142–5.

Tanner JM, Whitehouse RH and Takaishi M (1966a) Standards from birth to maturity for height, weight, height velocity and weight velocity: British children 1965, Part I. *Arch Dis Childh* **41**, 454–71.

Tanner JM, Whitehouse RH and Takaishi M (1966b) Standards from birth to maturity for height, weight, height velocity and weight velocity: British children 1965, Part II. *Arch Dis Childh* **41**, 613–35.

Whitehead RG and Paul AA (1985) Human lactation, infant feeding and growth: secular trends. In *Nutritional needs and assessment of normal growth*. Gracey M and Falkner F (Eds) Nestlé Nutrition Workshop Series No 7. Raven Press, New York.

7.4 Appendix 4: BMR equations and ready reference tables

7.4.1 BMR prediction equations

Prediction equations based on weight and height or surface area have been in use for many years. For reference, two of the most commonly used, those of Robertson and Reid (1952) and Harris and Benedict (1919), are given below.

However dietitians should note that these have now been superseded by newer equations and the following should be used in preference:

For clinical situations, the equations of Schofield *et al* (1985). See Section 1.12, the subsection on 'Calculation of the BMR'.

For healthy individuals, the modified Schofield equations given in the COMA report on Dietary Reference Values (DoH 1991), (see Section 2.1.2, the Subsection on 'Basal Metabolic Rate'). Ready reference tables of BMR based on these equations can be found in this section.

Calculation of the BMR from the standards of Robertson and Reid (1952)

1 The surface area of the patient is calculated using the formula:

$$M = W^{0.425} \times H^{0.725} \times 71.84$$

where M = surface area in m^2; W = weight in kg and H = height in cm.

Alternatively, a nomogram based on the above formula may be used (Fig. 7.3).

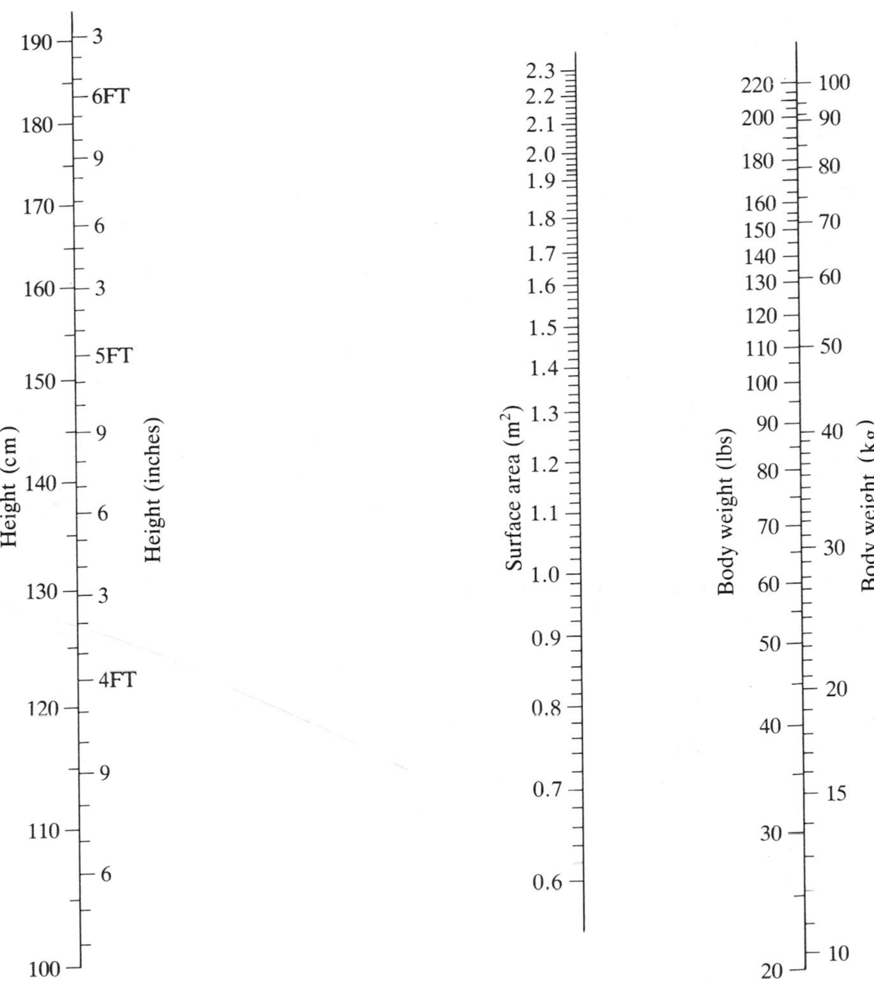

Fig. 7.3 Nomogram for determining body surface area (Dubois and Dubois 1916)

2 The surface area is then multiplied by the predicted standard metabolic expenditure for age and sex (Table 7.39).
3 The resulting figure is the basal metabolic requirement.

Calculation of the BMR using the Harris-Benedict equation

The following formulae will give an estimate of the BMR for disease-free individuals (kcal per 24 hours):

1 Males $= 66 + (13.7 \times W) + (5 \times H) - (6.8 \times A)$

2 Females $= 655 + (9.6 \times W) + (1.7 \times H) - (4.7 \times A)$

3 Infants* $= 22.1 + (31.05 \times W) + (1.16 \times H)$

where W = Body weight in kg; H = height/length in cm and A = age in years.

* This formula was derived from studies on infants under the age of two weeks.)

7.4.2 BMR ready reference tables

The following tables have been derived from the modified Schofield equations (Schofield *et al* 1985) and enable the BMR of an individual to be predicted from his/her weight and age, in either MJ (Table 7.40) or kcal (Table 7.41).

Table 7.39 Variation of basal metabolic rate per square metre body surface area for age and sex (Robertson and Reid 1952)**

Standard of ROBERTSON and REID (3–75 years)
Lancet **1**, 940 (1952)

Age	kcal per m² per hour		Age	kcal per m² per hour	
	Boys	Girls		Men	Women
3	60.1*	54.5*	17	39.7*	35.3
4	57.9	53.9	18	39.2	34.9
5	56.3	53.0	19	38.8	34.5
6	54.2	51.8	20	38.4	34.3
7	52.1	50.2	25	37.1	34.0
8	50.1	48.4	30	36.4	34.1
9	48.2	46.4	35	35.9	33.5
10	46.6	44.3	40	35.5	32.6
11	45.1	42.4	45	34.1	32.2
12	43.8	40.6	50	33.8	31.9
13	42.7	39.1	55	33.4	31.6
14	41.8	37.8	60	33.1	31.3
15	41.0	36.8	65	32.7	31.0
16	40.3	36.0	70	32.4*	30.7
			75	32.0*	—

* Extrapolated or based on fewer than 7 subjects.
** Alternative sets of standards have been devised by Fleish (1951) and Altman and Dittmer (1968)

Table 7.40 BMR Ready Reference table (MJ)

	Males					Females				
Wt kg	10–17 yrs	18–29 yrs	30–59 yrs	60–74 yrs	74+ yrs	10–17 yrs	18–29 yrs	30–59 yrs	60–74 yrs	74+ yrs
25	4.60	4.47	4.85	4.18	4.31	4.30	3.59	4.39	3.84	3.64
26	4.68	4.53	4.90	4.23	4.34	4.35	3.65	4.42	3.88	3.68
27	4.75	4.60	4.95	4.28	4.38	4.41	3.71	4.46	3.92	3.72
28	4.83	4.66	5.00	4.33	4.41	4.47	3.77	4.49	3.96	3.76
29	4.90	4.72	5.05	4.38	4.45	4.52	3.83	4.52	3.99	3.80
30	4.97	4.79	5.09	4.43	4.48	4.58	3.90	4.56	4.03	3.84
31	5.05	4.85	5.14	4.48	4.52	4.63	3.96	4.59	4.07	3.88
32	5.12	4.91	5.19	4.53	4.55	4.69	4.02	4.63	4.11	3.92
33	5.20	4.98	5.24	4.58	4.59	4.75	4.08	4.66	4.15	3.96
34	5.27	5.04	5.29	4.63	4.62	4.80	4.14	4.69	4.19	4.00
35	5.34	5.10	5.33	4.68	4.66	4.86	4.21	4.73	4.23	4.05
36	5.42	5.16	5.38	4.73	4.69	4.91	4.27	4.76	4.26	4.09
37	5.49	5.23	5.43	4.78	4.73	4.97	4.33	4.80	4.30	4.13
38	5.57	5.29	5.48	4.83	4.76	5.03	4.39	4.83	4.34	4.17
39	5.64	5.35	5.53	4.88	4.80	5.08	4.45	4.86	4.38	4.21
40	5.71	5.42	5.57	4.93	4.83	5.14	4.52	4.90	4.42	4.25
41	5.79	5.48	5.62	4.98	4.87	5.19	4.58	4.93	4.46	4.29
42	5.86	5.54	5.67	5.03	4.90	5.25	4.64	4.97	4.50	4.33
43	5.94	5.61	5.72	5.08	4.94	5.31	4.70	5.00	4.53	4.37
44	6.01	5.67	5.77	5.13	4.97	5.36	4.76	5.03	4.57	4.41
45	6.08	5.73	5.81	5.18	5.01	5.42	4.83	5.07	4.61	4.46
46	6.16	5.79	5.86	5.23	5.04	5.47	4.89	5.10	4.65	4.50
47	6.23	5.86	5.91	5.28	5.08	5.53	4.95	5.14	4.69	4.54
48	6.31	5.92	5.96	5.33	5.11	5.59	5.01	5.17	4.73	4.58
49	6.38	5.98	6.01	5.38	5.15	5.64	5.07	5.20	4.77	4.62
50	6.45	6.05	6.05	5.43	5.18	5.70	5.14	5.24	4.81	4.66
51	6.53	6.11	6.10	5.47	5.22	5.75	5.20	5.27	4.84	4.70

Table 7.40 *contd.*

	Males					Females				
Wt kg	10–17 yrs	18–29 yrs	30–59 yrs	60–74 yrs	74+ yrs	10–17 yrs	18–29 yrs	30–59 yrs	60–74 yrs	74+ yrs
52	6.60	6.17	6.15	5.52	5.25	5.81	5.26	5.31	4.88	4.74
53	6.68	6.24	6.20	5.57	5.29	5.87	5.32	5.34	4.92	4.78
54	6.75	6.30	6.25	5.62	5.32	5.92	5.38	5.37	4.96	4.82
55	6.82	6.36	6.29	5.67	5.36	5.98	5.45	5.41	5.00	4.87
56	6.90	6.42	6.34	5.72	5.39	6.03	5.51	5.44	5.04	4.91
57	6.97	6.49	6.39	5.77	5.43	6.09	5.57	5.48	5.08	4.95
58	7.05	6.55	6.44	5.82	5.46	6.15	5.63	5.51	5.11	4.99
59	7.12	6.61	6.49	5.87	5.50	6.20	5.69	5.54	5.15	5.03
60	7.19	6.68	6.53	5.92	5.53	6.26	5.76	5.58	5.19	5.07
61	7.27	6.74	6.58	5.97	5.57	6.31	5.82	5.61	5.23	5.11
62	7.34	6.80	6.63	6.02	5.60	6.37	5.88	5.65	5.27	5.15
63	7.42	6.87	6.68	6.07	5.64	6.43	5.94	5.68	5.31	5.19
64	7.49	6.93	6.73	6.12	5.67	6.48	6.00	5.71	5.35	5.23
65	7.56	6.99	6.77	6.17	5.71	6.54	6.07	5.75	5.38	5.28
66	7.64	7.05	6.82	6.22	5.74	6.59	6.13	5.78	5.42	5.32
67	7.71	7.12	6.87	6.27	5.78	6.65	6.19	5.82	5.46	5.36
68	7.79	7.18	6.92	6.32	5.81	6.71	6.25	5.85	5.50	5.40
69	7.86	7.24	6.97	6.37	5.85	6.76	6.31	5.88	5.54	5.44
70	7.93	7.31	7.01	6.42	5.88	6.82	6.38	5.92	5.58	5.48
71	8.01	7.37	7.06	6.47	5.92	6.87	6.44	5.95	5.62	5.52
72	8.08	7.43	7.11	6.52	5.95	6.93	6.50	5.99	5.65	5.56
73	8.16	7.50	7.16	6.57	5.99	6.99	6.56	6.02	5.69	5.60
74	8.23	7.56	7.21	6.62	6.02	7.04	6.62	6.05	5.73	5.64
75	8.30	7.62	7.25	6.67	6.06	7.10	6.69	6.09	5.77	5.69
76	8.38	7.68	7.30	6.72	6.09	7.15	6.75	6.12	5.81	5.73
77	8.45	7.75	7.35	6.77	6.13	7.21	6.81	6.16	5.85	5.77
78	8.53	7.81	7.40	6.82	6.16	7.27	6.87	6.19	5.89	5.81
79	8.60	7.87	7.45	6.87	6.20	7.32	6.93	6.22	5.92	5.85
80	8.67	7.94	7.49	6.92	6.23	7.38	7.00	6.26	5.96	5.89
81	8.75	8.00	7.54	6.97	6.27	7.43	7.06	6.29	6.00	5.93
82	8.82	8.06	7.59	7.02	6.30	7.49	7.12	6.33	6.04	5.97
83	8.90	8.13	7.64	7.07	6.34	7.55	7.18	6.36	6.08	6.01
84	8.97	8.19	7.69	7.12	6.37	7.60	7.24	6.39	6.12	6.05
85	9.04	8.25	7.73	7.17	6.41	7.66	7.31	6.43	6.16	6.10
86	9.12	8.31	7.78	7.22	6.44	7.71	7.37	6.46	6.19	6.14
87	9.19	8.38	7.83	7.27	6.48	7.77	7.43	6.50	6.23	6.18
88	9.27	8.44	7.88	7.32	6.51	7.83	7.49	6.53	6.27	6.22
89	9.34	8.50	7.93	7.37	6.55	7.88	7.55	6.56	6.31	6.26
90	9.41	8.57	7.97	7.42	6.58	7.94	7.62	6.60	6.35	6.30
91	9.49	8.63	8.02	7.47	6.62	7.99	7.68	6.63	6.39	6.34
92	9.56	8.69	8.07	7.52	6.65	8.05	7.74	6.67	6.43	6.38
93	9.64	8.76	8.12	7.57	6.69	8.11	7.80	6.70	6.46	6.42
94	9.71	8.82	8.17	7.62	6.72	8.16	7.86	6.73	6.50	6.46
95	9.78	8.88	8.21	7.67	6.76	8.22	7.93	6.77	6.54	6.51
96	9.86	8.94	8.26	7.72	6.79	8.27	7.99	6.80	6.58	6.55
97	9.93	9.01	8.31	7.77	6.83	8.33	8.05	6.84	6.62	6.59
98	10.01	9.07	8.36	7.82	6.86	8.39	8.11	6.87	6.66	6.63
99	10.08	9.13	8.41	7.87	6.90	8.44	8.17	6.90	6.70	6.67

Note: The deviation from the predicted value may be greater at the extremes of body composition. There is limited data on the BMR of individuals with body weights greater than 80 kg, and Schofield *et al* (1985) did consider it appropriate to include heavier weights in their look-up table. They are included here for ease of reference for those working in obesity clinics, although it is probable that the equations over-estimate BMR in the heaviest individuals.

Discussion on the use of these tables is given in Section 2.1.2

Table 7.41 BMR Ready Reference table (kcal)

	Males					Females				
Wt kg	10–17 yrs	18–29 yrs	30–59 yrs	60–74 yrs	74+ yrs	10–17 yrs	18–29 yrs	30–59 yrs	60–74 yrs	74+ yrs
25	1100	1070	1161	998	1031	1027	857	1054	917	869
26	1117	1085	1172	1009	1039	1040	872	1062	926	879
27	1135	1100	1184	1021	1048	1054	887	1070	935	889
28	1153	1115	1195	1033	1056	1067	901	1078	945	898
29	1170	1130	1207	1045	1065	1081	916	1087	954	908
30	1188	1145	1218	1057	1073	1094	931	1095	963	918
31	1206	1160	1230	1069	1081	1107	946	1103	972	928
32	1223	1175	1241	1081	1090	1121	961	1112	981	938
33	1241	1190	1253	1093	1098	1134	975	1120	991	947
34	1259	1205	1264	1105	1107	1148	990	1128	1000	957
35	1277	1221	1276	1117	1115	1161	1005	1137	1009	967
36	1294	1236	1287	1128	1123	1174	1020	1145	1018	977
37	1312	1251	1299	1140	1132	1188	1035	1153	1027	987
38	1330	1266	1310	1152	1140	1201	1049	1161	1037	996
39	1347	1281	1322	1164	1149	1215	1064	1170	1046	1006
40	1365	1296	1333	1176	1157	1228	1079	1178	1055	1016
41	1383	1311	1345	1188	1165	1241	1094	1186	1064	1026
42	1400	1326	1356	1200	1174	1255	1109	1195	1073	1036
43	1418	1341	1368	1212	1182	1268	1123	1203	1083	1045
44	1436	1356	1379	1224	1191	1282	1138	1211	1092	1055
45	1454	1372	1391	1236	1199	1295	1153	1220	1101	1065
46	1471	1387	1402	1247	1207	1308	1168	1228	1110	1075
47	1489	1402	1414	1259	1216	1322	1183	1236	1119	1085
48	1507	1417	1425	1271	1224	1335	1197	1244	1129	1094
49	1524	1432	1437	1283	1233	1349	1212	1253	1138	1104
50	1542	1447	1448	1295	1241	1362	1227	1261	1147	1114
51	1560	1462	1460	1307	1249	1375	1242	1269	1156	1124
52	1577	1477	1471	1319	1258	1389	1257	1278	1165	1134
53	1595	1492	1483	1331	1266	1402	1271	1286	1175	1143
54	1613	1507	1494	1343	1275	1416	1286	1294	1184	1153
55	1631	1523	1506	1355	1283	1429	1301	1303	1193	1163
56	1648	1538	1517	1366	1291	1442	1316	1311	1202	1173
57	1666	1553	1529	1378	1300	1456	1331	1319	1211	1183
58	1684	1568	1540	1390	1308	1469	1345	1327	1221	1192
59	1701	1583	1552	1402	1317	1483	1360	1336	1230	1202
60	1719	1598	1563	1414	1325	1496	1375	1344	1239	1212
61	1737	1613	1575	1426	1333	1509	1390	1352	1248	1222
62	1754	1628	1586	1438	1342	1523	1405	1361	1257	1232
63	1772	1643	1598	1450	1350	1536	1419	1369	1267	1241
64	1790	1658	1609	1462	1359	1550	1434	1377	1276	1251
65	1808	1674	1621	1474	1367	1563	1449	1386	1285	1261
66	1825	1689	1632	1485	1375	1576	1464	1394	1294	1271
67	1843	1704	1644	1497	1384	1590	1479	1402	1303	1281
68	1861	1719	1655	1509	1392	1603	1493	1410	1313	1290
69	1878	1734	1667	1521	1401	1617	1508	1419	1322	1300
70	1896	1749	1678	1533	1409	1630	1523	1427	1331	1310
71	1914	1764	1690	1545	1417	1643	1538	1435	1340	1320
72	1931	1779	1701	1557	1426	1657	1553	1444	1349	1330
73	1949	1794	1713	1569	1434	1670	1567	1452	1359	1339
74	1967	1809	1724	1581	1443	1684	1582	1460	1368	1349
75	1985	1825	1736	1593	1451	1697	1597	1469	1377	1359
76	2002	1840	1747	1604	1459	1710	1612	1477	1386	1369
77	2020	1855	1759	1616	1468	1724	1627	1485	1395	1379
78	2038	1870	1770	1628	1476	1737	1641	1493	1405	1388
79	2055	1885	1782	1640	1485	1751	1656	1502	1414	1398
80	2073	1900	1793	1652	1493	1764	1671	1510	1423	1408
81	2091	1915	1805	1664	1501	1777	1686	1518	1432	1418
82	2108	1930	1816	1676	1510	1791	1701	1527	1441	1428
83	2126	1945	1828	1688	1518	1804	1715	1535	1451	1437
84	2144	1960	1839	1700	1527	1818	1730	1543	1460	1447
85	2162	1976	1851	1712	1535	1831	1745	1552	1469	1457

Table 7.41 *contd.*

	Males					Females				
Wt kg	10–17 yrs	18–29 yrs	30–59 yrs	60–74 yrs	74+ yrs	10–17 yrs	18–29 yrs	30–59 yrs	60–74 yrs	74+ yrs
86	2179	1991	1862	1723	1543	1844	1760	1560	1478	1467
87	2197	2006	1874	1735	1552	1858	1775	1568	1487	1477
88	2215	2021	1885	1747	1560	1871	1789	1576	1497	1486
89	2232	2036	1897	1759	1569	1885	1804	1585	1506	1496
90	2250	2051	1908	1771	1577	1898	1819	1593	1515	1506
91	2268	2066	1920	1783	1585	1911	1834	1601	1524	1516
92	2285	2081	1931	1795	1594	1925	1849	1610	1533	1526
93	2303	2096	1943	1807	1602	1938	1863	1618	1543	1535
94	2321	2111	1954	1819	1611	1952	1878	1626	1552	1545
95	2339	2127	1966	1831	1619	1965	1893	1635	1561	1555
96	2356	2142	1977	1842	1627	1978	1908	1643	1570	1565
97	2374	2157	1989	1854	1636	1992	1923	1651	1579	1575
98	2392	2172	2000	1866	1644	2005	1937	1659	1589	1584
99	2409	2187	2012	1878	1653	2019	1952	1668	1598	1594

Note: The deviation from the predicted value may be greater at the extremes of body composition. There is limited data on the BMR of individuals with body weights greater than 80 kg, and Schofield *et al* (1985) did consider it appropriate to include heavier weights in their look-up table. They are included here for ease of reference for those working in obesity clinics, although it is probable that the equations over-estimate BMR in the heaviest individuals.

Discussion on the use of these tables is given in Section 2.1.2

References

Altman PL and Dittmer DS (1968) *Metabolism*. p. 345. Federation of American Societies for Experimental Biology, Bethesda.

Department of Health (1991) *Dietary Reference Values for food energy and nutrients for the United Kingdom*. Rep Hlth Soc Subj 41. HMSO, London.

Dubois D and Dubois EF (1916) Clinical calorimetry — a formula to estimate the approximate surface area if height and weight be known. *Arch Intern Med* **17**, 863–71.

Fleish A (1951) Le metabolisme basal standard et sa determination au moyen du 'metabocalculator'. *Helv Med Acta* **18**, 23.

Harris JA and Benedict FG (1919) *Biometric studies of basal metabolism in man*. Carnegie Institute, Washington DC.

Robertson JD and Reid DD (1952) Standards for the basal metabolism of normal people in Britain. *Lancet* **1**, 940–43.

Schofield WN, Schofield C and James WPT (1985) Basal metabolic rate — review and prediction, together with annotated bibliography of source material. *Hum Nutr: Clin Nutr* **39C**(Suppl 1), 5–96.

7.5 Appendix 5: Typical weights and portion sizes of common foods

The information in Tables 7.42 and 7.43 is intended as a guide for students and those inexperienced in assessing food intake. The values given have been derived from dietary survey data on healthy adults obtained by the Dunn Nutrition Centre, Cambridge, the former Nuffield laboratories of Comparative Medicine (now the Institute of Brain Chemistry and Human Nutrition), London and from information supplied by a number of dietetic departments.

In Table 7.42 columns 2 and 3, quantities of foods are expressed either as a typical portion (e.g. a serving of a vegetable) and/or by a convenient unit (e.g. a slice of bread). The weight in column 3 is that for the unit specified in column 2. The term 'typical portion' is a loose one and there will be considerable variation in the portion sizes consumed by individuals depending on age, sex and appetite. There will also be variation in portions consumed by an individual depending on appetite, activity, circumstances and the number of different items consumed at one eating occasion. The following spoon sizes have been used:

1 level teaspoon (tsp) = 5 ml
1 level dessertspoon (dsp) = 10 ml
1 level tablespoon (tbsp) = 15 ml

The portion weights in columns 4 and 5 are derived from a dietary study of families in Cambridge (Nelson, personal communication); 105 families provided 805 days of records from adult women, and 735 days from adult men. The portions eaten by women were cross-checked with those eaten by Cambridge mothers (73 mothers, 3185 days; Black, personal communication) and found to be similar. For many foods, the portions eaten by men and women were similar, but the men ate larger portions of meat and many cereal foods. Where too few portions of

Table 7.42 Typical unit weight/portion size of basic foodstuffs

Food	Unit	Unit weight (g)	Cambridge survey portion[1] Women (g)	Men[2] (g)
Cereal products				
Bemax			10	
Bran (wheat)			8	
Bread – large loaf	Thin slice	25		
– large loaf	Medium thick	33		
– large loaf	Thick slice	40		
– small loaf	Medium thick	20		
– wholemeal			60	65
– brown			55	75
– Hovis			55	70
– white			55	85
Rice, boiled	Portion	180	140	160
Spaghetti, boiled	Portion	200	190	240
Porridge			190	240
Breakfast cereals				
All Bran			30	20
Rice Krispies			30	35
Muesli	Portion	60	60	50
Porridge	Portion	180	190	240
Weetabix	2	35	35	35
Shredded Wheat	2	50		
Cornflakes	Portion	30	30	40
Biscuits, cakes and puddings				
Plain or semi-sweet	1	7		
Cream crackers	1	7		
Crispbread	1	8	20	20
Biscuits, digestive, plain			30	30
Biscuits, short sweet			25	25

Table 7.42 *contd.*

Food	Unit	Unit weight (g)	Cambridge survey portion[1] Women (g)	Men[2] (g)
Muffin	1	40		
Croissant	1	50		
Crumpet	2	80		
Scone	1	30		
Roll	1	40		
Currant bun	1	35		
Doughnut	1 medium	50		
Fruit cake	1 medium slice	75	70	100
Gingerbread	1 thick slice	60		
Sponge cake	Portion	55	50	60
Mince pie	1 medium	60		
Yorkshire pudding	1 small	30		
Cheesecake	Portion	150		
Milk puddings	Portion	120		
Ice cream	2 scoops	120–150		
Sponge pudding	Portion	150		
Soufflè	Portion	120		
Milk, dairy products, oils				
Milk				
in tea or coffee (2 tbs)		30	30	
in tea or coffee (1 tsp)		5		
glass		180	200	
Butter/margarine			12	16
thickly spread on 1 large slice		10		
thinly spread on 1 large slice		7		
thinly spread on 1 small slice		5		
Cream, single/double			30	45
in coffee	1 tbs	15		
on a dessert	2 tbs	30		
Cheese				
cottage	2 tbs	60	70	
Camembert	Portion	40	35	
Cheddar/Stilton	Portion	30		
cheese spread	Portion	20	20	
Cheddar			35	45
Edam type cheese			40	30
Stilton cheese			30	40
Yoghurt		125–150	140	140
Eggs – without shell	1 large	54		
without shell	1 medium	48		
without shell	1 small	40		
yolk only	Medium	17		
white only	Medium	31		
scrambled egg	1 egg	65		
fried egg	1 egg	50		
omelette	1 egg	60		
Cooking oil	1 tbs	18		
Cooking oil	1 tsp	5		
Meat and meat products				
Bacon, back, grilled	2 rashers	30		
streaky, grilled	3 rashers	30		
Bacon, gammon rashers, grilled			80	
Bacon, rashers, fried/grilled			35	
Beef, rump steak	Small	120		
Beef, rump steak	Large	250		
Beef, rump steak, fried			90	100
Beef, roast	3 slices	90	90	100
Lamb, roast		90	80	100
Pork/lamb chop	1 large	160		

Table 7.42 *contd.*

Food	Unit	Unit weight (g)	Cambridge survey portion[1] Women (g)	Men[2] (g)
Pork/lamb chop	1 small	100		
Pork chops, grilled			85	125
Pork, roast		90	85	125
Chicken/turkey, roast, meat only		100		
Chicken/turkey leg and bone		200		
Chicken, roast, meat only			80	130
Turkey roast, meat only			100	
Kidney, lamb	2	60		
Kidney, any kind			60	
Liver, lamb (fried)		90		
Liver, any kind			90	135
Corned beef	1 slice	30	50	65
Cold meats	2 slices	50		
Ham			40	40
Ham and pork, chopped			40	65
Luncheon meat			40	65
Tongue		60		
Black pudding		50	45	75
Paté — as starter to a meal		45		
— on bread		25		
Liver sausage			35	45
Frankfurters	2	60	55	
Salami	2 slices	30	30	
Sausages, grilled	2 large	80		
Sausage, chipolatas	4	80		
Sausages, grilled/fried			70	90
Beefburger	1	60		
Savaloy	1	80		
Pizza	7" diameter	200		
Pork pies	Large	300		
Pork pies	Medium	140		
Pork pies	Small	65		
Beef stew	Portion	200		
Chilli con carne	Portion	280		
Lasagne	Portion	300		
Cornish pasty	1 no.	170		
Sausage roll	1 no.	60		
Fish and fish products				
Cod/haddock/plaice, fried in batter	Portion	130	125	135
Cod, steamed	Portion		100	150
Herring, edible portion	1 small	90		
Kipper, baked	Portion	120	105	145
Mackerel, fried	Half a fish	90	95	
Pilchards/sardines		80	75	
Salmon (canned)		60	30	45
Sardines, canned in oil (fish only)			70	85
Tuna, canned in oil		60	70	85
Anchovies	3 thin fillets	12		
Shrimps, prawns	Portion	30	40	40
Fish fingers	2	50		
Fish cakes	2	120		
Vegetables and salad				
Beans — runner, boiled	Portion	75	75	75
— haricot, boiled	Portion	100	90	115
— baked in tomato sauce	2 tbs	40	115	160
Beetroot, cooked	Portion	40	40	40
Brussel sprouts, boiled	Portion	80	85	100
Cabbage, boiled	Portion	100	90	115
Carrots, boiled	Portion	70	60	80
Cauliflower, boiled	Portion	120	120	115

Table 7.42 *contd.*

Food	Unit	Unit weight (g)	Cambridge survey portion[1] Women (g)	Men[2] (g)
Celery	1 stick	60	45	50
Cucumber	1″	40	30	40
Leeks, boiled	Portion	80	80	80
Lettuce	Portion	25	25	30
Peas – garden	Portion	75	60	70
– chick	Portion	75	75	
– processed			85	90
Potatoes, typical portion of baked/chips/mashed/boiled		150	140	235
Potatoes, roast	Portion	120	110	170
Potatoes, chips			130	170
Potatoes, boiled	One	60		
Potatoes, chips	4 large	25		
Potatoes, roast	1 small	40		
Potatoes, mashed	1 heaped tbs	60		
Sweetcorn, tinned	2 tbs	60		
Swede	Portion	80	80	125
Tomatoes	1 medium	60	50	55
Fruit				
Apples, baking/eating			80	80
Apples	1 medium	120		
Apples	1 large	150		
Apricots, canned			100	
Avocado pear, without stone	Half medium sized	75		
Banana			70	70
Banana, peeled	1 small	70		
Banana, peeled	1 medium	100		
Currants, black (stewed with sugar)			25	
Dates	2	15	25	
Fruit, tinned/stewed	Portion	120		
Fruit juice	Small glass	100		
Gooseberries, stewed			100	
Grapes	10	60	55	
Grapefruit,	Half small	100	85	
Mandarin oranges, canned			100	
Melon	1 slice	120	105	
Orange, peeled	1 medium	120		
Oranges, raw			105	90
Peaches, canned			100	
Pears, canned			100	
Pineapple, canned			100	
Prunes, stewed with sugar			100	
Raspberries, canned			100	
Strawberries, raw		100	90	80
Tangerine	1 medium	60	45	30
Miscellaneous items				
Sugar	1 level tsp	5		
Sugar	1 rounded tsp	7		
Sugar	1 tbs	19		
Honey, in jars			15	
Jam/marmalade/honey	2 level tsp	15	20	
Peanut butter	2 tsp	15		
Syrup	1 tbs	20		
Treacle	1 tbs	20		
Mayonnaise	2 tbs	30		
Chocolate sauce	2 tbs	40		
White sauce	2 tbs	33		
Brown/tomato sauce	1 tbs	17		
Oxo cube	1	6		
Bournvita		15	7	
Cocoa powder		6	4	

Table 7.42 *contd.*

Food	Unit	Unit weight (g)	Cambridge survey portion[1] Women (g)	Men[2] (g)
Drinking chocolate			7	
Horlicks malted milk			10	
Ovaltine			7	
Instant coffee powder	1 tsp	2		
Soup	1 bowl	240		
Keg bitter beer			334	868
Lager, bottled beer			331	669
Stout, bottled			307	567
Cider, sweet			252	—
Beer/stout/cider	1 pint	568 ml		
	Half pint	284 ml		
Wine	1 glass	120–150 ml	163	256
Sherry/vermouth/port	Measure	60 ml	71	182
Spirits	1/6 gill	25 ml		
Vermouth	Measure	60 ml	68	122

Notes:
[1] The Cambridge Survey portion weight is a measure of how much on average was recorded as a single item. This might for example include several slices of bread, more than one biscuit or several pints of beer
[2] Where no weight is given for men, either men did not eat this food or data for both sexes were combined

Table 7.43 Typical weights of some manufactured food items

Foods	Weight (g)
Biscuits	
Bandit	20
Blue Riband	20
Cadbury's Chocolate Wheatmeal biscuit	10
Caramel chocolate covered wafer	25
Chocolate chip cookie	10
McVities	
Chocolate digestive	17
Digestive	15
Sports chocolate biscuits	22
Club (Jacobs)	25
Custard cream	15
Gingernut	10
Harvest crunch	18
Jaffa cake	12
Penguin	30
Rich tea (2)	15
Rich tea finger	5
Taxi	18
Trio chocolate biscuits	25
Wagon wheel	35
Yoyo	20
Butter puff	10
Cornish wafer	10
Cream crackers (2)	15
Tuc	5
Water biscuits (2)	15
Cakes	
Mr Kipling	
Cherry slice	38
Country slice	38
French fancy	30
Fruit pie	53
Jam tart	40
Lyons Harvest pie (family size)	300
Harvest pie (individual)	120
Harvest pie (small)	32
Iced tarts (1)	30
Caprice	15
Sainsburys	
Chocolate cup cake	40
Fruit pie (1)	55
Eccles cake	42
Jam tart	25
Lemon curd tart	25
Mince pie	50
Bird's Eye	
Chocolate eclair	35
Yoghurts/desserts	
St Ivel Shape	
– Natural	150
Fruit	125
Mr Men	150
Real	125
Yoplait	
Petits Filous	60
Chambourcy	
Nouvelle and Bonjour	125
Creme dessert	100
Black forest dessert	100
Caramel dessert	92
Eden Vale champagne sundae	125
Meat and meal products	
Harris cottage pie	180
Marks and Spencer minced beef and onion pie	190
Walls steak and kidney pie	180
Mattesons spreading pate	113
St Ivel pan bake pizza	500

contd.

Table 7.43 *contd.*

Foods	Weight (g)	Foods	Weight (g)
Fish		– medium packet	42
John West pink salmon	213 and 440	Polos (1)	1.5
John West tuna	99 and 198	Rolos (1 packet, 9 sweets)	46
Glenryck pilchards	425	Treets (1 packet)	42
Glenryck sardines	120		
		Chocolate	
Vegetables		Aero	42
Heinz baked beans		Banjo	47
large tin	450	Bounty (2 small bars)	58
medium tin	225	Bournville	50
small tin	150	Cadburys	
		Milk chocolate bar (small)	60
Crisps and nuts		Fruit and Nut	57
Crisps		Whole nut	55
Golden Wonder (small packet)	25	Creme egg	40
KP (small packet)	30	Caramac	20 and 38
KP Hula Hoops (small packet)	25	Crunchie	35
Marks and Spencer (large packet)	75	Double decker	50
Scampi fries (small packet)	25	Drifter	52
Walkers (small packet)	28	Flake	35
(medium packet)	50	Fry's chocolate cream	50
Nuts		Galaxy bar	70
Almonds (6 whole, shelled)	9	Harvest Crunch	18
KP almonds (small packet)	30	Jordans Original Crunchy bar	33
KP cashews	25	Kit Kat	
KP peanuts	50 and 100	4 finger	50
KP mixed nuts and raisins	50 and 125	2 finger	24
Golden Wonder mixed nuts and raisins	40 and 78	Lion bar	42
Sweets and Chocolate		Marathon	58
Sweets		Mars bar	
Buttered brazil (1)	9	– Normal size	68
Chews (1 packet)	30	– King size	100
Chewing gum (1 stick)	4	Milky way	32
Jelly babies (1 packet)	113	Marks and Spencer white chocolate bar	30
Maltesers (small packet, 18 sweets)	38	Prewetts bars	42
Minstrels		Star bar	45
– family packet (33 sweets)	90	Toffee crisp	40
– small packet (15 sweets)	40	Topic	53
New Berry fruit (1)	15	Twix (2 bars)	50
Smarties (1 tube)	32	Walnut whip	32
Pastilles		Wispa	35
– small packet	33	Yorkie bar	60

specific food items (codes) had been recorded to provide a reliable average portion weight, similar foods were grouped together, e.g. three kinds of liver. For fresh fruit, it was necessary to combine data from both sexes. 'Portions' here may include fractions or multiples of units. Thus the portion weight for bread is the average of the number of slices eaten on different occasions and not the weight of a unit slice.

Table 7.43 gives the average weights of some manufactured food items.

Further information on portion weights may be found in Crawley (1988), Bingham and Day (1987) and Davies and Dickerson (1991). The latter contains a useful introduction and discussion of the limitations of portion weights.

References

Bingham S and Day K (1987) Average portion weights of foods consumed by a randomly selected British population sample. *Hum Nutr: App Nutr* **41A**, 258–64.

Crawley H (1988) *Food portion sizes*. HMSO, London.

Davies J and Dickerson J (1991) *Nutrient content of food portions*. Royal Society of Chemistry, Cambridge.

7.6 Appendix 6: Composition of proprietary energy and nutrient supplements

Tables 7.44–7.55 give the 1992 composition of the following proprietary energy and nutrient supplements:

Table 7.44 Nutritional supplements: carbohydrate as the sole energy source.
Table 7.45 Nutritional supplements: fat or fat + carbohydrate as the sole energy source.
Table 7.46 Nutritional supplements: mainly protein with or without fat/carbohydrate.
Table 7.47 Multivitamin supplements.
Table 7.48 Single vitamin preparations.
Table 7.49 Mixed mineral supplements.
Table 7.50 Iron preparations.
Table 7.51 Potassium, sodium and zinc supplements.
Table 7.52 Calcium and phosphorus supplements.
Table 7.53 Vitamin and mineral supplements (prescribable).
Table 7.54 Substances used in vitamin preparations.
Table 7.55 Mineral salts used in pharmaceutical preparations.

These tables provide guidance on the range of products likely to be on the market. However, since this market changes rapidly, the exact composition and availability should be verified before any individual product is recommended or prescribed.

The tables also indicate whether or not a specific product is currently prescribable. Prescriptions should be marked 'ACBS' (Advisory Committee for Borderline Substances). Up-to-date information regarding their prescribability can be found in the *Monthly Index of Medical Specialities* (MIMS) or the *British National Formulary*.

The composition of proprietary enteral feeds can be found in Appendix 7, Tables 7.56, 7.57 and 7.58.

Table 7.44 Nutritional supplements: carbohydrate as sole energy source

		Composition per 100 g/100 ml		(February 1993)				
Product	Description	Unit size	CHO g	Energy kJ	Energy kcal	Sodium mmol	Potassium mmol	Prescribable?
Powders								
Caloreen (Clintec Nutrition)	Water-soluble dextrins	250 g bottle 5 kg tub	96	1674	400	<1.8	<0.3	Yes
Polycal (Cow & Gate Nutricia)	Maltodextrins Tasteless powder	400 g tin 900 g tin	95	1610	380	2.2	1.3	Yes
Polycose (Ross Labs)	Glucose polymers Tasteless powder	350 g tin	94	1596	380	4.8	0.3	Yes
Super Soluble Maxijul (SHS)	Maltodextrins Tasteless powder	140 g sachet 200 g tub 2.5 kg tub 25 kg tub	95	1500	360	2.0	0.1	Yes
Super Soluble Maxijul LE (SHS)	Maltodextrins Tasteless powder	100 g box 2.5 kg tub 25 kg tub	96	1536	365	0.01	0.01	Yes
Liquids								
Fortical (Cow & Gate Nutricia)	Maltodextrins in solution Four flavours	200 ml bottle	62	1050	246	<0.3	0.03	Yes
Hycal (SmithKline Beecham)	Glucose solution Sweet taste Four flavours	171 ml bottle	50	845	198	0.6	0.02	Yes
Liquid Maxijul (SHS)	50% dilution of Maxijul powder in water Four flavours	200 ml carton	50	800	187	≤1.0	≤0.1	Yes

Table 7.45 Nutritional supplements: fat or fat + carbohydrate as energy source

Product	Description	Unit size	Fat g	CHO g	Energy kJ	Energy kcal	Sodium mmol	Potassium mmol	Prescribable?
		Composition per 100 g/100 ml		(February 1993)					
Fat only									
Alembicol D (Alembic)	Coconut oil (MCT)	4 kg	100 50–60% C8 35–40% C10	—	3500	837	—	—	Yes
Calogen (SHS)	Emulsion 50% Arachis oil 50% water	250 ml 1000 ml	50 58% C18:1 21% C18:2	—	1850	450	0.9	0.5	Yes
Liquigen (SHS)	Emulsion 50% MCT oil 50% water	250 ml 1000 ml	50 81% C8 16% C10	—	1740	416	1.7	0.7	Yes
MCT oil (Cow & Gate Nutricia)	Fractionated coconut oil	1000 ml	100 56% C8 40% C10	—	3469	830	—	—	Yes
MCT Oil (Mead Johnson)	Fractionated coconut oil	950 ml	93 67% C8 23% C10	—	3250	775	—	—	Yes
Fat + carbohydrate									
Super Soluble Duocal (SHS)	Maltodextrins and vegetable oils Off-white powder	400 g tin	22.3 28% C8 7% C10	72.7	1988	470	≤0.2	≤0.1	Yes
MCT Duocal (SHS)	Maltodextrins and vegetable oils Cream coloured powder	100 g box	23.2 44% C8 39% C10	74	2042	486	1.3	0.09	No
Liquid Duocal (SHS)	Maltodextrins and vegetable oils White emulsion	250 ml bottle 1000 ml bottle	7.1 26% C8 4.5% C10	23.4	628	150	0.9	0.8	Yes
Duobar (SHS)	Palatable 'candy' bar; blend of fat and carbohydrate Two flavours	100 g bar	42	56	2450	600	0.43	0.51	Yes

Table 7.46 Nutritional supplements: mainly protein with or without fat/carbohydrate

Product	Description	Unit size	Protein g	Fat g	CHO g	Energy kJ	Energy kcal	Sodium mmol	Potassium mmol	Prescribable?
			Composition per 100 g/100 ml			(February 1993)				
Protein										
Casilan (Crookes)	Calcium caseinate powder	250 g	90	1.8	<0.5	1600	376	0.3	0.2	Yes
Super Soluble Maxipro HBV (SHS)	Whey protein supplemented with amino acids Powder	200 g tub 1 kg tub	80	6.0	<5 (lactose)	1662	393	5.6	12.0	Yes
Protifar (Cow & Gate Nutricia)	Modified skimmed milk powder	225 g tin	88.5	1.6	0.5 (lactose)	1575	370	1.3	1.3	Yes
Promod (Ross Labs)	Whey protein + Soy lecithin Powder	275 g tin	76	9.0	10	1788	424	9.9	25.3	Yes

Table 7.46 *contd.*

Product	Description	Unit size	Protein g	Fat g	CHO g	Energy kJ	Energy kcal	Sodium mmol	Potassium mmol	Prescribable?
		Composition per 100 g/100 ml				(February 1993)				
Protein + carbohydrate										
Forceval Protein (Unigreg)	Calcium caseinate with added vits + mins Powder Three flavours	300 g tin 15 g sachets	55	≤1	30	1540	366	<5.2	1.3	Yes
Provide (Fresenius)	Soya hydrolysate and maltodextrins in solution Three flavours	250 ml tetrabrik	3.6	<1.0	11	250	60	0.6 (Tropical fruit 2.6)	0.4 (Tropical fruit 3.2)	Yes
Protein + Fat + Carbohydrate Powders										
Build-up (Clintec Nutrition)	Skimmed milk pdr + vits/mins Natural + Four sweet and Three soup flavours	266 g sachet (Natural) 38 g sachets (Flavours) 40 g sachets (Savoury)	5.6	3.4	11.4	403	96	3.7	6.5	No
				NB FIGURES ARE PER 100 ml WHEN MADE UP AS DIRECTED BY MANUFACTURER						
Complan (Crookes)	Milk protein pdr + vits and mins	450 g carton 400 g	4	3.2	11.0	374	89	3.0	4.4	No
				NB FIGURES ARE PER 100 ml WHEN MADE UP AS DIRECTED BY MANUFACTURER						
Liquids										
Ensure (Ross Labs.)	Nutritionally complete liquid feed/ supplement Eight flavours	250 ml can	3.5	3.5	13.7	420	100	3.5	3.8	Yes
Ensure Plus (Ross Labs.)	Nutritionally complete energy-dense liquid feed/supplement Eight flavours	200 ml tetrapak	6.3	5.0	20.0	630	150	5.1	4.7	Yes
Fortimel (Cow & Gate Nutricia)	Nutritional supplement, high protein Six flavours	200 ml tetrapak	9.7	2.1	10.4	420	100	2.2	5.1	Yes
Fortisip (Cow & Gate Nutricia)	Nutritionally complete energy-dense liquid feed/supplement Seven flavours	200 ml tetrapak	5	6.5	17.9	630	150	3.5	3.8	Yes
Fresubin High Energy (Fresenius)	Nutritionally complete energy-dense liquid feed/supplement Three flavours	236 ml tetrapak	5.6	5.8	18.8	630	150	4.1	4.5	Yes
Liquisorb (E. Merck)	Nutritionally complete liquid feed/ supplement Four flavours	200 ml tetrapak	4.0	4.0	11.8	420	100	4.5 5.0 (Choc, banana, strawb)	4.5 6.0 (Choc)	Yes
Protein Forte (Fresenius)	Nutritional supplement high in protein Three flavours	200 ml tetrapak	10.0	2.5	9.5	420	100	3.9	3.8	Yes
Protein, Fat and Carbohydrate (Desserts/soups)										
Formance (Ross Labs)	Semi-solid dessert Three flavours	142 g can	4.8	6.8	23.9	739	176	7.4	6.0	Yes
Fortipudding (Cow & Gate Nutricia)	Semi-solid dessert Three flavours	150 g can	10.2	3.0	16.0	550	131	2.2	4.2–6.0	Yes

Table 7.46 *contd.*

Product	Description	Unit size	Protein g	Fat g	CHO g	Energy kJ	Energy kcal	Sodium mmol	Potassium mmol	Prescribable?
			Composition per 100 g/100 ml			(February 1993)				
Maxisorb (SHS)										
Desserts	Milk proteins + carbohydrates Powder reconstituted with water to make drink or dessert Three flavours	30 g sachet	40	20	30	1890	450	6.0	13.7	No
					NB FIGURES GIVEN ARE PER 100 G DRY PRODUCT					
Soups	Mainly soya proteins + milk proteins Powder reconstituted with water	30 g sachet	40	1.3	43	1400	333	87	14	No
					NB FIGURES GIVEN ARE PER 100 G DRY PRODUCT					

Table 7.47 Multivitamin supplements

(Compiled from MIMS, August 1992)	Abidec (Warner-Lambert)	BC 500 Whitehall Labs	Becozyme/Becosym (Roche)	Becozyme Forte (Roche)	Benerva compound (Roche)	Concavit capsules (Wallace)	Concavit drops	Concavit syrup	Dalivit drops (Eastern)
Dosing unit	per 0.6 ml	per tablet	per tablet or 5 ml	per tablet	per tablet	per capsule	per ml	per 5 ml	per 0.6 ml
		X	G	X	G	X	X	X	
Vitamin A (i.u.)	4000					5000	10 000	5000	5000
Vitamin D (i.u.)	400					400	800	400	400
Ergocalciferol (D_2)									
Vitamin E (i.u.)						2			
Tocopheryl acelate (mg)									
Vitamin K									
Acetomenaphthone (mg)									
Ascorbic acid (mg)	50					40	100	50	50
Na ascorbate (mg)		500							
Thiamin hydrochloride (mg)	1				1				
Thiamin mononitrate (mg)		25							
Thiamin (mg)			5	15		2.5	4	2	1
Riboflavin (mg)	0.4	12.5	2	15	1	2.5	2	1	0.4
Riboflavin sodium phosphate (mg)									
Pyridoxine hydrochloride (mg)	0.5	10							
Pyridoxine (mg)			2	10		1	2		0.5
Nicotinamide (mg)	5	100	20	50	15	20	25	12.5	5
Nicotinic acid (mg)									
Pantothenic acid									
Ca pantothenate (mg)		20				5			
Pantothenyl alcohol (mg)							4	2	
Cyanocobalamin (μg)		5				5	10	5	

Table 7.47 *contd.*

(Compiled from MIMS, August 1992)	Halycitrol (LAB)	Ketovite tablets	Ketovite liquid (Paines and Byrne)	Lipotriad (Lipomed)	Multibionta (Merck)	Orovite (SKB)	Orovite-7 (SKB)
Dosing unit	per 5 ml	per tablet	per 5 ml	per capsule or 1.67 ml	per 10 ml ampoule	per tablet or 12.5 ml syrup	per 5 g sachet
	X	P		X	P	X	X
Vitamin A (i.u.)	4600		2500		10 000		2500
Vitamin D (i.u.)	380		400				
Ergocalciferol/calciferol (D_2) (i.u.)							100
Vitamin E (i.u)							
Tocopheryl acelate (mg)		5			5		
Vitamin K							
Acetomenaphthone (mg)		0.5					
Ascorbic acid (mg)		16.6			500	100	60
Na ascorbate (mg)							
Thiamin HCl (mg)		1		0.33		50	
Thiamin mononitrate (mg)							1.4
Thiamin (mg)					50		
Riboflavin (mg)		1		0.33	10	5	
Riboflavin sodium phosphate (mg)							1.7
Pyridoxine HCl (mg)		0.33		0.33	15	5	2
Pyridoxine (mg)							
Nicotinamide (mg)		3.3		3.33	100	200	18
Nicotinic acid (mg)							
Pantothenic acid (mg)							
Ca pantothenate (mg)		1.16					
Pantothenyl alcohol (mg)				0.33	25		
Cyanocobalamin (μg)			12.5				
Hydroxocobalamin (μg)				1.66			
Folic acid (μg)		250					
Choline chloride (mg)			150				
Choline bitartrate (mg)				233			
Inositol (mg)		50		111			
Biotin (mg)		0.17					
Pro-lintane hydrochloride (mg)							
di-Methionine (mg)				28			
Dextrose (mg)							
Liver extract							

Table 7.47 *contd.*

(Compiled from MIMS, August 1992)	Parentrovite (Bencard) Intravenous high potency (IVHP)	Parentrovite (Bencard) Intramuscular high potency (IMHP)	Parentrovite (Bencard) Intramuscular maintenance (IMM)	Villescon liquid (Boehringer)
Dosing unit	per pair ampoules			per 5 ml
	P			PX
Vitamin A (i.u.)		As IVHP but without 1000 mg dextrose and with 140 mg benzyl alcohol	As IMHP but with 100 mg thiamin CHI and 80 mg benzyl alcohol	
Vitamin D (i.u.)				
Ergocalciferol/calciferol (D_2) (i.u.)				
Vitamin E (i.u.)				
Tocopheryl acetate (mg)				
Vitamin K (Phytomenadione)				
Acetomenaphthone (mg)				
Ascorbic acid (mg)	500			
Na ascorbate (mg)				
Thiamin HCl (mg)	250			1.67
Thiamin mononitrate (mg)				
Thiamin (mg)				
Riboflavin (mg)	4			
Riboflavin sodium phosphate (mg)				1.36
Pyridoxine HCl (mg)	50			0.5
Pyridoxine (mg)				
Nicotinamide (mg)	160			5
Nicotinic acid (mg)				
Pantothenic acid (mg)				
Ca pantothenate (mg)				
Pantothenyl alcohol (mg)				
Cyanocobalamin (μg)				
Folic acid (mg)				
Choline chloride (mg)				
Inositol (mg)				
Biotin (mg)				
Prolintane hydrochloride (mg)				2.5
dl-Methionine (mg)				
Dextrose (mg)	1000			
Yeast, dried (mg)				
Liver extract				

P = prescription only; X = not available on NHS; G = only generic equivalents available at NHS expense. FP10 prescriptions must be written in generic name

Table 7.48 Single vitamin preparations. Compiled from MIMS, (August 1992)

Preparation (manufacturer)	Availability	Vitamin	Dose
AT10 (Sterling Research Laboratories)		Dihydrotachysterol	0.25 mg per ml oily solution
Benerva (Roche)	G	Thiamin HCl	25, 50, 100 or 300mg per tablet
Cobalin-H (Paines and Byrne)	PG	Hydroxocobalamin	1000 μg per 1 ml ampoule
Comploment Continus (Napp)	X	Pyridoxine HCl	100 mg per tablet
Cytacon (Evans Medical)	X	Cyanocobalamin	35 μg per 5 ml
Cytamen (Evans Medical)	PG	Cyanocobalamin	1000 μg per 1 ml ampoule
Ephynal (Roche)		Tocopheryl acetate	10, 50 or 200 mg per tablet
Lexpec (RP Drugs)	P	Folic acid	2500 μg per 5 ml
Neocytamen (Evans Medical)	PG	Hydroxocobalamin	1000 μg per 1 ml ampoule
One-alpha (Leo)	P	Alfacalcidol (l α OHD_3)	0.25 or 1.0 μg per tablet;
Redoxon (Roche)	G	Ascorbic acid	25, 50, 200, 500 or 1000 mg per tablet
Refolinon (Farmitalia C E)	P	Ca folinate	15 mg per tablet
Ro-A-Vit (Roche)	P	Vitamin A acetate	50 000 i.u. per tablet
Rocaltrol (Roche)	P	Calcitriol ($1,25(OH)_2D_3$)	0.25 or 0.5 μg per capsule

P = prescription only; X = not available on NHS; G = only generic equivalents available at NHS expense. FP10 prescriptions must be written in generic name

Table 7.49 Mixed mineral supplements (per 100 g)

Mineral Composition per 100 g	Metabolic Mineral Mix (SHS)	Aminogran Mineral Mix (UCB Pharma)
Sodium (g)	3.96	4.0
(mmol)	172.2	170.0
Potassium (g)	8.3	8.3
(mmol)	212.3	210.0
Chloride (g)	1.8	—
(mmol)	50.8	—
Calcium (g)	8.2	8.1
(mmol)	204.6	200.0
Phosphorus (g)	5.96	6.0
(mmol)	192.4	190.0
Magnesium (g)	0.97	0.97
(mmol)	39.9	40.0
Iron (mg)	63.0	63.0
Zinc (mg)	48.0	48.0
Iodine (mg)	0.76	Tr
Manganese (mg)	5.7	4.0
Copper (mg)	13.0	13.0
Aluminum (μg)	Tr	Tr
Molybdeum (μg)	150.0	Tr
Chromium (μg)	—	—
Cobalt	—	Tr
Dose	1.5 g/kg/day (up to 5.5 kg), then 8 g/day up to 3 yrs adults 12 g/day	1.5 g/kg/day (up to 5.5 kg), then 8 g/day

Table 7.50 Iron preparations (Compiled from MIMS, October 1991)

	BC 500 with iron (Whitehall)	Fetol Spansule (SK and F)	Fetol Vit Spansule (SK and F)	Fetol Z Spansule (SK and F)	Feospan Spansule (SK and F)	Fergon (Winthrop)	Ferfolic SV (Sinclair)	Ferrocap (Consolidated)	Ferrocap F-350 (Consolidated)	Ferrocontin Continus (Asta Medica)	Ferrocontin Folic Continus (Asta Medica)	Ferrograd (Abbott)	Ferrograd C (Abbott)	Ferrograd Folic (Abbott)	Ferrous Gluconate	Ferrous Sulphate	Ferromyn Elix (Calmic)	Fersaday (Duncan Flockhart)	Fersamal (Duncan Flockhart)	Fersamal syrup (Duncan Flockhart)	Fesovit Spansule (SK and F)	Fesovit Z Spansule (SK and F)	Folex-350 (Rybar)	Folicin (Paines and Byrne)	Galfer (Galen)	Galfer FA (Galen)	Galfervit (Galen)
	per tablet	per capsule	per capsule	per capsule	per capsule	per tablet	per tablet	per capsule	per capsule	per tablet	per tablet	per capsule	per tablet	per tablet	per tablet	per tablet	per 5 ml	per tablet	per tablet	per 5 ml	per capsule	per capsule	per tablet	per tablet	per capsule	per capsule	per capsule
	X		X						P				X	P							X	X				P	X
Ferrous sulphate (mg)		150	150	150	150							325	325	325		200					150	150		200			
Ferrous fumarate (mg)	200							330	330									305	√	140			308		290	290	305
Ferrous gluconate (mg)						300	250								300												
Ferrous succinate (mg)																	106										
Ferrous glycine sulphate (mg)																											
Iron dextran complex (mg)																											
[Fe equivalent (mg)]		[47]	[47]	[47]	[47]	[35]	[30]	[110]	[110]	[100]	[100]	[105]	[105]	[105]	[35]		[37]	[100]	[65]	[45]	[47]	[47]	[100]	[60]	[100]	[100]	[100]
Thiamin mononitrate (mg)	25		2																		2	2					2
Riboflavin (mg)	12.5		2																		2	2					2
Nicotinamide (mg)	100		10																		10	10					10
Folic acid (μg)		500	500	500			5000		350		500			350									350	2500		350	
Pyridoxine hydrochloride (mg)	10		1																		1	1					4
Ascorbic acid (mg)			50										500								50	50					56
Sodium ascorbate (mg)	500																										
Calcium pantothenate (mg)	20																										
Calciferol (i.u.)																											
Calcium gluconate (mg)																											
Zinc sulphate (monchydrate) (mg)				61.8																		61.8					
[Zn equivalent (mg)]				[22.5]																		[22.5]					
Copper sulphate (mg)																								2.5			
Manganese sulphate (mg)																								2.5			

Table 7.50 *contd.*

	Givitol (Galen)	Imferon (Fisons)	Jelcofer (Astra)	Lepex (PR Drugs)	Meterfolic (Sinclair)	Niferex (Tillots)	Niferex tablets (Tillots)	Niferex-150 (Tillots)	Plesmet (Napp)	Pregaday (Duncan Flockhart)	Pregnavite Forte F (Bencard)	Slow-Fe (Ciba)	Slow-Fe Folic (Ciba)	Sytron (Parke-Davis)
	per capsule	per ml (2.5 and 20 ml ampoules)	per ml (1 ml ampoule)	per 5 ml syrup	per tablet	per 5 ml	per tablet	per capsule	per 10 ml	per tablet	per tablet	per tablet	per tablet	per 10 ml
	PX	P	P		P					P	PX		P	
Ferrous sulphate (mg)											84	160	160	
Ferrous fumarate (mg)	305				√					√				
Ferrous gluconate (mg)														
Ferrous succinate (mg)														
Ferrous glycine sulphate (mg)									√					
Iron dextran complex (mg)		√												
Iron sorbitol/citric acid complex			√											
Polysaccharide iron complex						√	√	√						
Sodium iron edetate														
[Fe equivalent (mg)]	[100]	[50]	[50]		[100]	[100]	[50]	[150]	[50]	[100]	[25.2]	[50]	[50]	[55]
Thiamin mononitrate (mg)	2													
Thiamin hydrochloride (mg)											0.5			
Riboflavin (mg)	2										0.5			
Nicotinamide (mg)	10										5			
Folic acid (μg)	500			2500	350					350	120		400	
Pyridoxine hydrochloride (mg)	4										0.33			
Ascorbic acid (mg)											13.3			
Sodium ascorbate (mg)	56													
Calcium pantothenate (mg)														
Vitamin A (i.u.)											1333			
Calciferol (i.u.)											133			
Calcium gluconate (mg)														
Calcium phosphate (mg)											160			
Zinc sulphate (monohydrate) (mg)														
[Zn equivalent (mg)]														
Copper sulphate (mg)														
Manganese sulphate (mg)														

P = Prescription only, X = not available on NHS

Table 7.51 Potassium, sodium and zinc supplements. Compiled from MIMS, October 1991

	Dioralyte (Rorer)	Kay-Cee-L (Geistlich)	Electrolade (Nicholas)	Kloref (Cox)	Leo-K (Leo)	Gluco-lyte (Cupal)	Nu-K (Consolidated)	Rehidrat (Searle)	Sando-K (Sandoz)	Slow-K (Ciba)	Slow sodium (Ciba)	Solvazinc (Thames)	Z-Span Spansules (Smith, Klein and French)
	per sachet	per ml	per sachet	per tablet	per tablet	per sachet	per capsule	per sachet	per tablet	per tablet	per tablet	per tablet	per capsule
Sodium chloride (mg)	470		236			200		440			600		
Sodium bicarbonate (mg)			500			300		420					
Sodium acid citrate (mg)	530												
Potassium chloride (mg)	300	75	300	140	600	300	600	380	600	600			
Potassium bicarbonate (mg)				455					400				
Potassium benzoate (mg)				50									
Glucose (g)	3.56		4.0			8.0		4.09					
Sucrose (g)								8.07					
Laevulose (g)								70					
Citric acid (mg)								440					
Betaine hydrochloride (mg)				740									
Zinc sulphate (mg)												200	
Zinc sulphate monohydrate (mg)													61.8

P = prescription only

Table 7.52 Calcium and phosphorus supplements. Compiled from MIMS, October 1991

	Cacit (Norwich Eaton)	Calcichew (Shire)	Calcidrink (Shire)	Calcimax (Wallace)	Chocovite (Torbet)	Citrical (Shire)	Osso pan 800 (Sanofi)	Sandocal 400 (Sandoz)	Sandocal 1000 (Sandoz)	Calcium Sandoz Syrup (Sandoz)	TitraCal (3M Health Care)			
	per tab	per tab	per sachet	per 5 ml X	per tab X			per tab	per tab	per 5 ml	per tab	per ml	per 20 ml X	
Calcium carbonate (mg)	1250	1260	2520			1260		700	1750		420			
Calcium chloride (mg)				120										
Calcium laevulinate (mg)				350										
Calcium gluconate (mg)					500									
Calcium lactate gluconate (mg)								930	2327					
Hydroxyapatite compound (mg)							830							
Calcium glubionate (mg)										3270				
Calcium lactobionate										2170				
Potassium phosphate (mg)												170.1		
Sodium phosphate (mg)												133.5		
Phosphoryl colamine (mg)													1000	
Sodium and phosphate (mg)														1936
Potassium hydroxide (mg)												14		
Sodium bicarbonate (mg)														350
Potassium bicarbonate (mg)														315
[Calcium mg]		[500]	[1000]			[500]		[400]	[1000]					
[Calcium mmol]	[12.5]							[10]	[25]					
[Phosphate mmol]												[2]		[16.1]
[Potassium mmol]												[1.5]		[3.1]
[Sodium mmol]												[1.5]		[20.4]
Citric acid (mg)								1189						
Sorbitol (mg)												1		
Glycine (mg)											180			
Calciferol (μg)					1.25									
Thiamin (mg)				0.5										
Riboflavin (mg)				0.125										
Pyridoxine (mg)				0.125										
Niacin (mg)				2										
Ascorbic acid (mg)				5										
Ca pantothenate (mg)				0.125										

X = not available on NHS.

Table 7.53 Combined vitamin and mineral supplements (prescribable)

	Forceval (Unigreg) Per capsule*	Forceval Junior (Unigreg) Per capsule**
Vitamin A (as β-Carotene)		
Retinol equivalent μg	750	375
Vitamin D_2 μg	10	5
Vitamin E mg	10	5
Vitamin K_1 μg	70	25
Thiamin mg	1.2	1.5
Riboflavin mg	1.6	1
Vitamin B_6 mg	2	1
Vitamin B_{12} μg	3	2
Vitamin C mg	60	25
Biotin μg	100	50
Nicotinamide mg	18	7.5
Pantothenic acid mg	4	2
Folic acid μg	300	100
Calcium mg	100	—
Iron mg	12	5
Copper mg	2	1
Phosphorus mg	77	—
Magnesium mg	30	1
Potassium mg	4	—
Zinc mg	15	5
Iodine μg	140	75
Manganese mg	3	1.25
Selenium μg	50	25
Chromium μg	200	50
Molybdenum μg	250	50

* Recommended dose (adults): 1 capsule/day
** Recommended dose (children): 2 capsules/day

Table 7.54 Substances used in vitamin preparations

Vitamin	Names	Formula	Molecular weight	Notes
Vitamin A	Vitamin A; retinol	$C_{20}H_{30}O$	286.5	Generally used in the form of esters
	Vitamin A acetate; retinyl acetate	$C_{22}H_{32}O_2$	328.5	1.15 g ≏ 1 g retinol
	Vitamin A palmitate; retinyl palmitate	$C_{36}H_{60}O_2$	524.9	1.83 g ≏ 1 g retinol
Vitamin B_1	Thiamine hydrochloride	$C_{12}H_{17}ClN_4OS\ HCl$	337.3	
	Thiamin mononitrate	$C_{12}H_{17}N_5O_4S$	327.4	
Vitamin B_2	Riboflavin	$C_{17}H_{20}N_4O_6$	376.4	
	Riboflavin sodium phosphate	$C_{17}H_{20}N_4NaO_9P\ 2H_2O$	514.4	1.37 g ≏ 1 g riboflavin
Vitamin B_6	Pyridoxine hydrochloride	$C_8H_{11}NO_3\ HCl$	205.6	
Vitamin B_{12}	Cyanocobalamin	$C_{63}H_{88}CoN_{14}O_{14}P$	1355.4	
	Hydroxocobalamin	$C_{62}H_{89}CoN_{13}O_{15}P$	1346.4	
	Liver extracts			No longer recommended for routine treatment
Other vitamins of the B group	Biotin	$C_{10}H_{16}N_2O_3S$	244.3	
	Folic acid; folacin; pteroylglutamic acid	$C_{19}H_{19}N_7O_6$	441.4	
	Calcium folinate	$C_{20}H_{21}CaN_7O_7\ 5H_2O$	601.6	
	Nicotinic acid; niacin	$C_6H_5NO_2$	123.1	
	Nicotinamide; vitamin PP	$C_6H_6N_2O$	122.1	
	Pantothenic acid	$C_9H_{17}NO_5$	219.2	Usually used as the calcium salt
	Calcium pantothenate	$(C_9H_{16}NO_5)_2Ca$	476.5	
	Dexpanthenol; pantothenol; pantothenyl alcohol	$C_9H_{19}NO_4$	205.3	
	Aminobenzoic acid; *p*-amino benzoic acid (PABA)	$C_7H_7NO_2$	137.1	
	Choline	$C_5H_{15}NO_2$	121.2	Used as acid tartrate, acid citrate or chloride
	Choline bitartrate; choline acid tartrate	$C_9H_{19}NO_7$	253.3	
	Choline chloride	$C_5H_{14}ClNO$	139.6	
	Choline dihydrogen citrate; choline acid citrate	$C_{11}H_{21}NO_8$	295.3	
	Inositol	$C_6H_{12}O_6$	180.2	
	Dried yeast (Contains >0.1 mg thiamin hydrochloride, >0.3 mg nicotinic acid; >0.04 mg riboflavin, also pyridoxine, pantothenic acid, biotin, folic acid, vitamin B_{12}, aminobenzoic acid and inositol per 1 g)			
Vitamin C	Ascorbic acid	$C_6H_8O_6$	176.1	
	Sodium ascorbate	$C_6H_7NaO_6$	198.1	
Vitamin D	Alfacalcidol; $1\alpha OHD_3$; 1α hydroxy cholecalciferol	$C_{27}H_{44}O_2$	400.6	
	Calcifediol; $25(OH)D_3$; 25 hydroxy cholecalciferol	$C_{27}H_{44}O_2\ H_2O$	418.7	
	Calcitriol; $1\alpha,25(OH)_2D_3$; 1,25 dihydroxy cholecalciferol	$C_{27}H_{44}O_3$	416.6	
	Cholecalciferol; vitamin D_3	$C_{27}H_{44}O$	384.6	
	Dihydrotachysterol	$C_{28}H_{46}O$	398.7	
	Ergocalciferol; calciferol; vitamin D_2	$C_{28}H_{44}O$	396.7	
Vitamin E	*d*-alpha tocopherol	$C_{29}H_{50}O_2$	430.7	1 mg = 1.49 units
	dl-alpha tocopherol	$C_{29}H_{50}O_2$	430.7	1 mg = 1.1 unit
	d-alpha-tocopheryl acetate	$C_{31}H_{52}O_3$	472.8	1 mg = 1.36 units
	dl-alpha tocopheryl acetate	$C_{31}H_{52}O_3$	472.8	1 mg = 1 unit
	d-alpha tocopheryl acid succinate	$C_{33}H_{54}O_5$	530.8	
Vitamin K	Phytomenadione; vitamin K_1	$C_{13}H_{46}O_2$	450.7	Natural vitamin K
	Acetomenaphthone	$C_{15}H_{14}O_4$	258.3	
Vitamin P	The name given to a substance claimed to increase the resistance of the capillaries and reduce their permeability to red blood cells. All substances claimed to have vitamin P activity are flavone derivatives. They include hesperidin, rutin and troxerutin			

Table 7.55 Some mineral salts used in pharmaceutical preparations

Salt	Formula	Molecular weight	Notes
Calcium glubionate	$(C_{12}H_{21}O_{12}, C_6H_{11}O_7)Ca\ H_2O$	610.5	
Calcium gluconate	$C_{12}H_{22}CaO_{14}\ H_2O$	448.4	1 g ≏ 2.2 mmol (4.5 mEq) Ca
Calcium hydrogen phosphate	$CaHPO_4\ 2H_2O$	172.1	Ca 23%, P 18%
Copper sulphate	$CuSO_4, 5H_2O$	249.7	
Ferric ammonium citrate	Complex		About 21.5% Fe
Ferrous fumarate	$C_4H_2FeO_4$	169.9	About 32.5% Fe
Ferrous gluconate	$C_{12}H_{22}FeO_{14}\ 2H_2O$	482.2	About 70 mg Fe in 600 mg dihydrate
Ferrous glycine sulphate	Chelate		About 40 mg Fe in 225 mg
Ferrous succinate	$C_4H_4FeO_4$	171.9	34–36% Fe
Ferrous sulphate	$FeSO_4\ 7H_2O$	278.0	About 60 mg Fe in 300 mg
Ferrous sulphate, dried	80–90% $FeSO_4$		About 60 mg Fe in 200 mg
Iodide, potassium	KI	166.0	1 g = 6 mmol (6 mEq) I
Iron dextran injection			About 50 mg Fe per ml
Iron sorbitol citric acid	Complex		About 50 mg Fe per ml
Sodium ironedetate	$C_{10}H_{12}FeN_2NaO_8\ 2H_2O$	385.1	
Hydroxyapatite	$3Ca_3(PO_4)_2, Ca(OH)_2$	1004.6	Used in a proteinaceous base, 1 g = 176 mg Ca and 82 mg P
Glycerophosphates	of Ca, Mn, K and Na		Have been widely used as 'tonic' but there is little evidence to support this
Manganese sulphate	$MnSO_4\ 4H_2O$	223.1	Use for their supposed effect in increasing the haematinic effect of iron in microcytic anaemia
Magnesium sulphate	$MgSO_4\ 7H_2O$	246.5	1 g ≏ 4.1 mmol (8.1 mEq) Mg
Magnesium sulphate dried	62–70% $MgSO_4$		
Potassium bicarbonate	$KHCO_3$	100.1	1 g ≏ 10 mmol (10 mEq) K
Potassium chloride	KCl	74.55	1 g ≏ 13.4 mmol (13.4 mEq) K
Potassium citrate	$C_6H_5K_3O_7\ H_2O$	324.4	1 g ≏ 9.25 mmol (9.25 mEq) K
Potassium sulphate	K_2SO_4	174.3	1 g ≏ 11.5 mmol (11.5 mEq) K
Sodium bicarbonate	$NaHCO_3$	84.01	1 g = 11.9 mmol (11.9 mEq) Na
Sodium chloride	NaCl	58.44	1 g = 17.1 mmol (17.1 mEq) Na
Sodium acid phosphate	$NaH_2PO_4\ 2H_2O$	156.0	1 g = 6.4 mmol (6.4 mEq) Na; 6.4 mmol (6.4 mEq) PO_4; 198.5 mg P
Zinc sulphate	$ZnSO_4\ 7H_2O$	287.5	1 g = 3.5 mmol (7 mEq) Zn; about 50 mg Zn in 220 mg
Zinc sulphate monohydrate	$ZnSO_4\ H_2O$		

Atomic weights: Ca = 40.08; Cl = 35.45; Cu = 63.55; Fe = 55.85; I = 126.9; P = 30.97; Mn = 54.94; Mg = 24.30; K = 39.10; Na = 23.0; Zn = 65.38.

7.7 Appendix 7: Composition of proprietary enteral feeds

The composition of proprietary enteral feeds is given in the following tables:

Table 7.56 Whole protein preparations.
Table 7.57 Peptide-based preparations.
Table 7.58 Amino acid-based preparations.

It should be noted that this data is given for guidance only. Both the formulation and availability of these products is likely to change over a period of time. The information given here must therefore be verified before being used in nutritional calculations.

Table 7.56 Proprietary enteral feeds: whole protein preparations

				Composition per 100 ml		(February 1993)					
Company	Product	Presentation	Unit size (Dilution)	Energy kJ	Energy kcal	Protein g	Nitrogen g	Sodium mmol	Potassium mmol	NPE:N ratio	Osmolality mosmol/kg water
Clintec Nutrition Ltd	Clinifeed:										
	– Iso	Liquid	375 ml can	420	100	2.8	0.45	1.52	3.8	200	338
	– Favour	Liquid	375 ml can 500 ml polythene Dripac®	420	100	3.8	0.6	3.0	2.8	146	388
	– 400*	Liquid	375 ml can (+ 125 ml)	336	80	3.0	0.48	1.9	3.3	142	293 (414 undil.)
	* Figures/100 ml when diluted according to manufacturer's instructions										
	– Protein* Rich	Liquid	375 ml can (+ 125 ml)	420	100	6.0	0.96	3.4	5.7	79	486 (700 undil.)
	* Figures/100 ml when diluted according to manufacturer's instructions										
	– Extra	Liquid	500 ml polythene Dripac®	559	133	6.65	1.06	2.1	3.3	102	360
Cow & Gate Nutricia Ltd	Nutrison/Nutrison Steriflo:										
	Pre-Nutrison	Liquid	**	210	51	2.0	0.31	1.7	1.7	135	140
	Standard	Liquid	**	420	100	4.0	0.63	3.5	3.5	133	290
	Energy Plus	Liquid	**	630	150	6.0	0.94	3.5	3.5	134	440
	Fibre***	Liquid	**	420	100	4.0	0.63	3.5	3.5	133	290
	Soya	Liquid	**	420	100	4.0	0.64	3.5	3.5	131	280
	Low Protein/ Low Minerals	Liquid	**	420	100	<1.2	<0.2	1.1	2.6	480	205
	Low Sodium	Liquid	**	420	100	4.0	0.63	1.1	3.5	133	230
	Paediatric (1–6 yr olds)	Liquid	200 ml bottle	420	100	2.7	0.4	2.5	2.1	223	245
	** Available in 1000 ml polypropylene bottles (Steriflo) or 500 ml glass bottles *** Dietary fibre content 1.5 g/100 ml										
Fresenius Ltd	Fresubin	Liquid	500 ml bottle 200 ml tetrapak	420	100	3.8	0.6	3.3	3.2	142	410
	Fresubin Plus F*	Liquid	500 ml bottle (Muesli) 200 ml bottle (Veg soup) 200 ml tetrapak (Muesli)	420	100	3.8	0.6	3.3	3.2	142	290 (Veg) 410 (Muesli)
	* Dietary fibre content 1.0 g/100 ml										
	Fresubin 750	Liquid	500 ml bottle	630	150	7.5	1.2	4.4	4.3	100	375

Table 7.56 *contd.*

Company	Product	Presentation	Unit size (Dilution)	Energy kJ	Energy kcal	Protein g	Nitrogen g	Sodium mmol	Potassium mmol	NPE:N ratio	Osmolality mosmol/kg water
			Composition per 100 ml (February 1993)								
E. Merck Ltd	Liquisorb	Liquid	500 ml bottle	420	100	4.0	0.63	4.5 (5.0 choc, banana, strawb)	4.5 (6.0 choc)	133	320 (400 vanilla/ banana/strawb/ choc)
	High Energy Liquisorb	Liquid	500 ml bottle	630	150	6.0	0.94	5.8	5.4	134	400 (neut) 450 (vanil/toffee)
	Liquisorbon MCT	Liquid	500 ml bottle	420	100	5.0	0.8	4.5 (5.0 choc)	4.5 (5.0 choc)	100	270 (neut) 390 (vanil) 430 (strawb/choc)
	Triosorbon	Powder	85 g sachet (+ 400 ml water → 470 ml)	357	85	3.4	0.55	3.6	3.6	129	250
Oxford Nutrition	Inmunonutril (contains arginine, glutamine, nucleotides & ω-3 fatty a.)	Powder	98 g sachet (in 400–420 ml)	420	100	5.0	0.9	3.6	2.1	89	376
	Protina G (contains glutamine, MCT, linoleic acid)	Powder	107 g (+ 425 ml → 500 ml)	420	100	4.6	0.7	0.74	1.6	116	218
	Protina MP (contains MCT, linoleic acid)	Powder	100 g (+ 330 ml → 400 ml) 85 g sachet (+ 280 ml → 340 ml)	462	110	6.9	1.0	2.5	3.8	82	355
Ross Labs	Ensure	Liquid	250 ml can 950 ml can 237 ml bottle	420	100	4.0	0.56	3.5	3.8	153	470
		Powder	400 g tin (56 g in 200 ml)								
	Ensure Plus	Liquid	250 ml can 500 ml bottle	630	150	6.25	1.0	5.1	4.7	125	590
	Osmolite	Liquid	250 ml can 500 ml bottle	420	100	4.0	0.68	3.8	3.8	122	277
	Enrich (+ fibre: dietary fibre content 2.75 g/100 ml)	Liquid	250 ml can	436	104	3.8	0.6	3.5	3.8	148	439
	Jevity (+ fibre: dietary fibre content 1.36 g/100 ml)	Liquid	500 ml bottle	420	100	4.0	0.68	3.8	3.8	122	310
	Two Cal HN	Liquid	237 ml can	842	200	8.4	1.36	5.7	6.2	124	690
	Pulmocare	Liquid	237 ml can	630	150	6.25	1.0	5.7	4.4	123	490
	Nepro (for dialysis patients)	Liquid	237 ml can	838	200	6.99	1.12	3.6	2.7	154	635
	Paediasure (1–6 yr olds)	Liquid	250 ml can	420	100	3.0	0.94	2.0	3.3	183	320
Scientific Hospital Supplies	Enteral 400	Powder	400 g (Dilute 1 in 5: i.e. 400 g up to 2000 ml)	370	88	2.68	0.43	2.4	2.8	180	269

Table 7.57 Proprietary enteral feeds: peptide based preparations

Composition per 100 ml prepared or as diluted per manufacturer's instructions (February 1993)

Company	Product	Presentation	Unit size (Dilution)	Energy kJ	Energy kcal	Protein g	Nitrogen g	Sodium mmol	Potassium mmol	NPE:N ratio	Osmolality mosmol/kg water
Clinitec Nutrition Ltd	Peptamen	Liquid	250 ml can (flavoured) 1 litre pouch	420	100	4.0	0.63	2.2	3.2	134	260
	Reabilan	Liquid	375 ml can 500 ml polythene Dripac®	420	100	3.15	0.5	3.04	3.21	175	350
Cow & Gate Nutricia Ltd	Peptison	Liquid	500 ml bottle	420	100	4.0	0.58	3.5	3.6	146	470
	Peptison Steriflo	Liquid	1000 ml polypropylene bottle								
	Pepti-2000 LF	Powder	126 g sachet (+ up to 500 ml)	420	100	4.0	0.58	2.0	3.63	146	490
Fresenius Ltd	Fresenius OPD	Liquid	500 ml bottle	420	100	4.5	0.7	4.4	3.2	117	500
E. Merck Ltd	Peptisorb	Liquid	500 ml bottle	420	100	3.75	0.6	6.0	3.0	142	400
	Peptisorbon	Powder	83 g sachet (+ 300 ml → 333 ml)	420	100	4.5	0.72	6.0	3.0	154	500
Scientific Hospital Supplies	Pepdite 2+	Powder	400 g tin (Dilute 1 in 5 i.e. 400 g up to 2000 ml)	357	85	2.76	0.44	1.82	2.64	167	351
	MCT Pepdite 2+	Powder	400 g tin (Dilute 1 in 5 i.e. 400 g up to 2000 ml)	369	88	2.76	0.44	1.82	2.64	174	389

Table 7.58 Proprietary enteral feeds: amino acid based preparations

Composition per 100 ml prepared or as diluted per manufacturer's instructions (February 1993)

Company	Product	Presentation	Unit size (Dilution)	Energy kJ	Energy kcal	Protein g	Nitrogen g	Sodium mmol	Potassium mmol	NPE:N ratio	Osmolality mosmol/kg water
Ross Laboratories	AlitraQ (Glutamine enriched)	Powder	76 g sachet (+ 250 ml → 300 ml)	426	100	5.27	0.8	4.4	3.1	94	575
	Perative	Liquid	237 ml can	554	131	6.68	1.07	4.6	4.4	97	385
Mead Johnson Nutritionals	Flexical	Powder	454 g tin (10 scoops + 207 ml → 250 ml)	418	100	2.25	0.36	1.5	3.2	253	550
Scientific Hospital Supplies	Elemental 028	Powder	100 g box (Dilute 1 in 5 i.e. 100 g up to 500 ml)	308	73	2.0	0.32	2.2	2.4	203	711 (flavoured) 496 (unflavoured)
	Neocate (for infants)	Powder	400 g tin (Dilute 15 g in 100 ml)	292	70	1.95	0.32	0.8	1.6	194	353

7.8 Appendix 8: Abbreviations used in dietetic practice

aa Amino acid(s)
AA Arachidonic acid
ACBS Advisory Committee for Borderline Substances
ACE Angiotensin converting enzyme
ACTH Adrenocorticotrophic hormone
AD Alzheimer's disease
ADH Antidiuretic hormone
ADI Acceptable daily intake
AGE Appropriate for gestational age
AIDS Acquired immunodeficiency syndrome
Al Aluminium
AMA American Medical Association
AN Anorexia nervosa
ANF Anti-nuclear factor
APACHE Acute physiology and chronic health evaluation (score)
ARC AIDS related complex
ARF Acute renal failure
ASBAH Association for Spina Bifida and Hydrocephalus
ATN Acute tubular necrosis
ATP Adenosine triphosphate
AV Arterio-venous

B_1 Thiamin
B_2 Riboflavin
B_6 Pyridoxine
BCAA Branched chain amino acids
bd Twice a day
BDA British Dietetic Association *or* British Diabetic Association
BHA Butylated hydroxyanisole
BHT Butylated hydroxytoluene
BIA Bioelectrical impedance analysis
BMA British Medical Association
BMI Body Mass Index
BMR Basal metabolic rate
BN Bulimia nervosa
BNF British Nutrition Foundation *or* British National Formulary
BP Blood pressure
BPA British Paediatric Association
BSE Bovine spongiform encephalopathy
BUN Blood urea nitrogen
Bx Biopsy

C Carbon
C3 Complement 3
C4 Complement 4
C18:2,n-6 Linoleic acid
C18:3,n-3 Alpha linolenic acid
C20:4,n-6 Arachidonic acid
C20:5,n-3 Eicosapentaenoic acid
C22:6,n-3 Docosahexaenoic acid
Ca Calcium *or* Cancer
CAPD Continuous ambulatory peritoneal dialysis
CAVHD Continuous arteriovenous haemofiltration
CCPD Continuous cyclic peritoneal dialysis
CCU Coronary care unit
Cd Cadmium
CD Crohn's disease
CDC Centers for Disease Control
CF Cystic Fibrosis
CHD Coronary heart disease
CHO Carbohydrate
cm Centimetre(s)
CMHT Community mental handicap team
CMV Cytomegalovirus
c/o Complaining of
Co Cobalt
CO Cardiac output *or* Carbon monoxide
CoA Coenzyme A
COAD Chronic obstructive airways disease
COMA Committee on Medical Aspects of Food Policy
COT Committee on Toxicity of Chemicals in Food
CPAG Child Poverty Action Group
CPN Central parenteral nutrition
CPSM Council for the Professions Supplementary to Medicine
Cr Chromium
CRF Chronic renal failure
CRP C-reactive protein
CSF Cerebrospinal fluid
CSO Central Statistical Office
CT Computed tomography
Cu Copper
cv Coefficient of variation
CVA Cerebrovascular accident (Stroke)
CVP Central venous pressure

d Day
D_2 Ergocalciferol
D_3 Cholecalciferol

DEXA	Dual energy X-ray absorptiometry
DoH	Department of Health
DHA	Docosahexaenoic acid
DHHS	Department of Health and Human Science (USA)
DHSS	Department of Health and Social Security
dL	Decilitre (100 ml)
DLW	Doubly-labelled water technique
DM	Diabetes mellitus
DNA	Deoxyribonucleic acid *or* Did not attend
DRV	Dietary Reference Value
dsp	Dessertspoonful
DSS	Department of Social Security
D&V	Diarrhoea and vomiting
DXT	Deep X-ray therapy
EAR	Estimated average requirement
EC	European Community
ECF	Extracellular fluid
ECG	Electrocardiogram
ED	Elemental diets
EDTA	Ethylene diamine tetra-acetic acid
EEG	Electroencephalogram
EFA	Essential fatty acid(s)
EHBA	Extra hepatic biliary atresia
EPA	Eicosapentaenoic acid
EPO	Evening primrose oil
ERCP	Endoscopic retrograde cholangiopancreatography
ESPGAN	European Society for Paediatric Gastroenterology
ESR	Erythrocyte sedimentation rate
ESRF	End stage renal failure
ET	Endotracheal
E:T ratio	Ratio of essential amino acids to total nitrogen
F	Fluorine
FA	Fatty acid(s)
FAC	Food Advisory Committee
FACC	Food Additives and Contaminants Committee
FAE	Fetal alcohol effect
FAO	Food and Agriculture Organization
FAS	Fetal alcohol syndrome
FBS	Fasting blood sugar
FDA	Food and Drug Administration
Fe	Iron
FFM	Fat-free mass
FHF	Fulminant liver failure
FOB	Faecal occult blood
FP10	Form used for the prescription of medicines in the UK
g	Gram(s)
Gamma GT	Gamma glutamyl transpeptidase
GBM	Glomerular basement membrane
GF	Gluten free
GFR	Glomerular filtration rate
GI	Gastrointestinal
GLA	Gamma linolenic acid
GN	Glomerulonephritis
GP	General Practitioner
GPX	Glutathione peroxidase
GRAS	Generally recognized as safe
GTT	Glucose tolerance test
GVHD	Graft-versus-host disease
HA	Health Authority
Hb	Haemoglobin
HB	Health Board
HBV	High biological value
HCO_3	Bicarbonate
HD	Haemodialysis
HDL	High density lipoprotein
HEA	Health Education Authority
HF	Haemofiltration
Hg	Mercury
HGH	Human growth hormone
HIV	Human immunodeficiency virus
HLA	Human lymphocyte antigen
HMG CoA	Hydroxymethylglutaryl Coenzyme A
HMSO	Her Majesty's Stationery Office
Ht	Height
HV	Health visitor
Hx	History
I	Iodine
IABP	Intra-aortic balloon pump
IBD	Inflammatory bowel disease
IBS	Irritable bowel syndrome
IBW	Ideal body weight
ICF	Intracellular fluid
ICU	Intensive care unit
IDD	Insulin dependent diabetic
IDDM	Insulin dependent diabetes mellitus
IDL	Intermediate density lipoproteins
IgA	Immunoglobulin A
IgE	Immunoglobulin E
IgG	Immunoglobulin G
IgM	Immunoglobulin M
IJO	Idiopathic juvenile osteoporosis
IL1	Interleukin 1
IL6	Interleukin 6
IM	Intramuscular
INR	International normalized ratio
ip	Intraperitoneal
IPD	Intraperitoneal dialysis
IQ	Intelligence quotient
ITU	Intensive therapy unit
iu	International units
IUGR	Intrauterine growth retardation

IV	Intravenous
IVH	Intravenous hyperalimentation
Jej Bx *or* Jb	Jejunal biopsy
JVP	Jugular venous pressure
K	Potassium
kJ	Kilojoule(s)
kcal	Kilocalorie(s)
kg	Kilogram(s)
l	Litre(s)
LAF	Laminar air-flow
LBM	Lean body mass
LBV	Low biological value
LBW	Low birth weight
L-CAT	Lecithin cholesterol acyltransferase
LCFA	Long chain fatty acids
LCT	Long chain triglycerides
LDL	Low density lipoprotein
LFT	Liver function tests
LNRI	Lower reference nutrient intake
m	Metre(s)
MAC	Medical Advisory Committee *or* Mid-arm circumference
MAFF	Ministry of Agriculture, Fisheries and Food
MAMC	Mid-arm muscle circumference
MAOI	Monoamine oxidase inhibitors
MCFA	Medium chain fatty acids
MCH	Mean cell haemoglobin
MCHC	Mean cell haemoglobin concentration
MCT	Medium chain triglyceride
MCV	Mean cell volume
mEq	Milliequivalents
mg	Milligram(s)
Mg	Magnesium
MID	Multi-infarct dementia
MIMS	Monthly Index of Medical Specialities
MJ	Megajoule(s)
ml	Millilitre(s)
mm	Millimetre(s)
mmol	Millimole(s)
Mn	Manganese
Mo	Molybdenum
MOFS	Multi-organ system failure
mosmol	Milliosmole(s)
MRC	Medical Research Council
MRI	Magnetic resonance imaging
MS	Multiple sclerosis
MSG	Monosodium glutamate
MUAC	Mid-upper arm muscle circumference
MUFA	Monounsaturated fatty acids
n-	Omega
N	Nitrogen
Na	Sodium
NACNE	National Advisory Committee on Nutrition Education
NADP	Nicotinamide adenine dinucleotide phosphate
NADPH	Reduced nicotinamide adenine dinucleotide phosphate
NAGE	Nutrition Advisory Group for Elderly People
NAS	No added salt
NBM	Nil by mouth
NCH	National Children's Home
NCHC	National Center for Health Statistics
NCT	National Childbirth Trust
NDC	National Dairy Council
NFS	National Food Survey
ng	Nastrogastric *or* Nanogram(s)
NHANES	National Health and Nutrition Examination Survey
NHS	National Health Service
Ni	Nickel
NIDD	Non-insulin dependent diabetic diabetes
NIDDM	Non-insulin dependent diabetes mellitus
NMES	Non-milk extrinsic sugars
NPE:N	Non-protein energy: nitrogen ratio
NRC	National Research Council
NSAIDS	Non-steroidal anti-inflammatory drugs
NS	Nephrotic Syndrome
NSP	Non-starch polysaccharide
NTD	Neural tube defect
N & V	Nausea and vomiting
OD	Overdose
OFG	Oro-facial granulomatosis
OPCS	Office of Population, Censuses and Surveys
osmol	Osmole(s)
OTC	Over the counter
OU	Open University
oz	Ounce(s)
P	Phosphorus
PABA	Para-amino benzoic acid
PAC	Pulmonary artery catheter
$PaCO_2$	Arterial carbon dioxide
PaO_2	Arterial oxygen
PAL	Physical activity level
PAR	Physical activity ratio
Pb	Lead
PCK	Polycystic disease of the kidney
PCP	Pneumocystis carinii pneumonia
PCR	Protein catabolic rate
PD	Peritoneal dialysis
PDUO	Previous day's urine output
PEEP	Positive end-expiratory pressure
PEG	Percutaneous endoscopic gastrostomy
PEM	Protein energy malnutrition

PENG	Parenteral and Enteral Nutrition Group
PG	Prostaglandin
Pi	Protease inhibitor
PKU	Phenylketonuria
PMH	Past medical history
PMT	Pre-menstrual tension
PN	Parenteral nutrition
PO_4	Phosphate
PPF	Plasma protein fraction
ppm	Parts per million
PPN	Peripheral parenteral nutrition
P/S ratio	Ratio of polyunsaturated to saturated fatty acids
pt(s)	Patient(s) *or* Pint(s)
PT	Prothrombin time
PTH	Parathyroid hormone
Pu	Passed urine *or* Peptic ulcer
PUFA	Polyunsaturated fatty acids
PWS	Prader-Willi Syndrome
Px	Prognosis
qds	Four times a day
RA	Rheumatoid arthritis
RAST	Radioallergosorbent test
RBC	Red blood cells
RBP	Retinol binding protein
RBS	Random blood sugar
RCP	Royal College of Physicians
RDA	Recommended daily amount *or* Recommended dietary allowance
RDI	Recommended daily intake
REE	Resting energy expenditure
r-HuEPO	Recombinant human erythropoietin
RME	Resting metabolic expenditure
RMR	Resting metabolic rate
RNA	Ribonucleic acid
RNI	Reference nutrient intake
RNIB	Royal National Institute for the Blind
RNMH	Registered nurse mental handicap
RQ	Respiratory quotient
RSC	Royal Society of Chemistry
RTA	Road traffic accident
Rx	Treatment
SAD	Seasonal affective disorder
SCI	Spinal cord injury
sd	Standard deviation
SDAT	Senile dementia of the Alzheimer type
se	Standard error
Se	Selenium
SFA	Saturated fatty acids
SFD	Small for dates
SFGA	Small for gestational age
SGA	Small for gestational age
SGOT	Serum glutamic-oxaloacetic transaminase activity
SGPT	Serum glutamic-pyruvic transaminase activity
SI	Systeme internationale *or* Statutory Instrument
SLE	Systemic lupus erythematosis
SRD	State Registered Dietitian
SRN	State Registered Nurse
Sx	Symptoms
T3	Tri-iodothyronine
T4	Thyroxine
TB	Tuberculosis
TBPA	Thyroxine binding prealbumin
TBW	Total body water
TCA	To come again
tds	Three times a day
TEE	Total energy expenditure
TF	Serum transferrin
TIBC	Total iron binding capacity
TLC	Total lymphocyte count
TNF	Tubular necrosis factor
TPN	Total parenteral nutrition
TSF *or* TST	Triceps skinfold thickness
TT	Thrombin time
TTO	To take out
Tx	Transplant
UC	Ulcerative colitis
U & E	Urea and electrolytes
μg	Microgram(s)
UHT	Ultra high temperature *or* Ultra heat treatment
μmol	Micromole(s)
Ur	Urea
UTI	Urinary tract infection
UVR	Ultraviolet radiation
V	Vanadium
VLCD	Very low calorie diet
VLDL	Very low density lipoprotein
VMA	Vanillymandelic acid
VO2 max	Maximum oxygen uptake
ω	Gamma
WBC	White blood cells *or* White blood count
W/H^2	Weight divided by height squared (Body Mass Index)
WHO	World Health Organization
WRVS	Women's Royal Voluntary Service
Wt	Weight
Zn	Zinc

#	Fracture
Δ	Diagnosis
∵	Because
1/52	One week
1/12	One month
1/1/12	One per month
1,25(OH)D	1,25 dihydroxy vitamin D
25(OH)D	25 hydroxy vitamin D
5-HIAA	5-hydroxyindoleacetic acid
5-HT	5-hydroxytryptophan

7.9 Appendix 9: Useful addresses

ACET (AIDS, Care, Education and Training), PO Box 1323, London W5 5TF. Tel 081–840 7879.

ACET (Scotland), PO Box 151, Edinburgh EH8 9NY. Tel 031–667 1978.

Action Against Allergy, 43 The Downs, London SW20 8HS.

Action for Blind People, 14–16 Vernay Street, London SE16.

ADA Reading Services, 6 Dalewood Rise, Laverstock, Salisbury, Wilts SP1 1SE. Tel 0722 26987.

Age Concern, Astral House, 1268 London Road, Norbury, London SW16 4ER. Tel 081–679 8000.

Alcohol Concern, 275 Gray's Inn Road, London WC1X 8QF. Tel 071–833 3471.

The Alfawap Trust Fund Ltd., 4 Woodchurch Road, London NW6.

Alzheimer's Disease Society, 158–160 Balham High Road, London SW12 9BN. Tel 081–675 6557.

Arthritis Care, 5 Grosvenor Crescent, London SW1X 7ER. Tel 071–235 0902.

Arthritis and Rheumatism Council for Research, Copeman House, St Mary's Court, St Mary's Gate, Chesterfield, Derbyshire S41 7TD. Tel 0246 558033.

Association of Breastfeeding Mothers, 26 Hearnshaw Close, London SE26 4TH. Tel 081–778 4769.

Association for Spina Bifida and Hydrocephalus (ASBAH), 43 Park Road, Peterborough PE1 2UQ. Tel 0733 555988.

Asthma Society and Friends of the Asthma Research Council, St Thomas' Hospital, Lambeth Palace Road, London SE1 7EH.

Avery Ltd., Foundry Lane, Smethwick, Warley, West Midlands B66 2LP. Tel 021–558 1112/2161.

BACUP (British Association for Cancer United Patients and their families and friends), 121/123 Charterhouse Street, London EC1M 6AA. Tel Cancer Information Service 071–608 1661.

BC Systems Ltd., 35 Harford Street, Trowbridge, Wilts.

Blackliners Helpline, PO Box 1274, London SW9 8EZ. Tel 071–738 5274.

Body Positive, 51b Philbeach Gardens, Earls Court, London SW5 9EB. Tel 071–835 1045.

Body Positive (Scotland), 37–39 Montrose Terrace, Edinburgh EH7 5DJ. Tel 031–652 0754.

Boots Company plc, Thane Road, Nottingham NG2 3AA. Tel 0602 506255.

The Braille Unit, HM Prison Wakefield, 5 Live Lane, Wakefield WF2 9AG. Tel 0924 387282.

The Braille Unit, Aylesbury Youth Custody Centre, HM Prison, Brerton Road, Aylesbury, Bucks. Tel 0296 24435.

Britannia Pharmaceuticals Ltd, Forum House, 41–75 Brighton Road, Redhill, Surrey RH1 6YS. Tel 0737 773741.

British Diabetic Association, 10 Queen Anne Street, London W1M 0BD. Tel 071–323 1531; Fax 071–637 3644.

British Dietetic Association, 7th Floor, Elizabeth House, 22 Suffolk Street, Queensway, Birmingham B1 1LS. Tel 021–643 5483.

British Geriatric Society, 1 St Andrew's Place, Regents Park, London NW1 4LB.

British Institute of Mental Handicap (BIMH), Wolverhampton Road, Kidderminster, Worcs DY10 3PP. Tel 0562 850251.

British Nutrition Foundation, High Holborn House, 52–54 High Holborn, London WCIV 6RU. Tel 071–404 6504; Fax 071–404 6747.

Campaign for People with a Mental Handicap (CMH) (*see* Values In Action).

CancerLink, 46 Pentonville Road, London N1. Tel 071–833 2451.

Cancer Relief Macmillan Fund, Anchor House, 15/19 Britten Street, London SW3 3TZ. Tel 071–351 7811.

Cantassium Company, 225–229 Putney Bridge Road, London SW15 2PY. Tel 081–874 1130.

Carers' National Association, 29 Chilworth Mews, London W2 3RG. Tel 071–724 7776.

Centre for Policy on Ageing, 25–31 Ironmonger Row, London EC1V 3QP. Tel 071–253 1787.

Cherlyn Electronics, King's Court, King's Hedges Road, Cambridge.

Child Poverty Action Group, 4th Floor, 1–5 Bath Street, London EC1V 9PY. Tel 071–253 3406.

Children's Liver Disease Foundation (CHILD), 138 Digbeth, Birmingham B5 6DR.

Clintec Nutrition, Shaftesbury Court, 18 Chalvey Park, Slough, Berks SL1 2HT.

Coeliac Society, PO Box 220, High Wycombe, Bucks HP11 2HY. Tel 0494 437278.

Coronary Prevention Group, 102 Gloucester Place, London W1H 3DA. Tel 071–935 2889.

Cow & Gate Nutricia Ltd, White Horse Business Park, Trowbridge, Wiltshire BA14 0XQ. Tel 0225 768381.

Crookes Healthcare Ltd, PO Box 94, 1 Thane Road West, Nottingham NG2 3AA.

CRUSE Bereavement Care, Cruse House, 126 Sheen Road, Richmond, Surrey TW9 1UR. Tel 081–940 4818.

Council for Professions Supplementary to Medicine, Park House, 184 Kennington Park Road, London SE11 4BU. Tel 071–582 0866.

Cystic Fibrosis Research Trust, 5 Blyth Road, Bromley, Kent BR1 3RS. Tel 081–464 7211.

Department of Agriculture and Fisheries for Scotland, Chesser House, 500 Gorgie Road, Edinburgh EH11 3AW.

Department of Health, Nutrition Unit, Wellington House, 133–155 Waterloo Road, London SE1 8UG. Tel 071–972 2000.

Dietary Foods Ltd, Cumberland House, Brook Street, Soham, Cambridgeshire CB7 5BA.

Disabled Living Foundation, 380–384 Harrow Road, London W9 2HU, Tel 071–289 6111.

Down's Syndrome Association, 155 Mitcham Road, Tooting, London SW17 9PG. Tel 081–682 4001.

Dunn Clinical Nutrition Centre, Hills Road, Cambridge CB2 2DH. Tel 0223 415695; Fax 0223 413 763.

Eating Disorders Association, Sackville Place, 44 Magdalen Street, Norwich, Norfolk. Tel 0603 621414.

EAST (Ecumenical AIDS Support Team), 3 Hamilton Terrace, Edinburgh EH13 1NB. Tel 0968 60253.

EC Commission, 8 Storey's Gate, London SW1P 3AT. Tel 071–973 1992.

Egerton Hospital Equipment Ltd, Farwig Lane, Bromley, Kent BR1 3TU. Tel 081–460 9878.

FACTS (Foundation for AIDS Counselling Treatment and Support, 23 and 25 Weston Park, Crouch End, London N8 9SY. Tel 081–348 9195.

Family Heart Association, Wesley House, 7 High Street, Kidlington, Oxford OX5 2DH. Tel 08675 70292.

Farley Health Products, Nottingham NG2 3AA. Tel 0602 507431.

The Food Commission, 102 Gloucester Place, London WC1. Tel 071–935 9078.

Food and Drink Federation, 6 Catherine Street, London WC2B 5JJ. Tel 071–836 2460.

Food Sense, (for publications from MAFF Food Safety Directorate), London SE99 7TT. Tel 081–694 8862.

Food Policy Research Department, University of Bradford, Bradford BD7 1DP.

Foresight (Association for the Promotion of Preconceptual Care), The Old Vicarage, Church Lane, Godalming, Surrey GU8 5PN.

Foundation for Education and Research in Childbearing, 27 Walpole Street, London SW3.

Fresenius Ltd, 6/8 Christleton Court, Stuart Road, Manor Park, Runcorn, Cheshire WA7 1ST. Tel 0928 579444.

General Designs Ltd, PO Box 38E, Worcester Park, Surrey KT4 7LX. Tel 081–337 9366.

HEADWAY. (*see* National Head Injuries Association.)

Health Education Authority, Hamilton House, Mabledon Place, London WC1H 9TX. Tel 071–387 9528.

Health Visitors Association, 50 Southwark Street, London SE1 1UN. Tel 071–378 7255.

Hermes Sweeteners, Boswell House, 37/38 Long Acre, Covent Garden, London WC2E 9JT.

HIV/AIDS Back-up Service, Health Education Department, 61 Grange Loan, Edinburgh EH9 2ER. Tel 031–447 6271.

HMSO Bookshop, 49 High Holborn, London WC1V 6HB. Tel 071–873 0011; Fax 071–831 1326.

HMSO Mail Order, HMSO Publications Centre, PO Box 276, London SW8 5DT.

HMSO Telephone orders, 071–873 9090.

Hyperactive Children's Support Group, c/o 59 Meadowside, Angmering, West Sussex BN14 4BW.

Ileostomy Association of Great Britain and Ireland, Amblehurst House, Chobham, Woking, Surrey GU24 8PZ.

Jacob's Bakery Ltd, Sutton's Business Park, Earley, Reading RG6 1AZ. Tel 0734 492400.

Joint Breastfeeding Initiative, Department of Health, Skipton House, 80 London Road, London SE1 6LW. Tel 071–972 2000.

Kabi Pharmacia, Therapeutics Division, Milton Keynes Energy Park, Davy Avenue, Knowlhill, Milton Keynes, Bucks MK5 8PH. Tel 0908 661101.

Kallo Foods Ltd, 129 Groveley Road, Sunbury-on-Thames, Middlesex TW16 7JZ. Tel 081–890 8324.

Kelgray Marketing Ltd, Kelgray House, Spindleway, Crawley RH10 1TH. Tel 0293 518733.

La Lèche League, PO Box BM 3424, London WC1N 3XX. Tel. 071–242 1278.

The Landmark, 47a Tulse Hill, London SW2. Tel 081–678 6686.

Leatherhead Food RA, Randalls Road, Leatherhead, Surrey KT22 7RY. Tel 0372 376761; Fax 0372 386228.

Listeria Support Group, c/o Mark Horvath, Worlingworth, Woodbridge, Suffolk IP13 7NZ.

Liver Support Group, Academic Department of Medicine, 10th Floor, Royal Free Hospital, London NW3 2QG.

London Association for the Blind, (*see* Action for Blind People).

The London Lighthouse, 111–117 Lancaster Road, London W11 1QT. Tel 071–792 1200.

Lothian Community Project (The Salvation Army), 77 Bread Street, Edinburgh. Tel 031–228 5351.

Mainliners Ltd, PO Box 125, London SW9 8EF.

Marsden Weighing Machine Group, 187 Cross Street, Sale, Manchester M33 1JG. Tel 061–962 1562.

Maternity Alliance, 59–61 Camden High Street, London NW1 7JL.

Mead Johnson (*see* Squibb).

Mecanaid Ltd, St Catherine's Street, Gloucester. Tel 0452 500200.

Mencap, 123 Golden Lane, London EC1Y 0RT. Tel 071–454 0454.

Merck E. Pharmaceuticals Ltd, Winchester Road, Four Marks, Alton, Hants GU34 5HB. Tel 0420 64011.

Migraine Trust, 45 Great Ormond Street, London WC1N 3HD. Tel 071–278 2676.

Milupa Ltd, Milupa House, Uxbridge Road, Hillingdon, Uxbridge, Middlesex UB10 0NE. Tel 081–573 9966.

Ministry of Agriculture, Fisheries and Food, Nobel House, 17 Smith Square, London SW1P 3HX. Tel 071–238 3000.

Motor Neurone Disease Association, PO Box 256, Northampton NN1 2PR. Tel 0604 22269.

Muscular Dystrophy Society, Natrass House, 35 Macauley Road, London SW4 0QP. Tel 071–720 8055.

Multiple Sclerosis Society, 25 Effie Road, Fulham, London SW6 1EE.

Multiple Sclerosis Unit, Central Middlesex Hospital Trust, Acton Lane, London NW10 7NS. Tel 081–453 2332/7.

National AIDS Helpline Tel 0800 567 123.

National Association for Colitis and Crohn's Disease (NACC), 98A London Road, St Albans, Herts AL1 1NX.

National Autistic Society, 276 Willesden Lane, London NW2 5RB. Tel 081–451 1114.

National Coaching Foundation, 4 College Close, Becket Park, Leeds LS6 3QH. Tel 0532 744802.

National Childbirth Trust, Alexandra House, Oldham Terrace, London W3 6NH. Tel 081–992 8637.

National Children's Home (NCH), Highbury Grove, London N1.

National Dairy Council, 5–7 Princes Street, London W1M 0AP. Tel 071–499 7822.

National Excema Society, Tavistock House North, Tavistock Square, London WC1H 9SR.

National Head Injuries Association (HEADWAY), 200 Mansfield Road, Nottingham NG1 3HX.

National Osteoporosis Society, PO Box 10, Radstock, Bath, BA3 3YB.

National Schizophrenia Fellowship, 28 Castle Street, Kingston upon Thames, Surrey KT1 1SS. Tel 081–547 3937.

National Society for Research into Allergy, PO Box 45, Hinckley, Leicestershire.

Nicholas Laboratories Ltd, 225 Bath Road, Slough, Berks.

Nutricia Dietary Products Ltd, 494–496 Honeypot Lane, Stanmore, Middlesex HA7 1JH. Tel 081–951 5155.

Nutrition Society, 10 Cambridge Court, 210 Shepherd's Bush Road, London W6 7NS. Tel 071–602 0228.

Open University, Walton Hall, Milton Keynes MK7 6AA. Tel 0908 274066.

Oxford Nutrition Ltd, PO Box 31E, Oxford OX4 3UH.

Parkinson's Disease Society, 36 Portland Place, London W1N 3DG. Tel 071–323 1174.

Partially Sighted Society, Queens Road, Doncaster DN1 2NX. Tel 0302 323132/368998.

The Poor Clares, Monastery of St Joseph, Lawrence Street, York YO1 3EB.

Positively Women, 5 Sebastian Street, London EC1V 0ME. Tel 071–490 5515.

Prader-Willi Syndrome Association (UK), 30 Follett Drive, Abbot's Langley, Herts WD5 0LP.

Procea, Alexandra Road, Dublin 1. Tel 010 353 1 741741.

Public Health Alliance, Room 204, Snow Hill House, 10–15 Livery Street, Birmingham B3 2PE.

Research into Ageing, 49 Queen Victoria Street, London EC4N 4SA.

Ross Laboratories (a Division of Abbott Laboratories) Abbott House, Norden Road, Maidenhead, Berks SL6 8JG. Tel 0628 773355.

Royal London Society for the Blind, 105–109 Salisbury Road, London NW6 6RH. Tel 071–372 1551.

Royal National Institute for the Blind (RNIB), 224 Great Portland Street, London W1N 6AA.

RNIB Production and Distribution Centre, PO Box 173, Peterborough PE2 0WS. Tel 0733 370777.

Royal Society of Chemistry, Thomas Graham House, Science Park,

Milton Road, Cambridge CB4 4WF. Tel 0223 420066; Fax 0223 423429.

Scientific Hospital Supplies (SHS), 100 Wavertree Boulevard, Wavertree Technology Park, Liverpool L7 9PQ. Tel 051–228 1992.

Scholl Consumer Products Ltd, 475 Capability Green, Luton, LU1 3LU.

SAM (Scottish AIDS Monitor), 64 Broughton Street, Edinburgh EH1 3SA. Tel 031–557 3885.

Scottish Health Education Group, Woodburn House, Canaan Lane, Edinburgh EH10 4SG. Tel 031–447 8044.

Scottish Home and Health Department, St Andrew's House, Edinburgh EH1 3DE.

Scottish Spinal Cord Injury Association (SSCIA), Unit 22, 100 Elderpark Street, Glasgow G51 3TR.

Searle Consumer Products Group, PO Box 53, Lane End Road, High Wycombe, Bucks HP12 4HL.

Seca Limited, Seca House, 40 Barn Street, Digbeth, Birmingham B5 5QB.

The Spastics Society, 12 Park Crescent, London W1N 4EQ. Tel 071–636 5020.

Spinal Injuries Association (UK), 76 St James Lane, London N10 3DF.

Sports Nutrition Foundation, National Sports Medicine Institute of the UK, c/o Medical College of St Bartholomew's Hospital, Charterhouse Square, London EC1M 6BQ. Tel 071–250 0493.

Sports Nutrition Service, Department of Physical Education and Sports Science, Loughborough University, Loughborough, Leics LE11 3TU. Tel 0509 263171 ext 4251.

Squibb ER & Sons Ltd, Bristol Myers-Squibb House, 141–149 Staines Road, Hounslow, Middlesex TW3 3JB. Tel 081–572 7422.

SSI Medical Services, Clinitron House, Ruddington Lane, Nottingham. Tel 0602 455355.

Standing Conference of Ethnic Minority Senior Citizens, 5 Westminster Bridge Road, London SE1 7XW. Tel 071–928 0095.

The Stroke Association, CHSA House, 123–127 Whitecross Street, London EC1Y 8JJ. Tel 071–490 7999.

Tak Tent, 132 Hill Street, Glasgow. Tel 041–332 3639.

Talking Books (RNIB), 224 Mount Pleasant, Wembley, Middlesex.

Talking Newspaper Association for the UK, 90 High Street, Heathfield, East Sussex TN21 8JD.

Tenovus Cancer Information Centre, 11 Whitchurch Road, Cardiff CF3 3JN. Tel 0222 619846.

Terrence Higgins Trust, 52–54 Grays Inn Road, London WC1X 8JU. Tel 071–831 0330.

Ulster Cancer Foundation, 40–42 Eglantine Avenue, Belfast BT9 6DX. Tel 0232 663281.

Ultrapharm Ltd, PO Box 18, Henley-on-Thames RG9 2AW. Tel 0491 578016.

Unigreg Ltd., Enterprise House, 181–189 Garth Road, Morden, Surrey SM4 4LL. Tel 081–330 1421; Fax 081–330 6812.

Values in Action (formerly Campaign for People with a Mental Handicap), Oxford House, Derbyshire Street, London E2 6HG.

The Vegan Society, 7 Battle Road, St Leonards-on-Sea, East Sussex TN37 7AA.

The Vegetarian Society, Parkdale, Dunham Road, Altrincham, Cheshire WA14 4QG.

Vitalia Ltd, Paradise, Hemel Hempstead, Herts HP2 4TF.

Whitworths, Victoria Mills, Wellingborough, Northants NN8 2DT.

Women's Therapy Centre, 6 Manor Gardens, London N7.

Wyeth Laboratories, Huntercombe Lane South, Maidenhead, Berks SL6 0PH Tel 0628 604377.

Index

Page numbers of sections are shown in **bold**